P9-DGW-098

DON'T GO
TO THE
COSMETICS
COUNTER
WITHOUT ME

A unique guide to over 35,000 products,
plus the latest skin-care research.

PAULA BEGOUN

Contributing Author: Bryan Barron
Editors: Sigrid Asmus, John Hopper, Jennifer Forbes Provo
Art Direction, Cover Design, and Typography: Erin Smith Bloom,
    Beginning Press
Printing: Publishers Book Services, Inc.
Research Director: Kate Mee
Research Assistants: Shira Druxman, Katherine Siergiej, Lori White

Copyright © 2003, Paula Begoun
Publisher: Beginning Press
        13075 Gateway Drive, Suite 160
        Seattle, Washington 98168

Sixth Edition Printing: January 2003

ISBN   1-877988-30-8
        10 9 8 7 6 5 4 3 2 1

All rights reserved. No part of this book may be reproduced or transmitted in any form or by any means, electronic or mechanical, including photocopying, recording, or by any information storage or retrieval system, without written permission from Beginning Press and/or Paula Begoun, except for the inclusion of quotations in a review.

This book is distributed to the United States book trade by:
Publishers Group West
1700 Fourth Street
Berkeley, California 94710
(510) 528-1444

And to the Canadian book trade by:
Raincoast Books Limited
9050 Shaughnessy Street
Vancouver, British Columbia, V6P 6E5 CANADA
(604) 633-5714

STAY UPDATED WITH PAULA'S WEB SITE
www.CosmeticsCop.com

What's New —
Learn about Paula's new products.

Special Features —
New best and worst products reviewed every month plus a new Dear Paula question.

Paula's FREE e-mail Beauty Bulletin —
Sign up for Paula's free bi-weekly bulletin and learn about specials, new products and reviews!

Specials —
Great deals every month.

Read
Find out about Paula's books, read Dear Paula columns, and check out product reviews.

Learn —
How can you best take care of your skin? What are some shortcuts for beautifully applied makeup? Find articles on these topics and more in our Learn section.

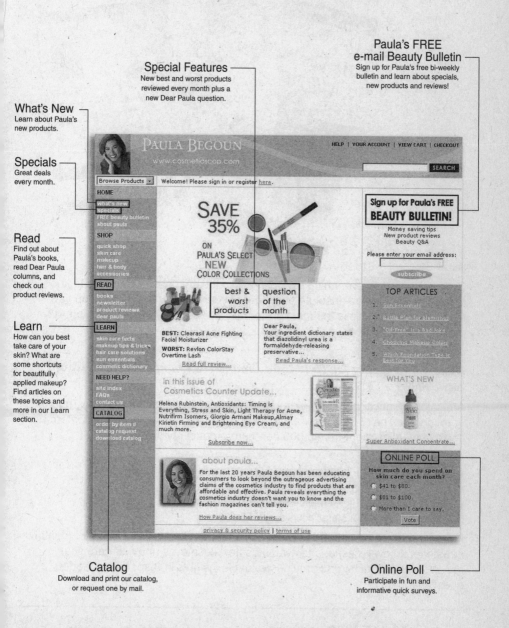

Catalog
Download and print our catalog, or request one by mail.

Online Poll —
Participate in fun and informative quick surveys.

ALSO BY PAULA BEGOUN...

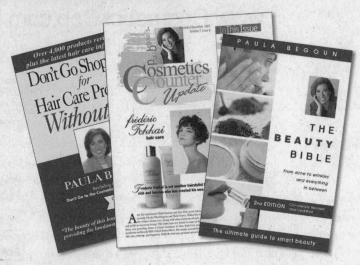

The Beauty Bible, 2nd Edition
Item # BB2 $18.95 US

Open your eyes to everything the cosmetics industry doesn't want you to know. Learn how to take the absolute best care of your skin and apply makeup flawlessly and easily. This is the most up-to-date and comprehensive book on skin care and makeup ever.

Don't Go Shopping for Hair Care Products Without Me, 2nd Edition
Item # HAIR2 $19.95 US

Are salon products better than drugstore brands? Is it possible to repair, nourish, or reconstruct hair? Find answers to all your hair-care questions in this informative book, containing more than 5,000 hair-care product reviews.

Cosmetics Counter Update Newsletter
Item # SUB, 1-year subscription (6 issues)
$18.75 to U.S., $26.25 to Canada, $33.75 to all other countries
Online subscription $12.50 (all countries)

Keep up with the constantly changing cosmetics industry with Paula's bi-monthly newsletter. In every issue, she evaluates new cosmetics and hair-care lines, reviews new products, and provides valuable insights in response to readers' questions.

800.831.4088 (U.S. and Canada) • **www.CosmeticsCop.com**

Beginning Press   •   13075 Gateway Drive, Suite 160   •   Seattle, WA 98168

FROM THE PUBLISHER

Paula Begoun is the best-selling author of *Don't Go to the Cosmetics Counter Without Me*, *The Beauty Bible*, *Don't Go Shopping for Hair Care Products Without Me*, and *Blue Eyeshadow Should Be Illegal*. She has sold millions of books, and has educated women about the facts and secrets the beauty industry doesn't want them to know.

Ms. Begoun is also a syndicated journalist with Knight-Ridder News Tribune Service, and her weekly "Dear Paula" column appears in newspapers across the country.

Paula is nationally recognized as a consumer advocate, covering the cosmetics and hair-care industries. She is called upon regularly by reporters and producers from television, newspapers, magazines, and radio as a cosmetics industry expert. She has appeared on hundreds of talk shows over the years, including *The View*, *Dateline NBC*, *Good Morning America*, *20/20*, *Today*, *Later Today*, *CBS Morning News*, *Canada AM*, and National Public Radio, and has made more than a dozen appearances on the *Oprah Winfrey Show*. Today, with the success of Paula's Web site, www.CosmeticsCop.com, women all over the world consider her the most reliable source for straightforward information about all their beauty questions.

In 1995, Ms. Begoun launched her own line of skin-care products, called Paula's Choice, and a few years later, created a makeup line, Paula's Select. This distinctive line of products is renowned for its effectiveness and affordability. While Paula is proud of her line, she realizes that there are vast numbers of product options for women to consider. As a result, she continues to provide her readers with substantiated and documented studies and analysis about skin-care and makeup products from other lines based on her extensive research and years of experience. The ratings in this edition show as many "happy faces" as "unhappy" and "neutral" ones. In her reviews and critiques, it is clear that Paula continues to maintain her evenhanded approach to offering readers an unprecedented assortment of choices for their cosmetic purchases.

PUBLISHER'S DISCLAIMER

The intent of this book is to present the author's ideas and perceptions about the marketing, selling, and use of cosmetics. The author's sole purpose is to present consumer information and advice regarding the purchase of makeup and skin-care products. The information and recommendations presented strictly reflect the author's opinions, perceptions, and knowledge about the subject and products mentioned. Some women may find success with a particular product that is not recommended or even mentioned in this book, or they may be partial to a skin-care routine Paula has reviewed negatively. It is everyone's unalienable right to judge products by their own criteria and to disagree with the author.

More important, because everyone's skin can, and probably will, react to an external stimulus at some time, any product could cause a negative reaction on skin at one time or another. If you develop skin sensitivity to a cosmetic, stop using it immediately and consult your physician. If you need medical advice about your skin, it is best to consult a dermatologist.

ACKNOWLEDGMENTS

There are no words that can adequately express the challenge and commitment required for writing a book of this scope and nature. The energy and resourcefulness needed to research, compile, review, write, and edit a 1000+ page book is an almost endless undertaking. If it were not for my co-writer Bryan Barron and research director Kate Mee, this book would not have been possible. Their perseverance and devotion to completing the project go beyond anything I could have hoped for. Not only did they meet deadline after deadline, they did it with an accuracy and exactness that exceeded my every expectation. Bryan and Kate bring new meaning to the concepts of proficiency and integrity. I am blessed to have these two people in my life. Without their feedback, patience, and contributions, this book would have been a very good idea but an absolutely unconquerable task.

DEDICATION

This book is dedicated to Steve Clark. Without Steve's consideration, encouragement, and patience over the past 17 years, my books would have never reached the audience they have. The fact that I have sold over 2 million copies is most certainly attributable to his confidence and belief in my work. Steve is a man of quiet integrity, compassion, generosity, faith, and astute business acumen. It has been my privilege to work with him. What I have learned from Steve continues to shape my life and career in a multitude of positive ways. I am eternally grateful.

TABLE OF CONTENTS

CHAPTER ONE—KNOWLEDGE IS BEAUTIFUL 1

CHAPTER TWO—HEALTHY SKIN: RULES TO LIVE BY 13

CHAPTER THREE—PRODUCT-BY-PRODUCT REVIEWS 31

Acne-Statin 79
Adrien Arpel's Signature Club A 80
Aesop 83
Ahava 86
Alexandra de Markoff 90
Almay 95
Aloette 104
Alpha Hydrox 110
Anna Sui 112
Annemarie Borlind 114
Arbonne 120
Artistry by Amway 127
Astara 132
Aubrey Organics 136
Aveda 142
Aveeno Facial Care 149
Avon 150
Avon beComing 165
Awake 172
B. Kamins Skin Care 179
Bain de Soleil 182
Banana Boat 183
bare escentuals 184
Basis 189
Bath & Body Works 189
BeautiControl 193
Beauty Without Cruelty 202
BeneFit 205
Bioelements 211
BioMedic 215
Biore 219
BioTherm 222
Black Opal 229
BlissLabs 233
Blistex 238

Bobbi Brown 239
Body & Soul 246
The Body Shop 249
Bonne Bell 260
Borghese 263
Burt's Bees 268
Calvin Klein 272
CamoCare 276
CARGO 279
Caudalie 281
Cellex-C 285
Cetaphil 289
Chanel 290
Chantal Ethocyn 302
Chantecaille 303
Christian Dior 307
Clarins 319
Cle de Peau Beaute 332
Clean & Clear by Johnson & Johnson 339
Clearasil 341
Clientele 342
Clinac 350
Clinique 350
Club Monaco 365
Complex 15 369
Coppertone 370
Corn Silk 372
Cover Girl 374
Crabtree & Evelyn 379
Darphin 380
Decleor Paris 388
Dermablend 394
Dermalogica 398
DHC 402
Diane Young 409
Differin 414
Doctor's Dermatologic Formula (DDF) 415
Dove 423
Dr. Dennis Gross, M.D. Skin Care 424
Dr. Hauschka 425
Dr. Jeannette Graf, M.D. 429
Dr. LeWinn's Private Formula 433
Dr. Mary Lupo Skin Care System 435
Elizabeth Arden 436
Elizabeth Grant 445

Ella Bache 448
Ellen Lange Skin Care 453
English Ideas & Lip Last 456
Epicuren 458
ERA Face Foundation 464
Erno Laszlo 465
Esoterica 471
Estee Lauder 472
Eucerin 490
Exuviance by Neostrata 491
FACE Stockholm 495
Fashion Fair 500
Flori Roberts 505
Gatineau 509
Giorgio Armani 511
Givenchy 514
Glymed Plus 518
G.M. Collin 521
Guerlain 526
Guinot 534
H$_2$0+ Skin Care 538
Hard Candy 542
Helena Rubinstein 545
Hydron 552
IGIA 555
Illuminare 558
Iman 560
I-Iman 564
Jafra 567
Jan Marini Skin Research 574
Jane 580
Jane Iredale 584
Jason Natural 587
Joey New York 594
Jurlique International 599
Karin Herzog Skin Care 603
Kiehl's 606
Kinerase 610
Kiss Me Mascara 611
Kiss My Face 611
L'Occitane 615
L'Oreal 618
La Mer 631
La Prairie 635
La Roche-Posay 645

Lac-Hydrin 647
Lancaster 647
Lancome 654
Laura Mercier 671
Linda Sy 676
Lip Ink 679
Liz Earle Naturally Active Skin Care 681
Lorac 682
Lubriderm 687
Lush 688
M.A.C. 692
Make Up For Ever 700
Marcelle 705
Marilyn Miglin 711
Mario Badescu 715
Mary Kay 721
Max Factor 727
Maybelline 731
M.D. Formulations 739
M.D. Forte 743
Mederma 745
Merle Norman 746
MetroGel, MetroLotion, and MetroCream 754
Moisturel 755
Morgen Schick 755
Murad 758
Nads Gel Hair Removal 762
NARS 763
Natura Bisse 768
Neostrata 776
Neutrogena 780
Neways Skin Care 790
Nivea Visage 792
Noevir 795
Noxzema 799
Nu Skin 800
Nutrifirm Isomers 808
N.V. Perricone, M.D. 809
N.Y.C. 815
Obagi Nu-Derm 817
Ocean Potion 819
Olay 820
Ole Henriksen Skin Care 824
Ombrelle 827
Origins 828

Orlane 839
Osmotics 845
Oxy Balance 848
PanOxyl 849
Parthena 849
Paula Dorf Cosmetics 855
Paula's Choice/Paula's Select 859
Peter Thomas Roth 867
Pevonia Botanica 874
Pharmagel 881
philosophy 883
pHisoDerm 888
Physician's Choice 889
Physicians Formula 893
Phytomer 901
Pola 906
Pond's 914
Posner 917
Prada Beauty 919
Prescriptives 923
Prestige Cosmetics 933
Principal Secret 935
ProActiv 940
PropapH 942
Purpose 942
Quo Cosmetics 943
Rachel Perry 946
Re Vive 948
Rejuveness 951
Rejuvenique 952
Remede 953
Reversa 958
Revlon 959
Rimmel 970
RoC 973
RoC in Canada 975
Sea Breeze 977
Sense Usana 978
Sephora 980
Serious Skin Care 982
Shaklee 989
Shiseido 992
Shu Uemera 1006
Sisley 1013
SkinCeuticals 1019

smashbox 1023
Sonia Kashuk 1027
Sothys Paris 1030
St. Ives 1036
Stila 1038
Stri-Dex 1043
Suave 1044
Sue Devitt Studio Makeup 1045
T. Le Clerc 1048
Thalgo 1051
Three Custom Color 1056
Tony & Tina 1058
Tri-Luma 1061
Trish McEvoy 1062
Trucco 1066
Ultima II 1069
University Medical Skin Care 1075
Urban Decay 1077
Uvavita 1081
Vaniqa 1083
Versace 1084
Vichy 1088
Victoria Jackson Cosmetics 1093
Victoria's Secret Cosmetics 1097
Vincent Longo 1100
Wet 'n' Wild 1104
Yon-Ka Paris 1107
Youngblood 1112
Yves St. Laurent 1114
Z. Bigatti 1120
ZAPZYT 1122
Zia 1123

CHAPTER FOUR—BABY'S SKIN-CARE PRODUCTS 1127

Arbonne Baby Care 1134
Baby Magic Baby Care 1135
Baby Powders 1135
Baby Wipe Products 1136
Bobbi Brown Baby Essentials 1137
Burt's Bees Baby Products 1138
California Baby 1138
Crabtree & Evelyn 1141
Diaper Rash Ointments 1142
Gerber Baby Products 1143

Johnson & Johnson Baby and Kids Products 1144
Kiehl's Baby Care 1145
Little Forest Baby Care 1146
Mustela Baby Products 1146
PEDIAM 1148

CHAPTER FIVE—MEN'S SKIN-CARE PRODUCTS 1149

Anthony Logistics 1152
Aqua Velva 1153
Aramis Lab Series 1153
Arbonne Skin Fitness 1155
Aveda Men's Skin Care 1156
Aveeno 1156
Biotherm Men 1156
The Body Shop Skin Mechanics for Men 1157
Burt's Bees Men 1157
California North Men's Skin Care 1158
Clarins Men's 1158
Clinique Skin Supplies for Men 1159
Colgate Shaving Care 1160
Crabtree & Evelyn for Men 1160
Edge Pro Gel 1161
Estee Lauder Pleasures for Men 1162
Gillette 1162
Kiehl's for Men 1164
Mary Kay Men's Skin Care 1165
Neutrogena Men 1165
Nivea for Men 1167
Old Spice 1167
Phytomen by Phytomer 1168
Ralph Lauren Polo Sport 1168
Shiseido Basala for Men 1169
Skin Bracer by Mennen 1169
Tend Skin 1169
Zirh Men's Skin Care 1169

CHAPTER SIX—THE BEST PRODUCTS SUMMARY 1171

CHAPTER SEVEN—COSMETICS DICTIONARY 1239

CHAPTER EIGHT—ANIMAL TESTING 1359

CHAPTER ONE

Knowledge is Beautiful

THIS IS THE LAST TIME

To the relief of some and to the dismay of others, I have decided that this will be the last edition of *Don't Go to the Cosmetics Counter Without Me* I am going to write . In many ways, this has been a very difficult and emotional resolution. After 22 years of writing books on the vagaries and marvels of the cosmetics industry, it is time to put the pen down—at least as far as my book writing is concerned. As you can imagine, I have a love/hate relationship with what I do. The physical burden and time involved in writing this kind of tome is nothing less than overwhelming. On the one hand, it is a fascinating business, to page after page uncover and reveal the web of secrets, missteps, and duplicity the cosmetics industry spins out of thin air and puts on exhibit for unsuspecting but captivated consumers. On the other hand, it is an endless battle that more than a thousand pages later I know I have lost. Even though I have seen significant changes in the industry and feel at least partially responsible for some of them, there are still countless egregious claims being made, substandard products being created, ads fashioned with misleading pictures or empty bravado, and unethical "scientific" research espoused as valid when it is anything but. And perhaps the worst part is knowing that millions and millions of women are seduced by all of it, wasting billions of dollars on hopes that are dashed until the next beauty magazine is read, infomercial is watched, or celebrity endorsement comes along. It is a struggle to deal with this insanity day in and day out. The frustration sometimes leaves me ranting in my office as my staff listens and offers commiseration, reminding me that my work isn't for naught. Yet at the end of every book, I never want to see another moisturizer, toner, mascara, or lipstick again for as long as I live! Well, OK, maybe not the moisturizer and mascara, but you get my point.

So, while I won't be writing any more books, I definitely do plan to carry on as the "cosmetics cop" by continuing my bimonthly newsletter *Cosmetics Counter Update* and my free biweekly online *Beauty Bulletin* (to subscribe, visit www.CosmeticsCop.com). These will provide ongoing reviews and analyses of new products, facts about the latest cosmetic ingredient fads, exposés of misleading product claims, and balanced information about how to best take care of your skin. That will be far less overwhelming for me and still allow me to provide you with information the rest of the cosmetics industry doesn't want you to hear.

BECOMING A COSMETICS COP

I often marvel at how I happened into this unusual occupation. It's not as if you can answer an ad for this kind of job, and clearly the cosmetics industry and beauty magazines aren't interested in hiring someone to do what I do. Yet, from the beginning, it was clear that there was a demand from consumers for this kind of information. With over 2 million books sold, I'm certainly glad I gave up my day job!

It all started in 1977, when I took my first job at a department-store makeup counter to supplement my income as a freelance makeup artist. As a young makeup artist in Washington, D.C., I had built up a list of celebrity clients and was doing quite well, both financially and professionally. I found the artistry of creating beautiful makeup styles for women intriguing, and the world of fashion and glamour thoroughly exciting. At the age of 24, I was thrilled with my career. My clients wanted only me, and they were some of the most powerful and formidable women in Washington. But, as with any business, it had its ups and downs, and once in a while it became necessary to supplement my income. A store at a mall in Silver Spring, Maryland, had an opening for a cosmetics salesperson. They hired me on the spot because, I was told, I looked the part, wearing nice makeup and dressing well. Amazingly (to me anyway) they weren't interested in my makeup experience.

Even back then, I knew something was awry with a substantial number of cosmetics and the advertising for them, particularly in the skin-care arena. Having struggled for years with oily skin and acne, I knew from personal experience that astringents didn't close pores, products claiming not to cause breakouts made me break out, and most products that promised to clear up acne only made my skin more red and irritated. I didn't yet know all the technical details of why this was so, but it was blatantly obvious that plenty of mascaras with claims of being flakeproof weren't, and that creams purporting to eliminate scarring and lighten "age spots" didn't. More often than not, the claims made about what the products would do rarely matched their performance. However, while it seemed unquestionable that much of the cosmetics industry was grossly misrepresenting its products, at the time I had no way to confirm my suspicions.

On my first day, I was assigned to work behind the counters for Calvin Klein (Klein had a makeup line then that lasted only a brief period; it was resurrected in 1999) and Elizabeth Arden. With no previous training or information about these lines, I was told to sell the products. I did the best I could. Unfortunately, my notion of how to help customers was completely different from that of the other salespeople and the line manager. My first mistake was telling several customers not to bother using an astringent because alcohol-based products wouldn't stop oil production, though it would add more skin problems to the mix by causing skin to become dry, red, flaky, and irritated. By the end of the second day, the woman working next to me was mortified. She called in the line representative, who made it clear that I should keep my personal opinions to myself and just sell the products. I said I would do my best. This was only my second day! Things had to get better, I thought. They didn't.

After I complained that the two lines I was assigned to didn't always have the best makeup colors or skin-care products for every woman I talked to, the cosmetics manager told me, "All the customer wants to know is what you tell her; the customers never ask questions, because they trust our products." Several disagreements later, I was out of a job.

Shortly after that incident, I read *The Great American Skin Game* by Toni Stabille. It changed my life. This landmark book conveyed in clear, concise terms the processes and techniques the cosmetics industry uses to sell hope to gullible and uninformed consumers. In fact, Stabille was largely responsible for proposing many present-day FDA regulations, including advertising guidelines, safety regulations, and mandatory ingredient lists. Her work confirmed what I had already reasoned must be true, and significantly changed the way I approached cosmetics.

Although it sounds a bit melodramatic, I couldn't continue selling something I knew to be a waste of money or bad for the skin. Consumers (including myself) deserved better. I wasn't anti-makeup—just the opposite—but I was (and am) anti-hype and against misleading information. As one newspaper reporter recently commented, "She's not Mother Teresa, but it does seem to be just Ms. Begoun against these huge cosmetics companies." Thus I took my first steps on a long career path—longer than I ever imagined—that went from owning my own cosmetics stores to working as a TV news reporter to owning my own publishing company, and back to owning my own skin-care and makeup company. With every step, my goal has been to do what it takes to find out and expose the truth behind the ads and the literally unbelievable claims thrown about by the cosmetics world. After all, one good sales pitch about an "exclusive patented secret" or a revolutionary new formula, and your pocketbook could easily be lighter—by $50 to $250 and up to $500—for a 1-ounce jar of standard cosmetic ingredients or for ingredients that can't possibly live up to the claims made for them.

I know that I can't stop the cosmetics industry from force-feeding consumers an endless stream of products and misleading or erroneous claims and information, but I also know there are enough women who are interested in seeing the other side of the picture to motivate me to continue to do what I do. Knowing the "rest of the story" can only help you feel and look more beautiful in the long run.

COSMETIC EXPOSÉ: A PRECARIOUS BUSINESS

What I do is controversial. I've known it almost since the beginning. Without question, every cosmetics company executive would be disturbed by someone challenging their claims and the quality of their products. Yet what I say or write is not unknown to those in the industry (at least not those involved in serious skin-care or makeup research and formulation). I draw my conclusions from many well-known cosmetics industry sources and a myriad of medical, alternative medicine, and biochemistry journals.

Three must-read sources for every cosmetics consumer are the FDA's Web site at www.FDA.gov and the medical research sites www.Medscape.com or www.pubmed.com. When it comes to trustworthy studies, the fundamental criterion is always to use published, peer-reviewed* research. This information is integral to my work, but I also spend a great deal of time interviewing cosmetics chemists, dermatologists, cosmetic ingredient manufacturers, biochemists, oncologists, and plastic surgeons. This accumulated research provides me with abundant sources of information that you may not get a chance to hear because the beauty magazines, infomercials, and cosmetics advertising leave out any information that their cosmetics advertisers don't agree with.

Despite the works I cite, I have been called everything from a charlatan to someone who has nothing more than a vendetta against the cosmetics industry, with no substantiation or proof backing up what I say. Yet I truly feel that it only takes a quick perusal of this book's *Cosmetics Dictionary,* Chapter Seven, to realize that I have substantiated every comment I make and that the fundamental research on which I base my evaluations is well-documented, with the specifics being detailed in my work.

Not surprisingly, I receive complaints (particularly from cosmetics salespeople) saying I hate all cosmetics except my own products. However, a quick flip through the pages of my book will easily reveal that I recommend hundreds and hundreds of other companies' products. How many cosmetics companies can make that claim? Can you imagine approaching the Estee Lauder counter and telling a salesperson you don't care for their moisturizers, but what do they recommend from Lancome or Chanel? The notion borders on ridiculous when you consider the air of superiority most lines love to exude, even when that line owns other lines in the same department.

Women who write to me often comment that they notice that the people who sell cosmetics usually find my work both awful *and* wonderful. They consider my book insightful and helpful when I recommend the products they sell, but if I suggest that some of the products in their line are a waste of money or potentially damaging to skin, then their opinion is that I don't know what I'm talking about and that I should mind my own business.

While those in the cosmetics industry protest that I don't like anything, paradoxically I also get letters from readers objecting to my long lists of "best products." I am consistently asked to narrow the field to my absolute ten favorites in each category. To help meet this wish, this edition includes a new rating (Paula's Pick, explained in Chapter Three), so you can look for the checkmark to help narrow down my list of the very best products.

I've also received criticism for making my recommendations too complicated and convoluted. How ironic! The cosmetics industry has no problem with their hundreds of lines and thousands of products all claiming identical miracles of one sort or another. And I'm the one making it complicated? Sigh.

---

*Note: Essentially, the peer-review process is a quality-control mechanism that medical, academic, technical, research, and professional journals follow to ensure that the articles they publish contain research and data that meet precise standards of objective and ethical scientific methodology.

Do I hate the cosmetics industry? Hardly. I am in constant awe of the spectacular quality and performance in relation to the multitude of remarkable skin-care and makeup products. What I do hate are the ludicrous claims, disproportionate prices, and the products that can hurt skin or mislead consumers into taking poor care of their skin.

What is difficult for me to comprehend is why so many women give carte blanche belief to what the cosmetics industry tells them. It doesn't seem to cause any doubts or raise any skepticism for women when cosmetics lines repeatedly have new miracle products every few months (but never tell us what was wrong or not as revolutionary with the previous products they once claimed were so spectacular for skin, because they almost always continue to sell them, too).

Lots of women can't wait to buy the products a celebrity claims to use or is selling, because it seems to be accepted as fact that being beautiful or famous means you must know about product quality or what is best for skin care and makeup. After the incessant hype and marketing distortion that accompany all of this, and despite the inevitable disappointment (if we weren't disappointed, the same lines wouldn't have to keep creating new antiwrinkle, acne, or myriad other skin-care items), we still buy whatever the next impressive ad or celebrity is selling—and repeat this pattern season after season, year after year.

There is a part of me that struggles with what I do. Not that I don't find the work rewarding, because I do. The wonderful feedback I get from thousands of readers touches me deeply in ways I can't even begin to describe. Despite that, it still isn't easy being the pariah of the cosmetics industry. I am truly dedicated to providing accurate and complete information about skin care and makeup to help you, the consumer, make educated, wise decisions about your purchases. You may not agree with me, but at least you will have someone else's voice in your ear saying, "Here is research or data showing this product won't work or is bad for skin" or "Consider that this other far less expensive product is better than the expensive one you're looking at" or "It isn't worth the money but at least the product is good for your skin"—and then you can make up your own mind about what works best for you. I believe this is far better than basing a decision on the thousands of never-ending, incessant claims that "our product cures or gets rid of (whatever you don't like about your skin)."

WHAT YOU DON'T KNOW ISN'T PRETTY

As was true for all previous editions of this book, this one covers many of the new lines that have appeared, and all the previously included lines have been entirely re-reviewed, critiqued, and balanced against current studies to make sure that the analysis reflects the most current research about ingredient efficacy, performance, and product integrity.

Do you need this book? If you've ever felt uncertain about a product, or too short of time or energy to figure out for yourself which foundations are too pink or too orange, which eyeshadows are too shiny or too difficult to use, which powders go on too chalky, which cleansers are too greasy, which toners are too harsh, what makes one moisturizer different from another, or how wrinkle creams differ, then yes, you need (and will benefit from) this book. As you read the various skin-care and makeup reviews, you will start to get a better understanding of how the cosmetics industry really works. I've also included a summary chapter of best finds and best buys, but don't jump to that one first. It is important to read the individual product assessments and criteria so you understand *exactly* what standards were used to evaluate each particular category.

For the makeup reviews, each product is described in terms of its reliability, value, texture, application, and effect. Within every category of product—foundations, mascaras, blushes, eyeshadows, concealers, powders, lipsticks, brushes, and pencils—I established specific criteria, and I evaluate the products using those criteria. For example, according to my criteria, a foundation meant for someone with oily skin should be matte, contain minimal to no greasy or emollient ingredients, blend easily, leave a smooth, even finish, and have no blatant breakout-triggering ingredients. All foundations must match skin tones exactly; they should not be any noticeable shade of orange, peach, rose, pink, or ash, because people are not orange, peach, rose, pink, or ash. I established similar criteria for mascaras, blushes, eyeshadows, concealers, pressed powders, lipsticks, and pencils. I relied on my more than 20 years as a professional makeup artist to help establish guidelines for the quality of a product and its application, along with comparing and contrasting hundreds of similar makeup products from different lines throughout the review process.

Skin-care products were evaluated almost entirely by analyzing the ingredient list and comparing the ingredients listed to the claims made about the product. If a toner asserts that it is designed for sensitive skin, it should not contain ingredients that irritate the skin. If a moisturizer claims it can hydrate the skin, it should contain ingredients that can do just that. In addition, I made a point of challenging the inflated claims made about myriad ingredients. I also explain why seemingly impressive-sounding ingredients might indeed benefit the skin or might hurt the skin, and I often elaborate on the validity or usefulness of a specific ingredient or combination of ingredients. In short, the skin-care reviews separate the state-of-the-art products from the so-so and "oh, no!" products found in line after line after line.

WHAT YOU AREN'T TOLD COULD FILL A BOOK

Cosmetics companies and cosmetics salespeople often attempt to defend their claims or products by using false or anecdotal information, particularly around the issue of ingredients. It is typical to hear the familiar refrain about how every product being sold is all natural and contains no chemicals or synthetic ingredients, a statement that presupposes that chemicals and synthetic ingredients are inherently bad for skin. For me to suggest that this is a completely bogus notion is an understatement: It is actually completely far-fetched. First, *everything*, from water to herbal extracts to fragrance and minerals, in a cosmetic is a "chemical." After a substance is extracted from a plant, preserved, and mixed with other "natural" and "unnatural" ingredients, the notion that it is still identical to what came from the ground is ludicrous. How many skin-care or makeup products are you willing to sprinkle on your salad anyway? Second, there is plenty of research establishing that many synthetic ingredients are superior for the health of skin and are distinctly preferred over botanical elements. Third—and this is a biggie—everything natural isn't good for the skin (think of poison ivy or ragweed), any more than everything synthetic is bad.

A particularly perilous omission from the world of beauty magazines and skin-care companies is information about ingredients that protect the skin from UVA radiation from the sun. To get complete UVA protection, there is overwhelming evidence to back up the efficacy of titanium dioxide, zinc oxide, avobenzone (also called Parsol 1789 or butyl methoxydibenzoylmethane) and, outside of the United States, Mexoryl SX (Sources: *International Journal of Pharmaceutics,* June 2002, pages 85–94; *Photodermatology, Photoimmunology, Photomedicine,* August 2000, pages 147–155; *Journal of the American Academy of Dermatology,* December 2000, pages 1024–1035; http://www.photo dermatology.com/sunprotection.htm; and *Skin Therapy Letter,* 1997, volume 2, number 5). Yet the majority of beauty magazines and most skin-care companies won't educate the consumer about this one. Why? Because a preponderance of the advertisers in beauty magazines don't reliably use those ingredients in their sunscreen products. Disagreeing with your advertisers is something beauty magazines can never do, at least if they want to stay financially secure.

I could go on, but I'll let the individual reviews speak for themselves. Substantiated information that sheds light on the dubious and erroneous claims asserted for thousands of products is what you will discover page after page in this book. It often isn't a pretty picture, but once you have the facts, both your skin and your budget will look a lot better.

TERMS YOU NEED TO KNOW

I am often asked, "How do they get away with it?" How do cosmetics companies get away with what appears to be nothing less than misleading and even lying to the public? First, you need to know that, according to the FDA, **cosmetics companies do not have to prove their claims or the efficacy of their products.** What's even more surprising is that the FDA also does not require safety documentation for cosmetics until *after* the product has been brought to market and the FDA starts receiving consumer complaints.

In essence what this lack of regulations means is that cosmetics companies get to say just about anything they want to about their products, and the claims absolutely do not have to be true or have any substantiated proof regarding what is being asserted. What is monitored to some extent are advertising claims, which are evaluated by the Federal Trade Commission (FTC, www.ftc.gov). Although the FTC has frequently cracked down on excessive and false claims made by cosmetics companies, this almost always takes place *after* the ads have run and *after* numerous consumers have fallen prey to another barrage of misleading or false promises.

The only part of the cosmetics industry that is strictly regulated for the consumer is the ingredient list. Since 1978, cosmetics companies have been required to divulge all the contents of their products, listed in the order of concentration from most to least. Unfortunately, the vast majority of consumers don't know how to read a cosmetic's ingredient list, which means they rely on the unregulated claims and assertions the marketing copy boasts about. Yet taking the time to decipher the ingredient lists is the only way to make a rational decision when it comes time to purchasing skin-care products.

To make it easier for you to become familiar with what you'll find on the ingredient lists, I have completely revised and updated the dictionary of cosmetic ingredients in Chapter Seven. Please refer to it when you don't know what an ingredient is or does, or when you hear a claim that a particular ingredient has some miraculous properties for skin. You will be amazed at how legitimate research rarely matches what a cosmetics company wants you to believe.

The following are a few of the more salient points you may not know regarding the marketing jargon, terms, and ingredients that get hyped and overhyped by the cosmetics industry, yet have little to no meaning when it comes to what you will actually be putting on your skin.

All Natural: This term denotes that the ingredients in a given product or product line were derived from plants or other organic material as opposed to being produced synthetically. While the "natural" implication resonates with consumers, it is a completely false concept. Natural claims are not regulated by the FDA. Although the FDA has tried to establish official definitions and guidelines for the use of terms such as "natural" and "hypoallergenic," its regulation proposals were overturned in court. Therefore, cosmetics companies can use the "all-natural" term on ingredient lists to mean anything they want, and almost always it means nothing at all. Many companies even claim their products are all natural when in fact they contain a preponderance of unnatural ingredients. Further, there is no convincing research showing that "natural ingredients" are better for skin than synthetic versions. And finally, when a plant product is added to a cosmetic, and is preserved, stabilized, and mixed with other ingredients, it loses most, if not all, of its natural orientation (Source: FDA *Consumer* magazine, May-June 1998; revised May 1998 and August 2000).

Hypoallergenic or Good for Sensitive Skin: These terms suggest to the consumer that the product is less likely to cause allergic reactions or skin sensitivities. However, there are no standard testing restrictions or regulations for determining whether a product qualifies as meeting this claim. A company can label their product as "hypoallergenic" or "good for sensitive skin" with no substantiation for the claim. This is also true for terms such as "dermatologist-tested," "sensitivity tested," "allergy tested," or "nonirritating." None of these terms are required to be based on any proof that they are better for your skin than products without these claims, because there are no standardized guidelines (Source: www.FDA.gov).

Alcohol-Free: This generally means that a product does not contain denatured alcohol, ethyl alcohol, methanol, benzyl alcohol, isopropyl (rubbing) alcohol, or SD alcohol, all of which are akin to grain alcohol, which is very drying and irritating for skin. However, many cosmetics may contain other "alcohol" compounds, such as cetyl alcohol, stearyl alcohol, cetearyl alcohol, or lanolin alcohol, also known as fatty alcohols; however, what these do is completely unrelated to grain alcohol's effect on skin. As is true for any skin irritant, the higher up on the ingredient list the alcohol is, the greater the risk of irritation. Grain-type alcohols that fall after or just before the list of preservatives rarely pose an irritation problem for skin.

Fragrance-Free: This indicates to the consumer that a product contains no perfume or fragrant ingredients. Despite this labeling, many products use fragrant plant extracts that can cause skin irritation or allergic reactions. Furthermore, fragrant ingredients (including fragrant plant oils and extracts) may be added to a "fragrance-free" cosmetic to mask any offensive odor originating from the raw materials used, but in such a small amount that they may not impart a noticeable scent. "Fragrance-free" can mean that a product does not exude a noticeable aroma, but it can still contain those types of ingredients. Either way, because "fragrance-free" is not a term regulated by the FDA, it ends up being meaningless information on a product's label—and one more reason why getting to know ingredients can be extremely helpful (Source: www.FDA.gov).

Noncomedogenic and Nonacnegenic: These terms are not regulated by the FDA and have no legal meaning. Again, any product can showcase these terms. In real life, the search for products that won't cause breakouts remains a struggle. Wouldn't it be nice if a product could live up to this claim? But given that almost all cosmetic ingredients can trigger breakouts for some people, the term is not only bogus, it can never really be true. Besides, we've all bought products labeled "noncomedogenic" that have made us break out (Source: www.FDA.gov).

Dermatologist Tested: No matter how impressive this sounds, as long as there are no published data stating otherwise, all this wording can mean is that a doctor applied the product to his or her skin or watched someone else do that and said they liked the product. It doesn't tell you anything about efficacy or how one product compares to any other product. A similar empty phrase that's often seen is "dermatologist approved" (Source: www.FDA.gov).

Laboratory Tested: A laboratory sounds so scientific—but any place a study is done can be referred to as a "laboratory" setting. Once you're past the scientific impression that term may give you, you realize that the testing issues are rarely logical, and that often the tests are engineered in advance to give the company precisely the results they paid for.

Patented Secrets or Patented Ingredients: There is no such thing as a patented secret. The very concept is an oxymoron. The only way to *obtain* a patent is to *divulge* the complete contents of the product and its intended use! There are also no patents that deal with proof of efficacy. All a patent can legally do is attribute to an ingredient or formulation the capability to be used for a specific purpose (such as wrinkles, acne, exfoliation, or skin-lightening). That has nothing to do with whether or not those ingredients can do anything at all. Patents also do not indicate quality, reliability, or usefulness of a product, nor does a patent mean that certain established ingredients can't be used by other companies for other purposes (Source: United States Patent and Trademark Office, www.uspto.gov).

I could go on and on, and I will over the next thousand-plus pages as I explain and cite sources explaining what works and what doesn't when it comes to skin-care products. The information I provide just restates everything the cosmetics industry already knows to be true (it's their information directly from their sources). I simply add what they won't tell you: what you absolutely need to know to make sensible, cost-effective decisions about what you put on your skin.

THE GOLD STANDARD: EXPENSIVE DOESN'T MEAN BETTER

The amount of money you spend on skin care has nothing to do with how your skin looks. And spending more money does not affect the status of your skin. What does affect the status of your skin are the products you use. An expensive soap by Erno Laszlo is no better for your skin than an inexpensive bar soap such as Dove (though I would suggest that both are potentially too irritating and drying for all skin types). On the other hand, an irritant-free toner by Neutrogena can be just as good as, or maybe even better than, an irritant-free toner by Orlane or La Prairie (depending on the formulation), and *any* irritant-free toner is infinitely better than a toner that contains alcohol, peppermint, menthol, essential oils, eucalyptus, lemon, or other irritants, no matter how natural-sounding the ingredients are and regardless of the price or claim. Spending less doesn't hurt your skin, and spending more doesn't necessarily help it. Simple, but true!

THEY'RE CHEATING ON YOU

The concept of brand loyalty is something many consumers feel comfortable with and are seeking. They reason (and this reasoning is reinforced by the cosmetics companies) that using only products from a single brand must be better for their skin, because products from a particular line must be specially formulated to work together. Therefore, mixing one brand of cosmetics with another is supposed to be like trying to fit a square peg into a round hole or mixing oil and water. I understand the reasoning behind this, but more often than not there is no valid reason to use skin-care or makeup products from just one company. Your skin and appearance will not suffer (and may actually improve) if you aren't monogamous with a single cosmetics company. Besides, when you stop to think about the other goods and services you purchase there really isn't much logic behind it. No one buys food products from just one company, and even doctors don't prescribe medications from only one company (and of course there's the fact that generic medications work as well as the brand names). These are cases where it's clear that brand loyalty would not be good for your health. But perhaps an even more convincing reason to ignore the concept of brand loyalty for cosmetics is because the cosmetics companies can't stay loyal to themselves.

The number of mergers and acquisitions that occur in the cosmetics industry is higher than ever before. In fact, over 75% of most department-store cosmetics lines are owned either by Estee Lauder or by L'Oreal. It's the cosmetics-world equivalent of the Hatfields versus the McCoys as these two powerhouse corporations battle for the consumer's attention (and dollars) every day. In an effort to summarize what is revealed about ownership throughout this book, I compiled the list below to show the more notable ownerships, and you may find it quite eye-opening.

Estee Lauder owns Stila, Aramis, Aveda, Clinique, Jane, Tommy Hilfiger Fragrances, Bobbi Brown, Prescriptives, M.A.C., Origins, Donna Karan Cosmetics, Jo Malone Perfumes, Bumble & Bumble, Kate Spade Beauty, and Creme de la Mer (Source: www.elcompanies.com).

L'Oreal owns Maybelline, Lancome, Helena Rubinstein, Kiehl's, BioMedic, Vichy, Biotherm, Giorgio Armani Parfums, Ralph Lauren Parfums, Shu Uemura, Ombrelle, Redken, Matrix, Garnier, and La Roche Posay (Source: www.loreal.com).

Procter & Gamble owns Cover Girl, Max Factor, Clairol, Olay, Noxzema, Pantene, and Vidal Sassoon (Source: www.pg.com).

Johnson & Johnson, in the realm of cosmetics and skin care-oriented medical products owns Neutrogena, Aveeno, Clean & Clear, PersaGel, RoC, Retin-A, and Renova (source: www.jnj.com).

Revlon owns Almay and Ultima II (Source: www.revlon.com).

Shiseido owns Cle de Peau, Decleor, NARS, and Sea Breeze (Source: Shiseido Annual Report, March 31, 2002, www.shiseido.co.jp/e/annual/html/anu92000.htm).

Beiersdorf owns La Prairie, Nivea, Basis, Eucerin, and Juvena of Switzerland (Source: www.beiersdorf.com).

CHAPTER TWO

Healthy Skin: Rules to Live By

A COMPANION TO *THE BEAUTY BIBLE*

Don't Go to the Cosmetics Counter Without Me is primarily a product review guide. It is meant as a source that tells you specifically what products live up to their claims, what products don't, and what products waste your money. There isn't room in this already overly expansive book to explain and describe why certain products do or don't work for your specific skin-care needs or what options there may be for treating a comprehensive variety of skin-care and makeup concerns. To understand how to take care of your skin, and what can and can't be done for different skin types, disorders, or problems (from acne to wrinkles, rosacea, psoriasis, skin discolorations, and everything in between) I encourage you to read my book *The Beauty Bible*, Second Edition. This 510-page book will help you take control of common and not-so-common skin woes and allow you to succeed in taking the best possible care of your skin, as well as show you time-tested ways to apply makeup creatively and beautifully for your lifestyle and preferences.

The Beauty Bible delves into all the issues that influence skin care and makeup. Over the past few years, the amount of documented and peer-reviewed research on skin-care and cosmetic ingredients has grown tremendously. Serious investigation has increased exponentially on all fronts—from antioxidants, anti-irritants, and the aging of skin, to why skin wrinkles, how skin heals, what the effects of hormones are on skin function, and how to treat blackheads and acne, not to mention a better understanding of how sun and oxygen destroy skin and why irritation is harmful for skin. Cosmetic dermatology and plastic surgery procedures have greatly improved, though the array of options has become more extensive and the risks more difficult to easily quantify and evaluate.

It is amazing how far the cosmetics world has advanced in understanding how skin behaves and reacts to environmental factors, to the passing of time, and to the products we put on it. Yet for all this progress, I am still shocked at how much has remained the same when it comes to misleading claims, poor formulations, products that contain ingredients that can hurt skin, and products that are priced with nothing more in mind than seducing women who are tempted by high prices because they are forever convinced that expensive means better. *The Beauty Bible* will help you put it all in perspective so the cosmetics industry can't waylay you from the real goal—taking great care of you skin. Then you can use this book to decide what products will best meet your needs and budget.

THE TRUTH WILL MAKE YOU BEAUTIFUL

A question I have been asked repeatedly over the years is: If the cosmetics industry's promises and claims are often disingenuous, if many companies operate under shared ownership, and if you can't rely on what the ads or products describe, then what is real? What is and isn't possible when it comes to treating your skin and skin-care needs? Although using the premises laid out in this book can prevent you from wasting money on overpriced or ineffective skin-care products, or stop you from being persuaded the next time you hear a sales pitch for a miraculous (or even semi-miraculous) sounding skin-care product or skin-care routine, you still need to know how to evaluate what to use and what to avoid for your own specific personal needs. The following is an overview to give you some insight on how to begin making decisions to create a skin-care routine that can help you achieve optimum benefits and results. Keeping these "rules" in mind and diligently following them will not only help you keep the craziness of the cosmetics industry in perspective, but also will result in healthy skin—and that's the truth.

GENTLY CLEAN YOUR SKIN. Research proving that you should clean the skin gently is now well-established. This is the basic first step for all skin types, from normal to oily, dry, blemish-prone, or sun-damaged. Nevertheless, no matter what your skin type, it is impossible and unhealthy to "deep-clean" skin. You can't get inside a pore and clean it out like a dentist with a drill. Even if you could get inside a pore and clean it out, the damage to the skin would negate any benefit of deep cleaning. (I know a blackhead looks like it's dirty, but dirt isn't what's making it look black!) Expensive water-soluble cleansers will not make your face any cleaner, nor are they necessarily any gentler than the less expensive water-soluble cleansers. In fact, the handful of standard cleansing agents used in cleansers is the same all across the cosmetics spectrum (Sources: *International Journal of Dermatology,* August 2002, pages 494–499; *Cosmetic Dermatology,* August 2000, pages 58–62; *Cutis,* December 2001, volume 68, number 5, supplemental; *Skin Research and Technology,* February 2001, pages 49–55; *Dermatology,* 1997, volume 195, number 3, pages 258–262; and *Journal of the American Medical Association,* April 1980, pages 1640–1643). Thankfully, overly drying cleansing agents are being used less and less, but there are still products that include them, especially bar soaps and bar cleansers, which are typically far more drying than water-soluble cleansers that use gentle cleansing agents.

__Essential Point:__ Find a gentle, water-soluble cleanser that doesn't dry out the skin or leave it feeling greasy and that can remove most types of eye makeup without irritating the eyes.

EVEN MINIMAL UNPROTECTED SUN EXPOSURE IS DAMAGING TO THE SKIN. Consumers clamor for the latest skin-care products that contain antioxidants, vitamins, plants, and a host of other exotics, yet all of that is meaningless if you aren't using an effective sunscreen every day of your life or are getting any amount of a tan from the sun. If you are exposed to the sun, even for as little as a few minutes every day—and that includes walking to your car, walking to the bus, or sitting next to a window during the day (the sun's damaging UVA rays come through windows)—regardless of the season, that exposure adds up over the years and it will wrinkle your skin, cause skin discolorations, and can result in skin cancer. If exposure that minimal can wrinkle the skin, imagine how much worse the impact of being in the sun for a long period of time can be and how ultimately detrimental sunbathing can be. No skin-care product except a sunscreen with an SPF of 15 or greater that has appropriate UVA-protecting ingredients of titanium dioxide, zinc oxide, avobenzone, or (outside of the United States) Mexoryl SX can help prevent that excessive and relentless damage from taking place. And you must apply sunscreen liberally! That means that using an expensive sunscreen can be dangerous if it discourages you from applying it generously. For more specifics about sun protection, including SPF ratings and UVA versus UVB protection, refer to Chapter Seven, *Cosmetics Dictionary*.

Essential Point: There is no such thing as a careful, safe, wrinkle-free, or non-skin-damaging suntan or unprotected sun exposure of any kind.

MANY SKIN-CARE PROBLEMS ARE CAUSED BY THE SKIN-CARE PRODUCTS SOLD TO PREVENT THEM. Most consumers would be shocked to learn that many of the products they buy to treat a specific skin condition actually can make matters worse. Overly emollient and too thick moisturizers can clog pores (even those products that claim to be noncomedogenic or nonacnegenic), products designed to control oily skin often contain ingredients that can make skin oilier (oil-free products often contain potential pore-clogging ingredients that don't sound like oils), and many skin-care products contain irritants that can cause a range of skin problems. Countless skin-care products, even from the most expensive lines, contain such irritating ingredients as fragrance, alcohol, peppermint, lemon, camphor, menthol, coltsfoot, arnica, and on and on. All of those ingredients can contribute to the very skin problems you are trying to eliminate from your face and your life.

Essential Point: Allergic, sensitizing, or irritating skin reactions are often caused by products that contain plant extracts, because many plant extracts, particularly fragrant ones, are inherently potent sources of skin problems.

DRY SKIN DOESN'T WRINKLE ANY MORE OR LESS THAN OILY SKIN—AND ALL THE MOISTURIZERS IN THE WORLD WON'T STOP WRINKLING. Oily skin may *look* less wrinkled, but that is only because oily skin has its own built-in moisturizer, namely the very oil produced by the skin's oil glands. Wrinkles, sagging, and skin discolorations are caused by a combination of events, but the primary culprits are sun exposure, genetic inheritance, sagging muscles (not from lack of exercise, but from the stretching and laxity that occur with use), facial trauma, loss of subcutaneous fat, and thinning of skin due to aging, but they are not caused by dry skin. That's not to say moisturizers (in their varying forms) can't do amazing things for skin, because they can, and there is more and more research showing this to be the case. Moisturizers with significant amounts of water-binding agents, state-of-the-art antioxidants, and anti-irritants can temporarily make skin look smoother, help skin function better, reduce the effects of sun damage, help improve texture and much, much more. However, the notion that this will somehow substitute for the work of a plastic surgeon or be enough to defend skin from further signs of aging is sheer fantasy.

Essential Point: What causes wrinkles to appear is *not* related to how dry or oily the skin may be. Wrinkles are caused by a number of factors, chiefly years of unprotected sun exposure and a person's own genetics.

IRRITATION IS BAD FOR SKIN AND MANY SKIN-CARE PRODUCTS CAN CAUSE IRRITATION. Your skin may become inflamed, dry, and blemished if you use too many scrubs (or overly abrasive ones), products that contain potentially irritating ingredients, or if you use more than one effective AHA or BHA product (please note that it is fine to alternate between one AHA and BHA product). Also, using topical prescription products (such as Retin-A or Renova) in conjunction with a too aggressive skin-care routine is just asking for trouble. Irritation is problematic for many reasons, but primarily because it inhibits the skin's immune response, reduces the skin's ability to heal, prevents cell growth, diminishes the skin's structure, and can in the long run break down collagen and elastin, the building blocks of skin. It is also important to understand that skin will not always tell you when it is being irritated. When skin is irritated, the damage taking place underneath the skin is not always reflected on the surface, yet problems are nonetheless taking place (Sources: *Skin Pharmacology and Applied Skin Physiology,* November-December 2000, pages 358–371; *Toxicology,* October 2000, pages 55–63; *Archives of Dermatologic Research,* November 1998, pages 615–620; and *Contact Dermatitis,* June 1998, pages 311–315). That means it is crucial that you pay attention to what you apply to your skin, so you can be informed about what is really going on beyond what you can see.

Essential Point: Irritation is a problem for skin health. The more sources of irritation you can eliminate, the better off your skin will be.

EXFOLIATE REGULARLY. Exfoliation is the process of removing the built-up outer layers of skin that haven't or won't come off on their own. Excess surface skin cells can be the result of sun damage, oily skin, overly emollient skin-care products holding down skin cells, or abnormally generated skin cells that adhere unevenly and tenaciously to the surface of skin. Exfoliation can be very important for many skin types. For dry skin, removing the excess layers of skin can help moisturizers absorb better, can generate collagen production, improve cell turnover, improve skin texture, and reduce the appearance of skin discolorations. Those with oily skin will find that regular exfoliation prevents clogged pores, can keep skin clear and even-toned, and can improve cell turnover. Perhaps the only skin type that cannot benefit from some form of exfoliation is extremely sensitive skin. Yet even very sensitive skin may be able to tolerate (and will benefit from) occasional, extra-gentle exfoliation. Among the most effective methods of exfoliation are topical scrubs, which can be as simple as using a washcloth or cosmetic cleansers that contain an abrasive material. However, research has established that salicylic acid (BHA), for normal to oily or blemish-prone skin, and alpha hydroxy acid (AHA) or polyhydroxy acid (PHA), for normal to dry skin, are not only effective exfoliants, but also increase collagen production, improve the overall health of the skin, increase cell turnover, and reduce the appearance of skin discolorations (Sources: *Cutis*, August 2001, pages 135–142; *Journal of the European Academy of Dermatology and Venereology*, July 2000, pages 280–284; *American Journal of Clinical Dermatology*, March-April 2000, pages 81–88; *Skin Pharmacology and Applied Skin Physiology*, May-June 1999, pages 111–119; *Dermatologic Surgery*, August 1997, pages 689–694, and May–2001 pages 1–5; *Journal of Cell Physiology*, October 1999, pages 14–23; and *British Journal of Dermatology*, December 1996, pages 867–875).

Essential Point: Regular exfoliation is beneficial for almost all skin types, particularly oily and dry skin.

BE WARY OF SKIN-CARE PRODUCTS THAT SMELL NICE OR HAVE PRETTY COLORS. I know the pretty blue or delicate pink shades of skin-care products are attractive, and a softly wafting fragrance from a cream or lotion can be appealing, but these fragrances and colors are often problematic and completely unnecessary in skin-care products. A great deal of research shows that fragrance is one of the primary skin irritants found in cosmetics (refer to the entry on fragrance in Chapter Seven, *Cosmetics Dictionary*). So why does almost every cosmetics company fragrance their products? Because consumer research (and marketing reports) have consistently and unequivocally shown that consumers, and women in particular, *want* their skin-care products to have a scent. The whole experience of using skin-care products (especially the pricey variety) is romanticized when it is associated with a seductive bouquet of scents (Sources: *Dermatology*, 2002, volume 205, number 1, pages 98–102; *Contact Dermatitis*, December 2001, pages 333–340; and *Toxicology and Applied Pharmacology*, May 2001, pages 172–178).

As for coloring agents, they may be great in a lipstick or foundation, but a blue or pink moisturizer is not great when the purpose of the skin-care product is to be absorbed into the skin.

Essential Point: Ingredients that add fragrance to a product, even natural fragrances, are notorious for causing allergic reactions or skin sensitivities.

DO NOT AUTOMATICALLY BUY SKIN-CARE PRODUCTS BASED ON THE NOTION OF AGE. Many products on the market are supposedly designed specifically for women who are in their 30s, 40s, or who are 50 or older. Before you buy into these arbitrary divisions, ask yourself why the over-50 group is always lumped together. Isn't it odd that women between the ages of 20 and 49 have skin that requires three or four categories, but that women over the age of 50 (often referred to as "mature skin") need only one? There are a lot of years between 50 and 90. According to this logic, someone who is 40 to 49 shouldn't be using the same products as someone who is 50, but someone who is 80 should be using the same products as someone who is 50. Skin has different needs based on how dry, sun-damaged, oily, sensitive, thin, blemished, or normal it is, all of which have little to do with age. Plenty of young women have severely dry skin, and plenty of older women have oily skin and breakouts (particularly those women experiencing perimenopausal or menopausal hormone fluctuations). Turning 40 or 50 does not mean a woman should assume that her skin is drying up and that she now must begin using overly emollient moisturizers or skin creams. And it definitely does not mean that the battle with blemishes is over.

**Essential Point:** Categorizing skin-care products by age groups is nothing more than a marketing device designed to sell products; it does not correlate at all with age-specific benefits to the skin.

DO NOT AUTOMATICALLY BUY SKIN-CARE PRODUCTS BASED ON YOUR SKIN TYPE. I know that statement sounds strange, but there are several reasons for this rule. It's not that skin type isn't important, but more often than not your skin type is not what you think it is. It's even possible that your skin type has been created by the products you are already using. Soap can severely dry the skin, overly emollient moisturizers can clog pores and cause blemishes, and alcohol-based toners can irritate the skin and cause dryness while doing nothing to change oil production (that can create classic combination skin). To know what your skin type really is, you must start from square one with the basics that won't alter or adversely affect your skin. That means using a gentle, water-soluble cleanser, an irritant-free toner (or a disinfectant if you break out) that contains effective water-binding agents, anti-oxidants, anti-irritants, or gentle detergent cleansing agents, an effective exfoliator (such as an AHA product if you have sun-damaged skin and/or a BHA product for breakouts), a sunscreen for daytime (which can be included in your moisturizer or foundation), and a well-formulated moisturizer at night (but only if you have dry skin or dry areas).

How do you know if you need a moisturizer? The first basic rule of thumb for those whose skin is not inherently dry is to begin by determining if other skin-care products are causing the dryness or flaking you're experiencing. If so, stop using those first before you decide to use a moisturizer.

For those with oily, combination, or blemish-prone skin, using a moisturizer, even if it's one of those claiming to be oil-free or specially formulated for oily skin, can cause more problems for you than it can possibly solve. If you still want the benefits of all the new antioxidants, water-binding agents, and anti-irritants, they can be obtained from a well-formulated toner or gel/serum-type product, which typically don't contain the unnecessary thickening agents (the ingredients that create lotion or cream textures) that can cause problems for oily or blemish-prone skin.

**Essential Point:** The intense cosmetics hype insisting that everyone needs a moisturizer is absolutely not true. (I discuss this at length in _The Beauty Bible._)

TREAT THE SKIN YOU HAVE TODAY, NOT THE SKIN YOU HAD LAST MONTH, LAST WEEK, OR YESTERDAY. Skin type can and will fluctuate. Skin-care routines based on a specific skin type don't take into consideration the fact that your skin changes according to the season, your emotions, the climate (humidity, dryness, cold, and heat all affect your skin), and your menstrual cycle. Pay attention to what your skin tells you it needs at any given time. This month you might need an extra-moisturizing sunscreen during the day, and a more emollient nighttime moisturizer. Next month you may only need a lightweight sunscreen or a foundation with sunscreen during the day and no moisturizer at night. The same is true for oily skin and breakouts. In fact, those dealing with breakouts may find that alternating their routine (such as using a disinfectant one evening and a BHA product the next) is necessary to balance the benefits with the potential side effects. But all of that doesn't mean you need new products every month—it just means you may need to use less of one item or more of another, adapting your routine flexibly according to your skin's current needs.

Essential Point: Don't hold fast to the idea that your skin fits squarely into and remains only one type—it changes, and so should your skin-care routine.

TEENAGERS ARE NOT THE ONLY ONES WHO HAVE ACNE. One of the biggest skin-care myths ever is that women over the age of 20 are not supposed to break out, and when they do, it is the exception to the rule. What a mistaken belief that is! Women in their 30s, 40s, and 50s can have acne just like teenagers, and the treatment principles remain the same.

Essential Point: Not everyone who has acne as a teenager will grow out of it, and even if you had clear skin as a teenager, that's no guarantee that you won't get acne later in life. You can blame this often maddening inconsistency on hormones!

BATTLING BLEMISHES OR ACNE IS NOT A MYSTERY, BUT IT DOES REQUIRE SPE-CIFIC TYPES OF PRODUCTS AND INGREDIENTS. Unfortunately, many cosmetics companies don't use those specific ingredients in their products for blemish-prone skin. As I wrote the reviews for this edition, I was flabbergasted that so few lines contain truly effective products for dealing with blemishes. This is one category of products where needless irritation is not the exception, but rather the unfortunate norm. The following is a very brief overview of how to win the battle against blemishes. For detailed information and specific battle plans, please refer to my Web site (www.CosmeticsCop.com) or *The Beauty Bible*.

The goals of effective blemish treatment are to reduce excess oil production, eliminate skin-cell buildup on the surface of skin and in the pore, and to kill the bacteria (*Propionibacterium acnes*) that cause the inflammation in the first place. This is best accomplished by using a gentle, water-soluble cleanser, exfoliating on the surface and in the pore lining with a pH-correct beta hydroxy acid (BHA) product, using a topical disinfectant (benzoyl peroxide is considered the most effective over-the-counter topical disinfectant), improving new skin-cell production (with topical prescription products such as azelaic acid or Differin), and absorbing excess oil from inside the pore. Blackheads and whiteheads are treated the same way, minus the disinfectant step. Note that these two specific skin maladies are not related to the presence of bacteria and do not respond to disinfectants the way acne does.

Essential Point: Battling blemishes requires experimenting to find the right combination of products, though a gentle cleanser, exfoliant, and topical disinfectant are the basics.

THERE ARE GREAT SKIN-LIGHTENING PRODUCTS AVAILABLE THAT CAN AFFECT THE APPEARANCE OF SUN-DAMAGED SPOTS. You can expect about a 20% to 40% improvement if you use skin-lightening products in association with an effective sunscreen (one with an SPF 15 or greater formulated with the UVA-protecting ingredients of avobenzone, titanium dioxide, or zinc oxide). Hydroquinone is the most commonly used skin-lightening agent because it has the most established research showing its ability to inhibit melanin production. It is available in 1% to 2% concentrations over the counter, and at 4% or higher concentrations from physicians. Along with sunscreen and hydroquinone, glycolic acid (an AHA) can also be extremely effective in achieving an overall reduction in skin discolorations.

Certain plants and plant extracts are also options, but they are not the best source for lightening skin. Arbutin is the most intriguing alternative to hydroquinone, yet even so it's arbutin's hydroquinone content that gives it its melanin-inhibiting properties (Sources: *Analytical Biochemistry,* June 2002, pages 260–268, and June 1999, pages 207–219; *Pigment Cell Research,* August 1998, pages 206–212; and *Journal of Pharmacology and Experimental Therapeutics,* February 1996, pages 765–769). Although the research describing arbutin's effectiveness is persuasive (even if almost all of the research was conducted on animals or in vitro), concentration protocols have not been established. That means we just don't know how much arbutin it takes to have an effect in lightening the skin. Therefore, choosing arbutin over hydroquinone (which does have long-standing concentration protocols) is a cross-your-fingers, hope-this-works proposition.

Mulberry extract, which contains arbutin, has one study showing it to have minimal effectiveness, though almost none when compared to the effectiveness of hydroquinone (Source: *Cosmetics & Toiletries,* 1997, volume 112, pages 59–62); plus, the study used a pure concentration of mulberry extract, not the minimal amounts that are present in cosmetics. Kojic acid, an extract from mushrooms, is another natural option, but it is not as effective as hydroquinone either. In addition, kojic acid is considered more irritating and unstable (Source: *Contact Dermatitis,* 1995, volume 32, number 1, pages 9–13).

There are also other plant extracts claiming to lighten skin, and while there are studies demonstrating some amount of effectiveness in vitro (meaning in a glass petri dish), there are no studies showing they can do this on human skin. Vitamin C, in the form of magnesium ascorbyl phosphate, has one study showing it to be an effective skin-lightening agent, but to have that effect the minimum required concentration was shown to be 10% (Source: *Journal of the American Academy of Dermatology,* January 1996, pages 29–33), and no cosmetics currently contain anywhere near that amount.

Regardless of which skin-lightening ingredient or product you decide to try, a well-formulated sunscreen used diligently, 365 days a year over exposed parts of the body, is absolutely the most effective way to prevent and reduce skin discolorations. Also, an effective AHA product (meaning one with a 4% to 10% concentration of AHA and with a pH of 3 to 4) can help encourage cell turnover, and that has been shown to improve skin discolorations, too.

Essential Point: When it comes to choosing the best ingredient for lightening sun-caused or hormone-induced skin discolorations, hydroquinone is the star of the show. No other skin-lightening ingredient has a more substantiated, successful track record.

STATE-OF-THE-ART ANTIOXIDANTS, WATER-BINDING AGENTS, AND ANTI-IRRITANTS HAVE AN ABUNDANCE OF RESEARCH SHOWING THEM TO BE EXTREMELY HELPFUL FOR ALL SKIN TYPES. I discuss these types of ingredients at length in my book *The Beauty Bible,* and it is a very lengthy and complicated discussion. That's because this aspect of skin care is probably near the top in importance when it comes to skin health and preventing and reducing the effects of sun damage and free-radical damage. Throughout this book, you will repeatedly see high ratings given to products that contain these types of ingredients.

Despite the benefit to skin these ingredients provide, you can ignore the special-effects battles the cosmetics industry is waging these days that set up antioxidants and water-binding agents against each other. Trying to decide which company has the best ones is a fool's game. There is absolutely no research showing any one ingredient to be "the best," though there are quantities of research showing that there are lots and lots of good ones, and no one company has a corner on any of these.

Essential Point: Dozens of antioxidants and water-binding agents have substantial value for skin. There is no single "best" option when it comes to choosing products that contain these ingredients, so don't get caught up in the hype. Refer to Chapter Seven, *Cosmetics Dictionary,* for specifics regarding antioxidants, water-binding agents, anti-irritants, and the various ingredients that provide benefits, as well as information concerning free-radical damage and sun damage.

THERE ARE NO COSMETICS THAT CAN ELIMINATE WRINKLES, NO MATTER HOW AWESOME THE CLAIMS SOUND, HOW EXOTIC THE INGREDIENTS ARE, OR HOW EXPENSIVE THE PRODUCT IS. According to the cosmetics industry, just about anything and everything cosmetics companies put in their products reduces, lessens, alleviates, diminishes, decreases, improves, enhances, restores (and on and on) the signs of aging or just wrinkles in general. With all the promises you find in line after line, and with product after product sounding the same, how do you as the consumer choose what to use? Typically, one or two ingredients are the hot ticket each season, with past favorites occasionally falling back into favor, or with new spins given to ingredients that have lost their panache with consumers. These might be collagen, AHAs, proteins, amino acids, DNA, milk lipids, elastin, emu oil, olive oil, myriad plants ranging from algae to ylang-ylang, metals such as copper, gold, or silver, or miscellaneous ingredients like Chinese herbs, bilberry, horsetail, melibiose, and more. And how many companies have jumped on the alpha lipoic acid, vitamin C, vitamin A, vitamin K, vitamin E, kinetin, or coenzyme Q10 bandwagon? Did I forget to mention aloe, chamomile, lavender, Dead Sea water, selenium, or transforming growth factors? The list is almost beyond comprehension. A quick look at the *Cosmetics Dictionary* in Chapter Seven will give you a daunting reminder of just how confusing, intricate, and overwrought an industry this is.

Sadly, most women buy into this insanity hoping that one or a combination of these options will finally be the winner. But how many secret, miraculous, antiwrinkle formulas can there be? Do we ever get tired of the onslaught? The answer seems to be no, we never get tired—which is why every month there's another cosmetic product or cosmetics company launched promising women perfect skin. And month after month, women predictably purchase another cache of products believing they've bought the answer that will erase their wrinkles. I imagine that many women must think: "It sounds so good, surely this must be it." Yet these products consistently fail to live up to their incredible claims.

The promises made for new miracle ingredients for skin care have a long history. There was the lemon craze in the late 1970s, the vitamin E hype from the early 1980s, the collagen and elastin frenzy from the mid 1980s, the retinol mania from the late 1980s (yes, the retinol being touted today is the same one that came and went in the late 1980s), the AHA mania from the early 1990s, and then the vitamin C hysteria of the late 1990s and kinetin into the millennium. At one point or another women thought all of these were the answers to their skin-care woes. Yet hundreds of these products were created and millions of units were sold—and women still had their wrinkles. It's not that vitamin E, vitamin C, retinol (vitamin A), collagen, elastin, or AHAs (to name a few) aren't good skin-care ingredients, because they are, but none of them are the fountain of youth we're being promised or that we're hoping for. For some driving reason, which social scientists may be better at ascertaining than I am, women seem to *need* to believe there is a magic potion out there that will restore their youthful appearance or get rid of any and all skin flaws. From that perspective, women will accept almost any sales pitch they're thrown as long as the promise is for miraculous results.

Essential Point: There is some interesting research behind many popular antiaging skin-care ingredients, but I haven't seen any legitimate research indicating that "the answer" or the fountain of youth has finally been found. Until this changes, the only product that can honestly call itself "antiwrinkle" is an effective sunscreen with UVA protection that's rated at SPF 15 or above.

CHOOSING A REALLY GREAT SKIN-CARE ROUTINE IS NOT AS COMPLICATED AS IT SEEMS. Most recommended skin-care regimens are at best unrealistic. They are either too complicated, too contrived, too irritating, or absurdly and unnecessarily expensive. Choosing a great skin-care routine isn't about the proverbial notion of getting back to basics either, because what is the definition of basic? Many women think of soap and water as basic, but the pH of most soaps can increase the level of bacteria on the skin, and the same ingredients that keep the bar in its solid form can clog pores. Bar soaps and bar cleansers can also be exceedingly drying and irritating, which is a serious problem for skin. Is sun protection part of getting back to basics? And what about exfoliation with an AHA or BHA or the use of a retinoid like Renova or Retin-A to improve cell production for those with sun-damaged skin? Choosing skin-care products doesn't have to be complicated, but it does have to address what is best for *your* skin, and, depending on your skin type, that's where things can get complicated.

As mentioned above, everyone needs a gentle cleanser. Beyond this, the only essentials are an effective UVA/UVB sunscreen with at least SPF 15 for daytime (this can come from your foundation, assuming you apply it evenly to your entire face) and a moisturizer for use over dry areas (including around the eyes) at night. Those three products form the cornerstone of a reliable skin-care routine. Of secondary importance are an AHA or BHA product for exfoliation and/or to help clear clogged pores, a disinfectant (if you are breaking out), and, for oily skin, an oil-absorbing mask. Optional products you may wish to add include a non-irritating toner, a silicone- or oil-based makeup remover, a specialty product (such as an eye gel, hydrating mask, or antioxidant serum), or a topical scrub.

Redundant or nonessential products include anything that contains unnecessary irritants, neck or bust creams and gels, lip-plumping products, anti-cellulite products, and de-puffing gels.

Depending on the condition of your skin, you may also be dealing with or considering topical prescription medicines. How these products fit into or will change your skin-care routine should be discussed with your physician or dermatologist.

Essential Point: Choosing a really great skin-care routine means doing what it takes to be good to your skin without wasting money or causing undue irritation, and buying only products that live up to their claims.

WHAT ABOUT ANTIWRINKLE PRODUCTS?

The bad news is that there are no skin-care products that get rid of wrinkles. I know the onslaught of claims the cosmetics industry asserts is overwhelming and convincing, but there is no reliable or published research showing any of it to be true. Or at least not the way we hope these products would work, and there is definitely nothing in the world of cosmetics that will do the job, especially when compared to the types of medical procedures performed by cosmetic surgeons or dermatologists. The good news is that there is a good deal of research showing a noticeable improvement with certain topical treatments that aren't medical procedures. Just don't expect miracles and don't get seduced by the endless frivolous promises flaunted for skin-care products.

One of the fundamental characteristics of sun damage is that the outer layer of the skin becomes thickened and yellow, while the underlying layer, where new skin cells are produced, becomes damaged, generating abnormal cell growth and hypermelanin production. The abnormal cell growth also results in malformed elastin, collagen deterioration, and distorted circulation of the blood and lymph systems. Regular use of sunscreen can slow this damage, allow for some improvement, and prevent further destruction. Topical tretinoin has been shown to partially reverse the clinical and histological (structural) changes induced by the combination of sunlight exposure and chronological aging. A formulation of tretinoin (as in Renova, Avita, Tazorac, or a generic tretinoin product) has been extensively investigated in multicenter, double-blind trials and has been shown to produce significant improvement with four to six months of daily use, when compared with application of the vehicle alone, as part of a regimen including sun protection and moisturizer use (Sources: *Cosmetic Dermatology,* December 2001, page 38; *Journal of Investigative Dermatology,* 2001, volume 111, pages 778–784; *Clinical and Experimental Dermatology,* October 2001, pages 613–618; *Clinical Geriatric Medicine,* November 2001, pages 643–659; and *Photochemistry and Photobiology,* February 1999, pages 154–157).

Alpha hydroxy acids (AHAs) have also been widely used for therapy of photodamaged skin, and these compounds have been reported to normalize hyperkeratinization (over-thickened skin) and to increase viable epidermal thickness and dermal glycosaminoglycans content. To sum this up, recent work has substantially described how the aging process affects the skin and has demonstrated that many of the unwanted changes can be improved by topical therapy (Sources: *Cutis,* August 2001, pages 135–142; *Journal of the European Academy of Dermatology and Venereology,* July 2000, pages 280–284; *American Journal of Clinical Dermatology,* March-April 2000, pages 81–88; *Skin Pharmacology and Applied Skin Physiology,* May-June 1999, pages 111–119; *Journal of Cell Physiology,* October 1999, pages 14–23; and *British Journal of Dermatology,* December 1996, pages 867–875).

There is every reason to consider using a combination of sunscreen (SPF 15 or greater with the UVA-protecting ingredients of avobenzone, titanium dioxide, and/or zinc oxide), topical tretinoin, and an AHA lotion, gel, or moisturizer as an effective approach for combating wrinkles. A wealth of research points to these as truly being as basic as it gets for your skin when it comes to battling wrinkles. From there, if you want to you can add a good moisturizer with potent antioxidants, which can also help, but exactly how much they help is yet to be established.

WHAT GETS RID OF BLEMISHES?

All of the steps described below address each of the factors that cause pimples. These are the best options for reducing oil production, for disinfecting the skin, for improving exfoliation, and for controlling hormonal activity, and are a potential cure for blemishes. Finding the combination that works best for you is the first goal; then you must focus on carrying out all the steps and carrying them out consistently.

Gentle cleansing. Using a water-soluble cleanser that gently cleans your skin without stimulating the oil glands, increasing redness, or creating dryness is standard for any skin-care routine because it makes an instant difference in the appearance and feel of the skin. It is also essential for reducing breakouts. Using cleansers that contain exfoliating agents, topical disinfectants, or oil-absorbing ingredients is not the best option, because the active ingredients would be on the skin for such a short time before they were washed away that they would have little to no chance of having any effect on skin. Save these ingredients for another step.

Exfoliating. Because blemishes occur inside the pore and involve oil production, an effective 1% to 2% salicylic acid (beta hydroxy acid, or BHA) product is a crucial over-the-counter starting point for exfoliating the skin. Salicylic acid dissolves lipids, which means it can penetrate the oil and exfoliate inside the pore, and as a plus, because it is related to aspirin, it has anti-inflammatory properties. I recommend using BHA in a gel, liquid, or extremely light lotion formula because these are unlikely to contain waxy thickening agents or emollients that can clog pores. Topical scrubs and alpha hydroxy acids (AHAs) can be helpful for surface exfoliation, but they can't affect oils in the pore lining, and it's essential to do that to deal with one of the root causes of a blemish.

Disinfecting. There aren't many options for disinfecting the skin. Alcohol (when used in the right concentrations) and sulfur can be good disinfectants, but basically they are too drying and irritating, causing more problems than they help, and that can generate more breakouts. Plant-derived disinfectants such as tea tree oil (melaleuca) are an option, but very few products currently being sold contain a high enough concentration to reliably kill bacteria. Benzoyl peroxide is still the best over-the-counter disinfectant for this purpose and is available in 2.5%, 5%, and 10% concentrations.

If benzoyl peroxide isn't effective, a topical antibiotic or even an oral antibiotic prescribed by a doctor may be the only option left to kill stubborn, blemish-causing bacteria, although an oral antibiotic should be a last resort. Oral antibiotics can indeed kill blemish-causing bacteria, but they also kill good bacteria in the body, often resulting in yeast infections and stomach problems. In addition, some of the acne bacteria *(P. acnes)* in your body can develop resistant strains in a short period of time, making the antibiotic you're taking ineffective.

Improving cell production. Tretinoins, Differin, and azelaic acid are prescription options for generating healthy cell growth that can change the shape of the pore, allowing for normal oil flow. This improvement can eliminate the environment that allows the blemish to develop.

Absorbing or controlling excess oil. Clay masks are an option for absorbing oil as long as they contain no irritating ingredients. Using milk of magnesia as a facial mask is a simple and effective way to absorb oil. Birth-control pills and hormone blockers can equalize hormones, reducing or eliminating the source of excess oil production. The pros and cons of taking these medications should be discussed with your physician.

When all else fails, and your breakouts persist after you've tried these over-the-counter and prescription options, then you can still try Accutane, which is the only medication that can essentially cure acne. This is the last option in any program addressing blemishes because it has serious side effects if a woman becomes pregnant while using it, plus other health concerns.

STEP UP TO A REALLY GREAT SKIN-CARE ROUTINE

The following is a realistic, viable skin-care routine that can be adapted for many skin types.

STEP 1

Even at night, when you're removing makeup, always wash your face with a gentle, water-soluble cleanser that rinses off completely and doesn't irritate the eyes. Your eye makeup should come off with the same water-soluble cleanser that cleans your face. If not, it may be necessary to use an eye-makeup remover.

Use only tepid to slightly warm water. Hot water burns the skin, and cold water shocks it. Repeated use of hot water, saunas, or Jacuzzis can cause broken capillaries to surface on the nose and cheeks, while also causing unwanted irritation that not only damages skin but also damages the skin's healing ability.

If you are wearing an ultra-matte foundation, you may need to use a washcloth to help remove makeup. This is an exception to the rule, but it may be necessary for these long-wearing, stubborn foundations that are very effective for oily skin types.

STEP 2

Exfoliating the skin helps unclog pores and removes dead skin cells, benefiting both dry and oily skin. There are two ways to exfoliate: with a mechanical exfoliant such as a scrub and with a chemical exfoliant such as AHAs or BHA. Many skin types need only one of these two types of exfoliant. Overexfoliating with scrubs and several AHA or BHA products is overkill, and I do mean kill. You only have so much skin, and too much exfoliation can cause damage and negate any of the positive effects you were hoping for. You can use a scrub after the face is cleansed or it can be used as your cleanser for Step 1.

Scrubs are a way to mechanically exfoliate the skin and are an option for some skin types, particularly those that tend to break out. However, mechanical scrubs must be used sparingly if you are also using an effective AHA or BHA because overexfoliating the skin is not helpful and can cause problems such as irritation or a rashlike breakout. There is also research showing that topical scrubs are not recommended for moderate to severe cases of acne. Mechanical exfoliation should be performed after you use your cleanser. The mechanical exfoliant can be a cosmetic cleanser that contains abrasive particles, but a plain washcloth (a clean one every time) also works very well as a topical scrub. One of my favorite scrubs is baking soda mixed with a gentle, water-soluble cleanser. While your face is still wet, pour a scant handful of baking soda into the palm of your hand. For a simple scrub, add a small amount of water to create a paste, gently massage your entire face with this paste, and then rinse generously with tepid water. You can also mix 1 or 2 teaspoons of baking soda with 1 or 2 tablespoons of a good, water-soluble cleanser such as Cetaphil Gentle Skin Cleanser, an alternative that is good for any skin type. How often you should exfoliate depends on your skin type.

For tips on applying an AHA or BHA product, see Step 5.

STEP 3 (OPTIONAL)

After your face is clean, as needed (but not every day) gently squeeze blackheads or blemishes that you want to remove. Blackheads usually don't disappear on their own; they can be stubborn even if you are using a good AHA or BHA product or Retin-A. For pimples, however, although they can heal on their own, relieving the pressure and removing the contents can help them heal faster and prevent further swelling, which can cause scarring. If you are shocked by this suggestion, that's OK; you don't have to do this, but it does help. This is what most facialists do best for your skin; however, it's cheaper to do it yourself. Many people worry about making matters worse. The only way to prevent that from happening is to NEVER, absolutely NEVER, oversqueeze. If the blemish or blackhead does not respond easily, stop and leave it alone. Moderate squeezing does not cause problems on the face; in fact, it is one of the best ways to clear blackheads and remove pressure from a swollen lesion. The problems occur when you massacre the skin by squeezing until you create scabs and sores. If you don't trust your own skill, a good facialist can provide this service and it can make a significant change in the appearance of your skin.

STEP 4

Toners are a step that follows the cleanser and scrub. Depending on your skin type and the product you choose, a toner can remove the last traces of makeup, help soothe skin, and add some good water-binding agents and antioxidants to the skin. For someone with normal to oily skin, a toner can substitute for a moisturizer and it can be the only "moisturizer" needed. For someone with normal to dry skin, a toner can be a good addition to your regular moisturizer. If you have acne or blemish-prone skin, the toner you use must be soothing or must contain an effective disinfectant to kill blemish-causing bacteria.

When your face is completely rinsed and dried, take a cotton ball and apply the appropriate toner for your skin type. Please keep in mind that toners (as well as any skin-care product that comes near your face or body) must be as irritant-free as possible. There are many irritant-free toners, but the more expensive ones are absolutely not worth their exorbitant price tags, especially when you consider that their basic ingredients are almost always the same as those in the less expensive versions.

STEP 5

This is the time to apply an AHA or BHA product. AHAs (preferably in the form of glycolic acid or lactic acid) and BHA (in the form of salicylic acid) are the most researched of all the exfoliants being sold in the world of skin care, so we know the most about their risks and performance requirements. AHAs are most effective in concentrations of 5% to

10% in a base with a pH of 3 to 4. BHA is most effective in concentrations of 1% to 2% in a pH of 3 to 4. (AHA and BHA products with an emollient base can double as moisturizers, or can be the only product your skin needs other than a cleanser and sunscreen.)

If you are using a topical retinoid such as Retin-A or Renova it would be applied now, either by itself, or after the AHA or BHA is applied. The same holds true if you are using MetroGel, MetroCream, or MetroLotion.

STEP 6

If you are breaking out, this would be the time to apply a topical disinfectant such as a 2.5%, 5%, or 10% benzoyl peroxide product. Note: If you are using Retin-A, Renova, or any topical retinoid, benzoyl peroxide cannot be applied at the same time.

STEP 7

During the day, every day, 365 days per year, it is essential to wear a sunscreen with an SPF of 15 that also provides UVA protection. You must be certain that the product you choose contains one of the following in the list of active ingredients: avobenzone (also called Parsol 1789 or butyl methoxydibenzoylmethane), zinc oxide, or titanium dioxide. If you have normal to dry skin, wear a sunscreen that comes in a moisturizing base (actually, most sunscreens come in a moisturizing base). If you have normal to oily skin, you do not need a moisturizer, but you still must wear a sunscreen with an SPF of 15 that provides UVA protection. In this instance, you can choose a matte foundation that includes an effective sunscreen. If you are using several skin-care products, in order not to dilute the effectiveness of the sunscreen, it must be the last product you apply to your skin. Let me repeat that: sunscreen should always be the last product you apply.

STEP 8

Moisturizing is the skin-care step most women obsess over, and the cosmetics industry is certainly glad they do. Loading up on moisturizers and antiwrinkle potions is big business. Yet, in truth, you only need to use a moisturizer if you have dry skin. In short, not everyone needs a moisturizer! The biggest myth you've been sold by the cosmetics industry is that there are wrinkle creams and moisturizers out there that will undo or prevent wrinkles. It just isn't true. Every month hosts of new antiwrinkle creams are launched with more promises and supposedly newfangled formulations. And every few months our hope is renewed—until the next round of misleading claims are thrown at us. Hundreds of great moisturizers in all price ranges are out there for skin, and also plenty of poorly formulated ones—and you may be shocked, reading the reviews, to find that some of the worst are the most expensive. Keep in mind, though, that using even the best-formulated moisturizer is meaningless if you are not diligent about sun protection. For specifics on how moisturizers were rated throughout this book, refer to Chapter Three, *Evaluating Skin-Care Products*.

SPECIALTY TREATMENTS

If you have melasma or chloasma, which are brown or ashen discolorations caused by sun damage or hormonal changes (usually the result of birth-control pills), then you may want to consider adding a skin-lightening product to your routine. These products should contain at least 1% to 2% hydroquinone (the percentages that are available over the counter), but may contain 4% or more, which are available only from physicians. This step would come after the toner and AHA or BHA product steps, but before the Retin-A, Renova, or sunscreen. This layering process can be tricky for some skin types, but it can prove to be quite effective in the lightening process. Please keep in mind that no lightening product of any kind works if you do not use an effective sunscreen day in and day out.

For other skin disorders, such as rosacea, psoriasis, severe dry skin, or wound and scar treatments, and more specifics regarding all skin-care concerns and options, refer to my book, *The Beauty Bible,* or search my Web site, www.CosmeticsCop.com.

CHAPTER THREE

Product-by-Product Reviews

How Products Are Rated

Rating a wide variety of cosmetic products is a rigorous, complex process. Setting up guidelines to distinguish and differentiate a terrible product from a great one, or a good product from one that's just mediocre, requires exact and consistently applied guidelines, and moreover guidelines that must be substantiated with published research and clear criteria. This is exactly what I've created for each product type that I review in this book.

First and above all, you need to know that I do not base any rating decision on my own personal experience with a product. In other words, just because I like the way a cleanser or a moisturizer feels on my skin doesn't mean that thousands of others will feel the same way about it. Personal feelings won't help you evaluate whether a product may hurt your skin or live up to any part of the claims showcased on the label. There are lots of online beauty chat rooms and bulletin boards, fashion magazines, and friends who love to share their personal experiences about the products they use. That might be interesting and entertaining, but it's important to recognize that lots of people like things that aren't good for them. Some people may like sun tanning or using products that contain irritating ingredients because they think it feels like it's "working." Most people have no idea what kinds of ingredients can damage skin. Even more to the point, these friendly sources of recommendations don't know that other products may perform equally as well if not better for a lot less money. If you're going to spend money on a product, why not find out first whether or not it can live up to its claims and what you can expect in regard to how it may or may not work for you based on formulary or comparison performance issues? That is what you will find out from the reviews in this book.

All of the ratings for the skin-care products in this book are based primarily on an individual product's formulation, using published, peer-reviewed studies about the ingredients in the product, and taking into consideration their possible resulting interaction with the skin. I also evaluate these formulas based on published cosmetics chemistry data about ingredient performance and consistency. From that I can assess a product's potential for irritation, dryness, breakouts, sensitivities, greasiness, and other issues of texture and performance.

Makeup products are evaluated more subjectively than skin-care products in regard to application, color selection, texture, and comparison to similar types of products from myriad other lines. Formulation is also a consideration for makeup products, predominantly for claims made in regard to skin care.

This rating process is more challenging than I can describe, because even if I think a company is absurdly overcharging for its products or is exceedingly dishonest in its claims and advertising, and no matter how unethical it seems to me, it does not prevent me from saying that a product of theirs is good for a particular skin type (though I do often say, "This is a good product but what a shame the price has to be so absurd and the claims so offensive!").

Overall, the evaluation process for this Sixth Edition of *Don't Go to the Cosmetics Counter Without Me* is the same as for previous editions. However, you will find one major difference that has had a direct impact on the product ratings: In this edition, I use a far more stringent standard for excellence for every category of product. Happy faces are no longer awarded to ordinary, perfunctory products with mediocre, standard, or even decent formulations. For example, if a product makes claims about containing anti-oxidants or anti-irritants, then it must contain a convincing amount of these ingredients. What you will notice is that far more products receive neutral ratings in this edition in comparison to previous editions.

Each cosmetics line is reviewed for several different elements. The first consideration is overall presentation and how user-friendly the displays or company literature are. For lines available at retail locations, I consider it an asset if their display units are set up with convenient color groupings, such as colors divided into warm (yellow) and cool (blue) tones, and are easily accessible. Skin-care and makeup products that are convenient to sample without the help of a salesperson are also rated high. For drugstore lines, colors must be easy to see, and samples or tester units are considered a bonus.

For infomercial and in-home shopping channel companies, my major criterion is the organization of their skin-care routines. Generally, ordering from sources like these means you are buying a set of products, not picking and selecting from what is being offered. If these prefabricated kits do not include an adequate sunscreen, or if the kit for someone with breakouts is only minimally different from the kit for dry skin, then the overall rating goes down dramatically (skin-care products with ingredients that are good for someone with dry skin are rarely suited for someone with oily, acne-prone skin).

I am also leery of any company's claim of being the best or having state-of-the-art formulations if they do not have a sunscreen of SPF 15 or greater with the UVA-protecting ingredients of avobenzone, titanium dioxide, or zinc oxide (and, outside of the United States, Mexoryl SX) as part of their daily skin-care regimen. Any company purporting to have worthwhile products or well-researched formulations could not possibly be telling the truth if they are not even aware of the well-known and easily accessible information on sunscreen ingredients (Sources: Food and Drug Administration at www.fda.gov and American Academy of Dermatology at www.aad.org).

The fundamental determination for each individual product's rating is based on specific criteria established for each product category. For every category, from blushes to eyeshadows, concealers, foundations, cleansers, toners, scrubs, moisturizers, facial masks, AHA products, brushes, and wrinkle creams, I've created specific standards that the products must meet to garner a happy, unhappy, or neutral (meaning unimpressive but not bad) face.

Makeup products are assessed mostly on texture (Was it silky-smooth or grainy and hard?), color (Was a wide range of colors available, and was there an adequate selection for women of color?), application (Could it be applied easily or was it difficult to spread or blend?), ease of use (Was the container poorly designed, were colors placed too close together in an eyeshadow set, was foundation put in a pump container that squirted too much product or didn't reach to the bottom of the jar?), and, finally, price.

Skin-care products are evaluated almost exclusively on the basis of content versus claim. If a product claims to be good for sensitive skin, it cannot contain irritants, skin sensitizers, drying ingredients, and so on.

I also asked the following questions to see if a product can measure up to its claims, based on established and published research:

1. **Given the ingredient list, and based on published research—not just what the cosmetics company wants you to believe—can the product really do what it promises?**

2. **How does the product differ from similar types of products?**

3. **If a special ingredient or ingredients are showcased, how much of them are actually in the product, and is there independent research verifying the claims for them?**

4. **Does the product contain problematic fragrances, plants, topical irritants, or other questionable ingredients that could cause problems for skin?**

5. **How farfetched are the product's claims?**

6. **Is the product safe? Are there risks such as allergic reactions, increased sun sensitivity, or poor sunscreen formulations, or potentially toxic ingredients?**

I wish I had the space to challenge and explain every single exaggerated claim and lofty explanation that accompanies the products listed in this book, but there is just not enough room (or time) to tackle that prodigious task. I cover most of the distortions and some of the hyperbole about products and ingredients in my book *The Beauty Bible,* Second Edition. Please refer to that as a source for understanding everything you need to know about taking care of oily skin, dry skin, wrinkles, and other special skin-care needs, as well as for a description of hundreds of skin-care ingredients and much more! You'll also find a great deal of additional helpful information on my Web site, at www.cosmeticscop.com.

WHAT CONSTITUTES LEGITIMATE RESEARCH?

The research quoted and cited throughout this book is taken almost exclusively from published and peer-reviewed medical and scientific journals, most of which are available online or in medical libraries. As important as this documentation is for the information I provide, perhaps even more significant is the "research" that I was not able to include in my assessments. When any cosmetics company claimed they had research demonstrating the effectiveness of their product, but the study was either not published, was proprietary (meaning it is not available to the public), or was otherwise not obtainable for review, the research was considered unacceptable. Just because a company says it has a "study" or did "laboratory testing" doesn't mean the results are scientifically valid, or have any relevance to overall efficacy. More often than not, the research conducted by cosmetics companies is little more than mere claim substantiation and not truly scientific evaluations.

For example, a preponderance of cosmetics ads and brochures state that they have studies showing astounding results according to what appears to be scientific research. What the consumer does not know, however, is that it doesn't take much to prove a product is effective! According to an article in *Cosmetics & Toiletries* magazine (December 1999, pages 52–53), "Skin moisturization studies using bioengineering methods are commonplace today. If data generated for a new test product demonstrate a statistically significant difference between the test product and untreated skin in favor of increased hydration, then claims indicating this to the consumer would be substantiated.... For example, [the claim] 'moisturizes your skin for up to 8 hours' would be substantiated by a study where a statistical difference was observed between the test product and untreated skin for up to 8 hours following application of the test product." All it takes to show the efficacy of a product is to apply it to one side of the face and leave the other side unmoisturized. In essence, using any moisturizer would show the same result.

While the FDA (at www.fda.gov) does not have regulations regarding cosmetics claim substantiation, there is nevertheless an entire industry of claim substantiation at work in the world of cosmetics. Some of this is due to the efforts of the Federal Trade Commission (www.ftc.gov) to crack down on misleading advertising, although budgetary limitations restrict much of their work. However, claim substantiation is growing in response to new European Union cosmetics legislation regarding animal testing, general substantiation of claims, and product safety (Source: 6th Amendment to the European Union Cosmetics Directive). This is because the EU guidelines call for more enforcement of product standards than guidelines in the United States. That means the U.S. cosmetics industry is fast and furiously establishing standards that basically meet regulatory rules, but give you no information that is helpful for evaluating how a product will affect your skin. Creative claim substantiation is fast becoming big business. Yet, tests like the one described above that compare dry, unmoisturized skin with dry skin that is moisturized and then proclaim that "our product works great!" are not very trustworthy, at least not from a consumer's viewpoint. It would be like doing a test that measures how drunk you can get by drinking a martini versus not drinking a martini—it provides no information at all because the result is already known: of course you don't get drunk when you don't drink! Likewise, of course, applying moisturizer to dry skin makes it look better than dry skin that isn't moisturized.

Anytime a study about a cosmetic product is mentioned, you need to ask yourself the following questions: How was the study conducted—was it peer reviewed, double blind, independent? Did the study have a broad enough scope to be significant (10 people is hardly a sweeping investigation)? Was there any independent corroborating research showing the same results? (Because one study showing great results is meaningless if it cannot be repeated by an unbiased independent source). Most important, who benefits from the study? And in particular, do the authors of the study stand to gain financially from the result of their study? All that information is vitally important and relates directly to the study's validity and credibility (Source: *Journal of the American Medical Association*, July 15, 1998, pages 225–226).

Very few consumers, or reporters for that matter, are aware of the large number of skin-care "research" laboratories whose only clients are cosmetics companies that want to use enticing statistics or want to validate incredible claims they can use as a marketing strategy. These research labs exist solely to provide pseudoscientific material for the cosmetics industry and these "studies" are never published. That way, if the marketing copy claims that a moisturizer provides an 82% increase in moisturization or a 90% increase in the skin's water content, the company may very well be able to point to a study that says this is true. Quoting these inconclusive, vague studies in a news story or ad can make them sound significant and meaningful, but in truth they are more often than not just hype and exaggeration generated exclusively to sell products. One of these claim-substantiation companies actually advertises its ability to deliver "creative claim generation/substantiation."

Here's a perfect example of how these feigned studies are performed. Let's take a typical claim about a moisturizer providing a large increase in the skin's moisture content. Without some basic information about how the study was conducted, that increase is meaningless. You can take almost anyone's skin, rub some alcohol on it or even just wash it with plain soap, then put on any moisturizer in the world, and the skin would reflect anywhere from an 82% to a 200% increase in moisture content. (In fact, you can soak in the bathtub for 30 minutes and come out with your skin well saturated with water and have a 500% increase in its moisture content.) Furthermore, perhaps the test included only five or ten women and compared only two products, one with an unknown formula. It may indicate that for this small group, brand A worked better than brand X—but what about how it worked compared with the 5,000 other moisturizers on the market? Maybe lots of those work just as well as brand A.

Such features are typical of these types of studies. At first glance, the study sounds impressive, yet it is virtually meaningless. It doesn't tell you anything about the product's effectiveness, or even whether that product is good for the skin (it turns out that a high moisture content isn't!), but it gives the cosmetics company statistics it can show off in its press releases.

I've seen this process at work firsthand, and it is disturbing. Whoever is paying the bill hires the research lab. The lab is handed the products and told what to look for and what kind of results are needed—for example, proof of moisturization, exfoliation, smoothness, reduction of wrinkles, or some other parameter. Then the lab goes about setting up a study to prove that position. Rarely are these studies done double blind, nor do they use a large group of women or show long-term results, and rarely (actually never) are the results negative. More to the point, these studies are never published. Yet consumers are led to believe this unverified information is factual when they read about it in editorials in magazines or newspapers.

Note: Double blind refers to a testing procedure designed to eliminate biased results, in which the identity of those receiving a test treatment is concealed from both the test administrators and the subjects until after the study is completed.

This same sleight of hand is used quite effectively in brochures and ads. Many cosmetics counters hand out impressively designed, scientific-looking brochures showing how well a product works on the skin. You might see, for example, a microscopic close-up of a patch of skin paired with an explanation of why it looks bad. Beside it is another close-up of the same patch of skin after the product is applied. See how wonderfully the product worked? The deception here is that you are not given enough "before" information. For example, if the woman had acne, what was she doing before to take care of her skin? Was she using products that clogged pores or aggravated breakouts? Had she never used any effective skin-care products for acne? In that case, any basic skin-care routine for acne could make a difference. And was this the single best result of the lot? Were there perhaps others who still had breakouts despite treatment? Or were the results just improved with computer savvy finesse (digitally retouched and changed) and have nothing whatsoever to do with the product? Just because information looks scientific doesn't mean it is.

I could go on and on about this kind of inadequate claim-substantiation business that takes place in the world of skin care and I do so numerous times throughout this book. What's important to remember is that phrases like "our studies show" or "our research establishes" or "our test results demonstrate" aren't worth the paper they are printed on unless you can see the entire study and can judge exactly how the research was carried out and whether or not the results are significant or senseless.

Next time you see stories about test results showing younger-looking skin, new cell growth, or any other claim that sounds too good to be true, regardless of who's making the claim, stop and think. Ask yourself how many times you've heard this "perfect skin in a bottle" message before. Is this "story" about only one study, or are there corroborating studies? Does it sound too good to be true? You may also want to ask yourself how many more times you are going to swallow another exaggerated claim about a skin-care product, or spend money believing that you've finally found the "best" product available. (Do you really believe that gorgeous, childlike model or photo-retouched celebrity in the picture looks like that because of the products being advertised?) Think about how many times you've been sucked in by a cosmetics ad, claim, or fashion magazine story, only to be disappointed again and again, until the next advertising campaign for a new product catches your attention.

DUE DILIGENCE

I can't stress enough how much time and effort my staff and I put into gathering our information. We are diligent about making sure we incorporate accurate and precise information or research for all of the products we review. To accomplish this, the first order of business with every edition is to contact every cosmetics company whose products I'm reviewing and ask them to please send whatever they can about their data or facts regarding their products and claims. Many more companies than ever before were forthcoming with information, including ingredient and product listings. Yet there were still a number of them who weren't willing to send us anything about their company or products, let alone details about the research or studies they use to substantiate their claims.

Let me state clearly that I am more than open to presenting any documented research that substantiates information contradicting something I've stated. I am more than willing to alter previously stated opinions and positions as new research comes to light showing that earlier information is no longer correct. For example, over the years I have changed my opinion on sunscreens with regard to the new research on UVA protection. I have modified my attitude toward antioxidants, too, given the growing body of literature establishing the positive effects of these ingredients for skin care. I have been more open to layering products when different active ingredients are needed, ranging from skin-lightening products to sunscreens and acne products. I could go on, but I want to be explicit about my desire to present the most up-to-date, currently published research that exists when it comes to skin-care formulations and makeup products.

I also want to thank the companies that did send me their information. While I may not agree with them on the quality of all their products or their advertising claims, their willingness to be forthcoming about their formulations and claims is appreciated.

The following companies were extremely helpful in providing information for the compilation of this book:

Aesop

Ahava

Alexandra de Markoff

Aloette

Alpha Hydrox

Annemarie Borlind

Aubrey Organics

Avon

Arbonne

Artistry by Amway

BeautiControl

Black Opal

Burt's Bees

Cetaphil

Clearasil

Cover Girl

Club Monaco

DHC

Dermablend

Dr. Mary Lupo
   Skin Care System

Ella Bache

Exuviance by NeoStrata

English Ideas/Lip Last

G.M. Collin

Jane Iredale

Jan Marini Skin Research

Linda Sy

Lip Ink

Liz Earle Naturally
   Active Skin Care

L'Oreal

Lubriderm

M.A.C.

M.D. Formulations

Mederma

Natura Bisse

Nu Skin

Ocean Potion

Ole Henriksen Skin Care

Ombrelle

Oxy Balance

PanOxyl

Paula Dorf Cosmetics

Peter Thomas Roth

pHisoderm

Pola

Rachel Perry

Rejuveness

Rejuvenique

Sense Usana

Stri-Dex

Tend Skin

Thalgo

Tony & Tina

Urban Decay

JUDGING A PRODUCT BY ITS LABEL

Many people wonder whether I can judge a skin-care product by its label. You may be thinking, "Wouldn't that be like judging a food just by the ingredients in it? What about tasting it for yourself?" Taste is necessary information, but it is also prudent to judge food by its ingredient list. It is no longer wise for any of us to consume any food without a clear understanding of how much fat, sodium, preservatives, coloring agents, or calories it contains, along with many other details pertinent to our health. Without that information, regardless of taste (and everyone has their own bias), you would never know what you were putting in your body. You could be causing yourself harm by eating more fat, calories, or salt than you should, leading to weight gain, cancer, high blood pressure, and so on. If you don't eat enough fiber, you could end up with gastrointestinal distress or other serious problems. If you aren't getting appropriate nourishment, you could become malnourished in some regard, and if you have food allergies or sensitivities, you could eat something that would be dangerous for you. How would you ever know what you were doing to yourself? The labels on food are every consumer's best friend, whether you're shopping at a discount grocery store or the fanciest gourmet shop.

Just as food labels are incredibly important, so are skin-care and makeup ingredient labels. If a skin-care product says it is good for sensitive skin or won't cause breakouts, but contains ingredients known to cause irritation or breakouts; that is essential information. If a skin-care product sells for $100 but contains the same ingredients as a product that costs $20, that is, to say the least, very important information. Perhaps even more significant, if a $100 product contains fewer or less effective ingredients than a $10 version, I think that is crucial consumer information. If a product claims to protect skin from the sun but it doesn't have an SPF 15 or greater and doesn't contain UVA-protecting ingredients, that is vital information regardless of price.

The ingredient list helps you sort through the jungle of choices. Besides, it is a far better starting point than basing decisions strictly on advertising mumbo jumbo or promises that are never delivered.

YOU WOULD BE SHOCKED

I wish there were some way I could teach every cosmetics consumer how to read an ingredient label. Once you became familiar with the chemical and Latin names of the ingredients listed and how they function, you would be stunned at how similar products in a particular category truly are. It's not that there aren't differences between products, but it's astounding how alike many products are. And I mean astounding. It is truly a marketing phenomenon when the cosmetics industry can convince women that there is a qualitative difference between a $10 cleanser and a $50 cleanser, or that a $60 sunscreen is far more advanced than one selling for $20, and so on for each product type. Even Dr. N.V. Perricone, author of the *The Wrinkle Cure* (a book describing Perricone's own unsubstantiated, non-scientific data regarding the treatment of wrinkles) and owner of the product line bearing his name, was quoted in the *New York Times* (Nov. 18, 2001, "The Skin Game with New Wrinkles") as saying "Promise them an unlined face, and you can sell them anything." This is exactly what he and hundreds of other companies are doing, selling empty promises that women fall for every time an ad proclaims the next answer for wrinkles.

· What I hope my book brings to light by the time you are done reading through the various lines and introductory chapters is that there are truly an amazing number of brilliant skin-care products being sold. However, if you are going to take truly beautiful care of your skin, you must also be aware that an alarming amount of misleading, overrated, and erroneous claims are being tossed about by companies who have no legal restrictions encouraging them to do otherwise. If you are seduced by price and advertising rhetoric, your skin and budget run the risk of being damaged, or, at the very least, being poorly taken care of. If you're not, you can gain some real benefits.

IRRITANTS AND COUNTER-IRRITANTS

For those of you who are familiar with my reviews, you may notice that I am now much more cautious about products that contain any amount of irritating ingredients, particularly those containing any form of grain alcohol (ethyl, ethanol, methanol, benzyl, or SD alcohol), as well as lemon, grapefruit, mint, peppermint, menthol, camphor, eucalyptus, ivy, fragrant oils, and overly drying or irritating detergent cleansing agents. My more exacting criteria in this area reflect the growing body of research indicating that irritation damages skin and hurts the skin's healing process (Sources: *Skin Research and Technology*, November 2001, pages 227–237 and *Microscopy Research and Technique*, volume 37, issue 3, pages 193–199). In the midst of our daily battle against sun damage, wrinkles, and the causes of breakouts, there is never a reason to unnecessarily irritate the skin with ingredients like these, which provide no benefit whatsoever for the face or body and can prevent the skin from healing.

It turns out that much of what we know about skin aging, wrinkles, and skin healing involves the skin's inflammatory reaction to sun exposure (ultraviolet radiation), pollution, and cigarette smoke. These elements trigger an inflammatory process leading to the accumulation of damage in the skin, in turn resulting in deterioration of collagen and elastin, depletion of disease-fighting cells, and free-radical damage (Sources: *Biogerontology*, 2001, volume 2, number 4, pages 219–229; *Ageing Research Reviews*, June 2002, pages 367–380; and *Journal of the International Union of Biochemistry and Molecular Biology*, October-November 2000, pages 279–289). Therefore, it never makes sense to use irritating ingredients on skin when they have no additional beneficial purpose (as topical disinfectants or certain exfoliants do). They would only hurt the skin and contribute to complications that make matters far worse for skin, not better.

What about counter-irritants? There is a misperception among many in the cosmetics industry, as well as among consumers, that ingredients considered to be counter-irritants, such as menthol, peppermint, camphor, eucalyptus, and mint, have anti-inflammatory or anti-irritant properties, and that is absolutely not true (Sources: *Archives of Dermatologic Research*, May 1996, pages 245–248; and Code of Federal Regulations Title 21—Food and Drugs, revised April 1, 2001, at 21CFR310.545, www.fda.gov). In fact, counter-irritants induce local inflammation as a way to relieve inflammation in deeper or adjacent tissues. In other words, they substitute one kind of inflammation for another. That is never good for skin. Both irritation and inflammation, no matter what causes them or how it happens, impair the skin's immune and healing response (Source: *Skin Pharmacology and Applied Skin Physiology*, November-December 2000, pages 358–371). And although your skin may not show it, or may not react in an irritated fashion, if you apply irritants to your skin the damage is still taking place and the effects are ongoing and add up over time (Source: *Skin Research and Technology*, November 2001, pages 227–237).

EVALUATING SKIN-CARE PRODUCTS

My reviews of skin-care products in each line are, with some exceptions, organized in the following categories: cleansers, eye-makeup removers, scrubs, toners, moisturizers (all kinds, regardless of the claim or type, such as eye or neck creams), alpha hydroxy acid or beta hydroxy acid exfoliants, specialty products, sunscreens, acne products, and facial masks. The criteria I used to evaluate the quality of the products in each of the different categories of skin-care products are explained below.

CLEANSERS: In reviewing facial cleansers, I am primarily interested in how genuinely water-soluble they are. Facial cleansers should rinse off easily, with or without the aid of a washcloth, and remove all traces of makeup, including eye makeup. Once a water-soluble cleanser is rinsed off, it should not leave the skin feeling dry, greasy, or filmy. And it should never burn the eyes, irritate the skin, or taste bad.

Removing makeup with cold cream–style, rinseable cleansers in lotion or cream form is an option for some women with extremely dry skin. In the past, I have been hesitant to recommend these because they do not remove makeup very well and they require heavy wiping and pulling of the skin to remove the makeup. However, for someone with dry skin, these can be the only good, soothing, nondrying products to clean the skin, when used along with a soft washcloth.

I do not recommend cleansers that contain concentrations of alpha or beta hydroxy acids (AHAs or BHA) or topical disinfectants such as benzoyl peroxide or triclosan. While these ingredients can be quite helpful in other skin-care products, in a cleanser they are rinsed down the drain before they have a chance to have a real effect on skin. It is also a concern that these ingredients can inadvertently get into the eye when rinsing the cleanser off the face. (I should mention that I have never found an effective cleanser that includes an AHA or BHA; either the amounts are too small or the base does not have an appropriate pH and neutralizes them. That means the AHA and BHA are useless in a cleanser, although some consumers no doubt are misled into believing they could have an effect on skin.)

EYE-MAKEUP REMOVER: It's not necessary to use a separate eye-makeup remover as an extra step. An effective but gentle, water-soluble cleanser should take off all your makeup, including eye makeup, without irritating the eyes. The problem with wiping off makeup is simply that you have to wipe and pull at your skin to get the stuff off. That repetitive pulling and wiping is not good for skin, particularly in the eye area. Another problem is the tendency for makeup to get wiped into the eye itself as opposed to splashed away, and that can cause irritation. Unless you are wearing waterproof mascara or can't get the knack of removing your eye makeup with a water-soluble cleanser, there are many reasons to avoid adding this step.

However, those women who find using a water-soluble cleanser ineffective for removing eye makeup can saturate a large cotton pad with eye-makeup remover, close their eyes, and very gently place the pad against the eyebrows and eyelids, holding it there for a few seconds. This way, they aren't tugging or pulling but instead are loosening and dissolving the eye makeup. Then they can follow with a water-soluble cleanser and more easily remove the makeup.

It is important to note that the vast majority of eye-makeup removers use many of the exact same ingredients found in water-soluble cleansers! In other words, many eye-makeup removers more often than not use a lightweight surfactant (detergent cleansing agent). In those instances, sticking with the water-soluble cleanser makes more sense. Other eye-makeup removers use either oils (plant or mineral) or silicones. These can help remove makeup without causing dryness, and for some skin types or personal preferences that can be beneficial.

Eye-makeup removers are one of the categories in which the products are nearly indistinguishable from one another. They are formulated so similarly that there are no surprises or real cautions needed.

EXFOLIANTS AND SCRUBS: With the advent of alpha hydroxy acids (AHAs) and the increased use of beta hydroxy acid (BHA; technical name, salicylic acid), there is less reason than ever before to use a mechanical exfoliant on the skin. Mechanical exfoliants are scrubs that remove skin cells as you rub particles over the skin. Even when the scrub particles are small and uniform in size, this procedure can still abrade the skin and be harsher than necessary, causing damage and affecting the skin's healing process. That means the major consideration for any topical scrub is that it has to be gentle on the skin and not rough or overly abrasive. It is also important that it rinses off easily without leaving any residue or greasy feel on the skin. Some women prefer the feeling of a scrub on their skin, but there aren't many scrubs that are any better than using plain baking soda mixed with Cetaphil Gentle Skin Cleanser for those with oily skin, or just a plain washcloth for that matter.

ALPHA/BETA HYDROXY ACID PRODUCTS: I expect products containing AHAs or BHA to be effective exfoliants. Though AHAs and BHA can also be effective as moisturizing ingredients, this is not what they do best for skin. Above all else, AHAs and BHA excel in exfoliating skin.

There is only one BHA (salicylic acid), but there are a variety of AHAs. The five major types of AHAs that show up in skin-care products are glycolic, lactic, malic, citric, and tartaric acids. Of these, the most commonly used AHAs are glycolic and lactic acids because of their special ability to penetrate the skin and because they have the most accumulated research on their functionality for skin. A search of the published literature for glycolic and lactic acids lists over 200 varying studies, while there are only a handful for the other three AHAs combined. A similar literature search for salicylic acid (BHA) reveals over 450 different published studies evaluating its effectiveness.

What glycolic, lactic, and salicylic acids can do is "unglue" the outer layer of dead skin cells. This helps to increase cell turnover by removing the built-up top layers of skin, allowing healthier cells to come to the surface. Removing this dead layer can improve skin texture and color, unclog pores, and allow moisturizers to be better absorbed by the skin. Both AHAs and BHA affect the top layers of skin, where they help to improve the appearance of sun-damaged skin, dry skin, and thickened skin caused by a variety of factors, including abnormal cell growth, smoking, and heavy moisturizers. A reminder: sun damage in particular causes the top layer of skin to thicken, creating a dull, rough texture and appearance on the surface of skin; AHAs nicely remove this thickened layer, revealing the more normal-appearing skin cells underneath (Sources: *Archives of Dermatologic Research*, June 1997, pages 404–409 and *Dermatologic Surgery*, May 1998, pages 573–577).

There is also a good deal of research showing that the use of glycolic acid (and most likely lactic acid) can improve the appearance of skin discolorations, increase collagen production, and reinforce the barrier function of skin (Sources: *Dermatologic Surgery*, May 2001, pages 429–433 and *American Journal of Clinical Dermatology*, March-April 2000, pages 81–88).

The fundamental difference between AHAs and BHA is that AHAs are water soluble, while BHA is lipid soluble (that is, oil soluble). This unique property of BHA allows it to penetrate the oil in the pores and exfoliate the built-up skin cells inside the oil gland. AHAs are not able to penetrate oil and so can't get through the fat content (sebum) of the skin and into the pores. Therefore, BHA is the best choice where blackheads and blemishes are the issue, and AHAs are more suitable for sun-damaged, thickened, or dry skin where breakouts are not a problem (Source: *Global Cosmetic Industry*, November 2000, pages 56–57).

I use very specific criteria to determine if an AHA or BHA product will be an effective exfoliant. I wish you could tell if it would be effective by reading the label, but that just isn't possible. There are no claims or promises on the product, or even the ingredient label, that will tell you whether you are purchasing an effective AHA or BHA product.

When it comes to AHAs and BHA, the crucial information comes in two parts. One is the type of ingredient and its concentration in the product, and the other is the pH of the product. AHAs work best at concentrations of 5% to 8% in a base with a pH of 3 to 4 (this is more acid than alkaline or neutral), and their effectiveness diminishes as the pH increases beyond 4.5. BHA works best at concentrations of between 1% and 2% at an optimal pH of 3, diminishing in effectiveness as the pH increases beyond 4. The effectiveness of both AHAs and BHA decreases as a product's pH increases and as the concentration of the ingredient decreases. This relationship is so central to the entire subject of exfoliation and cell turnover that it bears repeating: AHAs work best in a 5% to 8% concentration, in a product with a pH of 3 to 4; BHA works best in a 1% to 2% concentration, in a product with a pH of 3 to 4 (Source: *Cosmetic Dermatology*, October 2001, pages 15–18).

Salicylic acid (BHA), although it provides more penetrating exfoliation into the pore, is less irritating than AHAs because of its close relation to aspirin. Salicylic acid is derived from acetylsalicylic acid, which is the technical name for aspirin, and aspirin has anti-inflammatory properties. When applied topically on the skin, the salicylic acid in BHA products retains many of these anti-inflammatory effects.

AHA and BHA products can definitely smooth the skin, improve texture, unclog pores, and give the appearance of plumper, firmer skin (because more healthy skin cells are now on the surface). But the change isn't permanent; when you stop using them the skin goes back to the condition it was in before you started.

Products that contain AHA sound-alikes, including sugarcane extract, mixed fruit acids, fruit extracts, milk extract, and citrus extract, or BHA sound-alikes, such as wintergreen extract or willow bark extract, are not able to exfoliate skin, or do much of anything else (though willow bark may have anti-inflammatory properties), and, therefore, I rated products that contain these ingredients as not effective. You may think these are better because they appear to be a more natural form of AHA or BHA when you see these less technical, more familiar plant names on the label, but that perception is not reality.

As a general rule I do not recommend products that use both AHAs and BHA together because each has its specialized action, and that does not translate to all skin types. As mentioned previously, AHAs work on the surface of the skin and are best for sun-damaged skin that has developed a thickened outer layer, or for someone with dry skin who has a buildup of layers of skin that make the skin look dull and impede cell turnover. BHA can exfoliate on the surface of skin much like AHAs can, but BHA can also cut through the lipid layer of skin and, therefore, works better in the pore, helping skin to shed cells and loosen any plugs in the skin, improving the size and function of the pore. If you don't have breakouts, you don't need that kind of penetration; if you do have breakouts, AHAs may help to some extent, but the penetration from the BHA can be more effective.

One word of caution: Anytime you use a well-formulated AHA product that contains more than 5% AHAs, some stinging can occur, though this can diminish as the skin gets used to it. You should not let AHAs or BHA products come in contact with the eyes or any mucous membranes. It is also possible that you may have an irritation reaction or sensitivity to AHAs or BHA. Slight stinging is expected, but continued stinging is not; if the stinging continues, stop using it.

FACIAL MASKS: Many facial masks contain claylike ingredients that absorb oil and, to some degree, exfoliate the skin, which can be beneficial for someone with oily skin. The problem with many masks is that they often contain additional ingredients that are irritating or that can clog pores. Although your face may feel smooth when the mask is first rinsed off, after a short period of time you may experience problems created by the mask's drying effect. Even the few clay masks that contain emollients and moisturizing ingredients can still be too drying for dry skin and can cause oily skin to break out. There are also a range of masks that contain plasticizing (hairspray-like) ingredients that peel off the face like a layer of plastic. These take a layer of skin off when removed, and that can make skin feel temporarily smoother, but there is no long-term benefit to be gained.

The claims that clay from one part of the world or another, or from some part of the ocean or from a volcanic region is best for skin have no research of any kind showing that to be true. In essence, there isn't any research anywhere showing clay can do anything beneficial for skin other than absorb oil, and there is not a shred of research showing that plasticizing masks have any benefit whatsoever. Moreover, any skin-care step used occasionally simply can't have as much value as a better routine used daily.

Another type of facial mask that shows up is the kind with strictly moisturizing ingredients. These basically don't differ from other moisturizers except that they are thicker formulations. Calling the product a mask seems to make women feel like they are doing something special for their skin when, in actuality, they aren't. Despite all these shortcomings, which I point out in the individual reviews, there are masks in this book that did get happy faces, either because of their potential benefit for dry skin (if they contained reliable ingredients for this condition) or because of their absorbency for oily skin.

Overall, facial masks did not have any standout formulary considerations or miracles to offer. Therefore, masks are rated based on compatibility for each skin type. For dry skin the mask must have emollient properties and for oily skin absorbent ingredients.

TONERS: Toners, astringents, fresheners, tonics, and other liquids meant to refresh the skin or remove the last traces of makeup after a cleanser is rinsed off should not contain any irritants whatsoever. I evaluated these products primarily on that basis. Claims that toners can close pores or refine the skin are unachievable, so I ignore such language and look for toners that leave the face feeling smooth and soft, are able to remove the last traces of makeup, and do not irritate the skin. Toners that contain a good assortment of water-binding agents, anti-irritants, and antioxidants are rated as being optimal for all skin types (see information for each of these in the following section on "The Ingredients for Skin Care"). Toners that add plant oils to those preferred ingredients are rated best for normal to dry skin. Toners that add mild detergent cleansing agents with no emollients, but that also have water-binding agents, anti-irritants, and antioxidants are rated best for normal to oily skin.

Toners are always considered an optional step for most skin types, either to soothe skin after cleansing or to remove the last traces of makeup. For some skin types, a toner can be the only "moisturizer" the skin needs. Even for someone with dry skin, toners can be a great lightweight start to add extra water-binding agents and anti-irritant ingredients to the skin before applying a moisturizer.

MOISTURIZERS: Despite all the fuss, assertions, and price differences among anti-wrinkle, firming, antiaging, and "renewing" supplements and treatments that claim to restore youth to skin, in truth these products are nothing more than moisturizers. Regardless of the claims, none of these products can get rid of your wrinkles or restore even one minute of youth to your face or provide any other kind of unique benefit for skin. A plethora of these types of products are being marketed to women, but not one plastic surgeon is going out of business because of them.

As a general category, "moisturizers" were quite easy to review. Basically, despite the claims, moisturizers in one form or another keep the skin from looking and feeling dry—so I expect the same thing from all of them: They must contain ingredients that can smooth and soothe dry skin, keep water in the skin cell, and help maintain or reinforce the skin's protective barrier. Almost all other claims for this immense group of products are exaggerated and misleading, not to mention never-ending. Every month a new assortment is launched with new marketing copy to catch your attention.

One thing to keep foremost in your mind is that dry skin and wrinkles are not associated, so you cannot prevent, stop, or get rid of wrinkles by applying a moisturizer. But without question, dry skin looks and does better with a well-formulated moisturizer.

Another recurring myth espoused at cosmetics counters is that oily skin needs a moisturizer. In other words, you may be told that oily skin makes more oil because it is combating some form of underlying dryness. No part of that is true. Oil production is controlled and regulated by hormone production (Sources: *Clinical and Experimental Dermatology*, October 2001, pages 600–607; and *Seminars in Cutaneous Medicine and Surgery*, September 2001, pages 144–153). If dry skin could induce oil production, then everyone with dry skin would be oozing oil, but they aren't, because physiologically that isn't how skin works.

Lots of moisturizers boast that they can penetrate layers of skin cells better than others do, but that's a meaningless claim. Skin cells are quite permeable, so claims of penetrating layers of skin would be true for most products if they contain even one drop of water. Nonetheless, it is essential that some moisturizing ingredients be left on the surface of the skin to prevent the air from drinking up the water in your skin cells.

Apart from the redundant claims moisturizers make in regard to getting rid of wrinkles or firming skin, there are still significant distinct qualitative differences between products. Research on the function of antioxidants, anti-irritants, and water-binding agents that mimic the actual substances comprising the skin's intercellular matrix (the skin's own composition that binds skin cells together) shows that all these ingredients can potentially have a fundamental positive effect on skin. In this edition, more so than in earlier editions of my books, I rate favorably those moisturizers that have a preponderance of these ingredients. However, while these types of ingredients show incredible promise for preserving the health and balance of skin, there is no direct evidence or research showing that any specific antioxidant, anti-irritant, or water-binding agent is better than another, and there's also no research showing that they can get rid of wrinkles. The only "studies" that state otherwise are paid for or concocted by the companies showcasing those ingredients.

It is interesting to note that regardless of the claim, whether for firming, anti-wrinkling, restoring, repairing, cellular renewal, toning, and on and on, none of these products contain unique ingredients. Rather, they all share a range of overlapping, similar ingredients, so the "exclusive" claims become even more unbelievable.

Next, while there are multitudes of ingredients that are potentially helpful for skin, there are also a number that are a waste of time, or worse. These range from bee pollen to gold, plus animal extracts from thymus, spleen, and placenta, as well as many plant extracts that can be potential skin irritants, and I point out as many of these as I can in my reviews. If there is no research showing any of these are helpful for skin, then they are there for marketing purposes only and that doesn't help your skin.

Additionally, I was interested in the order the "good" or "hyped" ingredients were listed on the container. Just as with food labels, the ingredients present in the largest amounts are listed first. Often, the most interesting or the most extolled ingredients are so far down the list that the amounts of them in the product are practically nonexistent. Just because an ingredient appears on an ingredient label doesn't mean there's enough of it to have any impact on skin or to make a difference of any kind.

There are also moisturizers that claim to be great for combination skin because they are able to release moisturizing ingredients over dry areas and oil-absorbing ingredients over oily areas. This is categorically impossible. A product cannot hold certain ingredients back from the skin—where would they go? Imagine a lotion touching your skin and separating out so the ingredients for the oily parts get up and run over here and the ones for the dry area get up and head over there. It just isn't feasible in any way, shape, or form.

Note: Packaging can play a vital role when it comes to a product's efficacy and stability, particularly for products that contain antioxidants, plant extracts, skin-lightening agents, benzoyl peroxide, and vitamins. All of these active ingredients are negatively affected by air and light, and inappropriate packaging leaves the contents vulnerable to decomposition and deterioration. That means you should avoid containers that expose a product to light (via see-through or non-opaque material) or to air (such as a container with a large opening, especially jar containers with screw-off lids) because they allow maximum exposure to light and air every time they are opened (Source: FDA *Consumer* magazine, revised May 1995). I did not evaluate packaging for this edition of the book. However, it is something you should unconditionally take into consideration the next time you are thinking of spending money on any product, because if it is packaged in a see-through container or a jar it is unlikely that any of the "active" ingredients still retain any potency or efficacy. Instead, look for opaque or single-use units.

MOISTURIZERS FOR OILY SKIN: The only time to use a moisturizer is when you have dry skin; if you don't have dry skin, you don't need a moisturizer. For many with oily or combination skin the only moisturizer they may need is a toner with good water-binding agents, antioxidants, and anti-irritants. When a product, particularly a moisturizer, claims to be oil-free, noncomedogenic, or non-acnegenic, it often misleads consumers into thinking they are buying a product that won't clog pores. But those terms are not regulated by the FDA and have no legal meaning. A cosmetics company can use any or all of those terms without any qualifying ingredient listing or substantiation.

The term "oil-free" is probably the most misleading, as there are plenty of ingredients that don't sound like oils but can absolutely aggravate breakouts. Many cosmetics contain waxlike thickening agents that can clog pores. These ingredients are used in moisturizers because they duplicate the natural lipids (sebum or oil) in our skin, or prevent dehydration, and that's great. But if you have problems with the oil already being created in your pores, adding more of the same kind of substance will only make things worse. Despite the problems these ingredients can cause, they show up in lots and lots of so-called oil-free products.

While there is evidence that some specific ingredients can trigger breakouts, there are no absolutes. I wish there were, but there aren't. Several Web sites that showcase lists of comedogenic ingredients have created quite a stir among many women. The major source of information for these data appears to be *Dr. Fulton's Step by Step Guide to Acne,* published in 1983 by Harper & Row (though credit is not given on any Web site, they present the exact same information found in the book). At the time (and 1983 is a long time ago), Fulton's research on the causes of breakouts was unprecedented. Fulton applied cosmetics ingredients to rabbits' ears and waited to see what happened. As promising as this research was, it has never been repeated, and is rarely cited in later research (except when it suits a company's marketing agenda). There are many reasons why lists of this kind are unreliable.

First, the methodology involved pure concentrations of the ingredients, not the concentrations that are used in actual cosmetic formulations, which are usually only a fractional percentage. It also didn't address the issue of usage and application. For example, the exposure risks of specific ingredients are very different for a cleanser, which is left on the skin for a few seconds, and a lotion or liquid, which is left on the skin for hours. Beyond this, the research didn't look at the host of plant extracts or sunscreens in cosmetics that were introduced during the early '80s. To call this list out of date and inconclusive is an understatement!

I have to admit that I'm also to blame for some of the confusion. In my books I have included a list of ingredients that may cause breakouts. I based this list on the emollient or waxlike characteristics of the ingredients and on findings in more contemporary research when it was available. I warned against products that contain ingredient groups such as triglycerides, myristates, palmitates, and stearates, but it was probably not wise to include such a list because in some ways it is misleading. For example, isopropyl palmitate is a waxy thickening agent used to bind other ingredients together, has an emollient feel on skin, and is used most frequently in moisturizers for dry skin. On the other hand, ascorbyl palmitate is a stable form of vitamin C that is used in small amounts in skin-care products, and is not a problem for skin. That is only one example where the rule about palmitates doesn't hold water.

Further, depending on the ingredient, just because it is present in a formulation means nothing if it is toward the end of the ingredient list—while if it's the second, third, or fourth ingredient it may be problematic. However, that may not be true if there are many of these kinds of ingredients on a label and, therefore, they are all present in small amounts. Also, keep in mind that even the most notorious ingredients (such as isopropyl myristate) won't cause problems for everyone. Just because an ingredient *may* cause breakouts doesn't mean that it *will*.

Another point these kinds of lists can't account for is that there are thousands and thousands of cosmetic ingredients being used in skin-care and makeup products today! A lot of them are emollients, waxy thickening agents, or irritants that can cause skin problems. But whether they do or not is completely dependent on the amount used and the nature of the individual ingredient (some ingredients cause problems in far smaller amounts than other ingredients, while others cause problems in various combinations). A comprehensive list of all the ingredients and the potential effects of them and all the combinations of them would not only be impossible, but also would be nothing more than guesswork.

There are no easy answers for this one, but you can understand that trying to research, categorize, classify, and make absolute conclusions about 50,000 ingredients with an infinite number of possible combinations is just not humanly possible.

However, here are a few ideas to at least point you in the right direction. Because a thicker formulation is more likely to contain problematic ingredients, just as a highly emollient product can, it is far better for normal to oily skin types to use gel or "serum"-type products that leave out most if not all thickening agents. Moisturizers for oily skin are judged as being preferred for that skin type if they are lightweight and have minimal to no waxy or emollient ingredients of any kind listed near the beginning of the ingredient list (because these can theoretically clog pores).

Moisturizers marketed to those with oily or combination skin must meet similar standards, but in addition to a lack of thickening agents and emollients, I consider it beneficial if they do contain substantial amounts of antioxidants, water-binding agents, and anti-irritants because these types of ingredients are rarely problematic for skin.

DAY CREAMS VERSUS NIGHT CREAMS: There is no difference between what the skin needs during the day versus what it needs at night. The one big exception, and the only difference that needs to exist between a daytime moisturizer and a nighttime moisturizer, is that the daytime one should have an effective SPF (sunscreen) with UVA-protecting ingredients. Other than that, there are no formulation variances that make one preferable over the other. Many moisturizing formulations now have great sun protection, and that is the only way you should differentiate a daytime product from a nighttime version. All other claims on the label are rhetoric you should ignore.

EYE, THROAT, CHEST, NECK, AND OTHER SPECIALTY CREAMS, SERUMS, OR GELS: Buying a separate product for a special area of the face or body, whether it is in the form of a cream, gel, lotion, or serum, is altogether unnecessary. Almost without exception, the ingredient lists and formulations for these products are identical to other creams, gels, lotions, or serums identified as being only for the face. That doesn't mean there aren't some great specialty products out there for different skin types, but why buy a second moisturizer for the eye area when the one you are already using on the rest of your face is virtually identical?

The cosmetics industry makes a lot of money selling women extra products they don't need by dividing the body into different parts, each with purportedly different skin-care needs. Because of the relentless advertising pushing this erroneous concept, women stay tied to the belief that the eye area, throat, chest, legs, and hands all have different skin-care needs. Even more bothersome is the fact that most cosmetics companies give you a tiny amount of the so-called specialty products but charge you much more for them than for an equal amount of the face creams, despite the similarities. Paradoxically, what does show up frequently in eye-care products are irritating ingredients such as witch hazel, caffeine, and fragrance. So much for the eye area having special needs that special products can address! Moreover, many eye products don't contain sunscreen. If your well-formulated face moisturizer contains sunscreen but your eye product doesn't, then you would actually be damaging the skin around the eye by not using your face moisturizer because the eye product wouldn't protect from sun damage.

SUNSCREENS: Valid scientific research abounds demonstrating that wrinkles, skin damage, many skin discolorations, and possibly skin cancer are primarily a result of un-protected sun exposure (Source: *Mechanisms of Ageing and Development*, April 2002, pages 801–810). Clearly this subject has to do not only with cosmetics, but also with serious health issues. It is well established that the only true, first-line-of-defense antiwrinkle product is a well-formulated and carefully applied sunscreen. My Web site, www.cosmeticscop.com, as well as my book *The Beauty Bible*, Second Edition, both have extensive information on the wide variety of concerns, problems, and cautions regarding sunscreen formulations and application. Please refer to these for more specific information.

The main criterion I use to evaluate sun-care products is the SPF rating, with SPF 15 being the standard. SPF 15 or greater is considered the basic standard by the FDA, the American Academy of Dermatology, the American Academy of Pediatrics, and the National Cancer Institute. However, the SPF number only tells you how long you can stay in the sun without getting sunburned, which is caused by the sun's UVB rays. While that is helpful, it is only part of the protection you need. It is now known that most wrinkling, and possibly skin cancer, is a result of unprotected exposure to the sun's UVA rays. Because of the difference between UVA damage and UVB damage, and because there is still no UVA rating system, to be assured that you are getting adequate UVA protection, your sunscreen must contain one of three UVA-protecting ingredients listed as an active ingredient on the label. These active ingredients are avobenzone (also called Parsol 1789 or butyl methoxydibenzoylmethane), titanium dioxide, or zinc oxide (outside of the United States Mexoryl SX™ may also be used) (Sources: *Photodermatology, Photoimmunology, &*

Photomedicine, December 2000, pages 250–255 and *Photochemistry* March 2000, pages 314–320).

No sunscreens receive a happy face unless one of those UVA-protecting ingredie... listed on the active ingredient part of the ingredient list, and it has an SPF of 15 or greater.

Beauty Note: If you are using more than one product that contains sunscreen, such as an SPF 15 moisturizer and an SPF 8 foundation, it's the one with the higher SPF number that must contain UVA-protecting ingredients. However, it's important to realize that two sunscreens with different numbers do not add up to one big SPF number. In other words, an SPF 6 and an SPF 10 do not add up to an SPF 16. Yes, you would be getting an increased SPF value for protection, but there is no way to know what that increased protection would be. There is no way to know whether or not the formulations are complementary and whether the sunscreen ingredients are stable when combined. If you want to count on getting an SPF 30's worth of protection, you should look for one product that has that SPF number.

Synthetic sunscreen ingredients (only titanium dioxide and zinc oxide are considered to be mineral or "natural" ingredients) can be irritating to skin no matter what a product's label says. You have to experiment to find the one that works best for you. Although sunscreens that use only titanium dioxide or only zinc oxide as the active ingredient are considered almost completely nonirritating, they can still pose problems for someone with oily or acne-prone skin because their occlusive composition can clog pores and aggravate breakouts.

One More Beauty Note: Proper and diligent sunscreen application is of vital importance to obtain protection from the sun. Protection is determined not only by the SPF number and the UVA-screening ingredients the product contains, but also by how thickly and evenly the sunscreen is applied, and when, where, and how often it's re-applied. There is a mismatch between the expectation versus the reality of actual use (Sources: *Journal of Photochemistry and Photobiology*, November 2001, pages 105–108 and *American Journal of Clinical Dermatology*, 2002, volume 3, issue 3, pages 185–191). Keep in mind that an everyday liberal application of sunscreen, applied 20 minutes before you step outside (not once you get to the car, or get to the beach, or do anything—but before you leave the house) is the key element in getting the best protection possible. But within your skin-care routine, exactly when does sunscreen get applied? If you are applying several skin-care products, ranging from toners to acne medications to moisturizers, the rule is that the last item you apply during the day should be your sunscreen. If you apply sunscreen and then apply, say, your moisturizer or an acne product, you could inadvertently be diluting or breaking down the effectiveness of the sunscreen you've just applied.

Because applying sunscreen liberally is indispensable for the health of skin, all expensive sunscreens are potentially dangerous for skin because their cost could discourage liberal application. After all, how liberally would you apply a $50-for-1-ounce sunscreen to your face or body versus a product costing $20 for 2, 4, or 6 ounces?

SUNSCREENS FOR OILY OR COMBINATION SKIN: Sunscreens are a very tricky category for someone with oily or combination skin. It takes experimentation to find the one that will work best for you. The problem is that the ingredients used to suspend the active ingredients are not necessarily the best for oily skin. What I generally recommend is that someone with oily or combination skin select a foundation containing a well-formulated sunscreen. Then they can apply an appropriate lightweight moisturizer over dry areas or just use a well-formulated toner all over, which can be enough "moisturizing" for that skin type.

WATER-RESISTANT SUNSCREENS: The FDA's December 2002 regulations regarding sunscreen require companies to eliminate the use of the word "waterproof" as a valid claim. In truth, no sunscreen can really be "waterproof" because it must be reapplied if you have been sweating or immersed in water for a period of time. The only terms approved for use on sunscreens are "water-resistant" or "very water-resistant." This change reflects research data from studies that prove these products have only a limited ability to stay in place when people are in water or sweating. A product that is water-resistant means its labeled SPF value has been measured after application and then after 40 minutes of water immersion. To use the term "water-resistant", it must keep the same SPF value over that full time. A "very water-resistant" product means the SPF value on the label must remain intact after 80 minutes of water immersion (Source: www.fda.gov).

If you are swimming or sweating, you absolutely should use a sunscreen that's labeled water resistant or very water resistant and reapply it frequently. These sunscreens are formulated quite differently from regular sunscreens, using acrylate technology in their formulations, which helps them hold up remarkably well under water. Acrylate-type ingredients are, like hairspray, holding agents. These plasticizing ingredients form a film over the skin and can take a great deal of wear and tear in contact with water before the sunscreen protection is rinsed away.

SELF-TANNERS: All self-tanning products, whether you choose one made by Bain de Soleil, Clarins, Decleor Paris, or Estee Lauder, are created equal. The active ingredient in every one of these products is dihydroxyacetone, which is what turns the surface layer of skin brown. This ingredient acts on the skin cells and their amino acid content, causing a chemical reaction that temporarily gives the skin a darker color. These products are considered completely safe for skin (Source: *American Journal of Clinical Dermatology*, 2002, volume 3, number 5, pages 317–318).

Some self-tanners add a tint of color to help you see where you've applied the product, which can help you create a smoother, more even application.

Your personal preference as to how self-tanners make your skin appear actually has less to do with the product itself than with the nature of your own skin cells. The interaction between the active ingredient and your skin is controlled more by your body's chemistry than anything else.

You may not like the smell of one product versus another, but that is merely a function of the fragrance added to the product to mask the smell of the dihydroxyacetone. A masking fragrance might be pleasant, but it doesn't change how the product functions, and the natural odor of the product is transient. Where self-tanners do differ is in the amount of dihydroxyacetone present, although there is no surefire way to judge that from the ingredient list. However, you can assume that those self-tanners rated as light, medium, and dark have the correct corresponding amount of dihydroxyacetone. You can also assume that self-tanners without any stated level have a low to moderate concentration of dihydroxyacetone.

For more specific critiques of self-tanning products, you'll find the Web site www.sunless.com incredibly helpful, and I strongly recommend a visit.

ACNE PRODUCTS: From all the research I've seen, particularly in dermatological journals and literature from the American Academy of Dermatology, acne products need to deliver four categories of performance to deal with breakouts: (1) gentle cleansing (to reduce inflammation), (2) effective exfoliation, (3) disinfection, and (4) absorption of excess oil (Source: *American Journal of Clinical Dermatology*, 2001, volume 2, number 3, pages 135–141). I delve into this subject at length in my book *The Beauty Bible,* Second Edition, and on my Web site at www.cosmeticscop.com. I base my reviews for these types of products according to how they respond to these four important skin-care needs.

Cleansing: Using a gentle, water-soluble cleanser is standard for any skin-care routine, and it is equally necessary for those with blemish-prone skin. Often skin-care routines aimed at those with oily skin or acne use cleansers that are exceptionally drying or irritating, which can increase the inflammation of skin. Yet, as I've mentioned several times throughout this introduction, inflammation hurts the skin's healing process and that will make matters worse. Think about it this way: What color is acne? Red! So why use any product that makes skin redder? Inflammation can also increase the presence of acne-causing bacteria in the skin.

I also never recommend bar soap for acne or breakouts. Bar soaps of any kind are kept in their bar form by ingredients that can potentially clog pores. Research also shows that high-pH cleansers (soaps usually have a pH greater than 8) can increase the presence of bacteria in the skin (Source: *Cutis*, December 2001, Supplemental pages 12–19). To that end, gentle, water-soluble cleansers are rated high if they do not contain irritating or excessively drying ingredients.

Exfoliating: See the section above on "Exfoliants and Scrubs."

Disinfecting: To kill the bacteria in the skin that cause blemishes (*Propiobacterium acnes*), you need a reliable topical disinfectant (available over the counter) or topical antibiotic (available by prescription). There aren't many options when it comes to disinfecting the skin with over-the-counter products. The best over-the-counter topical disinfectant is either a 2.5%, 5%, or 10% benzoyl peroxide product (but only when no irritating ingredients are added).

Alcohol, when used in very high concentrations (more than 60%—thankfully, never found in skin-care products) and sulfur can be good disinfectants, but they are way too drying and irritating for most skin types and, therefore, are rarely used and are not recommended.

Other ingredients that repeatedly show up in products for problem skin, such as lemon, grapefruit, acetone, witch hazel, peppermint, menthol, eucalyptus, and camphor, have no effect at all on bacteria and cause unnecessary irritation and inflammation.

Tea tree oil (from the plant *Melaleuca alternifolia*) has some interesting research demonstrating it to be an effective antimicrobial agent. The *Journal of Applied Microbiology* (January 2000, pages 170–175) stated that "The essential oil of *Melaleuca alternifolia* exhibits broad-spectrum antimicrobial activity." For acne there is also some credible published information showing it to be effective as a topical disinfectant for killing the bacteria that can cause pimples (Source: *Letters in Applied Microbiology*, October 1995, pages 242–245). However, the crux of the matter for tea tree oil is: How much is needed to have an effect? The *Medical Journal of Australia* (October 1990, pages 455–458) compared the efficacy of tea tree oil to the efficacy of benzoyl peroxide for the treatment of acne. The study included 119 patients using 5% tea tree oil in a gel base versus a 5% benzoyl peroxide lotion. There were 61 patients in the benzoyl peroxide group and 58 in the tea tree oil group. The conclusion was that "both treatments were effective in reducing the number of inflamed lesions throughout the trial, with a significantly better result for benzoyl peroxide when compared to the tea tree oil. Skin oiliness was lessened significantly in the benzoyl peroxide group versus the tea tree oil group." However, while the reduction of breakouts was greater for the benzoyl peroxide group, the side effects of dryness, stinging, and burning were also greater—"79% of the benzoyl peroxide group versus 49% of the tea tree oil group."

At this time, however, there are no cosmetic products containing a sufficient concentration of tea tree oil to kill acne-causing bacteria. It appears that almost all of the tea tree oil products on the market contain little more than a 1% concentration, or they contain irritating ingredients that would negatively affect skin.

As a general rule, it would be better to begin with a 2.5% strength benzoyl peroxide solution to see if it is effective, rather than starting with the more potent, and somewhat more irritating, 5% or 10% concentrations. If those options don't work, the next step would be to see a dermatologist to investigate the options of a topical antibiotic in association with a topical retinoid such as Retin-A, Differin, Tazorac, or Avita. For more information on using topical antibiotics and retinoids along with other treatments for acne, please refer to my Web site www.cosmeticscop.com or my book *The Beauty Bible*, Second Edition.

Absorbing excess oil: There are many types of skin-care and makeup products designed to create a matte finish or oil-absorbing layer of ingredients on the skin. Although these products often work well to absorb excess oil and keep shine under control, none of them can stop oil production because oil production is primarily a result of your hormones, and that cannot be affected from the outside with cosmetics.

I often point out my concern that oil-absorbing ingredients like rice starch, corn-starch, and other food products are typically considered problematic for those who have breakouts. Food substances can get into pores and encourage bacteria production (after all bacteria thrive on organic substances), which is not the best when your goal is fighting off bacteria.

Clay masks are popular options for absorbing excess oil on the skin. While they can help, they often contain other ingredients that are skin irritants, can clog pores, or are too emollient for oily skin. I rate clay masks and other masks on whether or not they contain irritating or emollient ingredients that would not be appropriate for blemish-prone skin.

Beauty Note: For years I have recommended trying milk of magnesia (yes, like the Phillips' Milk of Magnesia that you take for indigestion) as a facial mask for acne or oily skin. It is by far one of the best ways to absorb oil. Milk of magnesia is nothing more than liquid magnesium hydroxide, which is known to soothe skin and reduce irritation, and it has incredible oil-absorbing properties. Magnesium absorbs more oil than clay, and clay has no disinfecting or soothing properties. How often you use the milk of magnesia has to do with how oily your skin is. Some use it every day; others, once a week. Only you and your skin can determine what frequency works best for you.

Beauty Note: Pore strips are not to be used for blemishes. In all their varying incarnations, pore strips are only meant to remove blackheads, and they do this only superficially and not very well. You place a piece of cloth with a sticky substance on it over your face, as you might do with a Band-Aid, wait a bit for it to dry, and then rip it off. Along with some amount of skin, blackheads are supposed to stick to it and come right out of your nose. There is nothing miraculous about these products, nor do they work all that well. The main ingredient on these strips is a hairspray-type ingredient. If the instructions are followed closely you can see some benefit in removing the very surface of a blackhead. In fact, you may at first be very impressed with what comes off your nose. Unfortunately, that leaves the majority of the problem deep in the pore. What concerns me most about pore strips is that they are accompanied by a strong warning not to use them over any area other than the intended area (nose, chin, or forehead) and not to use them over pimples or inflamed, swollen, sunburned, or excessively dry skin. It also states that if the strip is too painful to remove, you should wet it and then carefully remove it. What a warning!

Also, despite the warning on the package, I suspect most women will try these strips wherever they see breakouts. If I didn't know better, I know I would. The way these strips adhere, they can absolutely injure or tear skin. They are especially unsafe if you've been using Retin-A, Renova, Differin, AHAs, or BHA, are having facial peels, taking Accutane, or if you have naturally thin skin or any skin disorder such as rosacea, psoriasis, or seborrhea.

SKIN-LIGHTENING PRODUCTS: The surge in skin-care products making claims about lightening skin and depigmenting skin discolorations caused by sun exposure or hormonal changes is nothing less than astounding. Now that baby boomers are aging and brown patches are beginning to turn up on hands and faces (caused primarily by sun damage—they are not liver spots or age related at all), skin-lightening products are showing up in all sorts of skin-care lines. To convince consumers that a particular line has unique properties for fixing this problem lots of plant extracts are thrown into the mix, ranging from mulberry extract to kojic acid (extracted from a fungus grown on rice or soybeans).

Localized brown skin discolorations are caused by increased melanin production, or hyperpigmentation. Melanin, which is the pigment or coloring agent of skin, is created by melanin synthesis, a complex process controlled partly by an enzyme called tyrosinase. For topical treatments, according to an article in the *American Journal of Clinical Dermatology* (September-October 2000, pages 261–268), "[T]opical hydroquinone 2 to 4% alone or in combination with tretinoin 0.05 to 0.1% is an established treatment. Topical azelaic acid 15 to 20% can be as efficacious as hydroquinone…. Tretinoin is especially useful in treating hyperpigmentation of photoaged skin. Kojic acid, alone or in combination with glycolic acid or hydroquinone, has shown good results, due to its inhibitory action on tyrosinase. Chemical peels are [also] useful to treat melasma." However, kojic acid has proven to be an exceptionally unstable ingredient and as a result is being used less and less in reputable products.

Over-the-counter skin-lightening products often contain 2% hydroquinone, while 4% concentrations are available only from a physician. Hydroquinone is a strong inhibitor of melanin production (Source: *Journal of Dermatological Science*, August 2001, Supplemental pages S68–S75; and *Dermatological Surgery*, May 1996, pages 443–447), meaning that it lightens skin color. Hydroquinone does not bleach the skin (calling it a bleaching agent is a misnomer); it only disrupts the synthesis of melanin hyperpigmentation. Some concerns about hydroquinone's safety on skin have been mentioned, but research indicates that reactions are minor or a result of using extremely high concentrations (Source: *Critical Reviews in Toxicology*, May 1999, pages 283–330).

Hydroquinone can be an unstable ingredient in cosmetic formulations. Upon exposure to air or sunlight it can turn a strange shade of brown. It is thus essential, when you are considering a hydroquinone product, to be sure it is packaged in a nontransparent container that doesn't let light in and that minimizes the amount of exposure to air. Hydroquinone products packaged in jars or clear containers are not recommended because once opened they quickly become ineffective.

Plant-derived skin-care ingredients send out a definite siren call to consumers. Anyone developing "natural" alternatives to hydroquinone has an eager audience ready and willing to give them a try. To that end, arbutin, a hydroquinone derivative isolated from the leaves of the bearberry shrub, and cranberry, blueberry, and most types of pears, serves that purpose. Because of arbutin's hydroquinone content it can have melanin-inhibiting properties (Source: *Journal of Pharmacology and Experimental Therapeutics*, February 1996, pages 765–769). Although the research describing arbutin's effectiveness is persuasive (even if most of the research has been done on animals or in vitro), concentration protocols have not been established. That means we just don't know how much arbutin it takes to have an effect in lightening the skin. Moreover, most cosmetics companies don't use arbutin in their products because there are patents controlling its use in skin-care products for skin lightening. To get around this problem, many cosmetics companies use plant extracts that contain arbutin, such as bearberry. However, there is no research showing that the plant extract itself has any effect on skin color, and especially not in the tiny amounts that are present in cosmetics.

Vitamin C in the form of magnesium ascorbyl phosphate is considered stable and an effective antioxidant for skin. For skin lightening, there is only a single study showing it to be effective for inhibiting melanin production (Source: *Journal of the American Academy of Dermatology*, January 1996, pages 29–33). The study concluded that a moisturizer with a 10% concentration of magnesium ascorbyl phosphate "suppressed melanin formation…. The lightening effect was significant in 19 of 34 patients with chloasma or senile freckles and in 3 of 25 patients with normal skin." One study is not exactly anything to write home about, not to mention that at present there are no products on the market containing 10% magnesium ascorbyl phosphate. Most skin-care products that contain magnesium ascorbyl phosphate have less than a 1% concentration.

ROSACEA PRODUCTS: Although it is thought to afflict at least 30% of the Caucasian population, there are still only a handful of treatments for rosacea, and they are all available by prescription only. These include topical application of MetroGel, MetroCream, MetroLotion, and Noritate. The active ingredient in each of these is metronidazole, which is considered the primary treatment for rosacea (Source: *Skin Therapy Letter*, January 2002, pages 1–6). Occasionally, azelaic acid and oral antibiotics are also an option. Because you must experiment until you find what works best for your skin, all of these should be considered when developing your own battle plan for treating rosacea. (When considering an oral antibiotic you must also consider the risk of the microbe adapting to the antibiotic after prolonged use. If that happens, that specific oral antibiotic won't be effective to help deal with other types of infections you may encounter.)

Cosmetic skin-care products can help mitigate rosacea exacerbations, but there are no cosmetic products that can have an effect on the microbe that causes this skin disorder. Because redness, irritation, and skin sensitivities are part and parcel of rosacea itself, anything that makes these worse will cause more problems. In this regard, according to the National Rosacea Society (http://www.rosacea.org), gentle, nonirritating skin-care products are essential. Of course, I concur; and any skin-care products claiming to be helpful for rosacea must be completely irritant-free to receive a favorable rating.

INGREDIENTS FOR SKIN CARE

While I want to emphasize how extensive the misleading portrayals of skin-care products made by the cosmetics industry are, I also want to underscore that there are hundreds of great products for all skin types. When I describe my elation or enthusiasm about any product, I am also always careful to let you know what can really be expected and how out-of-line the price often is for what you are getting. So just because I think a formula can be amazing for dry skin, that doesn't mean I concur with its claims about firming, lifting, undoing or preventing wrinkling, reducing lines, fighting stress, erasing cellulite, and on and on and on….

Every skin-care product is evaluated on the basis of what ingredients it contains because its ingredients (and their potential effects) are the basis for whether a claim can be verified. Unlike my reviews in earlier editions of *Don't Go to the Cosmetics Counter Without Me*, I do not summarize the ingredient listing for every skin-care product in this edition. I wanted to include as many new lines as possible, and the repetitive "this product contains" listing—and from your letters that was not everyone's cup of tea—took up an incredible amount of space. Unless I feel that this kind of information is needed to help understand a product's performance, I provide just a general summary of the product's ingredients and then describe what it could and couldn't do. When I do list a product's ingredients, it is always in the order in which they appear on the ingredient list. I often comment about how a product compares to similar or better versions that cost much less. Of course, you will have to test for yourself how a specific product feels on your skin and how you react to its fragrance or lack thereof.

When I list a product's ingredients in the product reviews, I frequently use the phrase "contains mostly," often followed by one or all of the following terms: thickener or thickening agent, slip agent, water-binding agent, film-forming agent, scrub agent, absorbent, detergent cleansing agent or standard detergent cleanser, disinfectant, preservative, fragrance, plant extract or plant oil, vitamin, antioxidant, and anti-irritant. It was easiest to summarize groups of ingredients by using these general terms, but please read the following explanations of the terms before you read the reviews.

Beauty Note: When reading ingredient lists, remember that the closer a specific ingredient is to a **preservative** (such as methylparaben, propylparaben, ethylparaben, imidazolidinyl urea, or quaternium-15) or a **fragrance** (listed as fragrance or often as an individual essential oil like lavender or bergamot oil), or the closer it is to the end of the ingredient list, the less likely it is that there is a significant amount of it in the product. That means its impact, for better or worse, is negligible.

When I used the term "**thickeners**" to describe an ingredient, I'm referring to those components that add texture, thickness, viscosity, spreadability, and stability to a product. Thickeners are also vital for helping to keep other ingredients mixed together. **Thickening agents** often have a waxlike texture or a creamy, emollient feel, and can be great lubricants. There are literally thousands of ingredients in this category, and they are the staples of every skin-care product out there, regardless of the product's price or claims about "natural" ingredients.

Slip agents help other ingredients spread over or penetrate the skin and they also have humectant properties. Slip agents include propylene glycol, butylene glycol, hexylene glycol, methyl gluceth-10, polysorbates, and glycerin, to name only a few. They are as basic to the world of skin care as water.

Water-binding agents (also known as **natural moisturizing factors** or **NMFs**) are ingredients that help skin retain water and maintain its structural integrity. Skin is not in need of water so much as it is in need of substances that support the skin's own structure. **Humectants**, for example, attract water to skin and are one component of a moisturizer. But what good is getting water to the skin if the structure isn't there to keep the water from leaving? It turns out that skin cells usually have plenty of water if they don't become degraded or damaged. Once skin is irritated, overcleansed, exposed to the sun, dehydrated from air conditioning or heaters, and so on, the integrity of the skin surface is compromised. That means the substances that keep the skin cells bound together to create the surface structure we see as skin (the intercellular matrix) are depleted. This intercellular structure is made up of many different components, ranging from ceramides to lecithin, glycerin, polysaccharides, hyaluronic acid, sodium hyaluronate, sodium PCA, collagen, elastin, proteins, amino acids (of which there are dozens), cholesterol, glucose, sucrose, fructose, glycogen, phospholipids, glycosphingolipids, and glycosaminoglycans, to name just a few. All of these give the skin what it needs to keep skin cells intact. Just adding water is meaningless if the intercellular matrix is damaged or impaired. When a moisturizer does contain a combination of NMFs (water-binding agents), it reinforces the skin's natural ability to function normally and that temporarily reduces the presence of dry skin and allows the skin to create healthier skin cells and to repair itself from environmental onslaughts. I rate a moisturizer highly if it has a high number or a high concentration of NMFs.

There is no point in searching for one single mixture or "best" ingredient. Whether it's collagen, elastin, ceramide, hyaluronic acid—or whatever hyped ingredient is being pushed on you as the absolute best there is—realize that there isn't a best. Just like there isn't one "best" chocolate cake recipe, there isn't one best anything in the world of moisturizers. I wish there were, but the brilliance of cosmetics chemists and ingredient manufacturers lies in their ability to create and combine a profusion of ingredients to produce lots and lots of wonderful products. There are just too many great options to sum it up in any one ingredient or product. But I assure you, when a product lacks a good combination of important ingredients such as water-binding agents, antioxidants, or anti-irritants, I will let you know!

Abrasive or **scrub** ingredients are found in cleansing scrubs or in some facial masks meant to remove dead skin cells. The most typical scrub particles used are polyethylene, almond meal, cornmeal, ground apricot kernels, and almond pits. Polyethylene is the most common form of plastic used in the world and the most popular scrub agent. It is flexible and has a smooth, waxy feel. When ground up, the small particles are used in scrubs as a fairly gentle abrasive. Seashells (listed as diatomaceous earth on the ingredient label) are also used as abrasive substances in scrubs, but they can be extremely rough on skin.

Aluminum oxide (also listed as alumina), the same substance used in microdermabrasion treatments, is also starting to show up in scrub products. This substance can be extremely gritty and irritating for skin and is not recommended for regular use.

Absorbents are ingredients used in skin-care and makeup products designed to create a matte finish or oil-absorbing film layer on the skin. These absorbent materials are typically talc, silicates (such as magnesium aluminum silicate), clays, dry-finish silicones (usually cyclomethicone or phenyl trimethicone), nylon-12, and film-forming agents (hairspray-like ingredients), which can all absorb oil effectively. Some have drier finishes than others, but that depends on the specific formulation and the amount of the ingredient used. As I often point out, my concern about ingredients like rice starch, cornstarch, and other food products is that they are typically considered problematic for breakouts. Food substances can get into pores and encourage bacteria production, which is not the best when fighting off bacteria is the goal.

Film-forming agents are ingredients such as PVP (polyvinyl pyrrolidone), methylacrylate, and the polyglycerylacrylates presently being used in a vast number of moisturizers, wrinkle creams, and eye gels to help the skin look smoother. Film-forming agents are usually found in hairsprays and hairstyling products like gels and mousses because they place a thin, transparent, plastic-like layer over the hair (and skin). In the past, the kinds of film-forming agents used were problematic for some skin types; today, with the advent of new polymers, these ingredients do a good job of keeping moisture in the skin and are generally used in such tiny amounts that they are unlikely to be a problem for most skin types. They can also work to absorb oil in some formulations. When these film-forming agents are listed higher up on a product's ingredient list, they might be present at an amount that can leave a slightly tacky feeling on the skin.

Most skin cleansers include ingredients known as surfactants. Surfactant is a technical term that refers to a large number of ingredients that can cleanse as well as degrease. When cleansers contain surfactants as the primary cleansing agent, I use the phrases "**detergent-based**," "**detergent cleansing agent**," or "**standard detergent cleanser**." Ingredients in this category include cocoamidopropyl betaine, sodium laureth sulfate, TEA-lauryl sulfate, cocamide DEA, ammonium laureth sulfate, and ammonium lauryl sulfate, to name a few (though these tend to be the most typical). Because sodium lauryl sulfate, TEA-lauryl sulfate, and sodium C14-16 olefin sulfate are very strong detergent cleansing agents and are known for their irritation potential (Sources: *British Journal of Dermatology*, May 2002, pages 792–800 and *Toxicology in Vitro*, August-October 2001, pages 597–600), I warn against using a product that contains these ingredients when they appear in the first part of the ingredient list.

Preservatives, which are a fundamental component of every cosmetic product, are used in cosmetics to prevent bacterial and microbial contamination of the product. While there is definitely a risk of irritation from the inclusion of preservatives, the risk to skin and eyes from using a contaminated product is considered by many scientists to be even greater.

A group of preservatives known as formaldehyde donors or formaldehyde-releasing preservatives have garnered a reputation for being more problematic than other types of preservatives. Formaldehyde-releasing preservatives are commonly found in cosmetics (Source: *Contact Dermatitis*, December 2000, pages 339–343) and include quaternium-15, 2-bromo-2-nitropane-1,3-diol (trade name Bronopol), methyldibromo glutaronitrile, diazolidinyl urea, imidazolidinyl urea, and dmdm hydantoin. However, there is no research indicating that these ingredients pose a higher potential for irritation than other preservatives. In fact, studies have found no greater increase in skin reactions to formaldehyde-releasing preservatives than to other preservatives (Source: *British Journal of Dermatology*, March 1998, pages 467–476). In fact, there is a far greater risk to skin from a product without preservatives due to the potential for contamination and unchecked growth of bacteria, fungus, and mold.

There is a concern that formaldehyde-releasing preservatives, when present in a formulation with amines (such as triethanalomine—TEA; diethanalomine—DEA, or monoethanalomine—MEA), can form nitrosamines, which are carcinogenic substances that can potentially penetrate skin (Source: *Fundamentals and Applied Toxicology*, August 1993, pages 213–221). Whether or not that poses a health risk has not been established, and there is substantial disagreement among cosmetics chemists as to whether or not this is really a problem for skin. Many chemists suggest that going out of the house without a sunscreen or sitting in a bar exposing yourself to secondhand cigarette smoke poses more risk to the skin than any combination of skin-care ingredients ever could. However, you should be aware that there are those who consider this nonchalant attitude to be mere apologetics for and sidestepping around a very serious question. As a person who has looked at this issue for some time, I actually understand both viewpoints and have no definitive position to share. To that end, I leave the final decision to you. All you need to do is check the ingredient list of any product you are considering to determine whether it includes amines as well as the formaldehyde-releasing preservatives mentioned above.

When **fragrances** or **fragrant plant extracts** are listed among the ingredients, I indicate this clearly in the review. Fragrance and fragrant plant extracts are used in cosmetics either to mask the smell of a product's ingredients or to add a specific fragrance. My strong recommendation is that skin-care products not contain fragrance. Fragrances of all kinds, including essential oils, are irritants or skin sensitizers and serve little to no function for skin (Source: *Contact Dermatitis*, June 1999, pages 310–315).

An article in the January 24, 2000, issue of *The Rose Sheet* (a cosmetics industry newsletter) discussed an advisory report issued by the Scientific Committee on Cosmetic Products and Non-Food Products, a European Commission agency. The report stated that "Information regarding fragrance chemicals used in cosmetic products that have the potential to cause allergic reactions should be provided to consumers." According to the article, "It is seen that a significant increase in fragrance allergy has occurred and that fragrance allergy is the most common cause of contact allergy....." Pamela Scheinmann, MD, concurs with this conclusion in an editorial entitled "The Foul Side of Fragrance-Free Products" (Source: *Journal of the American Academy of Dermatology*, December 1999, page 1020). Scheinmann states that "Products designated as fragrance-free should contain no fragrance chemicals, not even those that have dual functions." She goes on to say that "hypoallergenic, dermatologist tested, sensitive skin, or dermatologist-recommended are nothing more than meaningless marketing slogans." Further research presented in the *American Journal of Contact Dermatitis* (June 1999, pages 310–315, and September 1998, pages 170–175) poses this same concern.

The cosmetics industry knows that most women emotionally and psychologically prefer cosmetics that smell nice, even if they say they want to avoid fragrance. But if a cosmetics company produces products without fragrance, you will instead get the scent of the ingredients, which are not in the least as appealing as an added sweet, floral, or citrus fragrance. This is why, in order to kill two marketing birds with one cosmetic stone, companies often list the fragrance components as essential oils or plant extracts rather than as fragrance or perfume on the label. As lovely as essential oils sound, they are still nothing more than fragrance. So while you may not see the word "fragrance" on the list, and you may approvingly think wintergreen oil, lemon oil, cardamom oil, ylang-ylang oil, or other oils sound pleasant and healthy, your skin may still respond disapprovingly.

The next time you admire the fragrant quality of a skin-care product you're about to apply to any part of your body or face, think twice. Similarly, aromatherapy shouldn't be a skin-care treatment, however therapeutic it is for the sense of smell and the emotions. Fragrance might be nice for your spirits, but it is a health risk for skin. And it doesn't matter if the source of the fragrance is essential oils or plant extracts; as far as the health of your skin is concerned, they are all the same.

Because of the risk of irritation, sensitivity, or allergic reaction to fragrant or volatile plant extracts, I would prefer that all skin-care products be fragrance-free. Nevertheless, women like their products to smell nice, and it's up to every woman to make her own decision on this matter. Even if I thought fragrance was OK in a skin-care product, fragrance is still a very tricky thing to comment on because smell is such a personal experience. Avoiding fragrance is easy to do by checking the ingredient label. But be alert: If you want to stay scent-free, you can't trust the term "unscented," because the product may still contain a masking fragrance. Of course, if fragrance (listed as "fragrance" on the ingredient label) or individual fragrant essential oils like lavender, cardamom, lemon, ylang-ylang, bergamot, and cinnamon, among others, are listed on an ingredient label, you know it has fragrance and you can choose what to do: either make your nose happy or make your skin happy; unfortunately, you usually can't do both.

A profusion of **plant extracts** are used in cosmetics, so many that it's impossible to list them all individually and explain their purpose or lack of purpose. As far as the world of cosmetics is concerned, if it grows, it can change skin. Yet there is no consensus on which plant is the most amazing. According to the various cosmetics companies, the plants they use have the most astonishing merits. When plants are an issue in a skin-care product, I point out the known benefits of those plants, such as antioxidant, anti-irritant, or antibacterial properties. I also explain when plants are a problem in cosmetics owing to their potential for causing irritation or a sensitizing reaction. There are times when plants have both the attribute of being potential irritants but also have antioxidant properties. In these instances I generally cite the irritation potential because there are so many plant extracts that have antioxidant properties without being irritating to skin.

Some plant oils, often referred to as **essential oils**, are highly fragrant, volatile oils and are almost always irritants or photosensitizers, and I indicate when this is the case. However, I attribute no superiority to one over another, because there is none. Essential oils are nothing more than a way to get fragrance into a skin-care product. The cosmetics industry knows that many women are aware that fragrance can be a strong source of skin irritation and sensitivities, so they use the term "essential oils" as a way to put fragrance in a product without saying "fragrance." Women may know that fragrance ingredients are bad, but they still want their products to smell nice. Caught between a rock and a hard place, the cosmetics industry came up with essential oils as a way around the dilemma. But the notion that plants can save the skin from wrinkles, stress, sun damage, scars, and a host of other skin ills is sheer fantasy and has no legitimate substantiation. That doesn't mean that natural ingredients can't be helpful, but they can't perform the miracles attributed to them by sales pitches, and fragrant oils such as clove, peppermint, citrus, ylang-ylang, cinnamon, coriander, and lavender, among many others, can cause irritation.

Nonfragrant plant oils or nonvolatile oils are almost always beneficial as emollients and lubricants. The debate whether or not emu, mink, sunflower, olive, canola, or any of myriad other oils or blends of oils is superior is a marketing game to showcase a product. There is research showing that some plant oils have antioxidant properties. But as more research is done in this field, especially over the past two years, it turns out that many plants have antioxidant properties of one kind or another.

I often list the exact name of any **vitamin** included in a product. Regardless of the individual vitamin—whether it is vitamin A, C, or E—vitamins in skin-care products can't feed the skin. However, many of them can work as antioxidants and theoretically that can benefit the skin.

Antioxidants are a fascinating part of many skin-care formulations. What makes antioxidants so intriguing is that they seem to have the ability to reduce and heal some effects of sun exposure and overall help skin heal. All of that is incredibly beneficial for cell turnover, maintenance, and reducing dehydration. I suspect that antioxidant research for skin will end up being even more fascinating over the next decade as we learn more about how these substances work and how their efficacy can best be applied to skin. In the meantime, even with all the research about antioxidants and their impact on skin, it's still not known how that relates to wrinkles.

Lots of antioxidants, such as selenium, superoxide dismutase, vitamin A (retinyl palmitate and retinol), vitamin C (ascorbyl palmitate and magnesium ascorbyl palmitate), beta-glucan, and vitamin E (tocopherol and tocotrienols), grape extract, green tea, curcumin, coenzyme Q10, and honey, to name the most common ones, are showing up in skin-care products these days. All of these and many, many more are excellent additions to skin-care products and moisturizers of all sorts.

Keep in mind that while antioxidants do have definite benefits, no basic amounts have been set for their effective use. Is 0.25% enough or 3% too much? *Is* there such a thing as too much? How long do they last on skin? When do you need to reapply? There are no answers anywhere to these questions. Until there is more information, it is safe to assume that antioxidants are a crucial aspect when it comes to skin care because the research in that regard is so overwhelming. A search for "antioxidants" on the National Library of Medicine Web site (www.ncbi.nlm.nih.gov/entrez/query.fcgi) produced over 80,000 published studies!

Anti-irritants are gaining more and more recognition and attention in skin-care formulations because of the mounting research showing that any kind of irritation and inflammation of the skin is damaging. Regardless of the source, sun exposure, pollution, stress, irritating skin-care ingredients, or environmental conditions, irritation and inflammation hurts skin. An abundance of research proves this, particularly in regard to inflammation and irritation impeding healing and repair of skin (Sources: *Skin Pharmacology and Applied Skin Physiology*, January-February 2001, Supplement 1, pages 87–91, and 2000, volume 13, number 6, pages 358–371). It would follow that anything you can do to reduce inflammation and irritation would be of great benefit to skin. Actually, a great deal of what we know about the effect of antioxidants on skin is due to their ability to reduce inflammation and irritation. Anti-irritants are impressive ingredients that are able to do just that: reduce inflammation and irritation on skin. An ever-increasing number of ingredients can perform this function and they do so quite nicely. When these types of ingredients—such as bisabolol, allantoin, burdock root, aloe, licorice root, green tea, or willow herb—are present in a product, I refer to them by the term "anti-irritant(s)."

Even plain **water** gets overhyped in skin-care products. Many products use an assortment of exclusive-sounding adjectives—deionized, purified, triple-purified, demineralized, fossilized—to describe what is nothing more than just plain water. These terms indicate that the water has gone through some kind of purification process or was taken from a specific water source, but that is standard for cosmetics. You will also find phrases such as "infusions of" or "aqueous extracts of" followed by the name of one or more plants. That means you're getting what I call "plant tea," or plant juice and water. Though descriptions like this indicate that you are getting mostly water and a hint of plant extract, they sound so pure and natural that they create the impression that they must be better for the skin. It turns out water is water. The kind of water used does not affect the skin or the final product. After the water is combined with other ingredients, its original status is unimportant.

Silicones are a remarkable, diverse, and ubiquitous group of ingredients that show up in over 80% of all cosmetic products being sold. Silicones may look, act, and have a feel reminiscent of oil, but these ingredients are not oils. Technically speaking, silicone as a chemical compound is related to fluid technology. Either way, regardless of the precise name, silicone is an elegant skin-care ingredient that has an exquisite, silky, somewhat slippery feel; it also has an affinity to skin and "dries" to an almost imperceptible finish. Its popularity in formulations reflects its versatility and the finish it gives products. For someone with oily or acne-prone skin, silicone is not necessarily a problem, because there are new silicone polymers that have oil-absorbing properties and can leave a soft matte finish on skin.

The daily use of **antibacterial ingredients** for purposes of general cleansing, as opposed to using them to treat acne or in other wound care, poses some problems for skin and for society. While cleanliness has merit, there are limitations to how clean a person can be. In the battle against germs and other loathsome microorganisms floating about our environment, the desire to wash with zest is valid (do not take that as a plug for Zest bar soap; I just couldn't resist the pun). We are also greatly influenced by news programs that ballyhoo the horror of bacteria being spread through less-than-scrupulous washing habits. It isn't surprising, then, to hear that sales of antibacterial soaps have increased dramatically over the past several years.

For the consumer, the problem for skin is that antibacterial soaps and cleansers contain **triclosan** or **triclocarban** (the most typical antibacterial agents used), and there is little to no independent scientific data published to suggest that using these products prevents infection. In addition, and even more problematic, is a finding that triclosan-resistant bacteria have recently been identified (Source: *American Journal of Infection Control*, October 2001, pages 281–283). Similar concerns were discussed in *Emerging Infectious Diseases* (2001, volume 7, issue 3, Supplemental pages 512–515). The article stated that "The recent entry of products containing antibacterial agents into healthy households has escalated from a few dozen products in the mid-1990s to more than 700 today. Antibacterial products were developed and have been successfully used to prevent transmission of disease-causing microorganisms among patients, particularly in hospitals. They are now being added to products used in healthy households, even though an added health benefit has not been demonstrated. Scientists are concerned that the antibacterial agents will select bacteria resistant to them and cross-resistant to antibiotics. Moreover, if they alter a person's microflora [the body's useful and functional bacteria], they may negatively affect the normal maturation of the T helper cell response of the immune system to commensal flora antigens; this change could lead to a greater chance of allergies in children." In other words, if we are too clean we actually prevent our bodies from developing healthy and natural immunities to many "germs" in our environment.

The April 19, 1999, issue of the *Journal of Biological Chemistry*, concluded that the ability of *E. coli* bacteria "to acquire genetic resistance to triclosan [the antibacterial agent found in many antibacterial hand creams and toothpastes] ... suggests that the widespread use of this drug will lead to the appearance of resistant organisms that will compromise the usefulness of triclosan."

Because of the limited research demonstrating the need for antibacterial products in daily skin care, these products are not recommended.

Benzoyl peroxide is considered the primary over-the-counter ingredient when a topical **antibacterial agent for acne** is needed in the treatment of blemishes (Source: *Skin Pharmacology and Applied Skin Physiology*, September-October 2000, pages 292–296). The amount of research demonstrating the effectiveness of benzoyl peroxide is exhaustive and conclusive (Source: *Journal of the American Academy of Dermatology*, November 1999, pages 710–716). Among benzoyl peroxide's attributes is its ability to penetrate into the hair follicle to reach the bacteria causing the problem (propiobacterium), and then killing them—with a low risk of irritation as long as no other irritating ingredients such as alcohol, menthol, peppermint, or citrus are added. It also doesn't pose the problem of bacterial resistance that some prescription topical antibacterials (antibiotics) do (Source: *Dermatology*, 1998, volume 196, issue 1, pages 119–125 and *Cutis*, February 2001, pages 25–27).

Benzoyl peroxide solutions range from 2.5% to 10%. For the sake of your skin, start with the less potent concentrations. A 2.5% benzoyl peroxide product is much less irritating than a 5% or 10% concentration, and it can be just as effective. It completely depends on how stubborn the strain of bacteria in your pores happens to be.

Despite benzoyl peroxide's superior disinfecting and penetrating properties, some bacteria just won't give up easily, and in those situations a different weapon may be necessary. That's when you should consider prescription topical disinfectants (topical antibiotics).

Alpha hydroxy acids and beta hydroxy acid: I do not recommend products that claim they have an association with AHAs or BHA but contain ingredients such as fruit extracts or sugarcane extracts. These may sound like they can work like AHAs or BHA, but they can't. There are a host of legitimate AHA ingredients, the two most popular and best researched being glycolic acid and lactic acid. While glycolic acid is indeed derived from sugarcane, assuming that sugarcane will net you the same result as glycolic acid would be like assuming you could write on a tree the way you can on paper. Paper is derived from wood but that doesn't mean you can write on the original wood. The same analogy holds true for lactic acid, which is derived from milk. If milk were as acid as lactic acid, you would not be able to drink it without serious stomach complications. It is important to remember that there is a vast difference between the isolated ingredient and the original form.

The only BHA is salicylic acid, and this performs best at a pH of 3 to 4 in a 1% to 2% concentration. Concentrations as low as 0.5% are available, but that amount is too small to be effective for most skin types. Because salicylic acid is derived from willow bark, many products use willow bark and claim they contain an effective form of BHA. Willow bark extract does contain salicin, a substance that when taken orally is converted by the digestive process to salicylic acid. But the process of converting willow bark to salicylic acid requires the presence of enzymes to take the salicin and turn it into salicylic acid, and that is most likely impossible topically. Besides, salicin, much like salicylic acid, is stable only under acidic conditions. The likelihood that willow bark in the tiny amount used in these products can mimic the effectiveness of salicylic acid is at best problematic, and in all likelihood probably impossible. However, willow bark may indeed have some anti-inflammatory benefits for skin, because in this form it appears to retain more of its aspirin-like composition. That is nice for skin but it definitely doesn't make willow bark better than other anti-inflammatories used in cosmetics, and it doesn't deliver the same exfoliating benefit as BHA.

For acne, salicylic acid not only penetrates into the pore (it is lipid soluble) but also has antibacterial properties. In Europe and Canada salicylic acid is considered a keratolytic (exfoliant) as well as an antibacterial agent.

The most well-researched AHA ingredients are glycolic acid and lactic acid. They are most effective in a base with a pH of 3 to 4 in a concentration of 5% to 10%. At a concentration over 10% there is a concern that the product would be too irritating for daily use in skin care (Source: *Cosmetic Dermatology*, October 2001, pages 15–18).

Just a reminder: Anytime you use a well-formulated AHA product that contains more than 5% AHAs, some stinging can occur; and you should not let the product come in contact with the eyes or any mucous membranes. Although slight stinging is expected, continued stinging is not. If the stinging does continue, you may have sensitivity to AHAs, and should discontinue use.

Though wearing sunscreen is always crucial it is even more imperative when using AHA or BHA products because these exfoliants remove surface layers of sun-damaged skin, leaving the skin even more vulnerable to the negative effects of the sun.

PLANTS: A GROWING QUESTION

Survey after survey indicates that women want products that are all natural. To appease the demands of the consumer, cosmetics companies profess that their products are indeed all natural. Yet, to the chagrin of cosmetic buyers everywhere, it turns out that there is no such thing as an "all natural" product. The term is not regulated by the FDA (www.fda.gov) and it only takes a cursory look at an ingredient label to notice that the preponderance of ingredients are decidedly unnatural.

To add insult to injury the cosmetics industry wants women to believe that a plant extract of any kind, short of rubbing broccoli or asparagus on our faces, must be good for skin and that synthetic ingredients must be bad. It doesn't matter if it's a completely unknown plant, if it grows, there must be an excellent reason to use it. It also doesn't matter that the plant ingredients make up less than 0.5% of the total product and the other unnatural ingredients account for more than 50% of the contents (with the rest being water). Regardless of these facts, the image of plants in cosmetics is an overpowering one for the consumer. Many cosmetics companies have made a religion out of plants, while others have turned it into a political issue. What is unquestionable is that, almost without exception, and to one degree or another, every company is on the bandwagon touting some miraculous leaf, stem, root, or bark.

But why use *Prunus persica* (peach extract) over *Hordeum distichon* (barley extract), *Betula alba* (birch extract) rather than *Brassica oleracea capitata* (cabbage extract), or *Cananga odorata* (ylang-ylang oil) instead of *Anthemis nobilis* (chamomile extract) or *Pseudopterogorgia elisabethae* (sea whip extract—actually this one is a marine invertebrate, but you get my drift)? There are literally hundreds and hundreds of plant extracts that can potentially be used in cosmetics. Do they all perform equally well? Or at all?

Not all plants that show up in cosmetics are beneficial for skin. There are many plant extracts that sound harmless, but the research indicates otherwise. For example, St. John's wort contains several components that are toxic on skin in the presence of sunlight (Sources: *Planta Medica*, February 2002, pages 171–173 and *International Journal of Biochemistry and Cell Biology*, March 2002, pages 221–241). *Ephedra sinica* is an extract from a Chinese herb also known as Ma huang that has a high tannin and volatile oil content and has been shown to have toxic properties (Source: *Toxicological Sciences*, August 2000, pages 424–430). Or take camphor, an aromatic substance obtained from the wood of a southeast Asian tree *Cinnamomum camphora*, which, when applied to the skin produces a cooling effect and dilates blood vessels, which in turn can cause skin irritation and dermatitis with repeated use (Sources: *British Journal of Dermatology*, November 2000, pages 923–929 and *Clinical Toxicology*, December 1981, pages 1485–1498). This list of problematic plant extracts will shock you as you read through the reviews in this book. So much for all plants being harmless and good for skin. There are literally hundreds and hundreds of plant extracts being used in cosmetics and most consumers blindly assume that all of these must hold some special benefit for their skin, when in truth that is not always the case.

The issue of natural versus synthetic is one I've written about extensively over the years. To sum it up succinctly, "natural" does not mean good and "synthetic" does not mean bad. Each group has its shortcomings and strengths, but I would no sooner accept any plant as automatically being good for my skin than I would walk naked through a patch of poison ivy assuming that because it's a plant, it must be OK.

"Natural" simply defines the source of the ingredient; it tells you nothing about the ingredient's effectiveness or risks. Menthol and peppermint may have a natural source, but both are serious skin irritants and a problem for skin. Ingredients like silicone and stearyl alcohol are synthetic but they are remarkably silky-soft ingredients, vital to a vast array of cosmetic formulations. Sodium lauryl sulfate is a detergent cleansing agent derived from coconut, but that doesn't make it good for skin.

"Synthetic" merely tells you that the ingredient was created in a laboratory (though technically that's true for plant extracts, too), and although that kind of origin may sound unhealthy, it often means that the resulting ingredient is going to be "purer" than a natural ingredient. Natural ingredients can be made up of hundreds of known and unknown ingredients and not all of those components may be good for skin. Plus, the ingredients it took to create the plant extract—the chemical processes used to extract the oil or other natural substance from the plant—are almost always completely synthetic and unnatural. After all, once that plant is processed and mixed into a moisturizer, it doesn't mean you'll want to eat that moisturizer for lunch.

None of this should be taken to suggest that plants have no benefits in skin-care products, because they do. But the notion that any plant, from grape to green tea and on and on, has any antiaging properties for skin is yet to be substantiated. Depending on the plant, it can have both a positive and negative effect on skin. Almost every plant extract contained in a product that is reviewed in this edition of my book are described with the accompanying research in Chapter Seven, *Cosmetics Dictionary*. Meanwhile, to imply that a pure tincture of a plant (or an extracted component of it) of the kind used in reported research can have the same effect on skin when mixed into a cosmetic in teeny, fractional amounts is, more times than not, a stretch of the imagination.

Having scoured the research regarding plant extracts, here's what I can report unequivocally:

1. **Most plant extracts in products have either minimal or no research establishing their efficacy for skin care when used in a cosmetic formulation.**

2. **When research does exist, it is usually for the pure plant extract, not for a watered-down version used in fractional amounts mixed into a cosmetic of some kind.**

3. **Most research that establishes a plant's efficacy doesn't take into consideration that plant extracts are highly unstable. Think about it: How long does a head of lettuce last in your refrigerator? The notion that a plant extract can last and remain effective long term in a skin-care product is most likely sheer fantasy.**

4. **While plants are unquestionably loaded with all kinds of substances that may be great when taken internally, the notion that all (or any) of those internal benefits can be achieved by application to the skin is unknown. There is either limited or no research establishing that rubbing a plant substance over skin is helpful for wrinkles or any other aspect of skin care (though many plants do have antioxidant properties). When taken orally, there are many reasons to consider plants or plant extracts for regular use.**

But for skin care their benefit is mostly theory, and in a skin-care product, the theory is a lot more diluted.

5. Almost without exception I rate the extracted active substance of the plant as having more efficacy potential than the plant. For example, bisabolol is the active anti-inflammatory component in chamomile (specifically *Matricaria recutita*). While chamomile in a pure concentration can have that type of effectiveness, the likelihood is that this effectiveness is lost when the plant extract is used in teeny amounts in skin-care products. However, when bisabolol is listed on the label, it means the product uses the isolated active ingredient in chamomile that has anti-inflammatory benefits, and that the skin has a better shot at gaining benefit.

Note: Many cosmetics contain between 5 and up to 75 different ingredients in their formulation. In addition, there is a consistent repetition of ingredients used within specific product lines and/or throughout different lines. It is thus impossible to include the analysis (the pros, cons, and hype) of every ingredient used for each of the thousands and thousands of products reviewed in this book. For details on specific ingredient, research documentation, and function considerations, please refer to Chapter Seven, *Cosmetics Dictionary* at the end of this book.

EVALUATION OF MAKEUP PRODUCTS

For each product category, I use a specific list of guidelines, considerations, and other factors to determine a product's performance, reliability, or value to skin.

FOUNDATIONS: My fundamental expectation for any foundation, regardless of type (liquid, pressed powder, loose powder, stick, or cream-to-powder), is that it not be any shade or tone of orange, peach, pink, rose, green, or ash—because there are no people with skin that color. Consistency, coverage, and feel are also important. All foundations, regardless of texture, must go on smoothly and evenly, not separate or turn color, and be easy to blend. Foundations that claim to be matte or ultra-matte must be truly matte, meaning no shine or dewy finish, and they must have the potential to last most of the day. Foundations that claim to moisturize must contain ingredients that can do that.

There is a new generation of shiny, iridescent foundations on the market today from many cosmetics lines. They come either in a sheer, moisturizing-type formula or with a slight amount of tint. What they provide is some iridescence or sparkle on the face. While I generally do not care for sparkly makeup, especially for daytime, these products are rated on ease of use, how well they last, how much they flake (controlling where the shine is placed is important—you don't want sparkles falling on your clothes), and how sheer and easy they are to blend.

FOUNDATIONS WITH SUNSCREENS: Foundations with sunscreens are held to the same standards as any other sunscreen, which means they must have at least an SPF 15 and must include a UVA-protecting ingredient as one of the active ingredients on the label. The only acceptable UVA-protecting ingredients are titanium dioxide, zinc oxide, and avobenzone (also called Parsol 1789 or butyl methoxydibenzoylmethane). In the reviews, you will notice that foundations with poor or inadequate sunscreens are criticized severely, but may still receive a happy face rating. In these situations, the performance of the foundations was considered excellent, but the foundation could not be relied on for sun protection and would require a well-formulated sunscreen to be worn underneath. For more details, see the information on sunscreens presented in the "Evaluating Skin-Care Products" section.

Beauty Note: Color suggestions for all makeup products are often based on tester units available at the cosmetics counter or on samples (including gifts with a purchase or discounted promotions), but mainly from products that were purchased. The color, shade, or tone of a particular product can fluctuate for a number of reasons. If I refer to a particular foundation as being "too peach" and you find that it's just right, it may be that we simply disagree, or it may be that the product I tested or bought was different from the one you ended up buying.

CONCEALERS: Concealers should never be any shade of orange, peach, pink, rose, green, or ash, and they should not slip into the lines around the eye. I look for creamy, smooth textures that go on easily without pulling the skin, don't look dry and pasty, and, perhaps most important, do not crease into lines. I generally do not recommend using concealers over blemishes, but there is rarely a problem with using most concealers on other parts of the face if they match the skin.

I don't recommend medicated concealers because they are rarely, if ever, "medicated" with ingredients or formulations that can affect breakouts. For medicated concealers to work, they would need to contain an effective exfoliant or an effective disinfectant, and I have yet to test one that meets those criteria and has a color that anyone would dare put on their face.

Despite claims a product may make for oily skin versus dry skin, please keep in mind that companies can make these claims regardless of what ingredients the product contains. In general, the thicker and greasier the product, the more likely it is to be problematic for oily, acne-prone skin. However, anything you apply over skin can cause problems. Just because a product does or doesn't contain oil is no guarantee one way or the other that it won't cause problems for the skin. There are also lots of ingredients that don't sound like oil that can cause problems for skin. Generally, a matte-finish product is best for oily skin, but that still won't ensure a lack of breakouts.

COLOR CORRECTORS: I am not a fan of color correctors in any form. Color correctors are usually a group of concealers you apply before you apply your foundation color. They generally come in shades of yellow, mauve, pink, or green. Color correctors are marketed as a way to change skin color, so that if your skin has pink undertones, a yellow color corrector is supposed to even that out. The only thing these products do is give the skin a strange hue. Does anyone think the colored layer isn't noticeable? That yellow or mauve layer then mixes with your foundation, giving it a strange color. Another problem with this kind of product is that it adds another layer on the skin, and the buildup of cosmetic ingredients on the face can be pore-clogging. A well-chosen foundation color and blush can easily provide the color balance you are looking for without adding another layer of strange makeup colors on the skin.

FACE POWDERS: Face powders come in two basic forms: pressed and loose. I evaluate them on the basis of whether they go on sheer, shiny, chalky, or heavy and whether they are too pink, peach, ash, or rose. I consistently give higher marks to powders that go on sheer and have a silky-soft texture with a natural beige, tan, or rich brown finish and that have no overtones of red, peach, orange, yellow, or green.

Talc is the most frequently used ingredient in powders in all price ranges, and it is one of the best for absorbing oil and giving a smooth finish to the face. Some companies make claims about their grade of talc being better than another company's. The issue of a grade difference cannot be proven and is irrelevant unless the product's feel and performance are affected.

Other minerals are used for the same purpose as talc, and though they may sound more exotic, they are not any better for the skin. Cornstarch or rice starch in powders do help create a beautiful texture and these are interesting substitutes for talc, but they can also be a skin concern because there is evidence that they can clog pores and cause breakouts. I try to screen for these in that regard.

When it comes to bronzing powders, I generally suggest using them as a contour color and not as an all-over face color. Darkening the face almost always makes for an overdone look. After all, if a foundation is supposed to match the skin, how can the use of a powder that darkens the skin be rationalized? The face will be a color decidedly different from the neck, and there will be a line of demarcation where the color starts and stops. Also, most bronzing powders are iridescent. Dusting a color over the face that is darker than your skin tone is bad enough, but why make it more obvious with particles of shine all over, particularly in daylight? The few bronzing powders without any hint of shine are rated highest.

There are numerous shiny powders being sold today, and I rate these products on ease of use, how well they last, how much they flake, and how sheer and easy they are to blend. Shiny powder as an oil-absorbent is never deemed a good idea because if the idea is to powder down shine, then applying more shine doesn't make sense. These products are an option for those who want to add sparkle to their all-over makeup appearance.

Powders are often designated by the cosmetics companies as being for dry or oily skin. Those designations are often bogus, however, with little if any real differences between the formulations. I rate a face powder as being good for oily skin if it contains minimal waxy or oily ingredients and has good absorbency without being heavy or thick on the skin.

There is absolutely no reason to spend a lot of money on powders. Regardless of formulation, there is nothing about price that differentiates one from the other. Some of the best powders, including those with sun protection, are also available at the drugstore.

Beauty Note: Talc is often criticized as an awful cosmetic ingredient that should be avoided. The concern about talc is not about how it is used in makeup, but, rather, when it is used in pure, large concentrations in the form of talcum powder. Part of the story dates back to several studies published in the 1990s that found a significant increase in the risk of ovarian cancer from vaginal (perineal) application of talcum powder (Sources: *American Journal of Epidemiology*, March 1997, pages 459–465; *International Journal of Cancer*, May 1999, pages 351–356; *Seminars in Oncology*, June 1998, pages 255–264; and *Cancer*, June 1997, pages 2396–2401). However, subsequent and concurrent studies cast doubt on the way these studies were conducted and on the conclusions they reached (Sources: *Journal of the National Cancer Institute*, February 2000, pages 249–252; *American Journal of Obstetrics and Gynecology*, March 2000, pages 720–724; and *Obstetrics and Gynecology*, March 1999, pages 372–376).

While more research in this area is being carried out to clear up the confusion, none of the research about the use of talc is related to the way women use makeup. There is no indication anywhere that there is any risk for the face when using products that contain talc. That means you need not avoid using eyeshadows, blushes, or face powders that contain talc. But it does mean you should consider not using talcum powder on your children or on yourself vaginally. If you still wish to avoid talc in makeup, it is easy enough to do by just checking the ingredient list.

FACE POWDERS WITH SUNSCREEN: There are a few pressed powders available that have a reliable SPF 15 or greater and that contain UVA-protecting ingredients. That is great news. However, I am concerned about the way women may use these products. While I don't doubt the validity of the SPF number, I worry that most women won't apply pressed-powder foundations liberally enough to get the amount of protection indicated on the label. If you lightly dust the powder over the skin, you will not be getting the SPF protection indicated on the label. You must be sure you apply the pressed powder in a manner that liberally, completely, and evenly covers the face. I feel that pressed powders are an iffy choice if they are the only product used for sun protection, though they are a great way to touch up your makeup during the day and reapply sunscreen at the same time!

BLUSHES: I consider it essential for blushes to have a smooth texture, to blend on easily, and to have a silky feel on the skin. Overall, I don't recommend shiny blushes. Although they don't make cheeks look as crepey or wrinkly as shiny eyeshadows do the eyes, sparkling cheeks look out of place during the day. Blushes that go on with a sheen or shine but do not sparkle I describe with a warning, but they receive a good rating if they go on evenly and smoothly and don't flake. This is more a matter of personal preference than a problem.

Cream blushes, cream-to-powder blushes, and liquid or gel blushes are rated on their blendability, whether they streak, how greasy or dry they feel, and how well they last. I also describe which cream blushes tend to work better over foundation and which ones perform better if applied directly on the skin.

EYESHADOWS: It won't surprise most of you who have read any of my previous books or newsletters to find out that I don't recommend eyeshadows of any intense shade of blue, violet, green, or red, whether they shine or not. Intense hues may be a personal preference, but I don't encourage anyone to use them. Makeup that speaks louder than you do may be kicky and fun, but it doesn't help empower a woman or help her be taken more seriously. If that's not your goal in life, ignore my color or shine recommendations.

Regardless of color or shine, I evaluate all eyeshadows on the basis of texture and ease of application. I point out which colors have heavy or grainy textures because they can be hard to blend and can easily crease. Eyeshadows that are too sheer or powdery are also a problem because the color tends to fade as the day wears on, and they can also be difficult to apply, flaking all over the place. I am also leery of eyeshadow sets that include difficult-to-use color combinations. Many lines have duo, trio, and quad sets of eyeshadows, with the most bizarre color combinations imaginable. Sets of colors must be usable as a set and coordinated in complementary colors; they should never paint a rainbow or kaleidoscope of color across the eye. However, if you are looking for a kaleidoscope, I've pointed them out; they just have an unhappy face next to them. Generally, it is best to buy eyeshadow colors singly, not in sets. That way you can be assured of liking all the colors you buy, not just two out of three or four.

Specialty eyeshadow products such as liquids, creams, powdery or creamy pencils, and loose-powder eyeshadows are evaluated on ease of use, blendability, staying power, and how well they work over and with other products. My reviews indicate a clear bias toward matte eyeshadow powders as opposed to any other type of eyeshadow. I find liquids and creams hard to control, and even more difficult to blend with other colors. Most of them also tend to crease easily, and almost always lose intensity throughout the day.

EYE AND BROW SHAPERS: Basically, all pencils, regardless of brand, have more similarities than differences. Most eye pencils, lip pencils, and eyebrow pencils are manufactured by the same company (meaning the same manufacturing plant) and then sold to hundreds of different cosmetics lines. Whether they cost $30 from Chanel or $7 from Almay, they are likely to be exactly the same product. Some pencils are greasier or drier than others, but for the most part there are few marked differences among them. Eye pencils that smudge and smear and eyebrow pencils that go on like a crayon—meaning thick and greasy—are always rated as ineffective, because they can get very messy as the day goes by.

(Keep in mind that whether an eye pencil smears along the lower eyelashes depends to a large extent on the number of lines around your eye, how much moisturizer you use around the eye area, the type of under-eye concealer you use, and how greasy the pencil is. The greasier the moisturizer or the under-eye concealer, the more likely any pencil will smear, and you can't blame that on the pencil.)

Liquid eyeliners are rated on how easily they are to apply and on how quickly they dry. The way these types of liners last throughout the day is also a consideration due to the fact that many liquid liners tend to flake and peel.

As a general rule, I do not recommend pencils for filling in the brow. Eyebrow pencil almost always looks harsh and artificial next to an eyebrow. I use only powder, and I encourage you to do the same. Any eyeshadow color that matches your eyebrow color as closely as possible can do the trick, applied with a tiny eyeliner or angle brush. The goal is to create a brow that is as natural looking as possible. Brow mascaras and eyeshadow or brow shadow work superbly together to fill in the brow. A handful of companies make a clear brow gel meant to keep eyebrows in place without adding color or thickness. This works well, but no better than hairspray on a toothbrush brushed through the brow.

LIPSTICKS AND LIP PENCILS: Every woman has her own needs and preferences when it comes to lipstick. Some women like sheer applications; others prefer glossy or matte finishes. Colors are also difficult to recommend because of the wide variation in taste. Given those limitations, I primarily review the range of colors and textures available, commenting on texture rather than critiquing it, because personal preference is vital to a final decision. The general groupings are glossy or sheer, creamy, creamy with shine or iridescence, matte, and ultra-matte. As a matter of preference, because of staying power and coverage, I give the highest marks to creamy or semi-matte lipsticks that go on evenly and aren't glossy, sticky, thick, or drying. The ultra-matte lipsticks (introduced first by Ultima II with its LipSexxxy and then made overwhelmingly popular by Revlon's ColorStay, which is virtually identical to the former) are unique because of their dry, flat finish and because they don't come off easily on coffee cups or teeth. They have since fallen out of favor for the very problems I originally commented on when they were first launched—they can chip and peel, and actually cause lips to feel drier and become more chapped.

I evaluate lip pencils according to whether they go on smoothly without being greasy or dry. Lip glosses are also evaluated based on their texture, application, and longevity.

MASCARAS: Mascaras should go on easily and quickly while building length and thickness. Mascara brush shapes have improved phenomenally over the years, although there are those that can still be awkward to use if they are too big or too small. Mascara should never smear or flake, regardless of price.

Whether or not mascaras smear is difficult to assess. No matter how well-formulated it is, no mascara can hold up to a heavy layer of moisturizer around the eyes. If you wear an extremely emollient moisturizer around the eyes and a lot of it, your mascara will smear.

I don't recommend waterproof mascaras except for swimming and for special occasions that likely will involve tears. All the pulling and wiping that is necessary to get waterproof mascara off isn't good for the skin and tends to pull lashes out. There are hundreds of waterproof mascaras out there, but only a few capture the best traits of non-waterproof mascaras while still being waterproof. Keep in mind that waterproof mascaras do not stay on any better than water-soluble ones, given that both break down in contact with emollients from moisturizers, sunscreens, under-eye creams, foundations, creamy under-eye concealers, and other specialty products applied around the eye.

Beauty Note: I should mention that I have a personal preference for mascaras that produce long, thick lashes. I admit that my own preference in this regard can get in the way of my evaluations, so understand that I get particularly excited about mascaras such as L'Oreal 3-D Lash Architect that builds thick, long lashes fast and easily without smearing or flaking, though with some clumping.

BRUSHES: Brushes are essential to applying makeup correctly and beautifully. Blush and eyeshadow brushes are offered by some of the major cosmetics lines, and all of the makeup artistry lines. Brushes are rated on overall shape and function as well as on the softness and density of the bristles. Eyeshadow or blush brushes with scratchy, stiff, or loose bristles are not recommended. As a rule, be cautious about buying brush sets because many include brushes you don't need or can't use.

UNDERSTANDING THE RATING SYSTEM

The following are the rating symbols for the products reviewed in this book. These simple, but succinct (albeit cute), symbols depict approval or disapproval of a specific product.

For those who are familiar with my reviews and ratings from past editions of my books and newsletters, this edition has incorporated a major shift in what constitutes an expensive and reasonably priced product and what constitutes a product that is well-formulated and state of the art.

☺ This smiling face indicates a great product that I recommend highly because of its performance or impressive formulary characteristics. The smiling face means the product is definitely worth checking into and potentially worth buying, especially considering that it is so reasonably priced.

☺ $$$ This symbol designates a great product that meets and/or surpasses the criteria set for that category of product. However, just because the product is well-formulated doesn't mean it is worth the money. Almost without exception there are always reasonably priced versions of a product that meet or exceed the same standards as the more expensive versions.

☺ This neutral face indicates an OK but unimpressive product, or an OK product that can cause problems for certain skin types. I often use this face to portray a dated or old-fashioned product formulation. That doesn't mean it's a bad product, but that it j isn't very interesting or is lacking some of the newer water-binding ingredients, antioxi dants, anti-irritants, emollients, or nonirritating ingredients for dry skin. I also use the neutral face to reflect a makeup product that isn't really bad, but that is completely unnecessary, ordinary, or in comparison to other products, not as well-formulated. Depending on your personal preferences, products rated with the neutral face may be worth checking out, but they're nothing to get excited about.

☺ $$$ This symbol indicates an ordinary, boring product whose excessive price makes it ludicrous to consider. For skin-care products, the rating reflects a lack of unique or interesting water-binding agents, anti-irritants, emollients, antioxidants, effective exfoliants, gentle cleansing agents, or combinations of those in a given formulation. For makeup, it reflects a performance that pales in comparison to other far better formulations, but that still can look OK when applied.

☹ For many reasons, this frowning face reflects a product that is truly bad for skin from almost every standpoint, including price, dated formulations, performance, application, and texture, as well as potential for irritation, skin reactions, and breakouts.

✓☺ PAULA'S PICK

✓☺ **Paula's Pick:** This is a new category I created for this edition of *Don't Go to the Cosmetics Counter Without Me*. One of the criticisms I've received over the years is that my lists at the end of the book for Best Products are too long and cumbersome. Women have asked me to narrow the list to just a handful. That's difficult to do because if a product is good I don't want to leave it out just to make my final listings more manageable to navigate. In searching for an ethical way to meet the needs of the reader and still review products fairly, I came up with what I think is a workable solution. When a product exceeds expectations and meets the criteria for a product in its category with minimal to no concerns I indicate that with a checkmark and happy face. In Chapter Six, those picks are then included as part of the Best Products summary by the same checkmark and happy face. Keep in mind that products with only a happy face and no checkmark do have value but are not extraordinary standouts in their category.

GENERAL REVIEW INFORMATION

Prices: Because the cost of drugstore cosmetics often fluctuates from store to store, and because cosmetics companies often change prices every six months, the prices listed in this book may not be up-to-date and may not match what you find when you are

as a basis for comparison, but realize that they may not precisely
you go shopping.

ormation: My staff and I diligently work to make sure all the infor-
ve is accurate and current. However, cosmetics companies frequently and
notice change or reformulate their products, sometimes in a minor way and
sometimes extensively. To keep abreast of these changes, which cannot be kept current in
a book, I report revisions and new product launches that occurred after this book went to
press in my newsletter, *Cosmetics Counter Update* and frequently in my free online *Beauty
Bulletin*.

Foreign names: For the most part, I give only the English names of foreign-pro-
duced products. The French and Italian names are pretty, but they don't tell you anything
about the product if you don't speak the language.

No endorsements: Neither the information nor the evaluations included in any of
my works are to be misconstrued as endorsements, nor do they represent a particular
company's sponsorship. None of the cosmetics companies paid me for my remarks or
critiques. All of the products listed in "Best Choices" or under Paula's Picks are just that,
choices and picks, with the final decision left to you.

Order of presentation: The cosmetics products are listed alphabetically by brand
name, so the order in which they appear does not represent my preference. There is no
implied winner among any of the cosmetics companies included in this book, and no one
line has all the answers or the majority of great products. Almost every line has its strong
and weak points.

Don't go shopping without me: I encourage you to take this book with you on shopping trips to the cosmetics counters or the drugstore. Then you will have all the information
you'll need readily at hand because there is no way you (or anyone) can remember the
details of each product, color, and brand. Do try to be discreet at the department-store
cosmetics counters—and don't be surprised if you find that using the book in clear view of
the salespeople makes them defensive or irritated. There are always risks when a consumer
comes prepared with information that disagrees with the salesperson's. I urge you to perse-
vere. Nothing will change at the cosmetics counters if you don't change first.

When we disagree: Please be aware that you may not and need not agree with all my
reviews to get some benefit from the information in this book. As you read my comments,
you may very well find yourself disagreeing with me. That is perfectly understandable and
as it should be, because the criteria you use to evaluate cosmetics may differ from mine.
Or, for any one of a dozen reasons (personal preference, different expectations, actual
usage such as once a week versus twice a day), a product I dislike may work well for you.
Or just the opposite can be true: you may hate a product I rate highly. What I cannot
account for is how millions of women will feel or react to a particular product. However,
you can learn whether your expectations about a product's efficacy are based on nothing
more than a placebo effect, or are based on a worthwhile formulation.

Why reviews in this edition may differ from reviews in previous editions: You may notice that in this edition the reviews of products have changed from those in previous editions. There are three major reasons why: (1) I have acquired new research that supports a different evaluation, (2) Other products in a category are significantly better and, therefore, the original evaluation of superior performance may be downgraded due to the comparison to superior formulations being sold, and (3) The company changed the product since I last tested it.

Beauty Note: For updates to this book, please visit my Web site at www.cosmeticscop.com.

THE REVIEWS A–Z

What I present in the following pages are merely guidelines, based on my extensive research and investigation about what works and what doesn't. If you decide to follow any of my suggestions, be aware that my recommendations are not a guarantee, but instead offer suggestions as to how to narrow down the endless options the cosmetics industry sells. It is my earnest desire to help you choose from this very crowded field so you can make the best choices possible. The final choice, of course, is yours.

ACNE-STATIN (SKIN CARE ONLY)

This small line of acne products has been around for years. How does Acne-Statin claim to deal with acne? Well, not very directly, that's for sure, because Acne-Statin doesn't list ingredients on its label. Thanks to a grandfather clause in the FDA's mandatory rules for listing ingredients, Acne-Statin doesn't have to list any of its nonactive ingredients because their formulations haven't changed since 1978 when the ingredient listing regulations for cosmetics became compulsory.

However, all products do have to list their active ingredients, and Acne-Statin does comply with that regulation. One of the cleansers contains 0.5% triclosan, which is a decent topical disinfectant, although there is no research showing it be effective for acne. The Acne Treatment Cream contains 0.5% salicylic acid, a good exfoliant but hardly special or unique to this line and not particularly effective at that low a concentration. What else comprises the other 99.5% in these two products is anyone's guess, but the thick consistencies make me suspect they contain ingredients that are probably not the best for someone prone to breakouts or with oily skin.

When I first wrote about this line in the First Edition of my book (1991) I challenged the claims this company made regarding its ability to heal or cure acne. It turns out the Federal Trade Commission (FTC) agreed with my original conclusions. According to a press release from the FTC on July 30, 1996 (http://www.ftc.gov/opa/1996/9607/karr2.htm), "Acne-Statin … has agreed to pay a $200,000 civil penalty to settle Federal Trade Commission charges that ads touting the product as an effective treatment for severe or cystic acne were deceptive. The claims also violate a 1979 order prohibiting Dr. Atida H. Karr from making unsubstantiated claims about the effectiveness or superiority of any acne preparation she markets, the agency alleges. Karr and her Beverly Hills, California, based companies sold Acne-Statin and currently sell the Acne-Statin Kit."

"The 1979 order prohibits Karr and her firms from advertising the effectiveness or superiority of any acne preparation unless the claims are supported by competent and reliable scientific or medical evidence. Karr paid $175,000 into a consumer refund account as part of the 1979 settlement of the initial case."

Since then Acne-Statin's claims have toned down to some extent, but they are still fairly sweeping for what ends up being nothing more than two fairly standard exfoliating and disinfecting ingredients (and not at particularly effective concentrations). But as consumers, we are given only advertising and hype to help us make a decision. The ingredient list, the only verifiable truth on any cosmetics label, is kept a secret. If the Acne-Statin products or any acne products for that matter were the only answer for acne, as the ads for Acne-Statin and other acne products often allege, who would have acne? Bottom line: The active ingredients listed here can't do what the product claims they can do, and moreover, despite the age of these formulations (they've been around for more than three decades), they haven't been updated either and the research about acne has certainly advanced since 1977. Because the ingredients for these products aren't listed, no ratings are given. For more information about Acne-Statin, call (877) 469-2263 or visit www.Acne-Statin.com.

Acne Treatment Cream *($24.95 for 4 ounces)* contains 0.5% salicylic acid (BHA) and preservatives, but no other ingredients are disclosed. Salicylic acid is a good exfoliant but the amount in this product isn't much and the pH is too high for it to be all that effective.

Cleanser/Moisturizer Lotion *($33.30 for 8 ounces)* has no ingredients listed. It performs like a rinseable cold cream, which may be an option for someone with normal to dry sensitive skin, but without a list of ingredients there is no way to know what you are really putting on your skin.

Sopstitute *($19.95 for 4 ounces)* the only ingredients listed are triclosan 0.5% and the product's preservatives. Triclosan is a good antibacterial agent used in many products, from oral hygiene to cleansers (Source: *Federation of European Microbiological Societies Microbiology Letter*, August 2001, pages 1–7). However, whether or not triclosan is effective for acne has not been researched.

Sun Statin SPF 16 *($19.95 for 4 ounces)* appears to be a very good sunscreen using titanium dioxide as the only active ingredient. This can feel heavy and occlusive (meaning it may cause breakouts) for someone with oily, blemish-prone skin.

ADRIEN ARPEL'S SIGNATURE CLUB A
(AVAILABLE ON HSN.COM ONLY)

Adrien Arpel's once successful department-store line has few locations left, yet the right for Arpel to use her name in any publicity or marketing ventures is owned by the original company with which she hasn't had any affiliation for years. After Arpel left her original line behind she started selling a new line of cosmetics on the Home Shopping Network (HSN), but she could not legally use her own name for endorsement purposes, hence her HSN line is called "Signature Club A by Adrien Arpel." It is interesting to note that whenever Arpel is on HSN, she is never introduced as "Adrien Arpel"; she is always introduced as just "Adrien." These days, the original Arpel line is sold primarily via mail order and in a handful of department stores in Canada and the United States.

Like most infomercial lines, Arpel promises that her Signature Club A by Adrien Arpel products will cure your skin-care woes, especially by erasing wrinkles. Arpel sells her products as miracles that deliver newly smooth, flawless skin with instant success. But there are no miracles to be found in this line. There are problems with many of the formulations, ranging from packaging that ensures active ingredients will not be active to an abundance of irritating ingredients.

Arpel also promotes the effectiveness of her Big "7" Wondercover Compact as being the only skin-perfecting makeup you need. It isn't, but what a sales pitch this greasy group of colors gets. For more information about Signature Club A, call (800) 933-2887 or visit www.hsn.com.

SIGNATURE CLUB A SKIN CARE

☺ $$$ **French Vanilla Meltdown, Cleansing Creme for Face & Eyes** *($18 for 4.5 ounces)* is just a wipe-off, cold cream–type cleanser with a tiny amount of vitamin A thrown in for effect. Even if the vitamin could help, you would be wiping it away before it had a chance to work. This can be an option for someone with dry skin, but it is easily replaced with far less expensive options. It does contain fragrance.

☹ **High-Potency Lemon Zest Meltdown Cleansing Creme for Face & Eyes** *($18 for 4.5 ounces)* is similar to the French Vanilla Meltdown above except that the lemon in this product is potentially irritating for the eyes and skin.

☺ **Alpha Hydroxy & Retinol Daily Face Wash** *($15.50 for 6 ounces)* is a standard, detergent-based, water-soluble cleanser that can be somewhat drying depending on your skin type. It has an assortment of AHAs and a minuscule amount of retinol, but the pH is too high for the AHA to be effective for exfoliation, and even if any of the ingredients were effective they would be rinsed off before they had a chance to have an effect. Plus, retinol is not stable in this kind of packaging. It does contain fragrance.

☹ **Daily Spa Toner with Caviar Extract** *($14 for 8 ounces)* contains alcohol and is too irritating and drying for all skin types.

☹ **Alpha Hydroxy & Retinol Oxygenating Tightening Toner** *($15.50 for 6 ounces)*. Between the salt and the mints that this product contains, the irritation for the face would be significant. What's even more absurd is that retinol is not stable in the presence of air, and so the oxygen in here (which is just hydrogen peroxide) makes this one self-defeating.

☹ **Alpha Hydroxy & Retinol Soft Resurfacing Peel** *($14.50 for 2 ounces)* contains mostly very thick, heavy waxes. Rubbing wax over the skin can take off skin cells, but it can also clog pores and cause breakouts. There are much better ways to exfoliate the skin than with this product. This kind of packaging also prevents retinol from being stable.

☺ **Alpha Hydroxy and Retinol Soft Scrub with Vanilla Bean** *($14.50 for 2 ounces)*. Another AHA product? But don't worry, the pH isn't right for the AHAs to be effective. This is a standard, water-soluble cleanser, and the scrub particles in it come from ground-up vanilla beans. This is an option for a topical scrub for someone with normal to dry skin.

☺ **The 5 Essentials Creme** *($24.95 for 4.5 ounces)* comes in a two-part container—Face Cream and Eye Cream—with one on top of the other. There is nothing essential about any of this. Without sunscreen, it leaves much to be desired for daytime use. The Face Cream is just a good moisturizer for dry skin, but it falls down on many aspects of the claims made about it. It's supposed to be an AHA product, but both the amount of AHA and the pH make it ineffective for exfoliation. It contains a small amount of retinol, but the packaging guarantees that the highly unstable retinol will decompose because the packaging is not airtight. It does have some good water-binding agents and emollients, but that's about it. The Eye Cream is almost identical, but for some impractical reason it contains several irritating plant extracts, including lemon, sage, lavender, and orange, which are probably there as fragrance additives.

☺ **$$$ Wrinkle Softening Stick with Vitamin C and Retinol** *($18 for 0.24 ounce)*. This lipstick-like moisturizer is greasy stuff and somewhat sticky, but it would work for dry skin. The pH and amount of AHA aren't right for it to be effective as an exfoliant. The vitamin C is OK, but the packaging allows the retinol to decompose because it isn't airtight.

☹ **High Potent-C Anti-Wrinkle Age Defying Capsules** *($26.50 for 0.5 ounce)* does contain vitamin C, but it uses ascorbic acid, which is not the most effective form (it is also considered to be irritating). The preferred form is magnesium ascorbyl palmitate. The product also contains some irritating ingredients that don't belong in a moisturizing-type product, including aluminum starch (octenylsuccinate) and ginseng extract.

☺ **$$$ Anti-Sag Extra-Firming Cream Duo with Caviar** *($28.50 for 2 ounces of Eye Gel and 2 ounces of Eye Creme)*. The Eye Gel is a good lightweight moisturizer, but there is nothing in this product that will live up to the anti-sagging claims. Without sunscreen, this product should not be used for daytime. The Eye Creme part is a good emollient moisturizer for dry skin but that's about it. Both products contain minuscule amounts of caviar, and while some fish eggs may be great to eat, none have any anti-sagging or firming benefit for skin.

☺ **Flower Acid Wrinkle Remedy Night Face Creme** *($23.50 for 2 ounces)* is a good moisturizer for dry skin, but there is no "flower acid" of any kind in here and there are no flower acids that can have any impact on skin.

☺ **Flower Acid Wrinkle Remedy Night Eye Ointment** *($15.50 for 0.75 ounce)* has a name that's far more exotic than this very standard, very thick, balm-style moisturizer for very dry skin could ever live up to.

☺ **Flower Acid Wrinkle Remedy Day Eye Creme** *($15.50 for 1 ounce)* is similar to the Night Face Creme above and the same basic comments apply.

☺ **Flower Acid Wrinkle Remedy Day Face Creme with Sunscreen SPF 20** *($15.50 for 2 ounces)* is a good in-part avobenzone-based sunscreen in a very standard moisturizing base.

SIGNATURE CLUB A MAKEUP

☹ **The Big "7" Wondercover Wheel** *($23.50)* is a group of seven concealers in colors that range from blue to mauve, peach, shiny beige, medium beige, and dark tan. This is a greasy mess that may be OK for very dry skin. Even so, if you place it around the eyes or other lined areas of the face it will easily crease and it tends to feel opaque and slippery on the skin. Mauve, peach, and blue only give the skin a strange cast. To cover face problems, all it takes is one concealer and one good foundation that doesn't crease.

☹ **Hide-A-Line Putty** *($19.50)* won't hide anything because no one's skin color looks like this shade of peach, and the greasy consistency will make it crease into lines and make them more noticeable.

☺ **$$$ Mistake Proof Blush** *($22.50)* is a mix of small, multicolored powder beads. It produces a slightly rose tone on the cheek. This one-color-fits-all concept doesn't work any better than one-size-fits-all clothes. If this isn't your color, it's a mistake. It has a silky application with some amount of shine.

AESOP (SKIN CARE ONLY)

Aesop is an Australian-bred line whose name is taken from the legendary Greek fabulist. The company espouses "modern survival of intelligent life forms" along with "morality and integrity in business." But most of all they are serious about plants. Their literature goes into great detail about why and how they use plants in their products in a way that most other so-called natural companies do not even attempt. If anything, Aesop is strangely forthcoming in its approach to using plant-based ingredients, be they essential oils or other plant components.

Aesop cautions pregnant women about using essential oils; provides detailed information about how their plant-based ingredients are harvested, selected, and processed; and even recommends patch-testing and sampling before purchasing a product. I agree that patch-testing is a sensible idea, particularly when it comes to volatile plant extracts— but remember, skin does not always tell us when it is being irritated. If you patch-test a product with potentially irritating plant extracts (and most of Aesop's products contain them), your skin may or may not visibly react—but the irritation these ingredients can cause may still be silently taking place.

In addition to Aesop's passionate belief in the goodness of plants, they are not shy about letting consumers know they are opposed to a host of other travesties, from animal testing and using petrolatum or mineral oil to the horrors of female genital mutilation (FGM) in Africa. Their principles and philosophies are certainly admirable, but before too long it makes you wonder if all of this politically correct posturing is meant to distract you from the fact that their products are quite ordinary and assuredly overpriced for what you get. Plus, almost every Aesop product contains fragrant plant oils, and despite the (mostly anecdotal) claims, these are nothing more than fragrance, and that's a problem for the skin.

Perhaps the most bewildering, inexplicable part of Aesop's skin-care advice is their up-front admission that daily sun protection is essential (particularly in Australia, the country with the highest incidence of skin cancer in the world), while a sunscreen is noticeably absent from their product lineup. They instead maintain that the only products they "prescribe" for the skin are cleanser, hydrating cream, and one "facial preparation," depending on the skin's needs and condition. Talk about contradictory! To make matters even more maddening, they justify the current lack of sunscreen by claiming their moisturizers "have an inherent SPF of 7," something that is absolutely not true. SPF is not something a product can have "inherently," either it has active sunscreen ingredients and has met FDA testing guidelines or it hasn't (Source: www.fda.gov).

When it comes to formulating sunscreens from available active ingredients, Aesop states that "we have not been able to satisfy ourselves that the data on currently available SPF ingredients does substantiate the claims of protection being made." Unbelievable! A quick search on Medline (National Library of Medicine, http://www.ncbi.nlm.nih.gov/entrez/query.fcgi) for sunscreen brings up over 3,000 studies from a vast array of professional, peer-reviewed journals. What more could they possibly want? This is a skin-care line whose irony and fiction make for interesting reading, similar to that of any fable, but that offers little help for your skin. For more information on Aesop, call (888) 223-2750 or visit www.aesop.net.au. **Note:** All of Aesop's products contain fragrance unless noted otherwise.

☺ **$$$ Amazing Face Cleanser** *($35 for 6.9 ounces)* is just a very standard, water-soluble cleanser. The "pure Australian water" in it sounds nice (although neither your skin nor the product care where the water came from), and it uses sodium laureth-3-sulfate and cocoamidopropyl betaine as the main cleansing agents. It also contains sea salt (sodium chloride), which gives it a slightly gritty feel, as well as fragrant plant oils, which, like all fragrant components, can be irritating. This can be an option as a light scrub for someone with normal to oily skin, but the only thing amazing about it is the name.

☺ **$$$ Fabulous Face Cleanser** *($35 for 6.9 ounces)* is a very good, though very basic, water-soluble cleanser using ammonium laureth sulfate as the main cleansing agent. Unfortunately, it also contains a good deal of fragrant plant extracts, which can be problematic for skin.

☺ $$$ **Purifying Facial Cream Cleanser** (*$35 for 6.9 ounces*) is a fairly gentle water-soluble cleanser that has plant oils along with detergent cleansing agents. It would be an OK option for someone with normal to dry skin. It also contains fragrant plant extracts, which can be problematic for most skin types.

☹ $$$ **Tea Tree Leaf Facial Exfoliant** (*$55 for 2.82 ounces*) is a curious mixture of walnut shell powder, clay, tea tree leaf powder, detergent cleansing agent, aloe, and grape seed extract. It's an option for a topical scrub, but walnut shells are rarely as smooth as synthetic scrub particles, so it can be rather abrasive on the skin. The tiny amount of "leaf powder" and "leaf particles" in this product have no known benefit for skin. This is not preferred to other far less expensive scrubs such as Aveeno Skin Brightening Scrub.

☹ **Facial Calming Shower** (*$25 for 3.53 ounces*) is an incredibly basic toner that contains sugarcane alcohol as the third ingredient (this amount of alcohol is problematic for skin) as well as small amounts of lavender, peppermint, and neroli extracts, and together that's enough to make this too irritating for most skin types.

☹ **Immediate Moisture Facial Hydrosol** (*$25 for 3.53 ounces*) is almost identical to the Facial Calming Shower above except this one uses rose and bergamot instead of lavender and peppermint. Nothing about this is immediate except potential irritation.

☺ $$$ **Oil Free Hydrating Mist** (*$37.50 for 3.35 ounces*) is alcohol-free and much gentler than the other Aesop toners, although this does contain a small amount of ylang-ylang, which smells great but has little benefit for skin. Other than that, the aloe, water-binding agent, glycerin, and anti-irritants make this a decent toner for normal to dry skin.

☹ $$$ **Camellia Nut Facial Hydrating Cream** (*$45 for 4 ounces*) is a richly emollient moisturizer for dry to very dry skin. It contains mostly plant oils, carrot juice, vitamin E, carrot oil, and fragrant plant oil. Orange flower and violet oils can be irritating and serve no purpose in these amounts other than to make the product smell appealing. The major concern is the lack of preservatives. Combining this many plant and food ingredients without preservatives means the product will not last for long before it becomes rancid. And at 4 ounces, it's likely going to be several months before you're done using this facial product (though it can certainly be used on any areas of dry skin). Aesop recommends storing this in the refrigerator immediately after opening, and I concur, but even with that it won't last more than a week or two before becoming spoiled.

☹ $$$ **Damascan Rose Facial Treatment** (*$60 for 0.88 ounce*) is an absurdly expensive mixture of plant, fruit, and vegetable oils, along with vitamin E and potentially irritating fragrant plant oils. This is recommended as an intensive hydrating treatment, but for the money you would be better off purchasing a combination of these oils (such as evening primrose and rose-hip oils) and making your own plant oil–based dry-skin treatment without the fragrance.

☹ $$$ **Fabulous Face Oil** (*$40 for 0.88 ounce*) is less expensive than the Damascan

Rose Facial Treatment above but would work just as well over dry skin. This contains mostly nut oils, plant oils, juniper oil (an irritant), vitamin E, and fragrant plant oil. Save your money by using plain olive, apricot kernel, or evening primrose oil instead.

☺ $$$ **Mandarin Facial Hydrating Cream** (*$45 for 4 ounces*) is a standard, but good, moisturizer for normal to slightly dry and dry skin that would be a better choice if it did not contain the irritants lemon peel oil, orange peel oil, and verbena extract. It lacks any state-of-the-art water-binding agents, antioxidants, or anti-irritants, making it much less interesting than many far less expensive moisturizers.

☺ $$$ **Primrose Facial Hydrating Cream** (*$45 for 4 ounces*) is similar to the Mandarin Facial Hydrating Cream above, though this one is slightly more emollient and contains a smaller amount of fragrant plant oils, using only tiny amounts of lavender, rosemary, and sage oils in place of the citrus peel oils. It's an OK option for normal to very dry skin, but it lacks any state-of-the-art water-binding agents, antioxidants, or anti-irritants, and that makes it much less interesting than many far less expensive moisturizers.

☹ **Chamomile Concentrate Anti-Blemish Masque** (*$40 for 1.8 ounces*) comes with an insulting price once you realize this is nothing more than water, clay, alcohol, more clay, plant oils, and irritating plant extracts. This will not help blemishes, but will dry out the skin and cause unnecessary irritation.

☹ **Primrose Face Cleansing Masque** (*$35 for 1.8 ounces*) is "recommended for deep cleansing of oily, combination, or open pores skin types," but is a rather confused product that contains a blend of clays, alcohol, slip agent, plant oils, preservative, and irritants like geranium and sage oils. This is bound to cause more problems for skin than it could ever hope to solve, and is easy to pass up.

☹ **Rosehip Seed Lip Treatment** (*$15 for 1.13 ounces*) is an ultra-pricey lip balm that feels smooth and light on the lips, but tends to dissipate quickly, meaning you'll be reapplying this frequently. If that's not enough of a deterrent, this also contains irritating tangerine and lavender oils, which are not what dry, chapped lips need.

☹ **Tuberose Lip Heal** (*$30 for 0.35 ounce*) is even more costly than the Rosehip Seed Lip Treatment above, and is simply a blend of plant oils and fragrant plant oils. To avoid unnecessary irritation, you can skip the tuberose and jasmine here and moisturize lips with wheat germ or almond oil that you could buy quarts of for far less at your local health food store.

AHAVA (SKIN CARE ONLY)

Ahava is the Hebrew word for love and also the name for this group of skin-care products imported from Israel. Other than the endearing title, the gimmick here is that Ahava products contain salts and minerals from the Dead Sea in Israel. So is your skin going to love these products containing Dead Sea water? Supposedly Cleopatra did, and of course she must have been a skin-care enthusiast or Mark Anthony wouldn't have risked everything for her. Isn't that a good enough reason to consider these for your skin-care routine? I hope not. Aside from the folklore, there is little truth behind the hype.

The Dead Sea in Israel is considered dead because nothing can live in it. Many environmental factors have contributed to making the Dead Sea one of the saltiest lakes in the world. Seawater from the Atlantic and Pacific Oceans has a 3% to 4% salt content; the Dead Sea has a 32% salt content, as well as a large concentration of minerals such as sulfur, magnesium, calcium, bromide, and potassium. If you haven't been to the Dead Sea, I can tell you that the aroma from the sulfur water is overwhelming. It is hard to imagine that anything so noxious would be considered a beauty treatment.

There are no clinical studies or research showing that Dead Sea minerals have any effect on wrinkles or acne. There are, however, several studies demonstrating that these minerals can have a positive effect on psoriatic skin (Sources: *Israel Journal of Medical Sciences*, November 2001, pages 828–832; *British Journal of Dermatology*, June 2001, pages 1154–1160; *International Journal of Dermatology*, February 2001, pages 158–159; and *Journal of the American Academy of Dermatology*, August 2000, pages 325–326). Psoriasis is a skin condition characterized by rapidly dividing, overactive skin cells. No one is quite sure how the Dead Sea minerals and salts affect psoriasis. One of the more popular theories regarding its benefit is that the mineral content of the water slows down the out-of-control cell division. Some of the research indicates that the benefit is cumulative and the results can last for up to five months.

It is important to point out that the benefits derived from Dead Sea minerals go beyond those that show up in cosmetics. Studies done by the Department of Medicine and Department of Epidemiology and Dermatology at the Soroka Medical Center of Kupat-Holim in Israel and Ben-Gurion University of the Negev found that "improvement [in skin] was found when patients soaked in two pounds (one kilo) for three baths per week, for a period of six weeks." That's a lot of Dead Sea water. If you are looking for Dead Sea water to heal wrinkles, which are completely unrelated to skin rashes, you're better off saving your money. Even if Dead Sea salts could benefit normal skin in some way, the amounts found in the Ahava products and other Dead Sea–oriented lines are infinitesimally small in comparison with the amounts used in the published studies.

Is there anything else in these products worth considering? Ahava products are about as standard and boring as they come. For more information about Ahava, call (800) 252-4282 or visit www.ahava.com. **Note:** All Ahava products contain fragrance unless otherwise noted.

☺ **$$$ Advanced Cleansing Milk for Normal to Dry Skin** *($24 for 8.5 ounces)* is just an overpriced cold cream–style cleanser. It can be an option for someone with dry skin but there are many far less expensive versions that would work as well if not better.

☹ **$$$ Advanced Facial Cleansing Milk for Oily Skin** *($24 for 8.5 ounces)* contains several emollient ingredients that would be a problem for someone with oily or combination skin. It also contains several potentially irritating ingredients that are a problem for all skin types, including nettle, balm mint, and coltsfoot. It also contains fragrance.

☺ **$$$ Advanced Gentle Mud Exfoliator for All Skin Types** *($24 for 3.4 ounces)* is a standard, detergent-based cleanser that uses synthetic scrub particles to exfoliate skin. This could work for someone with normal to dry skin. The emollients in this product make it inappropriate for someone with oily skin.

☹ **Dead Sea Mineral Glycerin Soap for Dry and Sensitive Skin** *($6 for 100 grams)* contains several problematic ingredients that could cause irritation or a sensitizing reaction, including cornstarch, sodium lauryl sulfate, and fragrance. None of these are good for any skin type.

☹ **Dead Sea Mineral Mud Soap for Oily and Problematic Skin** *($6 for 100 grams)* is almost identical to the Dry and Sensitive Skin version above and the same comments apply.

☹ **Dead Sea Mineral Salt Soap for All Skin Types** *($6 for 100 grams)* is almost identical to the Dry and Sensitive Skin version above and the same comments apply.

☺ **$$$ Deep Cleanser for All Skin Types** *($20 for 3.4 ounces)* is a standard, detergent-based cleanser that would work well for someone with normal to dry or combination skin; the plant oil in this product could be a problem for someone with oily skin. The claim that this is hypoallergenic has no substantiation, although this is one of the few products in the line that doesn't contain fragrance, something that all skin types can benefit from.

☺ **Eye Makeup Remover** *($18 for 6.8 ounces)* is an extremely standard, but good, detergent-based eye-makeup remover. It would work as well as any.

☹ **Advanced Facial Toner for Normal to Dry Skin** *($21 for 8.5 ounces)* is more a problem for what it doesn't contain. This toner has no water-binding agents, anti-irritants, antioxidants, or any single ingredient that can be helpful for skin. Not only isn't this advanced; it wasn't even advanced 20 years ago.

☹ **Advanced Facial Toner for Oily Skin** *($21 for 8 ounces)* is virtually identical to the Toner for Normal to Dry Skin above, except this one adds alcohol as the second ingredient, making it damaging to skin.

☺ **$$$ Advanced Eye and Neck Cream** *($40 for 1 ounce)* contains mostly water, thickeners, slip agent, water-binding agent, preservatives, silicone, vitamin E, vitamin A, more preservatives, and plant oil. Most of the good ingredients are listed well after the preservative, making this product far from advanced.

☺ **$$$ Advanced Mineral Beauty Serum for Very Dry Skin** *($60 for 1 ounce)* contains plant extracts such as sugarcane and sugar maple extract. These do not function in any way like alpha hydroxy acids do. This carob gum–based moisturizer offers little benefit for skin. It lacks antioxidants, water-binding agents, and anti-irritants. It does contain fragrance.

☺ **$$$ Advanced Moisturizer for Normal to Dry Skin** *($28 for 2.5 ounces)* is an OK moisturizer, but your skin deserves better than just OK.

☹ **Advanced Moisturizer for Oily Skin** *($28 for 2.5 ounces)* contains several problematic ingredients for any skin type, including nettle, balm mint, coltsfoot, and sage.

☺ $$$ **Advanced Moisturizer for Very Dry Skin** *($42 for 1.7 ounces)* is almost identical to the Moisturizer for Normal to Dry Skin above and the same comments apply.

☺ $$$ **Advanced Night Replenisher** *($48 for 1.7 ounces)* contains mostly water, thickeners, glycerin, emollient, antioxidants, anti-irritants, silicone, slip agents, preservatives, and fragrance. This would be a very good moisturizer for someone with normal to dry skin.

☹ $$$ **Advanced Nourishing Cream for Normal to Dry Skin** *($40 for 1.7 ounces)* won't nourish anyone's skin. It lacks many elements that would be helpful for skin. It is basically just water, thickeners, plant oil, a teeny amount of vitamin E, preservatives, and fragrance.

☹ $$$ **Advanced Mineral Beauty Masque for Very Dry Skin** *($35 for 3.4 ounces)* is basically just a mud mask with some emollients. It does contain a tiny amount of antioxidants and anti-irritant, which can be helpful for skin.

☹ $$$ **Advanced Mud Masque for Normal to Dry Skin** *($28 for 4.2 ounces)* is just a mud and clay mask. The pH of this mask isn't suitable to allow the salicylic acid to be effective as an exfoliant. For someone with very oily skin this may be helpful, but for someone with dry skin this would be an overly drying experience.

☺ $$$ **Advanced Mud Masque for Normal to Oily Skin** *($28 for 4.2 ounces)* is almost identical to the Masque for Normal to Dry Skin above and the same comments apply.

AHAVA TIME LINE

☹ $$$ **Age Defying 3D Essence Ampoules** *($80 for 30 vials)* arrives in packaging that is far more impressive than what you will find inside the capsules. They contain water, silicones, plant extracts, glycerin, more silicone, more plant extracts, and slip agents. Silicones feel good on skin, but the other ingredients aren't at all unusual, much less age-defying. The plant extracts are a mix of anti-irritants and irritants, so they in essence negate each other.

☹ **Age Defying All Day Moisture, SPF 15** *($35 for 1.7 ounces)* does not list its active ingredients, which means it is not in compliance with FDA regulations. Without knowing what active ingredients you are putting on your skin there is no way to know if you are getting full UVA protection.

☹ $$$ **Age Defying All Night Nourishment** *($45 for 1.7 ounces)* has plant extracts that are a combination of irritants and anti-irritants, which end up canceling each other out. This could have been a very good moisturizer for dry skin, but the irritating plant extracts make it more a waste of money.

☹ $$$ **Age Defying Continual Eye Treat** *($45 for 0.5 ounce)* is a good, lightweight, silicone-based moisturizer that would work well for normal to dry skin. Nothing in this product makes it better for the eye area. It contains a small amount of anti-irritants and water-binding agents.

☺ **$$$ Age Defying Optimizer Serum** *($72 for 1 ounce)* isn't much of a serum. It contains some irritating plants extracts that get in the way of the anti-irritant ingredients. What a waste.

ALEXANDRA DE MARKOFF

Alexandra de Markoff has had its share of ownership problems during the past several years, having been bought and sold numerous times. Since the previous edition of this book (Fifth Edition, 2001), it has remained under the ownership of Irving Rice. All of the past leapfrogging and varying owners have caused a lack of direction that has hurt the line, and the number of stores carrying it has declined. Yet de Markoff still prides itself on the one aspect of the line that has remained relatively constant since its debut decades ago: foundations.

When Countess Isserlyn Liquid Makeup debuted in 1926, it became an immediate hit for the Hollywood makeup artists who tended to the brightest movie stars of the day. The original Liquid Makeup was smooth, fluid, easy to apply, and richly pigmented— a far cry from the thick, greasy, or overly powdered pancake-style makeup that covered beautifully, but could cause problems for skin. Although the Countess Isserlyn product was an innovative product back in the late 1920s and into the 1930s, by today's standards it is way behind the times, and yet seemingly unwilling to play catch-up, especially when it comes to the shades, which are some of the poorest around. The de Markoff makeup is still around, ostensibly to cater to its steadfastly loyal older clientele. The foundations are undeniably rich, and that's great for dry skin—but the majority of the makeup offers textures and colors that have truly limited appeal and often outlandish prices. That may convey affluence and superiority in much the same way as Chanel or Dior, but these de Markoff products don't fulfill that illusion in reality. At least when you decide to pay top dollar at Chanel, you can be fairly confident you're getting a modern, workable product.

However, as was true in the previous edition of this book, there isn't much that's new here. There are no AHA or BHA products, and none of the sunscreens offer reliable UVA protection. In general, this line has limited appeal and, for the money, is relatively unimpressive. For more information about Alexandra de Markoff, call (800) 366-7470 or visit www.canyoncosmetics.com. **Note:** All Alexandra de Markoff products contain fragrance unless otherwise noted.

ALEXANDRA DE MARKOFF SKIN CARE

☺ **$$$ Balancing Cleanser** *($30 for 6 ounces)* is a mineral oil–based cleanser that also contains detergent cleansing agent, thickeners, and a group of fragrant oils. It may leave skin feeling greasy but it is an option for dry skin.

☺ **$$$ Comfort Cleanser with Rosemary and Mallow** *($42 for 4 ounces)* is a standard, mineral oil–based, wipe-off cleanser. This is a lot of money for mineral oil and standard thickening agents, though it is an option for dry to very dry skin. The cleanser also contains some good water-binding agents and antioxidants, but they would be wiped away before they had a chance to have benefit for skin.

☹ $$$ **Complete Foaming Cleanser with Ivy and Birch** *($30 for 6 ounces)* is a standard, detergent-based, water-soluble cleanser. Several of the cleansing agents are fairly drying and irritating, which makes this cleanser more of a problem than most of its kind. There are several fragrant oils in here, including clove oil and galbanum, which can be skin sensitizers.

☹ $$$ **Luxury Cream Cleanser with Aloe and Rosewater** *($40 for 6 ounces)* is a standard, cold cream–style, wipe-off cleanser. It does contain some good water-binding agents and antioxidants, but they would be wiped away before they had a chance to have benefit for skin.

☹ **Luxury Facial Cleansing Bar** *($20 for 4 ounces)* is a very overpriced, standard bar cleanser. The ingredients that keep bar cleansers in their solid form can clog pores and the cleansing agents can be drying for most skin types.

☹ **Moisturizing Face and Body Bar** *($15 for 4 ounces)* is a very overpriced, standard bar cleanser. Dove would work just as well as this one.

☺ **Gentle Eye Makeup Remover** *($18 for 4 ounces)* is a standard, detergent-based eye-makeup remover. It would work as well as any, though in its favor this one doesn't contain coloring agents or fragrance.

☺ $$$ **Professional Secrets Makeup Solvent** *($42 for 2 ounces)*. There is nothing secret in this product—it is just a standard, detergent-based eye-makeup remover, and I mean really standard, identical to almost everyone of its kind in this book. However, it won't be as gentle on the eyes as the Gentle Eye Makeup Remover above because this one contains fragrant plant extracts and coloring agents.

☹ **Fresh Solution Toner** *($28 for 7.5 ounces)* contains mostly water, slip agent, calamine, clay, witch hazel, plant extracts, water-binding agents, mineral salts, fragrant plant oils, and preservatives. This is a lot of money for what is essentially calamine lotion with a lot of fragrance. Calamine is zinc carbonate, which is considered a counter-irritant, but the purpose of a counter-irritant *is* to cause irritation.

☺ $$$ **Luxury Skin Toner** *($28 for 6 ounces)* is a very good, irritant-free toner with a handful of good water-binding agents and plant extracts that can be anti-irritants (a few of the plant extracts can be irritants, too, but these probably don't make up a significant portion of the content). It also contains coloring agents.

☺ $$$ **Advanced Daily Nourisher** *($75 for 2 ounces)* contains mostly water, plant extract, slip agents, thickeners, water-binding agents, plant oil, antioxidants, silicones, more slip agents, and preservatives. This would be a very good moisturizer for normal to dry skin.

☹ **Comfort Eye Gel** *($35 for 3 ounces)* is a lightweight gel that contains a poor mixture of plant extracts that are primarily skin irritants, including bergamot, lemon, and ginseng.

☺ **$$$ Compensation Skin Serum** *($68.50 for 2 ounces)* is a good, lightweight, silicone-based moisturizer for someone with normal to dry skin. It does contain antioxidants and some good water-binding agents, but the almost $70 price tag just doesn't make sense for what you get.

☹ **Countess Isserlyn Moisture 364 1/2, with SPF 15** (also **Mauve** and **Aqua**) *($47.50 for 1.8 ounces)*, in all versions, does not contain titanium dioxide, zinc oxide, or avobenzone for UVA protection, and is not recommended.

☹ **Vital 10 New Age Skin Complex SPF 6** *($68.50 for 2 ounces)* isn't vital, it's pointless. SPF 6 isn't adequate to protect the skin from sun, and it doesn't contain titanium dioxide, zinc oxide, or avobenzone for UVA protection.

☹ **Moisture Reserve Cream SPF 8** *($57.50 for 2.25 ounces)* does not contain titanium dioxide, zinc oxide, or avobenzone for UVA protection, and the SPF 8 is an unreliable number even for a full day of UVB sun-damage protection.

☹ **$$$ Daytime Moisturizer** *($47.50 for 4 ounces)* contains water, glycerin, alcohol, lanolin, fragrance, and coloring agents. This is an embarrassing formulation for any company to be selling at any price.

☹ **$$$ Fresh Moisture Lotion** *($50 for 4 ounces)* is an OK lightweight moisturizer for someone with normal to slightly dry skin. It contains a small quantity of antioxidants, but there are several fragrant oils in this product that can be a problem for skin.

☹ **Oil-Free Matte Moisture** *($40 for 4 ounces)* is a confused product. The second ingredient is talc, which can absorb oil, but the emollient thickening agents can be a problem for oily skin. A pressed powder would do a better job than this unnecessary product.

☺ **$$$ Skin Tight Firming Eye Cream** *($52.50 for 0.35 ounce)* won't firm skin, but it is very emollient—good for someone with dry skin. It does contain some good antioxidants and water-binding agents. The tiny amount of retinol in this product is easily replaced with far less expensive versions at the drugstore.

☹ **$$$ Sleep Tight Firming Night Cream** *($70 for 2.25 ounces)* is a good moisturizer for dry skin with several good water-binding agents, anti-irritants, and antioxidants. Unfortunately, it also has a long list of fragrant plant oils, of which several are strong potential skin sensitizers.

☹ **$$$ Subdual Spot Lightening Cream** *($45 for 2 ounces)* does contain bearberry and mitracarpe extracts that contain arbutin, a substance known for its skin-lightening properties. However, the amount of bearberry and mitracarpe is minuscule and not enough to have any impact on skin color.

☹ **$$$ Throat & Decolletage Cream** *($45 for 2 ounces)* contains nothing that makes it unique or special for the neck or throat area. It is a silicone-based moisturizer that contains some good water-binding agents, antioxidants, and anti-irritants, but it also contains several plant extracts that can be irritating for skin, including lime, clove oil, and jasmine.

☹ **Weekly Revitalizing Clay Mask, with Green Tea and Sage** *($32 for 2 ounces)* is a fairly standard clay mask that contains peppermint, which can be a skin irritant.

☺ $$$ Weekly Revitalizing Exfoliating Mask, with Pineapple and Papaya *($32 for 2 ounces)*. The plant extracts in this product are supposed to sound like they are related to AHAs and enzymes. They aren't, although they can be skin irritants.

☹ Weekly Revitalizing Moisture Mask, with Jasmine and Avocado *($32 for 2 ounces)* contains talc and mica, which aren't moisturizing in the least, as well as some irritating plant oils, including menthol, clove, and rose oil.

☹ Extra Help Gel for Lips *($22 for 1 ounce)* offers minimal help for dry lips. It has almost no emollients or skin-softening ingredients. It can put a film over the lips to make them look smooth temporarily, but it won't feel very good, particularly in the winter.

☹ Lip Conditioner Plus SPF 15 *($20 for 0.14 ounce)* doesn't contain the UVA-protecting ingredients of titanium dioxide, zinc oxide, or avobenzone, and is not recommended.

ALEXANDRA DE MARKOFF MAKEUP

FOUNDATION: There are a lot of poor shades to wade through here, with nothing suitable for darker skin tones. Thankfully, they are nicely organized on a revolving tester unit and numbered according to the shade's undertone. The #70s are mostly pink, the #80s are supposedly neutral (but there are still colors to watch out for), and the #90s have a golden undertone, with the exception of numbers 94 to 97, which are extremely rose and do not resemble real skin in the least.

☺ $$$ Sheer Illusion Lightweight Foundation *($37)* has a great whipped, creamy texture that blends on superbly and dries to a natural finish. Coverage is relatively sheer, so this is best for near-flawless normal to dry skin. Of the four shades, Light and Medium are the only ones to consider. **Countess Isserlyn Creme Makeup** *($47.50)* is an exceptionally thick, emollient foundation that is suitable only for very dry skin and for those who prefer medium to full coverage and a moist, satin finish. It blends on better than you might expect, but is very moist and slightly greasy. Of the 11 shades, 6 of them, including 71½, 72½, 76½, 86½, 92½, and 96½, are too glaringly peach, pink, or rose for most skin tones. Colors to consider are 8½, 88½, 91½, and 98½.

☺ $$$ **Countess Isserlyn Matte Makeup** *($47.50)* is hardly passable as matte; it does not contain water and has only a slightly lighter texture than the Creme above because it has silicone instead of mineral oil in the base. The silicone adds a lighter feel, but this foundation is meant for oily skin, and most would assuredly reject this as being too greasy and slick. Normal to dry skin would fare better, and this offers light to medium coverage. This is also a dual-phase formula, and the same separation issue applies here as for the Liquid Makeup below. You'll find some neutral colors within the 12 shades, but consider avoiding 71½, 72½, 76½, 86½, 91½, 196½, and 198½.

☹ **Countess Isserlyn Liquid Makeup** *($47.50)* comes in 20 shades and is oil-based. The formula is dual-phase, meaning the oil and pigments are separate and the product must be shaken vigorously to blend the two parts. Expect this separation to eventually translate onto the skin and cause streaking. Even though this can blend on smoothly and provides light to medium coverage, it leaves a slick, moist finish appropriate only for very dry skin. The following shades are undeniably too peach or rose for all skin tones: 71½, 72½, 76½, 86½, 88½, 89½, 91½, 94½, 95, 96, 96½, 97, and 97½.

☹ <u>CONCEALER:</u> **Disguise for Eyes** *($22)* comes in a tube with a wand applicator and has a rather greasy, silicone-based opaque texture that will surely crease. Of the three shades, only Neutral is a noteworthy option. **Countess Isserlyn Concealer** *($19.50)* has a very smooth cream texture and a greasy finish that gravitates into any lines around the eye. The colors are inadequate, and make this a problem for most skin tones. **Fresh Eye Cream** *($50)* is a concealer/eye cream hybrid that hardly conceals anything and leaves an unattractive rose cast on the skin. As an eye-area moisturizer, the formula is not what I would call elegant.

☺ $$$ <u>POWDER:</u> **Countess Isserlyn Loose Powdermist** *($40)* has the same pleasingly soft, dry texture found in numerous other talc-based powders in all price ranges. This one does lend more of an imperceptible finish to the skin, but that still doesn't justify the price. If opulent packaging appeals to you, be aware that it's what you're paying for with this one. **Countess Isserlyn Pressed Powdermist** *($35)* is talc-free and has a bit more coverage than the Loose Powdermist. This does have an elegant texture, but so do many other pressed powders that are much less expensive. The three shades for both Loose and Pressed Powdermist are workable.

<u>BLUSH:</u> ☹ **Outlasting Moisturizing Powder Blush** *($31.50)* has a great, smooth texture but all of the rich, vibrant colors take shine to new heights and are not recommended unless your goal is to make your cheeks as shiny and clownish as possible.

☺ $$$ **Outlasting Cream Blush** *($31.50)* is a traditional cream blush, meaning it is indeed creamy, with a dewy, moist, and sheer finish. The nine shades are fine, though a few are quite bold for blush— it's the price tag that's hard to applaud.

☹ <u>EYESHADOW:</u> **Disguise for Eyes Eyelid Foundation** *($27)* is nothing more than a semi-opaque, pale-pink liquid that claims to solve every eyeshadow pitfall. It just puts another layer on the eyelid that isn't necessary. The pitfall these eyeshadows try to make up for is de Markoff's greasy foundations, but that is better solved with a dusting of powder and not a concealer. If concealing were the objective, then a good concealer, which this line doesn't have, would be better. **Eye Defining Shadows** *($20)* are sold as single eyeshadows and almost every one of them is ultra-shiny, in colors that are makeup mistakes waiting to happen. The texture and application are acceptable, but not enough to redeem the negative points, especially for an older clientele.

<u>EYE AND BROW SHAPER:</u> ☹ **Eye Defining Pencil** *($18.50)* is a standard pencil with a princess-pleasing price that smears in no time. ☺ $$$ **Brow Defining Pencil** *($18.50)* is also standard and overpriced but does have a very nice, soft texture that applies easily and should stay put. There is a brow brush on the end to soften the line, and the seven available shades are very good for those who prefer brow pencil to powder. **Professional**

Secrets Liquid Eyeliner *($19)* has a good firm brush that is capable of drawing a thin line. The formula dries quickly and is quite tenacious. Caution: Heathered Taupe dries to an iridescent finish and Evergreen should be avoided if your goal is subtle sophistication.

LIPSTICK AND LIP PENCIL: ☺ $$$ Lasting Luxury Lipstick *($18.50)* makes the claim of having "unique liposomes that constantly release pigment and moisturizers." That's hard enough to swallow, but considering this lipstick's greasy texture, it's unlikely to stay on long enough for the liposomes to do much of anything anyway. Lip Defining Pencil *($18.50)* is a standard pencil with a creamy application and soft powder finish. Nothing exceptional, and not worth the imperious price tag.

☹ Undercolor for Lips *($26.50)* has a jaw-dropping price for what amounts to a sheer, silicone-based tint (a Clear version is also available) that smooths over the lips. This one claims to prevent lipstick from feathering and, unbelievably, that it will make any lipstick transfer-resistant—both of which it absolutely cannot do. It does help make lips smoother, but any longevity you experience will likely be coincidental!

MASCARA: ☺ $$$ Professional Secrets Mascara *($22)* builds decent length with a good amount of thickness and virtually no clumping, but for the money I wouldn't run out and make this my choice. There are far more impressive, less expensive mascaras available.

☹ Lash Amplifier *($22)* is clear mascara that is supposed to enhance the lashes, but it's no better than an extra coat of mascara. Besides, if the regular mascara is any good, why would it need an amplifier in the first place?

☺ BRUSHES: Brush Collection *($25)* seems value-priced, at least for a line like this. This nicely packaged set features an OK brush collection that may remind you of the brush sets of past "Free Gift with Purchase" promotions from Estee Lauder. They're serviceable, but not what I would call top-notch. The price is attractive, but high quality and craftsmanship are missing.

ALMAY

Almay has a long-standing reputation for being one of the few lines that is 100% hypoallergenic. Given that the FDA has never issued specific guidelines about which ingredients are likely to cause allergic reactions, this is an admirable marketing feat. Overall, with the launch of several new skin-care products, Almay has improved its product quality a thousandfold. There are some excellent cleansers, moisturizers, and sunscreens. This is definitely a line that has reinvented itself and for the better. For more information about Almay, call (800) 473-8566 or visit www.almay.com.

ALMAY SKIN CARE

☺ Dual Phase Eye Makeup Remover *($5.69 for 4 ounces)* is a very good silicone-based eye-makeup remover. It glides easily over the skin and leaves minimal to no greasy residue. It contains no coloring agents or fragrance.

☺ **Moisturizing Eye Makeup Remover Lotion** *($4.29 for 2 ounces)* is a standard, mineral oil–based makeup remover that works well to remove makeup but can leave a greasy film on the skin. As inexpensive as this is, plain mineral oil is even cheaper.

☺ **Moisturizing Eye Makeup Remover Pads** *($3.49 for 35 pads)* is identical to the Moisturizing Eye Makeup Remover Lotion, except that the pads are provided so you don't have to buy pads separately.

☺ **Moisturizing Gentle Gel Eye Makeup Remover** *($4.49 for 1.5 ounces)* is similar to the Moisturizing Eye Makeup Remover Lotion above only in gel form. The same basic comments apply.

☺ **Non-Oily Eye Makeup Remover Gel** *($4.49 for 1.5 ounces)* is a gentle, detergent-based eye-makeup remover that would work as well as any. This does not contain fragrance or coloring agents.

☺ **Non-Oily Eye Makeup Remover Lotion** *($4.29 for 2 ounces)* is similar to the Non-Oily Eye Makeup Remover Gel version above only in a liquid lotion form.

☺ **Non-Oily Eye Makeup Remover Pads** *($3.49 for 35 pads)* is identical to the Non-Oily Eye Makeup Remover Lotion above, except that the pads are provided so you don't have to buy pads separately.

ALMAY MILK PLUS SKIN-CARE LINE

Each one of the new Almay Milk Plus products has the following statement: "The Almay Hypoallergenic Standard: Fewer than 500 ingredients of the 9000 available for use in cosmetics meet Almay's performance standard. New ingredients are stringently tested before they may be included in Almay products." Almay's products may meet their standards but these are only Almay's standards and not exactly standards that would be developed using information published about problematic ingredients. For example, the Milk Plus products are not fragrance-free because they contain fragrant plant extracts (such as orange flower extract and clary extract) that can be sensitizing to some skin types. Several of the thickening agents used could be problematic for breakouts when used repeatedly by someone with blemish-prone skin. Perhaps the most confusing concept in regard to these products being hypoallergenic is the use of milk. Milk is not a benign ingredient for skin! If it is left on the skin it can be absorbed into the pore and encourage the production of bacteria, thus increasing the risk of breakouts.

☺ **Rinse-Off Facial Cream 2-in-1 Cleanser and Toner for Normal to Dry Skin** *($6.93 for 6.7 ounces)* is a standard, mineral oil–based, wipe-off cleanser that would work well enough for dry skin but can leave a greasy feel on normal to combination skin. There is nothing in this product that "tones" skin in the least. It does contain fragrance.

☺ **Foaming Facial Gel 2-in-1 Cleanser and Toner Normal to Oily Skin** *($6.93 for 6.7 ounces)* is a good, though standard, detergent-based cleanser for normal to oily skin and slightly dry skin. The teeny amount of witch hazel in it is probably not a problem for irritation or dryness, but because of the milk content this product must be rinsed off well to prevent the milk from being absorbed into the pore and stimulating growth of bacteria.

☺ **Nourishing Facial Lotion SPF 15 Normal to Oily Skin** *($10.93 for 4.2 ounces)* is a very good, avobenzone-based sunscreen that is best for normal to dry skin and not oily skin. The lotion contains mica, an ingredient that imparts a subtle shimmer on the skin. Milk left on the skin can stimulate bacteria growth. The pH of this product is 7, making the BHA (salicylic acid) ineffective as an exfoliant.

☺ **Nourishing Facial Cream SPF 15 Normal to Dry Skin** *($10.93 for 2 ounces)* is almost identical to the Nourishing Facial Lotion SPF 15 above only in cream form. The same basic comments apply.

☺ **Illuminating Eye Cream** *($10.93 for 0.5 ounce)* is a very good moisturizer for normal to dry skin. The only thing "illuminating" about this moisturizer is that it contains a good amount of titanium dioxide, which adds a slight whitening effect around the eye. This does contain fragrant plant extracts.

☺ **Skin Renewing Night Cream** *($10.93 for 2 ounces)* is a basic moisturizer, and although it contains BHA (salicylic acid), the pH of 6 makes it ineffective for exfoliation. It is not as interesting a formulation as the Illuminating Eye Cream above, which has far more innovative water-binding agents and antioxidants. This does contain fragrant plant extracts.

ALMAY KINETIN SKIN CARE

There is a "new" answer for your skin, or at least that's what Almay and The Body Shop want you to believe. Both companies have launched lines of skin-care products containing the ingredient kinetin. (The Body Shop's Skin ReLeaf products are reviewed in this book.) Almay wants you to believe kinetin will "rejuvenate" your skin, and The Body Shop, which has been eschewing claims about antiaging, is promoting their kinetin products as being about overall skin health. Either way, you probably want to know if this heavily hyped ingredient is worth your attention.

Originally, kinetin was launched in a product called Kinerase ($77 for 1.8 ounces), as well as in a product from Osmotics called Kinetin Cellular Renewal Serum ($78 for 1.7 ounces). Ironically, The Body Shop and Almay now have their versions for a fraction of the price. None of these companies reveals how much kinetin is in their products, but given that no one knows if any amount of it has any effect on wrinkles, if you are curious about kinetin, the cheap products contain the exact same ingredient as the expensive products.

All in all, for skin, kinetin is no more worth your attention than any other hyped skin-care ingredient, such as vitamin A, beta glucan, and vitamin C to niacinamide, copper, coenzyme Q10, mushroom extracts, and on and on. Kinetin definitely has antioxidant properties but whether or not it can stop skin from aging has not been published or independently demonstrated. For more information about kinetin please refer to Chapter Seven, *Cosmetics Dictionary*, at the end of this book.

Please note: All of the following products contain some unknown amount of kinetin. For the purposes of the reviews, the comments on kinetin in Chapter Seven, *Cosmetics Dictionary*, pertain to each product. I will only comment on the value of the product aside from the kinetin content. Most of Almay's kinetin line of products contain several vitamins, water-binding agents, minerals, and willow bark. The vitamins and minerals are decent antioxidants. The willow bark in them is chemically (and distantly) related to salicylic acid (BHA), but the process of converting willow bark to salicylic acid requires the presence of enzymes, and these enzymes are not present in skin. The chances that willow bark in the tiny amount used in these products can mimic the effectiveness of salicylic acid are almost next to none. However, willow bark may indeed have some anti-inflammatory benefits for skin because, in this form, it appears to retain more of its aspirin-like composition.

☺ **Skin Optimizing Cleanser** *($8.50 for 5 ounces)* is a standard, detergent-based, water-soluble cleanser that can be an option for normal to oily skin. It also contains a great deal of fragrance. The vitamins and minerals are fine as antioxidants but in a cleanser they would just be rinsed away.

☺ **Age Decelerating Daily Lotion SPF 15** *($18 for 4 ounces)* is a very good avobenzone-based sunscreen. It would work as well as any, which makes the price a bit hard to swallow, at least from a drugstore perspective. It does contain a teeny amount of vitamins and mineral components that can be good antioxidants and water-binding agents. This would be an option for someone with normal to slightly dry or slightly oily skin. It does contain fragrance.

☺ **Age Decelerating Daily Cream SPF 15** *($18 for 1.6 ounces)* is similar to the Lotion above only in cream form, and the same basic comments apply. The price difference between the Lotion and Cream appears to be a marketing maneuver, but then that's true for most all cosmetic pricing. This one is slightly better for normal to dry skin.

☺ **Repair & Rejuvenate Night Concentrate** *($18 for 1.7 ounces)* contains mostly water, silicones, thickeners, Vaseline (petrolatum), water-binding agents, slip agent, willow bark (anti-inflammatory), vitamins, plant oil, mineral oil, minerals, fragrant plant extracts, and preservatives. This appears to be a very good moisturizer for someone with normal to dry skin.

☺ **Anti-Wrinkle Booster Serum** *($18 for 0.3 ounce)* is a very good silicone-based moisturizer for someone with normal to dry skin.

☺ **Rejuvenating Eye Treatment** *($18 for 0.5 ounce)* is similar to the Anti-Wrinkle Booster above and the same basic comments apply.

☺ **De-Aging Neck & Chest Treatment** *($18 for 3.75 ounces)*. Are we supposed to believe the neck and chest have different needs than the face? They don't, but it doesn't matter anyway because the ingredients in this product are similar to the other Almay kinetin products, so the differentiation appears to be about marketing, not formulations. Keep in mind that this product does not have sunscreen and would be a problem for daytime if your neck and chest were exposed to the sun.

☺ **Kinetin Firming and Pore Refining Serum** *($17.99 for 1.9 ounces)* is a light-weight lotion that contains just about everything but the kitchen sink. This product contains soybean protein, kinetin, vitamins, minerals, plant extracts (a mix of irritants and anti-irritants), which adds up to a very good moisturizer for normal to slightly dry skin. The witch hazel distillate in it, rather high up in the ingredient listing, contains a good deal of alcohol, which may be drying for some skin types.

ALMAY MAKEUP

Almay's makeup selection offers some wonderful choices when it comes to foundation, concealers, and mascaras. In fact, their foundations offer one of the most neutral palettes at the drugstore, and the best of them contain effective sunscreens. Although testers are usually scarce, some larger drugstores do sell mini-sizes of Almay's newer foundations and concealers—worth a try if you find choosing a shade without testers as frustrating as I do. The mascaras run the gamut from superb to sub-par, while the blushes and eyeshadows are quite sheer and most are too shiny for daytime wear. Almay also has a fine selection of eye pencils and liners, while their lipstick selection offers some satisfying choices, including two with effective sunscreens. Most of the makeup is fragrance-free, but watch out for the fragrant plant extracts that show up in some of the foundations.

<u>FOUNDATION:</u>☹ ☺ **Wake-Up Call! Energizing Makeup SPF 15** *($9.99)*. The two different faces in the rating are not there by mistake, but are representative of several strong positives about this foundation and a couple of negatives that I just don't know how to put together to sum up in a single rating. The name sounds like a spa for the skin, with its showcased ingredients of botanicals, minerals, and the ever-present vitamin C. None of the ingredients are present in an amount capable of having any real impact on skin. What this makeup ends up being is a really nice, smooth-finish, lightweight liquid foundation with an in-part titanium dioxide sunscreen (it's an 8% concentration, which is just great!). Application can be a bit tricky to get the hang of because this has a lot of slip and can blend on slightly streaky if you're not careful. But once you get used to it the coverage is light to medium, with a soft, slightly powdery finish suitable for normal to oily skin. The ten available colors are truly superior, with options for very light but not very dark skin—the only one to consider avoiding is Caramel, which may be too peach for some skin tones. The only drawback of note is the inclusion of alcohol as one of the first few ingredients and menthol further down on the list. I suspect the alcohol is present as a solvent, but it has a distinctive alcohol smell and I'm concerned that it can pose a risk of irritation or flaking in the long run, while the unnecessary inclusion of menthol is a disappointment. What a shame, because the final look, shade selection, and sunscreen are just so impressive.

✓☺ **Skin Smoothing Foundation with Kinetin SPF 15** *($11.99)* has an elegant, lightly creamy texture, applies and blends beautifully, and offers sheer-to-light coverage and a slightly moist finish. Making a good thing even better, the sunscreen is pure titanium dioxide and zinc oxide, and almost all of the nine shades are stellar. Warm is slightly pink, while Caramel is too orange for most deep skin tones. If not for the potential unknowns of the topical use of kinetin, this wonderful foundation would be wholeheartedly recommended. However, the minuscule amount of kinetin used in this makeup is not likely to raise any red flags, and this is definitely worth a test drive if you have normal to dry or sensitive skin.

☺ **Amazing Lasting Sheer Makeup SPF 12** *($10.38)* is definitely sheer—actually it's beyond sheer to almost nonexistent. The titanium dioxide–based sunscreen is fine and the application smooth and even. The appearance is so sheer it would be hard to make a mistake with this stuff, but the tradeoff is you don't get any meaningful coverage. If you want transparent coverage with a slightly sticky texture (similar to Revlon's ColorStay foundations), with a decent SPF (though SPF 15 would be the best) and no moisturizing feel whatsoever, this one is a great option, but that is definitely a narrow range of requirements. Most of the ten colors are superior, just watch out for Pale, Naked, and Warm. **One Coat Light and Easy Liquid Stick Makeup SPF 15** *($12.49)* is a great option for foundation in stick form. It has a smooth, creamy application and a sheer, light powder finish. Almay has wisely added a superb titanium dioxide and zinc oxide sunscreen, and that means this formerly sheer makeup offers coverage that is more substantial than the previous version. There are 12 shades, and though all have a slight peach hue, most of them are still worth considering for some skin tones. Warm, Honey, and Caramel are too peach for most skin tones, while Mocha and Espresso are great options for darker skin tones. The one major drawback is that you can't see the colors, and the swatch on the package is no help at all—it's an amazingly poor representation at best—so again, choosing is all guesswork. This also has a built-in sponge tip for blending—a clever idea that's actually more of a contrivance, as it is too tiny to really be effective for a smooth, even application. As is true for most stick foundations, this one is best for normal to slightly dry or slightly oily skin.

☺ **Clear Complexion Light and Perfect Compact Makeup SPF 8** *($10.89)* has a too-low SPF (despite containing 12% titanium dioxide), but is a good cream-to-powder makeup whose eight mostly peach, orange, or rose-toned colors are not up to the standards of Almay's other foundations. With no testers around, and with such suspect shades, you're even more likely to get the color wrong. Light to medium skin tones may wish to consider Cream Beige or True Beige, but only if you're willing to wear a sunscreen underneath for real sun protection. **Amazing Lasting Makeup SPF 6** *($10.38)* comes awfully close to being amazing, at least in terms of staying power and color selection, but the titanium dioxide–based SPF 6 is a very unamazing number. Other than that, the eight colors, though limited to light and medium skin tones (except for Warm and Tan), are wonderfully neutral. This provides a dry, unmovable, ultra-matte finish. If the SPF was bumped up to 10 or 12 (15 would be superb), I would give this one a much better rating, but as is, for someone with oily skin (and that's who this makeup is really the best for) it would require an additional sunscreen underneath, thus negating the ultra-matte finish. **Skin Stays Clean Compact Makeup** *($12.89)* is a cream-to-powder foundation that claims somewhat indirectly that it can prevent breakouts (the label doesn't state that clearly but it is indeed implied and most consumers will read it that way). First, wearing foundation isn't all that clean in and of itself, plus the thickening agents and wax in this product can potentially clog pores, which can cause breakouts. Although this contains salicylic acid, the pH is too high for it to be effective. Having said that, this does have a great, smooth application that dries to a soft matte finish. It is an option for normal to partly dry or partly oily skin, and the ten colors are quite nice, except that you cannot see them without breaking open the box, so you're left in the aisle alone to guess your shade. One caution: This product also contains menthol, but I suspect that the amount is so small it shouldn't be a problem for the skin. Consider avoiding Warm, Tan, and Caramel—all are too peach or rose for most skin tones.

☺ **Skin Stays Clean Oil Free Foundation** *($10.89)* still contains menthol, and you will notice a burning sensation when you apply it anywhere near the eyes. There is no reason to put menthol into a skin-care product—it provides no benefit whatsoever—and that's why this foundation is not recommended. **Moisture Tint Sports Formula SPF 6** *($7.99)* has an extremely low SPF and is without adequate UVA protection. It might have passed muster as a standard tinted moisturizer if the two available colors weren't so outdated.

CONCEALER: ✔☺ **Amazing Lasting Concealer SPF 6** *($5.97)* is amazing. It doesn't crease and it goes on smoothly and evenly! There are only two colors available, but both are serviceable. For a greater selection of colors and an almost identical formula, check out Revlon ColorStay Concealer SPF 6. The sunscreen, though too low, is titanium dioxide.

☺ **Wake-Up Call! Energizing Concealer SPF 15** *($6.89)* has a great, in-part titanium dioxide–based sunscreen and ends up working well as a liquidy, light-to-medium-coverage concealer if you don't mind the slightly chalky finish and the slippery application. There are three colors to choose from, with Deep being too peach for most dark skin. The remaining two are best for those with light to medium skin tone. The fact that this is in a squeeze tube makes it difficult to control how much of it comes out, which can waste product, but it works well and doesn't crease. Definitely worth consideration!

☺ **Skin Smoothing Concealer with Kinetin SPF 10** *($6.99)* has a light, smooth texture and a soft matte finish that is well suited for crease-free application under the eye. The sunscreen is all titanium dioxide (almost 9%), but the SPF 10 is disappointing. There are only two shades, but one of them (Medium) is just too peach for most skin tones. **Cover-Up Stick** *($5.69)* is a good concealer that comes in two workable shades: Light and Medium. The lipstick-like applicator helps it go on creamy, but not greasy, and it tends not to crease in the lines around the eyes. Although the consistency may be too moist for someone with oily skin, this one is definitely worth looking into. This should not be used over blemishes, despite what it says on the label.

<u>POWDER:</u> ☹ **Clear Complexion Light and Perfect Pressed Powder** *($10.89)* is a good, talc-based powder, with a smooth finish, but mostly terrible color choices—Ivory, Sand, and Beige are a far cry from neutral, and will easily turn orange on oilier skin.

☺ **Skin Stays Clean Pore Minimizing Pressed Powder** *($10.89)* is a talc-based powder with an exceptionally silky, somewhat thick feel. It can work as well as any powder for coverage, but the claims for this one are disingenuous—how can Almay's "Clear Pore Complex" help keep oil out, when oil comes from within the skin? This powder features four shades, and two of them are great; Medium and Deep are too rose and orange for most skin tones. **Luxury Finish Loose Powder** *($9.19)* has a very satiny, light finish with a subtle shine. If you are using loose powder to reduce shine, this would not be the way to go about it. However, this can nicely set makeup and add a bit of a glow to dry skin. Avoid Beige, which is too peach for most skin tones.

☺ <u>BLUSH:</u> **Beyond Powder Blush** *($7.47)* has an extraordinarily silky feel, and applies beautifully. However, all of the colors go on extremely sheer and half of them have a sparkle that is quite evident in daylight. Still, this is an option for those with very pale to light skin tones who prefer very soft, warm-toned colors. The bronze tones are great tan colors, but way too shiny too look convincing on skin.

<u>EYESHADOW:</u> ☺ **Beyond Powder Eyeshadow** *($3.59 singles, $4.19 duos, $5.37 quads)* products have a silky, ultra-soft texture that is almost identical to the Beyond Powder Blush reviewed above. They apply and blend well, but almost all of the colors are shiny and many are pastel. All offer a sheer finish, so it takes some effort to build any intensity. The quads offer some beautiful color combinations, but at least one shade in each is very shiny. If shine doesn't bother you, they are an affordable option.

<u>EYE AND BROW SHAPER:</u> ✔☺ **Amazing I-Liner Liquid Liner** *($5.79)* is a very good liquid liner that goes on smoothly and easily, creating a thick, dramatic line without flaking or looking crinkled. I think you will find it identical in performance to many department-store liquid liners, and it's available in classic black or brown.

☺ **One Coat Gel Eye Color** *($6.49)* are thicker-than-standard pencils, and glide over the skin and impart soft, sheer color that is easy to blend. This starts off with a wet feel, then dries to a soft powder finish. Taupe and Khaki are excellent lighter colors if you want to experiment with something other than browns and blacks. Although these are innovative, they can still smudge without much provocation.

☺ **Amazing Lasting Eye Pencil** *($5.47)* is a standard pencil formula with a twist-up, no-sharpen pen applicator. It's nice but hardly amazing. **One Coat Gel Eye Pencil** *($5.69)* is a standard pencil that offers a slightly wet-feeling application, but it tends to drag and skip over the skin, which makes drawing a continuous line difficult. This sets to a relatively solid finish, but can be softened and blended if needed. The **Naturalist Eye Pencil** *($6.89)* is a standard "please sharpen me" eye pencil that has a smooth texture and soft powder finish, yet it still has lots of slip and can easily smudge. The color selection is very good, and although I still prefer matte powder shadow for lining, if you insist on pencils, this is as good an option as any pencil from the department store.

LIPSTICK AND LIP PENCIL: ✓☺ PureTints Protective Lip C[...] are great options if you want to combine sheer lip color with effecti[...] These in-part avobenzone-based lipsticks have a smooth, easy-glide, ge[...] a small but crowd-pleasing selection of semitransparent colors, as well a[...] less) option, which would be an excellent option for men—and the [...] neutral packaging resembles lip balm more than lipstick. The colors, though sheer, are not necessarily for guys. ✓☺ **Lip Vitality Smoothing Lipcolor with Kinetin SPF 15** *($8.69)* is an excellent creamy lipstick that veers a bit toward being greasy, but glides on easily and offers broad-spectrum sun protection thanks to its in-part titanium dioxide sunscreen. Kinetin is present, but it's a mere dusting, and of no significance. The medium coverage colors range from subtle to stunning, making this lipstick one more smart option in the growing list of lipsticks with effective sunscreens.

☺ **One Coat Lip Color** *($8.69)* is just a very greasy (yet comfortable) lipstick. It works well enough but doesn't go on any more reliably in one application than any other lipstick with the same glossy finish. **One Coat Lip Shine** *($6.99)* is a standard, but very emollient, slightly sticky and shiny lip gloss with a misleading name. If one-coat coverage is what you like, you can put on one coat of almost any lip product. If you like more, then you have to apply more. Simple, right? **Amazing Lasting Lip Liner** *($7.19)* is just a good, standard, automatic pencil with a small but workable selection of colors. I wouldn't call it amazing, but it is worth a try and the available shades are just fine.

☹ **One Coat Lip Cream SPF 15** *($8.69)* doesn't have adequate UVA-protecting ingredients and is otherwise just a fairly glossy, standard lipstick with a large range of colors. The finish is rather sheer, especially if you stick with just "one coat." **One Coat 3-in-1 Color Stick** *($8.69)* is a chunky, crayon-type pencil that can be used over the eyes and cheeks, but is essentially just for the lips. Almay's selection of shades does make for an interesting eyeshadow look, but the slightly greasy, sheer application can smear over the eye and just looks greasy on the cheeks. These pencils can be hard to sharpen and are not too practical, but for a monochromatic look they can be considered convenient.

☹ **Stay Smooth Anti-Chap Lipcolor SPF 25** *($9.19)* doesn't contain UVA protection and is not recommended for sun protection, but it does contain menthol, which can cause irritation and chapped lips, and that's not what I would call a smooth move. **Stay Smooth Anti-Chap Lip Liner** *($7.19)* has a name that its irritating performance can't live up to. Although this is indeed a smooth, automatic pencil, it burns and tingles on the lips for some time after it has been applied. There is no ingredient list on the product, but I suspect the tingling is more menthol coming back to wreak havoc and encourage chapping.

MASCARA: ✓☺ **One Coat Mascara Lengthening** *($6.19)* is superior mascara that applies beautifully and builds lashes that get decidedly thicker as opposed to longer. You will definitely get some length, but don't be fooled by the name—it makes lashes thick, too, and is definitely one to try!

☺ **One Coat Mascara Thickening** *($6.19)* builds much greater length than thickness, and applies much easier than it has in the past. By the way, for both of these mascaras, the "one-coat" term is meaningless. You will find it necessary to apply a few coats to get a truly defined, separated look, as is true for all mascara, no matter the price or quality. **Longest Lashes Mascara** *($6.19)* is fine mascara, but not as good as the Thickening and Lengthening versions above. **Super Rich Mascara** *($6.19)* is perfect if all you need is a reliable lengthening mascara. Thickness is scarce, but this goes on lightly and cleanly, lasts well, and is easily removed.

☹ **Stay Smooth Mascara** *($6.19)* is really a packaging gimmick rather than a unique mascara formulation. This one does stay on well during the day and applies easily, building decent length, but it also tends to clump a bit. To help smooth out those clumps there is a built-in lash comb. It's cute and can be of help, but mascara that didn't clump would be more helpful. **One Coat Color and Curl Mascara** *($6.19)* is just OK. You'll notice little to nothing in terms of curl, and minimal thickness. With some effort (way more than "one coat"), you'll get long lashes with a soft, natural appearance that doesn't flake or clump. But the large, curved brush is not all that easy to use. **Stay Smooth Waterproof Mascara** *($6.19)* builds some length and definition but makes the lashes stick together and look almost brittle. It is waterproof, but there are other choices that are far more flattering. **The Insider!** *($6.19)* is supposed to nourish lashes and make them stronger. It can't do that anymore than hair-care products can do it for your tresses. This is just mascara and an OK one at that. With effort, it does build decent, though not exciting, length, but no thickness. For a softer mascara look it works fine and it doesn't smear or clump. **Amazing Lash Waterproof Mascara** *($6.69)* isn't amazing, although it is waterproof. It builds sparse length, no thickness, and is only worth considering if you want a very sheer waterproof mascara.

☺ **Amazing Lash Mascara** *($6.19)* remains average mascara, and one that falls short of the performance you get from Almay's best mascaras. This doesn't clump or smear, but the end result is nothing to write home about. **One Coat Thickening Waterproof Mascara** *($6.19)* is not one-coat mascara in the least. It can take many coats and then you still won't look like you have any lashes. Plus, the lashes tend to clump together when wet—not the best look from waterproof mascara.

ALOETTE

Clearly aloe is at the heart of Aloette's formulas. How is it as a cosmetic ingredient? It may have some benefit for the skin as an anti-irritant, but not a great deal more. There is no real evidence that aloe vera helps the skin in any significant way. An article in the *British Journal of General Practice* (October 1999, pages 823–828) stated that "Topical application of aloe vera is not an effective preventative for radiation-induced injuries.... Whether it promotes wound healing is unclear.... Even though there are some promising results, clinical effectiveness of oral or topical aloe vera is not sufficiently defined at present." Similarly, the *American Journal of Clinical Dermatology* (2002, volume 3, number 5, pages 341–348) stated that "The data for aloe vera gel … indicate that [there is no] compelling evidence of effectiveness." However, there is also research that has isolated certain components of aloe vera and demonstrated that these have some effectiveness for wound healing and as an anti-irritant (Sources: *Journal of Ethnopharmacology*, December 1999, pages 3–37 and *Free-Radical Biology and Medicine*, January 2000, pages 261–265). So, banking on pure aloe being helpful for skin is obviously not an absolute. Pure aloe probably can be soothing and nonocclusive, but whether or not it can have the same effect mixed in a cosmetic has not been proven—or even studied for that matter.

In the summer of 2000, Aloette revamped its product line and for some products those changes have been for the better. What is interesting to me about the changes is that I received a great number of complaints from Aloette salespeople and executives regarding my comments on their original product line. They insisted I was wrong and that these products were the best products ever. If they were the best ever, then why did they reformulate them? It seems that somewhere along the line management got the idea that the Aloette formulations were exceptionally dated and that aloe alone wasn't enough for skin care. Several of the new formulations include good water-binding agents, plant oils, and anti-irritants (and not just aloe), though some of the products still include alcohol and irritating plant extracts. There are definitely some inexpensive options to consider in this line, but there are also ones to stay away from. For more information about Aloette, call (905) 336-6590 or (800) 256-3883 or visit www.aloettecosmetics.com. **Note:** All Aloette skin care products contain fragrance unless otherwise noted.

ALOETTE SKIN CARE

☺ **$$$ Essential Cleansing Oil** (*$16 for 2 ounces*) contains, as the name implies, several non-fragrant plant oils: safflower, sesame, peanut, sunflower, olive, avocado, and wheat germ oils. This can leave a somewhat greasy film on the face, though it can be an option for very dry skin. While the mix of oils seems interesting, you could get the same effect with a single oil from your kitchen cabinet for far less money.

☺ **Foaming Citrus Cleanser** (*$13.50 for 6 ounces*) is a standard, detergent-based, water-soluble cleanser that would be an option for someone with normal to oily skin.

☺ **Hydra-Cleansing Emulsion** (*$13.50 for 6 ounces*) contains emollients and gentle detergent cleansing agents, which can be good for someone with normal to dry skin. The balm mint and fragrant oils are disappointing in what would have otherwise been a good cleanser.

☺ **Gentle Citrus Scrub** (*$14 for 4 ounces*) can work as a scrub using almond meal as the abrasive. It is an option for normal to oily skin but the clay in here makes it slightly tricky to rinse off, though it does leave the skin feeling soft. Keep in mind that plain almond meal you mix in with any cleanser you're using can do the same thing.

☹ **Skin Refining Toner** *($14 for 8 ounces)* is basically just water, glycerin, aloe, preservatives, plant extracts, fragrant plants oils, and coloring agents. The plant extracts are a mix of irritants and anti-irritants.

☹ **Oil Control Toner** *($14 for 8 ounces)* lists alcohol as the second ingredient as well as camphor and lime peel further down the list. All of those add up to drying and irritating the skin, which won't control oil in the least.

☺ **Nutrition Vitamin Complex** *($17 for 8 ounces)* contains mostly aloe, glycerin, slip agents, water-binding agents, antioxidants, fragrant plant oils, and preservatives. This would have been superior without the fragrant plant oils, but other than that, this could be a good toner for most skin types.

☺ **Sensitive Skin Toner** *($14 for 8 ounces).* At least this product leaves out the fragrant plant oils. But it still uses fragrance and coloring agents, which doesn't make it better for sensitive skin in the least. This is an otherwise good toner with glycerin, water-binding agents, and plant extracts for normal to dry skin.

✔☺ **Line Control Eye Gel** *($12.50 for 0.5 ounce)* includes nothing that will change one wrinkle on your face, but it is a good, lightweight moisturizer for slightly dry skin. It contains mostly water, water-binding agents, glycerin, thickener, antioxidants, and preservatives. It does contain fragrant plant extract.

☺ **Maximum Moisture Complex** *($20 for 2.3 ounces)* contains mostly water, aloe, thickeners, glycerin, plant oil, emollients, silicone, water-binding agents, plant extracts, fragrance, and preservatives. The plant extracts are a mix of anti-irritants and irritants, so they negate each other and it's disappointing. Still, this can be an option for someone with normal to dry skin.

☺ **Nutri-C Moisture Cream** *($15.50 for 3 ounces)* is a good moisturizer for normal to dry skin. It does contain fragrant plant oils.

☹ **Nutri-Moisture Lotion** *($15.50 for 3 ounces)* is a standard moisturizer that contains mostly water, thickeners, plant extracts, water-binding agent, fragrance, and preservatives.

☺ **$$$ Time Restore Firming Serum** *($45 for 1 ounce).* The alcohol in this product is almost too high up on the ingredient list for comfort, but assuming it's present in just a teeny amount this could be a very good, lightweight moisturizer for someone with normal to slightly dry or combination skin. The rosemary extract in it can be a good antioxidant but it is also potentially a skin irritant.

☹ **Visible Aid** *($12.50 for 2 ounces)* is a rather ordinary moisturizer that contains mostly aloe, water, thickeners, lanolin, plant oil, fragrance, and preservatives. That would work for normal to dry skin but it lacks many elements needed for healthy skin.

☹ **SPF 24 Lotion** *($13 for 4 ounces)* does not contain the UVA-protecting ingredients of titanium dioxide, zinc oxide, or avobenzone, and is absolutely not recommended.

☹ **After Sun Lotion** *($11 for 7 ounces)* is a good basic, though rather ordinary, moisturizer that would not be as helpful for skin as pure aloe vera gel from the health food store.

☺ **Self Tanning Lotion** *($18 for 4.5 ounces)* is a good, though standard, self-tanner. As is true for all self-tanners, this one uses dihydroxyacetone to affect the color of skin.

☹ **Sun Defense Body Mist, SPF 4** *($13 for 4 ounces)*, with an SPF 4, is an affront to good skin care. This is tantamount to a product advertising its ability to cause wrinkles and sun damage.

☹ **Perfect Lift Kit** *($39.95)* includes **Perfect Lift Powder** *(1.25 ounces)* and **Perfect Lift Activator** *(2 ounces)* and combines egg white with cornstarch, some plant extracts, and glycerin. This persistent, long-standing cosmetic chicanery has been around forever. Egg white and cornstarch can't lift skin or get rid of wrinkles—though if they could you could easily whip this up in your kitchen for substantially less.

☺ **Skin Renewal Mud Masque** *($14 for 4 ounces)* is actually quite a good clay mask for someone with normal to oily skin because it includes some water-binding agents and a small amount of plant oil to keep it from being too drying.

☹ **Soothe n' Smooth Lip Balm/Lip Scrub** *($24.50 for 0.58 ounce)* are sold together. The **Lip Scrub** is just a scrub that uses ground-up plastic as the exfoliant. The **Lip Balm** is just a standard Vaseline- and mineral oil–based balm that would be a lot better for lips without the irritating peppermint oil it contains.

ALOETTE ALOEPURE SIMPLY CLEAR

☺ **Clarifying Face Wash** *($13 for 4 ounces)* is a very good, though very standard, detergent-based cleanser that would work well for someone with normal to oily skin. The teeny amounts of glycolic, lactic, and salicylic acids in it aren't enough to have an effect on skin, though even if the concentrations were higher the pH of 5 is too high for these ingredients to have any exfoliating properties. This does contain fragrant oils.

☹ **Clarifying Deep Action Toner** *($13.50 for 4 ounces)* is mostly water and witch hazel with a small amount of detergent cleansing agents. Witch hazel's primary component is alcohol and that can be irritating and drying for skin. It does contain fragrant oils.

☹ **Acne Treatment Lotion** *($13.50 for 0.5 ounce)* could have been a potentially effective AHA lotion, but the fragrant citrus oils high up on the ingredient listing are problematic for all skin types. Further, the pH of 5 is too high for it to be effective as an exfoliant.

☺ **Clarifying Moisture Balance** *($13.50 for 2 ounces)* contains AHAs, but the amount isn't large enough and the pH of 6 isn't low enough for it to be effective as an exfoliant. This won't balance skin in the least, but it is a good, soft-matte finish moisturizer that would work well for someone with normal to combination skin.

ALOETTE MAKEUP

Referred to as Color Blends, this well-rounded collection presents some viable options for foundation, loose powder, blush, pencils, lipstick, and brushes. Although it doesn't offer as many different formulas and textures as most other lines, you will find most of the makeup performs quite well, and is definitely on par with the best options at drugstores and department stores. The mascaras are bland and the eyeshadows aren't as smooth and hassle-free as many others, but these are minor shortcomings in a line that has a much longer list of pros than cons.

FOUNDATION: ☺ **Oil-Free Liquid Makeup** *($12.50)* has a very light texture and smooths effortlessly over skin, drying to a natural semi-matte finish. Coverage is in the sheer to light range, and the assortment of ten shades is mostly wonderful, offering some great options for very light to medium skin tones. The following shades look quite neutral in the bottle, but quickly turn pink, peach, or rose on the skin: Soft Ivory, Golden Dawn, Natural Linen, and Deep Sable, and are not recommended. **Creme-to-Powder Foundation** *($14)* is classic cream-to-powder makeup, with a smooth, slightly thick texture that applies evenly and dries down to a soft powder finish. This works well for sheer to medium coverage, and is best for normal skin with no dry areas because this type of foundation will only emphasize the dry areas. There are four shades, which is somewhat limiting, but they're all worthy options. Medium may be too rose for some skin tones.

☺ **Bronze Wash** *($12.50)* is an OK liquid bronzer option that comes in one shade, a reddish-tan. It's not as universally flattering as many other bronzers, but is worth considering for light to medium skin tones. **Heavenly Sheen** *($9)* is a sheer liquid highlighter that comes in a tube with a wand applicator. It's lightweight and dries to a matte finish, but in feel only—this has a subtle sparkling effect that may work for evening, but can look distracting in daylight.

☺ **CONCEALER:** The **Concealer** *($10)* comes in a pot and has a very thick, slightly greasy texture that performs better than expected. It blends on surprisingly well and has a natural, creamy finish with excellent coverage and only a slight tendency to slip into lines. Of the three shades, Light is workable for fair to light skin, Medium is OK but slightly pink, and Dark is just too peach for most skin tones.

POWDER: ☺ **Fresh Finish Loose Powder** *($15)* has a delicate, very silky texture and smooth finish that would be appropriate for normal to dry skin. Oily skin will likely need a powder that has a drier texture. Among the five talc-based shades, all except Light are good, and there are options for darker skin, too.

☹ **Fresh Finish Pressed Powder** *($14)* has a slick, waxy texture and a very sheer finish. There are many other pressed powders that have a more pleasant texture than this one, and to top it off, Aloette's version has a cloyingly sweet fragrance.

BLUSH: ✓☺ **Cheek Color Powder** *($12.50)* comes in a stunning array of colors, from the palest pastel pink to the deepest red. This product has a splendid soft texture that goes on evenly and lasts. The majority of colors have a satin-matte finish, but the following shades have visible shine: Raspberry Sorbet, Boysenberry, Golden Sand, and Satin Rose. Women of color, take note—there are some lovely options here!

☺ **EYESHADOW:** **Custom Eyesilks** *($15.50 duo sets)* have a soft, slick texture that is similar to the Fresh Finish Pressed Powder above. These eyeshadows are sheer and go on a bit creamy, which means they will not last the day if you're prone to eyeshadow fading or creasing. The color selection is sizable, but over half of the shades are shiny or unbecoming colors like Bright Pink, Royal Purple, and Tiger-Stripe Orange. The following shades are beautiful and matte: Eggshell, Black Onyx, Taupe, Apricot, Rich Cocoa, Soft Charcoal, and Rich Chocolate. A nice feature with these is that you can choose which colors you want and add them to a single or duo compact.

EYE AND BROW SHAPER: ☺ **Eye Definer** *($7)* pencils are just standard eye pencils that have a firm texture and slightly creamy finish. As far as pencils go, these don't break the mold, but the price doesn't break the bank! **Water-Resistant Brow Definer** *($12)* is an OK automatic brown pencil that has a stiff application and slightly sticky finish that is indeed waterproof. Almost identical to this is the **Waterproof Eyeliner** *($10)*, which does hold its own under water but won't hold up if you're prone to oily eyelids.

✓☺ **Liquid Eyeliner** *($12.50)*. If any liquid eyeliner can be called easy, this is the one. Featuring a built-in, expertly shaped felt-tip applicator, it allows you to lay down a thin to thick line of color with quick precision. The formula dries fast and lasts—if you prefer liquid liner, what more could you want?

LIPSTICK AND LIP PENCIL: ✓☺ **Lip Color** *($9.50)* has a plush, creamy texture and a beautiful, opaque application. The color range offers something for everyone, including classic neutrals and bold, bright hues. **Waterproof Lipliner** *($10)* is a standard, but very good, automatic lip pencil that comes in a small but pleasing selection of colors. For those who require it, this really is waterproof.

☹ **Lip Sheen** *($8.50)* is an incredibly thick, sticky clear lip gloss that is flavored with spearmint. My lips are still tingling, and that's not a good sign!

On the more gimmicky side, Aloette offers their ☺ **Lip Modifier** *($9.50)* and **Lip Difference** *($9.50)*. The Lip Modifier is simply a standard lipstick that adds a golden peach shimmer to any lipstick. The Lip Difference is simply a colorless emollient lipstick that claims to control lipstick bleeding and smearing, but instead only adds to these woes—just like any other lip balm would.

☺ **MASCARA: Color Blends Lash Color** *($8.50)* appears to be one formula, but it comes with different brushes, although this is not indicated on the packaging. Both brushes make for an average lengthening mascara that cleanly applies the color. You won't see any thickness, but these do last very well and are easy to remove.

✓☺ **BRUSHES: Professional 7-Piece Brush Set** *($66.50)* is wonderful. Each brush is well-designed, appropriately dense, and luxuriously soft. This is a practical set as well, and includes all the necessary brushes to apply full makeup. My only (minor) gripe is that the blush brush is cut to resemble a contour brush. However, it still works well to sweep blush over the cheekbones.

☺ **$$$ SPECIALTY:** If you're sold on Aloette's makeup, you may want to consider using their **Makeup Planner** *($66.50)*, which is basically a binder with a detachable makeup bag inside, as well as pockets for brushes and plastic "pages" that allow you to arrange your eyeshadows, blushes, pressed powder, and cream-to-powder foundation. This is a practical, sleek way to organize and transport your makeup.

ALPHA HYDROX (SKIN CARE ONLY)

Alpha Hydrox Lotion and Alpha Hydrox Face Creme were two of the more effective and reasonably priced alpha hydroxy acid products that first appeared on the market when the AHA craze exploded back in 1992. While other companies often hedge when telling you how much AHA their products contain, Alpha Hydrox is one of the few companies that is more than forthcoming about their contents. The AHA in these products is glycolic acid, which is considered one of the best (aside from lactic acid), and the pH of the products is at a level that makes AHAs effective. If you are interested in trying an AHA in a moisturizing or gel base, this is a great place to start. The prices and the product quality, as far as the AHA content is concerned, are excellent. A few words of caution: While the AHA formulations are reliable they have not been updated since this line was launched more than a decade ago. Regrettably, they contain minimal to no antioxidants, anti-irritants, or water-binding agents. Further, to capitalize on the success of its showcase AHA products, Alpha Hydrox introduced several additional products to its line. It did add a good retinol moisturizer but the other moisturizers and the fade gel are disappointing. There are some interesting and reasonably priced products to check out, but aside from the AHAs, these lack many state-of-the-art ingredients. For more information about Alpha Hydrox, call (800) 447-1919 or visit www.alphahydrox.com.

☺ **Facial Moisturizing Cleanser** *($5.99 for 5 ounces)* is a basic, mild cleanser that contains a decent (though small) assortment of water-binding agents. In a cleanser, ingredients like that tend to be washed away, so they serve little purpose. Nonetheless, this is still a good cleanser that would work well for most skin types. It does contain fragrance.

☺ **Foaming Face Wash for All Skin Types** *($5.57 for 6 ounces)* is a standard, detergent-based, water-soluble cleanser that can be good for someone with normal to oily skin, but may be too drying for other skin types.

☹ **Toner-Astringent for Normal to Oily Skin** *($5.99 for 8 ounces)* contains alcohol and menthol, and that makes it too irritating and drying for all skin types.

☺ **AHA Creme 8% AHA Facial Treatment for Normal Skin** *($9.29 for 2 ounces)* is a very good and effective AHA exfoliant in a standard moisturizing base for normal to dry skin types.

☺ **AHA Enhanced Creme 10% AHA Facial Treatment, for Dry to Normal Skin** *($8.41 for 2 ounces)* is similar to the 8% AHA Facial Treatment above, only this one contains more AHA; the same basic comments apply.

☺ **AHA Lotion 10% AHA Facial Treatment, for Dry Skin** *($9.29 for 6 ounces)* is similar to the 10% AHA Facial Treatment above, only this one is in a very standard lotion base.

☺ **AHA Sensitive Skin Creme, 5% AHA Facial Treatment** *($9.29 for 2 ounces)* is similar to the Enhanced Creme 10% above, only this one has half the amount of AHA, which does make it better for sensitive skin, though the pH of 5 makes it somewhat ineffective for exfoliation.

☺ **Extra Strength AHA Oil-Free Formula, 10% AHA Facial Treatment** *($9.29 for 1.7 ounces)* is virtually free of any ingredients that could clog pores and is a very good option for an AHA exfoliant for someone with normal to oily skin. This does contain a good anti-irritant.

☹ **SPF 15 Moisturizing Daily Lotion** *($8.29 for 4 ounces)* does not contain the UVA-protecting ingredients of avobenzone, titanium dioxide, or zinc oxide, and is not recommended.

☺ **Multi-Performance Eye Therapy Creme** *($9.29 for 0.5 ounce)* is a good, though ordinary, moisturizer for normal to dry skin.

☺ **Night Replenishing Creme for Normal to Dry Skin** *($8.29 for 2 ounces)* is a good, though exceptionally standard, moisturizer for someone with normal to dry skin.

☺ **Oxygenated Moisturizer** *($12.29 for 2 ounces)* contains oxidized corn oil (which usually means an oil is rancid, but go figure), but the notion that this can release oxygen to the skin in any way is a stretch of the imagination. Even if it were possible, it doesn't answer the question about oxygen causing free-radical damage. This is a good standard moisturizer for dry skin, and the claims about oxygen being beneficial for skin care are not valid.

☺ **Under Eye Renewal** *($12.99 for 0.5 ounce)* is a mineral oil–based moisturizer whose third ingredient is talc, which means any hydrating or emollient capacity is minimal at best. This also contains peroxidized corn oil, listed as TriOxygen C, which is claimed to promote healing of skin, increased circulation, and stimulation of collagen owing to its release of oxygen into the skin. Yet the clinical studies (performed by NeoTeric, the parent company of Alpha Hydrox) failed to address the fact that releasing oxygen into the skin causes free-radical damage, something that does not in the least support any type of healing or collagen stimulation. Further, studies show the damage peroxidized lipids (oils) can have on the body (Source: *Antioxidant and Redox Signaling*, Fall 1999, pages 339–347). This moisturizer does have a nice assortment of antioxidants and water-binding agents, but adding talc and "oxygen" makes it shortsighted for an under-eye product, or for any other part of the face for that matter.

☺ **Retinol Night ResQ Anti-Wrinkle Firming Complex** *($11.99 for 1.05 ounces)*. If you are interested in finding out if all the talk about retinol is true (I'm referring to the notion that retinol, a form of vitamin A, can work just as well as the active ingredient in Retin-A or Renova), for content, price, and the correct packaging to ensure stability, this is one of the better options you will find!

☹ **Fade Cream** *($8.29 for 3.5 ounces)* could have been a very good 2% hydroquinone-based skin lightener in a fairly standard moisturizer base for normal to dry skin, but the packaging (in a jar) means the hydroquinone will be unstable after opening because of exposure to air.

☺ **Purifying Clay Masque 4% AHA Facial Masque, for Normal to Oily Skin** *($8.35 for 4 ounces)* is a standard clay mask with a small amount of AHA, but the pH is too high for it to be effective as an exfoliant. Regardless, keep in mind that you don't need more than one effective AHA product. Using several is just overkill—after all, you only have so much skin that needs to be exfoliated. And it's best to use only one effective AHA product on a regular basis, rather than in a face mask you use once or twice a week. It contains some potentially irritating plant extracts.

☹ **Lasting Lip Treatment, SPF 8 Sunscreen, All-in-One Care** *($3.85 for 0.35 ounce)* doesn't contain avobenzone, titanium dioxide, or zinc oxide, and the SPF 8 is not reliable for all-day protection, so this product is not recommended.

☹ **Vanishing Blemish Solution** *($8.29 for 0.5 ounce)* contains 2% salicylic acid (BHA) but the pH of 5 makes it ineffective for exfoliation and the second ingredient is alcohol and that makes it a poor choice for any skin types.

ANNA SUI (MAKEUP ONLY)

If you aren't familiar with Anna Sui, it may be because her more unconventional clothing designs, described by *Women's Wear Daily* as "…overt, hip fashions that manage to be both saucy and sweet," are not exactly what you would call mainstream. Although her unique designs have been part of the New York fashion scene since 1980, her skincare and color collection is still relatively young, having been launched in 1999 and 2001, respectively. What do Anna Sui's fashion eccentricities bring to her makeup line? Basically what you'll find is a lot of style and romanticized sass with questionable substance. Sui's makeup line can only be described as floral-tinged gothic. Her all-black, scallop-shelled containers and black tester units look like they would be right at home on the vanity of Morticia Addams (this is not the "Chanel" black-lacquer look). I'm not quite sure who this line is supposed to appeal to—the glitter and many of the unconventional colors may speak to experimental teenagers, but career-oriented women are likely to pass by this line in favor of more classic, straightforward options. Yet even though clothing design is clearly still Sui's strong suit, her makeup collection has made some notable strides since it was last reviewed, especially with foundations and brushes. Granted, the glittery gimmick products still outnumber (and assuredly outshine) the best finds, but this line should not be entirely overlooked anymore. For more information about Anna Sui, call (800) 826-3186 or visit www.annasuibeauty.com

FOUNDATION: ☺ $$$ **Fluid Foundation** *($35)* is a sheer-coverage, silky-smooth, light matte foundation that would be fine for normal to oily skin. It blends out smoothly and the colors have been greatly improved and expanded to include seven light to dark neutral shades and one iridescent option, which can be a choice for evening shimmer.

☺ **Compact Powdery Foundation** *($25 for powder cake; $8.50 for compact)* is a standard, talc-based pressed powder with slightly more coverage than standard pressed powders, so it can be used as a foundation. There are six excellent shades, including some great options for very light skin tones. Pressed-powder foundations are best for normal to slightly dry skin, and this particular formula contains synthetic wax as the second ingredient, which can be a problem for those with a tendency toward breakouts.

☺ $$$ <u>POWDER:</u> **Face Powder** *($33)* has only three colors, and all of them are shiny. This is definitely overpriced for what amounts to nothing more than a standard, talc-based loose powder. The shine negates the intended effect of powdering, which is to take down shine and set makeup—and the lavender shade is just plain odd. **Pressed Face Powder** *($23.50)* is an average, talc-based powder that has a thicker, drier texture than Sui's Compact Powdery Foundation and features an odd assortment of colors. The shades are divided into Accent, Nuance, or Base colors, but that only slightly helps determine how you use them. The only colors to consider for powdering the face are #700, #701, #702, and #703, although these all have a slight shine. Many of the others are either too yellow, white, lavender, or green (these are supposed to be for nuance or accent but they don't do anything except add a strange color to the skin). A few of the colors can work as blush, but are not preferred over considerably less expensive options. The puff that comes with this powder is ridiculously small for practical use.

<u>BLUSH:</u> ☺ $$$ **Blush Face Colors** *($22)* offers a small but passable selection of brighter blush tones that have a soft, smooth texture and sheer application—these do not go on as intense as they appear. For those concerned with shine, all of these do have a touch of shimmer. ☹ $$$ **Face Color Stick** *($22)* is a twist-up, cream-to-powder makeup stick divided into Accent, Conceal, and Highlight colors. These all have a light, smooth texture, but only #700 is an option for a concealer. Shades #302, #400, and #500 would make decent blush colors if you prefer this texture and finish.

☹ $$$ <u>EYESHADOW:</u> The **Eye Color** *($17)* has a slightly grainy, powdery texture that would ensure it flakes onto the skin while you're applying it. The colors are quite sheer, but they tend to deposit color unevenly. After looking at the available colors, I'm not sure any other criterion was followed except for making sure every shade had lots of shine and glitter. **Eye Gloss** *($17)* is a greasy, non-sticky, but sparkly, product that is supposed to add a "wet look" to the eye. If you really want to try this, Vaseline would produce the same smeary, messy effect used over any iridescent eyeshadow you already own. **Creamy Eye Color** *($17)* is a very glittery eyeshadow that comes in a tube with a wand applicator. Although the blendable texture is non-greasy and not sticky, the intense shine will enter the room before you do!

<u>EYE AND BROW SHAPERS:</u> ☹ **Eyeliner** *($16)* is a chubby pencil with a creamy, incredibly smear-prone formula. This borders on greasy and is not recommended. **Glitter Eye Liner** *($16)* is identical to the pencil above, only these are infused with large flecks of glitter. The application and end result are not what I would call pretty.

☺ $$$ **Liquid Eye Liner** *($19)* is a very good liquid liner that features a fine brush to facilitate application. This formula dries quickly and stays put—the only drawback is that five of the six shades are shiny. Shade #500 is a matte taupe/brown hue, and worth a try if you don't mind the price.

<u>LIPSTICK AND LIP PENCIL:</u> ☺ $$$ The **Lipsticks** *($19)* have a greasy feel and high-shine, semi-opaque finish. So as not to break the pattern, many of the lipsticks have

glitter galore, although there are some good red and red-brown shades to consider. **Gloss Lipstick** *($19)* has a very smooth, slick texture and a glossy, iridescent finish. It's fine for lightweight, sheer color. ☺ **Lip Gel** *($13)* is a fairly standard tube gloss with a thick, sticky texture and very glossy finish. The sheer colors offer still more glittery options for your consideration. **Lip Tint** *($15)* is simply clear lip gloss in a pot. It has the same thick, sticky texture as the Lip Gel. **Ring Rouge** *($12)* is sheer lip color packaged in a mini compact that's attached to a black plastic ring. The juvenile, yet Gothic, packaging is unappealing, and there are some real "Why bother?" colors, making this one easy to pass up.

☹ $$$ **Lip Gloss** *($18)* comes in a tube with a wand applicator, and is similar to the products above, but is more tenacious and sticky. **Lip Liner** *($16)* is a standard pencil that comes in a good range of colors, but is quite creamy. This is an option, but should not be relied on for helping lipstick stay where it's supposed to!

☺ $$$ <u>MASCARA:</u> Sui's **Mascara** *($19)* lengthens and defines lashes nicely, but there are dozens of other superlative mascaras available that outperform this one for far less money. Avoid the clear, glittery mascara unless you don't mind it flaking into your eyes or onto your skin.

☺ $$$ <u>BRUSHES:</u> The **Brushes** *($12–$50)* have come a long way since I last reviewed this line! Gone are the odd, impractical, and cutesy tools and in their place is a small but stellar collection of makeup brushes. There are seven options, and with the exception of **Brow Comb #07** *($12)*, all of them are worth a look. The **Blush Brush** *($32)* is soft and dense but cut straight across, which is not the most foolproof way to apply powder blush. Still, this may appeal to some and is worth auditioning.

☺ <u>SPECIALTY:</u> Perhaps the biggest attention-getter here is the huge assortment of $$$ **Nail Colors** *($13)*, which tend to be the focus of the line's visual presentation. There are over 50 colors, with most having the same glitter content and the unusual, edgy colors you find in lines like Hard Candy or Urban Decay.

Blotting Paper *($10 for 100 sheets)* is standard, oil-blotting sheets that work well to absorb excess oil. These are a bit smaller than normal, but would work well stashed in a micro-sized evening bag.

ANNEMARIE BORLIND (SKIN CARE ONLY)

Annemarie Linder is a German-born businesswoman whose extensive product line was first developed after she found that the only things that worked to cure her persistent acne were herbal extract treatments. After a stint at cosmetology school, and "exhaustive research into the effects of herbs on human skin," she opened her first skin clinic in East Germany, circa 1947. Her first products were not launched until 1951, but by 1958 her business was so successful that it attracted a bit too much attention from the then-Communist East German government, thus necessitating a hasty move to the West. A meeting with herbal remedy manufacturer Hermann Borner led to the formation of Annemarie

Borlind—and a vast skin-care line built on the premise of "the finest natural ingredients with the strictest quality control standards."

The Borlind line uses rhetoric that preaches nothing less than all-natural, with claims and product descriptions that capitalize on organic farming, environmental awareness, and rigorous testing to ensure hypoallergenic products are made with pure ingredients, all accompanied by the allure of "European elegance." They even claim to use all-natural preservatives, which isn't true in the least, as these products contain methylparaben and phenoxyethanol, decidedly unnatural substances. While these products do have a fair number of plant-based extracts, they also have their share of ingredients that are standard throughout the cosmetics industry, like dioctyl sodium sulfosuccinate, caprylic/capric triglyceride, cetyl palmitate, and glyceryl stearate, none of which has a natural profile.

Despite these inconsistencies, the best reason to consider Borlind's products is that they do tend to contain a good assortment of plant extracts known for their anti-irritant or antioxidant properties. That doesn't necessarily make these products better, but for those with a penchant for natural this line is one to keep in mind.

(An interesting piece of herbal history: The official German Commission E Monographs have been at the forefront in attempting to organize, categorize, and control the use and efficacy of herbal preparations. While there is strong criticism about the information in the monographs, they are considered by many to be a good basic resource for a description of herbs and their uses.)

The Borlind line features a parade of noticeably repetitive products, separated into subcategories for varying skin types and concerns. According to Borlind, everyone needs moisturizers—day creams and night creams—and sunscreen is needed only when one is sunbathing. This antiquated advice is still common among many European-bred lines, despite the fact that you would be hard pressed to find a dermatologist or oncologist who would agree with this dangerous and damaging skin-care advice. Although Borlind's brochures do suggest choosing a day cream with antioxidants in order to gain sun protection, antioxidants alone will not stop UV light from inflicting its harm on the skin—to think otherwise is dangerous for your skin and your health. If anything, today's research is showing that antioxidants are a potent additive to traditional sunscreens because they boost the effectiveness and stability of the *active* sunscreen agents. But those active ingredients must be on your skin in the first place. Antioxidants in any form are never substitutes for active UVA- and UVB-protecting ingredients.

Other fallacies abound throughout this line, the most absurd being Borlind's contention that special eye-care products are needed after the age of 20, that all women over 30 have dry, parched skin, and that a cleanser is more effective when it is removed with a washcloth or sponge. (This last bit of advice does make sense for unrinseable cold cream–style cleansers, which is true for this line, as only one of Borlind's cleansers is truly water-soluble.)

There are some good products to consider here, including some that use nonirritating plant extracts that have proven benefits for skin. But be prepared to shore up your finances, roll up your sleeves, and wade through lots of thick, confusing underbrush before you get to a sensible routine for your skin. For more information about Annemarie Borlind, call (800) 447-7024 or visit www.borlind.com. **Note:** All Annemarie Borlind skin-care products contain fragrance unless otherwise noted.

ANNEMARIE BORLIND COMBINATION SKIN SERIES

☺ **$$$ Combination Cleansing Gel** *($32.54 for 5.07 ounces)* is a basic, relatively gentle, water-soluble cleanser. It does contain minute amounts of witch hazel and silver chloride (an antiseptic, though with repeated use it can cause silver toxicity), but they are unlikely to pose a problem for skin in such small amounts. Although there are those who believe that silver salts are somehow beneficial for healing skin, the notion is not supported by published research.

☹ **Combination Facial Toner** *($36.50 for 5.07 ounces)* contains alcohol as the second ingredient, and even though Borlind states that it is plant alcohol, it's still ethyl alcohol—the very same type that can be very irritating to skin when used in this amount.

☺ **Combination Light Day Essence** *($36.61 for 1.7 ounces)* is basically just water and plant oil along with a synthetic sunscreen agent (not listed as active and, thus, not reliable for sun protection). The rest of the formula is fairly standard, though there are some good water-binding agents and antioxidants, but they likely are present in too small an amount to make much difference. This would be OK for patches of dry skin, but should be kept away from oily areas, especially if breakouts are an issue. This does contain fragrance.

☺ **Combination Night Cream** *($36.61 for 1.7 ounces)* is nearly identical to the Light Day Essence above, minus the sunscreen ingredient, and the same basic comments apply.

ANNEMARIE BORLIND LL BI AKTIV REGENERATION SERIES

The LL Series is for mature skin over 30, but exactly what is meant by "mature skin"? Although mature skin commonly refers to skin that is showing signs of wrinkles and discoloration, there are plenty of women over age 30 whose skin looks just great, especially if they have been diligent about sun protection. In contrast, women in their 20s who have spent years in the sun or on tanning beds often look older than they actually are. Moreover, the term "mature skin" still doesn't tell you if your own skin is dry, oily, sensitive, has acne, rosacea, dermatitis, or is in any other condition. Mature isn't a skin condition of any kind, just a marketing concept exploiting a fear of wrinkles.

☺ **$$$ LL Cleansing Milk** *($33.75 for 5.07 ounces)* is a standard, wipe-off cleansing lotion that uses the same emollients and thickeners that show up in dozens of other cold cream–style cleansers. This contains an interesting assortment of soothing and irritating plant extracts (which basically cancel each other out), though they are all present in such tiny amounts as to be almost insignificant anyway. This would be an OK option for normal to dry skin, but you will need a washcloth to remove this completely. It does contain fragrance.

☹ **LL Blossom Dew Gel** *($38.75 for 5.07 ounces)* would have been an excellent nonirritating toner if it did not contain alcohol. This does contain lactic acid, but there's too little of it to have an effect as an exfoliant.

☺ **$$$ LL Day Cream** *($49 for 1.7 ounces)* is a very good, emollient moisturizer for dry skin. It does contain a tiny quantity of witch hazel and sage, but the amounts are too low to make them a problem for most. Please remember that without a sunscreen this cream is not appropriate for daytime use unless you are willing to wear a reliable sunscreen with it.

☺ **$$$ LL Decollete Cream** *($47.50 for 1.7 ounces)* contains nothing that makes this a specialized product for the chest area (that's what decollete refers to)—it is merely a plant oil–based moisturizer that would be just fine for dry skin anywhere on the body. This does contain small amounts of lemon, rosemary, and horsetail, but likely not enough to be a problem for the skin. It contains mostly water, thickeners, plant oils, water-binding agents, anti-irritants, vitamins, preservatives, and fragrance.

☺ **$$$ LL Liposome Emulsion** *($65 for 1 ounce)* would have been an excellent moisturizer for normal to dry skin, but with alcohol as the third ingredient this is bound to be too potentially irritating for most skin types. What a shame, as this emulsion has a great formula that leaves out other irritating plant extracts altogether.

☹ **LL Moisturizing Ampoules** *($49 for 7 vials)* contain even more alcohol than the Liposome Emulsion above, making the product too irritating for most skin types.

☺ **$$$ LL Night Cream** *($49 for 1.7 ounces)* is a good emollient moisturizer for dry skin.

☺ **$$$ LL Regeneration Ampoules** *($49 for 7 vials)* contain essentially a good combination of plant oils, emollient, soothing agents, vitamins A, B, C, and E, and fragrance. There is no reason to spend this much money for plant oils, which you can purchase and use separately over dry skin. It does contain farnesol, which Borlind claims can get rid of wrinkles. It can't. There is minimal research demonstrating farnesol's effect in reducing pancreatic cancer in mice, but there is no evidence that this translates to a positive effect on skin.

☺ **$$$ LL Wrinkle Cream** *($41.75 for 1 ounce)* is a very rich, emollient moisturizer that would take very good care of dry skin. Do not expect more than a temporary improvement in the appearance of wrinkles, just as with any other moisturizer. This does contain very small amounts of witch hazel, horsetail, and alcohol—but the amounts are too small to be a matter of concern for skin.

☺ **$$$ LL Moisturizing Mask** *($49 for 1.7 ounces)* is a very good moisturizer that is quite similar to the other moisturizers in this series. This does contain tiny amounts of alcohol and balm mint, but likely not enough to be cause for concern.

☹ **LL Vital Cream Mask** *($55.75 for 1.7 ounces)* is nearly identical to the Moisturizing Mask above, save for some extra plant extracts; however the addition of menthol and camphor means this should be avoided.

ANNEMARIE BORLIND ROSE DEW HYDRO-STIMULANT SERIES

☺ **$$$ Rose Cleansing Milk** *($24 for 5.07 ounces)* is an emollient, oil-based, cold cream–style cleansing lotion that does not rinse away without the aid of a washcloth. It would be a good option for dry to very dry skin. It does contain fragrance.

☹ **Rose Facial Toner** *($29 for 5.07 ounces)* is an alcohol-based toner and is too irritating for all skin types. Without the alcohol, this would have been a contender for a fairly gentle toner.

☺ **Rose Day Cream** *($36.50 for 1.7 ounces)* is similar to other moisturizers in the Borlind line, meaning it is basically a combination of water, thickeners, plant oils, glycerin, vitamins, and plant extracts—both irritating and non-irritating, but present in such minute amounts that their effect (positive or negative) is inconsequential. Why this one costs several dollars less than the LL Day Cream above is a mystery as it's not different in any significant way. Because this does not contain sunscreen it cannot be relied on alone to provide protection for daytime use.

☺ **Rose Night Cream** *($37.75 for 1.7 ounces)* is almost identical to the Rose Day Cream above and the same basic comments apply.

ANNEMARIE BORLIND SYSTEM ABSOLUTE SERIES

The Absolute Series is meant to be "an extra dimension in skin care for the mature skin." This group of products contains a "magical" seaweed extract known as superphycodismutase, which Borlind maintains strengthens the immune system of the skin. This special seaweed is carefully harvested off the coast of Brittany. As I have mentioned in the past, seaweed (algae) contains a worthwhile antioxidant for skin, but all other claims, whether they're about the skin's immune system or vanquishing wrinkles, are unfounded. The association between a plant's ability to survive in its own habitat and how it will affect skin is completely unrelated and there is no research showing that superphycodismutase has any benefit for skin.

☺ **$$$ Absolute Cleanser** *($46.50 for 5.07 ounces)* is an emollient; cold cream–style lotion cleanser that's similar to the other cleansers in the Borlind line, and can be an option for dry skin. It requires the aid of a washcloth or tissue to get it off. This rather simple formula does not warrant the high price tag.

☹ **Absolute Beauty Fluid** *($82.50 for 1.7 ounces)* is an inordinately overpriced alcohol-based toner. If not for the alcohol, this would be a very good, non-irritating toner for all skin types—but that price tag!

☺ **$$$ Absolute Day Cream** *($98 for 1.7 ounces)* is amazingly similar to, but remarkably more expensive than, many of the other moisturizers in the Borlind line and would work equally as well.

☺ **$$$ Absolute Firming Fluid** *($50 for 0.5 ounces)* contains mostly plant oils, thickeners, some algae, water-binding agents, preservatives, and fragrance. This would be a fine (though very overpriced) option for dry skin.

☺ **$$$ Absolute Night Cream** *($98 for 1.7 ounces)* is similar to, but slightly richer than, the Absolute Day Cream above and the same basic comments apply.

☹ **Absolute Serum Decollete** *($95 for 1.7 ounces)* claims it can counteract the aging effects of loss of elasticity and tone in the chest area by strengthening and firming bust tissue as well as tissue in the neck area. Nothing in here is capable of stopping a loss of elasticity, especially not when a skin irritant like alcohol is the second ingredient, and no effective sunscreen is included. In essence, this is just one of the many Borlind moisturizers repackaged, and with a similar formulation accompanied by a different name and price tag.

ANNEMARIE BORLIND YOUNG BEAUTY PEACH SERIES

The two products below are recommended by Borlind for those with younger skin, and actually claim to "provide insurance against premature aging of the skin." Without an effective sunscreen, don't count on this being insurance of any kind—peaches and avocado are no substitute for a reliable sunscreen if your concern is forestalling wrinkles.

☺ **$$$ Peach Skin Cleansing Cream** *($16.75 for 3.4 ounces)* contains peach kernel oil, but is otherwise basically indistinguishable from the other cleansers in this line. It would be an OK option for normal to dry skin, and will not rinse well without the aid of a washcloth.

☺ **$$$ Peach Skin Facial Cream** *($16.75 for 1.7 ounces)* is a very good moisturizer for dry skin that avoids using even small amounts of irritating plant extracts, which is a bonus in comparison to several of the other Borlind products. I should also mention that this formula is remarkably similar to almost every other Borlind moisturizer—and notice the huge cost difference between this and the others!

ANNEMARIE BORLIND YOUNG BEAUTY U SERIES

☺ **$$$ U Cleansing Milk** *($20.75 for 5.07 ounces)* is not an appropriate cleanser for "troubled skin." Someone with blemishes would do well to avoid cleansing lotions that contain pore-clogging thickeners and plant oils as this one does. This would be an OK option for normal to dry skin that is not prone to blemishes, though this does contain small amounts of irritating plant extracts.

☹ **U Facial Toner** *($21 for 5.07 ounces)* does not break the tradition of the other Borlind toners, as this one is also alcohol-based and not recommended for any skin type. This one also contains witch hazel, camphor, and balm mint, which will not help blemished skin in the least.

☺ **U Day Cream** *($19.75 for 1.7 ounces)* is a fairly standard moisturizer with a less interesting assortment of ingredients than others in this line. It is absolutely not recommended for use over blemishes or blemish-prone areas. Contrary to the claim, there are no "infection-fighting" ingredients in here that could have even a minor impact on blemish-causing bacteria. The absence of sunscreen in this cream also means that another product would have to be layered over it for protection, and that would only add to the woes of someone with blemish-prone skin.

☹ U Night Cream *($17.75 for 1.7 ounces)* is the last thing blemish-prone skin needs! Who thought it was a good idea to use an emollient cream that contains several plant oils, lanolin, beeswax, and zinc oxide? This is a good moisturizer for very dry skin that is being marketed to the wrong skin type.

ANNEMARIE BORLIND ZZ SENSITIVE SERIES

The most significant aspect of the ZZ Series is the claim that these products do not contain preservatives, at least not synthetic preservatives. However, the plant extracts in them—yarrow extract, balm mint extract, horsetail extract, and wild thyme extract—have no ability to adequately inhibit mold, fungus, staph, or other microbial contaminants that are typical to cosmetics. The slight astringent properties these may have are more irritating than helpful when used on a regular basis. The vitamin C and vitamin E in this product have minimal effects as preservatives. I am skeptical when any company makes claims about products that don't contain preservatives. Either they are telling the truth, which means these products pose a risk of contamination in a short period of time, or they aren't telling the truth and you don't have anything to worry about. The final determination is yours.

☹ ZZ Sensitive Cleansing Milk *($19.35 for 5.07 ounces)* is another emollient, cold cream–style cleanser that is not easily rinsed off and would need the help of a washcloth. It would not be a good choice for those with sensitive skin, as several of the plant extracts are potentially irritating for skin.

☹ ZZ Sensitive Facial Toner *($25 for 5.07 ounces)* is yet another alcohol-based toner that adds insult to sensitive skin injury by also including sage, balm mint, horsetail, and wild thyme extracts.

☺ $$$ ZZ Sensitive Day Cream *($24.70 for 1.7 ounces)* needs a sunscreen to be suitable for daytime, but it is the potentially irritating plant extracts that make this problematic for sensitive skin. Other than that it is similar to many of the Borlind moisturizers, so the others are just as good an option.

☺ $$$ ZZ Sensitive Night Cream *($24.70 for 1.7 ounces)* is a standard, emollient moisturizer that is similar to many of the Borlind moisturizers and would be suitable for dry to very dry skin.

ARBONNE

Like many in-home sales lines from Nu Skin USA to Shaklee, Arbonne boasts more about what its products do not contain than about what they do. That isn't necessarily good or bad, but I happen to like some of the ingredients Arbonne warns against. Much of their literature states that things such as mineral oil, lanolin, and collagen are *not* used in any

Arbonne products. I disagree strongly with Arbonne's argument that mineral oil, petrolatum, and collagen are inherently bad for the skin because (they claim) their molecular structure is too large to be absorbed into the skin, and therefore they can clog pores, cause blemishes, and interfere with skin respiration. The molecular structure of many other cosmetic ingredients, including elastin, mucopolysaccharides, waxes, and other thickeners are also too large to permit absorption into the skin. Yet one of the best ways to prevent dehydration is to keep air off the face, and one of the best ways to do that is with a cosmetic ingredient with large molecules like this that work as a barrier between your skin and the air. If everything were absorbed into the skin, what would be left on top to keep air off the face? Mineral oil, petrolatum, and collagen are not so totally occlusive that the skin suffocates; they simply protect it from the air. Besides, just because a cosmetic ingredient can be absorbed into the skin doesn't mean it won't clog pores. Quite the contrary: once inside the pore, the ingredient is trapped and can't easily be washed or wiped away.

I do agree with Arbonne's recommendation against alcohol because of its drying and irritating effect on the skin. If only the company excluded all other irritants, such as witch hazel and certain plant extracts, the line would be even better. What is most frustrating is that Arbonne includes several problematic plant extracts in their products, including comfrey, watercress, St. John's wort, and peppermint (refer to Chapter Seven, *Cosmetics Dictionary*, for more detailed information). Not to mention that several of the sunscreen products don't contain UVA-protecting ingredients or appropriate SPF ratings (Sources: http://www.photodermatology.com/sunprotection.htm and *Skin Therapy Newsletter*, 1997, volume 2, number 5).

I could go on, but to sum it up, despite my reservations, Arbonne has some good products to consider. However, the rather misleading marketing language is not convincing. None of the natural-sounding ingredients in the world can keep you from reacting to an irritating preservative or fragrance or from breaking out due to cosmetic waxes such as stearic acid or myristyl myristate. For more information about Arbonne International, call (800) ARBONNE (272-6663) or visit www.arbonne.com.

ARBONNE SKIN CARE

☺ $$$ **Cleansing Cream** *($16 for 2 ounces)* is a safflower oil–based, cold cream–style cleanser. There would be little difference between this and just using plain safflower oil from your kitchen cupboard. It can leave a slight greasy film on the skin, though this would work well for dry skin. It does contain a fragrant plant extract.

☺ $$$ **Cleansing Lotion** *($15 for 3.25 ounces)* is similar to the Cleansing Cream above and the same comments apply.

☹ **Snap! 2 in 1 Eye Makeup Remover Pads** *($18.50 for 60 pads)* is a standard, detergent-based eye-makeup remover. The eyebright extract in this product has no research showing it to have any benefit for the eyes or skin, but comfrey, the third ingredient, can be a significant skin irritant.

☹ **Facial Scrub** (*$17.50 for 2 ounces*) is a standard scrub, but ground-up nuts are not the best way to exfoliate because they can be scratchy against skin, and the peppermint in here can add to the irritation.

☺ **Awaken Rejuvenating Mist** (*$14 for 4 ounces*) is a very good toner for all skin types. It contains mostly water, slip agent, water-binding agents, anti-irritants, preservatives, and fragrant oils.

☺ **Reactivate Rejuvenating Mist** (*$14 for 4 ounces*) contains a strange mix of anti-irritants and irritating plant extracts (pepper, jasmine, and nutmeg).

☺ **Unwind Rejuvenating Mist** (*$14 for 4 ounces*) is similar to the Reactivate version above, only with different fragrant and potentially irritating plant extracts.

☹ **Freshener** (*$19 for 8 ounces*). The witch hazel and horsetail plant extract in this product are potential skin irritants and are not very refreshing for skin to say the least.

☹ **Toner** (*$19 for 8 ounces*). Witch hazel, peppermint, and lemon are very irritating and drying for all skin types.

☺ **Moisture Cream Normal to Dry Skin** (*$19 for 2 ounces*) is a good standard moisturizer for dry skin that contains mostly water, plant oils, thickeners, plant extracts, vitamins, fragrant plant extract, and preservatives. The plant extracts are a mix of anti-irritants and irritants. Without sunscreen, this moisturizer should not be worn for daytime.

☹ **Moisture Cream Normal to Oily Skin** (*$19 for 2 ounces*) is similar to the Normal to Dry Skin version above except that this one also contains peppermint oil, a completely unnecessary skin irritant. Aside from the potential irritation, the plant oils and emollients in this moisturizer are inappropriate for oily or combination skin.

☺ **Night Cream for Normal to Dry Skin** (*$21.50 for 2 ounces*) is similar to the Moisture Cream Normal to Dry Skin above, and the same comments apply.

☹ **Night Cream for Normal to Oily Skin** (*$21.50 for 2 ounces*) is almost identical to the Moisture Cream for Normal to Oily Skin above, and the same comments apply.

☺ **Phyto Prolief** (*$30 for 2.5 ounces*) contains mostly water, plant oils, thickeners, glycerin, progesterone, anti-irritants, vitamin E, silicone, and preservatives. Applying progesterone to the skin raises medical concerns, and it should not be promoted under the guise of skin care. There is no way to know how much progesterone you are applying and whether or not it is even warranted. The evening primrose oil in this product has no research substantiating that it is effective for premenstrual syndrome (Source: *Journal of the American College of Nutrition*, February 2000, pages 3–12). While this can be a good moisturizer, I give it a neutral rating because of health concerns regarding the random topical application of hormones and their potential effect on the body (Source: *Journal of Steroid Biochemistry and Molecular Biology*, April 2002, pages 449–455).

☺ **Rejuvenating Cream for All Skin Types** (*$31 for 2 ounces*) contains mostly water, plant oils, thickeners, water-binding agents, anti-irritants, and a small amount of antioxidants. This would be a good moisturizer for someone with normal to dry skin.

☺ **Skin Conditioning Oil** *($16.50 for 1 ounce)* is a blend of several plant oils as well as aloe vera, vitamins, some plant extracts that are good anti-irritants, and water-binding agent. For someone with very dry skin, this would be a nice extra for problem areas, but for the most part any plant oil from your kitchen cabinet would work as well for far less money. This does contain fragrant oils.

☹ **Lip Protector SPF 15** *($5.50 for 0.12 ounce)* doesn't contain the UVA-protecting ingredients of avobenzone, zinc oxide, or titanium dioxide, and is not recommended.

☺ **Self Tanner for Face and Body** *($16.50 for 4 ounces)* is similar to all self-tanners, using dihydroxyacetone to affect the color of skin. This one would work as well as any.

☹ **Take Cover Face SPF 15** *($15.50 for 2 ounces)* doesn't contain the UVA-protecting ingredients of avobenzone, zinc oxide, or titanium dioxide, and is not recommended.

✓☺ **Take Cover for Face and Body SPF 30+** *(18.50 for 4 ounces)* contains zinc oxide as one of the active ingredients, which makes it a good option for a sunscreen. It also contains a good complement of water-binding agents, antioxidants, and soothing agents, making this a good sunscreen for normal to dry skin.

☺ **Mild Masque** *($17.50 for 5 ounces)*. For a clay mask, this is indeed fairly mild, but it is still just a clay mask. It can leave the skin feeling soft, but it could also make extremely dry skin feel even drier.

☹ **Extra Strength Masque** *($17.50 for 5 ounces)* is a fairly standard clay mask. Someone with oily skin won't be pleased with the oil in this product, but the amount is so tiny as to have almost no effect. The cornmeal in it can be rough on the skin.

☹ **$$$ Thermal Fusion Enzyme Masque** *($20.50 for 2.5 ounces)* contains mostly water, plant oils, papain, vitamins, thickeners, and preservatives. There is little to no research showing papain to have any effect topically on skin, though theoretically it can be an exfoliant.

ARBONNE CLEAR ADVANTAGE

☺ **Arbonne Clear Advantage Acne Wash** *($15.50 for 4 ounces)* is a standard, detergent-based cleanser that would work well for someone with normal to oily skin. The 1% salicylic acid, however, would be washed away before it had a chance to have an effect on skin, plus the pH of this product is too high for it to be effective as an exfoliant. The peppermint can be a skin irritant.

☹ **Arbonne Clear Advantage Refining Toner** *($15.50 for 4 ounces)* contains several potentially irritating ingredients, including witch hazel, lemon, and peppermint. Note that the AHA-sounding plant extracts in this product have no exfoliating properties.

☹ **Arbonne Clear Advantage Acne Lotion** *($16.50 for 2 ounces)* contains 1% salicylic acid in a silicone base, but the pH of this product isn't low enough for the BHA to have exfoliating properties. This also contains peppermint, which can be a skin irritant.

☺ **Arbonne Clear Advantage Skin Support Dietary Supplement** *($18.50 for 60* *tablets; 30-day supply)*. Whether or not the vitamins and herbs in this supplement (vitamin A, vitamin B6, pantothenic acid, zinc, L-lysine, burdock, and sarsaparilla) have any effect on acne has limited supporting research. If you are taking additional vitamin supplements, please check the total amount of vitamin A you are getting because there is a risk of taking too much vitamin A, which can be toxic. Please refer to www.drweil.com to make sure that your supplements meet established safety guidelines.

ARBONNE BIO-HYDRIA HYDRATING TREATMENT SYSTEM

☺ $$$ **Bio-Hydria Gentle Exfoliant** *($23.50 for 2 ounces)* is a mechanical exfoliant, but the plant extracts in it are mostly irritants (comfrey, St. John's wort, birch leaf, watercress, and ginseng), which doesn't help skin in the least. The scrub particles are fairly gentle, but there are better options for exfoliating skin than this.

☹ **Bio-Hydria Alpha Complex SPF 8** *($35.50 for 2 ounces)* has a dismal SPF, doesn't contain the UVA-protecting ingredients of avobenzone, zinc oxide, or titanium dioxide, and is absolutely not recommended.

☺ $$$ **Bio-Hydria Extreme** *($35 for 2 ounces)*. The plant extracts in this product are mostly irritants (comfrey, St. John's wort, birch leaf, watercress, and ginseng), which doesn't help skin in the least, so it's disappointing, given that the rest of the moisturizing formulation is impressive.

☺ $$$ **Bio-Hydria Eye Cream** *($24.50 for 0.75 ounce)* is similar to the Extreme version above and the same comments apply.

☺ $$$ **Bio-Hydria Naturesomes** *($39 for 0.95 ounce)* is similar to the Extreme version above, except that it contains more problematic plant extracts; the same basic comments apply.

ARBONNE BIO-MATTE OIL-FREE

☺ $$$ **Bio-Matte Oil-Free Cleanser** *($16.50 for 2 ounces)* is a good, detergent-based, water-soluble cleanser that would work well for most skin types. The plant extracts in this product are a strange mix of irritants and anti-irritants, which doesn't help skin in the least, but they would all be washed down the drain before they could cause problems anyway. It does contain fragrance.

☹ **Bio-Matte Oil Free Toner** *($15.50 for 4 ounces)* contains witch hazel, balm mint, and ivy, which makes it too potentially irritating for all skin types.

☹ **Bio-Matte Oil Free Moisture for Day, SPF 8** *($20.50 for 2 ounces)* has an embarrassingly low SPF, doesn't contain the UVA-protecting ingredients of avobenzone, zinc oxide, or titanium dioxide, and is not recommended.

☹ **Bio-Matte Oil Free Moisture for Night** *($20 for 2 ounces)* contains several ingredients that are problematic for someone with oily skin (isopropyl palmitate and triglyceride—great for dry skin though) and several of the plant extracts can be irritants. This is a mediocre moisturizer for someone with dry skin, and it has more problems than benefits.

ARBONNE NUTRIMIN C WITH BIO-HYDRIA

☺ $$$ **NutriMin C Night Cream with Bio-Hydria** *($62.50 for 2 ounces)* is mostly water, plant oils, thickeners, water-binding agents, silicone, antioxidants, preservatives, and soothing agents. The plant extracts are potentially irritating and photosensitizing, but the amount is so small it can't have much impact on skin. This is a very good moisturizer for someone with normal to dry skin.

☺ $$$ **NutriMin C Lift with Bio-Hydria** *($36 for 3.3 ounces)* is similar to the Night Cream above only in a gel-lotion form. The same basic comments apply, although this would work well for someone with normal to slightly dry or combination skin.

☹ $$$ **NutriMin C Night Serum with Bio-Hydria** *($39 for 1 ounce)* is supposed to contain AHAs, but sugarcane extract is not AHA and the lactic acid is present at a concentration of only about 2%, which is too small a concentration for it to be effective as an exfoliant. The salicylic acid in this product (about 0.5%) could potentially exfoliate, but overall the pH of this product is too high for it to be effective for that purpose. Besides, several plant extracts in it can be irritants, including lemon, orange, ginseng, watercress, and comfrey.

ARBONNE MAKEUP

Arbonne's latest makeup renovation is called About Face, and along with the new name come several new products and reformulations that do bring this line more up to speed with other makeup collections. The color palette is divided into warms, cools, and neutrals and although I don't agree with all of Arbonne's classifications, this system is helpful for choosing colors. The biggest improvements are to the textures of the foundations, blushes, eyeshadows, and lipsticks. Everything is smoother, more elegant, and easy to blend. What's not so great is the lamentable SPF 8 of both foundations, the profusion of shiny blushes and eyeshadows, greasy concealers, mediocre mascara, and fairly peach or pink powders. Arbonne continues to warn against the horrors of using mineral oil and talc in cosmetics, and wants you to know that their lipsticks do not contain tallow; but then none of the lipsticks I review in this entire book contain any tallow (or any form of it). Regardless of the purity-this or botanical-that claims, this line has its share of both positives and shortcomings. Ironically, the positives are largely due to the synthetic (yet essential) ingredients that Arbonne downplays, while the negatives often result from the choice of problematic plant extracts.

☺ $$$ <u>FOUNDATION:</u> **About Face Line Defiance Makeup SPF 8** *($26)* is purported to "literally and visually lift" skin, but the ingredients in this lightweight formula cannot suspend sagging skin even a little bit. Yet that's no reason not to consider this ultra-silky foundation that offers a natural matte finish and light to medium coverage. The in-part titanium dioxide–based sunscreen is present in too low an amount to provide daytime protection, but if you're willing to pair this with a higher SPF product and have normal to slightly dry skin you should be pleased with this one. Of the 15 shades, the following are too pink, peach, or rose for most skin tones: 3N, 4C, 5C, 6N, 10N, 11C, and 12C. **About Face Luminous Color Wand SPF 8** *($24)* also contains an in-part titanium dioxide–based sunscreen, but why Arbonne stopped at SPF 8 is a frustrating mystery. This stick foundation has a smooth, creamy texture that blends wonderfully and provides sheer to light coverage and a natural satin finish that those with normal to dry skin will appreciate. The 15 shades showcase some great light and dark options, and are identical to the ones above, including the shades to avoid.

☹ <u>CONCEALER:</u> **Cream Concealer** *($12)* is one of the greasiest concealers I've seen, yet it's enduring appeal can only mean that enough women are willingly putting up with it despite the availability of superior options that blend on well and do not crease. The one-size-fits-all color is too pink to pass as neutral. **Peach Concealer Pencil** *($10.50)* is a standard creamy pencil whose fleshy peach color won't look convincing on most skin tones. This product is a favorite of actress-cum-health and diet book author Marilu Henner, and I can only surmise that her exposure to really good concealers has been limited.

<u>POWDER:</u> ☺ **$$$ About Face Translucent Finishing Powder** *($22)* is a soft, sheer talc-based loose powder packaged in a tube with a powder brush on the end. Pressing a button on the opposite end shoots a small amount of powder onto the brush, and a cap is included so this is a practical on-the-go option. If only the two fairly peach shades were better, this would be easier to recommend. **Bio-Matte Oil-Free Personalizer** *($21.50)* is a pressed powder that's only available in a strange shade of green. This contains mostly clay, oat flour, and wheat starch. While it does have a dry finish, the green builds a strange color on the skin, and the oat flour and wheat starch are not the best idea for preventing breakouts—it's sort of like feeding the bacteria that cause the problem.

☺ **$$$Translucent Pressed Powder** *($16.50)* has a smooth, dry texture that makes this a sensible option for de-shining the face. The two shades are not the most versatile, but they're better than the Finishing Powder above.

☺ <u>BLUSH:</u> **About Face Blushers** *($12.50 for pan; $3 for Custom Color Compact)* have an exquisite texture that applies evenly and imparts soft color that can be built up for more intensity. However, every shade is shiny and the cheek sparkles just don't communicate sophisticated daytime makeup. For evening glamour, these are contenders!

☺ <u>EYESHADOW:</u> **About Face Eye Shadows** *($10 per shade; $3 for Custom Color Compact)* have an enviable texture that is identical to the Blushers above. These cling well, blend smoothly, and build color with ease. Again, the shine speaks louder than the wonderful texture, and most of these shades are shiny enough to emphasize wrinkles or crepey skin. The almost-matte options include Shy, Subtle, Suede, Diva, Reckless, Linen, and Sugar Beet.

☺ <u>EYE AND BROW SHAPER:</u> **About Face Eye Pencil** *($15)* is a standard, but very good, pencil that glides on and tends not to smudge or smear. If only the colors weren't so iridescent—on older skin these will only exaggerate an imperfect lashline.

<u>LIPSTICK AND LIP PENCIL:</u> ☺ **About Face Lipstick** *($15)* f͞ ͏˜ ͏ˆ a gorgeous

selection of shades, each with a creamy texture and slight glossy finish. These full-coverage lipsticks contain a plant-based fragrance that is not for the allergy-prone. **About Face Sheer Shine Duos** *($15)* is a dual-ended wand lip gloss that has a decent, minimally sticky feel and soft, sheer colors. There's nothing wrong with this gloss, but the price is steep for what you get.

☺ **About Face Lip Pencil** *($10)* is a standard pencil whose colors are decidedly vivid, but this is too creamy to prevent lipstick from feathering, and the colors tend to bleed.

☹ <u>MASCARA:</u> **About Face Lash Duos** *($18)* is a dual-ended mascara that has **Lash Colour Mascara** on one end and **Thick-It Lash Enhancer** on the other. The mascara itself is unspectacular and makes lashes feel brittle, while the Enhancer is nothing more than a colorless lash primer that does make a difference, but not nearly enough to make this worth choosing over dozens of other less expensive mascaras.

<u>BRUSHES:</u> ✓☺ **9-Piece Precision Brush Set** *($35)* is a jaw-dropping value when you consider that most other lines charge two to three times more for such quality makeup brushes. The essential brushes that make up the bulk of this collection are all wonderfully soft and well-shaped. The non-essential brushes serve as extras you likely will not use, but these can be removed so you can store preferred additional brushes in the attractive non-leather pouch.

☺ $$$ <u>SPECIALTY:</u> **About Face Colour Sets** *($101.50)* are pre-selected color kits that feature two eyeshadows, one blusher, a lipstick, lip pencil, lip gloss, eye pencil, and mascara. If you're sold on Arbonne makeup, these kits aren't the best thing to dive into, since each one features at least one poor color or odd color combination. You do get free eye-makeup remover pads, but that's not much consolation when you could spend less and coordinate better by choosing your own shades.

Custom Colour Palette *($18)* is a faux leather tri-fold makeup carrier that has room for every single Arbonne blush and eyeshadow. If the holders could be adapted to fit different size colors from other lines, this would make sense. As is, you'd have to be completely sold on Arbonne makeup to make this a useful purchase.

ARTISTRY BY AMWAY

A lot of people are selling Amway products throughout the world, and unless you have been living in a shell or on a mountaintop, it's likely that by now someone has approached you with the opportunity to either share in the theoretical wealth or at least become a customer. Talk about company loyalty! As one Amway sales representative said to me, "Why would the company make anything that wasn't wonderful?" Obviously, no cosmetics line is perfect, or they wouldn't discontinue "old" products and introduce "new" ones as this line has done, particularly for makeup. Company loyalty for those selling Amway is actually a little scary and the controversies surrounding it have mythic proportions. Type "Amway" and "cult" into any search engine and a few thousand hits are returned.

A shopping experience accompanied by a risk of needing to be deprogrammed; now that really is different.

If you want to shop in the privacy of your own home and enjoy being able to test the products, there are things to consider when taking a look at Amway's skin-care and makeup lines. I hope this doesn't mean I've unleashed a monster on any of you who have an Amway representative in your area, because you will be recruited to become an Amway salesperson with declarations of making lots of money even while you sleep. Make it clear from the beginning that you are interested only in buying products and not in becoming an Amway representative. That's not going to help really; but it's worth a try.

To shop Amway online is a tricky experience, at least in comparison to almost any other Internet commerce site. According to an article in *Forbes* (June, 26, 2001) "Quixtar is the online offspring of $5 billion, Grand Rapids, Mich.-based Amway Corp. Launched by the company at the height of the Internet stock craze in September 1999, Quixtar's business model is virtually identical to Amway's, only it's Web-enabled. IBOs [independent business owners] gather in cult-like meetings and chat rooms on the Web, and introduce friends, family, and co-workers to the password-protected Quixtar Web site where they can buy thousands of the same mostly overpriced health, beauty and household products that Amway sells. Things like Time Defiance, a $62 wrinkle-fighting cream that promises to 'turn back the clock' while you sleep. Or a Queen ten-piece stainless steel cookware set that sells for $700."

When it comes to their skin-care products, Artistry insists that they test their products extensively, but there is no published research or complete documentation (other than claims and snippets of data) forthcoming from the company. Further, as is true with many cosmetics companies, there are problematic ingredients in several products. What is a positive turn for Artistry is that their sunscreen formulations have improved and now include UVA-protecting ingredients.

Overall this line is not a bargain in the least—for many of the products, prices are right up there with the high-end department-store brands. For more information about Artistry by Amway, call (616) 787-6000 or (800) 992-6929 or visit www.amway-usa.com or www.quixtar.com.

ARTISTRY BY AMWAY SKIN CARE

☺ **Clarifying Foaming Cleanser for Normal to Oily Skin** (*$17.20 for 4.4 ounces*) uses TEA-lauryl sulfate as the second ingredient, which is potentially irritating and sensitizing for all skin types.

☹ **Clarifying Astringent Toner for Normal to Oily Skin** (*$16.60 for 8.1 ounces*) is an exceptionally standard, alcohol-based toner that is too irritating and drying for all skin types.

✔☺ **Clarifying Balancing Moisturizer for Normal to Oily Skin SPF 15** (*$24.45 for 2.5 ounces*) has been reformulated and now includes zinc oxide as one of the active ingredients. It is a silicone-based moisturizer with good antioxidants and water-binding agents. This is an excellent sunscreen for normal to slightly oily or dry skin. (Zinc oxide can be too occlusive for oily skin types.) It does contain fragrance.

☺ **Moisture Rich Vitalizing Cleansing Creme for Normal to Dry Skin** *($17.20 for 4.4 ounces)* is a very basic, cold cream–style cleanser that contains mostly thickening agents and plant oils. It needs to be wiped off, and that can leave a slight greasy residue on the skin. This can be an option for someone with dry skin. It also contains coloring agents and fragrance.

☻ **Moisture Rich Refreshing Toner for Normal to Dry Skin** *($19.30 for 8.1 ounces)* contains several potentially irritating plant extracts (orange and lemon), which make it a problem for all skin types. The sugarcane and sugar maple extracts are unrelated to AHAs and have no exfoliating properties. This is disappointing, because this toner contains several very good water-binding agents.

✓☺ **Moisture Rich Moisturizer for Normal to Dry Skin SPF 15** *($24.45 for 2.5 ounces)* has been reformulated and now includes UVA-protecting avobenzone as one of the active ingredients. It also contains some excellent water-binding agents and antioxidants. It would indeed work well for someone with normal to dry skin.

☺ **Delicate Care Cleanser for Sensitive Skin Types** *($17.20 for 4.2 ounces)* is a cold cream–style cleanser that would be good for someone with dry skin or sensitive skin, though it does take a washcloth to help it get makeup off. It doesn't contain fragrance, coloring agents, or irritating plant extracts, which would have been a good idea for all the Artistry skin-care products to adopt. For the money it is actually almost identical to Neutrogena's Extra Gentle Cleanser ($7.29 for 6.7 ounces).

☹ **Delicate Care Toner for Sensitive Skin Types** *($19.30 for 8.45 ounces)* lists the third ingredient as benzyl alcohol, which is a skin irritant and not something I would recommend for any skin type, much less someone with sensitive skin.

✓☺ **Delicate Care Calming Moisturizer for Sensitive Skin Types** *($24.45 for 2.5 ounces)* is a very good moisturizer for dry skin that contains some excellent water-binding agents and antioxidants. It does not contain coloring agents or fragrance.

☺ **Eye & Lip Makeup Remover** *($12.80 for 4 ounces)* is a standard, silicone-based makeup remover that also contains plant extracts (anti-irritants) and detergent-based cleansing agents. It will work as well as any. It does not contain fragrance or coloring agents.

☺ $$$ **Exfoliating Scrub** *($23.10 for 3.4 ounces)* is a mineral oil– and petrolatum-based cleanser that contains some synthetic scrub particles (ground-up plastic). It will exfoliate the skin gently, but the mineral oil and Vaseline and several of the thickening agents are not appropriate for someone with oily or blemish-prone skin.

✓☺ $$$ **Alpha Hydroxy Serum Plus** *($43.15 for 1 ounce)* is an AHA-containing, gel-like lotion with about a 6% concentration of lactic acid and a pH of 4 with good water-binding agents and antioxidants, as well as no coloring agents or fragrance. That makes it a good AHA solution—but the price is over the top for what you get.

☺ $$$ **Advanced Daily Eye Creme** *($20.25 for 0.5 ounce)* is a very good moisturizer for dry skin with great water-binding agents and vitamin E as the antioxidant. There is nothing about this product unique for the eye area.

✓☺ $$$ **Time Defiance Nighttime Renewal Creme** *($63.05 for 1.7 ounces)* is supposed to be "the first and only antioxidant complex designed to delay signs of aging caused by free radicals...." While there is a vast body of research (only in animal studies) showing antioxidants to be helpful for skin, how all that affects wrinkles has not been demonstrated on people. Still, not one ingredient in this product is unique to Amway's Artistry line; they all show up in lots of skin-care products and lots of skin-care products use other potent antioxidants over and above these. However, there are indeed good antioxidants in this product as well as excellent water-binding agents. This moisturizer is an excellent option for normal to dry skin, but all the other claims are unsubstantiated.

☺ $$$ **Time Defiance Nighttime Renewal Lotion** *($63.05 for 1.7 ounces)* is similar to the Creme version above and the same comments apply, though this one is better for normal to slightly dry skin because this formula base is primarily silicone and film-forming agent.

☹ $$$ **Bright Idea Illuminating Essence** *($52.50 for 1 ounce)* is supposed to be a skin lightener for sun-damaged discolorations, though it is unlikely to perform that way. This product contains bearberry extract, which primarily has antibacterial properties for skin. However, bearberry also contains arbutin, which has been shown to inhibit melanin. Still, it only does that in its pure form, not as a plant extract, and especially not in the trivial amount found in this product.

☹ **Blemish Control Acne Treatment** *($13.10 for 0.53 ounce)*. The primary ingredient in this product is alcohol and that makes it too drying and irritating for all skin types.

☹ $$$ **Hydrating Masque** *($18.80 for 2.6 ounces)* is an emollient, though standard, facial mask for someone with dry skin. It contains mostly water, thickeners, Vaseline, plant oils, preservatives, and coloring agents. It's really more of an ordinary moisturizer than a mask.

☹ $$$ **Deep Cleansing Masque** *($17.75 for 3.3 ounces)* is a standard clay mask that also contains a small amount of alcohol, but probably not enough to be a problem for the skin. It does contain fragrance.

☹ **Vitamin C + Wild Yam Treatment** *($38.60 for 0.34 ounce)* may contain wild yam, but wild yam does not contain progesterone or anything else that would act like progesterone. According to *The PDR Family Guide to Natural Medicines & Healing Therapies*, Physician's Desk Reference, 1999, wild yam "is used in the production of artificial [synthetic] progesterone but it will not yield the hormone in the absence of a chemical conversion process that the body can't supply." It has no effect on skin. Ascorbic acid, the form of vitamin C used in this two-step product, can be an effective antioxidant but it can also be a skin irritant.

☺ **Self Tanning Lotion** *($18.20 for 4.23 ounces)*. Just like all self-tanners, this product uses dihydroxyacetone as the ingredient to affect skin color. This one works as well as any.

☹ **Matte Finish Gel** *($11.99 for 0.53 ounce)* is just a combination of three dry-finish silicones. It can feel soothing and soft on skin but without any antioxidants, water-binding agents, or anti-irritants, this is more of a hair-care product than a skin-care product.

ARTISTRY BY AMWAY MAKEUP

FOUNDATION: ☺ **Absolute Oil Control Foundation SPF 15** *($24.25)* is a good liquid foundation with a fairly matte finish that has light to medium coverage. It can be an option for someone with normal to oily skin. It does contain zinc oxide as one of the sunscreen agents, which is great, but don't count on this product to control seriously oily skin in the least. The colors to avoid, because they are too peach, pink, or rose, are Honey Beige, Shell Bisque, Warm Amber, and Cappuccino. **Versatile Matte Pressed Powder Foundation** *($18.20)* is really a standard, talc-based pressed powder that has a silky-smooth feel, though it can appear a bit too powdery if you have dry skin. Using it wet is an option but it can look streaky and uneven so be careful. All but one of the shades are excellent; only Shell Bisque may be too peach. Amway considers these both pressed powders as well as an option for foundation, but they are best as pressed powders. **Self-Defining Sheer Foundation SPF 15** *($22.45)* doesn't contain the UVA-protecting ingredients of titanium dioxide, zinc oxide, or avobenzone, so you can't rely on the SPF for complete sun protection. It is a liquid foundation with a soft matte finish and light coverage. Many of the colors do look like real skin so this is an option for normal to slightly dry or slightly oily skin, but only if you wear a good sunscreen underneath.

☹ **Featherlight Maximum Coverage** *($23.25)* may be good for someone with dry skin, but it tends to be greasy and very thick; there is nothing featherlight about it. Most of the colors have a slight peach tone, but it's only slight, so they may be an option for some skin tones.

☹ **CONCEALER: Enhancing Concealer** *($14.55)* is a stick concealer with four decent shades, though it does tend to crease into lines around the eyes. **Ultimate Coverage Concealer** *($16.85)* comes in a squeeze tube and has three shades.

☺ **$$$ POWDER:** The **Loose Powder** *($17.50)* is a standard, talc-based powder with three good color choices, though three is definitely a limited selection. It has a dry, smooth finish.

☹ **EYESHADOW AND BLUSH:** Amway's eyeshadows and blushes come in individual tins that are placed into a compact that you purchase separately, either a **Two Pan Compact** *($11.25)* or a **Four Pan Compact** *($12.85)*. That means you can create your own makeup-collection compact that includes blushes and eyeshadows. It's a nice idea. The prices given below for the Powder Blush and Eye Colour are for the tins only, without a compact. The handful of **Powder Blush** *($11 refills)* colors have a silky texture that goes on soft and even, and they all have some amount of shine, as do the **Eye Colour** (*$7.30 refills*) eyeshadows, which have a lovely soft texture and go on smoothly and evenly. Even the so-called matte eyeshadows have shine.

☺ <u>EYE AND BROW SHAPER:</u> **Softstick for Eyes** (*$12.40*) are standard pencils in seven good shades, though these aren't all that soft. One end of the stick has a sponge applicator to soften hard lines. A brow pencil called **Softstick for Brows** (*$9.35*) is available in five colors identical to the pencils for eyes. **Fine Liner** (*$13.45*) is just a standard tube liquid liner that goes on smoothly and doesn't chip or flake; it comes in only two shades.

<u>LIPSTICK AND LIP PENCIL:</u> ☺ **Perfect Moisture Lip Colour** (*$12.90*) lipsticks are standard creamy lipsticks with a slight glossy finish. The color selection is decent. **Lip Sheer Colour SPF 15** (*$12.90*) are standard, glossy-finish lipsticks, but the SPF 15 doesn't include UVA-protecting ingredients. **SoftStick for Lips** (*$11.10*) are just standard lip pencils with a creamy application and a good color selection, but they do require sharpening.

☺ **Jumbo Lip Pencil** (*$12.50*) is a very soft lipstick in pencil form. This one may be too soft, can smush down to nothing fairly quickly, and isn't the most reliable option for applying lipstick or lipliner.

☺ <u>MASCARA:</u> **Smudgeproof Mascara 200** (*$14.50*) builds decent length and thickness quite quickly and doesn't smudge or smear.

☹ **Waterproof Mascara 200** (*$14.50*) builds great length and some amount of thickness, but it isn't all that waterproof. It can start coming off after a few splashes with water, and it easily smears even when you aren't wet.

☹ <u>BRUSHES:</u> The **Cosmetic Brush Set** (*$32.95*) is disappointing and shockingly overpriced for what you get. It comes with six brushes, of which three are OK; the other three are not worth the money. The powder brush is fine, but the bristles are a little too loose, so the powder can be hard to control on the face. The eyeshadow and angle brushes are also OK and usable. The eyebrow/eyelash comb is like those found everywhere; an old toothbrush would work equally well. The lipstick brush is a good six inches long and wouldn't fit easily in most makeup bags; the smaller, retractable lipstick brushes are much better. Finally, the blush brush is too small to be suited to anyone's cheeks.

ASTARA (SKIN CARE ONLY)

You may have heard about Astara as a line Hollywood stars clamor after and it does get some play in fashion magazines. Astara's Web site states that their products were previously only available "in high-end resort spas, day spas, salons, and medical facilities." Of course you would never want to sell your products in low-end locations because that wouldn't generate any business when your prices are this high, and image is everything in the realm of beauty. Besides, if you can get celebrities interested in what you sell, it is almost always a sure thing that regular consumers will soon want to know what they're missing.

Many cosmetics companies have a tag line or motto accompanying the name of their line that describes a key quality or attribute of the products they sell. Astara's is Conscious Skin Care. Initially I really liked the concept of consciousness (i.e., awareness) about skin care. That can only be a good thing, right? But what Astara means by "Conscious Skin Care" is that their "...products possess a dynamic life-force energy radiation that is absorbed by our skin externally, and by our bodies internally. This has a powerful effect in the repair, regeneration, and long-term maintenance of our skin's appearance outwardly, and in the health and longevity of our cells inwardly." And they mean it. Astara believes their products are in essence alive, and they prove that via something called Kirlian electrophotography. According to Astara, this type of photography "is one way of measuring and seeing the life-force energy radiating from a living organism or material. If a life-force does not exist, there will be no visible radiation coming from the subject being photographed. On the other hand, the more alive the subject is the greater will be its visible energy field and its capability to affect other life beneficially." They even have pictures to prove it (though I suspect you can do just about the same thing with Photoshop these days right on your computer).

I have no way to evaluate this claim anymore than I can comment on cosmetics being sold to bring you spiritual fulfillment and, as a result of that fulfillment, to attain great skin. Believing that skin-care products, plants, or people radiate a life force you can take a picture of sounds like trusting the appearance of a magician's trick. Though it isn't a magician's trick at all. A quick review of photography techniques indicates that it's not difficult to generate this kind of "aura-appearing" picture. The photography experts I talked to explained how you could take aura-radiating pictures of just about anything. I wonder if everyone's products are alive? But mostly I wonder why anyone believes this stuff. What's certainly true is that there is no research anywhere (not even in alternative medical literature) substantiating any of these claims, though it seems to cost a good deal of money to buy products that generate a life force.

It isn't surprising that Astara's claims are about keeping skin eternally young ("slows aging effects in the skin"), reducing free-radical damage, and containing "highly natural ingredients." Also, while this line's products definitely appear to have an abundance of plant extracts, the ingredient listings on the labels don't comply with FDA regulations and therefore cannot be taken at face value. For example, Astara's brochure states that their "...products typically contain enough chemical preservatives to have a three-year shelf life," yet there are no preservatives of any kind included on their ingredient labels. Plus, the order of the ingredients is misleadingly separated into self-created categories, with something they call "carrier oils" in one versus "essential oils" in the other, making the "essential oils" look more prominent than other ingredients. Perhaps the most egregious claim, and one of serious concern, is Astara's assertion that their "...moisturizers provide natural antioxidant UV ray protection including at the cellular level where it counts most." That's a dangerous claim. Not only are their products void of sunscreen ingredients, there are not even any SPF ratings. There is no research anywhere showing that antioxidants can come even close to reproducing the protection attained by a sunscreen with an SPF of 15 or greater and with UVA-protecting ingredients.

You will find some very good, albeit highly fragranced, moisturizers with excellent antioxidants and water-binding agents in this line, and a fairly gentle cleanser. But you will have to look elsewhere for reliable sun protection (the cornerstone of healthy skincare, especially if you really want any hope of "slowing aging") or products for oily or blemish-prone skin (oils and emollients on blemish-prone skin will make matters worse, not better). Those with sensitive skin will also find many of the plant extracts to be over the top for their skin type as well. Basically, this line is more about belief than actual product quality, with fiction winning out over fact, yet that is what so much of the skin-care industry is about these days. For more information about Astara, call (877) 4-Astara or visit www.astaraskincare.com. **Note:** All Astara products are highly fragranced.

☺ $$$ **Botanical Cleansing Gele** *($26 for 4 ounces)* is a standard, detergent-based cleanser that contains some good water-binding agents. The plant extracts are a mix of irritants and anti-irritants and cancel each other out. Note: This contains bergamot oil, which can be a problem for skin; refer to Chapter Seven, *Cosmetics Dictionary*, for specifics.

☺ $$$ **Daily Refining Scrub** *($28 for 4 ounces)* is an abrasive scrub using diatomaceous earth, a technical name for a particular type of rock high in sea-life skeletons. It is an option, though over-priced, for normal to oily skin.

☺ $$$ **AHA Nutrient Toning Essence** *($26 for 4 ounces)* does contain about a 3% concentration of lactic acid, but the pH isn't low enough for it to be effective as an exfoliant. There are some very good antioxidants and water-binding agents, but this also contains some irritating plant oils.

☺ $$$ **Botanical Eye Treatment** *($48 for 1 ounce)* is a silicone- and film-forming agent–based emollient gel moisturizer that contains some very good plant oils, antioxidants, water-binding agents, and anti-irritants, and does not include many of the irritating plant extracts and oils found in many of the other Astara products.

☺ $$$ **Anti-Oxidant Light Moisturizer** *($42 for 2.2 ounces)* is a very good, though highly fragranced, moisturizer for normal to dry skin. It contains very good plant oils, antioxidants, emollients, water-binding agents, and anti-irritants. However, the exposure of the product via its jar packaging reduces the stability of the antioxidants in it.

☺ $$$ **Microcluster Anti-Oxidant Infusion** *($72 for 2.2 ounces)* is similar to the Anti-Oxidant Light version above and the same comments apply.

☺ $$$ **Anti-Oxidant Rich Moisturizer** *($52 for 2.2 ounces)* is similar to the Anti-Oxidant Light version above and the same comments apply.

☺ $$$ **Facial Serum for Mature Skin** *($48 for 0.5 ounce)*, like all of Astara's Facial Serums, is mostly a mix of plant oils—including almond, jojoba, evening primrose (which has anti-inflammatory properties), carrot, and a tiny amount of vitamin E. Added to this standard, but good, mix of emollient plant oils are some extremely fragrant and potentially irritating plant oils that include fennel, patchouli, sage, sandalwood, ylang-ylang, myrrh, and rose. Some of those plant extracts may have antibacterial or antifungal properties and some have been shown to repel insects, but there is no existing research showing any other benefit for skin. There is a lot to be said for a placebo effect, and if you're going to spend this kind of money on skin-care products you might just find benefit from what amounts to putting perfume and plant oil on your skin. For specifics regarding each of the plant oils found in these products, refer to Chapter Seven, *Cosmetics Dictionary*.

☺ $$$ **Facial Serum for Dry Skin** *($48 for 0.5 ounce)* is similar to the Facial Serum for Mature Skin, and the same basic comments apply.

☺ $$$ **Facial Serum for Sensitive Skin** *($48 for 0.5 ounce)* is similar to the Facial Serum for Mature Skin, and the same basic comments apply.

☺ $$$ **Facial Serum for Normal Skin/T-zone** *($48 for 0.5 ounce)* is similar to the Facial Serum for Mature Skin, and the same basic comments apply.

☺ $$$ **Facial Serum for Oily Skin** *($48 for 0.5 ounce)* is similar to the Facial Serum for Mature Skin, and the same basic comments apply.

☹ $$$ **Facial Serum for Blemished Skin** *($48 for 0.5 ounce)* is similar to the Facial Serum for Mature Skin, and the same basic comments apply. This does contain some plant oils that have some antibacterial and antifungal properties, but there is no research showing these oils to be effective against the bacteria that cause blemishes. Plus the emollient oils in here can be a problem for this skin type. Note: This contains bergamot oil, which can have serious complications for skin; refer to Chapter Seven, *Cosmetics Dictionary*, for specifics.

☺ $$$ **Activated Sea Mineral Mask** *($39 for 1.9 ounces)* is an emollient mask with clay and plant oils and small amounts of seaweed. The plant extracts in here that are meant to sound like AHAs (sugarcane and sugar maple) have no exfoliant properties; and the menthol is a skin irritant.

☹ $$$ **Blue Flame Purification Mask** *($37 for 2.2 ounces)* is a standard clay mask with some good antioxidants, though the plant extracts are a mix of irritants and anti-irritants. The tiny amount of tea tree oil isn't enough for it to be effective as a disinfectant.

☺ $$$ **Golden Flame Hydration Mask** *($39 for 1.9 ounces)* is a very good, emollient, gel-style mask that would be a good option for normal to dry skin.

☹ $$$ **Green Papaya Nutrient Mask** *($37 for 2.2 ounces)* contains China clay, which is just another name for kaolin, a standard clay used in most facial masks being sold. It also contains papain and an enzyme derived from papaya, but there is no research showing papain to be effective for exfoliation in a cosmetic formulation.

☹ $$$ **Violet Flame Enzyme Mask** *($37 for 2.2 ounces)* is similar to the Green Papaya version above only it is supposed to be more potent. However, concentration values don't bear that out. The same basic comments for the Green Papaya Mask apply here as well.

AUBREY ORGANICS

If you haven't heard of Aveda, Zia Natural Skin Care, Rachel Perry, or Aubrey Organics, you haven't been paying attention to the world of natural, health food store cosmetics, which of course is fine by me. The products manufactured under the names of this group of "natural" notables contain enough plants and herbs to make me wonder how anything can still be growing on this earth. These gurus of the "natural" skin-care and makeup craze sell a plethora of foliage-based concoctions that are supposed to deliver every woman's deepest desire for her face—namely, flawless skin. Of course, none of their formulas are the same. Each company has its own "natural" recipes that guarantee wrinkle-free, acne-free, smooth, even-toned, glowing skin.

If there is any such thing as a "natural" true believer, Aubrey Hampton is indeed one. His books *Natural Organic Hair and Skin Care* (Organica Press, 1987) and *What's in Your Cosmetics?* (Odonian Press, 1995) articulately express his convictions. Foremost is his philosophic position regarding his products: "For almost 30 years I have collected herbs from around the world and combined them in 100% natural hair- and skin-care products. I make my natural shampoos, conditioners, soaps, lotions, masks, and so forth the way my mother taught me almost 50 years ago—without chemicals, using herbs known to be beneficial to the hair and skin." And yes, every plant is a miracle and every synthetic ingredient that he doesn't use is bad.

If Hampton is relying on information that is over 50 years old, people using his products are in a lot of trouble. What we know about sun protection we've only learned about over the past few years, and cell turnover, the life-and-death process of every skin cell, is a recent discovery, too. The whole complex physiology of skin (the formation of the intercellular layer and its functions), along with the nature of skin disease, are continually being investigated. Data regarding the exact chemical and biomolecular structure of skin fill volumes with new research, revealing astonishing information that has altered everything we once thought to be true about the skin. It's nice to think Mom knew it all, but I wouldn't make a skin-care decision based on such obsolete and fanciful thinking any more than I would a decision about my computer.

Hampton also lauds his position on animal testing: "I don't believe in animal testing and never use it. None of my products are formulated with data obtained from animal testing, and yet I know they're safe to use because they contain ingredients that have been used for hundreds, sometimes thousands, of years by people all over the world. That's the best track record, don't you think?"

Well, I don't think so in the least. As nice as all that sounds, in some ways it's actually dangerous. By his own admission, Hampton has only anecdotal past history to go by, and that is just too risky for my taste. "Natural" powders laced with "natural" lead were used by fashionably correct women centuries ago, causing necrotic skin and sometimes death. And what about sun exposure, which causes skin cancer and pervasive wrinkling? No one knew about that until very recently. So much for history being an arbiter of good health. Furthermore, while I abhor animal testing, scientists over the past 20 years have ascertained the benefits of most new skin-care ingredients, from water-binding agents and the new anti-irritants to AHAs, BHA, Retin-A, and sunscreens that provide UVA protection, mostly based on animal research. If Hampton is truly telling us that he ignores all that information, his products would be risky to use and some of the most dated in the industry.

Another Hampton phobia, shared by many other "natural" eccentrics in the world, has to do with petrochemicals. (I assume Hampton doesn't drive a car, take a taxi, or fly anywhere.) He states, "Petrochemicals, [which] are infinitely cheaper and much more convenient for mass manufacturers to use ... [and make] our hair and skin suffer as a result. What's worse, the long-term effects of these harsh chemicals on both the body and the environment are still unknown...."

Suggesting that all petrochemicals are harsh and all plants are good is as uninformed as thinking that eating any plant you encounter in the wild won't kill you because it is natural. Besides, petrochemicals have a decidedly natural source: they come from decomposed plant and animal life! But I've belabored these subjects before. More to the point is the Aubrey Organics arsenal of skin-care recommendations.

One of the steps in Hampton's skin-care routine is steaming the face. "Applying steam is an excellent way to detoxify and deep-cleanse your skin. Pour boiling water into a heat-proof glass bowl and add 4 tablespoons of Face Flowers [an Aubrey Organics product]." Nowhere does Hampton mention what kind of toxins are sweated out of the skin, nor does he discuss the potential for damage from overheating the face, such as causing surfaced capillaries to occur or making them look worse.

I am also very skeptical of the way Hampton handles his skin-care ingredient lists. They make no mention of standard cosmetic preservatives, and the ones that are listed—vitamins C, A, and E—have their own stability problems, with vitamin C being the most unreliable. Further, given that there are myriad types of vitamins A, E, and C, and there is no ingredient called "coconut fatty acid" (there are dozens of these, each with their own pros and cons), there is truly no way to make sense of these misleading ingredient labels. This concern was echoed in an industry newsletter, *The Rose Sheet* (March 15, 1999), which stated that Aubrey Organics was "in violation of catalog mislabeling and Good Manufacturing Practices.... [The] FDA investigators also determined several Aubrey products ... bear labeling that is not in compliance." In fact, because Aubrey's labels are blatantly not compliant with CTFA (Cosmetic, Toiletry, and Fragrance Association) or FDA labeling regulations, reviewing this line with any modicum of accuracy is a long shot, because there is no way to know what is really in these products and what is going on your face.

Ironically, many of Aubrey's products contain PABA, a synthetic sunscreen ingredient that has long since been set aside by cosmetics formulators because it poses a high risk of irritation and sensitizing skin reaction.

Setting aside my continuing concern about the farfetched hype and unsubstantiated claims surrounding "natural" products (though Hampton is one of the few who seems to glory in the lack of real evidence), I must point out that Aubrey Organics is one of the most reasonably priced "natural" skin-care lines around, almost to the point of being cheap! If you are one of the myriad "natural" skin-care seekers out there, this line won't hurt your pocketbook. Of course, I question what it can really do for skin, but that's what my reviews will reveal. For more information about Aubrey Organics, call (813) 877-4186 or (800) 237-4270, or visit www.aubrey-organics.com.

AUBREY ORGANICS SKIN CARE

AUBREY ORGANICS DRY SKIN #1

☹ **Facial Cleansing Cream** (*$14.75 for 8 ounces*) lists alcohol as the second ingredient and that can be drying and irritating for all skin types. The typical detergent-based cleanser in this product is standard in the industry, only here it has a less technical (and mislabeled) name, "coconut fatty acid." Coconut fatty acid goes by many less-friendly names, from tridecyl cocoate to cocamidopropylamine oxide, but if they were on the label then it would start sounding like everyone else's products and it would be so much harder to convince people that you were all natural. This cleanser can be drying for most skin types.

☹ **Jojoba Meal and Oatmeal Mask and Scrub** (*$8 for 4 ounces*) contains the same detergent cleansing base and alcohol as the Facial Cleansing Cream above and the same comments apply. It also contains oatmeal flakes, which can be lightly exfoliating. The plant oils are good emollients, but the alcohol and cleansing agents can be drying.

☹ **Rosa Mosqueta and English Lavender Facial Toner** (*$9.25 for 8 ounces*) lists alcohol as the second ingredient, and all the plants in the world can't change how irritating that is for skin. However, several of the plant extracts in this product are either skin irritants or have potential photosensitizing or toxic reactions on skin, including peppermint, coltsfoot, nettle leaf, St. John's wort, watercress, horsetail, arnica, and lemon.

☹ **Rosa Mosqueta Rose Hip Moisturizing Cream** (*$15.50 for 4 ounces*) contains problematic plant extracts and an incomplete ingredient listing that doesn't follow FDA or CTFA regulations.

AUBREY ORGANICS COMBINATION DRY SKIN #2

☹ **Facial Cleansing Cream** (*$12 for 8 ounces*) is similar to the Facial Cleansing Cream for dry skin above and the same comments apply.

☹ **Sea Buckthorn and Cucumber with Ester-C Moisturizing Mask** (*$8 for 4 ounces*) is a topical scrub in an unknown base that includes alcohol.

☹ **Sea Buckthorn and Cucumber with Ester-C Facial Toner** (*$9.25 for 8 ounces*) is over the top with irritating ingredients, including alcohol, witch hazel, peppermint, coltsfoot, St. John's wort, watercress, lemon peel oil, balm mint, and arnica.

☺ **Sea Buckthorn and Cucumber with Ester-C Moisturizing Cream** (*$15.50 for 4* *ounces)* includes plant oils and a fatty-acid base (of unknown origin) along with shea butter. That isn't appropriate over oily areas, though it can be an option for normal to dry skin. Now if we only really knew (as the FDA regulations call for) what's in here, you could be assured you knew what you were really putting on your skin.

AUBREY ORGANICS NORMAL SKIN #3

☹ **Facial Cleansing Lotion** *($14.75 for 8 ounces)* is almost identical to the Facial Cleansing Cream for dry skin above, only this one is in lotion form. The same concerns apply.

☺ **Green Tea and Green Clay Rejuvenating Mask** *($9 for 4 ounces)* is a standard clay mask that includes glycerin, plant extracts, and thickeners. It would work as well as any clay mask for someone with oily skin.

☹ **Green Tea and Ginkgo Facial Toner** *($9.25 for 8 ounces)* lists alcohol and several plant extracts that are potentially serious irritants and sensitizing ingredients for skin.

☹ **Green Tea and Ginkgo Moisturizer SPF 10** *($15.50 for 4 ounces).* The SPF 10 claim is completely without regard for the recommendations of the National Cancer Institute or the American Academy of Dermatology for sunscreen needing to be at least SPF 15. Plus, it does not contain the UVA-protecting ingredients of titanium dioxide, zinc oxide, or avobenzone, and it is not recommended.

AUBREY ORGANICS COMBINATION OILY SKIN #4

☺ **Facial Cleansing Lotion** *($14.75 for 8 ounces)* is just detergent cleansing agents with some plant extracts (some irritating) and plant oil (also some that are irritating).

☺ **Blue Green Algae with Grape Seed Extract Soothing Mask** *($8.75 for 4 ounces)* is almost identical to the Green Tea and Green Clay Rejuvenating version above and the same comments apply. Some of the plant extracts in this product are potential skin irritants.

☹ **Blue Green Algae with Grape Seed Extract Facial Toner** *($9.25 for 8 ounces)* is almost identical to the Green Tea and Ginkgo Facial Toner above and the same warnings apply.

☹ **Blue Green Algae with Grape Seed Extract Moisturizer SPF 10** *($15.50 for 4 ounces)* is similar to the Green Tea and Ginkgo Moisturizer SPF 10 version above and the same warnings apply.

AUBREY ORGANICS OILY SKIN #5

☹ **Natural Herbal Facial Cleanser** *($14.75 for 8 ounces)* contains several irritating ingredients that are not helpful for oily skin or any skin type. Alcohol, eucalyptus, camphor, and menthol can cause redness and a sensitizing skin reaction that can hurt the skin's healing response.

☺ **Natural Herbal Seaclay with Goa Herb Oil Balancing Mask** *($8.50 for 4 ounces)* is a standard clay mask with some plant extracts. The peppermint oil in it can be a skin irritant.

☹ **Natural Herbal Facial Astringent Oily Skin** *($9.25 for 8 ounces)* is almost identical to the Green Tea and Ginkgo Facial Toner above and the same warnings apply.

☹ **Natural Herbal Maintenance Oil Balancing Moisturizer** *($13 for 2 ounces)* contains several irritating ingredients that won't balance anyone's skin. Alcohol, balm mint, coltsfoot, and nettle are a problem for all skin types.

AUBREY ORGANICS SENSITIVE SKIN #6

☹ **Facial Cleansing Lotion** *($14.75 for 8 ounces)* contains several ingredients that are completely inappropriate for sensitive skin, or any skin type for that matter, including St. John's wort, coltsfoot, and lemon peel.

☹ **Vegecol with Organic Aloe and Oatmeal Soothing Mask** *($8.50 for 4 ounces)* contains several ingredients that are inappropriate for sensitive skin, or any skin type for that matter, including alcohol, St. John's wort, coltsfoot, and lemon peel.

☹ **Vegecol with Organic Aloe Alcohol-Free Facial Toner** *($9.25 for 8 ounces)*. Thankfully this is alcohol-free, but it does contain witch hazel, which is part alcohol. It also contains lavender water, and that can be a skin irritant.

☹ **Vegecol with Organic Aloe Moisturizing Cream** *($13 for 2 ounces)* contains several ingredients that are inappropriate for sensitive skin, or any skin type for that matter, including alcohol, St. John's wort, coltsfoot, and lemon peel.

MISCELLANEOUS AUBREY ORGANICS PRODUCTS

☺ **Herbessence Makeup Remover** *($6.95 for 2 ounces)* is just plant oil; sweet almond oil, jojoba oil, wheat germ oil, avocado oil, and macadamia nut oil, among others and fragrance. You would do just as well using plain sweet almond oil you buy from the health food store.

☺ **Sparkling Mineral Water Herbal Complexion Mist** *($7.25 for 4 ounces)* is just water, aloe, and some irritating plant extracts (balm mint, fennel, and musk oil). Forgo the plants and just get some pure aloe from the health food store. Mixed with water, that will do the same thing for skin without the added irritation.

☹ **Natural AHA Fruit Acids with Apricot Toning Moisturizer** *($19.95 for 4 ounces)* is similar to many of the products Aubrey sells, with no regard to skin type. The alcohol, lavender, peppermint, coltsfoot, nettle, sage, St. John's wort, watercress, lemon, ivy, arnica, and lemon peel are all serious problems for skin.

☹ **Vegecell Nightime Hydrator with Green Tea** *($15.75 for 1 ounce)* has all of the same problems as the Apricot Toning Moisturizer above and the same concerns apply.

☺ **$$$ Lumessence Rejuvenating Eye Cream with Liposomes** *($22.50 for 0.5 ounce)* has the potential for being a good moisturizer for skin, but the ingredient list does not meet CTFA or FDA regulations and so this product cannot be relied on to take care of your skin.

☺ **Rosa Mosqueta Night Crème with Alpha Lipoic Acid** *($17.50 for 1 ounce)* has the same problem as the Lumessence Rejuvenating Eye Cream above and the same comments apply.

☺ $$$ **Sea Buckthorn Rejuvenating Serum with Ester-C** *($15.75 for 0.36 ounce).* Assuming that the ingredient list is somewhat accurate, this is just jojoba oil and some form of vitamin C. That can be helpful for dry skin.

☺ **Rosa Mosqueta Rose Hip Seed Oil** *($12.50 for 0.36 ounce)* is just rose-hip oil, a good emollient with antioxidant properties. However, that is also true for the olive oil in your kitchen cabinet for a lot less money.

☺ **Collagen Therapeutic Cream Moisturizer** *($13 for 2 ounces)* has the same problem as the Lumessence Rejuvenating Eye Cream above and the same comments apply.

☹ **Amino Derm Gel Clear Skin Complex** *($7.95 for 2 ounces)* contains several ingredients that are problematic for skin, including alcohol, watercress, sage, lemon, calamine, and ivy.

☹ **Natural AHA Fruit Acids with Apricot Exfoliating Mask** *($19.95 for 4 ounces)* lists the second ingredient as alcohol, which make this a problem for skin. The plant extracts in this product are not all that natural, nor do they have exfoliating properties in this formulation due to the low pH and too small concentration.

☺ **After Sun Natural Tanning Maintenance Moisturizer** *($10.75 for 8 ounces).* If you use most of the Aubrey sun products you will need a lot more than this to take care of the damage caused by the absence of good sun protection. This has the appearance of being a good moisturizer for normal to dry skin, but the ingredient listing does not comply with CTFA or FDA regulations so there is no way to know what you are really putting on your skin. Several of the plant extracts in this product are potential skin irritants.

☹ **Sun Shade Ultra 4 Tanning Cream SPF 4** *($7.25 for 4 ounces),* with its SPF 4, is completely without regard for the National Cancer Institute or the American Academy of Dermatology recommendations for sunscreen needing to be at least SPF 15. Plus, it does not contain the UVA-protecting ingredients of titanium dioxide, zinc oxide, or avobenzone, and it is not recommended. This is like asking for wrinkles and sun damage to hit you in the face.

☹ **Saving Face SPF 10 Spray** *($8 for 4 ounces)* poses similar concerns to the SPF 4 version above and the same comments apply.

☹ **Sun Shade Ultra 8 Tanning Cream SPF 8** *($7.25 for 4 ounces)* poses similar concerns to the SPF 4 version above and the same comments apply.

☹ **Rosa Mosqueta Sun Protection Herbal Butter SPF 12** *($7.25 for 4 ounces).* This version does contain titanium dioxide, but an SPF 15 is critical and basic to good skin care.

☹ **Sun Shade Ultra 12 Tanning Cream SPF 12** *($7.25 for 4 ounces).* This version does contain titanium dioxide but an SPF 15 is critical and basic to good skin care.

☹ **Swimmers Moisturizer SPF 15** *($8.75 for 4 ounces)* does not contain the UVA-protecting ingredients of titanium dioxide, zinc oxide, or avobenzone, and it is not recommended.

☺ **Sun Shade Ultra 15 Tanning Cream SPF 15** *($7.25 for 4 ounces)* is a good in-part titanium dioxide–based sunscreen that would work well for someone with normal to dry skin (it contains several plant oils).

☺ **Green Tea Sunblock for Children SPF 25** *($8.50 for 4 ounces)* is a decent sunscreen with part titanium dioxide that would work well for someone with dry skin (it contains several plant oils and emollients). However, there is nothing in it that makes it any more appropriate for children than adults.

☺ **Titania Full Spectrum Sunblock SPF 25** *($8 for 4 ounces)* is a decent sunscreen with part titanium dioxide that would work well for someone with dry skin (it contains several plant oils and emollients).

AUBREY ORGANICS MAKEUP

Perhaps the two best words to describe the small assortment of makeup from Aubrey Organics are "Don't bother," but "What were they thinking?" is a close second. Available as single products or in preselected kits, what you'll find are a selection of loose powders and sheer lip tints. The ☹ **Natural Translucent Base** *($18.65)* and ☹ **Silken Earth** *($6.05, or $18.40 for the kit)* powders are designed to be used as foundation, highlighter, contour, and blush, but the gritty texture of each and the incredibly dry finish make them all poor candidates—not to mention that each one contains cinnamon powder. That may smell nice and it certainly is natural, but it's nevertheless problematic for skin.

The ☹ **Natural Lips** *($6.95, or $14 for the kit)* products are simply sheer lip tints that come packaged in glass jars. The colors are very soft and pretty, but they all contain enough peppermint oil to sound the irritation alarm for lips.

Last, the ☹ **Natural Cosmetic Brush** *($3.95)* is inferior to almost any other powder brush you'll find for sale, and while the ☹ **Natural Cosmetic Sponge** *($3.95)* is a true sea sponge, it is awkward to use and tends to soak up any liquid makeup before it can be smoothed onto the face. The sponge's uneven, large pores tend to make loose powder application a messy chore.

AVEDA

Aveda, a part of the Lauder Corporation since 1997, has softened its approach. In their original rallying cry against unnatural ingredients, particularly petrochemicals, Aveda's brochure once posed the question, "Would you moisturize with petroleum? Enjoy the sweet smell of methyl-octine-carbonate? [Or] accentuate your eyes with a coat of tar? That's just what you do with many mainstream health and beauty products. Aveda's products are grown from a simple premise: what you put on your body should be as healthy and natural as what you'd put into it." Today, plants are still the focus, but—as has been true from the beginning—a quick look at Aveda's ingredient listings reveals many components that aren't edible in the least. Who would want to eat isostearyl benzoate, polyglyceryl-6 deoleate, diazolidinyl urea (a formaldehyde-releasing preservative), or octyl methoxycinnamate (a synthetic sunscreen ingredient)? I could go on, but you get my drift.

Beyond the claims made about these products, one aspect that is a consistent draw for many consumers is the fragrance of Aveda's products. As a bystander in an Aveda store, it is interesting to see how many customers are lured in by the smell alone, and often make a purchasing decision based on that single criterion. As nice as that sounds, in the end it only shortchanges the consumer. Regardless of whether or not a product's fragrance is natural or synthetic, the potential for irritation and a host of other problems is still there. In fact, many of the "essential" oils used in Aveda products have a known history of unpleasant side effects, including allergies and dermatitis. Aveda would truly like you to believe that it is in fact the flower and plant essences in its products that are doing the "work." Alas, one only has to look at the ingredients to realize that Aveda uses many of the same industry-standard ingredients as everyone else. Many of the "special" ingredients merely contribute to the fragrance of the products, which isn't helpful for skin, and isn't enough to ensure a great (or even good) product. It has also been well established that once many of these "organically derived" plants and oils are purified and processed for use in cosmetics, they retain very little of their original benefit.

Jumping on the tourmaline bandwagon is a Lauder maneuver (as in their Creme de la Mer line), and if you are interested in that trendy ingredient, the products Aveda is offering are far less expensive. Aside from the struggle with Aveda's marketing claims, I do think that Aveda has some good products to consider. I also want to applaud Aveda for demonstrating such concern for the environment and animals. In many ways, Aveda has been an industry leader in the effort to streamline packaging and to use recycled materials. Now if it would only turn down the "natural" rhetoric and focus on ingredients that don't irritate or cause problems for skin, then for sure we would all be able to see the forest for the trees! For more information about Aveda, call (800) 328-0849 or visit www.aveda.com.

AVEDA SKIN CARE

☺ **Purifying Cream Cleanser** *($17 for 5.5 ounces)* is a lightweight, slightly emollient, standard, detergent-based cleanser that would work well for someone with normal to dry or combination skin. Several of the plant extracts can be potential irritants, but they are probably present in a scant enough quantity so as to not affect skin.

☺ **Purifying Gel Cleanser** *($17 for 5.5 ounces)* is a good, though very standard, detergent-based, water-soluble cleanser that is best for most skin types except someone with dry skin. The lavender and rosemary extracts can be skin irritants.

☺ **Pure Gel Eye Makeup Remover** *($15 for 3.7 ounces)* is a standard gel-type, gentle detergent-based eye-makeup remover. The rosewater and lavender in it aren't the best for the eye area.

☹ **Exfoliant** *($17 for 5.5 ounces)* could have been a good BHA (salicylic acid) exfoliant except that it contains alcohol as the second ingredient as well as other plant extracts that can be skin irritants.

☹ **Skin Firming/Toning Agent** *($17 for 5.5 ounces)* is a simple rosewater toner with a water-binding agent and more fragrant oils. This is more of a fragrance than a skin-care product and it's potentially irritating for all skin types.

☹ **Toning Mist** (*$17 for 5.5 ounces*) contains a host of irritating ingredients, including alcohol and peppermint. Aveda recommends this for oilier skin, but this is best avoided by any skin type, unless irritation is the goal!

☺ **All Sensitive Cleanser** (*$18 for 5.5 ounces*) is a standard, detergent-based, water-soluble cleanser. It can be drying for some skin types and the plant extracts (cardamom and sandalwood) are hardly good for sensitive skin.

☺ **All Sensitive Toner** (*$18 for 5.5 ounces*) is definitely not appropriate for sensitive skin, as several plant extracts in it can be skin irritants—including sandalwood, cardamom, vetiver, and barberry—though other plant extracts can be antioxidants. Aside from the plants, this could have been a good basic toner that contains plant tea, glycerin, water-binding agents, anti-irritants, slip agents, detergent cleansing agents, and preservatives.

☺ **All Sensitive Moisturizer** (*$30 for 5.5 ounces*). Several of the plant extracts in this product can be a problem for sensitive skin, including vetiver, cardamom, and sandalwood. Other than that, this is just a very basic, ordinary moisturizer for normal to dry skin that lacks interesting water-binding agents and antioxidants.

☺ **$$$ Firming Fluid** (*$32 for 1 ounce*) contains some good vitamins that can be antioxidants and water-binding agents. This is a good, lightweight moisturizer for normal to slightly dry skin, but it has no ingredients that can firm skin.

☺ **Hydrating Lotion** (*$28 for 5 ounces*) is a good, rather ordinary moisturizer for normal to dry skin that lacks antioxidants and state-of-the-art water-binding agents.

✓☺ **$$$ Night Nutrients** (*$38 for 1 ounce*) is a silky, silicone-based moisturizer that also contains several emollient plant oils and some vitamins that have antioxidant properties. This would be a good moisturizer for dry to very dry skin. Although it will not rejuvenate the skin from daily damage and it can't feed skin (as the label claims), it is one of the few Aveda products that are aroma- and fragrance-free, an idea that would have been far better if it were adopted for their entire lineup, not just for this one product.

☺ **$$$ Pure Vital Moisture Eye Creme** (*$25 for 0.5 ounce*) is a good moisturizer for someone with normal to dry skin, but most of the really interesting ingredients (antioxidants and water-binding agents) are at the end of the ingredient list and don't add up to much.

☺ **$$$ Tourmaline Charged Hydrating Creme** (*$30 for 1.7 ounces*). This relatively standard moisturizer has its share of plant extracts, but thankfully ones like huang qi, a vasodilator that can cause surface capillaries, are present in such minute amounts they aren't much of an issue. Aveda's claim for this product is that the tourmaline crystals (and there's less than 0.1% of them) "galvanize marine and plant ingredients to highest efficacy." There is no known efficacy on skin for minuscule amounts of plankton and algae. By the way, the process of galvanizing has to do with coating iron or steel with a layer of zinc to prevent it from rusting. There is no way to coat plants with tourmaline, nor is there any reason to do so.

☺ **$$$ Tourmaline Charged Protecting Lotion SPF 15** (*$38 for 1.7 ounces*) is a very good moisturizer with several excellent water-binding agents and antioxidants, plus it has a good SPF 15 with a small amount of titanium dioxide (less than 1%). It would have been far better had that amount been greater to truly protect skin from UVA damage.

☺ $$$ **Tourmaline Charged Eye Creme** *($30 for 0.5 ounce)* is supposedly based on Ayurvedic principles of medicine. The Aveda line has always been loosely based on Ayurvedic ideals, but the company for the most part has played this down because the philosophy is just too complicated. Possibly the recent popularity of other lines boasting Ayurvedic principles has brought Aveda back to its original marketing concept. (For more information on Ayurveda, please refer to Chapter Seven, *Cosmetics Dictionary*.) Regardless of whether or not skin-care products can balance doshas or dhatus is anyone's guess; there is truly no research anywhere supporting any aspect of this concept for skin care. Still, this silicone-based moisturizer would be good for normal to dry skin. It contains mostly silicones, water, glycerin, tourmaline (a semiprecious gemstone), plant extracts, antioxidants, water-binding agents, thickeners, fragrance, and preservatives.

✓☺ **Daily Light Guard SPF 15** *($16.50 for 5 ounces)* is an in-part titanium dioxide–based sunscreen that would be very good for someone with dry skin and it's far better formulated than the far more expensive Tourmaline SPF 15 version above.

☹ **Bio-Molecular Perfecting Fluid** *($28 for 1 ounce)* lists alcohol as the fourth ingredient, making it unnecessarily irritating for all skin types. The lactic acid and salicylic acid in this product could have been good exfoliants for skin.

☺ $$$ **Balancing Infusion for Dry Skin** *($18 for 0.33 ounce)* is a blend of several plant oils that would benefit dry skin nicely. However, given that these are just plant oils, you'd be better off using almond oil, olive oil, or canola oil from your kitchen cabinet; you'd get the same results and not have to deal with the irritation from the fragrance this product contains.

☹ **Balancing Infusion for Oily Skin** *($18 for 0.33 ounce)* contains 0.5% salicylic acid as well as jojoba oil, plant oil, and silicone. Even if this product had the right pH to work as an exfoliant (it doesn't), the jojoba oil can be too emollient for oily skin types.

☺ $$$ **Balancing Infusion for Sensitive Skin** *($18 for 0.33 ounce)*. For real balancing, what would have been preferred is for Aveda to leave out all the irritating plant extracts. Other than that, this is just an emollient with some plant extracts, plant oil, and vitamins. It would work well for someone with dry skin.

☺ $$$ **Deep Cleansing Herbal Clay Masque** *($19 for 4.5 ounces)* is as standard a clay mask as it gets. Although this mask has enough emollients to make it more "comfortable" than many other clay masks, the emollients are more suited to normal to dry skin than oily skin. Clay is not cleansing in the least, though it can absorb oil from skin.

☺ $$$ **Intensive Hydrating Masque** *($19 for 5.5 ounces)* dries to a thin "plastic" layer over the skin and it can be somewhat soothing for normal to dry skin. It contains a "tissue respiratory factor," described on the label as biofermentation of corn. Fermentation in this instance means the action of bacteria on corn. The bacteria breaks down the corn, resulting in the release of gases such as hydrogen sulfide and carbon dioxide. It sounds better when you don't know what it really is, doesn't it? And none of this helps skin breathe.

☹ **Lip Saver SPF 15** *($7.50 for 0.15 ounce)* doesn't contain the UVA-protecting ingredients of avobenzone, titanium dioxide, or zinc oxide, and is not recommended.

☺ **Sun Source** *($16.50 for 5 ounces)*, like all self-tanning products, uses dihydroxyacetone to turn skin a shade of brown, but this doesn't work any better than far less expensive versions.

AVEDA MAKEUP

Aveda's makeup collection presents some very good options when it comes to foundations, concealers, and powders, but falls disappointingly short of its past reputation with blushes and eyeshadows, as most of the shades are intensely shiny or are simply odd, difficult-to-work-with colors. The ubiquitous pure plant essences are incorporated here as well, but, not surprisingly, you will see a bevy of standard, often non-plant-derived ingredients making up the backbone of these formulas. Aveda's well-edited brush collection is worthy of consideration before you move on to the higher-priced department-store brush collections, and their lipsticks, though flavored with potential irritants, are still beautiful.

FOUNDATION: ☺ **Cooling Calming Cover Sheer Face Tint** *($18)* is Aveda's version of a stick foundation, only with a stay-put finish. The texture of water-to-powder formulas like this makes them suitable for normal to oily skin, as they go on rather wet and quickly dry to a light matte finish with light to medium coverage, depending on your blending. Aveda's is a bit tricky because once it dries it has no slip. That means any streaks or uneven blending stay that way all day (if you get it right, that can be great for someone with oily skin). But keep in mind that any attempts to even out mistakes will only make matters worse. If you get this blended on well, it provides sheer to light coverage in six very good colors. Only Walnut Veil may be too peach for some skin tones. There is nothing for very light or very dark skin tones. **Base Plus Balance** *($18)* is a very good foundation for normal to slightly dry or slightly oily skin. The colors are, for the most part, neutral, and the application is smooth. Thanks to the talc it contains, this foundation leaves a semi-matte finish. However, oilier skin types will find this formula rather heavy and any breakthrough shine will be noticeable shortly after application. The only color to watch out for is Praline, which can turn slightly orange. There are shades for very light and darker skin tones. ✓☺ **Dual Base Minus Oil** *($19.50 without compact, $30 with)* is an excellent pressed-powder foundation that goes on lighter than most. It is supposedly good for both wet and dry use, but to avoid streakiness use it dry and blend it well. The seven colors are all quite workable and soft; only Bronze can be too orange on the skin. This base can be layered for an ultra-matte, full-coverage look. It's not the most natural, but for some skin types this may be an option. ✓☺ **Moisture Plus Tint SPF 15** *($25)* is an ultra-sheer foundation that offers an excellent titanium dioxide sunscreen!

The color selection is superb, with five excellent "real skin" shades. This formula is best for normal to dry skin, as it contains several emollients that would not please oily or breakout-prone skin. The coverage is truly sheer, with excellent blendability.

☺ <u>CONCEALER:</u> **Conceal Plus Protect** *($13.50)* goes on and on about the vitamins and botanical essences it contains, as do most of the Aveda makeup products. Yet there aren't enough of them in any of the formulations to really make much, if any, difference for your skin. This concealer does go on smoothly and covers well, with minimal to no chance of creasing, but may need to be layered for very dark circles or redness. The application is more cream-to-powder than cream, so any drier areas will look cakey or flaky unless moisturized first. The color selection is workable, with only Sequoia being questionable.

<u>POWDER:</u> ☺ $$$ **Pressed Powder Plus Antioxidants** *($17.50 without compact, $28.50 with)* and **Loose Powder Plus Replenish** *($17 in tub with puff)* are standard, talc-based powders with a silky, dry, translucent finish. The color selection is mostly beautiful and the application sheer and soft. Avoid the Loose Powder in Sheer Teak, as this is bound to be too yellow for most medium skin tones. **Color Plus Definition** *($15)* is loose, shimmery powder that comes in a generous-sized tub. For those who don't mind the out-and-out shine and messy application, these are worth a look.

<u>BLUSH:</u> ☺ **Blush Minus Mineral Oil** *($13 for blush tablet; compacts sold separately)* has taken somewhat of a disappointing, though no doubt crowd-pleasing turn, as many of the suitable matte options have vanished and been replaced by shiny to glittery hues. These still have a soft, sheer texture that blends well, but the only colors worth considering are Nutmeg, Rose Quartz, Lotus, and Paprika. If you don't mind shiny cheeks, the rest of the palette can be considered. ☺ $$$ **Cooling Calming Color** *($18)* is identical to the Cooling Calming Cover Sheer Face Tint foundation reviewed above, except that these colors are blush or highlighting shades. The same problems for blending and streaking exist for this version as well. You can use this one on the cheeks or eyes. Of the four colors available, only Honeysuckle Tint is matte, and the rest are softly shiny. This formula is best for normal to oily skin types.

☺ **Color Plus Shimmer** *($14.50)* is a sheer, shimmery liquid/cream highlighter. The color is an attractive pink-gold tone, but the shine is not what I would call soft and subtle, so use this sparingly and only if you prefer high-wattage shine.

☹ <u>EYESHADOW:</u> **Shadow Plus Vitamins** *($10 for eyeshadow tablet; compacts sold separately)* have taken an ultra-shiny, pastel-toned turn for the worse. The few remaining matte shades are wonderfully neutral and soft, with more of a translucent coverage and minimal to moderate intensity. What a shame Aveda has joined the sparkly, glittery eyeshadow bandwagon with such unbridled abandon. **Onecolor Plus Two** *($14)* is an assortment of the chubby pencils that show up in almost every Lauder-owned makeup line. These feature two colors, one on each end, and are certainly clever. Just like other jumbo pencils, these can drag and pull the skin. Aveda says they are for eyes, lips, and cheeks, and that can be an option, but the texture is too dry for lips and too creamy to function for long as an eyeshadow, liner, or blush. Add all of this to the fact that these need regular sharpening and you are looking at a clever inconvenience.

☺ **EYE & BROW SHAPER:** **Eye Liner Minus Petro Waxes** *($11)* are nothing special, just a nice selection of standard pencils with an appropriate dry finish. For the pencil devotee, these should please. By the way, almost none of the pencils being sold in the United States contain "petro" waxes, meaning "petroleum derived." However, there is nothing bad about petroleum-derived ingredients; after all, their origin—oil from the ground—is a source that's about as natural as it gets.

LIPSTICK AND LIP PENCIL: ☺ **Lip Satin Plus Fresh Essence** *($14.50)* is a beautiful collection of creamy lipsticks that do offer more staying power than many others in this class. Some shades are quite iridescent, but the reds and neutrals have excellent color and coverage. There are some sheer colors as well, identified as **Lip Sheer Plus Fresh Essence.** If you are at all sensitive to peppermint, cinnamon, or anise (they can be sensitizing on skin) beware: all of these lipsticks are flavored with them. **Lip Satin Plus Uruku** *($14.50)* is Aveda's attempt at an "all natural" lipstick. Although uruku is indeed a plant pigment used to make annatto and other colors, one only has to read the ingredient list to see that these stack up the same as any other pigmented lip product—meaning that the same standard, unnatural-sounding pigments are right there with the uruku, offering their unsung color support. ✔☺ **Brilliant Lip Shine** *($11.50)* is a slick, non-sticky lip gloss that produces a dazzling, clear shine without resorting to glitter. It comes in a tube with an angled tip, so application is a breeze.

☺ **Lip Gloss Minus Lanolin** *($11.50)* is typical lip gloss in a pot—nothing remarkable—and comes in a very limited color selection seemingly aimed at a younger crowd. Unless you are sensitive to lanolin, avoiding it as an ingredient in lip products does not make much sense because it is excellent for dry skin. Also, reports that lanolin is a common skin sensitizer have proven to be unfounded.

☺ **MASCARA:** **Mascara Plus Rose** *($11)* seems to have undergone an improvement since it was last reviewed. Although still not what I would consider must-have mascara, this does produce copious length and decent thickness with less tendency to clump or smear than past versions. The main problem is the wet, almost too-heavy application—but if you're patient with this and desire dramatic lashes, it's worth a try. **Mosscara** *($14)* claims its conditioning formula is helped by the inclusion of Iceland moss, yet there is not enough moss in it to cover a twig, let alone condition lashes. This is an ordinary mascara formula that produces average length and OK thickness, but it's hardly exciting or worth considering over the best Maybelline or L'Oreal mascaras.

BRUSHES: Aveda's brush collection is mostly superb, with many worthwhile, affordable options. The brushes use pony or sable hair, and their thickness (density) and shape are excellent. Of particular note are the ✔☺ **Powder Brush** *($27.50),* which is not too big or too small or floppy; the **Blush Brush** *($25),* which is cut to fit the contours of the face; and the **Eyeshadow Brushes** *($14, $13, and $12, depending on size)*, which are more rounded as opposed to tapered and offer greater ease for deft blending of shadows. The **Lip Brush** *($15.50)* has a handle most would find inconvenient, although it may be an option for concealer application. The ☺ **Eyeliner Brush** *($10)*, **Angle Brush** *($10.50)*, and **Brow & Lash Brush** *($8)* are less impressive but still functional.

AVEENO FACIAL CARE (SKIN CARE ONLY)

Depending on what section of the drugstore you shop, you may have noticed that Aveeno now offers skin-care products for adults and the one for babies. This current expansion isn't surprising given that Aveeno, well-known for their oatmeal bar soaps, was purchased by Johnson & Johnson in 1999. J&J's influx of money has now created some new products that have some amount of interest for your skin. This isn't an exciting line, but it does have a good cleanser, a sunscreen, and a retinol moisturizer. It is also interesting to note that the trademark Aveeno oatmeal is nowhere to be found. What they included instead is a soy extract. J&J-sponsored studies say that soy can help all sorts of skin problems, from oil control to enhancing skin elasticity and reducing skin discolorations. As wonderful as that sounds, the study results from Johnson & Johnson were less enticing, with 25% showing moderate improvement, 8.5% showing marked improvement, and 4.3% completely cleared of skin discolorations. However, given that a lot of women experience improvement of their skin color over a period of time with the application of almost any good skin-care routine, these numbers are really ho-hum. Overall, the Aveeno line shouldn't be dismissed outright, but in comparison to other J&J lines at the drugstore, such as RoC and Neutrogena, these new Aveeno products add little to the mix. For more information about Aveeno, call (877) 298-2525 or visit www.drugstore.com.

☺ **Acne Treatment Bar** *($2.89 for 3 ounces)* contains 1% BHA in a bar cleanser, but the pH is too high for the BHA to be effective as an exfoliant. Bar cleansers can be drying, though this one is gentler than most; it could work for someone with normal to oily skin who doesn't have blemish-prone skin.

☺ **Balancing Bar for Combination Skin** *($2.99 for 3 ounces)* is almost identical to the Acne Treatment Bar above minus the salicylic acid. The same basic comments apply.

☺ **Moisturizing Bar for Dry Skin** *($2.39 for 3 ounces)* is almost identical to the Balancing Bar above and the same comments apply.

☺ **Skin Clarifying Cleanser** *($7.99 for 6.7 ounces)* is a decent, though standard, detergent-based, water-soluble cleanser that would work well for most skin types except those with very dry skin. It does contain fragrance. The amount of soy derivative (PEG-16 soy sterol) added here is not only teeny, but there is no research showing that this version has any positive effect on skin. Soy extract can have antioxidant and anti-inflammatory properties, but it's not any better than many other plant extracts.

☺ **Skin Replenishing Cleansing Lotion** *($7.99 for 6.7 ounces)* is a very good cleanser for normal to dry skin, though it may take a washcloth for your skin to feel completely clean of makeup. This one is fragrance-free, which is great, but then it makes me question why fragrance was added to the other products in this line.

☺ **Skin Brightening Daily Scrub** *($6.99 for 5 ounces)* is a standard, detergent-based scrub that uses ground-up plastic as the abrasive, a fine option for normal to oily skin types. The claims that this will improve skin tone, texture, and clarity can be made by almost any well-formulated scrub, and even more so by a well-formulated AHA or BHA product. Exfoliating does help skin look better, but mechanical exfoliation like this is not considered as reliable or as effective as exfoliation with AHAs or BHA.

☺ **Skin Clarifying Toner** *($7.99 for 6.7 ounces)* is an OK alcohol-free toner, but it leaves much to be desired in terms of advantages for the skin. It contains mostly water, slip agent, cleansing agents, a soy derivative, preservative, fragrance, and water-binding agents. The teeny amount of water-binding agents is disappointing, as with this toner your skin would be getting more fragrance than good skin-care ingredients.

☺ **Radiant Skin Daily Moisturizer** *($13.99 for 4 ounces)* contains mostly water, thickeners, water-binding agents, silicone, shine (mica), film-forming agent, fragrance, and preservatives. This is a good basic moisturizer for normal to dry skin, but to be exciting it really needs more antioxidants and water-binding agents.

☺ **Skin Brightening Daily Moisturizer** *($14.99 for 1 ounce)* is a good, retinol-type moisturizer that adds vitamin C to the mix as an extra incentive to make it appear more interesting than the other retinol products out there. If you want to try a retinol product with vitamin C this would be the one to consider. It also contains a very small amount of soybean extract, but don't count on that providing any "plant estrogen" benefit for your skin, even though it is a good antioxidant. This does contain fragrance. Some good water-binding agents would have made this a far more interesting product.

✓☺ **Skin Brightening Daily Moisturizer SPF 15** *($14.99 for 1 ounce)* is similar to the version above, only this one adds a good sunscreen with avobenzone! That makes it an excellent alternative for daytime use over any of the other retinol products on the market. It does contain fragrance.

✓☺ **Radiant Skin Daily Moisturizer SPF 15** *($13.99 for 4 ounces)* is similar to the Skin Brightening Daily Moisturizer above, only minus the retinol, though the same basic comments apply.

AVON

Avon has gone to great lengths over the past few years to modernize its products and move its image from the "Avon Calling" of the 1970s ad campaign to its current direction of "Let's Talk Avon." The ads embody Avon's attempt to appeal to savvy, beauty-conscious women who prefer the attraction and "department store quality" makeup. For the most part, Avon is succeeding, as it continues to be one of the top-volume cosmetics companies in the world.

The most telling transformation is Avon's Web site, www.avon.com. It is state-of-the-art for online cosmetics shopping, including accurate ingredient listings and easy navigation. Add to this the improvement in the quality of its skin-care products and Avon is a player to contend with in the world of cosmetics. The complaint that still lingers for Avon is its sales force. Though they try hard, most of them are little more than order-takers. In fact, most of the representatives I talked to were quite honest about how much they didn't know about makeup or skin care, or the specifics about the products they were selling. None of the Avon women I spoke to even had samples or testers. And there is often a great deal of confusion about what products are available during a given "campaign." If you have the wrong book or the products aren't up on the Web site, you're out of luck. That's not just confusing, it's frustrating.

Adding to the confusion is the astonishing number of Avon products. I doubt that any salesperson could keep track of them all anyway, or afford to. In addition, most of the women who work for Avon do it part-time, to earn extra money, not as a major source of income. (The average sales representative earns about $5,000 a year, top sellers earn about $10,000, and only the rare exceptions earn more than $20,000 a year.) That constitutes a sales force whose main interest is not necessarily Avon. (Avon does guarantee 100% satisfaction, and it is true to that policy.)

However, if you know what you want, there are some incredible bargains, particularly the water-soluble cleansers and moisturizers for dry skin. Just keep in mind that there are also plenty of poorly formulated and lackluster products that aren't a bargain at any price.

By the way, Avon's line of AHA products, called Anew, went through quite an overhaul that has eliminated the reliability of these products. While it now offers more products than ever before, for the most part the AHA content is missing, and some of the sunscreen additions contain no UVA protection. That isn't an improvement in the least.

I must praise Avon's commitment to consumer information. The operators at its ordering number—(800) 233-2866—and its consumer information center number—(800) 445-2866—were quite helpful. No matter how many products I requested, ingredient lists for them were provided without hesitation or question. Thank you, Avon, for great customer service. Avon's Web site is www.avon.com.

AVON SKIN CARE

AVON ANEW SKIN CARE

☺ **Anew Perfect Cleanser** (*$11 for 5.1 ounces*) isn't perfect, it is merely a standard, gentle, detergent-based, water-soluble cleanser that can be good for most skin types. It does contain a small amount of fragrant oils, which can be skin irritants, but that is true for all fragrance additives.

☺ **Anew Ultra Cream Cleanser** (*$14 for 5.1 ounces*) is more of a wipe-off cleanser than anything else. It would work well for someone with normal to dry, sensitive skin, but it won't take off makeup very well and you'll need a washcloth to really clean your face. For the money, try Neutrogena's Extra Gentle Cleanser ($7.29 for 6.7 ounces).

☺ **Anew Clarifying Essence** *($14.50 for 5.1 ounces)* is an exceptionally ordinary toner of water, glycerin, and a teeny amount of yeast, which may have antioxidant properties. All in all this is very basic and very boring.

☹ **Anew Advanced All-in-One Self-Adjusting Perfecting Lotion SPF 15** *($16 for 1.7 ounces)* doesn't contain the UVA-protecting ingredients of titanium dioxide, zinc oxide, or avobenzone, and is not recommended.

☹ **Anew Advanced All-in-One Self-Adjusting Perfecting Cream SPF 15** *($16 for 1 ounce)* has the same basic problems as the Lotion version above and the same comments apply.

☹ **Anew Biologie + Skin Optimizer SPF15** *($18 for 1.7 ounces)* doesn't contain the UVA-protecting ingredients of titanium dioxide, zinc oxide, or avobenzone, and is not recommended.

☹ **Anew Clearly C 10% Vitamin C Serum** *($20 for 1 ounce)* contains mostly alcohol, which is clearly drying and a skin irritant. It does contain ascorbic acid, a form of vitamin C, but that is considered one of the more irritating and least stable forms of this vitamin when it comes to antioxidant properties.

✓☺ **Anew Force Extra Triple Lifting Day Cream SPF 15** *($22 for 1.7 ounces)* comes with claims that your face "will see a 60% improvement in fine lines and wrinkles in one week." If that happens in just a week, in two to three weeks you should be wrinkle-free! Aside from the hype, this ends up being a decent moisturizer with a good SPF that includes avobenzone as one of the active ingredients. What makes this product unique, along with a few other Anew products, is Avon's trademark ingredient trioxaundecanediouc acid (also known as oxa acid). A patented ingredient, oxa acid is supposed to be effective as an exfoliant and to perform better than AHAs without irritation. The only research supporting this notion is a very long, rambling patent held by Avon. What makes it confusing is that while one complaint about AHAs is that the low pH required to make them effective for skin can cause irritation, it seems that oxa acid, according to the patent, has the same problem: "…in treating skin conditions [oxa acid] has been found to be affected by the pH of the composition … preferably in the pH range between 3.5 and 4.0." That's the same range that makes for effective use of AHAs. Nonetheless, if you wanted to give another exfoliant a try, this is one to consider, though the pH is definitely higher than the patent for this ingredient suggests. It also contains mostly water, glycerin, vitamin C, thickeners, silicones, water-binding agents, vitamins, plant oil, film-forming agent, preservatives, and fragrance.

✓☺ **Anew Force Extra Triple Lifting Day Lotion SPF 15** *($22 for 1.7 ounces)* is almost identical to the cream version above, only in lotion form, and the same basic comments apply. It does contain fragrance.

☺ **Anew Force Extra Triple Lifting Night Cream** *($22 for 1.7 ounces)* won't lift anything and this isn't the best product in the Anew lineup, but it is a good basic moisturizer for normal to dry skin.

☺ $$$ **Anew Force Extra Triple Lifting Eye Cream** *($18 for 0.5 ounce)* is almost identical to the Night Cream above, only with more silicones and a teeny amount of good water-binding agents, so it is probably far better for skin all over the face than the Night Cream. The teeny amount of caffeine in it won't wake up the eye area.

☺ $$$ **Anew Instant Eye Smoother, SPF 15** *($16.50 for 0.5 ounces)* is a very good, in-part titanium dioxide–based sunscreen that would work well for any part of the face. It contains mostly silicones, film-forming agent, glycerin, thickeners, water-binding agents, plant extracts, more silicones, and preservatives. The silicones give this a silky feel and it would work well for normal to dry skin. The plant extracts may have antioxidant properties but the amount is too tiny to be of much significance.

✓☺ **Anew Perfect Eye Care Cream SPF 15** *($13.50 for 0.53 ounce)* is a product containing about 1% AHAs in a base with a pH of 6, which makes it a poor exfoliant, but that's good news for the eye area. This is just a good in-part titanium dioxide–based SPF 15 product with some great antioxidants and water-binding agents, making it a good moisturizer for dry skin.

☺ **Anew Line Eliminator Dual Retinol Treatment** *($16 for 1 ounce)* contains mostly water, glycerin, vitamin C, thickeners, silicones, pH balancer, retinol, vitamin E, preservatives, and fragrance. This definitely contains retinol, and if you're interested, this is as good an option as any in the same price range as products from L'Oreal's Line Eraser to Cetaphil with Retinol, though the latter is fragrance-free.

☺ **Anew Luminosity Skin Brightener SPF 15** *($20 for 1.7 ounces)* is a good, avobenzone-based sunscreen for normal to slightly dry skin. That makes it a mediocre moisturizer for normal to dry skin (assuming the amount of alcohol is so minor it would not be irritating for skin). It also contains a form of AHA but only about 2%, which isn't enough for it to work as an exfoliant (though it acts as a good water-binding agent). The plant extracts of bilberry, licorice, and mulberry are supposed to reduce brown patches, but the research on these and their effects is minimal, especially as ingredients in a cosmetic (as opposed to their pure form). What this product does contain is a good group of antioxidants, anti-irritants, and water-binding agents. It also contains fragrance.

☹ **Anew Positivity Cooling Flash Relief** *($12.50 for 1 ounce)*. With alcohol, menthol, and ginseng being the first ingredients, you will get a cooling sensation but you will also get dryness and irritation. There is no evidence that soy or black cohosh applied topically on skin can have any effect on menopausal or peri-menopausal symptoms.

✓☺ **Anew Retroactive Eye Age Reversal Serum** *($18 for 0.4 ounce)*. The claim that this is a "revolutionary eye serum deliver[ing] powerful age-reversing ingredients" is great marketing but simply not true. There is nothing particularly unique about this Serum that separates it from other well-formulated moisturizers in this line or others. It is a very good moisturizer for normal to slightly dry skin. It contains mostly water, film-forming agent, glycerin, slip agents, antioxidant, water-binding agents, and anti-irritants. That's great but not age-reversing.

✔☺ **Anew Positivity Empowering A.M. Fortifier, SPF 15** *($20 for 1 ounce)* is a very good in-part avobenzone-based sunscreen that also contains water, silicones, thickeners, lactic acid, plant extracts, vitamins, water-binding agents, more thickeners, fragrance film-forming agent, and preservatives.

☺ **Positivity Recharging P.M. Replenisher** *($25 for 1 ounce)* has over 57 ingredients, so you might hope something in here could live up to the promise of reducing hot flashes for those having warm moments in their middle years. But this 2% AHA product won't do it. The plant extracts are nice but have no effect on the hormonal rush or change in skin texture that a lack of estrogen can cause. Several of the plant extracts (particularly soy and black cohosh) do contain phytoestrogens (meaning a plant source of estrogen), but the minuscule amounts in this product do not have any potential for estrogenic effects on the skin. Positivity also contains saw palmetto. There is some anecdotal information that saw palmetto can have an estrogenic effect, but that is unlikely, and is highly improbable when applied topically. This is also replete with good water-binding agents, anti-irritants, and antioxidants, which is great for skin. If you ignore the trappings for the over-50 set and have dry skin you won't be disappointed.

☺ **$$$ Anew Pure O2, Oxygenating Youth Complex SPF 15** *($24 for 1.7 ounces)* is a good, in-part avobenzone-based sunscreen that is dispensed as a mousse, although the propane and isobutane (the propellants that drive the mousse out of the container) are not a source of oxygen. And there are no other oxygen or oxygen-releasing ingredients in this product. But that's actually good news, because oxygen is not a skin-friendly ingredient. The whole basis for the antioxidant craze is using them to keep oxidative substances—one of which is oxygen—off the skin. Adding more oxygen to the skin would cause far more problems than it could possibly help. The interesting assortment of antioxidants this moisturizer contains are what could have made it really special, but the butane and propane gases used to create the mousse-like delivery system would most likely make the antioxidants unstable. Other than being a decent (albeit overpriced) sunscreen, this is a good, lightweight, silicone-based lotion that would work OK for someone with normal to slightly dry skin. The light lotion formula makes it suitable even for someone who tends to break out. It does contain fragrance.

☺ **Anew Retroactive Age Reversal Cream** *($24 for 1.7 ounce)*. If only the name of this product were true, then all plastic surgeons would have to close up shop tomorrow! This is just a good moisturizer for normal to dry skin, nothing more, nothing less. It has a good blend of water-binding agents and silicones but that's about it. Some great antioxidants and anti-irritants would have been far more impressive. It does contain coloring and fragrance.

☺ **Anew Skintrition Multi-Vitamin Skin Primer** *($16 for 1.7 ounces)*. If you were looking for every vitamin and mineral under the sun, this product contains them (well, almost). The amounts are negligible, but no one has any information about how much the skin needs of any of this stuff anyway, so you may as well hedge your bets with this one. This lightweight, silicone-based moisturizer would be good for normal to slightly dry skin and it competes nicely with Estee Lauder's Nutritious Bio Protein ($45 for 1.7 ounces) and Origins' Night-A-Mins ($28.50 for 1.7 ounces). Avon's version contains mostly water, silicones, slip agents, salt, thickener, lots of vitamins and minerals, plant oil, preservatives, and fragrance.

☺ $$$ Anew Dramatic Smoother Facial Mask *($14 for 2.5 ounces)* is a standard clay mask with a small amount of alcohol and an even smaller amount of glycolic acid. The alcohol is drying but the amount is probably insignificant, plus the glycolic acid is ineffective for exfoliation.

☺ $$$ Anew Line Eliminator Lip Complex *($10 for 0.33 ounce)*. Nothing in this product will eliminate one line on your face. This is just a good lip emollient that contains mostly water, glycerin, thickeners, Vaseline, retinol, vitamin C, silicones, film-forming agent, preservatives, and fragrance. Retinol and vitamin C can be helpful for skin but the amounts are negligible.

AVON CLEARSKIN

☹ Clearskin Deep Pore Cleanser *($5.29 for 5.1 ounces)* lists the fourth detergent-cleansing agent as sodium lauryl sulfate, which makes it potentially too irritating for all skin types. There are lots of good cleansers of this type to be found that don't include problematic ingredients.

☹ Clearskin Extra Strength Cleansing Pads *($4.29 for 42 pads)* contain alcohol and menthol, which makes the product too irritating and drying for all skin types, especially sensitive skin.

☹ Clearskin Medicated Gel Wash *($5.29 for 5.1 ounces)* is a detergent-based cleanser with 2% salicylic acid. In a cleanser, the effectiveness of the salicylic acid would just be washed away, plus the main cleansing agent, sodium C14-16 olefin sulfonate, can be very drying and irritating.

☹ Clearskin Cleansing Scrub *($4.29 for 2.5 ounces)* is OK as a scrub, but the plant oil is not great for anyone with oily skin, and the menthol and alcohol are irritating for all skin types.

☹ Clearskin Extra Strength Astringent Cleansing Lotion *($4.29 for 8 ounces)*. The primary ingredient is alcohol (it's listed even before the water), which makes it too drying and irritating for any skin type.

☹ Clearskin Anti-Shine Treatment *($5.29 for 1.7 ounces)* is similar to the Extra Strength Astringent Cleansing Lotion above and the same comments apply.

☹ Clearskin Overnight Acne Treatment *($5.29 for 2 ounces)* contains alcohol as the second ingredient, which makes it too irritating and drying for all skin types.

☹ Clearskin Clay Mask *($3.99 for 3.4 ounces)* is a standard clay mask with alcohol and cornstarch, two very problematic ingredients for acne-prone skin.

☹ Clearskin Targeted Blemish Remover *($5.29 for 0.5 ounce)* lists its two primary ingredients as alcohol, plus it also contains peppermint, which makes it too drying and irritating for any skin types. Ouch!

AVON PORE-FECTION LINE

☺ **Pore-fection Cleanser** *($7 for 6.7 ounces)* is a standard detergent-based cleanser that also contains clay, which can leave the skin feeling smooth but slightly difficult to rinse off the skin.

☹ **Pore-fection Mattifier** *($8 for 1.7 ounces)*. The second ingredient listed is alcohol, which makes it too drying and irritating for any skin type. Plus, despite the claim, it does contain ingredients that can potentially clog pores.

☹ **Pore-fection Mask** *($8 for 3.4 ounces)* is similar to the Pore-fection Mattifier above and the same comments apply.

MISCELLANEOUS AVON PRODUCTS

☺ **Keep It Clean! Multi-Vitamin Cleanser** *($6 for 6.7 ounces)*. The fourth listed detergent cleansing agent is sodium lauryl sulfate, which is potentially too irritating for all skin types. There are lots of good cleansers of this type to be found that don't include problematic ingredients.

☺ **Forgive & Forget Eye Makeup Remover Pencil** *($5 for 0.10 ounce)* is a clever idea: a waxy, silicone-based pencil that can remove makeup. This isn't the most sanitary way to deal with eye-makeup removal. How would you keep the pencil clean? An eye-makeup remover or oil on a cotton swab you toss away after you use is far better for your eyes.

☺ **Moisture Effective Eye Makeup Remover Lotion** *($3.50 for 2 ounces)* is just water, mineral oil, Vaseline, some thickeners, and preservatives. This would work, but so does plain mineral oil or plain Vaseline.

☺ **Perfect Wear Makeup Remover** *($4.50 for 2 ounces)* is a very standard, but very good, silicone-based eye-makeup remover. It can take off makeup and doesn't leave a greasy film on the skin. It does contain fragrance.

☹ **Keep It Fresh! Multi-Vitamin Toner** *($6 for 5.1 ounces)* lists the second ingredient as alcohol, which isn't refreshing in the least, but instead just drying and irritating.

☹ **7 Day Wonder Intensive Skin Moisture Ampoules** *($35 for 7 ampoules; 1 week supply)*. The only wonder about this product is why a chemist could think alcohol would be appropriate as one of the primary ingredients in a moisturizer.

✓☺ **Age Block Environmental Protection Cream, SPF 15** *($12.50 for 1.7 ounces)* is a very good, in-part avobenzone-based sunscreen. It has a fairly standard moisturizing base that also includes some antioxidants and water-binding agents. It would work well for normal to dry skin. It does contain fragrant plant extracts.

✓☺ **Banishing Cream Skin Lightening Treatment** *($8.50 for 2.5 ounces)* is a very good 2% hydroquinone-based skin-lightening product. It lacks any other interesting ingredients, but with its melanin-inhibiting properties it would do the job.

☺ **Basics Face Cream, Rich Moisture** *($4.99 for 3.4 ounces)*. Calling this basic is an understatement! It is little more than water, slip agent, alcohol, thickeners, plant oil, lanolin oil, fragrance, and coloring agents. Your skin deserves a lot more than this.

☺ **Basics Face Cream, Vita Moist** *($4.99 for 3.4 ounces)* is just water, mineral oil, Vaseline, thickeners, a teeny amount of antioxidants, preservatives, and fragrance. The price is the only good thing about this product. For dry skin it would work, but the health of your skin calls for more than this.

☺ **Botanisource Comforting Moisture Cream** *($9.50 for 1.7 ounces)* is actually a very good, silicone-based moisturizer that would work well for someone with normal to dry skin. It contains some excellent water-binding agents, antioxidants, and anti-irritants. Some of the plant extracts can be skin irritants and it contains fragrance.

☹ **Botanisource Eye Comfort Gel** *($7.50 for 0.5 ounce)* contains several plant extracts that can be good anti-irritants and also some good water-binding agents. However, witch hazel (the second ingredient) can be a skin irritant, and the salicylic acid is not best for the eye area.

☺ **Dramatic Firming Cream for Face and Throat** *($12 for 1.7 ounces)* is a very good moisturizer for any part of the body if you have dry skin. Regrettably, the arnica can be a skin irritant if it is used repeatedly.

☺ **$$$ Eye Block Environmental Protection Cream** *($9.50 for 0.5 ounce)* is a good in-part avobenzone-based sunscreen that also contains a good assortment of antioxidants and some water-binding agents. Of concern is the fourth ingredient, which is alcohol. I suspect it isn't enough to be a problem, but there is no way to be sure.

☹ **Hydrofirming Day Cream SPF 15** *($11.50 for 1.7 ounces)* doesn't contain the UVA-protecting ingredients of titanium dioxide, zinc oxide, or avobenzone, and is not recommended, which is a shame because it contains an excellent array of water-binding agents, antioxidants, and anti-irritants.

☹ **Hydrofirming Day Lotion SPF 15** *($11.50 for 1.7 ounces)* is similar to the Hydrofirming Day Cream above and the same comments apply.

✓☺ **Hydrofirming Night Cream** *($11.50 for 1.7 ounces)* contains mostly water, glycerin, Vaseline, thickeners, plant oils, plant extracts, antioxidants, water-binding agents, silicones, fragrance, and preservatives. This is an excellent moisturizer for normal to dry skin.

✓☺ **Hydrofirming Eye Cream** *($9.50 for 0.5 ounce)* is similar to the Hydrofirming Night Cream above and the same basic comments apply.

☺ **Lighten Up Plus Undereye Treatment** *($15 for 0.5 ounce)* is a very good moisturizer for dry skin that contains mostly water, silicones, slip agent, water-binding agents, Vaseline, antioxidants, plant oil, and preservatives. However, the vitamin K (phytonadione) in it has no research showing it can be effective for dark circles.

✓☺ **Moisture 24 Long-Lasting Hydrating Cream** *($11 for 1.7 ounces)* won't last any longer on the skin than any other well-formulated moisturizer in the Avon lineup. This one contains good emollients, water-binding agents, and antioxidants and is an excellent option for dry skin. It does contain fragrance and coloring agents.

☺ **Moisture Therapy Extra Strength Cream** *($5.99 for 5.3 ounces)* is a very basic and rather boring moisturizer for dry skin.

☹ **Multi-Boost Daily Vitamin Moisturizing Cream, SPF 15** *($8 for 2.5 ounces)* doesn't contain the UVA-protecting ingredients of titanium dioxide, zinc oxide, or avobenzone, and is not recommended.

☺ **Nurtura Replenishing Cream** *($9 for 1.7 ounces)* is a good basic moisturizer for normal to dry skin.

☺ **Refraiche Me Restorative Moisturizing Lotion** *($20 for 1.7 ounces)* contains several plant extracts that are potentially irritating, including balm mint and rosemary. It also contains plant extracts that are anti-irritants. This is more confusing than moisturizing.

☺ **Ultimat-E Vitamin E Cream** *($8 for 1.7 ounces)* is a silicone-based moisturizer that definitely contains some vitamin E, and a teeny amount of water-binding agents. It also contains about 3% glycolic acid, but the pH of this cream isn't appropriate for it to be an exfoliant. This can be an OK moisturizer for normal to dry skin. It does contain fragrance.

☹ **Virtual Lift Instant Results Serum** *($12 for 1 ounce)* lists the second ingredient as alcohol, and that won't lift anything, though it can cause irritation and dryness.

☹ **Deep Cleansing Warming Mask** *($7.50 for 2.5 ounces)* contains peppermint oil, which doesn't deep clean, though it can cause irritation.

☹ **Magic Matte Oil-Absorbing Films** *($5.99 for 50 films)* are films of plastic (polypropylene) with some mineral oil. That isn't magic and this has minimal oil-absorbing properties.

☹ **Super Hydrating Cooling Mask** *($7.50 for 2.5 ounces)*. The cooling effect from this mask comes from a form of menthone (a primary constituent of peppermint) that can be a skin irritant.

☹ **Moisture Therapy Moisturizing Lip Treatment SPF 15** *($1.49 for 0.15 ounces)* does not contain the UVA-protecting ingredients of titanium dioxide, zinc oxide, or avobenzone, and is not recommended.

☺ **On Everyone's Lips Daily Lip Refiner** *($8.50 for 0.5 ounce)* is a good, silicone-based moisturizer that also contains some antioxidants and water-binding agents. This would work well for slightly dry skin, but there is nothing in it that makes it unique for the lip area.

AVON SKIN-SO-SOFT

☹ **Skin-So-Soft Bug Guard Plus Moisturizing Lotion, SPF 30** *($12 for 4 ounces)* does not include the UVA-protecting ingredients of titanium dioxide, zinc oxide, or avobenzone, and is not recommended.

☹ **Skin-So-Soft Bug Guard Plus, Moisturizing Lotion, SPF 15** *($12 for 4 ounces)* is similar to the SPF 30 above and the same comments apply.

☺ **Sun-So-Soft Self-Tanning Lotion** *($7.99 for 4.2 ounces)*. As is true for all self-tanners, this one uses dihydroxyacetone to affect skin color. It would work as well as any.

☹ **Sun-So-Soft SPF 8 Sunscreen Spray Lotion** *($7.50 for 4.2 ounces)* does not include the UVA-protecting ingredients of titanium dioxide, zinc oxide, or avobenzone, plus the SPF is below the standards set by the American Academy of Dermatology and the National Cancer Institute. This product is not recommended.

☹ Sun-So-Soft SPF 15 Lip Balm *($1.50 for 0.15 ounce)* does not include the UVA-protecting ingredients of titanium dioxide, zinc oxide, or avobenzone, and is not recommended.

✓☺ $$$ Sun-So-Soft SPF 25 Sunscreen Stick *($7.50 for 0.42 ounce)* is a very good, in-part avobenzone-based sunscreen. It also contains some good water-binding agents and antioxidants. However, it can feel sticky on the skin. It does contain fragrance.

☺ Sun-So-Soft SPF 40 Sunscreen Lotion for Kids *($9 for 4.2 ounces)* is a very good, in-part avobenzone-based sunscreen that would work well for normal to dry skin. There is nothing in this product that makes it better for children than adults. It would be far more interesting for all skin types if it contained good antioxidants and water-binding agents.

☺ Sun-So-Soft Sunscreen Lotion SPF 15 *($8.50 for 4.2 ounces)* is similar to the SPF 40 Sunscreen Lotion for Kids above and the same comments apply.

☺ Sun-So-Soft Sunscreen Lotion SPF 30 *($8.50 for 4.2 ounces)* is similar to the SPF 40 Sunscreen Lotion for Kids above and the same comments apply.

AVON MAKEUP

The best reason to consider several of Avon's makeup products is price. Avon continues to offer a full assortment of value-priced makeup that is often advertised for even less than the suggested retail prices that appear below. If you find a great product here, there is every reason to expect a bargain, particularly if you shop from Avon's user-friendly Web site. There are always special promotions, free gifts, and other enticements that are sure to appease those who can't fathom buying a lipstick or blush and not getting something extra, even if it is an unnecessary item. (Do any of us really need another tote bag?)

What's disconcerting about Avon's makeup is that the products are a mix of clear winners and poor losers. There isn't much middle ground here, and for the most part you will either be pleased or perturbed with your selection. Avon excels with most of their foundations (though there are a fair number of must-avoid shades), most of the blush options, all of their powders and concealers, and their lipsticks. The line disappoints with mediocre to inferior eyeshadows, liquid liner, eye pencils, and mascaras. Since few Avon representatives have a variety of makeup testers or color samples, you're left to base your decision on the opinion of the salesperson, your own judgment, or a picture of the color—which is not always the best way to go. For one thing, these methods don't help you determine how a product will feel and perform once it is on the skin. However, Avon does have a brilliant and easy return policy, especially if you make your purchase online. For those of you who feel confident choosing shades without seeing and trying them in person, this may be a non-issue. Others can look at Avon's return policy as security that Avon stands by its claim of "If you're not happy, we're not." Now if only they would take that slogan and direct it toward improving the underachieving elements of their makeup selection, this line would be considered a must-shop!

FOUNDATION: ☺ **Incredible Finish Foundation SPF 8** *($7)* has an in-part titanium dioxide–based sunscreen, but a woefully low SPF number. This comes in a tube and has a slightly runny texture and a slick feel. It applies smoothly and leaves a natural matte finish. If you have normal to slightly oily skin and prefer light coverage, this is an option. There are 16 shades available, but almost half of them are too rose or pink for most skin tones. Avoid Natural Cream, Blush Beige, Natural Fawn, Honey Beige, Beautiful Bronze, Toast, and Cappuccino. **Hydra Finish Stick Foundation SPF 8** *($9)* is a water-to-powder stick foundation that has the requisite cool, wet application and dries quickly to a reasonably solid powder finish. Although the texture is light, it will take practice before you can easily obtain a streak-free application. It is a suitable option for those with normal to oily skin who wish to use a stick foundation and want sheer coverage, but a separate sunscreen must be applied with it because the SPF of 8, even if it is a titanium dioxide–based sunscreen, is too low for adequate protection. The 16 shades provide options for very light and dark skin tones. The following colors are too peach, pink, or rose for most skin tones: Natural Cream, Honey Beige, Warmest Beige, Rich Honey, Blush Beige, Almond Beige, and Natural Fawn. Toast and Cappuccino are excellent for dark skin tones. **Face Lifting Moisture Firm Foundation Cream Souffle** *($9)* is a light, creamy foundation that would work well for someone with dry skin. It doesn't lift skin anywhere, but it does blend smoothly and provides light to medium coverage. There are 16 shades, and some of them are decent options, but consider avoiding the following colors: Natural Fawn, Soft Bisque, Ivory Beige, Rich Honey, Warmest Beige, Honey Beige, Almond Beige, Blush Beige, Toast, and Beautiful Bronze.

☺ **Beyond Color Illuminating Radiance Vitamin C Foundation SPF 12** *($11)* comes in a jar and has a moist, foamy, whipped-cream appearance and feel. Although the formula is prone to separation, it does blend easily over the skin and leaves a satin-matte finish. It also contains a sunscreen that is part titanium dioxide, which is good, but SPF 12 falls short of the desired SPF 15 benchmark for long-wearing and reliable sun protection. Nonetheless, if you combine this with an additional sunscreen product (pressed powder or moisturizer) it is an OK option for normal to slightly dry skin seeking medium coverage. There are 16 shades, and although there are some good options for light and dark skin tones, half of them should be avoided. Natural Cream, Ivory Beige, Warmest Beige, Rich Honey, Blush Beige, Honey Beige, and Beautiful Bronze are too pink, peach, or rose for almost all skin tones. **Perfect Match Wet/Dry Powder** *($9)* will only be a perfect match if your skin tone resembles one of the six merely OK colors. This is a standard, talc-based powder foundation that has a silicone base, so it applies easily without looking too thick. Wet application tends to harden the powder cake, making this unusable if you later wish to apply it dry. The light-coverage matte finish is a decent option for normal to slightly oily skin. **Invisible Light Illuminating Makeup Base** *($10)* is a standard, silicone-based primer that contains mica and imparts a subtle shine on the skin. Avon suggests using this under makeup or alone to create "instant perfection." This won't perfect the skin but is fine as a lightweight moisturizer to use under foundation, and the shine is essentially covered when this is used in tandem with a foundation.

☹ **Perfect Wear All-Day Comfort Foundation SPF 10** *($9)* does have a titanium dioxide–based sunscreen, but the too-low SPF 10 makes it a poor choice for a day's worth of sun protection. This is Avon's version of a stay-put foundation, and it does work OK, although the texture leaves much to be desired, having a dry feel and an almost sticky finish. Also, all of these colors have some amount of sparkle. What is shine doing in a product meant to have a matte, transfer-resistant finish? **Beyond Color Vertical Lift Foundation SPF 8** *($12)* has a reliable titanium-dioxide–based sunscreen but an unimpressive SPF, so it should not be trusted for daily protection. Basically, this is just a very lightweight, sheer, silicone-based foundation with a matte, almost staining finish, which would be fine except that the colors are some of the worst I've seen in a long time. For the most part, all of the 15 shades are too peach or pink to consider, and I mean *really* peach or pink. The only ones worth considering are Natural Cream, Classic Ivory, Honey Beige, Toast, and Rich Honey. **Clear Finish Great Complexion Foundation** *($8)* contains 2% salicylic acid (BHA), but the pH of 5 prevents it from having exfoliating properties. Still, this does have a lightweight texture and leaves a soft matte finish that normal to oily skin should appreciate. There are 16 shades; the ones to steer clear of due to overtones of peach, rose, or pink are Soft Bisque, Ivory Beige, Beige, Blush Beige, Natural Fawn, Honey Beige, Beautiful Bronze, and Natural Cream. **Invisible Finish Tinted Smoothing Gel** *($5.50)* is a silicone-based cream designed as a line and wrinkle filler. It has a liquid-cream texture that dries quickly to a grainy powder finish and leaves noticeable sparkles and an unattractive white cast in its wake. Don't count on this for any sort of visible wrinkle reduction, or anything positive for that matter.

CONCEALER: ☺ **Incredible Finish Concealer** *($4.50)* has a creamy, blendable texture and provides light to medium coverage with a natural finish. Creasing should be minimal, and the seven colors are fairly good, particularly the three lightest options. ✔☺ **Perfect Wear Total Coverage Concealer** *($5.50)* comes in a glass jar and has an initial thick feel, but winds up being a light-textured cream-to-powder concealer that offers excellent coverage. The seven shades are quite good, though Medium Neutral can be too rose. This is one to consider for dark circles! ✔☺ **Precise Coverage Concealing Stick** *($5)* is a cream-to-powder concealer in a twist-up tube. This has a great smooth texture that blends well, but it also dries fast to a matte finish with minimal risk of creasing. Of the seven shades, Medium, Light Neutral, and Extra Deep are too orange or pink to recommend.

☺ **Clear Finish Great Complexion Concealer Acne Treatment** *($7.50)* contains 2% salicylic acid, which is great for advanced exfoliation—yet the pH of this concealer is too high to allow that to occur. However, this is a worthwhile matte finish concealer that applies easily and stays put. Due to the BHA, I would not recommend using this in the immediate eye area or on the eyelids, but it works well over other areas of discoloration or on blemishes. Of the seven shades, the only ones to avoid are Extra Deep and Medium Neutral—both are too peach for most skin tones.

☺ <u>POWDER:</u> **Incredible Finish Loose Powder** *($7.50)* is a talc-based powder that goes on smoothly but has a thicker feel than many of today's drier, featherlight powders. The four shades are all excellent, and this is an option for normal to dry skin. ✓☺ **Incredible Finish Pressed Powder** *($7.50)* is also great for normal to dry skin. This talc-based powder possesses a suede-smooth texture that applies evenly without looking heavy or chalky. The seven shades are beautiful. **Clear Finish Great Complexion Pressed Powder** *($8.50)* claims it can keep skin clear, but that is wishful thinking for what amounts to soft-textured, dry-finish pressed powder with 0.6% salicylic acid. When present in such a small amount, salicylic acid isn't of much use, and the pH of a powder is simply too high for it to have any effect on skin. However, the seven shades are beautiful, and there are options for light and dark skin tones.

<u>BLUSH:</u> ☺ **True Color Powder Blush** *($7.50)* has a sheer, silken texture and a pleasant mix of matte and soft shine colors. The shiny hues could work for an evening look, but the following colors are too iridescent for daytime wear: Antiquity, Mad About Mauve, Lilac Dusk, Rose Lustre, Golden Glow Light/Medium, and Golden Glow Dark.

✓☺ **Split Second Blush Stick** *($7.50)* is an exceptional cream-to-powder blush that effortlessly glides over the skin and blends out to a soft, sheer matte finish. This does require expedient blending before it dries in place. It works best if you dab on the color in dots and then blend with a sponge or clean fingers. The color selection is slightly marred by one too many iridescent shades, but there are enough great colors so that it's worth a test run if you prefer this type of blush.

☺ **Illuminating Stick** *($7.50)* is a sheer, creamy, twist-up highlighter that imparts an incredibly soft shine to the skin. This is one you could get away with wearing during the day and not end up looking like you're adorned with sparkles!

☹ **Go With the Glow All Over Face Color** *($5)* is a cream blush that comes in a squeeze tube, and it definitely takes some effort to apply successfully. This has a very thick, toothpaste-like texture, but does blend well over the skin and imparts soft, transparent color and a powder-dry finish. If you're willing to tolerate the extra effort it takes to get this out of the tube (and can control how much comes out), this is worth a look. It comes in six attractive colors, though Elegant is too shiny for daytime wear.

<u>EYESHADOW:</u> ☺ **True Color Powder Eyeshadows** *($3.50 singles; $4.25 duos; $6 quads)* have a soft, blendable texture that applies nicely, though it takes some effort to build intensity. The number of matte shades in each category has decreased, which is disappointing—however, what remains in the Powder Eyeshadow Singles and Duos are worth a look. Each quad set has at least one shiny shade, but the color combinations are attractive.

☹ **Luminous Liquid Eye Color** *($6)*. Who thought that ultra-shiny, but sheer, liquid eyeshadow would be a good idea? Even women who covet shiny lids will likely not want to put up with this product's spotty application, slow drying time, and tendency to crease. To make matters worse, this breaks up and looks terrible on the skin as the day goes by. **Glimmer Lights Eyeshadow** *($6)* are creamy, wax-based, shiny eyeshadows that not only come in some awful colors but also will crease before you're out the door. **Perfect Wear All Day Comfort Eyeshadow** *($6.50)* are wind-up cream-to-powder eyeshadows that have been reformulated to offer a smoother application and drier finish. However, the majority of the colors are outright shiny, and the iridescence tends to flake off on the skin throughout the day. **Beyond Color Triple Benefit Eyeshadow** *($6.50)* calls itself "shadow perfected," but I think a more accurate term would be "shadow rejected." How this ultra-slick cream eyeshadow with high-wattage shine can have even one benefit for the user is beyond me—even minor wrinkles will be more apparent once this is applied.

EYE & BROW SHAPER: ☹ **Perfect Wear Eye Liner** *($5.50)* is an automatic pencil that has a creamy, slightly sticky texture and that tends to fade quickly and smear with little provocation. **Glimmerstick Eye Liner** *($5)* and **Glimmerstick Brow Definer** *($5)* have identical formulas, and both come in automatic, retractable pencils, feel slick, and are too creamy to last for long, particularly as eyeliner. If you prefer pencils, there are better ones available in this price range from Revlon, L'Oreal, and others. **Color Glide Liquid Eyeliner** *($5)* is an awful liquid liner that applies a thick line of spasmodic color that sets quickly but can smear, chip, and flake throughout the day.

☺ **Brow Powder** *($6)* comes in three very good talc-based matte finish colors. Each shade goes on sheer, which can be a plus if you're new to using a powder for brow defining. Seasoned brow veterans will likely find this too time-consuming compared to a more pigmented matte powder eyeshadow. **Eyewriter Liquid Eyeliner** *($6)* is a fountain pen-style liquid eyeliner that goes on intense with an easy-glide, tapered brush. The one drawback is that it's all too easy for the color to smudge before it's dried—and this doesn't dry as quickly as many others. **Ultra Luxury Eyeliner** *($4)* has an attractive price for a standard pencil that applies easily and offers a smooth, dry finish. Strangely, this is still prone to mild smearing as the day wears on. **Big Color Eye Pencil** *($5)* are standard chunky pencils that have a smooth, silicone-enhanced application and a soft, slightly creamy finish. Every color is quite shiny, but if that's your thing these do hold up reasonably well. **Ultra Luxury Brow Liner** *($4)* is an ordinary brow pencil that has the typical stiff, dry texture, but it is easier to apply than most. The price is right, and this is one to consider if you prefer brow pencil to powder.

LIPSTICK AND LIP PENCIL: ☺ **Beyond Color Nutralush Plumping Lipstick SPF 12** *($8)* goes on and on about how its collagen-enriched Superplump Complex creates "visibly fuller, smoother, younger-looking lips," but it ends up being just a standard, but good, opaque creamy lipstick. As far as plump, full lips are concerned, you won't be mistaken for Julia Roberts or Angelina Jolie, and don't expect lips to get any younger, especially since the sunscreen lacks adequate UVA protection. **Ultra Color Rich Renewable Lipstick** *($6.50)* is available in three formulas and finishes. The **Velvet Mattes** are not matte in the least but do offer an elegant, creamy-opaque texture. The **Satin** leans to the greasy side of creamy, and is not for anyone who battles with lipstick feathering into lines around the mouth, while the **Sheer SPF 15** is simply a glossy lipstick with transparent colors. The SPF 15 is great, but it doesn't contain the UVA-protecting ingredients of titanium dioxide, zinc oxide, or avobenzone, and cannot be relied on for adequate sun protection. **Brilliant Moisture Lipcolor** *($6.50)* brags about how its rich moisturizers keep lips soft for 24 hours and, given that this is a fairly straightforward cream lipstick formula, I suppose that's true—provided you keep reapplying this lipstick over the course of a day. This does have a comfortably smooth texture and offers full coverage with a creamy finish. **Glazewear Liquid Lip Color** *($5)* is a very good, full-coverage lip gloss that has a slick application and a non-sticky, glossy finish. The color range presented here is gorgeous. The **Lip Artist Color Collection** *($7.50)* features four creamy lip colors and one shimmery lip color in one compact. There are five different sets, and all of them are well coordinated. Each compact also includes a lip brush, which works OK but isn't as elegant as many others—still, at this price, that's a minor quibble.

☺ **Ultra Luxury Lip Liner** *($4)* has a great price for a standard pencil that isn't too dry or too creamy for precision. The well-edited color selection makes this even more worthwhile! **Glimmerstick Lip Liner** *($5)* has a slightly too-soft texture, but otherwise works well for a silicone-based, automatic, retractable lip pencil. The Glimmer Clear shade works reasonably well to keep lipstick from bleeding into lines around the mouth.

☺ **Beyond Color Nutralush Lip Conditioner SPF 12** *($8)* is fine for an emollient lip balm, but does not contain avobenzone, titanium dioxide, or zinc oxide, and is not recommended for sun protection. **Perfect Wear Double Performance Lipstick** *($8)* is Avon's ultra-matte lipstick, but it is not all that matte. Rather, it has a very slick texture and a slightly creamy finish. These lipsticks do have a lot of stain, which makes for longer wear. More than half of the colors are frosted, while the rest have an opaque, flat finish.

☹ **Perfect Wear Ever Glaze Lip Ink** *($8)* is Avon's version of Max Factor's Lipfinity ($12.49), and it ends up being no competition for that formidable long-wearing lipstick. The Lip Ink is primarily water, film-forming agent, glycerin, and pigment. Avon claims this leaves a semi-matte finish, but it actually leaves an opaque, dry finish that only feels drier the longer it is on. To remedy this, you can apply **Perfect Wear Ever Glaze Lip Gloss** *($7)* over the color without causing it to smear or come off. Just like Lipfinity's Moisturizing Top Coat, this extra step significantly enhances comfort and provides a glossy finish. However, the Lip Ink gradually peels and flakes off and tends to collect in the corner of the mouth, so it looks as if you have just eaten a big handful of cookies, but have forgotten to use a napkin. In trying to reach the next plateau of long-wearing lipstick, all Avon has provided is a short-term-wear ultra-matte lipstick that is tolerable only if used with the lip gloss, which is sold separately.

<u>MASCARA:</u> ☹ **Extreme Volume Flexicoat Maximizing Mascara** *($6)* has a tongue-twisting name that makes this sound like *the* mascara for women with short or sparse

lashes. This ends up being a disappointment, building merely OK length and thickness while flaking and smearing easily.

☺ **Incredible Lengths Long and Strong Mascara** *($6)* builds excellent length and decent thickness without clumping. This does smear a bit before it dries if you're not careful, but otherwise it's a winner. ✓☺ **Curl-Ascious Maximum Curling Mascara** *($6)* is my favorite Avon mascara. The no-nonsense formula is adept at adding length and some thickness, and lends a soft curl to the lashes as it dries. It does not go on too heavily, and builds evenly—so you're left with nicely defined lashes that never look clumpy or spiked.

☺ **Wash-Off Waterproof Mascara** *($6)*. The best thing about this lackluster mascara (and the only reason to consider it) is that it really is waterproof. If you're after length and thickness that will prompt shameless eyelash fluttering, look elsewhere.

☺ **Astonishing Lengths Lengthening & Defining Mascara** *($7)* is a very good clump-free lengthening mascara, although it tends to flake, so recommending this is iffy. What would really be astonishing is if Avon's mascaras were as good as those from comparably priced L'Oreal or Maybelline.

AVON beComing

Avon launched its Avon beComing department-store brand of skin-care and makeup products in August 2001. The company had originally intended to unveil the new line at Sears stores across the country, and had to work fast to find alternate locations when Sears announced it was eliminating almost everything from the cosmetics departments in their retail outlets and catalog. After some negotiating, J.C. Penney was selected as the new home for the Avon beComing line of products, with the hopes of opening in many, if not all, of their 1,600 locations over a period of time. Whether or not that ever takes place is yet to be seen. This line has had an incredibly shaky beginning that it may not be able to overcome.

According to a press release for beComing, it is a line meant to speak to a woman's "aspiration and self-actualization." How a skin-care and makeup line can accomplish this is a bit of mystery, but then the world of cosmetics is often more about astute positioning than real differences between products. Possibly the diversity of the line will speak louder than anything else. Avon wants beComing to add baby products, new-mother products, aromatherapy, sports products, vitamins, and fragrances. This isn't such a daunting task for Avon when you consider the stable of over 1,000 products they maintain in their other product lines and the fact that they are one of the largest cosmetics companies in the world. For more information on beComing locations, call (866) IBECOME or visit www.ibecome.com and www.avon.com.

AVON beComing SKIN CARE

☺ **All Gone Cleansing Makeup Remover** *($12 for 3.4 ounces)* is a fairly standard, wipe-off makeup remover than can leave a slightly greasy film on the skin. This can be an option for dry skin, though wiping off makeup is not best for the skin. The teeny amount of grapefruit extract present means it won't be a skin irritant. It does contain fragrance.

☹ **Clean Gesture Hydrating Foam Cleanser** *($12 for 6.8 ounces)* is a foaming cleanser that uses potassium hydroxide as the main cleansing agent, and that makes this a fairly alkaline cleanser that can be too drying and irritating for most skin types.

☺ **Cool Current Purifying Gel Cleanser** *($12 for 6.8 ounces)* is a standard, detergent-based cleanser that would work well for normal to oily skin. It contains fragrance.

☹ **Gone with a Wipe Instant Cleansing Cloths** *($12 for 45 wipes)* lists alcohol as the second ingredient, and with that the only thing that will happen instantly is a feeling of dryness followed by eventual irritation.

☹ **Get Clear Refreshing Mist** *($12 for 5 ounces)* is basically just glycerin and a detergent cleansing agent along with some plant extracts. The cleansing agent can be fairly drying and the orange and grapefruit extract can be irritating. There are better toners for skin than this.

☺ **Get Supple Hydrating Mist** *($12 for 5 ounces)* is basically just glycerin and rose water, along with some good antioxidants and water-binding agents. For a toner this is a very good option for most skin types, though the rose water can be a skin sensitizer.

☺ **Get Vital Rejuvenating Mist** *($12 for 5 ounces)* contains mostly water, glycerin, slip agent, ginseng, water-binding agents, plant extracts, film-forming agent, fragrance, and preservatives. If ginseng isn't a problem for your skin this can be a good toner for most skin types.

☺ **$$$ Soothing Booster** *($20 for 0.5 ounce)* is a very good, serum-style moisturizer that is meant to be worn under one of the other moisturizers in the line. It ends up being little more than a thick toner with some good antioxidants. It isn't necessary. Most of beComing's moisturizers have plenty of good antioxidants, so it makes me wonder if adding this to the mix suggests Avon doesn't trust the quality of their moisturizers. It contains mostly water, slip agents, glycerin, antioxidants, fragrance, and preservatives. This can be an option for normal to slightly dry skin or for slightly oily skin with dry areas, but it lacks a good assortment of water-binding agents.

☺ **$$$ Detoxifying Booster** *($20 for 0.5 ounce)* is similar to the Soothing Booster above, and the same comments apply.

✓☺ **$$$ Hydrating Booster** *($20 for 0.5 ounce)* is similar in style to the Soothing Booster above, only with a more impressive selection of water-binding agents and plant oils, which makes it better for someone with normal to dry skin. It still isn't necessary to add this step, but worn alone it is a good lightweight moisturizer for normal to slightly dry or combination skin. It does contain fragrance.

☹ **Equalizing Booster** *($20 for 0.5 ounce)* lists alcohol as the third ingredient, so this is probably too irritating and potentially drying for all skin types.

☹ **Retexturing Booster** *($20 for 0.5 ounce)* is similar to the Equalizing Booster above, and the same comments apply.

✔☺ $$$ **Skinfusion Revitalizing Complex SPF 15** *($40 for 1.7 ounces)* is a good, in-part avobenzone-based sunscreen. It contains a couple of good antioxidants and water-binding agents that are in several other Avon moisturizers that cost far less than this overpriced version.

✔☺ $$$ **Skinfusion Renewal Complex Night** *($40 for 1.7 ounces)* is a very good moisturizer for dry skin. It contains mostly water, antioxidants, thickeners, glycerin, Vaseline, more thickeners, silicone, retinol, water-binding agents, plant extracts, film-forming agent, fragrance, and preservatives. Retinol won't renew skin but it can be a good antioxidant.

☺ **Luminous Transfirm Contouring Treatment** *($35 for 1.7 ounces)* is supposed to "Instantly, reveal renewed brilliance and achieve precision contouring over time with this age-proof treatment. Transfirm's 3-D Sculpting Complex and advanced age-fighting factors visibly firm and contour in as little as three days, giving skin a virtual mini-lift." I guess if it doesn't work for you in three days you can always return it. If you don't want to waste your time, what you end up getting, aside from the typical tired claim of an age-free, lifted face, is a silicone-based moisturizer for normal to dry skin that contains some very good water-binding agents, anti-irritants, a small amount of antioxidants, and subtle shine. The shine is the luminous part, but that is hardly transfirming. This is a good moisturizer with over-inflated, exaggerated claims.

☹ **Brighter Days Moisture Lotion SPF 15** *($15 for 1.7 ounces)*; **Brighter Days Intensive Moisture Cream SPF 15** *($15 for 1.7 ounces)*; and **Brighter Days Light Moisture Lotion SPF 15** *($15 for 1.7 ounces)* do not contain the UVA-protecting ingredients of avobenzone, zinc oxide, or titanium dioxide, and are not recommended.

☺ **Resist the Elements SPF 15 Sunscreen Body** *($13.50 for 2 ounces)* is a very good in-part avobenzone-based sunscreen in a good moisturizing base for normal to dry skin.

✔☺ **Resist the Elements SPF 30 Sunscreen Face** *($13.50 for 2 ounces)* is similar to SPF 15 Sunscreen Body above and the same comments apply. This one does contain an impressive mix of antioxidants.

☹ **Resist the Elements Protective Lip Balm SPF 15** *($5 for 0.15 ounce)* does not contain the UVA-protecting ingredients of titanium dioxide, zinc oxide, or avobenzone, and is not recommended.

☺ $$$ **Eye Wish Super Firming Complex** *($22 for 0.5 ounce)*. With aluminum starch octenylsuccinate as the fourth ingredient, this ends up being a rather matte-finish and fairly nonmoisturizing eye product. It does have small amounts of water-binding agents at the end of an exceptionally long list of ingredients, which is nice, but that still won't change the problem of the more primary ingredient. I would recommend the other more-moisturizing options from this line for the eye area.

☺ $$$ **Pack Your Bags De-Puffing Eye Gel** *($24 for 0.5 ounce)* is an interesting mix of soothing agents, anti-irritants, antioxidants, water-binding agents, and some plant extracts that may be irritants. All in all, this has far more positives than negatives for normal to slightly dry skin, but there is nothing in this product that will reduce puffiness under eyes.

☺ **Evening Retreat Moisture Cream** *($20 for 1.7 ounces)* is a very good moisturizer for normal to dry skin that contains mostly water, silicones, thickeners, glycerin, antioxidants, water-binding agents, plant extracts, mineral oil, fragrance, and preservatives.

☺ **Evening Retreat Intensive Moisture Cream** *($20 for 1.7 ounces)* is similar to the Retreat Moisture Cream above but with Vaseline as the third ingredient, which makes it more appropriate for dry to very dry skin.

☹ **Evening Retreat Light Moisture Lotion** *($20 for 1.7 ounces)* is similar to the Retreat Moisture Cream above but in lotion form. The second ingredient in this product is a synthetic sunscreen ingredient, octyl methoxycinnamate, and it's completely out of place in a nighttime moisturizer. It's a good sunscreen ingredient, but a poor moisturizer.

☺ **$$$ Off Line Anti-Wrinkle Quick Click** *($24 for 0.5 ounce)* has a clever name, and is a decent, serum-style moisturizer that contains several good antioxidants and water-binding agents in a silicone-base. It would work well for someone with normal to slightly dry skin. It does contain fragrance.

☹ **See Spot Go Acne Treatment** *($15 for 0.33 ounce)* contains salicylic acid, which would be an option for breakouts, except that the second ingredient is alcohol, which makes it too drying and irritating for all skin types.

☹ **Matte About You Anti-Shine Solution** *($15 for 1.7 ounces)* lists alcohol as the second ingredient; added to that, the inclusion of grapefruit extract can make this too irritating for all skin types.

☹ **$$$ Liphoria Maximum Lip Conditioner** *($9.50 for 0.1 ounce)* is a good, but basic, lip moisturizer that is somewhat more like spackle than an emollient for lips. It does have a small amount of interesting water-binding agents, but overall your lips won't feel all that conditioned.

AVON beComing MAKEUP

The Avon beComing line picks up some steam when it comes to makeup. Titled beComing Radiant, the line generally offers some very good, inexpensive options. There are only three foundations, which seems minimal from a powerhouse like Avon, but they are impressive, and you can be assured there will likely be more formulas in the not-so-distant future. The lipsticks offer a bevy of color choices, with mostly satisfying formulas, and the mascaras are also worth considering.

Where the makeup loses momentum is with the plethora of shiny blushes, eyeshadows, and substandard eye pencils that leave much to be desired when it comes to texture and application. Instead of bucking the shine trend, Avon has chosen to add still more iridescent options to the burgeoning pile. If this line was targeted more to teens than thirty-somethings and baby boomers, I would be more willing to concede the shiny makeup point. But shimmering eyelids and glitter-flecked cheekbones are not what I would call the most "becoming" way to enhance "aspiration and self-actualization" or to empower any modern, professional woman. Not to mention that shiny eyeshadow makes skin look more wrinkly, not less.

FOUNDATION: ☺ **Pure Brilliance Perfect Balance Foundation SPF 8** *($15)* has a very smooth, slick texture—so you'll get lots of movement with this light-textured foundation, which can make blending a bit trickier than usual. However, once it dries it imparts a lovely soft matte finish and provides sheer to light coverage. The sunscreen is part titanium dioxide, but the SPF number is far from brilliant, so you'll still need a separate, adequate sunscreen (meaning SPF 15) with this. Despite the lack of the basic SPF requirement, this foundation is a big improvement over Avon's other foundations sold at kiosks in malls, online, or by catalog. What is most impressive and a step forward are the colors. Of the 15 shades, almost all are beautifully neutral! The only ones to avoid due to overtones of pink or peach are Porcelain, Warm Beige, Wheat, Sand, and Cinnamon. There are shade options for very light skin and dark (but not very dark) skin, too!

✓☺ **Bases Covered Cream to Powder Compact SPF 15** *($15)* is a real find for those who prefer cream-to-powder makeup. It has an exquisite silky, weightless texture that applies and blends easily, offering sheer to light coverage and an in-part titanium dioxide–based sunscreen with an adequate SPF. Cream-to-powder makeups work best on normal to slightly oily skin—and this one will definitely accentuate any dry areas once it has dried to its soft matte finish. Of the ten mostly excellent shades, the only real duds are Porcelain (too pink for most light skin) and Honey (too red for most darker skin tones).

✓☺ **Redefine Airbrush Foundation SPF 10** *($19.50)* is an amazing foundation despite its litany of misleading claims. To begin, Avon calls this an "age-proof foundation" that contains a "3-D Airbrush Complex" that works to camouflage lines, wrinkles, and imperfections. Redefine goes further still, touting natural extracts like shitake mushroom and soy protein to further enhance this already great cocktail. There is nothing in this formula that can age-proof your skin, nor will this do a thing when it comes to firming, lifting, or hiding every line on your face. Yet it will provide a silky, light to medium coverage courtesy of a superior smooth texture that must be felt to be believed. This dries to a soft matte finish that would be appropriate for normal to slightly dry or slightly oily skin. The 15 shades are wonderfully neutral, and the only ones to avoid are Caramel, Cinnamon, Toast, Warm Beige, and Wheat. Aside from the inflated claims, my only other gripe is that Avon stopped at an SPF 10, which is substandard for daytime protection, though the active ingredient is titanium dioxide.

CONCEALER: ☺ **Hide the Evidence Concealing Quick Stick** *($14)* has an adorably appealing name—it's a shame the product performance isn't as foolproof as it sounds. It's packaged in a pen-style container, where you click the base to feed product into the waiting nylon brush tip—a clever idea if you can successfully control how much product is released. It has a soft, creamy texture that does cover well, but blending takes time, and it stays slightly creamy on the skin. That means some creasing will be inevitable, so if you have pronounced lines under the eyes you will want to avoid this product. There are three skin-tone shades as well as one pink tint titled Illuminator and a Yellow Corrector (which isn't nearly as yellow as most), and all but the Illuminator are worthwhile options.

✔☺ $$$ **Beyond Color Line Diminishing Concealer SPF 15** *($6)* has a wonderful creamy, cushiony texture that blends like a dream and sets to a satin finish with only a slight chance of creasing. The in-part titanium dioxide–based sunscreen and four excellent colors make this a slam-dunk choice the next time you're shopping for concealer. The only caveat is that coverage can take some time to build. If you have deep discolorations or very dark circles, this concealer is not the ideal choice.

<u>POWDER:</u> ✔☺ **Smooth Finish Pressed Powder** *($14)* is a fine-textured, talc-based powder that glides on the skin and does not look dry or powdery. There are seven shades, and five of them are great colors with a matte finish. The other two (Radiant and Luminous) are too shiny for daytime wear, but would be options for evening shimmer.

☺ **Shimmer Color** *($6.50)* features small pots of loose, very shiny powder. Although these come in salt-shaker containers, they can still be messy, and this much shine is just distracting. It should be considered only for the occasional gossamer glow for evening— if you don't mind getting it all over your clothes, too, as these don't cling to skin very well.

<u>BLUSH:</u> ☹ **Cheek Color** *($6.50)* is a liquid lotion blush that only comes in two shades, both of which are quite sheer and shiny. These have an undesirable sticky finish, and are a step down from many other liquid and cream blushes available from other lines.

☺ **Added Brilliance Powder Blush & Highlighter** *($14)* is a good concept—pairing an attractive blush color with a lighter shade in the same tonal family. However, Avon waved the shine wand over this product, too, and it only ends up being half of what it could be. The enticing range of blush colors, most of which are very sheer and workable, are matte, while the complementary highlighter shades are glaringly shiny. If the idea of shimmery cheekbones appeals to you, there are more subtle options than this, such as Revlon's Sleek Cheeks Creme Blush Duo ($9.49).

☺ **Light De-Light** *($13)* is a water-to-powder blush stick that has a cool, wet feel on the skin. These sticks can be tricky to blend, and work best over smooth, even-textured skin. The six sheer shades all have a soft shimmer—it's not nearly as obvious as the shimmer of the Added Brilliance Powder Blush & Highlighter above—but they're still best reserved for evening makeup.

<u>EYESHADOW:</u> ☺ **Three Cheers Multi-Look Eye Color** *($14)* are a collection of eyeshadow trios that each contain two powder-based and one cream eyeshadow to be used as a highlighter. Although most of the color combinations are workable, every trio has one shiny powder eyeshadow, and the cream highlighter is ultra-shiny. These go on very sheer and take a while to build any intensity, making them even easier to pass up. **Dynamic Duo Eyecolor & Liner** *($12)* features one shiny powder eyeshadow coupled with shiny powder eyeliner. The shine is fairly subdued, but still enough to enhance an eyelid or underbrow area.

☹ **Eye Color** *($6.50)* are pots of cream-to-powder eyeshadows that come in a most unbecoming array of pastel, cotton-candy hues, and these are primed for maximum shine. Is anyone over the age of 30 really looking for more of this type of product?

EYE AND BROW SHAPER: ☺ **Defining Moment Eye Liner** *($9)* is a too-creamy pencil that won't stay in place for very long, although it does glide on easily. If you use pencils and prefer to smudge them before they smudge on their own, these are worth a look, but please consider avoiding Plum, Blue Kohl, and Emerald. **Double Up Eyeshadow and Eye Liner Duet** *($12)* is a dual-sided automatic pencil that features a sheer, iridescent cream eyeshadow on one end and a very good retractable eye pencil on the other. The poor eyeshadow half makes this whole thing only half as good as it could have been.

☺ **Defining Moment Liquid Liner** *($12)* has a great, flexible brush and applies smoothly and without skipping. The formula dries quickly and then really stays put—no chipping or flaking. Avoid Sapphire, Code Blue, and Golden Bronze if your goal is a sophisticated eye design.

☺ LIPSTICK AND LIP PENCIL: **Liphoria Full Satin Lipcolor** *($9.50)* has a creamy-opaque, slick texture with a slightly greasy finish. These won't induce any euphoria, but you will undoubtedly be impressed with the over 40 shades, from the palest pink to the richest plumy browns. **Lasting Desire Matte Wear Lipcolor** *($9.50)* is not matte in the least. In fact, it's now getting to the point where so many creamy, even greasy lipsticks are being billed as matte that when women finally try on a real matte lipstick they dislike it instantly, and go back to matte-in-name-only lipsticks like this one. These have a slightly less greasy texture than the Liphoria, but there are significantly fewer shades. **Double Up Lipstick and Lip Liner Duet** *($12)* comes with an opaque, nicely creamy lipstick on one end and a very good automatic, retractable lip pencil on the other. This is a convenient product if you happen to like the color combinations, but for some reason, the lipliner color is noticeably darker than the lipstick shade. **Sheer Impact Sheer Shine Lipcolor SPF 15** *($9.50)* is a transparent, slick lipstick with a glossy finish. The SPF 15 is nice but it doesn't contain the UVA-protecting ingredients of titanium dioxide, zinc oxide, or avobenzone, and cannot be relied on for sun protection. For soft, fleeting color these work well. **Shining Moment Lip Gloss Quick Click** *($12)* is packaged identically to the Hide the Evidence Concealing Quick Stick above, only this dispenses a sheer, shimmery lip gloss. Although the texture of Lip Gloss Quick Click is not too sticky, it is easy to dial up too much gloss, and once that happens, there's no putting it back. Still, this is a decent option for gloss if you prefer applying it with a brush. **3-D 3-in-1 Gloss** *($12)* comes in a compact and offers a smooth, non-sticky texture and very sheer, iridescent colors. It's fine as far as gloss goes. **Lip Color** *($6.50)* products are large pots of sheer, shimmery lip color. They're more of a very soft lip tint than a full-on lipstick, and would be a fine option for an understated look. **Defining Moment Lip Liner** *($9)* is a standard, creamy lip pencil that is slightly creamier than most, so don't expect this to help keep most lipsticks in place. The available colors are well-edited and the pencil has a brush at one end for blending the color.

<u>MASCARA:</u> ☺ **On the Fringe All Purpose Mascara** *($11)* is an excellent lengthening mascara that applies quickly and easily with no clumps. It stays on well and removes easily with a water-soluble cleanser.

✔☺ **Swim Wear Waterproof Mascara** *($11)* is an excellent mascara that is not only waterproof but also builds significant length and enough thickness to distinguish itself from most other waterproof mascaras. It also leaves lashes soft, and is relatively easy to remove.

AWAKE

This Japanese-owned cosmetics company has been around since 1995. The company's philosophy is to blend "Japan's technological expertise and its tradition of spiritual aesthetics with US latest fashion trends to create the most advanced skin care and fashionable color." If this represents Japan's cosmetics expertise, they have a ways to go—if I were you I'd stick with Sony. That's because, when it comes to skin care, Awake needs to wake up to some basic information about irritation and skin sensitivity. Their claim that these products are hypoallergenic is inexcusable. The cleansers are fairly strong, lots of the products contain potentially irritating or sensitizing plant extracts, and several contain alcohol.

Some of the comments made about the products defy logic: "skin rejuvenates by retaining oxygen and protecting cells from free radicals." But oxygen causes free-radical damage and therefore cannot protect skin from the very thing it actually generates. Awake's brochure explains that "glycine is an amino acid that makes up 33% of collagen" and implies that glycine can thus somehow affect the production of collagen in skin. It can't. Protein is a complex structure made up of an intricate network of amino acids, and triggering just one won't get the collagen to change. The technology for these products is not advanced in the least and actually leaves much to be desired. There is nothing in these products that many lines don't do better for far less. For more information about Awake, visit www.awakecosmetics.com.

AWAKE SKIN CARE

☹ **Cleansing Sheets** *($5 for 10 sheets)* lists alcohol as the second ingredient, which makes these too irritating and drying for skin.

☺ **$$$ Clear Cream Wash for Dry Skin** *($28 for 4.2 ounces)* is a standard, detergent-based, water-soluble cleanser that could work OK for normal to oily skin, but the cleansing agents and several plant extracts can be irritating and sensitizing for the skin.

☺ **$$$ Clear Cream Wash for Oily Skin** *($28 for 4.2 ounces)* contains fairly drying cleansing agents that can be too irritating for most skin types, including oily skin. It also contains some potentially irritating plant extracts.

☺ **$$$ Clear Gel Wash for Combination Skin** *($28 for 4.2 ounces)* is similar to the Cream Wash for Dry Skin version above and the same comments apply.

☹ **Deep Purity Clay Wash** *($30 for 4.2 ounces)* is a detergent-based cleanser that uses ground-up plastic as the scrub particles. That would be all right for normal to oily skin, but this also contains sulfur, which makes it deeply irritating.

☹ **Deep Purity Fluid Cleanse** *($36 for 6.7 ounces)* contains alcohol as the third ingredient. The rest is mostly silicone, and together that adds up to a "Why bother?"

☹ **Deep Purity Smoothing Wash** *($40 for 4.2 ounces)* is a standard, detergent-based cleanser that uses ground-up plastic as the exfoliant. It also contains some potentially irritating plant extracts, including coltsfoot, grapefruit, lemon, and lime extracts.

☹ **Deep Purity Smoothing Gel** *($36 for 2 ounces)* lists alcohol as the second ingredient. Ouch!

☺ $$$ **Point Makeup Remover (Eye and Lip)** *($15 for 2.1 ounces)* is basically just plain mineral oil with some film-forming agent, slip agent, plant extracts (some can be skin irritants), and preservatives. If you want this kind of product, your pocketbook would be far happier with just plain mineral oil!

☹ **Lotion Refresher** *($25 for 6.3 ounces).* Several of the plant extracts in this product can be irritating or sensitizing for skin, including ivy, rosemary, watercress, lemon, pine cone, and sage.

☹ **Lotion Exfolizer** *($30 for 3.3 ounces)* lists alcohol as its second ingredient, which makes it a problem for all skin types.

☺ $$$ **Aroma Facial Oil** *($40 for 0.67 ounce)* is just silicones, synthetic fragrance, thickener, macadamia oil, and vitamin E. This can be good for dry skin, but it lacks many components that could make it really worthwhile for skin.

☺ $$$ **Direct Nutrition** *($65 for 1 ounce)* is just a good, basic moisturizer for normal to dry skin that would work well, but it is absurdly overpriced for what you get. Avon has moisturizers with more interesting formulations than this one.

☺ $$$ **Hydro-Force Oil-Free Treatment** *($45 for 1.7 ounces)* is a very good, lightweight moisturizer for normal to slightly dry skin. It is a simple formulation that contains some good antioxidants and water-binding agents.

☹ **Hydro-Plus Eyes** *($45 for 0.7 ounce)* contains far too many irritating ingredients, including alcohol, lemon, ginseng, pine cone, and sage, to make this a benefit for skin, particularly in the eye area.

☹ **Nano Essence AX** *($60 for 0.8 ounce)* is similar to the Hydro-Plus above and the same basic comments apply.

☹ **Nano Lotion White** *($40 for 2.1 ounces)* lists alcohol as its second ingredient, which is a problem for all skin types and doesn't help to lighten skin.

☺ $$$ **Serum Up-Sign Face Essence** *($70 for 1.4 ounces)* is a lightweight moisturizer that contains mostly water, slip agent, thickeners, glycerin, plant oil, anti-irritants, antioxidants, more plant oils, and preservatives. This would work well for someone with normal to oily skin.

☺ $$$ **Skin Renovation** *($95 for 1 ounce)* is a good, lightweight moisturizer for normal to slightly dry skin, but it won't renovate anything and the price is the only thing really significant about this product. The yeast in it won't provide oxygen to the skin as claimed, and the serine, an amino acid, won't affect collagen in skin. Still, this does have some very good water-binding agents and a tiny amount of antioxidants.

☺ $$$ **Skin Renovation Eye** *($90 for 0.7 ounce)* is a basic moisturizer that has some good water-binding agents and vitamin E (antioxidant), but that's about it. It would make your eyes sting if you knew how truly overpriced this product is.

☺ $$$ **Skin Renovation Serum 14** *($180 for 14 ampoules; total 0.62 ounce)*. I'm almost speechless at what an immense waste of money this product is. Not only doesn't it contain anything that can change one wrinkle on your skin, but there are also a lot of products for far less that have better formulations. This contains mostly water, slip agents, water-binding agents, plant oil, thickeners, and preservatives. It is a good lightweight moisturizer, but that's it, and I mean that's *all*.

☺ $$$ **Vital Express** *($60 for four 0.14-ounce capsules)* contains vitamin C (magnesium ascorbyl palmitate) with some slip agents and silicone, but that's about it. If you want vitamin C, this is an option, but it won't help skin any more than other forms of vitamin C in products available for far less, and the dent in your pocketbook for what you get is painful.

☹ **True-Matte Fresh** *($40 for 2.1 ounces)* lists alcohol as its first ingredient, and it also contains lemon, menthol, ivy, sage, and pine cone extracts, making it a very expensive way to irritate the skin.

☺ $$$ **Gentle Day Protection SPF 16 Sunscreen** *($30 for 1 ounce)* is a very good, pure titanium dioxide–based sunscreen in a very basic moisturizing base. The cost would discourage liberal application and it takes liberal application to achieve the SPF number on the label of any sunscreen product. Several of the plant extracts are potential skin irritants. This product does nothing that Neutrogena's Sensitive Skin UVA/UVB Block SPF 17 ($8.99 for 4 ounces) or Sensitive Skin UVA/UVB Block SPF 30 ($8.99 for 4 ounces), will do.

☺ $$$ **Eye Concentrate Mask** *($50 for 0.7 ounce and 20 sheets)*. What makes this product unique is that you get a really small vial of a lotion and 20 sheets of a material that you soak with the lotion. You then place the sheets on the face and they become clear. You are supposed to believe that the sheets are like skin and that they help heal and cure whatever is taking place in your skin. What a concept! But the sheets aren't like skin in the least and the ingredients don't add up to much. It does contain soybean extract, which can be an antioxidant and possibly soothing for skin, but the estrogenic effects of soy when taken orally cannot be achieved by applying soy topically to the skin.

☹ **Pop-Out Mask** *($15 for 24 pieces)* is an expanding sponge material that becomes a full sheet when soaked with Awake's Lotion Refresher or Lotion Whitener. This just absorbs and wastes a lot more product than your skin needs.

☹ **Sebum Clear Mask** *($40 for 2.1 ounces)* lists a hairspray ingredient (film-forming agent) first on its ingredient list, alcohol is third, and the plant extracts can be skin irritants. So, in general, this product is clearly more of a drying irritant than anything else.

☺ $$$ **Skin Renovation Mask** *($80 for 2.2 ounces; 8 single-use containers)* is a good emollient mask with some good emollients, anti-irritants, and antioxidants. However, there is absolutely nothing in this mask that isn't easily replaced with a well-formulated moisturizer used every day, and for a lot less money than this overpriced concoction.

☹ **Smooth Clear Mask** *($40 for 2.8 ounces)* is almost identical to the Sebum Clear Mask above and the same comments apply.

☺ $$$ **Vital Express Mask** *($50 for 4 ounces; 12 sheets)* is just some slip agent and vitamin C and E. That can be good for skin, but lots of less pricey products contain these along with a longer list of good water-binding agents and anti-irritants.

☹ **Cool On Matte Mask** *($40 for 2.8 ounces)*. The second ingredient in this product is alcohol along with a small amount of menthol, which can feel cool but can also cause dryness and irritation, and this is a problem for all skin types.

☹ **Lip Repair EX, SPF 18** *($18 for 0.10 ounce)* doesn't contain the UVA-protecting ingredients of titanium dioxide, zinc oxide, or avobenzone, and is not recommended.

AWAKE MAKEUP

The makeup collection from Awake remains relatively unchanged since the previous edition of this book. The biggest news (if you can call it that) is the launch of Stardom, a makeup subcategory within the Awake line that boasts "advanced formulas and unique textures that illuminate your complexion, and polished shades that flatter your features." Aside from the stand-up-and-take-notice bright-red packaging, there is little reason to get excited about Stardom. Almost all of the products are simply new twists on the shimmer theme, offering such minor departures from the norm as "holographic" finishes and shiny eyebrow powder. The ad copy is enticing, but Stardom's promise of glitz and glamour can be had elsewhere for far less, and often with longer-lasting results.

Awake asserts that it uses specially treated pigments in its makeup to "reduce irritation." Treated pigments are by and large the standard throughout the cosmetics industry, and are chiefly used to make colors more stable, thus enhancing their longevity. Awake uses this claim with the angle that its cosmetics are more suited to sensitive skin, but there is no proof for this assertion. Regardless of the claims and Awake's unnecessary Stardom line, you will find some excellent makeup options, with the foundations, powder blush, and Volumizing Mascara being the real attractions.

$$$ **FOUNDATION:** ☺ **Skin Renovation Fluid Makeup** *($55)* won't renovate anything, but it does have a creamy texture, soft natural finish, and medium coverage. This formula is best for normal to dry skin, and the eight shades offer mostly neutral options. Nutmeg is too peach and Toast too orange, but the remaining shades are worth considering. ✓☺ **Skin Renovation Powder Makeup** *($48)* is a talc-free powder foundation with a gorgeous soft texture that is almost creamy, and it applies splendidly. Coverage

is seamless and light, and of the ten shades the only one to shy away from due to a peach overtone is Camel. ✔☺ **Hydro-Touch Foundation SPF 18** *($40 with compact, $30 for refills)* is a wonderful water-to-powder makeup with a wet, cool application that dries to a matte finish capable of sheer to light coverage. This one requires deft blending, as the formula tends to dry quickly into place and is then not easy to move. Water-to-powder foundation (as opposed to cream-to-powder) works best on normal to oily skin. This has an in-part titanium dioxide–based sunscreen, which is a boon for those with oily, blemish-prone skin who are trying to use as few products as possible on the face. There are nine mostly neutral shades, including options for very light skin tones. Peach and Sand can be too peachy for most, while Bronze is a great tan shade for medium to dark skin. **Oil Free Foundation** *($32)* is a very sheer, liquidy foundation that has a smooth, weightless texture and a soft, natural finish. For those who prefer slight coverage and have normal to slightly oily skin, this is an option and blends out effortlessly. Of the eight shades, three are too orange or peach to recommend: Peach, Sand, and Beige. There are some very light shades to consider, but nothing suitable for darker skin. ☺ **Fine Finish Foundation** *($38 with compact, $28 refill, $4 for sponge)* is Awake's rendition of a wet/dry powder foundation, but it's nothing more than a mica- and talc-based pressed powder. It does have an incredibly smooth, silky texture. This would be best for normal to slightly dry skin or slightly oily skin, as the emollient feel this imparts would not be great over oily skin and the powder part can be drying for dry skin types. As usual, wet application of this type of foundation can produce streaks and an uneven finish, but used dry it is beautiful. Of the eight shades, Sand and Beige are too peach for most skin tones.

☹ **$$$ CONCEALER: Concealer** *($18)* comes in a compact; it has a rather tacky feel and a slightly greasy application, but it does dry to a natural matte finish with minimal risk of creasing. The one drawback is that this only provides moderate coverage, and if you layer more on to get the results you may need, it can end up looking heavy or dry. The three shades are quite workable, though Ecru can be too peach for most skin tones. **Spot Concealer** *($20)* has a pointed, sponge-tip applicator that dispenses the concealer onto the skin. It claims to contain a unique ingredient that "vaporizes upon application on skin" while a "highly emollient ingredient prevents dryness and creasing." Since there is no ingredient list for this product (a big FDA no-no), you're left to guess as to how such two very different-sounding claims can work in concert with each other. Either way, this somewhat thick, matte-finish concealer blends out nicely (though it can leave a thick, choppy finish if you aren't careful). This can cover blemishes, but no better than many other concealers. There are only two colors, a definite shortcoming, but both are OK options for light to medium skin tones. **Stardom W Concealer** *($26)* is sold as a pre-foundation pore and wrinkle filler, but the effect you get from this dual-sided silicone-based product is short-lived at best. Calling this a concealer is a misnomer, as the pale peach and opalescent pink shades provide no coverage and leave a soft finish that doesn't do much to fill in lines or pores. **Stardom Face Color Palette** *($36)* has an out-of-this-world cream-to-powder texture and features four color-correcting shades in one compact. How small amounts of pale yellow, bronze, white, and pale blue can do much to correct anything is beyond me, and the shiny finish these have will only draw attention to what you want to downplay. As a shimmery highlighter or contour, these shades work, but you can achieve the same effect for far less.

POWDER: ☺ $$$ **Loose Powder** *($28)* is a standard, talc-based powder that has a very silky texture and a sheer finish. The cumbersome container can make applying this even messier than it usually is for loose powder. The six colors offer some beautiful neutral to yellow tones for fair to medium skin.

☹ $$$ **Nuance Veil** *($35)* is a talc- and wax-based pressed-powder compact with four colors swirled together in either a pale flesh tone or a bronzer. Both versions come off as a single color on the skin and have a subtle shiny finish.

☺ $$$ BLUSH: The powder **Blush** *($18)* comes in ten predominantly warm-toned shades and with a lovely, soft texture. The shiny shades to watch out for are Amber Glow and Day Lily. Shy Camel is an excellent shade for contouring.

EYESHADOW: ☹ $$$ **Multidimension Eye** *($36)* is a set of three eyeshadows in a split-pan compact. Two of the colors are powders, the third is cream-to-powder. All of the shades are sheer and quite shiny, and although the texture is smooth the color combinations are hardly amenable to an understated look. **Eye Shadow** *($17)* is a large collection of single, somewhat powdery shadows, all with a supremely smooth texture. Over half of the shades are shiny, and there are a number of pastel blues and greens to ignore, but the lingering matte shades are worth a try.

☹ **Stardom Eye Gloss** *($18)* is a glitter-infused liquid eyeshadow that features sheer colors and a slightly grainy texture that takes far too long to blend, and then doesn't stay put. This is a truly pointless product that even those hooked on glitter will find infuriating,

EYE AND BROW SHAPER: Both the ☺ $$$ **Eye Pencil** *($16)* and the ✔☺ **Brow Pencil** *($16)* are standard fare, with a dry texture and a soft powder finish that tends not to smear. The Brow Pencil is very easy to apply, and is worth considering if you prefer pencil to powder. ☺ $$$ **Liquid Eye Liner** *($20)* is a decent liquid liner with a flexible, fine-tipped brush—but there is no logical reason to spend this much on liquid liner with all the superb options available from L'Oreal and Maybelline. ☺ $$$ **Stardom Eye Brow** *($26)* is one of the only sensible Stardom products. It features two brow colors in a compact, a sheer creamy shade and a coordinating brow powder. Why these have a soft shine is strange, but even stranger is the claim that the gingko extract in it "stimulates blood circulation in delicate skin tissue above the eye," something that the tiny amount of it in the product assuredly does not do (nor would you really want it to). This is more gimmicky than practical, but it can work to create a softly groomed, defined brow, and the colors are flattering.

LIPSTICK AND LIP PENCIL: ✔☺ **True-Rich Lipstick** *($22)* has a great smooth texture that feels light and creamy on the lips. This provides full-coverage color and a soft, glossy finish. If you want to splurge on Awake lipsticks, start here. ☺ $$$ The standard **Lipstick** *($17.50)* is very creamy and smooth, with medium to sheer coverage and a slightly glossy finish. The color selection is quite nice, but overall there is nothing about these that makes them preferable to any other (far less expensive) lipsticks, though Awake does its best to convince you otherwise. **HydroSheer for Lips** *($20)* is a standard sheer lipstick with a glossy finish. The marketing language makes it sound like an epiphany for lips, but you won't find this much different from any other sheer lipstick you've tried. **Stardom Lipstick** *($20)* is a small collection of dazzlingly packaged shimmer lipsticks, each with a greasy texture and glossy finish. The colors are pretty, but the formula is not as nice as the True Rich Lipstick above. **Lip Palette** *($12)* is a mini-compact with six lip colors that are fairly creamy and have a slightly glossy finish. If you don't mind having to apply your lip color with a brush all the time, this is an option, but you only get a tiny amount of each color. **Lip Gloss** *($18)* is basic gloss with a brush applicator and a pleasant, minimally sticky texture, but it's nothing to consider over anything you may find at the drugstore for a quarter of the price—plus the brush tends to splay. **Stardom Gloss for Lips** *($18)* are dual-sided pot glosses that have a lightweight, slick texture that isn't the least bit sticky. The color combinations are unconventional, but they're bound to appeal to someone. The **Lip Pencil** *($16)* is as standard as they come, and it needs to be sharpened. It does have a creamy texture that is almost too soft for a controlled, fine line.

     ☹ $$$ **Lipscape** *($18)* includes a small group of silky, powdery colors that can be used on lips, cheeks, or eyes. These are mostly shiny and yet claim to leave a matte texture, so don't be fooled.

     <u>MASCARA:</u> ✔☺ $$$ **Volumizing Mascara** *($17)* is an excellent mascara that builds incredible length and thickness without clumping or smearing. Few department-store mascaras can rival those from Lancome, but this one achieves that feat!

     ☹ **Lengthening Mascara** *($17)* has small fibers in the formula that are supposed to help with lengthening, but they don't help much in that regard. And if you get the wand too close to the eye the small fibers can easily fall off and get into the eye, causing irritation. Add to that the fact that this produces paltry length and no thickness and it's easy to ignore.

     ☹ **Stardom Mascara** *($25)* is an absurdly overpriced two-part mascara that features a base coat and a top coat. The base has a standard curved mascara brush that allows ample lengthening, but builds no thickness. It also tends to make lashes look spiky and sticks them together, too, so you look like you have fewer lashes than you really do. The top coat is just a mascara comb that adds little to the base coat other than a second step. Save money, time, and frustration by choosing any L'Oreal mascara over this one.

     ☹ $$$ <u>BRUSHES:</u> The brushes *($15–$40)* at Awake are well intentioned, but most of them are either absurdly small or too big to work with on a variety of face shapes and features. If price is not a concern, the following are the best ones to consider: **Retractable Lip Brush** *($15)* has an excellent full, but tapered, cut; **Eyebrow Brush** *($20)* is firm without being scratchy; and **Eye Shadow #3 Brush** *($18)* is adequately sized for detailed work.

B. KAMINS SKIN CARE

When a line of facial products refers to itself as "Baby Boomer Skin Care" you have to admire them for being so direct. No mixed messages here as to who their target market is! So who is B. Kamins? He is Ben Kaminsky, and according to the company's press release, he "is a leading Canadian chemist [who] has headed a team of expert chemists, dermatologists, and pharmacists in search of a solution to oxidation and wrinkling of aging skin. Kamins questioned how living matter, specifically certain Canadian maple trees *(Acer saccharum)* could survive and thrive for hundreds of years in a cold, unforgiving climate. After more than 30 years of research, Kamins has developed a patent pending method of extracting and purifying a biological compound from these vital maple trees. The result of this extraction is Bio-Maple™ compound, found exclusively in B. Kamins products."

As it turns out, maple, in whatever form, is not the answer to your wrinkle woes. How plants manage to thrive in sunlight and the elements while our skin and body functions can't take it for very long is the essence of antioxidant research. But no one knows which antioxidant is the most effective one, or how any of that relates to the appearance of our skin over the long term (not to mention that the biological functions of plants and humans are completely different). Given the intense research going on in the world of antioxidants (ranging from vitamin E to selenium, grape, and everything in between), we now know that there are many reasons to consider a wide variety of skin-care ingredients, from vitamin C, beta-glucan, vitamin A, and superoxide dismutase to green tea and grape seed extract, and on and on. All of these and more are backed by a formidable amount of research, especially when compared to the minimal amount of research carried out on the maple that is used in the B. Kamins products.

On a closer look at this line, however, it seems that while Kaminsky was researching maple trees he overlooked the research about sun protection, and his line actually has products with an SPF 8 and an SPF 12, both without UVA-protecting ingredients (though there is one sunscreen that contains avobenzone and has a good SPF). Kaminsky explains the use of a lower SPF based on the need to only include ingredients that the skin needs, and feels that if you are not going to be in the sun for long periods of time you don't need a higher SPF. However, given that UVA light comes through windows, and given that no one knows in advance how long they are going to be in the sun on any given day, the safest thing for your skin is to follow the SPF 15 minimum recommendation of the American Academy of Dermatology and the National Cancer Institute.

Kaminsky also suggests he has the answer for rosacea because "there is virtually no topical treatment" available. However, there's a great deal of research establishing many successful treatments for rosacea, particularly prescription treatments such as Noritate and MetroLotion. I have seen no research on the B. Kamins products or their ingredients showing that they can have any effect for this condition, and given that some of these formulations include irritating ingredients (ranging from fragrance and alcohol to menthol and mint), there is little reason to believe these will be of help.

There are some interesting products to consider in this line, but choose carefully because there is far more hype than substance in these formulations. For more information about B. Kamins, call (888) B-KAMINS or visit www.bkamins.com.

☺ $$$ **Botanical Face Cleanser** *($32 for 8.5 ounces)* is an OK cleanser that can be rinsed off, but you would need the help of a washcloth to remove all your makeup.

☺ $$$ **Vegetable Skin Cleanser** *($32 for 8 ounces).* There are no vegetables in this product (at least not the real kind, unless you plan on putting sodium oleth sulfate, among others, on your salad). Rather, this is a very standard, detergent-based cleanser that would work well for normal to oily skin. This one is fragrance-free.

☺ $$$ **Vitamin Face Cleanser** *($42 for 8 ounces)* is a plant oil–based, wipe-off cleanser that is more of a cold cream than anything else. It also contains ground-up nutshells so it works like an exfoliant, just a rather greasy one (this can definitely leave a film on the skin), but it may be an option for someone with very dry skin. This does contain fragrance.

☹ $$$ **Flower Water Treatment Spray** *($42 for 8 ounces)* is water, maple extract, slip agent, preservatives, and fragrance. This is a lot of money for maple extract (an antioxidant) and water.

☹ **Hydrogen-Ion Moisturizing Toner for Dry Skin** *($32 for 8 ounces).* The amount of hydrogen ions present in a water solution is a way to measure the acidity of any substance. The way it works is that the higher the concentration of hydrogen ions, the more acidic the solution and the lower the pH, while the fewer hydrogen ions are present the more alkaline a substance is (with a higher pH). But this is only a very fancy way of saying this product is acid balanced, just like most skin-care products are these days. Aside from the technical lingo, this toner contains menthol, which can be a skin irritant. It also has lactic acid, but the pH of 4.5 is too high for it to be effective as an exfoliant (while the company states that this toner is not intended as an exfoliant, that is what lots of women would expect from that ingredient in the list).

☹ **Hydrogen-Ion Moisturizing Toner for Oily Skin** *($32 for 8 ounces)* contains alcohol as the second ingredient, as well as mint and menthol. This is a problem for irritation and dryness for all skin types! For an explanation of the term "hydrogen ion", see the review for the Toner for Dry Skin above.

☹ **Hydrogen-Ion Moisturizing Toner for Normal or Combination Skin** *($32 for 8 ounces).* The menthol and balm mint make this product potentially too irritating and drying for all skin types. For an explanation of the term "hydrogen ion", see the review for the Toner for Dry Skin above.

☺ $$$ **Booster Blue Rosacea Treatment** *($59 for 1.7 ounces)* contains mostly water, slip agent, sunscreen agent (though this product has no SPF rating), maple extract, thickeners, plant oil, preservatives, silicones, water-binding agent, anti-irritant, and coloring agents. Despite the claims that maple extract is good for rosacea, there is no research showing that to be the case. And aside from that, this version contains nothing that would make it more useful for rosacea than the other products in the B. Kamins line. The tiny amount of bisabolol (an anti-irritant) can have some efficacy, but there is no research showing it can have that effect for rosacea. It does have a blue tint but that won't camouflage redness!

☺ $$$ **Cellular Renewal Serum** *($59 for 1.7 ounces)* contains mostly water, plant extracts, film-forming agent, thickeners, water-binding agents, maple extract, preservatives, and fragrance. This is a good, lightweight moisturizer for normal to dry skin, but there is nothing in here for cellular renewal. The plant extracts are just floral water and have no exfoliating properties. There is no research showing that lemon, sugar cane, orange, or bilberry have exfoliating properties of any kind.

☹ $$$ **Revitalizing Booster Concentrate** *($59 for 1.7 ounces)* contains mostly water, slip agent, UVB sunscreen agent (though this product does not have an SPF rating), maple extract, thickeners, plant oil, preservatives, silicones, and vitamins. This rather ho-hum formulation isn't boosting in the least. If you're looking for maple, the Cellular Renewal Serum above is just fine and a more interesting formulation for skin.

☹ **Day Cream for Dry to Normal Skin, SPF 15** *($59.50 for 2.2 ounces)* does not contain the UVA-protecting ingredients of titanium dioxide, zinc oxide, or avobenzone, and is absolutely not recommended.

☹ **Day Lotion for Oily Skin SPF 8** *($59 for 1.7 ounces)* has a woefully inadequate SPF rating and doesn't contain the UVA-protecting ingredients of titanium dioxide, zinc oxide, or avobenzone. It is not recommended.

☺ $$$ **Maple Treatment Cream, SPF 15** *($88 for 2 ounces)* is a good, in-part avobenzone-based sunscreen in a very standard, Vaseline-based moisturizing base. For this amount of money it should be loaded to the hilt with antioxidants and water-binding agents. Alas, very little of those are found in this product. Keep in mind that you must apply sunscreen liberally to get any benefit from using it. If an expensive sunscreen discourages you from liberal application it can be a serious problem for the health of your skin.

☺ $$$ **Eye Cream** *($52 for 0.6 ounce)* contains mostly water, vitamin E, thickeners, maple extract, water-binding agents, silicones, soy extract, plant oil, and preservatives. This is a very good moisturizer for dry skin, though it won't change a wrinkle. If you want soy for your skin, Aveeno has the same ingredient that's in this one, and for far less money! But the notion that soy can change skin function is no more a reality than the notion that maple extract can.

☹ $$$ **Menopause Skin Cream** *($102 for 1.6 ounces)* is similar to the Eye Cream above, only this one has a more interesting mix of water-binding agents and antioxidants. It also contains salicylic acid, but the product's pH is too high for it to be effective as an exfoliant. This ends up being a good moisturizer with a form of menthol added to the mix to make the skin feel cool. That won't stop a hot flash but it can end up being irritating to skin. This does contain fragrance.

☺ $$$ **Night Cream for All Skin Types** *($78 for 2.2 ounces)* is similar to the Menopause Skin Cream above only minus the menthol, which makes it a far better moisturizer for normal to dry skin. This product is not appropriate for all skin types; the oils in it would not make someone with oily skin happy.

☺ $$$ **Sunbar Sunscreen SPF 30, Fragrance** and **Fragrance-Free** (*$29 for 4 ounces*) are very good, but very overpriced, sunscreens in an exceedingly ordinary moisturizing base that includes both avobenzone and titanium dioxide. (This is a very good combination for UVA protection that is acceptable outside of the United States, but it is not FDA approved for use in the United States.) That's great, but other sunscreens at the drugstore can provide similar protection for far less, and given that a liberal application is essential to receive the benefit of the SPF, think about how liberal you're going to be with this one given the price.

☹ $$$ **Diatomamus Earth Masque for Dry to Normal Skin** (*$38 for 4.6 ounces*). The name refers to earth or clay containing skeletons of diatoms. By any name, this ends up being just a good clay mask with some plant oils. The form of menthol used can be a problem for irritation, but given that masks don't stay on very long it shouldn't be much of problem. It does contain fragrance.

☹ $$$ **Diatomamus Earth Masque for Oily or Combination Skin** (*$38 for 4.6 ounces*) is similar to the Dry to Normal Skin version above, only without the oils, which does make it better for oily skin. The form of menthol used still makes this one problematic.

BAIN DE SOLEIL (SUN CARE ONLY)

This line of sunscreen products is so far behind in meeting any of the basic standards set by the American Academy of Dermatology, the National Cancer Institute, or the American Academy of Pediatrics, that it is tantamount to a sham that it is being sold under the category of sunscreens. Bain de Soleil is owned by Schering-Plough. For more information on Bain de Soleil, call (908) 298-4000 or visit www.baindesoleil.com.

☺ **Oil-Free Protecteur Sunscreen Spray, SPF 25** (*$8.99 for 4 ounces*) is a good, in-part avobenzone-based sunscreen in a rather mundane, and barely moisturizing formula.

☹ **Oil-Free Protecteur Sunscreen Lotion, SPF 35** (*$8.99 for 4 ounces*) is a good, in-part avobenzone-based sunscreen in a base of alcohol and film-forming agent. This can be irritating and drying for the skin.

All of the following products either do not contain the UVA-protecting ingredients of titanium dioxide, zinc oxide, or avobenzone or have an inadequate SPF rating that would give a terribly false sense of protection that could result in serious skin damage. They are absolutely not recommended.

☹ **Luminessence Sunscreen SPF 4** (*$8.99 for 3.5 ounces*); **Luminessence Sunscreen SPF 8** (*$8.99 for 3.5 ounces*); **Oil-Free Faces Sunscreen, SPF 15** (*$8.99 for 2 ounces*); **Orange Gelee Sunscreen SPF 4** (*$8.99 for 3.12 ounces*); **Orange Gelee Sunscreen SPF 8** (*$8.99 for 3.12 ounces*); **Orange Gelee Sunscreen SPF 15** (*$7.99 for 3.12 ounces*); **Tanning Mist SPF 4** (*$8.99 for 3 ounces*); **Tanning Mist SPF 8** (*$8.99 for 3 ounces*); **Tropical Deluxe Sunfilter, SPF 4** (*$6.99 for 4 ounces*); **Tropical Deluxe Sunscreen SPF 4** (*$5.99

for 4 ounces); **Sunfilter with Self Tanner** *($6.99 for 4 ounces)*; and **Mega Tan Sunscreen with Self Tanner SPF 4** *($5.99 for 4 ounces)*.

All of the following products, like all self-tanners, use dihydroxyacetone to affect the color of skin. They would work as well as any.

☺ **Auto-Bronzant Self Tanning Creme, Dark** *($8.99 for 3.12 ounces)*; **Auto-Bronzant Self Tanning Spray, Dark** *($8.99 for 3.5 ounces)*; **Auto-Bronzant Self Tanning Spray, Deep Dark** *($8.99 for 3.5 ounces)*; **Faces, Tinted Self-Tanning Creme for All Skin Tones** *($8.99 for 2 ounces)*; **Radiance Eternelle Self Tanning Creme, Dark** *($13.99 for 3.2 ounces)*; **Radiance Eternelle Self Tanning Creme, Medium Dark** *($13.99 for 3.2 ounces)*; **Streakguarde Self Tanning Creme, Dark** *($8.99 for 3.12 ounces)*; **Streakguarde Self Tanning Creme, Dark, Dark** *($8.99 for 3.12 ounces)*; and **Streakguarde Self Tanning Creme, Deep Dark** *($8.99 for 3.12 ounces)*.

BANANA BOAT (SUN CARE ONLY)

The fact that many of Banana Boat's products aimed at sun protection do not contain effective UVA-protecting ingredients means that this sun care line cannot be trusted for sun protection. Over the past two years they have added products that meet the industry standard, yet they've left the poorly formulated ones still on the shelves for unsuspecting consumers to stumble upon. Another problem, even for the sunscreens that do offer state-of-the-art protection, is that none of Banana Boat's products list nonactive ingredients. As a result there is no way to really know what you are putting on the skin. Therefore, the ratings below are strictly about sun protection and not about what other benefits or problems these products may pose for the skin. For more information about Banana Boat, call (800) 723-3786 or visit www.bananaboat.com.

☺ **VitaSkin Lotion Facial Care SPF 30** *($9.99 for 5.7 ounces)* is a good, in-part avobenzone-based sunscreen.

☺ **VitaSkin Lotion SPF 15** *($9.99 for 6 ounces)* is a good, in-part avobenzone-based sunscreen.

☺ **VitaSkin Lotion SPF 30** *($9.99 for 6 ounces)* is a good, in-part avobenzone-based sunscreen.

☺ **VitaSkin Lotion SPF 50** *($9.99 for 6 ounces)* is a good, in-part zinc oxide–based sunscreen.

☺ **Ultra Sunblock Quick Dry Spray SPF 30** *($8.99 for 6 ounces)* is a good, in-part avobenzone-based sunscreen.

☺ **Sunblock Spray Lotion SPF 48** *($8.99 for 6 ounces)* is a good, in-part titanium dioxide–based sunscreen.

☺ **Active Sport Sunblock Gel SPF 30** *($8.99 for 6 ounces)* is a good, in-part avobenzone-based sunscreen.

☺ **Baby Block Sunblock Lotion SPF 50** *($8.99 for 4 ounces)* is a good, in-part titanium dioxide–based sunscreen. There is nothing in this product that makes it preferred for babies. If anything, the synthetic sunscreen agents can be too irritating for a child's skin.

☺ **Kids Sunblock Spray Lotion SPF 48** *($8.99 for 6 ounces)* is similar to the Baby Block above and the same comments apply.

All of the products in the following paragraph either do not contain the UVA-protecting ingredients of titanium dioxide, zinc oxide, or avobenzone, or have an inadequate SPF rating that would give a terribly false sense of protection that could result in serious skin damage.

☹ **Dark Tanning Lotion SPF 4** *($7.99 for 8 ounces)*; **Dark Tanning Oil Spray SPF 4** *($7.99 for 8 ounces)*; **Active Sport Quick Dry Sunscreen Spray SPF 25** *($8.49 for 6 ounces)*; **Faces Plus Sunblock SPF 23, Normal/Combination Skin** *($8.99 for 4 ounces)*; **Kids Sunblock Lotion SPF 30** *($8.99 for 8 ounces)*; **Kids Quik-Blok SPF 25** *($9.99 for 8 ounces)*; **Maximum Sunblock Cream SPF 50** *($8.99 for 4 ounces)*; **Quik Blok Sunblock SPF 25** *($9.59 for 8 ounces)*; **Protective Tanning Oil SPF 8** *($7.99 for 8 ounces)*; **Protective Tanning Oil SPF 15** *($7.99 for 8 ounces)*; **Sport Sunblock Lotion SPF 15** *($8.99 for 6 ounces)*; **Sport Sunblock Lotion SPF 30** *($8.99 for 6 ounces)*; **Sunblock Lotion SPF 15** *($8.99 for 8 ounces)*; **Sunscreen Lotion SPF 8** *($8.99 for 6 ounces)*; **Ultra Sunblock Lotion SPF 30** *($8.99 for 6 ounces)*; and **Aloe Vera Sun Screen Lip Balm SPF 15** *($1.59 for 0.15 ounce)*.

The products in the following paragraph, like all self-tanners, use dihydroxyacetone to affect the color of skin. They would work as well as any.

☺ **Sunless Tanning Creme, Soft Medium** *($7.99 for 3.75 ounces)*; **Sunless Tanning Creme, Deep Dark** *($7.99 for 3.5 ounces)*; and **Sunless Tanning Spray Soft Medium and Deep Dark** *($5.99 for 3.75 ounces)*.

☹ **VitaSkin Lotion Daily** *($9.99 for 12 ounces)* is a good, but very standard, moisturizer for dry skin. It contains mostly water, thickeners, silicones, vitamins A and E, film-forming agents, and preservatives.

bare escentuals

Bare escentuals, with all its cosmetics boutique appeal, started as a store concept quite similar in style to Aveda, The Body Shop, and Garden Botanika. Given the financial instability these kinds of cosmetic boutiques have experienced, bare escentuals progressed into the world of home shopping television. That world is QVC, where the bare escentuals bareMinerals makeup and Cush skin-care products are sold. QVC reaches lots of women with the rapturous praise it uses to sell everything. As a result, many women want to know if bareMinerals works as amazingly and purely as the spokesperson asserts. Of course, nothing ever works as well as they say in ads, though the powders are unique in their coverage, application, and simple formulation, and, depending on your point of view, they are an interesting way to apply face and eye makeup. See the reviews below for details.

I should mention that there is nothing particularly cushy about Cush. It has a marine life angle that is clever, but how many seafaring people have you met with wrinkle-free skin? Algae and other sea-plant life, just like plant life all over this planet, can have some antioxidant and anti-inflammatory properties. That is great for skin, but it isn't a miracle or unique to this line. What is problematic are the peppermint oil and other fragrant plant oils in almost every product. Add to that the lack of sunscreens (poorly formulated or otherwise) and it's like asking for sun damage and wrinkles to happen sooner rather than later. Cush is a line you can easily avoid.

In the fall of 2001, M.D. Formulations (reviewed in this book) and bare escentuals merged, thus marrying a line with a clearly medical orientation to an all-natural, new age–aimed company. If you happen into a bare escentuals boutique, you will find spa-styled products radiating aromatherapy and bouquets of plant extracts side-by-side with the ultra-serious, nonfragranced line of skin-care products called M.D. Formulations. Exactly how this marriage will affect either product line is yet to be seen, but I will certainly report any changes in my newsletter, *Cosmetics Counter Update*, as they occur. For more information about bare escentuals, call (800) 227-3990 or visit www.bareescentuals.com or www.qvc.com. **Note:** All bare escentuals skin-care products contain fragrance.

bare escentuals CUSH SKIN CARE

☺ **Deep Sea Foaming Seaweed Cleanser** *($20 for 6.5 ounces)* is a detergent-based cleanser that would have been a great consideration for normal to dry skin, except it contains sage oil, lavender oil, and peppermint oil, and while these all may smell nice they are irritating and sensitizing for skin.

☹ **Equilibrium Sea Facial Tonic** *($20 for 6.5 ounces)* is mostly algae, water, witch hazel, and fragrance (sandalwood oil, lavender oil, and peppermint oil), which offer no benefit for skin, though the risk of irritation is fairly good.

☺ **Eye Makeup Remover** *($14 for 4.4 ounces)* is an exceptionally standard eye-makeup remover that uses gentle detergent cleansing agents. This one, thankfully, does not contain fragrance or fragrant plant oils.

☺ **Turning Tide Fresh Face Exfoliator** *($36 for 2.3 ounces)* is a scrub that uses diatomaceous earth (crushed-up rock created from skeletal remains of sea life) as the abrasive material. That could be good for exfoliation, but the fragrant plant oils are a problem for skin.

☹ **Nutritious Marine Moisturizer** *($32 for 2.1 ounces)* is an OK moisturizer with vitamins that is missing some interesting water-binding agents. In addition, the vitamins, which are good antioxidants, are listed after the fragrance, amounting to very little content.

☹ **$$$ Life Source Time Peeling Serum** *($36 for 1 ounce).* The witch hazel and peppermint oil in this product are potential skin irritants. Though the glycolic acid, at about 4% to 5%, would have been good as an exfoliant, the pH is too high for it to be very effective in doing that job.

☺ $$$ **Detox Mask** (*$28 for 5.5 ounces*) won't detoxify any part of your skin or pores. It's just a very fragrant mask of clay and thickening agents. Some of the plant extracts have antioxidant properties, but they are minimal in comparison to the fragrant plant extracts that can be skin irritants.

☺ **bareVitamins Skin Rev-er Upper** (*$21 for 2.3 ounces*) contains about 1% salicylic acid in a lightweight, silicone-based moisturizer. It contains some good water-binding agents, antioxidants, and anti-irritants, and is fragrance-free, which makes this one of the better-formulated products in this line. Unfortunately, the pH of the product is too high for the salicylic acid to be helpful for exfoliation.

☺ **Faux Tan** (*$22 for 4.5 ounces*) uses dihydroxyacetone as the ingredient to affect skin color, the same as all self-tanners. This one would work as well as any. It does contain fragrance.

☺ **Buzz Latte Lip Balm** (*$8 for 0.25 ounce*) is an emollient lip balm that would work well for dry lips.

bare escentuals MAKEUP

All of the bareMinerals powders, whether for foundation, eyeshadow, brow color, or blush, are loose powders that are applied with a brush. The color line is known as i.d., and calls itself "the purest cosmetic collection in the world." The products boast that they don't contain fragrance, oil, binders, preservatives, emulsifiers, or any other problematic ingredients, but that turns out not to be the case. Bismuth oxychloride is a major ingredient in all the powder formulations and it can cause skin irritation, while the other minerals can be drying. Aside from the overstated claim about natural this and purity that, loose powders are as messy as it gets in terms of your vanity (countertop, not ego) and your makeup bag. The powder just gets all over the place! Additionally, while there are softer neutral shades, and some fairly exotic shades as well, all are mildly to extremely shiny and make any amount of crepey skin look more so. The face powder does provide some amount of opaque coverage, but the shine and the thickness can be a bit much. The eyeshadows and blushes apply in a somewhat lighter way, though they still provide good coverage. If you find the loose powder makeup concept and the shine intriguing, these are an option, but I feel safe in suggesting they will end up as one of those cosmetics whims that you never use more than a few times.

☺ <u>FOUNDATION</u>: **bareMinerals foundation** (*$25*) is the loose-powder foundation that put bare escentuals on the map and it is the backbone of this makeup line. This talc-free, mica-based powder has a soft, almost creamy texture and an undeniably shiny finish. The titanium dioxide and bismuth oxychloride lend this powder its opacity, medium coverage, and slightly thick finish. Eight shades are available in the handful of bare escentuals stores, and five of these are also sold on QVC. The shades tend to lean a bit too far into the rose and peach zones, but not enough to avoid them. Still, if this type of foundation with all of its trappings appeals to you, Jane Iredale's Amazing Base SPF 20

($35.50) offers a smoother formula, an effective titanium dioxide–based sunscreen, and more neutral colors—not to mention a pressed-powder option for those who don't want to deal with the fallout from loose powder! The **Bisque multi-tasking makeup** *($18)* has a description that makes it sound like the Wonder Woman of makeup, seemingly able to tackle any cosmetic whim or need with one sweep of a brush. This is merely a pale, slightly shiny pigmented powder whose formula is nearly identical to the bareMinerals foundation above. It works as a highlighter or eyeshadow base, but so does a good matte finish concealer—and with a lot less mess and more precision, too!

The Reviews B

POWDER: ☺ $$$ **bareMinerals mineral veil** *($19)* is a talc-free loose powder with a softer and lighter consistency than the bareMinerals foundation, and sans the shine! It has a sheer, but dry, powder finish, and is best for someone with normal to oily skin. This is cornstarch-based, so avoid it if you're prone to or are battling blemishes.

☹ $$$ **Warmth color** *($20)* is a sheer, slightly shiny bronzing powder that comes in an attractive tan color but is simply not worth the expense, considering the number of impressive pressed-powder bronzers that cost less and are much easier to apply and blend than this one. The **Facial sculpting kit** *($42)* is a three-piece collection that includes two matte loose powders and a brush. The Emphasize It powder is a pale yellow shade used to highlight, and the Chisel It is an appropriate soft brown contour color that can be used to define and add structure to the face. The brush is soft and dense but improperly sized, and most women will find it too big to use on the underbrow area and way too small to contour under the cheekbones and onto the temple area. Besides, why deal with the messiness of loose powders when there are countless pressed-powder options? If you are up for the task and don't mind paying too much, this can work to achieve a more sculpted face.

☹ $$$ BLUSH: **bareMinerals blush** *($18)* has the same basic texture as the loose foundation, and the comments about it being messy and hard to control apply here, too. There are some matte shades of this product, and the application is soft and relatively even once you've mastered how much loose color to pick up on your brush for best results. Although it's hard for me to encourage this option, I'm sure some women will love it. **All over face color** *($20)* is identical to the Warmth Color above, only this one is a pale rose shade that is best used as blush. Dusting this loose powder all over your face would only make you look mildly sunburned. This has a minimal shine that is not distracting in daylight.

☺ EYESHADOW: **bareMinerals eyeshadow** *($12)* is similar to the blush and foundation reviewed above, though the eyeshadows have a much silkier, lighter texture. All of the colors are slightly shiny, though there are some great neutral shades. I still don't get the advantage of going for this kind of messy, flaky application, but for some women it is an option. **bareMinerals glimmer** *($13)* is the same as the bareMinerals foundation and blush except that these are ultra-shiny and have a grainier texture due to the high amount of mica. Any flaking will be extremely obvious. **Liner Shadow** *($12)* is a matte, loose-powder eyeshadow that features richly pigmented hues. This is impossible to use dry without it flaking into your eye or onto the skin. Wet application is preferred (if not essential) for getting this to go on smoothly and to apply precisely.

EYE AND BROW SHAPER: ☺ **Eye pencil** *($10)* is a standard, twist-up eye pencil that comes in one color. Luckily, that color is black, and this is an option, though no more special than pencils you can buy at the drugstore. ☹ **Brow color** *($11)* is loose powder for the brows that comes in six suitable colors, though this is an incredibly untidy way to shape and define your brows. Why anyone would choose this over a pressed matte brow powder (or eyeshadow) is something I cannot comprehend. After using the Brow color, you can set the powder with ☺ **Brow finishing gel** *($12)*. This standard, clear brow gel works as well as any, and can double as a clear mascara for those seeking minimal lash enhancement.

☺ **LIPSTICK AND LIP PENCIL:** The **Lipstick** *($15)* has a creamy, opaque, slightly glossy finish. The rose-geranium fragrance is subtle, but can be problematic for those allergic to plants. **Lip Quickies** *($15)* are simply sheer, iridescent lipsticks that are sold as "quick-change artists" that can alter the look of your existing lipstick. Most women know that any lipstick (or liner and gloss) used over one color will produce a variation on that shade that results in a "new" color. What's the big deal here? **Lip gloss** *($14)* is a standard non-sticky wand lip gloss, nice but ordinary. **Lip liner** *($11)* is a standard, twist-up lip pencil that comes in a limited number of shades.

☹ **MASCARA:** The **Mascara** *($15)* has been reformulated and, although it is no longer a terrible mascara, it isn't great either. The spiral brush allows you to build satisfactory length and some thickness, but the lashes tend to stick together and take on a bent appearance, which you then must correct with a lash comb. There are better mascaras at the drugstore that sell for half the price.

☺ **BRUSHES:** The **Brushes** *($12–$24)* are for the most part soft and easy to use, although they are offered in sizes that may or may not be your preference for application. For example, there are two eyeshadow brushes, one that is rather oversize and the other that is almost too small. I would prefer two brushes in sizes right between these.

The **Face Brush** *($22)* is a great size and quite soft, and the **Retractable Face Brush** *($30)* is a sleek, practical option for on-the-go powdering. Avoid the **Lash Comb** *($10)*, which features metal teeth that can be severely damaging if you inadvertently scratch your eye. If you prefer using a lash comb, stick with the safer versions that have plastic teeth. The **Travel Makeup Brush Kit with Bag** *($111)* includes six makeup brushes, a small mirror, and a clutch-style nylon bag. If the majority of these brushes were more practically shaped, this might be worth considering—but other lines have superior brush sets that cost less than this.

☺ **SPECIALTY:** **Showgirl body glow** *($20 for 8.8 ounces)* is a lightweight, glycerin-based lotion that contains a good deal of mica for an iridescent finish. A showgirl would indeed like this, as would anyone who likes making a statement with sparkling skin.

BASIS (SKIN CARE ONLY)

For information on Basis, call (800) 227-4703 or visit the Basis section at www.drugstore.com.

☹ **All Clear Bar** *($2.29 for 4 ounces)* contains a small amount of triclosan, a good disinfectant. However, there is growing concern about the need for antibacterial agents and the rising bacterial resistance to this kind of product. In addition, this cleanser contains several ingredients that could be drying and irritating, particularly for the face, including sodium xylenesulfonate, lemon, sage, lime, and sodium lauryl sulfate.

☺ **Cleaner Clean Face Wash** *($4.99 for 6 ounces)* is a standard, water-soluble cleanser that could work well for someone with normal to oily skin. It does contain fragrance.

☺ **Comfortably Clean Face Wash** *($4.99 for 6 ounces)* is a standard, water-soluble, detergent-based cleanser that can be quite good for someone with normal to oily skin. It does contain fragrance.

☹ **Sensitive Skin Bar** *($2.29 for 4 ounces)* is a fairly standard bar cleanser that contains ingredients that can be irritating or problematic for sensitive skin. Although the Vaseline and plant oil can mitigate that problem, why use any problematic ingredients to begin with?

☹ **Vitamin Bar** *($1.99 for 4 ounces)* does have a teeny amount of vitamins in it, but even if they could have an effect on skin they would be washed down the drain before they had a chance. This is nothing more than a standard bar cleanser with ingredients that can be too drying for most skin types.

☺ **So Refreshing Cleansing Towelettes** *($4.99 for 30 cloths)* is just a standard, detergent-based makeup remover presoaked on towelettes. It works, though fragrance-free baby wipes do the same thing without the fragrance and less expensively.

☺ **Facial Cleansing Cloths, Individually Wrapped** *($4.99 for 20 cloths)* is identical to the So Refreshing version above and the same comments apply.

BATH & BODY WORKS

In their general appearance, the Bath & Body Works stores are similar to their neighboring mall competitors—The Body Shop, H2O Plus, and Origins. In addition to the wafting fragrance and herbal-natural influence they share, all of these stores have open, inviting display units and encourage product testing. Bath & Body Works takes this approach a step further with a notably friendly environment and a take-your-time demeanor. The stores are overflowing with farmer's baskets full of highly scented shower gels and body lotions, while white, wooden, and overstocked shelves line the walls. You half expect to see someone in a red and white gingham apron serving hot apple pie "Fresh From America's Heartland"! There's even a sink so you can experiment with products and then wash them off—a nice touch!

In 2000, Bath & Body Works discontinued their entire facial skin-care line and went to work revamping their product offerings. It turns out they missed some vital information about skin-care products. Several products contain significant skin irritants, and one of the sunscreens doesn't have UVA-protecting ingredients. This isn't much of an improvement, but then there's always next year! For more information about Bath & Body Works, call (800) 395-1001 or visit www.intimatebrands.com.

BATH & BODY WORKS SKIN CARE

☹ **Balancing Cleanser** (*$8 for 6 ounces*) lists the main detergent cleansing agent as sodium lauryl sulfate, which makes this too irritating for all skin types.

☺ **Completely Clean Facial Cloths** (*$8 for 20 cloths*) uses a gentle detergent cleansing agent in a rather standard formulation with nicely soft cleansing cloths. However, this is no different than using a makeup remover with cotton pads, or even fragrance-free baby wipes for that matter. This does contain fragrance.

☺ **Completely Clean Foaming Face Wash** (*$8 for 6 ounces*) is a very good, though very standard, detergent-based cleanser that would work well for someone with normal to oily skin. It does contain some irritating plant extracts but the amount is negligible and, therefore, has little risk for skin. It does contain fragrance.

☺ **Hydrating Facial Cleanser** (*$8 for 6 ounces*) is a fairly standard, cold cream–style cleanser that also contains some detergent cleansing agents. This would work well for someone with normal to dry skin. It does contain fragrance and coloring agents.

☺ **Oil-Control Cleanser** (*$8 for 5.25 ounces*). There isn't one ingredient in this product that can control oil in any way, shape, or form. It is just a basic cleanser with standard detergent cleansing agents that is good for normal to oily skin. It does contain fragrance.

☺ **Soothing Eye Makeup Remover** (*$7 for 4 ounces*) is a standard, detergent-based eye-makeup remover that isn't soothing in the least, but it will remove makeup. It does contain fragrant plant extract.

☹ **Smoothing Facial Scrub** (*$8 for 4 ounces*) uses TEA-lauryl sulfate as the main cleansing agent, and adds menthol, which makes this too irritating for skin.

☹ **Balancing Facial Toner** (*$8 for 8 ounces*) is primarily witch hazel, which can be a skin irritant, and some plant extracts that are a mix of anti-irritants and irritants.

☺ **Hydrating Facial Toner** (*$8 for 8 ounces*) is primarily water, glycerin, and fragrance, making this a boring toner for normal to dry skin.

☹ **Oil-Control Facial Toner** (*$8 for 8 ounces*) contains sulfur as the third ingredient. That can't control oil, but it can irritate the skin, as can several other ingredients in this poorly formulated toner.

☹ **Balancing Lotion with SPF 15** (*$12 for 2.75 ounces*) doesn't contain the UVA-protecting ingredients of avobenzone, zinc oxide, or titanium dioxide, and is not recommended.

☺ **Hydrating Day Creme with SPF 15** (*$12 for 2 ounces*) is a good, in-part avobenzone based sunscreen in a rather ordinary moisturizing base.

☺ **Hydrating Night Cream** *($12 for 2 ounces)* is a good moisturizer for normal to dry skin with some good emollients, water-binding agents, and a teeny amount of antioxidants. It does contain fragrance.

☺ **Illuminating Face Lotion** *($20 for 1 ounce)* contains mostly water, silicones, glycerin, water-binding agents, thickeners, antioxidants, fragrance, and preservatives. The only illuminating part of this product is the mica, which adds shine particles to this well-formulated moisturizer.

✓☺ **Nourishing Eye Cream** *($12 for 0.5 ounce)* is a good basic moisturizer for normal to dry skin. It does contain some good water-binding agents, emollient, and antioxidants.

☹ **Oil-Control Lotion** *($12 for 2.75 ounces)* lists its second ingredient as witch hazel distillate, which can be a skin irritant, and that won't help control oil in the least.

☺ **Skin Renewal Serum** *($20 for 1 ounce)* is a good, silicone-based moisturizer that would work well for normal to dry skin. It contains a small amount of water-binding agents and antioxidants. It does contain fragrance.

☺ **Soothing Eye Gel** *($12 for 0.5 ounce)* is just glycerin, thickening agents, preservatives, and fractional amounts of plant extracts and vitamin C.

☹ **Blemish Control Gel with 0.5% Salicylic Acid** *($8 for 0.75 ounce)* does contain a tiny amount of salicylic acid, but the amount of irritating fragrant plant oil (rosewood, orange, and peppermint) makes it a problem for all skin types.

☺ **Oil Absorbing Tissues** *($3 for 75 tissues)* are reliable papers for gently absorbing oil from skin.

☺ **Purifying Facial Mask** *($12 for 4 ounces)* is a standard clay mask that also contains scrub particles. It can be an option as a mechanical exfoliant and mask but that won't purify anything, it's just exfoliating. It does contain a small amount of menthol, which is present in such a small amount that it has minimal risk of being a skin irritant.

BATH & BODY WORKS MAKEUP

Bath & Body Works makeup collection has been diminished and retooled to cater to the younger clientele who are drawn to shiny, glittery makeup much the same way ants are to a picnic. Sadly, some of the best products (foundations, concealers, and powders) have been eliminated, while the shine-fest continues unabated. If what's left appeals to you (and there are still some choice picks here), the store's makeup tester unit is very user-friendly and you're free to play to your heart's content.

☺ <u>BLUSH:</u> **First Blush Cheek Color** *($10)* still has a great, velvety-smooth texture and sheer, even application, but now every one of the 13 beautiful shades has a soft shine. Although the shine with some of the colors is quite subtle, it can still make cheeks look too showy for daytime wear.

☺ <u>EYESHADOW:</u> **Catch My Eyeshadow** *($10)* presents a large range of colors, and all of them have a subtle to intrusive shine and a sheer application that necessitates some effort to build intensity. The texture and application of the eyeshadows has improved, so if shine catches your eye, take a look at these. **Aqua Stick Cooling Eyeshadow** *($12)* has a cool, wet-feeling application and dries to a soft powder finish that leaves behind a semi-opaque layer of intense shine. These do stay put, but the shine will put the spotlight on less-than-taut eyelids.

<u>EYE AND BROW SHAPER:</u> ☹ **Defining Moment Eye Liner** *($7)* has a smooth, slightly creamy texture that tends to cause a spotty application, and over half of the colors are iridescent.

☺ **Eye Drama Liquid Liner** *($7)* has a suitably firm brush that is only capable of drawing a thick line. This doesn't dry as quickly as other liquid liners, but once it does it stays on. All of the colors except Coal are quite shiny—which teenagers will be drawn to, but adults should approach with caution, especially if the goal is sophisticated makeup.

☺ <u>LIPSTICK AND LIP PENCIL:</u> **Feel Good Lip Color** *($10)* leans just to the greasy side of creamy, but does offer an impressive range of full-coverage, mostly iridescent colors. Don't expect much longevity from these—the colors have little to no stain. **See-Thru Lip Color SPF 15** *($10)* is simply a greasy, sheer lipstick that offers no significant UVA protection. Almay's PureTints SPF 25 ($4.89) is a far better option for sheer color and effective sun protection. **Jewel Finish Lip Polish** *($10)* is a silicone-based liquid lip color that provides sheer, often sparkly, color and a glossy finish. **Extended Stay Lasting Lip Color** *($10)* is a standard creamy lipstick with a decent stain and some very good full-coverage colors. These do have a slightly glossy finish. **Color Splash Lip Pen** *($15)* is more about the innovative packaging than what's inside. This is a standard, sticky lip gloss in a pen-style tube that feeds color into a brush as you click the base. Why this is priced several dollars more than the Bath & Body Works regular lipsticks doesn't make much sense. **Color Kissed Lip Gloss** *($5.50)* is a fairly thick, standard, sticky lip gloss that features a wand applicator. **To the Point Lip Pencil** *($6.50)* has some great colors and is an attractively-priced standard pencil with a smooth application and soft, dry finish.

☹ <u>MASCARA:</u> **All Out Volumizing Mascara** *($10)* produces some length but minimal thickness. Not only does it take lots of effort to make its mark, it also smears shortly thereafter. **All Out Lengthening Mascara** *($10)* is one of the most do-nothing mascaras you're likely to come across. Enhanced length is negligible, and this somehow manages to *de*-emphasize lashes.

<u>BRUSHES:</u> The Bath & Body Works makeup star performers are the decently soft, affordably priced ☺ **Brushes** *($7–$13)*. For the most part each one has a workable shape and applies color well. The **Powder Brush** *($9.50)*, **Blush Brush** *($8)*, and **Large Eyeshadow Brush** *($8)* can be a bit too big for some faces; the **Small Eyeshadow Brush** *($5.50)* works well for applying lid and underbrow color, and the ✔☺ **Retractable Powder Brush** *($13.50)* is a superior brush for on-the-go powder touch-ups.

BEAUTICONTROL

BeautiControl, now owned by Tupperware, tries very hard to be all things to all women. The company not only gives you information about skin care and makeup application when you book a free consultation with one of the sales representatives, but also analyzes your wardrobe and tells you which colors look best on you and which clothing styles complement your body shape. Unfortunately, as always, you must depend on the expertise of the salesperson, and we all know how that can work out.

Overall, the skin-care line has improved, and now has some really excellent new moisturizers and cleansers, and the line's AHA products are, for the most part, well formulated. What is particularly disturbing is that the skin-care routines don't include sunscreen. The Sunlogics lineup is a pathetic selection of inadequate sun protection, at least as far as the standards of the American Academy of Dermatology and the National Cancer Institute are concerned, plus only one of the products contains UVA-protecting ingredients. One word of caution: The company claims that your skin type and product needs are determined by a "precise, scientific … dermatologist-tested, proven Skin Condition Analysis." There is nothing precise or scientific about it. Little pieces of sticky paper the company calls "sensors" are stuck on different cleansed areas of your face. What comes off on these strips determines the products you are to use. But, depending on the time of day or time of month you are tested you will receive different evaluations, which makes sense: no one's skin is the same in the morning as it is at the end of the day or at different times of the month. Also, be aware that the sensors can irritate skin. Skin isn't static: it changes with the seasons, your menstrual cycle, stress, and your environment. The idea is cute, but I wouldn't choose skin-care products based on this analysis alone.

These products are more than reasonably priced, but regrettably you have to pick and choose carefully to avoid making mistakes. For more information about BeautiControl, call (800) BEAUTI-1 or (800) 872-0601 or visit www.beauticontrol.com. **Note:** All BeautiControl skin care products contain fragrance unless otherwise noted.

BEAUTICONTROL SKIN CARE

BEAUTICONTROL ALL CLEAR SKIN PRODUCTS

☺ **All Clear Skin Wash** (*$12 for 6 ounces*) is a standard, detergent-based, water-soluble cleanser that would be great for normal to oily skin. It does contain a tiny amount of salicylic acid (BHA), but the pH is too high for it to be effective as an exfoliant.

☹ **All Clear Skin Scrub** (*$13 for 4 ounces*) contains synthetic (plastic) scrub particles suspended in alcohol, slip agents, thickeners, and fragrance. Alcohol as the second ingredient makes this potentially irritating and drying for all skin types.

☹ **All Clear Skin Solution** (*$15.50 for 6 ounces*) is merely 2% salicylic acid suspended in alcohol and witch hazel. It could be an option for a good exfoliating BHA product (it has a pH of 3) if the alcohol weren't there. The exfoliation from the salicylic acid can be irritating enough for the skin without the presence of the alcohol.

✓☺ **All Clear Outta Sight Nighttime Clearing Complex** *($14 for 1 ounce)* is a very good, though very standard, 2.5% benzoyl peroxide topical disinfectant that is definitely helpful for breakouts.

☹ **Pore Smoother** *($12 for 1 ounce)* contains peppermint as the second ingredient and alcohol as the fourth. That won't smooth anything, but it can easily cause irritation and dryness.

☺ **All Clear Skin Moisture** *($14 for 4 ounces)* is a good BHA exfoliant for someone with normal to slightly dry or slightly oily skin, but there are emollients present that can be a problem for someone with blemish-prone skin.

BEAUTICONTROL CELL BLOCK-C AND MICRODERM PRODUCTS

☺ $$$ **Cell Block-C New Cell Protection SPF 20** *($30 for 0.95 ounce)* is a very good in-part avobenzone-based sunscreen that would work well for someone with normal to dry skin. It contains a good mix of water-binding agents but only a teeny amount of antioxidant.

✓☺ $$$ **Cell Block-C PM Cell Protection** *($30 for 0.95 ounce)* is a very good moisturizer for normal to dry skin with some very good water-binding agents, anti-irritants, and antioxidants.

✓☺ $$$ **Microderm Eye-X-Cel Daily Therapy Creme** *($19 for 0.5 ounce)* contains mostly water, thickeners, slip agent, water-binding agents, antioxidants, film-forming agent, anti-irritants, and preservatives. This is a very good moisturizer for normal to dry skin.

☹ **Microderm Oxygenating Firming Gel** *($29.50 for 2 ounces)* is a good, lightweight moisturizer that would work for normal to slightly dry skin. It won't firm anything, and thankfully it isn't oxygenating in the least. In fact, it contains a good antioxidant, superoxide dismutase, high up on the ingredient list. What it lacks are some good water-binding agents.

☹ $$$ **Microderm Tight Eyed Eye Firming Complex** *($30 for 0.75 ounce)* contains a good mix of water-binding agents and anti-irritants in a very lightweight moisturizing base that could be an option for someone with normal to slightly dry skin. The lemon and balm mint, for fragrance, are probably not a problem. Alcohol is high up on the ingredient list so that could be drying and irritating for the skin. It does contain shine and coloring agents.

☹ **Microderm Tight Fix Facial Firming Complex** *($35 for 1 ounce)* lists alcohol as the second ingredient, and there are also some other irritating plant extracts. This could create more problems for skin than it can help.

BEAUTICONTROL REGENERATION PRODUCTS

☹ $$$ **Platinum Regeneration Skin Renewing Serum** *($60 for 1.8 ounces)* is a standard silicone-based moisturizer that contains about 3% AHA with an effective pH of 3. However, the 3% AHA concentration isn't a platinum standard by any means. It does contain small amounts of water-binding agents, antioxidants, and anti-irritants, but this isn't all that exciting.

☺ **Platinum Regenation Eye Serum** *($30 for .6 ounces)* is a good moisturizer for normal to dry skin that contains a very good mix of antioxidants and anti-irritants. The teeny amount of AHAs and the pH of 5 make it ineffective for exfoliation.

☺ **Regeneration Face and Neck Creme** *($32 for 2 ounces)* is a very basic, though very good, 4% to 5% AHA product using lactic acid as the exfoliating agent. It is an option for exfoliation, but it doesn't regenerate anything, and it doesn't work any better than Alpha Hydrox's 5% AHA product.

☺ **Regeneration 2 Face and Neck Creme** *($32 for 2 ounces)* is almost identical to the Regeneration Face and Neck Creme above, except that this one contains about a 6% to 7% AHA concentration, and the same comments apply.

☺ **Regeneration Face and Neck Cream, Oily Skin** *($32 for 2 ounces)* is a silicone-based, 4% to 5% AHA gel/lotion. It would work well for most skin types, and this one contains a small amount of water-binding agents, which makes it better formulated than almost every other Regeneration product.

☺ **Regeneration 2 for Oily Skin** *($32 for 2 ounces)* contains about 8% AHA (primarily lactic acid with trace amounts of tartaric and citric acid) in an effective pH and can be an option for someone with normal to dry or slightly oily skin. It is in a lightweight, silicone base with standard thickening agents and fragrance. As a good AHA exfoliant, this product has no advantage over those from Alpha Hydrox at the drugstore.

☹ **Regeneration Blemish Duo** *($14.50 for 0.11 ounce of Blemish Gel and 0.12 ounce of Blemish Cover-Up)* is a tube with Oil-Free Blemish Cover-Up, which is nothing more than a concealer (it comes in two colors, neither of which matches most skin tones) at one end and Blemish Gel, which is mostly alcohol, at the other. The alcohol is too drying and irritating for all skin types and won't help reduce blemishes. The Duo does contain salicylic acid (BHA), but to really combat blemishes, the ideal duo should have been an exfoliant (the BHA) and a topical disinfectant.

☹ **Regeneration Extreme Repair** *($30 for 4.5 ounces)* isn't extreme in the least. The third ingredient is urea, which was once a very popular exfoliant, but subsequent research shows that glycolic acid and lactic acid are far more useful for that purpose and have a wider range of benefit (from collagen production to cell regulation). This product also contains a tiny amount of lactic acid, but not enough for it to have much benefit as an exfoliant. The rest of the ingredients are just thickening agents and silicone, making this extremely boring for skin and easily replaced with products available at the drugstore from Eucerin, which has urea-based exfoliant lotions.

☺ **Regeneration Gold** *($56 for 1.8 ounces)* is an AHA product with about an 8% concentration of AHA dispensed in a mixture that is part lotion and part gel. The packaging is attractive, but that holds no advantage for skin. It's still just an AHA exfoliant with some thickening agents, film-forming agent, anti-irritants, fragrance, and water-binding agents. It's a good option, but this isn't exactly the "gold" standard for AHA formulations.

☺ $$$ **Regeneration Gold Eye Repair** *($25 for 0.5 ounce)* is an OK moisturizer for normal to slightly dry skin. This does contain soy flour, but that has no estrogenic effect when applied topically. It also includes only about 1% AHA and a truly insignificant amount of BHA, but even if there were more, the pH is too high for this to be effective as an exfoliant. At least there are some good water-binding agents and a minimal amount of anti-irritants.

☺ $$$ **Regeneration Time to Go** with **Retinol** *($35 for 1 ounce)*. This contains a small amount of retinol in a good moisturizing base that includes some interesting water-binding agents and anti-irritants, but if you're looking for retinol in a product, the L'Oreal Line Eraser Pure Retinol Concentrate ($12.49 for 1 ounce) and Alpha Hydrox Retinol Night ResQ Anti-Wrinkle Firming Complex ($11.99 for 1.05 ounces) also contain retinol and for far less.

☺ $$$ **Regeneration Gold Lip Therapy** *($20 for 0.12 ounce)* is just a standard emollient "lipstick." The pH is too high for the teeny amount of AHA or BHA to be effective as exfoliants. It does have a tiny amount of good water-binding agents and anti-oxidant, but barely enough to have any impact on skin.

BEAUTICONTROL SKIN EQUATIONS, THE SENSITIVE SKIN LINE

☺ **Gentle Wash** *($14 for 5.7 ounces)* is indeed a very good, gentle, detergent-based cleanser that would work well for most skin types, though not those with very dry skin.

✓☺ **Calming Rinse** *($15.50 for 5.7 ounces)* is a very good, irritant-free toner that contains mostly water, slip agent, silicone, anti-irritants, water-binding agents, and preservatives.

✓☺ **Relaxing Moisture** *($16 for 4 ounces)* is a very good moisturizer for normal to dry skin that contains some good water-binding agents, anti-irritants, and antioxidants.

BEAUTICONTROL SKIN LOGICS FOR COMBINATION SKIN

☺ **Chamomile Balancing Cleansing Lotion for Combination Skin** *($14 for 8 ounces)* is a very standard mineral oil–based cleanser that also contains some detergent cleansing agents. It can be a good option for someone with dry skin. The fragrant extracts in it smell nice but can be a problem for skin, as is true for all fragrance.

☺ **Balancing Scrub for Combination Skin** *($14.50 for 3 ounces)* is a standard, detergent-based scrub that uses synthetic particles (ground-up plastic) as the abrasive. This works as well as any scrub for most skin types except dry skin.

☹ **Balancing Tonic for Combination Skin** *($14 for 8 ounces)* is an interesting combination of anti-irritant and irritating plant extracts. Primarily it is just water, witch hazel, and glycerin. The witch hazel contains alcohol and that can be irritating and drying for most skin types.

☺ **Balancing Moisturizer** *($16 for 4.5 ounces)* is a good emollient moisturizer for normal to dry skin that includes some good water-binding agents. But there are several plant extracts in it that can be potential skin irritants and the emollient (lanolin, plant oils, and mineral oil) can be a problem for oily areas.

BEAUTICONTROL SKIN LOGICS FOR DRY SKIN

☺ **Mild Rosemary Cleansing Fluide for Dry Skin** *($14 for 8 ounces)* is a mineral oil– and lanolin oil–based cleanser that must be wiped off. This is a very standard cold cream–type cleanser that can leave a slight film on the skin. For ultra-dry skin it may be an option. It does contain fragrant citrus extracts.

☺ **Renewing Scrub/Masque** *($14 for 3 ounces)* is a detergent-based, water-soluble cleanser that contains synthetic scrub particles (ground-up plastic). This would work well for most skin types but not for someone with dry skin.

☺ **Moisturizing Toner** *($14.50 for 8 ounces)* is a good toner for most skin types. It contains mostly water, slip agents, water-binding agents, preservatives, fragrant plant extracts, and coloring agents.

☹ **Essential Moisture Lotion** *($16 for 4.5 ounces)* is a very good emollient moisturizer for normal to dry skin. It contains mostly water, plant oils, mineral oil, thickeners, vitamins, fragrant plant extracts, and preservatives.

BEAUTICONTROL SKIN LOGICS FOR OILY SKIN

☺ **Purifying Cleansing Gel** *($12 for 8 ounces)* is a very good and very standard detergent cleanser that can be good for normal to oily skin.

☹ **Almond Clarifying Scrub/Masque** *($14.50 for 3 ounces)* is a standard clay mask that also contains apricot seeds and almond meal along with thickening agents, preservatives, fragrance, and coloring agents. It is a fairly scratchy scrub and the thickening agents aren't the best for blemish-prone skin.

☹ **Clarifying Tonic** *($14.50 for 8 ounces)* is an alcohol-based toner that can be quite irritating and drying for all skin types. It also contains benzalkonium chloride, an antimicrobial that has no research showing it to have any effect against the acne-causing bacteria *Propionibacterium acnes*.

☹ **Oil-Free Moisture Supplement** *($16 for 4.5 ounces)* is a silicone-based moisturizer that has some good water-binding agents, but it also has several plant extracts that can be potential skin irritants. It can't absorb oil and the problems don't outweigh the small benefits.

☹ **Oil Control Serum** *($12 for 1 ounce)*. Nothing in this product can control oil, although the potato starch can encourage bacteria growth. The thickening agents are also problematic for oily skin, particularly the isopropyl palmitate.

BEAUTICONTROL SPECIALTY PRODUCTS

☹ **Skin Hydrator Anti-Ash Creme** *($13 for 4.5 ounces)* is just a very good, Vaseline-based moisturizer for very dry skin. There is nothing in here that can affect the color of skin.

✔☺ **Skin Lightening Complex** *($25 for 1 ounce)* is a very good, though very basic, 2% hydroquinone moisturizer. It also has about 2% glycolic acid, which isn't enough for it to be effective as an exfoliant. When used in conjunction with the diligent daily application of a sunscreen, hydroquinone can inhibit melanin production.

☺ **Lash & Lid Bath** *($9.50 for 4 ounces)* is a very standard, but good, detergent-based, water-soluble, wipe-off eye-makeup remover and it is a definite option for those wanting to wipe off eye makeup. It does not contain fragrance and that's a plus.

✔☺ **$$$ Lip Apeel** *($16 for 1.25 ounces of Lip Balm and Lip Peel)* is a two-part product (peel and balm) that helps peel dry skin off the lips and then places a thick gloss on them afterward. The peel is a bit of wax, clay, and silicate that can indeed rub off dead skin. The balm is simply a very emollient, thick lip gloss of castor oil, petrolatum, and lanolin. It does the trick and is an excellent option for preventing chapped lips.

☹ **Herbal Hydrating Mist** *($9 for 8 ounces)* contains arnica, a potent skin irritant, and is not recommended. What a shame, because otherwise this could have been a good toner for most skin types.

☺ **Protective Services** *($15 for 1 ounce)* contains 0.5% hydrocortisone, along with some plant extracts that can be anti-irritants, though it also contains guarana, which can be a skin irritant. However, the hydrocortisone is an active pharmaceutical ingredient and can indeed reduce skin inflammation, though it should only be used short term because repeated application can cause skin to thin and collagen to break down. This is a nice formulation, but there is no extra benefit to be gained by using this rather than Lanacort or Cortaid from the drugstore.

☺ **Corticure Comfort Lotion** *($17 for 3 ounces)* contains half the amount of cortisone as the Protective Services above, and the same basic comments apply.

☹ **Demarkable Dermal Smoothing Lotion** *($35 for 4.5 ounces)* contains nothing different from many of the BeautiControl moisturizers. There is nothing in this product that can affect scarring or stretch marks, and it is a misleading waste of time.

BEAUTICONTROL SUNLOGICS

☹ **Sunlogics Tanning Mist SPF 8** *($14 for 8 ounces)*, with an SPF 8, is without regard for the National Cancer Institute or the American Academy of Dermatology recommendations for sunscreen needing to be at least SPF 15. Plus, this does not contain the UVA-protecting ingredients of titanium dioxide, zinc oxide, or avobenzone, and, therefore, is not recommended. This is like asking for wrinkles and sun damage to happen.

☹ **Sunlogics Sunless Tanning Lotion, SPF 6** *($14.50 for 4.5 ounces)*. This product is similar to the Mist SPF 8 above, and the same comments apply.

☹ **Sunlogics UV Lip+Eye Stick SPF 15** *($9.50 for 0.06 ounce)* doesn't contain the UVA-protecting ingredients of avobenzone, zinc oxide, or titanium dioxide, and is not recommended.

☺ **Sunlogics Waterproof Sunblock SPF 30** *($15 for 4.5 ounces)* is a good, in-part avobenzone-based sunscreen in a fairly ordinary moisturizing base. It would be an option for someone with normal to dry skin.

☹ **Sunlogics Bronzer** *($12 for 0.35 ounce)* is not a self-tanner, it is just a matte-finish, lightweight, tinted cream that also contains talc, cornstarch, zinc stearate, mineral oil, and lanolin, which makes it an inappropriate formula for just about every skin type.

BEAUTICONTROL MAKEUP

BeautiControl makeup has about as many strong points as weak points. Almost every makeup category has its share of winners and, for lack of a better word, losers. Several products, such as the blushes and eyeshadows, have exemplary textures and wonderful applications that are marred by too much shine and unflattering colors. There are a couple of great foundations, too, but the extensive color range needs to be edited to improve the poor color choices, particularly for warm skin tones. (BeautiControl tends to want to put warm skin tones in peach shades, and that includes foundation.) In terms of warm and cool tones, the makeup selection clearly favors cool tones; that means if you're "typed" as a warm tone, your makeup options are limited. Try as they might, the BeautiControl image tools for makeup and skin care work best as suggested guidelines, not as mandates. For women who truly feel clueless about where to begin with makeup, however, the image tools can be a somewhat helpful starting point. Just be careful you don't treat this color and wardrobe information as anything other than a suggestion, and not as tenet.

<u>FOUNDATION:</u> ☺ **Perfecting Wet/Dry Finish Foundation** *($20.50)* is a standard, talc-based pressed powder that has a decent color selection and covers softly and smoothly. The texture and finish are great. It's supposed to be able to diffuse light in order to minimize lines, but it can't do that. Most of the 24 colors are reliable and neutral, with the light to medium shades faring best. The only colors to avoid are Peaches & Cream, Bisque, Golden Honey, Toffee, Nutmeg, Dark, and Bronze. **Color Freeze Liquid Makeup SPF 12** *($20)* is an excellent matte-finish foundation that is great for oily skin types. The SPF 12 is below SPF 15 and shouldn't be relied on for all-day protection, but it does contain titanium dioxide. This is definitely an option and one of the better foundations of this type. The only colors to avoid are Peaches & Cream, Bisque, Golden Honey, Toffee, Mocha, Nutmeg, Dark, and Bronze.

☺ **Sheer Protection Oil-Free Liquid Foundation** *($11)* is a lightweight foundation that provides light to medium coverage and has a soft matte finish. All of the shades are divided into cool and warm tones, but most are too pink or peach. Someone with warm skin tones should not wear a vivid peach foundation, nor should someone with cool skin tones wear a vivid pink foundation. Another caution: There are definitely ingredients in this product that could trigger breakouts and that you might want to avoid. The only colors to consider are Nude, Natural, Alabaster, Buff, and Porcelain Beige. The other colors are too pink, rose, orange, or peach to look convincing in daylight. **Secret Agent**

Wrinkle Deflector *($15)* is a sheer iridescent lotion that has a pink undertone and is designed to be used under foundation to diffuse wrinkles and add a glow to the skin. This doesn't work the way you may hope it does, and is one more in a growing pile of shiny foundation-hybrid products that does add "glow," but that doesn't change the appearance of one wrinkle on your face.

☹ **Perfecting Creme to Powder Finish Foundation** *($13)* is a very thick, greasy foundation that does have a powder finish, but it never loses its greasy feel. Its claim to be waterproof is pretty accurate, but it is almost cleanser-proof, too, and it can easily clog pores if you're not careful. There are many other cream-to-powder foundations that are more modern and they're readily available at drugstores or department store. **Creme Sheer Protection Foundation** *($12.50)* is more like a creamy pancake makeup and is very greasy, containing mineral oil, heavy wax, and lanolin, which is a lot for anything but dry skin to handle. The six colors tend to be on the peachy side.

<u>CONCEALER:</u> ☹ **Extra-Help Concealer** *($5.50)* blends on easily and provides good to medium coverage, but it is fairly greasy and can crease into lines around the eyes moments after being applied and continue to do so the rest of the day. The Light and Medium shades can be too peach for most skin tones. **Color Perfectors** *($12)* are standard, lipstick-style skin-color correctors that come in three shades: Mint, Yellow, and Mauve. They can't change skin tone convincingly, they layer on more makeup than any woman needs, and they can wreak havoc when you apply a foundation. **All Clear Blemish Duo** *($14.50; $9 for Blemish Gel refill)* is a two-part product that includes a lightweight concealer and clear blemish gel with 2% salicylic acid and a pH of 3. A clever idea, but both concealer shades are too pink (not the shade you want to place over an inflamed, red blemish) and the blemish gel is alcohol-based, which is too irritating for skin.

☺ **Secret Agent Undercover Line Smoother** *($12)* is a stealthy tool that can work to some extent to fill in minor wrinkles. It's a thick silicone cream that has a soft, spackle-like effect on the skin, but how long it lasts depends on how deep your wrinkles are and how expressive your face is. This is worth a try if you're curious about the effect.

<u>POWDER:</u> ☹ **Loose Perfecting Powder** *($10.50)* is a standard, talc-based powder that has a soft, dry texture, but it contains benzaldehyde, a highly toxic ingredient that is best avoided.

☺ **Sun Faux You Bronzing Powder** *($15)* is a wonderfully soft pressed-powder bronzer that sweeps on easily and does not streak. It has a matte finish and attractive tan color that works best on fair to light skin. **Secret Agent Private Detective Pressed Powder** *($15)* claims to contain light-deflecting particles for a youthful glow and flawless appearance, but this is just a standard, but good, talc-based pressed powder with a silky, dry matte finish and three superb colors.

☺ <u>BLUSH:</u> The **Unbelievable Blush** *($13.50)* shades all have some amount of shine, but not enough to be a problem for most skin types. (Someone with oily skin may not be happy with it, though.) The colors are beautiful and the texture is soft and smooth. Note:

The Reviews B

the colors are fairly vivid and pastel, and there aren't many neutral shades. If you're not one to shy away from blush, you will be pleased with these colors.

☺ <u>EYESHADOW:</u> **Sensuous Shadows** *($9 for singles, $13.50 for trios)* come in singles or compacts with three shades, but some of the combinations are poor, and the colors range from barely shiny to very shiny; if you have any lines on your eyelids, shine will make them look worse. The singles offer a better way to pick and choose the colors you want, although shine still reigns supreme. **Shadow Control Creme** *($7)* does help to keep your eyeshadow on, without creasing, for the entire day. There are four colors, but, like the eyeshadows, they are all shiny.

<u>EYE & BROW SHAPER:</u> ☺ **Eye Defining Pencils** *($7.50)* and **Eye Brow Pencils** *($12)* are standard pencils that come in a dated range of colors (too many blues and teals, though the brown, gray, and black tones are fine). They tend to be on the dry side, which makes them a little harder to apply, but they also tend to last longer. The Brow Pencils have a smoother texture than most and are worth considering if you prefer pencils to powder. **Color Freeze Eye Liner** *($9.50)* comes in a twist-up container and has better staying power than the Eye Defining Pencils. **Brow Powder** *($15)* comes with two matte pressed brow powders per pan, and these apply well and enhance the brows nicely. Having two colors to work with isn't mandatory, but for those who want to customize, these tone-on-tone shades work well together.

☹ **Secret Agent Licensed to Fill Lip Primer** *($12)* is a solid white, silicone- and wax-based lipstick that is designed to fill in lines and enhance fullness. Although this formula can go the distance to prevent some lipsticks from feathering, it tends to apply unevenly and balls up or flakes off. Great name, though! **Brow Control Creme** *($7)* comes in a squeeze tube that you apply to a mascara-like wand and then roll through the brow. I like making brows look fuller, but this is a messy option. Similar products come with the brush inside, so the color is evenly distributed.

<u>LIPSTICK & LIP PENCIL:</u> ☺ **Lasting Lip Color** *($9)* is a very creamy, slightly greasy lipstick that doesn't last very long, but the color selection is attractive. The colors are divided into tonal families, as well as creams and frosts, which helps prevent the accidental purchase of an iridescent lip color if that's not what you're looking for. **Color Freeze Lip Color** *($10)* performs just like all the other ultra-matte lipsticks, only this one is so soft in the tube it smushes and deteriorates with the least amount of pressure. It isn't a bad product, just not an improvement in price or performance over Revlon ColorStay Lipstick. **Regeneration Gold Volumizing Lip Color** *($15)* claims it is "full-treatment lip color" that helps "repair lips, increase fullness, and give lips a more contoured look with special dimension pigments." And all of this should happen within two weeks! Not to burst anyone's bubble, but this is just a lightweight, semi-opaque creamy lipstick that glides on and has disappointing staying power. As for the special dimension pigments, these are simply mica suspended in emollients, and indistinguishable from most other iridescent lipsticks. This is not a bad lipstick, just one with overinflated claims.

☺ **$$$ LipSTICK System** *($38.50 for both the Color ON and Shine ON—they are also sold separately)* is BeautiControl's version of a semi-permanent lip stain. The **Color ON** *($18.50)* is a deeply pigmented, semi-permanent lip stain. This alcohol-based formula burns as you apply it, and dries in a flash, laying down a thin but rich layer of pure color. Next up is the **Shine ON** *($10)*, which is a clear, silicone-based lip gloss that allows for shiny, comfortable wear without removing the color. To remove this very tenacious product, you can use the **Color OFF** *($10)*, which is nothing more than alcohol (functioning as a solvent to break up the lip color), water, glycerin, and gel-based thickeners. All in all, this expensive three-part system will provide a full day's (and sometimes into the next day) worth of lasting color. However, for the money and a less irritating experience, I still recommend Max Factor Lipfinity or Cover Girl Outlast over this.

✓☺ **Lip Control Creme** *($7)* is excellent. It prevents even greasy lipstick from feathering into the lines around the mouth; however, it would be even better if it came in an easier-to-use applicator so you wouldn't have to spread it with your finger or a lipstick brush.

☺ **Lip Shaping Pencils** *($7.50)* are just standard pencils in a nice array of colors and that need to be sharpened. **Color Freeze Lip Liner** *($9.50)* is a twist-up container that does have better staying power than the Lip Shaping Pencils.

☹ **Clear Lip Gloss** *($9)* is a standard, wand-applicator lip gloss that has a thick, sticky texture. It's fine as far as gloss goes, if you can tolerate the stickiness.

MASCARA: ☹ **Spectaculash Waterproof Mascara** *($8.50)* comes off easily with water and cleanser, and it doesn't smear after a long day. It would be great mascara if it could build long, thick lashes, but it can't. It's just OK.

☹ **Spectaculash Thickening Mascara** *($9)* is not what I would call spectacular in the least. It creates minimal length and doesn't make lashes all that thick, but it is waterproof. There are better, easier-to-find waterproof mascaras available than this one.

BEAUTY WITHOUT CRUELTY (SKIN CARE ONLY)

Many companies proudly boast that they do not test their products on animals. Nonetheless, despite the fact that they don't test their finished products on animals, there isn't a company selling a sunscreen or using vitamins or myriad plant extracts in their products that doesn't know about the efficacy of these ingredients based on recent or current animal testing. While it is wonderful that companies like Beauty Without Cruelty do not test their products on animals, as is true for many companies, a good many of their formulations are based on the results of animal research. If Beauty Without Cruelty does excel in one area, it is that none of their products are sourced from animals, which is somewhat unique in the industry and definitely a plus for vegans. But it would be naïve to believe that any company can stay abreast of what is and isn't healthy for skin without the animal testing of the ingredients in their products.

Much like the rest of the cosmetics industry, Beauty Without Cruelty makes elaborate claims about the benefits of its plant extracts. And, as is also the case for many cosmetics companies, they use plant extracts that are both irritants and anti-irritants. For the most part the products are a mixed bag; there is a good sunscreen, and some decent cleansers, but some of the moisturizers are excellent and deserve a closer look. Beauty Without Cruelty is typically distributed in health food stores and can be found in some drugstores. You can also order direct by calling (800) 227-5120 or online at www.avalonnaturalproducts.com. They also offer a makeup line, but its distribution is extremely limited and haphazard across the United States, and, therefore, it is not reviewed in this edition.

☺ **Extra Gentle Facial Cleansing Milk** *($9.95 for 8.5 ounces)* is a fairly fragrant, plant oil–based, cold cream–style cleanser. It can be an option for normal to dry skin, but the plant extracts are far better for your olfactory sense than your skin.

☹ **Herbal Cream Facial Cleanser** *($7.95 for 8.5 ounces)* is a detergent-based, water-soluble cleanser that also contains some plant oils. This could have been a good cleanser for normal to dry skin, but the number of potentially problematic plant extracts are hard to ignore.

☺ **3% Alpha Hydroxy Facial Cleanser Normal/Oily Skin Types** *($7.49 for 8.5 ounces)* is a standard, detergent-based, water-soluble cleanser that can be very good for someone with normal to oily skin. The AHA concentration of 3% isn't sufficient for it to be an exfoliant, plus in a cleanser it would just be washed down the drain before it had a chance to have any effect. This does contain fragrance, and several of the plant extracts can be skin irritants.

☹ **Vitamin C Facial Cleanser** *($7.95 for 8 ounces)* contains several irritating plant extracts and TEA-lauryl sulfate as the main cleansing agent, which makes it a problem for all skin types.

☹ **Extra Gentle Eye Makeup Remover** *($5.95 for 4 ounces)* is a fairly standard, detergent-based eye-makeup remover, though the tea water contains some witch hazel (and that contains alcohol), which may be a problem for the eye area.

☹ **Extra Gentle Facial Smoother** *($7.95 for 4 ounces)* can be an OK facial scrub that uses jojoba wax beads and almond meal as the abrasives, which makes it fairly gentle. Be aware that a few of the plant extracts in it can be skin irritants.

☺ **Balancing Facial Toner for All Skin Types** *($7.95 for 8.5 ounces)* is a good, almost irritant-free toner that contains a nice assortment of water-binding agents, anti-irritants, and teeny amounts of vitamins that can be antioxidants. Some of the plant extracts can be a problem for sensitive skin types.

☹ **Renewal Moisture Cream 8% Alpha Hydroxy Complex for All Skin Types** *($13.95 for 4 ounces)*. The claim about 8% AHA in this product is dubious at best. Plus the label indicates it contains an "alpha hydroxy acid complex," which is not compliant with FDA guidelines for listing ingredients. But none of that matters, because the pH is too high for it to be effective for exfoliation. The plant oils in it would not be appreciated by all skin types.

☺ **All Day Moisturizer Normal/Dry Skin** *($13.95 for 2 ounces)* doesn't contain a sunscreen, which makes it a poor choice for all day, but it can be a very good, emollient nighttime moisturizer for someone with dry skin. However, it does contain fragrance and several of the plant extracts can be skin irritants.

✓☺ **Green Tea Nourishing Eye Gel** *($14.49 for 1 ounce)* is a very good lightweight moisturizer for normal to slightly dry skin that can be used over the entire face. This does not contain fragrance, and has a great array of water-binding agents, antioxidants, and anti-irritants.

✓☺ **Maximum Moisture Cream Benefits Dry/Mature Skin** *($14.49 for 2 ounces)* is a very good moisturizer for someone with very dry skin because it contains excellent emollients, water-binding agents, antioxidants, and anti-irritants. It does contain fragrant plant extracts.

☺ **Oil-Free Facial Moisturizer** *($12.49 for 2 ounces)* contains several plant extracts that can be skin irritants. However, it could be a good lightweight moisturizer for someone with normal to slightly dry skin, though it lacks many of the interesting components of the Green Tea Nourishing Eye Gel above (the Eye Gel would be a far better option for someone with normal to oily skin).

✓☺ **SPF 15 Daily Facial Lotion, Benefits All Skin Types** *($9.49 for 4 ounces)* is a very good, titanium dioxide–based sunscreen that would work great for someone with normal to dry skin. The plant oils and emollients in it, however, would not be suitable for all skin types.

☹ **Vitamin C SPF 15 Moisture Plus** *($14.95 for 4 ounces)* doesn't contain the UVA-protecting ingredients of titanium dioxide, zinc oxide, or avobenzone, and is not recommended.

✓☺ **Vitamin C Renewal Cream** *($18.95 for 2 ounces)* is a good emollient moisturizer for normal to dry skin. It does contain a stable form of vitamin C (magnesium ascorbyl palmitate) that's a good antioxidant, as well as some excellent water-binding agents and anti-irritants, but don't count on that renewing anything.

✓☺ **Vitamin C Vitality Serum** *($24.95 for 1 ounce)* is similar to the Renewal Cream above only in a light lotion form, and the same basic comments apply. This is a better option for someone with normal to slightly dry skin.

✓☺ **Vitamin C Revitalizing Eye Cream** *($24.95 for 1 ounce)* is similar to the Vitality Serum above and the same comments apply.

☺ **Purifying Facial Mask** *($8.95 for 4 ounces)* is a standard clay mask that is as good an option as any for absorbing oil. It does contain fragrance.

beComing (SEE AVON beComing)

BENEFIT

BeneFit was developed by twins Jean Danielson and Jane Blackford, whose brief claim to fame was a stint as the Calgon twins back in the 1960s. They opened their first cosmetics store in San Francisco around 1976. When BeneFit was purchased by the LVMH group, also the parent company of the Sephora chain of stores, BeneFit traded a bit of its independence, but vowed to stay true to the zany irreverence that put it on the map. Fortunately the change hasn't eroded Benefit's makeup philosophy, which is outrageously fun, or its product arsenal, which is centered on impossibly cute names and a lexicon aimed at teenagers. BeneFit single-handedly started the trend of selling makeup and skin-care products with ultra-cute appellations for less than ultra-cute prices. "Zaparella, feared foe of the Evil Blemish, sweeps night skies" and "Do the bags under your eyes look like carry-ons? Unload those bags …" are hardly your typical scientific, elegance-laden cosmetics selling points. You'll find the standard promises of curing wrinkles and blemishes here right along with a large dose of misleading and erroneous information. Cuteness aside, most of these products simply can't do what they say. The blemish products contain irritating ingredients that can make breakouts worse; products claiming not to contain fragrance blatantly contain extremely fragrant plant oils plus plant extracts that are all potential skin irritants; and the label describes several decidedly unnatural ingredients as being natural. Here is one of the more maddening examples: "… moisturize or you'll break out more!" Sorry! Moisturizers cannot prevent breakouts in any way, shape, or form.

The strong points of this product line lie in the excellent, reasonably priced brushes and a vast collection of lipsticks with a color range that would satisfy everyone from a debutante to a malcontent. The rest of the line tries its best to entice you, and I must admit the products are almost irresistible, but does anyone really need seven products to take care of the lips? However, there's nothing here that is worthy of too much attention or that can't be found in many other lines that offer the shine and glitz of BeneFit along with a healthy dose of real-world shades and exemplary textures.

For more information about BeneFit, call (800) 781-2336 or visit www.benefit cosmetics.com.

BENEFIT SKIN CARE

☺ $$$ **All Types Skin Wash** *($16 for 4 ounces)* is about as close a knockoff of Cetaphil Gentle Skin Cleanser as I've seen. At least they're on the right track for a sensitive-skin cleanser, but they're charging a lot more than Cetaphil.

☹ **Fantasy Mint Wash, for Combo/Oily Skin** *($24 for 4 ounces)* contains spearmint, which can be a skin irritant, especially for the eyes, for all skin types. This product also contains emollients that would be problematic for combination and oily skin.

☺ **Clean Sweep** *($14 for 4 ounces)* is a very standard, detergent-based eye-makeup remover. It will indeed wipe off your eye makeup.

The Reviews B

☺ **Make Up Remover and Brush Cleaner Baby!** *($21 for 12 ounces)* is a standard, detergent-based cleanser that would be an option for someone with normal to oily skin.

☺ **Pineapple Facial Polish** ($24 for 5.5 ounces), thankfully, contains only a minuscule amount of pineapple and kiwi, so they have no irritating impact on skin. This is just a standard scrub that uses jojoba beads as the exfoliant in a base of glycerin and thickeners and is an option for normal to dry skin.

☹ **Azulene Toner** *($16 for 4 ounces)*. Several of the plant extracts in this product can be skin irritants, including witch hazel, arnica, ivy, pellitory, and rose oil. Azulene is a chamomile extract, but it is used primarily as a coloring agent in cosmetics and has few of chamomile's anti-irritant properties.

☹ **Rosewater Toner** *($14 for 4 ounces)* is just witch hazel and fragrance. It lacks any benefit for skin. There isn't an antioxidant, anti-irritant, or water-binding agent in sight.

☹ **Alpha Clean 5% AHA** *($20 for 4 ounces)* doesn't list the form of AHA used, which doesn't meet FDA requirements for ingredient listings. Plus the scrub particles are scratchy and potentially irritating. Even if the AHA were effective, it would just be washed down the drain in this strangely formulated cleanser.

☺ **Alpha Smooth 5% AHA Toner** *($20 for 4 ounces)*. The pH is low enough for it to be an effective exfoliant but the source of the AHA is not listed, so not only does the ingredient label not meet FDA standards, but also you can't rely on it for information about what you're putting on your skin.

☺ **$$$ Seven %** *($38 for 1 ounce)* doesn't contain a low enough pH to be an effective exfoliant. Again, the label doesn't indicate what kind of AHA is used, so this is definitely not in compliance with FDA regulations. Other than that, this is a good, though rather basic, moisturizer for normal to dry skin.

☺ **Daily Hyaluronic Crème for Seriously Sensitive Skin** *($22 for 2 ounces)* is a good emollient cream for someone with dry skin. This does contain some very good water-binding agents, plant oils, and some antioxidants, which is great, but the pollen and fragrance make this inappropriate for someone with sensitive skin.

☹ **$$$ Dr. Feel Good** *($24 for 0.85 ounce)* is supposed to be worn either alone or over makeup to "smooth pores and fine lines leaving skin silky, flawless and matte to the touch." And because it contains vitamins A, C, and E, "it repairs skin without a prescription." Wow! Who wouldn't want this product? It turns out that Dr. Feel Good is an extremely thick pot of wax resembling a thick lip balm or clear shoe polish more than anything else. I guess you could also call this product spackle, because that is exactly how it works. The wax melts over the skin and then fills in the flaws (at least somewhat). I didn't notice a difference in my wrinkles, but over the long haul I would be very concerned about clogged pores because this is really thick, heavy stuff.

☺ **Eye Lift** *($25 for 1 ounce)* is a good, lightweight moisturizer for normal to slightly dry skin, but nothing about it will lift the eye. It contains mostly water, silicone, glycerin, antioxidants, and preservatives. At least this one doesn't contain fragrance!

☺ $$$ **RePair Aromatherapy, for Sun Damage** *($32 for 1 ounce)* contains no ingredients that can repair sun-damaged skin. This is a very misleading product that insinuates that you can get sun damage and then reverse it, when you can't. It is just hazelnut oil with some fragrance. Skip the fragrance, which is a problem for skin, and just buy some hazelnut oil from the health food store and use that.

☹ **ReEyedrate Aromatherapy, for Eyes** *($32 for 1 ounce)* is almost identical to the RePair version above except that this one contains different fragrant extracts. The same basic comments apply.

☹ **Boo-Boo Zap** *($16 for 0.25 ounce)* contains mostly water, two types of alcohol, witch hazel, and camphor. This doesn't help blemishes in the least; in fact, it can cause more irritation and redness and make skin dry and inflamed. Ouch!

☹ **Buh-Bye! Nighttime Blemish Blaster** *($21 for 0.25 ounce)* is a blemish product that contains Vaseline as the third ingredient. Unbelievable! But it's just one of the many problems for this product. It also contains pineapple juice and eucalyptus oil, which can be irritating and won't help blemishes, plus sanguinaria (bloodroot) extract, which has some antimicrobial properties but it's unlikely that it has any impact on blemishes or is effective in the teeny amount used in this product.

☺ $$$ **Shrink Wrap Mask, for Combo/Oily Skin** *($26 for 2 ounces)* is a good mask of aloe, water-binding agents, fragrance, and preservatives. This would work well for someone with normal to dry skin or combination skin.

☺ $$$ **Smoooch** *($18 for 0.25 ounce)* is just a very good, though standard, clear lip moisturizer in a tube applicator. It would work as well as any.

☺ $$$ **Aruba in a Tuba Ultra Sunless Tan** *($22 for 5 ounces)* is a sunless tanner that uses the exact same active ingredient to turn the skin brown that all other sunless tanners use: dihydroxyacetone. It would work as well as any, but I just love the name of this product.

BENEFIT MAKEUP

FOUNDATION: ☺ $$$ **PlaySticks** *($30)* is a strictly cream-to-powder foundation in stick form that must be blended quickly because it dries to a powder finish almost immediately, and it does have a soft matte finish in the long run. Coverage can go from light to medium and the drier finish makes this suitable for normal to slightly oily skin only, but it won't hold up as the day goes by for those with very oily skin. Each of the seven colors is soft and neutral. **I Am Rebel SPF 15** *($26)* bills itself as a "defiantly different tinted moisturizer," but it ends up being as standard as they come. The Rebel comes in a generous-size tube and has a creamy, somewhat thick texture that blends down to a natural finish with sheer coverage. I suppose the "different" angle comes into play with the inclusion of an in-part avobenzone-based sunscreen; although that's a plus, it's hardly defiant! The only real drawback with this product is that it is only available in one color, a soft yellow-toned neutral shade that would be best for light to medium skin.

☺ $$$ <u>CONCEALER:</u> **Boi-ing** *($18)* is "100% industrial strength" and it does provide fairly opaque coverage. However, contrary to claims, the cream-to-powder texture may not last through the day without fading or creasing, and the three colors available are slightly pink or peach. Still, this may work for some skin tones. **Ooo La Lift** *($18)* is an "instant eye lift!," or so BeneFit would like you to believe. This is just a pale pink liquid highlighter with a smooth texture and a slight shine. There is absolutely nothing in it to support the "depuffing and firming" claims.

☹ **It-Stick** *($16)* is a thick pencil concealer intended to "whisk away creases" and expression lines. There is only one color, a pale peach, which won't work on most skin tones, and the creamy texture dries to an unflattering chalky finish.

☹ **Eye Bright** *($16)* is a pale pink, slightly greasy pencil meant to be used on the dark inner corners of the eyes. It is completely unnecessary because any neutral-shade concealer can do the same without the somewhat odd pink tint.

<u>POWDER:</u> ☹ **Get Even** *($24)* is a standard, talc-based pressed powder with three shades that range from yellow to cantaloupe. This is supposed to invisibly get rid of shine and discoloration, but the yellow- and orange-tone powder on the face is hardly invisible; all it does is alter the color of your foundation to a strange, unattractive hue.

☺ $$$ **Hoola** *($26)* is an overpriced, but excellent, bronzing powder. If you don't mind parting with this much moola, you'll find that Hoola has a smooth texture, matte finish, and an attractive tan color that would be very flattering on fair to medium skin.

<u>BLUSH:</u> ☹ **Color Wash** *($24)* is a group of loose powders in blush-like colors that are an exceedingly messy and inconvenient way to use blush. With so many excellent blush options at other counters, this is a total waste of time and money.

✓☺ $$$ **BeneTint** *($26)* is a simple, rose-tinted, liquid cheek color that, while sheer, is only good on flawless, smooth skin. This can be used as a lip stain, and is relatively long-lasting in that capacity. If you prefer liquid blush, this is one of the best. ✓☺ **Glamazon** *($26)* is virtually identical to the BeneTint, but this is a sheer (though liquidy) believable bronze tint. If your skin is perfectly smooth and even, it will work well. ✓☺ **Cheekies** *($20)* is billed as a "satin cream blush," which is an accurate description. It comes packaged in a metal tube, which is a viable option for dispensing a cream blush. It applies easily and blends well—a little goes a long way—and the four worthwhile colors are vibrant but can also go on sheer. Whether or not you'll get much use from the "blending sponge on a stick" that comes with this blush depends on your patience, though it's easier to apply with a regular makeup sponge or your fingers.

☺ $$$ **Nine One One** *($18)* is a soft, brownish pink tint in a tube applicator meant to be used for the eyes, lips, and cheeks. It has a slightly sticky texture and a creamy finish that works best on the lips. If you're prone to breakouts, the greasiness isn't best for the cheeks, and if you have any problem with eyeshadows creasing, this will make matters worse.

<u>EYESHADOW:</u> ☺ $$$ **Creaseless Creme Eyeshadow** *($14)* has a creamy, slick feel and a soft powder finish. These actually do a great job of not creasing, but the colors,

though sheer and relatively easy to apply, are almost all shiny. I would say it's easier to start off with a powder in the first place, but if you are interested in cream eyeshadows this is a definite option: **Powder Eyeshadow** *($12)* has a relatively smooth but dry texture and does offer a handful of sophisticated matte shades. They tend to go on sheer, so building intensity will take some effort. The shiny shades are not as easy to work with as those from lines like Stila or Lorac. **FY … eye** *($20)* is an overpriced, peach-toned eyeshadow base that adds a subtle, strange tone to the eye area. This manages to stay slick on the skin but has a powdery finish. Again, your foundation or matte concealer will do fine instead. The **Cowgirls Eye Shadow** *($18)* includes ultra-slick, cream-to-powder eyeshadows that feature neutral but shiny home-on-the-range-hues. **She Shells** *($18)* are cream-to-powder eyeshadows housed in a seashell compact. If the type of packaging appeals to you, that's what you're paying for—what's inside is neither exceptional nor even user-friendly.

☹ **Show-offs** *($16)* are small vials of iridescent loose powder that are pretty to look at but messy to apply. For intense shine, wasted money, and sloppy application, these are hard to beat. **Swingin' Sweetie Eye Sparkle** *($14)* are small pots of very shiny, loose-powder eyeshadow. Both the color and shine are potent enough, but why put up with such a messy product when there are countless pressed-powder eyeshadows (including shiny ones)?

☹ **Lemon Aid** *($18)* is an unnecessary pale yellow eyeshadow base that has a thick texture; it does not work as well as a neutral foundation for minimizing discoloration.

<u>EYE & BROW SHAPER:</u> ☺ $$$ **Babe Cakes** *($16)* are standard cake eyeliners that go on wet and then dry to a dramatic, shiny finish. **Sketching Kohl Pencils** *($15)* are standard pencils that have a soft, creamy, ready-to-smudge texture. Application is easy, but you might as well resign yourself to some amount of smudging before the day is done.

☹ **Bad Gal, Gilded,** and **Mr. Frosty** *($16)* are standard chunky pencils that are all shiny and creamy enough to consistently smear.

☺ **Eye Pencils** *($12)* go on well, with a slightly dry texture. They're standard but nice, and there's a good assortment of soft colors.

☹ $$$ **Brow Zings** *($22)* are brow colors that are a cross between a waxy pencil and a dry brow powder. They are meant to tame brows, but they can make them look matted. Brow Zings are sold with a stiff, scratchy mini brow brush and a tiny pair of tweezers. For longevity and ease of use, Brow Zings are not preferred over a good matte powder eyeshadow.

☹ $$$ **She-Laq** *($24)* is a thick, alcohol-based liquid with hairspray ingredients that is meant as a sealant for lipstick, eyeliner, or brow color. This should not go anywhere near the eye, as the irritation potential is just too high. Otherwise, it's just an expensive variation on brow gel.

<u>LIPSTICK & LIP PENCIL:</u> BeneFit's ☺ **Lipstick** *($14)* has a great selection of colors. Although they are unspecified (which is confusing), there are creams that are

indeed creamy with a glossy finish, and mattes that are almost matte, but do have a slightly creamy finish. The shade selection is quite varied, and many of the shade names are a hoot! **Lip Gloss** *($14)* has a slippery, almost non-sticky texture and most of the colors are opaque. Nice, but overpriced. **Dancing Darlings Lip Sparkle** *($16)* are just standard lip glosses in pots with a handful of colors heavily infused with sparkles. For glittery lips at a premium price, these will do. ☺ $$$ **BeneTint Lip Balm SPF 15** *($18)* is a standard, castor oil–based lip gloss that does not contain adequate UVA protection. It's fine as a lip gloss, with a texture that is not too sticky and a sheer, cherry-red color that would work well on a variety of skin tones. **She Shells Lip Cremes** *($18)* are slick and glossy lipsticks in a compact. They're fun to look at but not fun to pay for. **Cowgirls Lip Creme** *($18)* is just semi-opaque, glossy lipstick in a compact. The neutral colors will work for most skin tones. **Charge It!** *($16)* is a pot of copper-colored lip gloss infused with lots of sparkles, for those whose lips must glisten with come-hither allure as they plunk down their credit cards.

☺ **Depth Charge** *($14)* and **Light Switch** *($14)* are lipsticks you apply over other lipsticks that you want to make lighter or darker. Basically, they are light and dark lipsticks just to the greasy side of creamy, and, like any light or dark lipstick, they will change the color of a lipstick you want to alter.

☺ **Lip Pencil** *($12)* has a rich, creamy texture but is otherwise standard and ho-hum. **Sketching Silk Lip Pencil** *($15)* has a less creamy texture than the regular lip pencil and is fine as far as standard pencils go. ☺ $$$ **Smoooch** *($18)* is simply lip balm in a tube. It's emollient and feels nice, but why spend this much for something so boring and basic when many other lines have identical versions for far less? **De-groovie** *($22)* is supposed to prevent lipstick from feathering. It does an OK job, but just OK.

☹ **Lip Plump** *($16)* is a lightweight concealer for lips that gets almost as much beauty press as the BeneTint. It slightly, and I mean slightly, fills in the lines on your lips, but breaks down almost immediately after you apply your lipstick, meaning that the difference is barely discernible. I have a feeling this is a one-time-only purchase for most women.

MASCARA: BeneFit's ☺ **Mascara** *($14)* is still just OK mascara; it applies nicely and tends to not smear, which is always a plus. It can work for lengthening, but don't expect much thickness. There is also clear mascara that could work as a brow gel.

☹ **Lash Lovies** *($18)* is cream mascara in a toothpaste-style aluminum tube that includes a mascara wand on the side of the tube. All in all this mascara is more trouble to apply and maintain than it's worth. You do get to choose from four truly outrageous colors—purple, turquoise, cranberry, and mint green—but you can get outrageous mascara colors from lots of other lines (Hard Candy and Urban Decay to name two) without the tricky, hard-to-use packaging.

BRUSHES: There is much to like about BeneFit's ✔☺ **Brushes** *($11–$27)*, including the down-to-earth prices. Most of these are beautifully shaped and appropriate for a variety of looks. Check them out if you happen to see them! There are really only two to avoid: ☹ **Get Bent Eyeliner** *($13)* has a fun name and it is bent, but the brush itself is long and splays too easily to get a controlled line, and **Sheer Powdering** *($16)*, which is a sparse, fan-shaped brush whose purpose has never been adequately explained to me, and whatever the intended effect is, it can surely be created with a more traditional brush. The ☺ **Blush Brush** *($21)* is nicely cut but almost too sparse for controlled application. Still, test this yourself if the price fits your budget.

☺ $$$ <u>SPECIALTY PRODUCTS:</u> Because BeneFit's image emphasizes fun and frivolity, you'll find quite a few additional products that can be a brief departure from the norm for special occasions. **Lightning** *($20)* is an intense, golden shimmer body lotion. **Flamingo Fancy** *($20)* is almost identical to Lightning, only it has a coral-bronze shimmer color. **Classic Kitten**, **Kitten Shops New York City**, and **Kitten Goes to Paris** *(all $24)* are nothing more than adorably packaged, shiny, talc-based loose powders for the body, incredibly overpriced, but decidedly sexy. **High Beam** *($18)* comes in a nail-polish bottle and is applied to the face in a similar manner. It is just a shiny moisturizer that dries to a matte finish, leaving the shine behind. **Moon Beam** *($18)* is a golden pink liquid shimmer product that will add subtle, but still noticeable, shine wherever it is applied.

☺ $$$ **Glamourette Refillable Makeup Ensemble** *($38 for complete set; $11 for blush and powder refills; $9 for lipstick refills)* is a prime example of how BeneFit takes cleverness to new heights, though not always with stellar results. Case in point: this set of makeup, which resembles a small black lacquered hand-held mirror, but houses pressed powder, blush, and a mini lipstick. Dollar for dollar, you're obviously paying for the elaborate packaging and fancy presentation—what's inside is best described as below average. The talc-based pressed powder and blush are unusually dry, applying too sheer and often unevenly, while the lipstick is just a tiny version of a standard, slightly greasy formula. The concept and execution are darling, but the ooo's and ah's stop there.

BIOELEMENTS (SKIN CARE ONLY)

You may have seen this line of skin-care products being sold at the salon where you get your hair cut or nails done. It is very attractively packaged and uses all the current buzzwords that the cosmetics industry loves to bandy about. The brochure states, "Your skin is a mirror that reflects your inner well-being. Visible surface problems like premature wrinkles, dryness, excess oil, irritation, and blemishes are often visual reflections of deeper, below-the-surface imbalances. These imbalances occur when your body is thrown out of sync by the normal everyday challenges of air pollution, chemicals, the sun, poor nutrition, or emotional upsets.… [This] stress[es] your system's inner balance."

That sounds great, but none of it is true. The aging process is much more complicated than this sermon on inner peace and health lets on. The one thing it is right about is that the effects of the sun are potent, but for all that Bioelements has only one decent sunscreen, the rest lack UVA-protecting ingredients or are have an SPF of less than 15. Even more disappointing is the Acne Clearing System, which is unlikely to do anything other than cause irritation and redness. The rest of the products are on the hokey side, as are the claims that you can give extra oxygen to the skin to slow down visible signs of aging, or detoxify the skin with antioxidants. For more information on Bioelements, call (800) 533-3064 or visit www.bioelements.com.

☺ $$$ **Decongestant Cleanser** *($21.50 for 6 ounces)* is a standard, detergent-based, water-soluble cleanser. It would be good for someone with oily to combination skin. It does contain a fragrant plant extract that can be problematic for skin.

☺ $$$ **Moisture Positive Cleanser** *($21.50 for 6 ounces)* is more of a cold cream–type cleanser than can be good for someone with dry skin, though it doesn't remove makeup well without the help of a washcloth. It does contain fragrant plant extracts that can be problematic for skin. However, to save money and forgo the fragrance, Neutrogena's Extra Gentle Cleanser ($6.06 for 6.7 ounces) is almost identical for almost a third the price.

☹ **Twice Daily Bar Gentle Non-Soap Cleanser** *($17.50 for 5 ounces)* is one expensive bar cleanser and does not differ in any significant way from bar cleansers from Neutrogena or Dove. It is indeed far gentler than regular soap, but the detergent cleansing agents can still be drying and irritating. The ingredients that keep it in a bar form can also potentially clog pores. It does contain a good deal of fragrance.

☹ **Makeup Dissolver, Oil-Free Formula for Your Eyes** *($19.50 for 6 ounces and a sponge)* lists witch hazel and a fragrant plant extract as the first ingredients, and these can be skin irritants, especially around the eye area.

☺ $$$ **Measured Micrograins** *($24 for 2.5 ounces)* is a standard scrub that uses little pieces of polyethylene (plastic) as the scrub particles. It does contain fragrant plant extracts, some of which can be problematic for skin.

☺ **Equalizer** *($20 for 6 ounces)* is an OK, but very ordinary, toner for most skin types. Some of the plant extracts it contains can be potent skin irritants, including ginseng, watercress, rose, ylang-ylang, and sumac.

☺ $$$ **Absolute Moisture** *($29.50 for 2.5 ounces)* is an exceptionally ordinary moisturizer that lacks antioxidants and anti-irritants. It does contain some good plant oils but only a teeny quantity of water-binding agents. What is absolute about it is that it's not worth the money.

☹ **Beyond Hydration Moisturizer** *($29.50 for 2.5 ounces)* contains several problematic plant extracts, including peppermint, sage, sumac, and ginseng. There is never a good reason to put unnecessarily irritating ingredients on the skin, especially not when the goal is moisturizing.

☺ **Crucial Moisture** *($29.50 for 2.5 ounces)*. There is nothing crucial or even very interesting about this product, as it lacks even one state-of-the-art moisturizing ingredient.

☹ **Eye Area with AlphaBlend** *($35 for 1 ounce)*. The pH of this product makes it a poor exfoliant, and the third ingredient is alcohol. Together that makes it an absurd product to use on the face, much less in the eye area.

☺ $$$ **Immediate Comfort 1% Hydrocortisone Lotion** *($27 for 1 ounce)* is a version of other over-the-counter cortisone creams such as Lanacort and Cortaid. Given the similarity, it's up to you to choose whether you want to spend $3 for 1 ounce or $27 for 1 ounce for almost identical products. However, hydrocortisone is an active pharmaceutical ingredient and can indeed reduce skin inflammation, though it should only be used short term because repeated application can cause skin to thin and can promote the breakdown of collagen. This is a nice formulation but it offers no extra benefit over Lanacort or Cortaid from the drugstore.

☺ $$$ **Jet Travel** *($35 for 1 ounce)* is a silicone-based moisturizer that contains a small amount of water-binding agent and that's about it. There are no other interesting ingredients for skin in this product.

☹ **Oxygen Cocktail** *($35 for 1 ounce)* contains something called tissue respiratory factors, which is a trade name for a form of yeast suspended in alcohol. There is only one independent study showing it to have some wound-healing benefits (Source: *Journal of Burn Care Rehabilitati*on, March-April 1999, pages 155–162), but the study used the pure form, not the form that's used in a cosmetic formulation. Further, this product contains hydrogen peroxide, a potent generator of free-radical damage, which isn't helpful for skin and may be problematic if used consistently.

☹ **Oxygenation** *($48 for 1 ounce)* contains hydrogen peroxide, a potent generator of free-radical damage. That isn't helpful for skin and may be problematic if used consistently.

☹ **Quick Refiner** *($40 for 3 ounces)* lists its second ingredient as alcohol and that won't refine anything, although it can cause dryness and irritation.

☺ $$$ **Recovery Serum** *($52 for 1 ounce)* is a good, silicone-based moisturizer for normal to dry skin that contains some very good water-binding agents.

☺ $$$ **Stress Solution** *($35 for 1 ounce)* is more of a toner than anything else. It contains mostly water, glycerin, water-binding agent, anti-irritants, preservatives, and fragrance.

✓☺ $$$ **Urban Detox** *($35 for 1 ounce)* is similar to the Stress Solution above only with the addition of superoxide dismutase, a potent antioxidant, and is preferred over the Stress Solution version. It does contain fragrance.

☹ **T-Zone Monitor** *($35 for 1 ounce)* contains lemon, sage, and eucalyptus, which are all skin irritants that will only hurt skin, not help it.

☹ **Everyday Protector SPF 8** *($29.50 for 6 ounces)* is not recommended due to the low SPF. According to the American Medical Association and the National Cancer Institute, SPF 15 is the minimum SPF number for preventing sun damage.

☹ **Sun Diffusing Protector SPF 15** *($29.50 for 6 ounces)* doesn't contain the UVA-protecting ingredients of titanium dioxide, zinc oxide, or avobenzone, and is not recommended.

☺ $$$ **Serious Self Tanner for Face and Body** *($31 for 6 ounces)* is a standard self-tanner that uses the same ingredient every other self-tanner does, dihydroxyacetone, to affect the color of skin.

✓☺ $$$ **Year-Round Protector SPF 30+ Moisturizer** *($45 for 2.5 ounces)* is a very good, though overly expensive, in-part titanium dioxide–based sunscreen. It also contains some very good antioxidants and water-binding agents. It does contain fragrance.

☹ $$$ **Cremetherapy Very Emollient Mask** *($25 for 2.5 ounces)*. Because there are so many emollient plant oils in this product and so little clay, it could be a fine mask for someone with dry skin. What a shame that it also contains several irritating plant extracts, including peppermint, sage, ginseng, and sumac.

☹ **Kerafole Deep Exfoliating Mask** *($45 for 2.5 ounces)* contains several irritating plant extracts, including lavender oil, lemon, orange, and clove, and very standard emollients and thickening agents. This is steeply overpriced and is not recommended.

☺ $$$ **Restorative Clay Active Treatment Mask** *($23.50 for 2.5 ounces)*. If you have dry skin and want to try a clay mask, the oils in this one can help soften the drying effects of the clay, but all in all this is just a standard clay mask that won't restore anything.

☹ $$$ **Instant Emollient** *($12.50 for 0.14 ounce)* is more of a clear, fragrant lipstick than anything else. It's emollient, but also greasy and heavy.

☺ $$$ **Pigment Discourager** *($21 for 0.5 ounce)* is a standard 1% hydroquinone skin-lightening product. Hydroquinone can improve skin discolorations, but not without the help of a sunscreen or a skin exfoliant. Plus there are far less expensive products like this available, and most contain 2% hydroquinone, a more effective concentration.

☹ $$$ **Bioelements Actives** *($2)* are tiny bottles of plant extracts or minerals suspended in a base combining alcohol and silicone. These can be added to whatever product you buy from Bioelements. However, none of the plant extracts or minerals can live up to even a modicum of the claims associated with them. This is a very cute gimmick, but overall its appearance is far more impressive than its effect.

BIOELEMENTS ACNE CLEARING SYSTEM

☹ $$$ **Spotless Cleanser, Salicylic Acid Acne Treatment** *($38.50 for 3 ounces)* is a standard, detergent-based cleanser that also contains 2% salicylic acid. Salicylic acid is an effective exfoliant, but in a cleanser product it would just be washed down the drain. The teeny amounts of pineapple and papaya extract have no exfoliating properties for skin. This is extremely overpriced for what you get.

☹ $$$ **Active Astringent, Salicylic Acid Acne Medication** *($38.50 for 3 ounces)*, with only 0.5% salicylic acid, has minimal exfoliating properties. Most of the plant extracts in it can be skin irritants.

☹ **Acneplex Daytime Treatment Gel** *($46 for 1 ounce)* is similar to the Active Astringent above, but has a 2% concentration of salicylic acid. That can be more effective, but with witch hazel as the primary ingredient, along with some of the plant extracts including lime and grapefruit, this can be a skin irritant.

☹ **Poreplex Night Treatment Gel** *($46 for 1 ounce)* contains 3% sulfur. Sulfur is a good topical disinfectant for fighting blemishes, but it is also extremely irritating, in the long run causing more problems than it helps.

✓☺ **$$$ Breakout Control** *($35 for 1 ounce)* is a very good 2.5% benzoyl peroxide topical disinfectant in a nonirritating base that can be effective for acne. However, there are many products containing the same concentration and similar nonirritating base for far less than this.

☹ **Amino Mask, Sulphur and Salicylic Acid Acne Treatment** *($46 for 2.5 ounces)* contains 3% sulfur, and the same comments apply as for the Poreplex Night Treatment Gel above. Because the pH of this product is over 8, the salicylic acid is not effective for exfoliation. This product also contains peppermint and cedar, which have no benefit for acne; they are only skin irritants.

BIOMEDIC (SKIN CARE ONLY)

Note: As this book goes to press BioMedic was in the process of merging product lines with L'Oreal-owned La Roche-Posay. Please refer to the review for La Roche-Posay in this book for information about that merger.

BioMedic is a line of skin-care products being marketed to dermatologists because dermatologists are selling skin-care products these days, lots of them. Not surprisingly, the number of lines marketed to dermatologists has increased more than 100% over the past ten years. But there is nothing medical about the products being sold at a doctor's office (or any products for that matter). Every skin-care and makeup line being sold at doctors' offices comes under the FDA's guidelines regulating cosmetics, and that means they legally don't have to provide accurate or viable claim substantiation. Just like the products sold by the rest of the industry, these contain ingredients that only need to be approved for cosmetic or over-the-counter use.

The benefit touted by physicians in defense of their selling skin-care products is their expertise: Who else, they say, is better able to prescribe products for someone's skin? I find that a plausible argument, except when I see the price tags and the types of products these doctors are selling. When a physician sells expensive sunscreens that have formulas and efficacy similar to drugstore brands, knowing that this might mean they will be improperly applied (that is, liberal application is essential for achieving the protection indicated on the label and if it's expensive, the consumer is less likely to apply it liberally), I simply don't buy the premise of "better recommendations." Besides, when doctors recommend their product lines by filling a prescription, when similar or identical products are available over the counter or from other lines for far less, that's a conflict of interest.

BioMedic has made one major change during the past year; they have eliminated much of the misleading information that I took issue with in the previous edition of this book. That is a welcome relief! What remains is a mixed bag of standard products, products with irritating ingredients, and some well-formulated options for skin care.

BioMedic's true claim to fame is its MicroPeel, which carries a bit more panache and allure. MicroPeel is a light, acid-type peel with AHA concentrations ranging between 15% and 30% (as opposed to deeper peels with concentrations of 50% to 70%). The light acid peels can be performed by an aesthetician, and as with all AHA peels there can be immediate benefits, although these light peels are not long-lasting. Even the BioMedic brochure states that "only the advanced chemical peels [TCA or phenol] effectively treat wrinkles. In no way do we feel the results of the BioMedic MicroPeel Procedures are equivalent to that of an advanced [deep] peel." That is true and completely honest. Because the results are fleeting, many aestheticians and doctors perform these peels in sets of four and six. I am concerned about the repetitive deep irritation and the limited duration of the benefits. I often wonder why women would get light AHA peels (15% to 30%) instead of the higher-concentration versions or other peels, or even laser resurfacing, which is longer-lasting and needs to be done only once every several years.

For more information about BioMedic, call (800) 736-5155 or visit www.biomedic.com.

☹ **Gentle Cleansing Gelee** *($10.95 for 6 ounces)* uses TEA-lauryl sulfate as the main detergent cleansing agent, which has the potential for being a skin irritant for all skin types.

☹ **Gentle Cleansing Bar** *($4.95 for 4 ounces)* is a standard, sodium tallowate–based bar cleanser similar to many. It can be drying for many skin types and the tallow can potentially cause breakouts.

☺ $$$ **Purifying Cleanser** *($26.95 for 6 ounces)* is a standard, detergent-based, water-soluble cleanser that can be good for normal to oily skin. It contains a tiny amount of AHA (less than 1%), which is not enough for it to be effective as an exfoliant.

☹ **Micro Massage Exfoliating Wash** *($14.05 for 6 ounces)* uses crushed rock as the abrasive, which can be too abrasive for some skin types. It also contains several fragrant plant oils that make this extremely fragrant and a risk for irritation.

☺ **Gentle Soothing Toner** *($14 for 6 ounces)* is as standard a toner as you will find. It is just water, slip agent, glycerin, soothing agents, and preservatives. It lacks many elements such as water-binding agents or antioxidants that could make it a great option for skin.

☺ $$$ **Conditioning Eye Cream** *($23.95 for 0.5 ounce)* is a good moisturizer for normal to dry skin that contains some good antioxidants and water-binding agents. It also contains sugarcane and maple extract and citrus extract, which have no benefit for skin and cannot perform like AHAs.

☺ **Conditioning Cream** *($24.95 for 2 ounces)* is a very standard 8% glycolic acid moisturizer. The low pH makes it very effective for exfoliation, but the other ingredients are no different from what you would find at the drugstore in Alpha Hydrox's AHA products for a lot less.

✓☺ $$$ **Extra Rich Moisturizer** *($31 for 1 ounce)* is a very good emollient moisturizer for dry skin that includes plant oil, water-binding agents, antioxidants, and anti-irritants. It does contain fragrant plant extract.

☹ **Hydrating Fluid** *($21.95 for 2 ounces)* is overflowing with fragrant and irritating plant oils, which are a problem for all skin types.

☺ **Gentle Soothing Cream** *($16.95 for 1 ounce)* contains hydrocortisone, which is an active pharmaceutical ingredient that can indeed reduce skin inflammation, though it should only be used short term because repeated application can cause skin to thin and cause the breakdown of collagen. There is absolutely no extra benefit from using this rather than Lanacort or Cortaid from the drugstore.

☺ **Hydro Active Emulsion** *($22.95 for 2 ounces)* is a very good moisturizer for normal to slightly dry skin that contains antioxidants, silicones, and a tiny amount of water-binding agents.

☺ $$$ **Damage C Control** *($32 for 0.5 ounce)* has a very good concentration of magnesium ascorbyl phosphate, which is considered a very stable and effective form of vitamin C, along with other antioxidants. One concern is the small amount of sulfur in this product, which gives the product a pH that is potentially irritating. Overall though, for a good vitamin C product, this definitely delivers.

☺ $$$ **Ultra C Protection** *($45.95 for 1 ounce)* is similar to the Damage C Control above except that Ultra C is in a silicone base and has no irritating ingredients of any kind. Vitamin C is good for skin, but it isn't everything. This is a one-note product that would be far more interesting with a blend of skin-friendly ingredients.

☹ $$$ **Maximum C** *($12.95 for 0.25 ounce)* uses ascorbic acid as the main source of vitamin C. That can have antioxidant properties, but it is considered a potential skin irritant as well. This would not be preferred over the Ultra C above.

☺ $$$ **Retinol Creme 15** *($30.95 for 1 ounce)*; **Retinol Creme 30** *($30.95 for 1 ounce)*; **Retinol Creme 60** *($30.95 for 1 ounce)*. Retinol is the technical name for vitamin A, and there is limited evidence demonstrating that retinol can have an effect similar to tretinoin (a derivative of vitamin A and the active ingredient in Retin-A, Renova, Tazorac, and Avita) on skin. The problem is that, in the skin, tretinoin (all-*trans* retinoic acid) is the form of vitamin A that can affect actual cell production by binding to the tretinoin receptor sites on the cell. Retinol needs to be converted to tretinoin in the skin if it is to do the same thing. Theoretically, retinol can become tretinoin in the skin, but the process isn't direct. Retinol can be absorbed into the skin and if certain enzymes are present it could then be converted to tretinoin. After retinol does get into skin, the question is whether it is converted into tretinoin, and the research results on this are conflicting (Sources: *Journal of Investigative Dermatology*, 1998, volume 111, pages 478–484; *Journal of Investigative Dermatology*, 1997, volume 109, pages 301–305; and *Skin Pharmacology and Applied Skin Physiology*, November-December 2001, pages 363–372). For more specifics, refer to Chapter Seven, *Cosmetics Dictionary*. The BioMedic products' contain 0.15%, 0.3%, and 0.6% respectively. Whether or not those are effective amounts, and whether or not more is best is not clear, but this is one of the few companies that is upfront about their concentrations.

☺ $$$ **Hydrating Serum** *($56.25 for 3 ounces)* is a good lightweight moisturizer for normal to oily skin containing mostly water, water-binding agents, thickener, and preservatives.

☺ $$$ **Gentle Moisturizing Emulsion SPF 20** *($17.95 for 2 ounces)* is a good, in-part avobenzone-based sunscreen for normal to dry skin. It is in a fairly standard, emollient base with a teeny amount of antioxidants at the end of the ingredient list.

☺ $$$ **Facial Shield SPF 20** *($19.95 for 2 ounces)* is a good, in-part avobenzone-based sunscreen for normal to oily skin in an otherwise boring formulation. It lacks any water-binding agents, antioxidants, or anti-irritants.

☹ **Lip Shield SPF 15** *($10.95 for 0.12 ounce)* doesn't contain the UVA-protecting ingredients of titanium dioxide, zinc oxide, or avobenzone, and is not recommended.

☺ $$$ **Pigment Shield SPF 18** *($19.95 for 2 ounces)* is a very good, zinc oxide–based sunscreen in an extremely standard emollient base that would work well for someone with normal to dry skin.

☺ **Self Tan** *($22.95 for 4 ounces)*, like all self-tanners, uses dihydroxyacetone to affect the color of the skin. This one would work as well as any.

☹ **Conditioning Gel** *($18.95 for 2 ounces)* does not indicate how much hydroquinone this product contains, a lack that makes it problematic to know exactly how effective it can be. However, the second ingredient is alcohol, and that is too drying and irritating for skin and not conditioning in the least.

☹ **Conditioning Gel Plus** *($24.95 for 2 ounces)* is almost identical to the Conditioning Gel above and the same basic comments apply.

☹ **Pigment Control** *($18 for 0.5 ounce)* lists its second ingredient as alcohol, which is drying and irritating for skin. That doesn't help skin in the least. The kojic acid has some ability to inhibit melanin production, but it is an extremely unstable ingredient.

☹ **Conditioning Solution** *($18.95 for 6 ounces)* contains alcohol as the second ingredient as well as eucalyptus oil, which is drying and irritating for all skin types.

☺ **Gentle Healing Ointment** *($11.95 for 1.76 ounces)* is just Vaseline, mineral oil, wax, glycerin, and soothing agent. There is absolutely no benefit in using this over plain Vaseline.

☺ **Phospholipid Gel** *($20.95 for 2 ounces)* lists its second ingredient as glycolic acid, and in a base with a pH of 4 that makes it an effective exfoliant for skin. The other parts of this formulation are very basic and boring. There is nothing about this product that makes it any better than Alpha Hydrox's less expensive glycolic acid products.

☺ **Phospholipid Lotion** *($20.95 for 2 ounces)* is similar to the Phospholipid Gel above and the same basic comments apply.

✓☺ $$$ **High Density Gel** *($23.95 for 0.5 ounce)* is a very good lightweight moisturizer for normal to slightly dry skin that contains mostly water, film-forming agent, glycerin, silicones, water-binding agents, antioxidants, and preservatives.

☹ **Acne Control** *($20 for 0.5 ounce)*. While this product does contain salicylic acid, it contains alcohol as the primary ingredient. Alcohol is drying and irritating for all skin types and this product is not recommended.

☺ **AntiBac Lotion** *($18.95 for 1 ounce)* is a good, though basic, salicylic acid lotion

The Reviews B

that has a pH of 4, which makes it an effective exfoliant. However, this product does not specify the concentration of salicylic acid content so there is no way to know exactly what you are putting on your skin.

☺ **Antibac Acne Wash** *($17.95 for 6 ounces)* is a standard, detergent-based cleanser that contains about 2% salicylic acid, although the pH of the cleanser is too high for it to be effective for exfoliation.

☹ **Antibac Protection** *($22.95 for 1 ounce)* is a silicone- and alcohol-based serum. That's a poor way to disinfect acne, because alcohol is not effective against the bacteria that cause it; instead, it is drying and irritating for all skin types.

✓☺ **$$$ Antibac Spot Treatment** *($16.95 for 0.5 ounce)* is a very good 2.5% benzoyl peroxide topical disinfectant for acne. Thankfully, this one contains no other irritants and it is even fragrance free.

☺ **$$$ Pure Enzyme Mask** *($19.95 for 1 ounce)* contains bromelain, papain, and cysteine. There is no research showing that these enzymes have benefit for skin.

☺ **Extra Mild Protection** *($21.95 for 2 ounces)* is just silicones and preservatives. These can feel soothing for skin, but it contains no other ingredients that are beneficial, and the skin deserves more than this when it comes to protection.

BIORE (SKIN CARE ONLY)

Many skin-care lines are launched with a specific gimmick to grab the consumer's attention, and Biore is in this category. The gimmick is ☺ **Biore's Pore Perfect Deep Cleansing Strips** *($5.99 for 6 nose strips)*. This product is supposed to instantly clean pores. All you do is place a piece of cloth with an incredibly sticky substance on it over your nose, as you might do with a Band-Aid, wait 15 minutes for it to dry, and then rip it off. Along with some amount of skin, blackheads are supposed to stick to it and come right out of the skin on your nose. What does this miracle product contain? The main ingredient on the strip is polyquaternium-37, a film-forming hairspray ingredient—so it's basically a piece of gauze with a form of hairspray on it.

What has me most concerned about these so-called Cleansing Strips is that they are accompanied by a strong warning not to use them over any area other than the nose and not to use them over inflamed, swollen, sunburned, or excessively dry skin. It also states that if the strip is too painful to remove, you should wet it and then carefully remove it. What a warning!

You may at first be impressed with what comes off your nose. (Well, there is no question: you will be impressed.) Most people do have some oil sitting at the top of their oil glands (most of the face's oil glands are located on the nose), and whether you use these strips or a piece of tape, black dots and some skin will be removed. Is that helpful? Only momentarily, but if you use the Biore product, the plastic-forming agent can get into the pores and possibly cause breakouts and irritation.

Also, despite the warning on the package, most women will try these strips wherever they see breakouts. If I didn't know better, I know I would. The way these strips adhere, they can absolutely injure or tear skin and cause spider veins to surface. They are especially unsafe if you've been using Retin-A, Renova, AHAs, or BHA; having facial peels; or taking Accutane; or if you have naturally thin skin or any skin disorder such as rosacea, psoriasis, or seborrhea.

Biore's brochure claims this product can pull an entire blackhead plug out of the skin. It can't. If you could grab a blackhead out of the skin, your skin would be left with an empty hole (and there is nothing in this product that will close it up), but that's not what happens. Instead, just the top layer of the blackhead is removed, and then the blackhead returns because the source of the problem was never corrected. Nothing was done to reduce irritation, exfoliate skin cells, help keep oil flow normal, or close the pore. What about the rest of Biore's products? This line is based on these strips and little else. Biore is being sold in drugstores across the country. For more information about Biore, call (888) BIORE-11 or visit www.biore.com.

☹ **Blemish Fighting Cleanser** *($5.99 for 5 ounces)* is a standard, detergent-based, water-soluble cleanser that would be an option except that the fourth ingredient is alcohol, and that can be drying and irritating for skin. This also contains a minimal amount of BHA (0.5%), but the pH of this cleanser makes it ineffective as an exfoliant.

☺ **Cool Action Cream Cleanser** *($5.99 for 5 ounces)* is a cold cream–style cleanser that can be difficult to rinse from the skin. It definitely doesn't "deep clean." This would have been a decent option for someone with normal to dry skin, but the inclusion of menthol, the only thing "cool" about this product, makes it too irritating for all skin types. It does contain fragrance and coloring agents.

☹ **Facial Cleansing Cloths** *($6.99 for 34 cloths)* contain mostly alcohol, and that's too drying and irritating for all skin types.

☺ **Foaming Cleanser** *($5.99 for 5 ounces)* is a very good, though very standard, detergent-based, water-soluble cleanser for someone with normal to oily skin.

☹ **Warming Deep Pore Cleanser** *($6.99 for 5 ounces)* does feel warm, but heat on the skin has no benefit for breakouts. If anything, the heat can make already red-looking blemishes even redder.

☺ **Mild Daily Cleansing Scrub** *($5.99 for 5 ounces)* is a standard, detergent-based, water-soluble cleanser that uses synthetic scrub particles (polyethylene, a form of plastic) as the abrasive. This would work as well as any for most skin types. It does contain fragrance and coloring agents.

☹ **Pore Perfect Toner** *($5.99 for 5.5 ounces)* has three different types of alcohol in it, including the alcohol in witch hazel, and there's even some menthol just in case your skin needed even more irritation.

☹ **Deep Pore Toner** *($4.99 for 5.5 ounces)*. The only thing deep about this is the irritation the alcohol and menthol can cause.

☺ **Balancing Moisturizer for Normal to Dry Skin** *($7.99 for 3.5 ounces)* contains mostly water, glycerin, silicone, vitamin E, thickeners, teeny amounts of water-binding agents, preservatives, and fragrance. This is an OK moisturizer for normal to dry skin, and it's cleverly dispensed from an aerosol container.

☺ **Balancing Moisturizer, Oil Free** *($7.99 for 3.5 ounces)* won't balance anything, and actually feels rather sticky and tacky when applied. The foam dispenser is cool, and that's the only thing of interest in this otherwise lightweight and basic moisturizer.

☹ **Blemish Bomb** *($6.99 for 10 packets)* contains mostly alcohol, which makes it a bomb for the skin, not for blemishes.

☹ **Blemish Double Agent** *($6.49 for 0.75 ounce)* is a 2% salicylic acid (BHA) solution that unfortunately contains a whole lot of alcohol and some menthol. Plus, the pH is just barely low enough to be effective for exfoliation.

☹ **Pore Perfect Ultra Strip** *($6.49 for 6 strips)*. Aside from the lack of research that these can have any benefit for skin, this version contains menthol, adding the risk of *more* irritation (ouch!) by using them.

☹ **Self-Heating Mask** *($5.12 for 6 packets)* is a standard clay mask that does get warm when applied to the skin, but the heating effect doesn't help skin—if anything, heat can make inflamed skin look more red and irritated.

☹ **Self-Heating Moisture Mask** *($5.99 for 6 packets)* is similar to the Self-Heating Mask above only without the clay. This is fairly emollient and could be useful for dry skin, but the heating effect can be problematic for skin.

☹ **Beyond Smooth Daily Face Moisturizer, Normal to Dry** *($6.99 for 4 ounces)* is a rather ordinary moisturizer with some problems to watch out for. First, because it doesn't contain sunscreen it wouldn't be for use during the day. It also lacks interesting water-binding agents, antioxidants, and anti-irritants, which makes it exceedingly ordinary and out of date in comparison to other products. It does contain a small amount of vitamin E, which is nice, but that's the only "special" part of the formula. This moisturizer uses ginger root extract to supposedly make "recurring facial hair softer, finer, and less visible" in six weeks. Although I could find no published research showing ginger root to have any effect as a hair lightener or hair-growth inhibitor, it is interesting to note that ginger root does show up in countless hair-*growth* products aimed at thinning hair or baldness—yet these hair-growth claims are unsubstantiated as well. Ginger root has not been shown to have any effect whatsoever on hair, much less having less or more of it, though it does have a long history of internal use and is believed to be beneficial for such conditions as sore throats, digestive upset, headaches, and motion sickness.

☹ **Beyond Smooth Daily Face Moisturizer, Normal to Oily** *($6.99 for 4 ounces)* is quite similar to the Normal to Dry version above only minus some of the thickening agents. That can be better for normal to oily skin, but basically this is still just a boring moisturizer.

BIOTHERM (SKIN CARE ONLY)

BioTherm is one of the many companies owned by L'Oreal USA and has a vast array of products. In many ways this line isn't as elegant or interesting as L'Oreal or Lancome (also owned by L'Oreal). Though BioTherm's claims are wrapped around the exotic spa concept, the products are far from unique or specially formulated. One ingredient BioTherm does use to gain your attention is something they call "biotechnological thermal plankton." Plankton are microscopic plants and animals that are adrift in fresh and salt water. They come in many forms, including one-celled amoebas, tiny jellyfish, fish larvae, and some forms of algae. I imagine the thermal reference is that they were somehow heated before being stuck in some of these products. What can plankton do for your skin? That's anyone's guess, because there is no research showing it to have any benefit for skin. However, if thermal plankton is supposed to be so remarkable, why doesn't this amazing ingredient show up in other L'Oreal product lines? This kind of marketing two-step is one of the characteristic runarounds of the cosmetics industry.

BioTherm also showcases some minerals in several of their products, namely zinc, copper, and manganese gluconate. Each has interesting benefits, but given the trace amounts that are present in these products it is unlikely they have much impact.

"Naturally purifying extracts" is another phrase BioTherm likes to use. While these products do indeed contain a handful of plant extracts, they are neither purifying, nor essential, nor are the products predominantly "natural." Actually, a strong point for BioTherm is that it uses minimal amounts of plant extracts, which reduces the risk of allergens and irritation. Several of the products do contain decent antioxidants, including vitamin E and superoxide dismutase, and, for distribution outside of the United States, it has excellent suncare products. In the long run, this line has more strengths than weaknesses; there are some very good cleansers, well-formulated moisturizers and toners, and some good masks. For more information about BioTherm, call (212) 818-1500 or visit www.biotherm.com. **Note:** All BioTherm products are highly fragranced.

BIOTHERM ACNOPUR

☹ **Acnopur Pore-Unclogging Purifying Foam, Acne Prone Skin** *($14.50 for 5 ounces)* contains a tiny amount of triclosan, a disinfectant typically found in hand cleansers. There is no research showing that triclosan is effective against the bacteria that cause acne. This cleanser also contains clay, but that can be tricky to rinse off. It also contains peppermint. All in all, this adds up to a fairly standard, though somewhat drying and potentially irritating, cleanser.

☹ **Acnopur Clarifying Exfoliating Lotion, Acne Prone Skin** *($14 for 8 ounces)* lists alcohol as the second ingredient, and it also contains peppermint oil, which makes it too drying and irritating for all skin types.

☺ **Acnopur Moisturizing Regulating Care, Acne Prone Skin** *($21 for 1.7 ounces).*

Aside from the peppermint oil, which is an irritant, this is an OK, silicone- and clay-based 2% salicylic acid product, though the pH is almost too high for it to be effective.

☹ **Acno Pur Emergency Anti-Acne Treatment** *($11.50 for 0.5 ounces)* lists alcohol as the second ingredient and includes peppermint, making it likely that you'll need emergency repair from the dryness and irritation this can cause.

BioTherm Biopur

☺ **Biopur Pure Cleansing Gel** *($15.50 for 5 ounces)* is a decent, though truly standard, detergent-based, water-soluble cleanser that would work well for most skin types.

☺ **Biopur Purifying and Balancing Mask** *($16.50 for 2.5 ounces)* is a standard clay mask, except that this one contains wheat starch, which can be problematic for people prone to breakouts.

☺ **$$$ Biopur Double Purifying Exfoliator** *($16.50 for 2.5 ounces)* is a standard, detergent-based, water-soluble cleanser that uses synthetic scrub particles (polyethylene—ground-up plastic) as well as ground-up rock as the abrasives. This can be an option for oily skin.

☺ **BioPur Mattifying Astringent Lotion** *($14.50 for 8 ounces)* is an OK, relatively irritant-free toner that would work well for oily skin.

☺ **BioPur Matte Hydrating Fluid** *($21 for 1.7 ounces)* is a silicone-based moisturizer that has a very matte finish on the skin. It contains a teeny amount of salicylic acid, but the pH is too high for it to be effective as an exfoliant. Without any significant water-binding agents, antioxidants, and anti-irritants, this ends up being unhelpful for skin.

☺ **BioPur Clarifying Balancing Night Gel** *($21.50 for 1.7 ounces)* is a lightweight, silicone-based moisturizer that contains a small amount of water-binding agents and antioxidants. It contains a teeny amount of salicylic acid, too, but the pH is too high for it to be effective as an exfoliant. It would be a rather standard option for normal to slightly dry skin.

☺ **BioPur Emergency Anti-Imperfection** *($11 for 0.5 ounce)* is more spackle than anything else, containing mostly water, titanium dioxide, clay, slip agent, emollients, thickeners, film-forming agent, preservatives, and fragrance.

☺ **BioPur Matte Hydrating Fluid SPF 15** *($25 for 1.7 ounces)* is an OK, though extremely basic, sunscreen with a small amount of titanium dioxide as one of the active ingredients. It is an option for someone with normal to oily skin. This does contain salicylic acid, but the pH of this formula is not low enough for it to be effective as an exfoliant.

☹ **BioPur Ultra-Matte T-Zone Essence** *($15.50 for 0.5 ounce)*. The amount of alcohol in this product can make skin feel temporarily degreased, but in the long run ends up causing more problems for skin.

BioTherm Biosensitive

☺ **Biosensitive High Tolerance Fluid Cleansing Milk** *($20 for 5 ounces)* is mostly glycerin and thickening agents and a tiny amount of detergent cleansing agent. It is a very basic, but good, cleanser for normal to dry skin. It would require a washcloth to help get makeup off.

☺ **Biosensitive Self-Foaming Gentle Cleanser** (*$19 for 5 ounces*) is a standard detergent-based cleanser that would work well for most skin types. It also contains something called vitreoscilla ferment, a bacteria culture, but there is no research indicating this to be of any help for skin. There is nothing about this cleanser that makes it unique for sensitive skin types.

☺ $$$ **Biosensitive Calming Thermal Spring Spray** (*$20 for 5 ounces*). The microscopic amount of plankton in here is barely worth mentioning.

☺ **Biosensitive Calming Thermal Spring Spray** (*$14.50 for 5 ounces*) is a very ordinary toner of water, glycerin, preservatives, and fragrance. The fractional amount of plankton in this product has no benefit for skin.

☺ **Biosensitive Calming Regulating Daily Cream** (*$23 for 1.7 ounces*) is a good emollient moisturizer for someone with normal to dry skin. Unfortunately, the interesting ingredients are listed well after the preservative, meaning the amount is barely detectable.

☹ **Biosensitive Calming Regulating Oil-Free Lotion SPF 12** (*$30 for 1.7 ounces*) doesn't contain the UVA-protecting ingredients of titanium dioxide, zinc oxide, or avobenzone—and is not recommended.

☺ $$$ **Biosensitive Yeux Calming Eye Cream** (*$24 for 0.5 ounce*) is an OK, but ordinary, emollient moisturizer.

☺ $$$ **Biosensitive Hydrating and Soothing Concentrate Masque** (*$20 for 2.53 ounces*) is a good basic emollient mask that holds little advantage or benefit over a well-formulated moisturizer.

BIOTHERM BIOSOURCE NORMAL TO COMBINATION SKIN

☺ **Biosource Foaming Cleansing Gel** (*$15.50 for 5 ounces*) is a detergent-based, water-soluble cleanser that would work well for normal to oily or normal to slightly dry skin types.

☺ **Biosource Enriched Cleansing Foam** (*$15.50 for 5 ounces*) uses fairly drying and irritating cleansing agents. It would be an option only for oily skin. The teeny amounts of zinc, copper, and plankton included in this product have no effect on skin.

☺ **Biosource Invigorating Cleansing Milk** (*$15.50 for 8 ounces*) is a very ordinary mineral oil–based cleanser that also contains small amounts of detergent cleansing agents. This would be an option for someone with normal to dry skin, though it may require a washcloth to make sure it comes completely off the skin. The fractional amounts of minerals and plankton are not enough for even a few skin cells to notice, and the mineral oil would not make someone with combination skin happy.

☺ **Biosource Clarifying Exfoliating Gel** (*$14.50 for 2.5 ounces*) is a gentle, detergent-based cleanser that uses polyethylene (ground-up plastic) as the exfoliant. That can be effective for most skin types. The mineral and salt components have some antibacterial and anti-irritant properties, but in a cleanser their effect would be washed down the drain.

☺ **Biosource Invigorating Toner** *($14.50 for 8 ounces)*. The mixture of good ingredients and potentially irritating ingredients makes this a confused product for the skin.

☺ **Biosource Invigorating Toner, Normal or Combination Skin** *($14.50 for 8 ounces)* has some good water-binding agents and antioxidants, but the witch hazel can be a skin irritant.

☹ **Aquasource Ultra Cool Hydrating Water Gel** *($25 for 1.7 ounces)*. What a shame alcohol is the second ingredient and peppermint is one of the plant extracts (which explains the cool—read "irritating"—impact on skin) because there are some good water-binding agents in this product.

☺ **$$$ Aquasource Intensely Moisturizing Mask, for Normal /Combination Skin** *($20 for 2.53 ounces)*. With the fourth ingredient being palm oil, this ends up being a bit too emollient for oily areas of skin. It also contains an absorbent, which is fine for oily areas but not for dry areas. This does contain some very good water-binding agents and antioxidants, but overall doesn't really add much benefit to skin over what an appropriate moisturizer would.

☹ **Biosource Clean Skin Peel-Off Mask** *($23 for 2.53 ounces)*. With alcohol as the second ingredient, this mask poses an irritation potential that is a problem for all skin types.

BIOTHERM BIOSOURCE DRY SKIN

☺ **Biosource Softening Cleansing Milk** *($15.50 for 5 ounces)* is a mineral oil–based cleanser that also contains several detergent cleansing agents and other emollients. This would be an option for someone with normal to dry skin.

☺ **Biosource Enriched Cleansing Foam, for Dry Skin** *($15 for 5 ounces)*. The clay and detergent cleansing agents in this foam aren't the best for dry skin, though this may be an option for someone with normal to oily skin.

☺ **Biosource Softening Exfoliating Cream** *($14.50 for 2.5 ounces)* is a mineral oil–based cleanser that uses a small amount of crushed rock as the exfoliant. It can be an option as a topical scrub for normal to dry skin.

✓☺ **Biosource Softening Toner** *($14.50 for 8 ounces)* is an excellent toner that contains water-binding agents, anti-irritants, and antioxidants. This is a great option for all skin types.

☺ **$$$ Aquasource Intensely Moisturizing Mask, for Dry Skin** *($20 for 2.53 ounces)* is virtually identical to the Aquasource Intensely Moisturizing Mask, for Normal/Combination Skin above and the same comments apply.

☺ **Aquasource Oligo-Thermal Moisturizing Gel** *($25 for 1.7 ounces)* is a decent emollient moisturizer that would work well for normal to dry skin. Alcohol is high up on the ingredient listing, which can be a problem for some skin types.

BIOTHERM DETOX

☺ **Hydra-Detox Cleansing Foam** *($18 for 5 ounces)* contains ground-up pumice as the second ingredient, and contains detergent cleansing agents. That makes this a fairly abrasive scrub that won't detoxify anything. Even if you could detoxify the skin, the only research for this points to the need for potent antioxidants of a kind that this and all the detox products in this group lack. The plant extracts in this product are described as having effects related to those of AHAs, but they have no such exfoliating properties.

☹ **Hydra-Detox Moisturizing Detoxifying Wipe-Off Lotion** *($16.50 for 4.2 ounces)* lists alcohol as the second ingredient, making this otherwise well-formulated toner too irritating and drying for all skin types.

☺ $$$ **Hydra-Detox Yeux Moisturizing Eye Gel** *($25 for 0.5 ounce)* is just an OK moisturizer with potentially irritating plant extracts, including the caffeine, and none of that is detoxifying in the least.

☺ **Hydra-Detox Daily Moisturizing Cream** *($35 for 1.7 ounces).* There is nothing in this product that will purge toxins from your skin. This is just a good emollient moisturizer that contains some water-binding agents and antioxidants. It also contains plant extracts that are meant to sound as if they perform like AHAs, but they have no exfoliating properties. In addition, the salicylic acid that is present can't exfoliate skin because the pH of the cream is too high for it to be effective for that purpose.

☺ **Hydra-Detox Daily Moisturizing Lotion** *($35 for 1.7 ounces).* The third ingredient listed is alcohol, which is problematic for any moisturizer. That is a shame because this contains a very good blend of antioxidants and water-binding agents without the useless AHA-wannabes in the Hydra-Detox Daily Moisturizing Cream above.

☺ $$$ **Hydra-Detox Moisturizing Mask** *($20 for 2.53 ounces)* is an OK emollient moisturizer that contains tiny amounts of water-binding agents and antioxidants. It also contains some alcohol, which makes it potentially irritating for skin.

BIOTHERM D-STRESS

☹ **D-Stress Nuit Relaxing Night Care Anti-Fatigue Radiance Gel Normal to Combination Skin** *($35 for 1.7 ounces).* With alcohol as its third ingredient, the benefits of the antioxidants and water-binding agents in this product are wasted.

☺ **D-Stress Fortifying Anti-Fatigue Radiance Cream Dry Skin** *($28.50 for 1.7 ounces)* is a very good emollient moisturizer that would be an option for someone with dry skin. It contains mostly water, shea butter, silicones, a small amount of antioxidants, water-binding agents, preservatives, and coloring agents.

☹ **D-Stress Fortifying Anti-Fatigue Radiance Serum** *($33.50 for 1 ounce)* lists its second ingredient as alcohol, and that isn't revitalizing, though it can be drying and irritating.

☹ **D-Stress Relaxing Night Care Anti-Fatigue Radiance Fluide Normal to Oily Combination Skin** *($35 for 1.7 ounces)* is similar to the Serum above and the same comments apply.

The Reviews B

☺ **D-Stress Relaxing Night Care Anti-Fatigue Radiance Cream Dry Skin** *($35 for 1.7 ounces)* is a good emollient moisturizer that contains mostly water, shea butter, slip agent, silicones, thickeners, water-binding agents, plant oil, film-forming agents, vitamin E, preservatives, and fragrance. It does contain a tiny amount of salicylic acid, but the pH isn't low enough for it to be effective as an exfoliant.

☺ **$$$ D-Stress Yeux Anti-Fatigue Eye Care** *($26 for 0.5 ounce)* is a silicone-based moisturizer that contains more mica (sparkle) than beneficial ingredients. Still, this does contain a very good blend of antioxidants and water-binding agents and adds up to a very good moisturizer for normal to dry skin.

☹ **D-Stress Relaxing Radiance Moisture Mask** *($20 for 1.7 ounces)* lists alcohol as the second ingredient and this product is not recommended.

BioTherm Age Fitness

☺ **Age Fitness Active Revitalizing Age Treatment SPF 15, for Dry Skin** *($35 for 1.7 ounces)* is a very good in-part avobenzone-based sunscreen in a very good emollient base that would indeed be good for someone with normal to dry skin.

☺ **Age Fitness Active Revitalizing Age Treatment SPF 15, for Normal to Combination Skin** *($35 for 1.7 ounces)* is similar to the Dry Skin version above except that this one includes alcohol, which isn't helpful for any skin type. However, the sunscreen and other ingredients in this product are quite good for skin.

BioTherm Special Needs

☺ **Biocils Soothing Eye Make-up Remover** *($14 for 4.2 ounces)* is a standard eye-makeup remover with slip agents and detergent cleansing agents. It does contain fragrance.

☺ **Biocils Waterproof Eye Make-up Remover** *($14.50 for 4.2 ounces)* is a silicone-based eye-makeup remover and it works well to remove waterproof makeup.

☹ **Skin Firming Contour Gel Draine Up Lifteur** *($33.50 for 1 ounce)* contains alcohol as the second ingredient, which isn't firming in the least, although it can be drying and irritating for skin.

☺ **Anti-Wrinkle and Firming Cream, Dry Skin** *($31 for 1.7 ounces)* is an extremely ordinary mineral oil- and Vaseline-based moisturizer that lacks any unique state-of-the-art skin-care ingredients.

☹ **Tensing Wrinkle and Firming Essence** *($35.50 for 1 ounce)* contains alcohol as the second ingredient, which makes it a problem for all skin types.

☺ **$$$ Reducteur Rides Anti-Wrinkle and Firming Eye Cream** *($30 for 0.5 ounces)* is an OK, basic moisturizer for normal to slightly dry skin, but there is nothing in it capable of fighting wrinkles. The absorbent ingredients in this product make it a problem for dry skin. Vitamin E is a good antioxidant but that won't affect wrinkling, and the small amount of soybean protein is just a good water-binding agent and possible antioxidant, it imparts no estrogenic benefits for skin.

☺ **Reducteur Rides Anti-Wrinkle and Firming Cream for Face and Neck** *($37 for*

1.7 ounces) is similar to the Firming Eye Cream above only without the absorbent ingredients, which makes it better for dry skin.

☺ $$$ **Retinol Smoothing Anti-Wrinkle Care** *($35.50 for 1 ounce)* contains retinol in a good, but ordinary, emollient base. If you are interested in trying a retinol product, this is one to consider, but L'Oréal's Line Eraser Pure Retinol ($12.89 for 1 ounce) is almost identical and is less than half the price.

☺ $$$ **Retinol Eye & Lip** *($35 for 0.5 ounce)* is similar to the Retinol Smoothing version above and the same basic comments apply.

BioTherm Densite

BioTherm Densite is another group of BioTherm antiwrinkle products, I guess because the other 50-plus antiwrinkle, firming, and antiaging creams BioTherm sells must not work.

☹ $$$ **Densite Lift Firming Lift Serum** *($42 for 1.01 ounces)* lists alcohol as the second ingredient, which is problematic in a moisturizer. It has the requisite antioxidants and water-binding agents, along with a little shine, but the basic formulation leaves much to be desired.

☹ $$$ **Densite Lift Redensifying Anti-Wrinkle Care (Dry Skin)** *($39 for 1.76 ounces)* is a very emollient, Vaseline-based moisturizer that contains a small amount of antioxidants and water-binding agents. Not bad, but not great.

☹ $$$ **Densite Lift Yeux Redensifying Anti-Wrinkle Eye Care** *($30 for 0.52 ounce)* is a silicone-based, emollient moisturizer with minimal water-binding agents and antioxidants, which isn't eye opening in the least.

☹ $$$ **Densite Lift Redensifying Anti-Wrinkle Care Normal and Combination Skin** *($39 for 1.76 ounces)* is almost identical to the Redensifying Anti-Wrinkle Eye Cream above and the same comments apply. There are several ingredients in this moisturizer that would be a problem for combination skin, including Vaseline and shea butter.

BioTherm Suncare

✓☺ **Aquasource UV SPF 15** *($25 for 1.7 ounces)* is a very good, in-part titanium dioxide–based sunscreen. It also contains several very good antioxidants and water-binding agents.

☺ **UV Protect SPF 25** *($14.50 for 1 ounce)* is a very good, in-part titanium dioxide–based sunscreen in a rather ordinary emollient base.

☺ **High Protection Sun Block SPF 30** *($15 for 1.7 ounces)* is a very good, in-part titanium dioxide–, avobenzone-, and Mexoryl SX–based sunscreen in a rather ordinary emollient base. It does contain fragrance. (This formulation is only available outside of the United States.)

☺ **High Protection Sun Block SPF 25** *($15 for 1.7 ounces)* is similar to the High Protection Sun Block SPF 30 above and the same comments apply.

☺ **Sun Block Lotion High Protection SPF 25** *($15 for 5 ounces)* is a very good, in-part titanium dioxide–, avobenzone-, and Mexoryl SX–based sunscreen in a rather ordinary matte-finish base. (This formulation is only available outside of the United States.)

☺ **Protective Lotion SPF 15** *($15 for 5 ounces)* is a very good, in-part titanium dioxide– and Mexoryl SX–based sunscreen in a rather ordinary emollient base. (This formulation is only available outside of the United States.)

☹ **Moisturizing Sun Gel Oil Free SPF 15** *($15 for 5 ounces)* is a very good, in-part titanium dioxide– and Mexoryl SX–based sunscreen in an alcohol-based gel. That makes it too irritating and drying for the skin. (This formulation is only available outside of the United States.)

☺ **Special Wrinkle Sun Block SPF 15** *($15 for 1.7 ounces)* is a very good, in-part titanium dioxide–, avobenzone-, and Mexoryl SX–based sunscreen in a rather ordinary matte-finish base. Nothing about this product makes it more helpful for wrinkles than any other well-formulated sunscreen. (This formulation is only available outside of the United States.)

☺ **Bronze Magic Express Self Tanner, Face SPF 15** *($15 for 1.7 ounces)*. Do not rely on this for sun protection because it doesn't contain the UVA-protecting ingredients of titanium dioxide, zinc oxide, or avobenzone. It uses dihydroxyacetone, the same ingredient in all self-tanners that affects the color of skin.

☹ **Anti-Drying Protective Lip Treatment SPF 8** *($10 for 1.7 ounces)* does not contain the UVA-protecting ingredients of titanium dioxide, zinc oxide, or avobenzone, and the SPF 8 is below what is recommended by the American Academy of Dermatology. This product is not recommended.

BLACK OPAL

Black Opal is a cosmetics line aimed at African-American women. The skin-care products, although reasonably priced, have some problems. They were supposedly designed by a dermatologist, but either the dermatologist didn't do all the chemistry homework necessary to design a skin-care line or there were terrible oversights. What's missing are effective sunscreens, and what's present are too many irritating ingredients and extremely dated toner and moisturizer formulations. There is little here of benefit for any skin type or, for that matter, any skin color.

For more information about Black Opal, call (800) 625-6725 or visit www.cherylburgess.com.

BLACK OPAL SKIN CARE

☹ **Blemish Control Complexion Bar** *($3.50 for 3.5 ounces)* contains peppermint, camphor, eucalyptus, and menthol in a standard tallowate-containing bar cleanser. Those ingredients are too drying and irritating for all skin types and that can make acne worse, not better.

The Reviews B

☹ **Blemish Control Wash** *($5.95 for 6 ounces)* contains sodium lauryl sulfate, a strong skin irritant, as the main detergent cleansing agent. This cleanser also contains several other serious skin irritants, including camphor, menthol, eucalyptus oil, and peppermint oil. This product is absolutely not recommended.

☹ **Daily Fade Cleanser** *($5.95 for 5 ounces)* uses sodium C14-16 olefin sulfonate and sodium lauryl sulfate as the main detergent cleansing agents, which can be too irritating and drying for all skin types. And nothing in this product can fade or change skin color.

☺ **Oil Free Cleansing Gel** *($5.95 for 6 ounces)* is a standard, detergent-based, water-soluble cleanser that can be good for someone with oily skin. It does contain fragrance.

☹ **Pre-Fade Complexion Bar** *($3.50 for 3.5 ounces)* is a standard tallowate-based bar cleanser that can be too drying and irritating for all skin types.

☹ **Blemish Control Astringent** *($5.95 for 6 ounces)* contains mostly alcohol, but it also has arnica, menthol, eucalyptus, peppermint, and camphor, which makes this a serious source of irritation.

☺ **Purifying Astringent** *($5.95 for 6 ounces)* won't purify anything. It is just an exceedingly ordinary toner that contains mostly water, glycerin, and fragrance with some plant extracts.

☹ **Daily Fade Lotion SPF 15** *($8.95 for 2 ounces)* doesn't contain the UVA-protecting ingredients of titanium dioxide, zinc oxide, or avobenzone, and is not recommended.

☺ **Oil Free Moisturizing Lotion** *($5.95 for 1.75 ounces)* is an OK, though ordinary, moisturizer for someone with normal to slightly dry skin.

✓☺ **Advanced Dual Complex Fade Gel** *($11.95 for 0.75 ounce)* is a standard 2% hydroquinone gel with about 7% glycolic acid in a pH that makes it effective for exfoliation. Hydroquinone in this concentration can inhibit melanin production and the glycolic acid can help with cell turnover. However, without diligent use of a well-formulated sunscreen no skin-lightening product can be effective. This is an option for someone with normal to oily skin.

☺ **Advanced Dual Phase Fade Creme** *($11.95 for 1.75 ounces)* contains several ingredients that have some research showing effectiveness for inhibiting melanin production, including mulberry and licorice extract and vitamin C. However, the amount of these ingredients in this product is not sufficient for them to have that effect on skin. This is, however, a well-formulated moisturizer for someone with normal to dry skin.

☹ **Advanced Dual Phase Fade Creme with Sunscreen** *($11.95 for 1.75 ounces)* does contain 2% hydroquinone for skin lightening, but it doesn't contain the UVA-protecting ingredients of titanium dioxide, zinc oxide, or avobenzone for sun protection, and it is not recommended.

☹ **Blemish Control Gel** *($5.95 for 0.35 ounce)* contains resorcinol, an effective topical disinfectant. However, research has shown resorcinol to be overly irritating for skin, and as a result it is rarely used nowadays for treating blemishes. Besides, this gel also contains camphor, menthol, eucalyptus oil, and peppermint oil, which serve no purpose for skin except to create irritation and dryness.

BLACK OPAL MAKEUP

Black Opal's makeup has basically remained the same since the previous edition of this book, and continues to offer women of color the richly pigmented products they need to perform beautifully (and show up) on deep skin tones. You'll find a respectable, but small, selection of lipsticks and pencils, but the eyeshadows, blushes, and lip glosses have gotten more and more garish and gimmicky, and have consequently become harder to recommend. That's a shame, as this line used to have such stellar matte blush and eyeshadow choices. Where Black Opal really excels is with its foundations. The textures and finishes may not be universally appealing, but the shades are in line with true skin tones, with very few to avoid. The selection isn't as big as Prescriptives or M.A.C., but for the money this is a color line that women with medium to very dark skin tones on a budget should definitely investigate.

FOUNDATION: Without testers, it is hard to recommend the Black Opal foundations, though if you shop this line from a drugstore that allows cosmetics to be returned, you may want to take a chance on two or three shades. Some drugstores sell sample sizes of Black Opal foundations, but this does not appear to be a widespread option for this line, so it's more or less touch and go.

☺ **Cream Stick Foundation SPF 8** *($7.99)* comes in a stick form and looks like it would go on quite greasy, but in fact just the opposite is true. It goes on smooth and then dries to a soft, matte finish. It does tend to stay in place once it's on, so blending and removing this can be tricky. Ten colors are available, and most are quite good. The colors to avoid are Cinnamon Toast, Hazelnut, and Carob—these are too orange or red for most dark skin tones. This would be appropriate for normal to slightly dry or slightly oily skins not prone to breakouts, but the sunscreen is not to be relied on for all-day sun protection.

☹ **Cream to Powder Foundation SPF 8** *($7.99)* not only doesn't provide any UVA protection, but the colors are either too orange, red, or peach for most darker skin tones, and the consistency of this will cause the shades to turn color on oilier skin.

☺ **True Color Maximum Coverage Foundation** *($7.99)* is a silicone-based, stay-put foundation that offers truly opaque coverage and a soft matte finish, yet doesn't leave a heavy after-feel. The six shades are mostly excellent, but watch out for Heavenly Honey, which is too peach for most skin tones. **True Color Liquid Foundation Oil Free** *($7.99)* goes on quite smooth and sheer, drying to a matte finish. It can feel very dry on the skin and is, therefore, best for oily skin. The eight shades are mostly good options, but avoid Cinnamon Toast, Hazelnut, and Beautiful Bronze, which are too orange or rosy red for most dark skin tones. **Perfecting Powder Makeup SPF 8** *($7.99)* has a too-low SPF and lacks adequate UVA protection, but is nevertheless a decent cream-to-powder foundation. It tends to blend on a bit thick, but smooths nicely over the skin and offers a matte finish. Of the five shades, the only ones to watch out for are Heavenly Honey and Carob.

☺ **CONCEALER: Flawless Perfecting Concealer** *($3.79)* is a lipstick-style concealer that comes in four workable shades. It has a thick, creamy texture that covers well and leaves a minimal powder finish. The four shades are slightly orange but may work for some skin tones, and creasing shouldn't be a major problem. This is not the type of concealer you would want to use over blemishes.

POWDER: ✓☺ Oil Absorbing Pressed Powder *($7.99)* is a standard, talc-based powder that now comes in an expanded selection of colors. This has a silky texture that blends on easily and the colors tend to not turn ash, which is a major plus for darker skin tones. Cafe Au Lait, Cappuccino, Powdermedium Gold, Powderdark Cocoa, and Powderlight Caramel can all be too peach or red for most skin tones, but Rich Mocha, Powdermedium Brown, Classic Espresso, and Light Sand are great options. ☺ **Color Fusion Pressed Powder** *($7.99)* comes in one "shade," which is actually several colors swirled together in a mosaic pattern that come off as one sheer brown color on the skin. It's nearly identical in formula and application to the Oil-Absorbing Pressed Powder above and may indeed work for some skin tones, but save your receipt. **Color Fusion Bronzer** *($8.99)* is similar in appearance to the Color Fusion Pressed Powder above, but the Bronzer comes in matte and shimmer options, with the matte strongly preferred even though it is not deep enough for truly dark skin tones. Try this if you have medium skin and want a good matte bronzing powder.

☹ **Deluxe Finishing Loose Powder** *($7.99)* is talc-based and still has an unfriendly assortment of peach and rosy red shades that are best avoided.

☹ **BLUSH: Color Fusion Blush** *($8.99)* tries to please all skin tones by combining fragments of peach, rose, red, pink, purple, and plum tones in one compact. It ends up as more of a contrivance, and the color you get is no substitute for Black Opal's discontinued single-color blush options.

☹ **EYESHADOW: Duo Eyeshadow** *($4.79)* are all very shiny or are infused with brightly colored shiny particles that tend to flake off on the skin. These require precise blending, as they tend to grab on the skin and are hard to move. And there are some truly dated color combinations. Black Opal also offers mosaic and swirled single **Eyeshadow** *($4.79)* options, but these are more artifice than art, and not what I would consider practical or easy to use. **Eyeshadow Trios** *($4.79)* come in strange color combinations and do not have dividers, so the colors spill over onto each other.

☺ **EYE AND BROW SHAPER: Phat Eye Pencil** *($4.99)* is a standard pencil that applies nicely but can smear unless it's set with powder. **Precision Eye Definers** *($3.49)* are standard pencils with a mix of traditional and bold colors. Please keep in mind that royal blue and bright purple pencils tend to detract from rather than enhance the shape of the eyes.

☺ **LIPSTICK AND LIP PENCIL: Matte Plus Moisture Lipstick** *($5.69)* is also labeled as Matte Lipstick and isn't all that matte, but actually rather creamy with an almost glossy finish. The bold color selection is small, but wonderful for darker skin tones. **Lipstick** *($5.29)* is a very good creamy lipstick with a soft glossy finish. The small selection of shades still offers such gorgeous rich tones! **True Tone Vitamin Rich Lipstick** *($5.49)* is more emollient than matte, but it's not the least bit greasy. Again, the shade selection is on par with the needs of deeper skin tones. **Simply Sheer Lipstick SPF 15** *($5.29)* is, as the name implies, a simply sheer, fairly glossy lipstick. The sunscreen does not contain UVA-protecting ingredients and should not be relied on for sun protection. **Patent Lips Liquid Lipstick** *($5.49)* is an exceptionally sparkly, semi-opaque lip gloss in a tube with a wand applicator. It has a thick texture that can feel sticky, but it's also more tenacious than standard lip gloss. **Lip Gloss** and **Swirl Lip Gloss** *($3.79)* are very greasy glosses that come in pots and feature some excellent deep, mostly iridescent colors. **Dual Lip Gloss** *($5.29)* gives you two glossy colors in one package. This has a pleasantly smooth, minimally sticky texture and sheer, sparkly colors that work on most skin tones, dark or otherwise. **Precision Lip Definer Pencil** *($3.79)* is a standard "must be sharpened" lip pencil with some great colors to complement dark lipsticks.

☺ <u>MASCARA:</u> **Lash Defining Mascara** *($3.99)*, after all these years, still has one of the strangest brush shapes I've ever seen for mascara. It definitely doesn't aid in making lashes remarkably longer. This takes a while to build marginal length or thickness, and it doesn't clump or smear, but that brush is not deserving of a happy face.

BLISSLABS

The way Bliss came to be one of the more successful and well-known spa locations around is an intriguing story. Marcia Kilgore, a native of Canada, was a student at New York's Columbia University, but when her tuition plans fell through she had no choice but to fall back on her one marketable skill, personal training. Though her venture was blossoming she was routinely troubled by her complexion, and ended up enrolling in a skin-care course where the seeds of a future empire were planted. Kilgore developed a knack and passion for facials, and soon she was on her way to becoming a beauty guru among Manhattan's social elite and celebrities. As Kilgore expanded from a one-room spa to a small business, word spread of her talents, and in July 1996 Bliss was established with the goal of offering "super-effective treatments in an uncontrived 'no-attitude' atmosphere."

What immediately set Bliss apart from the then relatively quiet spa business was Kilgore's sense of irreverence and openness, and her commitment to skill and jazzed-up product formulations that are seemingly right on the pulse of what consumers are looking for, namely natural botanicals, exotic scents, and anything and everything that can duplicate (as closely as possible) the spa experience at home.

In 1999, Bliss entered a partnership with luxury goods conglomerate Louis Vuitton-Moet-Hennessey (LVMH), and Kilgore has seen her business continue to skyrocket as new spa locations have opened and dozens of new products have been created. The BlissLabs product line is now widely distributed in department stores, through the BlissOut catalog (circulation: eight million), and also at the LVMH-owned beauty emporium Sephora.

Until very recently, the Bliss products primarily consisted of staple spa items and included everything from cuticle creams to body scrubs and all manner of body masks, accompanied by an endless parade of spa accessories, again with the goal of bringing the luxurious spa experience home. Now with the launch of Spa-Strength Skin Care, Bliss is aiming at the facial-care category. According to www.blissworld.com, Spa-Strength Skin Care spent "two years in the lab and after tankerloads of testing, BlissLabs French-bred chemistry team has unleashed a range of formulas that perfectly fit our do-it-yourself pampering profile."

After all the spin has been spun, is there a legitimate reason to seriously consider this line? Once you get past the notion that "flash-distilled" fruit water is somehow beneficial for skin, or that ingredients like lemon and grapefruit are more a problem for skin than a help, the answer is yes and no. On the one hand, these are hardly what could be considered breakthrough products. The majority of them are standard formulations whose subtle varia-tions show up in almost every modern skin-care line. Yet that does not make them poor products. What hurts this line is the very thing that hypes it, namely, the presence of certain plant extracts and botanicals that sound like cure-alls but are actually problematic for skin. Although these ingredients are not present in every product, they show up often enough that the caution is warranted. Not surprisingly, all of the products contain fragrance.

What is disturbing, and "after tankerloads of testing," too, is to find BlissLabs carry-ing on about the antiaging properties of their Spa-Strength Skin Care line when there's not a sunscreen to be found. (In two years of research they couldn't come up with a sunscreen formulation?) But then again, this is still the cosmetics industry, and in spite of BlissLabs's boastings, such blatant omissions are par for the course. Actually, the main BlissLabs line does have a decent sunscreen (included in this review), but it's not included as part of the Spa-Strength routines. For more information about BlissLabs, call (888) 243-8825 or visit www.blissworld.com.

BLISSLABS SKIN CARE

☺ **Fully Loaded Cleansing Milk for Dry Skin** *($23 for 8.5 ounces)* is a light, cold cream–style cleanser that would work well for dry skin. The lotion texture feels soft on the skin and this should work well to remove makeup, but it's not the easiest to rinse away, and you may need a washcloth to get it all off. It does contain fragrance and coloring agents.

☺ **Fully Loaded Skin Finishing Rinse for Dry Skin** *($18 for 8.5 ounces)* is a good toner for dry skin that contains mostly water, glycerin, plant oils, slip agents, preserva-tives, water-binding agent, fragrance, and coloring agents. This is hardly fully loaded, as it lacks an array of antioxidants, anti-irritants, or water-binding agents.

☺ **Fully Loaded Moisture Lotion for Dry Skin** *($36 for 1.7 ounces)* is almost iden-tical to the All Around Eye Cream reviewed below; the only difference is the price. So you have to ask, what myth about product placement is convincing you that this version can't be used around the eyes?

☺ **Low Fat Cleansing Milk for Oily Skin** *($23 for 8.5 ounces)* is similar to the Fully Loaded Cleansing Milk for Dry Skin above, only this one has somewhat fewer emollients and adds some irritating plant extracts. This is not the best option for oily skin, though it could be an option for normal to dry skin.

☹ **Low Fat Rinse for Oily Skin** *($18 for 8.5 ounces)* contains alcohol, lemon, caffeine, horse chestnut, camphor, grapefruit, and menthol, which are exceptionally irritating and drying and have no effect on reducing oil production. Even more confusing in this jumble of ingredients are plant oils that would add to the woes of someone struggling with oily skin. This product does contain niacinamide for which there is some research indicating it can be helpful for reducing breakouts, but the study demonstrated that 4% niacinamide was necessary to achieve that benefit and this product contains less than 0.5%.

☹ **Low Fat Moisture Lotion for Oily Skin** *($36 for 1.7 ounces)* contains denatured alcohol as the second ingredient, along with lemon, grapefruit, camphor, and menthol, all irritating to skin and with no balancing benefit for any skin type. This product also contains a small amount of mineral oil, which isn't the best for oily skin. The amount of niacinamide is too minuscule to have any effect on skin.

☺ **Middleweight Cleansing Milk for Normal Skin** *($23 for 8.5 ounces)* is similar to the Low Fat Cleansing Milk for Oily Skin above and the same basic comments apply. It does contain fragrance.

☺ **Middleweight Finishing Rinse for Normal Skin** *($18 for 8.5 ounces)* is similar to the Fully Loaded Skin Finishing Rinse for Dry Skin above, only this one has orange fruit extract as the second ingredient, which makes it potentially sensitizing for many skin types. That's disappointing, because all of the other ingredients would work well for normal to dry skin.

☺ **Middle Weight Moisture Lotion for Normal Skin** *($36 for 1.7 ounces)* is simply a lighter version of the Fully Loaded Moisture Lotion for Dry Skin above. This one contains orange fruit extract, which smells nice but can be a skin irritant, especially when used in this amount (it's the second ingredient).

☺ **Quiet Type Cleansing Milk for Sensitive Skin** *($23 for 8.5 ounces)* claims it is for sensitive skin, which I guess is why they left out the citrus irritants that are present in the Low Fat and Middleweight cleansers above, an idea that would have been better for those skin types as well. However, this still contains fragrance, something best left out of any skin-care product for sensitive skin. This remains a good cleanser for dry skin, quite similar to Neutrogena's Extra Gentle Cleanser ($7.29 for 6.7 ounces) for far less.

☺ **Quiet Type Finishing Rinse for Sensitive Skin** *($18 for 8.5 ounces)* is similar to the Fully Loaded Skin Finishing Rinse for Dry Skin above and the same basic comments apply. This would be an OK gentle toner for normal to dry skin. This does contain fragrance and coloring agents, not the best for sensitive skin types.

☺ **Quiet Type Moisture Lotion for Sensitive Skin** *($36 for 1.7 ounces)* is almost identical to the All Around Eye Cream below and the same basic comments apply.

☺ **$$$ All Around Eye Cream** *($26 for 0.5 ounce)* is a good moisturizer for normal to dry skin, though there is nothing about this that makes it better for the eye area. The amount of antioxidants and water-binding agents isn't exciting, but they are present.

The **BlissLabs Task Masks** are all blends of diatomaceous earth, which is a relatively absorbent, fine-grained powder composed of soil and minute shellfish skeletons. It can be somewhat abrasive, which doesn't make sense for all skin types. Further, the base for all of these masks is identical and so it's probably too absorbent for normal to dry skin. These also contain algin, a seaweed-derived, gel-like substance that is more of a thickener than anything else. However, most algae do have benefit as antioxidants. The same is true for the form of vitamin C in these products. Of course, how any of that relates to wrinkles in unknown.

☺ **$$$ Bilberry & C Task Mask** *($45 for 10.5 ounces)* contains the above-mentioned ingredients, plus buffering agents, bilberry extract, coloring agents, and fragrance. Nothing about this mask will "stimulate antiaging activity." Bilberry extract can be a good antioxidant, but the tiny amount present (plus the fact that all masks are washed off) makes any benefit limited at best.

☹ **Breakout Busting Task Mask** *($45 for 10.5 ounces)* is similar to the Bilberry Mask above, only this one contains menthol and a teeny amount of tea tree oil. The menthol can be irritating and there isn't enough tea tree oil here for it to have any impact as a disinfectant.

☺ **$$$ Exfoliating Task Mask** *($45 for 10.5 ounces)* is similar to the masks above, except that this one contains papaya extract. At its best, papaya is a relatively unstable exfoliant (though there is no research demonstrating this to be true when used in a cosmetic formulation), and it's no match for a well-formulated AHA or BHA product.

☹ **Instant Lifting Task Mask** *($45 for 10.5 ounces)* is similar to all the masks above, only this one adds spirulina (a type of blue-green algae for which there is research showing established benefits when taken orally, but there is no research indicating benefits when it is used topically). But it also contains menthol, and that doesn't lift anything, though it can be a skin irritant.

☺ **$$$ Lighten Up Task Mask** *($45 for 10.5 ounces)* is the most worthwhile mask in the bunch. This one has nonirritating plant extracts and, thankfully, no fragrance or coloring agents. Unfortunately, none of the ingredients present have the same potent skin-lightening abilities as hydroquinone, kojic acid, or certain forms of vitamin C (notably magnesium ascorbyl palmitate or ascorbyl phosphate). Whatever effect it has is further reduced by the fact that any skin-lightening agent needs to be left on the skin for a much longer period of time than the few minutes a mask is left on if it is to have the intended effect.

☺ **Lid and Lash Wash** *($22 for 8.5 ounces)* is an exceptionally standard detergent-based eye-makeup remover. It's a fairly gentle formula that would have been even better if they had not included fragrance. There is nothing in here that is, to quote the BlissOut

The Reviews B

catalog, "puff-trouncing," though it resembles almost every eye-makeup remover of this ilk being sold.

☺ **Sunban Lotion SPF 30** *($21 for 4.2 ounces)* is an effective blend of sunscreen agents (though 1% titanium dioxide is cutting it close when it comes to significant UVA protection) in a standard moisturizing base. This would be best for normal to dry skin, and it is fragrance-free.

BlissLabs Makeup

BlissLabs makeup is practically in love with itself. Rarely have I read such fawning descriptions about such everyday items as foundation and lip gloss. The most bewitching adjectives are used to provide tantalizing details on each shade, with words like "captivating," "commanding," and "incredibly pretty" vying for your attention. Each shade of every product sounds so wonderfully perfect it's hard to imagine not owning (and wearing) them all. Yet doing so isn't likely to produce the results hinted at in each color's portrayal because this is just ordinary makeup. Yes, these will work to enhance and define your features—but no better (and sometimes worse) than countless products from other lines, most of which are available at drugstores for less than half of BlissLabs's fee. You won't be completely disappointed by BlissLabs makeup, but the difference between the embellished claims and actual performance is bound to be a sobering reality check.

☺ **$$$ FOUNDATION: Skin Twin Liquid Complexion Perfection with SPF 12 Protection** *($35)* has a tongue-twisting name and an SPF that is marginally low for daytime protection, not to mention that this one does not contain titanium dioxide, zinc oxide, or avobenzone for sufficient UVA protection. What a shame, because this has a soft, light texture that feels great on normal to dry skin. Skin Twin offers sheer to light coverage in five mostly excellent colors—only Naked is slightly peach—but knowing you would need to pair this with an effective sunscreen makes this tough to recommend.

☺ **$$$ POWDER: Skin Twin Pressed Powder** *($25)* is a great pressed powder that is available in three truly neutral tones. The smoothness and silkiness are here, but for the money this isn't worth choosing over pressed powders from Sonia Kashuk or Almay.

☺ **BLUSH: blissglows** *($15)* are very sheer cream-to-powder blushes that come in sleek translucent compacts. These leave a soft, minimally moist finish and have a touch of shimmer, but not enough to be distracting. If you're interested in this type of blush, Revlon, L'Oreal, and Avon sell similar versions for less. Note: Grappa is a not a blush tone; it's a white highlighter with a soft shimmer.

☺ **$$$ EYESHADOW: blisslids** *($17)* have a velvety texture and smooth, clingy application that blends on sheer. The small collection of shades offers mostly nude-to-neutral options, each with a soft to obvious shine. If you're looking for intensity, look elsewhere. Otherwise, if you don't mind the shine, these are worth a try.

EYE & BROW SHAPER: ✔☺ **Powder Brows** *($16)* is a standard brow pencil whose performance is better than standard. This has a smooth application that deposits soft, powdery color that lasts. The three shades are beautiful, but there is no option for redheads. ✓☺ **Lidstick** *($15)* looks like traditional eye pencils, but these apply with ease and have a soft powder finish that adds significant longevity. Although these softly shiny pencils can't outlast a matte powder used as an eyeliner, if you're pencil-prone, these are tough to beat.

LIPSTICK AND LIP PENCIL: ☺ **$$$ lips stick** *($17)* is a standard chubby lip pencil that has a creamy application and slightly glossy finish. The colors are semi-sheer and mostly attractive, but this has an unpleasant waxy smell that's more pervasive than it should be. The **blissgloss** *($18)* is a very standard pot-type lip gloss that has a thick, sticky texture and transparent colors. The price is bizarre given the ordinary formula. **Lip liner stick** *($15)* is a standard creamy pencil that surpasses most of the competition only in price.

☺ **$$$ blissbalm** *($18)* is a simple wax- and emollient-based lip gloss that will take good care of dry lips. The clear and sheer pink shades are scented with vanilla, which will undoubtedly be attractive to many consumers, though it has no benefit for the lips.

☺ **$$$ MASCARA:** Supposedly, **Blisslash** *($16)* was "long in the lab and extensively tested," so you could reasonably expect this mascara to be top-notch. But maybe BlissLabs was going for middle of the road, as this unexceptional formula builds decent length, but barely any thickness or oomph. It's not a terrible mascara, but certainly pales in comparison to less expensive options from Maybelline, Almay, L'Oreal, and Jane.

BLISTEX (LIP CARE ONLY)

How this small line of lip products has achieved the status of being the solution for cold sores or chapped lips eludes me! These lip products contain enough irritating ingredients to chap anyone's lips. Lots of lip products claim to be medicated, but "medicated" is a dubious term at best, with no regulated meaning. As Blistex and other companies choose to define medicated it means the products contain camphor, peppermint oil, eucalyptus, or menthol, but these are not medicines for dry lips; they make dry skin worse and can cause irritation. Products like Blistex can include 0.5% phenol, a potent disinfectant, but phenol is strong stuff and can actually trigger some serious problems, the least of which are dryness and irritation. It is not something I would recommend for anything but extremely limited use. Even more lamentable is that this popular line of lip products has several sunscreen products for the lips, but not one of them includes UVA-protecting ingredients. For more information about Blistex, call (630) 571-2870 or visit www.blistex.com.

All of the following products either do not contain the UVA-protecting ingredients of titanium dioxide, zinc oxide, or avobenzone or have an inadequate SPF rating that would give a terribly false sense of protection that could result in serious skin damage. They are absolutely not recommended.

☹ **Complete Moisture, SPF 15** *($1.99 for 0.15 ounce)*; **Daily Conditioning Treatment SPF 20** *($1.50 for 0.25 ounce)*; **Fruit Smoothies, SPF 15** *($3.49 for 3-pack of*

0.30-ounce tubes); ☹ **Herbal Answer Stick, SPF 15** ($1.99 for 0.15 ounce); F
swer Tube, SPF 15 ($1.99 for 0.15 ounce); **Lip Balm SPF 15** (Regular, Berry,
($1.29 for 0.15 ounce); **Lip Tone SPF 15** ($1.59 for 0.15 ounce); **Silk and Shine, SPF 15**
($2.39 for 0.13 ounce); and **Ultra Protection, SPF 30** ($2.15 for 0.15 ounce).

☹ **Medicated Lip Ointment** ($1.99 for 0.21 ounce) contains menthol, camphor,
and phenol in a base of Vaseline and alcohol. Everything but the petrolatum is too irritating for the lips—or any part of the body, for that matter.

☹ **Lip Medex** ($0.86 for 0.25 ounce) is similar to the Lip Ointment above, only this
one has large quantities of the irritating ingredients.

☺ **Lip Revitalizer** ($0.95 for 0.25 ounce). The second ingredient is carvone, a flavor-
ing ingredient and fragrance. That can taste good but it can also be a skin irritant.

BOBBI BROWN

Bobbi Brown has been one of the most quoted and referred-to makeup artists in
fashion magazines and on television for several years now, and her handiwork has graced
the faces of countless models and celebrities. Brown's product line, which was launched
over ten years ago with a small collection of brown-based lipsticks, established her reputation as the source of the natural neutral palette. Shortly thereafter, Brown launched
foundations and these have become the mainstay of her makeup collection. Although the
first round of colors were noticeably yellow, the shades have been tweaked and since then
have ranked among some of the more reliable range of foundation shades in the business.
In fact, since Estee Lauder purchased Bobbi Brown in 1995, the line has seen tremendous
growth. What started out as a small makeup line has evolved into a large line with a
diverse array of products.

Lauder's influx of money has allowed Brown to continually expand the line. One
growth spurt was the revamping of the entire skin care line in September 2002; out with
the old and in with the new. Leaving behind glycolic acid (AHA) and salicylic acid (BHA)
products along with some fairly irritating plant extracts in some of the cleansers, Brown's
latest offerings do have some improvements, but overall, especially in comparison to the
products of other Lauder-owned cosmetics companies, they just aren't as impressive as
you would expect. Brown's products aren't bad by any means, it's just that they weren't
improved as much as they could have been. While Brown's new products do contain
some good water-binding agents, antioxidants, and anti-irritants, they aren't unique in
any way. Both Lauder (the more expensive matriarch) and Clinique (the less pricy younger
sister) offer far better options with more varied formulations for different skin types and
an abundance of state-of-the-art water-binding agents and antioxidants.

A new slant for Brown is the claim that most of the products are "dermatologist
tested," but a quick call to the company revealed that there are no test results to be had.
According to the FDA (FDA *Consumer* magazine, May 1995, www.fda.gov) "...label
claims that a product is 'dermatologist-tested,'... carry no guarantee that it won't cause

reactions. [The] FDA tried to publish regulations [in 1975] defining hypoallergenic to mean a lower potential for causing an allergic reaction.... In addition, we were going to require that companies submit information to FDA establishing that in fact their products were hypoallergenic.... However, two cosmetic manufacturers, Almay and Clinique, challenged the proposed regulations in court, claiming that consumers already understood that hypoallergenic products were no panacea against allergic reactions. In July 1975, the U.S. District Court for the District of Columbia upheld FDA's regulations, but the two companies appealed. On Dec. 21, 1977, the U.S. Court of Appeals for the District of Columbia reversed the district court's ruling."

Without regulations and without test results that state why the products deserved the blessings of any dermatologist (or what standards or comparisons were used), the claim of "dermatologist-tested" is meaningless. Aside from the claims, there are some options here to consider, but nothing to get all that excited about. For more information about Bobbi Brown call (212) 572-4200 or visit www.bobbibrowncosmetics.com.

BOBBI BROWN SKIN CARE

☹ **Exfoliating Cream Wash** *($22 for 3.4 ounces)* is an emollient, plant oil–based cleanser that contains several irritating plant extracts including arnica, grapefruit, and eucalyptus. Other than that, it's just a very ordinary cold cream–style cleanser that also contains clay, which makes it more confusing than exfoliating given that clay is best for oily skin and the emollients in here are best for dry skin.

☺ **$$$ One-Step Cleanser and Long-Wear Makeup Remover** *($22 for 3.4 ounces)* contains mostly thickeners, plant oils, glycerin, and preservatives. This basic cold cream–style cleanser is an option for normal to dry skin.

☺ **$$$ Purifying Gel Cleanser** *($22 for 4.2 ounces)* is a standard, detergent-based cleanser that can be an option for someone with normal to oily skin. It does contain fragrance.

☺ **$$$ Rich Cream Cleanser** *($22 for 4.2 ounces)* is a very basic, though emollient, Vaseline-based cleanser. This is little more than cold cream, but it is an option for normal to dry skin. It does contain fragrance.

☺ **$$$ Extra Balm Rinse** *($50 for 6.8 ounces)* is a lot of money for what is essentially just glycerin, olive oil, orange oil, slip agents, and a teeny amount of antioxidant, which adds up to cold cream. There are far less expensive ways to remove the last traces of makeup.

☺ **$$$ Eye Makeup Remover** *($18.50 for 3.4 ounces)* is a very standard detergent-based eye-makeup remover similar to almost every other one of this ilk, and it would work just as well, though there are far cheaper versions. It does contain fragrance.

☺ **$$$ Soothing Face Tonic** *($22 for 6.7 ounces)* is a decent toner that would work well for most skin types. It contains mostly water, slip agents, glycerin, plant extracts, water-binding agents, fragrant plant extract, and preservatives. The plant extracts are a nice mix of anti-irritants.

☺ **$$$ Extra Soothing Balm** *($50 for 0.5 ounce)* is a fairly basic emollient balm containing mostly thickeners, emollient, vitamin E, plant oils, fragrant oils, preservatives, and coloring agents. The plant oils are a nice mix of soothing agents and antioxidants, but hardly unique or worth this inflated price tag.

☺ **$$$ Hydrating Eye Cream** *($32.50 for 0.5 ounce)* is a very good emollient moisturizer for normal to dry skin that contains mostly water, plant oils, silicone, thickeners, water-binding agents, antioxidants, and preservatives. This is nice, but not as interesting as alternatives from Clinique or Lauder that are available for less money and have more state-of-the-art formulations. This is fragrance free.

☺ **$$$ Hydrating Face Cream** *($38 for 1.7 ounces)* is similar to the Hydrating Eye Cream above only this one contains fragrance. The same basic comments apply.

☺ **$$$ Hydrating Face Lotion SPF 15** *($38 for 1.7 ounces)* is a good, in-part, titanium dioxide–based sunscreen in a lightweight moisturizing base. It contains a good mix of antioxidants and anti-irritants, but only a tiny amount of water-binding agents, which is disappointing. In many ways, this is quite similar to Clinique's Weather Everything Environmental Cream SPF 15 ($18.50 for 1 ounce) and Lauder's Day Wear Super Anti-Oxidant Complex SPF 15 ($37.50 for 1.7 ounces).

☺ **$$$ Intensive Skin Supplement** *($50 for 1 ounce)* is a very good, silicone-based lotion that contains a good mix of antioxidants, anti-irritants, water-binding agents, and preservatives. The small amounts of vitamin C and mulberry root are probably not present in a high enough concentration to have an effect on melanin production.

☺ **$$$ Extra Moisturizing Balm SPF 25** *($75 for 1.7 ounces)*. I had to double check the price tag on this balm twice to be sure I was seeing clearly, I was. This in-part avobenzone-based sunscreen contains some emollients, plant oils, fragrance, anti-irritants, antioxidants, tiny amount of a water-binding agent, and preservatives. It is a very good sunscreen for dry skin, but the cost doesn't jive with what you're getting. Keep in mind that sunscreen must be applied liberally if you are going to net any benefit from it. How liberally are you going to apply a $75 sunscreen that won't last more then a couple of weeks if you're applying it correctly? The only extra about this product is the cost, not the benefit for skin.

☺ **$$$ Shine Control Hydrating Face Gel** *($38 for 1.7 ounces)* contains mostly water, silicones, film-forming agent, anti-irritants, water-binding agents, vitamin E, and preservatives. This is a good lightweight moisturizer for normal to slightly dry skin, but there isn't anything in it that will "control" oil, though it does have a matte finish.

☺ **$$$ Sunless Tanning Gel for Face and Body** *($27.50 for 4.2 ounces)* contains dihydroxyacetone, the same ingredient that all self-tanners use to affect the color of skin. This one would work as well as any, and offers no advantage over versions sold at the drugstore, from Coppertone to Bain de Soleil.

☹ **SPF 15 Lip Balm** *($15.50 for 0.12 ounce)* does not contain the UVA-protecting ingredients of titanium dioxide, zinc oxide, or avobenzone, and is not recommended. It also contains menthol and peppermint, which can be skin irritants.

BOBBI BROWN MAKEUP

According to Brown's Web site, a woman's true beauty style is not about following the latest runway trend or creating a cookie-cutter face. Rather, it's about wearing makeup that's self-enhancing. While that statement is indeed admirable and empowering, it neglects the fact that Bobbi Brown *is* a trendsetter, as her anticipated seasonal looks attest. It was trendiness that was the backbone of Brown's now-defunct ColorOptions line.

This line really excels in its original offerings of superior foundations, true matte blushes and eyeshadows, and all of the other basics that are essential to a woman's classic makeup wardrobe. All of these are certainly worth checking out and they win this line high marks.

FOUNDATION: ☺ **$$$ Foundation Stick** *($35)* bills itself as "foundation and concealer in one." It falls short on both counts, especially in comparison with Brown's other foundations. This is fairly emollient and could easily crease into lines around the eyes or mouth. The coverage is light to medium with a creamy finish, making this best for normal to dry skin. Most of the colors are quite neutral and not nearly as yellow as they originally were. The 12 shades present options for light and darker skin, but avoid Walnut (too red) and Warm Natural (too peach). Natural and Golden may be too peach for some skin tones, but are still worth considering.

☺ **$$$ Oil-Free Even Finish Makeup SPF 15** *($35)* is a replacement for Brown's former Oil-Free Foundation. Whether or not you think it is an improvement depends on what you liked or didn't like about the original version. In contrast to the original Oil-Free Foundation (which I preferred), this formula has a sunscreen, although because it lacks the reliable UVA-protecting ingredients of titanium dioxide, zinc oxide, or avobenzone it cannot be relied on for adequate protection. This version does have a lighter, slightly smoother texture than its predecessor, but also offers a less substantial matte finish and less initial coverage. Application is easier than before, but if you need more than light coverage you may want to consider other options. There are 12 shades available, including options for darker skin tones, and almost all of them are beautiful. The only ones to consider avoiding are Warm Natural, Golden, and Walnut. This is worth a look if you have normal to slightly dry or slightly oily skin and don't mind wearing a separate effective sunscreen underneath.

☺ **$$$ Moisture-Rich Foundation SPF 15** *($38)* has a wonderfully soft, creamy texture that blends beautifully and dries to a natural finish. Coverage is in the light to medium range and the 12 shades are almost impeccable—the only ones to watch out for are Golden, which is quite yellow, and Walnut, which is slightly red. There are even some excellent dark tones, along with traditional options for light skin tones. The major drawback is the lack of adequate UVA protection from the sunscreen, which is dismaying. Of lesser importance is the fact that this is housed in a pump bottle, which is not the most economical method for dispensing foundation, because you tend to pump out more than you need and there's no getting it back in the bottle. However, if you have normal to dry skin and are willing to wear a separate sunscreen underneath this, it is worth checking out. **Fresh Glow Cream Foundation** *($35)* is best for normal to slightly dry or slightly oily skin. This has a whipped texture and a thicker consistency, but blends on better that you might expect. The coverage is medium to full, with a semi-matte finish, meaning those with very dry skin expecting a rich foundation will not be happy with this one. Avoid these colors: Warm Natural, Golden, and Walnut. The lighter colors are excellent, and Espresso is beautiful on very dark skin.

☺ $$$ **Oil-Free Even Finish Compact Foundation** *($38)* is a silicone-based creamy compact makeup that applies and blends beautifully. Rather than a traditional cream-to-powder finish, this one has a very slightly moist, natural finish that is flattering on normal to dry skin. This sheer to medium coverage formula would be too rich for those with breakout-prone skin. Of the 12 shades, the only ones to consider avoiding are Warm Natural, Golden, and Walnut. This can double as concealer, and its texture is preferable to Brown's Creamy Concealer.

✓☺ $$$ **SPF 15 Tinted Moisturizer** *($35)* has been reformulated because, according to the counter personnel I spoke with, Bobbi Brown wasn't satisfied with the colors. If you were a fan (and there were many) of the previous version, you will notice only minor changes in terms of texture, application, and finish. The SPF 15 still offers UVA protection with an in-part titanium dioxide–based sunscreen, and the formula is now more silicone-based, so it has a lighter feel on the skin. The five colors are mostly exceptional—only Deep is too orange for most skin tones. For effective sun protection, sheer color, and a beautiful finish, this is highly recommended.

<u>CONCEALER:</u> ☺ $$$ **Concealer Kit** *($35)* is a revision of Brown's former Professional Concealer, though it isn't much better than the original. This is now a two-part product, with a creamy, thick, crease-prone concealer nestled on top of a small jar of loose powder. I suppose this will seem handy for some, but it adds little to the appeal of this product. The pros for the concealer are excellent coverage and reliable colors—only Bisque and Beige are too peachy pink to pass muster. The lightest shade, Porcelain, is a great color for very fair skin, but it is coupled with a Pure White powder that can look ghostly on the skin. The rest of the ten shades come paired with Brown's Pale Yellow powder, which can be too yellow for some skin tones. The **Creamy Concealer** *($25)* is also available alone, but it's sobering to realize you're paying an extra ten dollars for a tiny container of loose powder and mini powder puff!

☺ $$$ **Blemish Cover Stick** *($20)* has a creamy, slightly greasy texture that is not what I would recommend using over a blemish. This stick concealer contains too many ingredients that can be problematic for use on breakout-prone skin. However, its natural finish and good coverage make it a winner for use on dark circles or other discolorations. The six shades nicely represent light to dark skin tones, and the only one to be cautious with is Warm Honey, which is slightly yellow-orange.

☺ $$$ <u>POWDER:</u> Bobbi Brown's loose **Face Powder** *($29)* is a standard, talc-based powder that has an airy, silky texture and a dry finish. The colors are a mixed bag: half are just too orange or yellow (sallow) to recommend. If you're considering trying one of these, proceed with caution and double-check the color in natural light. **Pressed Powder** *($26)* is virtually identical to the loose powder, with the same colors and same warnings. For both powders, avoid Sunny Beige, Golden Orange, and carefully consider Pale Yellow. **Sheer Finish Loose Powder** *($30)* is a talc-based powder that has the requisite soft, dry texture and—true to its name—a sheer application, with six mostly attractive colors. What is frustrating and rather shocking about this powder is that it costs more than Brown's regular Loose Powder and offers 75 percent less product (0.25 ounce versus 1 ounce)! If you must have Bobbi Brown Powder, there is no reason to choose this one over the regular Face Powder above because both have a similar application and appearance on skin. **Sheer Finish Pressed Powder** *($28)* is also talc-based and has the same basic texture, finish, and color selection as the Loose Powder version above. Although overpriced, it is an option for a soft, matte-finish pressed powder.

☺ $$$ <u>BLUSH:</u> The powder **Blush** *($19)* features gorgeous colors that apply and blend evenly with a smooth matte finish. The only colors to think twice about are Rose, Blushed, and Soft Pink, which are all shiny. **Cream Blush Stick** *($25)* is a sheer, slightly greasy cream blush that remains creamy on the skin. Blending takes some time, and this is really best for flawless normal to dry skin, as it is too greasy for oily skin types. The only color to be careful with is Warm Peach, which can be too orange for most skin tones. **Bronzing Stick** *($28)* has the same texture as the Cream Blush Stick, but the Bronzing Stick has great bronze tones that are an option if you want to create a sun-kissed look. All three shades are quite sheer, with no shine to be found! **Bronzing Powder** *($26)* would be a better choice for normal to oily skin types than the Bronzing Stick. The powder is richer in pigment and it is easier to apply and to control the intensity because you apply it with a brush. All three shades are beautiful and only slightly shiny.

<u>EYESHADOW:</u> Bobbi Brown's ☺ $$$ **Eye Shadows** *($18)* have a silky, smooth-blending texture and most of the colors are beautifully matte. There are some great choices for darker skin tones, and many of these shades would work well for lining the eyes or defining the eyebrows. The only colors to consider avoiding are Navy and Moss. **Shimmer Eye Shadow** *($18)* is at least named accurately, because there are three very shiny cream-to-powder eye colors. The shine is soft, making these wearable for a special evening look.

☹ $$$ **Shimmer Wash Eye Shadow** *($18)* is a collection of sheer to intense iridescent colors that are set apart from the matte colors on the tester unit, making them easy to avoid. They apply easily, but the shiny particles tend to flake on the skin—not the desired effect, but a reality nonetheless.

☹ **Cream Shadow Stick** *($20)* is a creamy eyeshadow in a roll-up stick form. These may be an option for some, but they tend to go on choppy and are difficult to blend out evenly. Plus, the texture of this starts smooth, but once it has set, it remains sticky!

<u>EYE & BROW SHAPER:</u> ☺ $$$ **Creamy Eye Pencil** *($20)* is a standard needs-sharpening pencil that definitely has a creamy texture. It tends to have a sticky finish, and

is not for someone who dislikes eyeliner smudging. Check out Brown's excellent matte eyeshadows for lining instead.

✓☺ $$$ **Long Wear Gel Eyeliner** *($18)*, which comes in a glass pot and needs to be applied with an eyeliner brush. This is sort of a hybrid between using a powder eyeshadow and liquid liner. The product applies slightly wet, has a fair amount of slip, and then "sets" to a solid powder finish. If you can master the application, you'll find this to be quite a tenacious product. Still, if you're prone to eyeliner fading or smudging, this is a unique product that is a must-try. ✓☺ $$$ **Natural Brow Shaper** *($16.50)* is a great way to groom and shade your eyebrows with natural-looking color. This is truly best for the brows only; it applies well and dries quickly, yet the bristles on the brush aren't long enough to reach down to the roots of any gray hair you may wish to conceal. The colors aren't the best for very dark brown or black hair, but there is a nice range for lighter hair shades, including redheads. A Clear version is also available.

LIPTSICK & LIP PENCIL: This is where Bobbi Brown began, and although the color palette is exceptional, the formulas are pretty standard. The ☺ $$$ **Lip Color** *($18)* is strictly a cream lipstick with nice opaque coverage and great colors, most of which are brown-based. **Lip Shimmer** *($18)* is basically the same as the Lip Color above, only with iridescence. Besides the shine, the colors include more mauve and plum options. **Lip Stain** *($17)* is more of a gloss in lipstick form than anything else, and these are too sheer to leave any trace of a stain. Nice colors, though. **Cream Lip Gloss** *($18)* features ten beautiful colors (they really are exquisite), but otherwise it's a standard opaque lip gloss that has a traditional thick, sticky texture and the requisite wet, glossy finish. If paying top dollar for lip gloss doesn't bother you, it would be wise to start here! **Shimmer Gloss Stick** *($18)* is heralded as an innovative product that combines the look of gloss and the convenience of lipstick application. Although this very glossy lipstick has a slick texture that's completely non-sticky, it's hardly unique. However, extra points are earned for the beautiful colors, each laced with iridescence.

☺ $$$ **SPF 15 Lip Shine** *($17.50)* is a creamy, shiny lipstick that is overpriced for what you get and the sunscreen has no UVA-protecting ingredients. The **Lip Gloss** and **Shimmer Lip Gloss** *(both $18)* are extremely overpriced, standard, sticky glosses with a poor brush that tends to splay after a few uses; the Shimmer version just adds sparkle. **Crystal Lip Gloss** *($15)* is a very thick, sticky and syrupy gloss that comes in a squeeze tube. This will provide a high shine to the lips, but the thick feel is less than pleasant. **Art Stick** *($25)* is a copycat version of everyone else's jumbo pencils for lips and cheeks. This is too greasy to work well as cheek color because application can be streaky and blending tricky. As a lipstick, it may be OK, but at this price a regular lipstick is far easier and doesn't need to be sharpened. The four available colors are neutral and workable. **Creamy Lip Liner** *($20)* is a standard pencil that comes with a lip brush on one end, which is a nice convenience. This is almost identical in texture and application to the Creamy Eye Pencil above, and that's just fine for lips as long as you don't have a problem with lipstick feathering.

☹ **Lip Balm SPF 15** *($15.50)* does not contain the UVA-protecting ingredients of avobenzone, titanium dioxide, or zinc oxide—but does contain irritating peppermint oil—and is absolutely not recommended.

☹ **Lip Tint SPF 15** *($15)*. Given the various lip glosses Brown's line features, this addition without adequate UVA protection was hardly necessary. The sheer, slightly sticky lip gloss has a minty flavor and barely-there colors that just aren't exciting given the price.

☺ **$$$ <u>MASCARA</u>: Defining Mascara** *($16)* is Bobbi Brown's original mascara that does an excellent job with lengthening and tends to not clump or smear. **Thickening Mascara** *($16)* is not thickening in the least, but could work for a natural, defined lash look if you don't mind the large brush. The Plum shade is quite purple and best avoided. **Lash Lustre Waterproof Mascara** ($16) is a very good mascara that builds some length but very little thickness. It is indeed waterproof, but the brush tends to stick the lashes together while you're applying it, so be careful. **Lash Glamour Lengthening Mascara** *($19)* is a lightweight, sheer mascara that darkens lashes without adding any length. It doesn't clump, but does add some thickness. This is a repackaged, renamed version of Brown's LashTint Mascara in a Tube.

☺ **$$$ <u>BRUSHES</u>:** Brown's **Brushes** *($18.50–$62.50)* are quite nice, with well-tapered edges and dense bristles. The Concealer and Eyeliner brushes are superb. As an added bonus, all of the brushes are available in either a travel (4-inch) or professional (6-inch) length. There are some to carefully consider, and some to ignore altogether. One to ignore is the **Loose Powder Brush** *($62.50)*, which for this amount of money should be perfect, but it's too floppy and soft to apply powder well. The same holds true for the **Blush Brush** *($42.50)*, also too floppy and soft for controlled application. The **Brow Brush** *($18.50)* is very stiff and scratchy, and the **Contour Brush** *($29)* and **Eye Shader Brush** *($26)* are both too big for most women's eye area, again making control and placement of color an issue. The rest of the collection is worth a look for some nice additions or extras for your makeup toolkit.

Conditioning Brush Cleanser *($16.50 for 3.4 ounces)* is nothing more than standard, gentle shampoo that will nicely clean your brushes, but it can easily be replaced with much less expensive options from L'Oreal, Johnson & Johnson, or Neutrogena.

<u>SPECIALTY ITEMS:</u> The number of accessories available has grown to the point where they certainly deserve a belated mention. From **Professional Brush Cases** *($27.50–$40)* to **Makeup Palettes** *($22.50–$25)*, a variety of **Makeup Bags** *($30–$75)*, and the well-designed **Beauty Kit** *($67.50)*, there are some valid, somewhat pricey, options for organizing and traveling with your cache of makeup.

BODY & SOUL (MAKEUP ONLY)

Nestled among familiar cosmetic lines such as Shiseido and Christian Dior at Sephora you'll find this comparatively small, but nevertheless complete, makeup collection. Body & Soul's initial lure is its retro 1940s-inspired packaging. The bottles, compacts, and some untraditional containers have an elegant, artful flair that you can almost picture on the vanities of Veronica Lake or Rosalind Russell. The concept behind Body & Soul is "to offer vintage-inspired makeup in modern formulations to put the romance back into beauty." Assuming by romance they mean intimacy with another person, I fail to see how any woman would feel any more romantic using these cosmetics over anyone else's. Feminine or familiar would be better choices, especially for those of you who remember watching your mother or grandmother poised at her vanity, beautifying herself with the magic contents of several attractive bottles and jars. Yet within the black-lacquered compacts adorned with images of classic glamour gals lie some intriguing products to consider. A key strong point for this line is the neutral color palette of its foundations and powders, as well as their blushes (which, fittingly for the era it harkens back to, are called "Rouge"). The lipsticks and brushes are of admirable quality as well, though the prices are certainly present-day dollar amounts!

The main problem with this line is the inclusion of a small amount of sparkly particles in every blush, eyeshadow, and in both powders—even the brow powder. Many of these shades are beautiful and suitable for many skin tones, yet if you're looking for matte finishes, the soft sparkle here is bound to disappoint. However, if you want to step down from "Hey, look at me!" iridescence to a low-key ladylike glimmer, this is a good place to start. And if your first introduction to the world of makeup occurred about the same time *Casablanca* graced the silver screen, this line's accoutrements will no doubt inspire nostalgia!

For more information about Body & Soul, call Sephora at 1-877-737-4672 or visit www.bodyandsoul.com.

☺ $$$ **FOUNDATION:** ✔☺ **Beauty Make-Up** *($35)* is a basic foundation formula that provides a soft and lightly creamy texture and moist application suitable for normal to dry skin. This claims full coverage, but unless you're willing to pile it on, medium coverage is what you'll have to settle for. The seven colors are stunning—the only one to view suspiciously is No. 6, which leans a bit too much toward peach for some medium skin tones. ✔☺ **Two-in-One Face Powder** *($35)* is a standard pressed-powder foundation that has a fine-textured, silky application and light coverage. The talc-based formula is on par with others in its class, such as Lancome's Dual Finish ($31), and the nine shades are exceptional.

☹ **CONCEALER: Cover-Up** *($18)* is a creamy, lipstick-style concealer that really does seem like a 1940s makeup transplant. Concealers have evolved too well since then for it to make sense to consider this retro, slightly greasy, sparse coverage, crease-prone product—though the four shades are very good.

POWDER: ☺ $$$ **Loose Face Powder** *($30)* comes housed in a painted aluminum saltshaker container that Body & Soul claims is "suitable for collecting." The artwork is reminiscent of cocktail party glamour, but is that enough to make you want to hold on to this when it's empty? The talc-based powder has a fluffy, light texture and sheer matte finish that is laced with a tiny amount of sparkly particles. The four shades are neutral and understated, and great for light to medium skin tones. **Perfect Face Powder** *($32)* is also talc-based and shares the same traits as the Loose Face Powder, except that this has a drier finish. The four shades are excellent, and the compact is tailor-made to be noticed as you apply touch-ups in public.

☺ $$$ **Glitz Powder** *($30)* is a light golden tan shimmer powder with a touch of pale pink that creates a soft glow on the skin. It isn't as clingy as many other shiny powders, so flaking can be a problem.

BLUSH: ☺ $$$ **Rouge** *($16.50)* has a cushiony-soft texture and clean, sheer application that is very attractive on skin. This pressed-powder blush comes in a range of tastefully understated colors, each made with the same sparkly bits that show up in the face powders above.

☹ **Cream Rouge** *($28)* is almost double the price of the regular Rouge, yet not nearly half as nice. This is a substandard cream-to-powder blush stick that tends to go on thick and roll off in little pieces as it's blended. Each shade is iridescent, though not distractingly so. **Face Glow** *($28)* is an emollient, gel-textured stick blush that imparts very sheer color and a slightly sticky, glossy finish. This has been done before, and better.

☺ $$$ **EYESHADOW:** Body & Soul's **Eyeshadow** *($16.50)* has a soft, slightly dry texture that tends to go on thick and color-true. It's a bit difficult to blend and soften, so if you decide to try these and want a natural look, begin with as sheer an application as possible. The range of shades is impressive, including some beguiling matte neutrals, though these do have a subtle sprinkling of sparkles.

EYE AND BROW SHAPER: ☹ **Eye Liner** *($16)* is a very standard pencil that applies smoothly but is too soft and creamy to stay put. This pencil includes a built-in sponge tip for smudging, though it will smudge on its own unless it's set with powder eyeshadow.

☺ $$$ **Brow Powder** *($16.50)* is a pressed powder that features four very good colors and a soft, smooth application. Why Body & Soul needed to infuse these otherwise fine powders with sparkles is beyond my comprehension.

☺ $$$ **LIPSTICK AND LIP PENCIL:** **Lipstick** *($18)* comes in a chic, hourglass-shaped aluminum tube and has a texture that is just to the greasy side of creamy. The shade range presents both classic and contemporary colors, and includes some great reds.

☺ $$$ **Lip Glow** *($16.50)* is lip gloss in a pot, and this one has a fine middle-of-the-road texture—it's not too thick and not too sticky. There are some beautiful colors to choose from here, too! **Eternal Lips** *($20)* is a dual-sided lip gloss that shares the same basic formula as the Lip Glow, but you get the convenience of a wand applicator. The color selection and overall finish of the Lip Glow is still more appealing than this gloss, even in its moderne-style package. **Lip Liner** *($16)* is a standard, but good, lip pencil that has a soft texture and relatively tenacious stain. The pencil comes equipped with a lip brush, and again, the color selection is great.

☺ $$$ **MASCARA:** **Mascara** *($18.50)* calls its black shade "Drama" and its brown shade "Mink" and that's about the only unique aspect of this completely lackluster formula. You will be able to build some clump-free length with repeated effort, but nothing that warrants this price.

☺ $$$ <u>BRUSHES:</u> The makeup **Brushes** *($20–$55)* include some great and mediocre options, though even the less-than-impressive brushes still perform nicely. The **Powder Brush** *($55)* and **Blush Brush** *($45)* are well-shaped, but not as soft or dense as they could be, so application isn't as flawless as you would expect at this price. The other five brushes include excellent eyeshadow, liner, and brow brushes. Also available is a **Mini-Brush Set** *($85)* that includes all seven travel-sized makeup brushes and a satin Body & Soul–embossed pouch for storage. If the majority of brushes here appeal to you, this is a worthwhile investment.

☹ $$$ <u>SPECIALTY:</u> **Glitz Moisturizer** *($35)* is a lightweight, overpriced moisturizer that imparts a sheer, golden shimmer on the skin. This seems dated compared to most other shiny lotions, but perhaps that was the intention.

THE BODY SHOP

The Body Shop has been quite a saga over the years, but remains a leader in the boutique-style cosmetics world. From its inception The Body Shop's main goal has been to let you know that they are not only about beauty and natural ingredients but also about saving the environment and ending cruelty to animals. But they are also about shopping and with reasonable prices and tester units open for experimenting, it is an affable environment. There isn't much room to spread out and the mirrors are awkward, but the sales pressure is low-key.

While The Body Shop's political message has remained the same, the product lines have been reinvented over the past two years. The major product overhauls mean you won't find many of the same products still there from just two years ago. If you have not been in one of their stores for awhile, I can almost guarantee you will be bombarded by dozens of new offerings for pampering every inch of your skin and hair. Of course, whenever I see a cosmetics company undertake such a steady, consistent revamping of their product line, I wonder how they go about explaining such obvious changes to customers who all along were under the impression the former products were the very best.

The Body Shop has big plans for global expansion, including increasing the number of stores in the United States from 300 to 1,000 within the next few years, and increasing the number of new stores in the United Kingdom by at least 150 (Source: *The Rose Sheet*, March 4, 2002). This bevy of new product launches (with lots more on the way) is without a doubt a gamble that The Body Shop hopes will pay off, or it will be forced to rethink its product lineup yet again. In the end, the strength of the products and whether or not the consumer spends his or her money on them will decide The Body Shop's fate. For more information about The Body Shop and Colourings, call (800) 541-2535 or visit www.usa.the-body-shop.com. **Note:** All Body Shop skin-care products contain fragrance unless otherwise noted.

THE BODY SHOP SKIN CARE

THE BODY SHOP SKIN DEFENSIVES

The Body Shop's new Skin Defensives line is meant to be amazing for skin because it uses a tidal-zone seaweed known as the Sea Tangle, which survived the catastrophic *Amoco Cadiz* oil spill off the coast of Brittany in France. I suspect that if a plant can make it through an oil spill it must somehow be good for your skin, but exactly how that translates to taking care of skin The Body Shop doesn't explain. I have seen no research anywhere indicating that seaweed of any kind is *the* answer for skin, but even so, in the amounts used in these products, it is barely detectable, much less readily available for helping the skin. Overall, this group of products is lackluster and doesn't add much to The Body Shop's lineup. While I might agree with Anita Roddick (the line's founder) about there being no magical potions for the face, lots of truly great options for skin are still out there and they can make an impressive difference for skin. These just aren't in that category.

☺ $$$ **Skin Defensives Cleansing Face Wash** (*$15 for 3.4 ounces*) is a decent, standard, water-soluble cleanser for normal to dry skin. It does contain fragrance.

☹ $$$ **Skin Defensives Hydrating Freshener** (*$15 for 3.4 ounces*) is a product that needs to find a really good reason why water, propylene glycol, preservatives, fragrance, and the teeniest amount of seaweed possible have any benefit for skin. This one is as disappointing as it gets, with no benefit whatsoever when it comes to taking care of skin.

☹ **Skin Defensives Moisture Cream SPF 10** (*$18 for 1.7 ounces*) has no UVA protection and an SPF 10, and that makes this a rather offensive, as opposed to defensive, product for skin!

☺ **Skin Defensives Night Treatment** (*$20 for 1 ounce*) is standard as far as moisturizers go, although it would be good for dry skin.

☹ $$$ **Skin Defensives Exfoliating Mask** (*$18 for 1.75 ounces*). There is nothing particularly exfoliating about this mask, but the absorbent can be helpful for oily skin, though the product is truly overpriced for what you get.

☹ $$$ **Skin Defensives Intense Moisture Mask** (*$18 for 1.75 ounces*) is a standard clay mask. Clay is not moisturizing in the least, but for a clay mask this is as good as any.

THE BODY SHOP RE-LEAF WITH KINETIN

Both Almay and The Body Shop have launched lines of skin-care products that feature the ingredient kinetin. (The Body Shop's Skin Re-Leaf products are reviewed below.) Almay wants you to believe kinetin will "rejuvenate" your skin and The Body Shop, which has been eschewing claims about antiaging, is promoting their kinetin products as being about overall skin health.

All in all, for skin, kinetin is no more deserving of your attention than any other hyped skin-care ingredient, from vitamin A to beta glucan, vitamin C, niacinamide, copper, coenzyme Q10, mushroom extracts, and on and on. Kinetin definitely has antioxi-dant properties, but whether or not it can stop skin from aging has not been independently demonstrated or verified by published research. For more information about kinetin, refer to Chapter Seven, *Cosmetics Dictionary*.

Please note: All of the following products contain some unknown amount of kine-tin. For the purposes of the review, the comments on kinetin in Chapter Seven, *Cosmetics Dictionary* pertain to all products that contain kinetin. I comment only on the value of the product aside from the kinetin content. Also, The Body Shop's Re-Leaf series all contain spearmint, which can be a skin irritant.

☺ **Skin Re-Leaf Illuminating Face Treatment with Kinetin** *($25 for 1.4 ounces)* contains mostly water, silicone, slip agent, thickeners, plant oil, anti-irritant, emollient, vitamin E, fragrant plant oils, fragrance, and preservatives. This would be a good mois-turizer for someone with normal to dry skin. The spearmint can be a skin irritant.

☺ **Skin Re-Leaf 24-Hour Treatment Lotion with Kinetin** *($25 for 1 ounce)* con-tains mostly water, silicone, slip agent, thickeners, plant oil, anti-irritant, emollient, vitamin E, fragrant plant oils, fragrance, and preservatives. This would be a good, though basic (except for kinetin), moisturizer for someone with normal to dry skin. The spearmint can be a skin irritant.

☺ $$$ **Skin Re-Leaf Daily Eye Treatment with Kinetin** *($20 for 0.4 ounce)* is an OK moisturizer for normal to dry skin. This one does not contain fragrance. It does contain *Paullinia cupana*, an herb that contains two to three times the amount of caffeine normally found in coffee beans. While there are companies that maintain caffeine can brighten the eye area, I've seen no research substantiating this. Meanwhile there *is* evi-dence that caffeine can be a skin irritant.

☺ $$$ **Skin Re-Leaf Illuminating Eye Treatment with Kinetin** *($15 for 0.25 ounce)* is similar to the Daily Eye Treatment above and the same basic comments apply. The illumination in this version is from mica, which adds a teeny amount of pink shine to the skin. Other than that, it adds no benefit over the Daily Eye Treatment above.

☺ **Skin Re-Leaf Protective Hand Treatment with Kinetin** *($15 for 3 ounces)* is a good, though ordinary, moisturizer for dry skin. The spearmint and orange oils in it can be skin irritants. This product claims to be a "water-resistant formula [that] stays on even after washing hands." While I found that to be slightly true, keep in mind that because this product doesn't contain sunscreen it is a poor option for daytime (when you would probably be washing your hands most often).

THE BODY SHOP SKIN ESSENTIALS

The Skin Essentials collection consists of facial products based on chamomile, soy, calendula, or grape seed. Each of these plant ingredients has merit for skin as an antioxi-dant or anti-irritant, which can be great for skin. Unfortunately, these products don't contain much of these ingredients, and most are almost negligible.

☹ **Chamomile Moisturizing Eye Supplement** *($16 for 0.5 ounce)* is a lightweight, silicone-based moisturizer that would have been an OK option for normal to slightly dry skin if witch hazel (which should not go anywhere near the eye area) weren't so prominent on the ingredient list and alcohol weren't lagging very far behind.

☺ **Chamomile Soothing Eye Cream** *($15 for 0.5 ounce)* contains less witch hazel than the Eye Supplement above. This rather light, silky-feeling moisturizer contains mostly water, silicones, glycerin, thickeners, plant oils, mica (adds shine), plant extracts, and preservatives. This lacks any antioxidants or interesting water-binding agents.

☺ **Soy & Calendula Gentle Cleanser, for Dry/Sensitive Skin** *($10 for 6.7 ounces)* is a standard, plant oil–based, cold cream–style cleanser, but it would need the aid of a washcloth to rinse it completely and to take off all your makeup. This would be a good option for dry skin.

☺ **Soy & Calendula Daily Soothing Moisture Cream, for Dry/Sensitive Skin** *($12 for 1.7 ounces)* contains a mere dusting of calendula, as it is listed well after the preservatives. This does feature a good amount of soybean oil, along with standard emollients and thickening agents, plus other dry skin–friendly plant oils and water-binding agents. It is an option for those with normal to dry skin. This does contain fragrance.

☺ **Soy & Calendula Extra Rich Night Cream, for Dry/Sensitive Skin** *($15 for 1.7 ounces)* is almost identical to the Soy & Calendula Daily Soothing Moisture Cream above, except this has a silkier texture courtesy of the silicone it contains as its second ingredient. Otherwise, the same comments apply.

☺ **Soy & Calendula Soothing Supplement, for Dry/Sensitive Skin** *($15 for 1 ounce)* is nearly identical to the Soy & Calendula Daily Soothing Moisture Cream above, except this one has a slightly lighter, more fluid texture. This does contain fragrance. Despite the name this product contains only a minute amount of calendula extract. It does contain fragrance.

✓☺ **Grapeseed Daily Hydrating Moisture Cream, for Normal to Dry Skin** *($12 for 1.7 ounces)* is a very good emollient moisturizer for dry skin, not unlike the Soy & Calendula products above, except that it contains a good amount of grape seed oil that has antioxidant properties and several water-binding agents. This does contain fragrance.

✓☺ **Grapeseed Extra Rich Night Cream, for Normal to Dry Skin** *($15 for 1.7 ounces)* is a very good, silky-textured moisturizer for dry skin that contains mostly water, silicone, grape seed oil, thickeners, slip agent, plant oil, water-binding agents, preservatives, fragrance, and more preservatives.

☺ **Grapeseed Moisture Rescue Supplement, for Normal to Dry Skin** *($15 for 1 ounce)* is similar to, but not as interesting or well-formulated as, the two Grapeseed moisturizers above, which have far more impressive ingredients. This is really a superfluous product whose name makes it sound essential even though it's actually just a basic moisturizer with grape seed oil in disguise as a "treatment" product. It lacks interesting water-binding agents and soothing agents.

THE BODY SHOP TEA TREE COLLECTION

Tea tree oil, also known as melaleuca, has disinfecting properties that have been shown to be helpful for breakouts. According to the *Healthnotes Review of Complementary and Integrative Medicine* (http://www.healthwell.com/healthnotes/Herb/Tea_Tree.cfm) and the *Medical Journal of Australia* (October 1990, pages 455–458), 5% tea tree oil and 2.5% benzoyl peroxide are both effective in reducing the number of blemishes, but the benzoyl peroxide showed significantly better results than the tea tree oil. Skin oiliness was lessened significantly in the benzoyl peroxide group versus the tea tree oil group. However, the tea tree oil had somewhat less irritating side effects. Regrettably, while tea tree oil is an option for treating blemishes, only one of The Body Shop's products claims to contain a 15% concentration, the rest all have less than even a 1% concentration, which means they are unlikely to have any effect on breakouts.

☹ **Tea Tree Oil Soap** *($3.70 for 3.5 ounces)* is a standard soap with a tiny amount of tea tree oil. This can be too drying and irritating and that isn't helpful for blemishes.

☺ **Tea Tree Oil Facial Wash** *($10 for 8.4 ounces)* is a standard, detergent-based, water-soluble cleanser with a small amount of tea tree oil.

☹ **Tea Tree Oil Daily Foaming Facial Wash** *($10 for 5 ounces)* is a standard detergent-based cleanser that contains peppermint oil, which makes it potentially too irritating for all skin types.

☺ **Tea Tree Oil Facial Scrub** *($10 for 3.7 ounces)* is a standard, detergent-based cleanser that is minimally abrasive. It also contains cornstarch, which can be a problem for blemish-prone skin.

☹ **Tea Tree Oil Freshener, for Oily or Blemished Skin** *($10 for 8.4 ounces)* contains a good amount of alcohol, which can cause unnecessary irritation, and that won't help breakouts in the least.

☹ **Tea Tree Oil** *($6 for 0.34 ounce)*. The Body Shop claims this is a 15% concentration of tea tree oil, which would make it more effective for disinfecting blemishes, but the alcohol concentration is far greater than the tea tree oil (which is the second ingredient), and that makes this fairly irritating and drying for all skin types. It is not recommended.

☹ **Tea Tree Oil Blemish Pads** *($8 for 30 pads)* lists the third ingredient as alcohol, which makes it too drying and irritating for all skin types. The amount of tea tree oil is barely detectable.

☹ **Tea Tree Oil Blemish Stick** *($6 for 0.8 ounce)*. Even if the tiny amount of tea tree oil here could help breakouts, the alcohol in this product would just cause irritation and dryness.

☺ **Tea Tree Oil Facial Moisture Concentrate for Oily or Blemished Skin** *($8.50 for 1.7 ounces)* is a very ordinary, silicone-based moisturizer that offers little benefit for any skin type. The tiny amount of tea tree oil in this product is too small for it to work as a disinfectant for breakouts.

☺ **Tea Tree Oil Facial Mask** *($8 for 4.8 ounces)* is a standard clay mask that contains several emollients that would be a problem for someone with blemishes, though it could be an option for someone with dry skin. It does contain a teeny amount of tea tree oil, but not enough to work as a disinfectant for blemishes.

THE BODY SHOP VITAMIN C PRODUCTS

☺ **Vitamin C Hydrating Cleanser** *($14 for 8 ounces)* contains a teeny amount of vitamin C in a cold cream–type, plant oil–based cleanser that needs to be wiped off. It is an option for normal to dry skin, but if you're looking to get vitamin C on your skin, this trace amount isn't the way to do it. It does contain fragrance and citrus oils that can cause skin irritation.

☺ **Vitamin C Energizing Face Spritz** *($8 for 4 ounces)* is a toner that does contain a stable form of vitamin C along with some slip agents and preservatives. It would take a far more interesting mix of ingredients to garner a better rating. However, if all you want is vitamin C, this one will do. It does contain fragrance.

☺ **Vitamin C Intensive Night Repair** *($18 for 1.25 ounces)* is ascorbic acid in a silicone base. Ascorbic acid can be a good antioxidant, but the acid component makes it potentially irritating for skin.

✓☺ **Vitamin C Protective Daywear Moisturizer with SPF 15** *($12 for 2.5 ounces)* is a good, in-part titanium dioxide–based sunscreen that would work well for someone with normal to dry skin. It does contain a small amount of vitamin C and water-binding agents.

✓☺ **Vitamin C Super Charged Serum** *($20 for 1 ounce)* is a good, emollient, silicone-based, serum-style moisturizer that also contains some good antioxidants and water-binding agents. This is a very good option for someone with normal to dry skin.

☹ **Vitamin C Stimulating Mask** *($16 for 2.5 ounces)* could have been a good emollient facial mask for dry skin, but the only thing stimulating in it is the menthol, and that can be a problem for skin.

THE BODY SHOP VITAMIN E PRODUCTS

☹ **Vitamin E Cleansing Bar** *($50 for 3.5 ounces)* is a standard bar cleanser that can be too drying and irritating for all skin types. The amount of vitamin E present is insignificant.

☺ **Vitamin E Cream Cleanser** *($10 for 6.8 ounces)* is a very standard, cold cream–style cleanser that can work well for someone with normal to dry skin. It does contain fragrance and coloring agents and an insignificant amount of vitamin E.

☺ **Vitamin E Face Mist** *($10 for 3.2 ounces)* is a very ordinary toner made of water, slip agent, glycerin, emollient, vitamin E, fragrance, and preservatives.

☺ $$$ **Vitamin E Facial Day Lotion SPF 15** *($12 for 2.5 ounces)* is a very good in-part titanium dioxide–based sunscreen for normal to dry skin. Yet, aside from the sunscreen, this is just a very basic water-and-wax formulation, and the amount of vitamin E is negligible. There are far better and far less expensive sunscreen formulations to consider (with good antioxidants, water-binding agents, and anti-irritants in them, too) than this ho-hum version.

☺ **Vitamin E Illuminating Moisture Cream** *($12 for 1.7 ounces)*. The amount of vitamin E in this cream is hardly worth mentioning and it lacks any state-of-the-art moisturizing ingredients. It is emollient, but very ordinary. The only thing illuminating is the mica that adds shine to the product.

☹ **Vitamin E Moisture Cream** *($12 for 1.8 ounces)* is as dated a formula as you can get in a moisturizer. It contains mostly water, thickeners, lanolin, fragrance, preservatives, and coloring agents.

☺ **Vitamin E Nourishing Night Cream** *($12 for 1.7 ounces)* is an exceedingly mundane formulation for dry skin that contains mostly water, glycerin, plant oil, silicones, thickeners, emollient, vitamin E, preservatives, fragrance, and mica.

☺ **Vitamin E Under Eye Cream** *($12.50 for 0.5 ounce)* is a good emollient moisturizer for normal to dry skin, though there is nothing in this product that makes it preferred for the eye area. This does contain a small amount of shine.

☹ **Vitamin E Lip Care SPF 15** *($4.50 for 0.15 ounce)* does not contain the UVA-protecting ingredients of avobenzone, zinc oxide, or titanium dioxide, and is not recommended.

THE BODY SHOP SUN PRODUCTS

☺ **Aloe & Chamomile Oil Free Face Lotion SPF 25** *($12 for 2.5 ounces)* is a very good, in-part titanium dioxide–based sunscreen in an otherwise standard moisturizing base with a slight matte finish. It would be an option for normal to slightly oily skin.

☺ **Aloe & Chamomile Sun Protection Body Lotion SPF 25** *($15 for 5.7 ounces)* is a very good, in-part titanium dioxide–based sunscreen in an otherwise standard, matte-finish base. It would be an option for normal to dry skin.

☹ **Sesame Oil Sun Protection Body Spray SPF 12** *($15 for 6.7 ounces)* does not contain the UVA-protecting ingredients of titanium dioxide, zinc oxide, or avobenzone, and is not recommended. Moreover, the SPF 12 is below the SPF 15, which is the minimum recommended by the National Cancer Institute.

☺ **Shea Self-Tanning Lotion SPF 15** *($15 for 6 ounces)* is a very good, in-part avobenzone-based sunscreen in an otherwise ordinary moisturizing base for normal to dry skin.

☺ **Shea Sun Protection Facial Stick, SPF 30** *($6.50 for 0.6 ounce)* is a very good in-part zinc oxide–based sunscreen in an otherwise ordinary and greasy lipstick-like formulation.

MISCELLANEOUS BODY SHOP PRODUCTS

☺ **Chamomile Makeup Wipes** *($10 for 30 wipes)* uses standard detergent cleansing agents that make this product almost identical to baby wipes, but you can get baby wipes fragrance-free, and this version contains fragrance.

☺ **Seaweed Purifying Facial Wash, for Normal to Oily Skin** *($10 for 3.4 ounces)* is an extremely basic, detergent-based cleanser that would work well for normal to oily skin.

☺ **Peachy Clean Exfoliating Wash** (*$10 for 3.4 ounces*) uses ground-up peach pits as the abrasive in an otherwise ordinary detergent-based cleanser. It can be an option for someone with normal to oily skin.

☺ **Honey & Oat 3-in-1 Scrub Mask** (*$12 for 3.6 ounces*) is a thick, oat bran–based mask that contains clay and honey along with several emollient thickening agents. This is really an unnecessary product, but it's harmless enough for those with normal to dry skin to consider as a creamy facial scrub. Mixing plain oat bran with your cleanser would have the same effect, and it would be much easier to rinse from the skin. It does contain fragrance.

☺ **Chamomile Eye Make-up Remover, for All Skin Types** (*$12 for 8.4 ounces*) is a standard, detergent-based eye-makeup remover that would work as well as any. This does contain fragrance.

☺ **Chamomile Gentle Eye Makeup Remover Gel** (*$10 for 3.4 ounces*) is a silicone-based eye-makeup remover that can easily remove waterproof makeup without leaving a greasy film behind on the skin.

☺ **Soothing Eye Makeup Remover Gel** (*$10 for 3.38 ounces*) is a silicone-based eye-makeup remover that also contains a small amount of detergent cleanser. It easily removes waterproof makeup without leaving a greasy film behind on the skin.

☺ **Seaweed Purifying Toner** (*$9 for 6.75 ounces*) lacks any helpful or interesting ingredients for the skin, while the witch hazel can be a skin irritant.

☺ **Aloe Vera Daily Soothing Moisture Cream, for Dry/Sensitive Skin** (*$12 for 1.7 ounces*) is an OK moisturizer for dry skin, but overall, quite mundane.

☺ **Carrot Moisture Cream** (*$12 for 1.8 ounces*) contains mostly water, plant oil, thickeners, silicone, preservatives, fragrance, vitamins, and coloring agents. The teeny amounts of carrot oil and vitamins are insignificant.

☹ **Elderflower Eye Gel** (*$8 for 0.5 ounce*) contains witch hazel and alcohol and little else, and it is not recommended for any area of the face.

☺ **Hydrating Moisture Lotion, for Normal to Dry Skin** (*$16 for 3.38 ounces*) is a good emollient moisturizer that contains mostly water, plant oil, thickeners, silicone, water-binding agents, antioxidant, preservatives, and fragrance.

☺ **Seaweed Daily Shine Control** (*$12 for 1.7 ounces*) is just silicone and clay, which won't absorb oil any better than a pressed powder. It does contain menthol and that can be a skin irritant. The teeny amount of seaweed in here barely deserves mentioning.

☺ **Mineral Gentle Exfoliating Mask** (*$12 for 2.5 ounces*) is a standard clay mask that also contains silicone, plant oils, and ground-up rock. That is exfoliating, but it isn't exactly gentle. It can be an option for someone with normal to dry skin, but be careful. It does contain fragrance.

☺ **Natural Oceanic Clay Ionic Mask** (*$17 for 4.2 ounces*) is just clay, preservatives, and fragrance. It doesn't get much more basic than this, though it can be an absorbent for someone with oily skin.

☹ **Warming Mineral Mask, for All Skin Types** *($12 for 5.1 ounces)* includes cinnamon and ginger oil and that can make skin feel warm—but they are also skin irritants. This mask uses a zeolite as the absorbent earth mineral.

😐 **Blue Corn Mask** *($12 for 4.2 ounces)* is a standard clay mask, period. The corn powder can be an absorbent, but it can also be problematic for blemishes. It does contain fragrance.

☺ **Cocoa Butter Lip Care Stick** *($4.50 for 0.15 ounce)* is an excellent emollient lip balm that contains mostly plant oils, emollients, vitamin E, and anti-irritant.

☺ **Facial Blotting Tissues** *($10 for 2 packs, 65 sheets each)* absorb oil and are an option for touch-ups during the day.

😐 **Hemp Facial Moisturizer, for Dry/Very Dry Skin** *($12 for 1.7 ounces)* is an exceptionally standard moisturizer for dry skin.

😐 **Hemp Intense Moisturizing Serum** *($12 for 0.43 ounce)* is just silicones, hemp seed oil, fragrance, and a fractional amount of vitamin E. This is not intense in the least, but it is boring and relatively a waste of time for skin.

😐 **Hemp Lip Conditioner** *($6.50 for 0.12 ounce)* is a standard castor oil– and wax-based lip balm that also contains plant oil. This does contain fragrance.

☺ **Hemp Lip Protector** *($6.50 for 0.30 ounce)* is a good, but basic, lip balm of plant oils, thickeners, lanolin, plant oil, silicones, fragrance, and a teeny amount of antioxidants.

☹ **Speak Out on Family Violence Lip Care Stick SPF 15** *($5 for 0.15 ounce)*. The Body Shop donates $1 from every Lip Care Stick purchased to support the National Domestic Violence Hotline. While that is an admirable cause, this product is not one that will help you in the least. There are no UVA-protecting ingredients of titanium dioxide, zinc oxide, or avobenzone, and it is not recommended. I strongly recommend you donate the $5 you would have spent on this product directly to the cause at http://www.ndvh.org.

THE BODY SHOP MAKEUP

August 2002 saw the reintroduction of The Body Shop's makeup after a brief absence that included selling the last remnants of their former Colourings line at rock-bottom prices. This new collection has sleek, eco-friendly packaging and the new display unit puts testers within easy reach and provides ample lighting, mirrors, and even a bit of counter space. Despite the snazzy window dressing, this color line remains one you may not even want to window shop. It's not that the products are bad—quite the contrary. Although there are some missteps here, I was really hoping that this reincarnation would keep pace with the rest of the cosmetics industry or at least bring back the former glory of Colourings. Instead, The Body Shop makeup is typical of what they offered over the last couple of years, and that isn't exciting in the least. I wouldn't dismiss this line altogether, because there are some excellent, though limited, options for foundations, pencils, improved brushes, and creamy lipsticks. The prices are reasonable, too, but they're no bargain when you discover the average to disappointing performance from the majority of this makeup. If The Body Shop wants to compete with the many superior color products at drugstores and department stores, it needs to put on a far better show than this to earn applause.

FOUNDATION: ☺ Oil-Free Face Base SPF 8 *($15.50)* is a liquid foundation that has a spreadable lotion texture that offers sheer coverage and a natural, slightly moist finish. This formula is best for someone with normal to slightly dry skin. Of the six shades, three should be avoided: 02 (slightly pink), 04 (slightly peach), and 06 (very peach). The SPF of the in-part titanium dioxide–based sunscreen is just too low for significant daytime protection. If you're looking for excellent sun protection from a foundation, consider **Moisture Face Base SPF 15** *($15.50)*, especially if you have normal to dry skin. This in-part zinc oxide–based sunscreen has a thick but remarkably smooth application that has significant slip, but eventually blends to a light coverage, dewy finish. There are nine mostly good shades, including an option for dark skin (shade 14) that doesn't turn ashy. Avoid the too-peach 06 and 08, as well as shade 12. **All in One Face Base** *($15.50)* is a holdover from the Colourings line and remains a standard, but smooth, talc-based powder foundation. This comes in only four shades, which aren't the most neutral around, but it goes on sheer and will work for fair to light skin tones. For best results, use this dry instead of wet. **Skin Re-Leaf Kinetin Tinted Moisturizer** *($18)* has an amazing, almost fluffy cream texture that feels great and blends superbly over normal to dry skin. The three sheer coverage shades are for fair to light skin only, and each has an understated shine and contains a minuscule amount of kinetin.

☺ **Tea Tree Oil Foundation SPF 15** *($15)* has a very light texture that belies the fact that it looks thick in the bottle. If you're looking for a sheer coverage foundation with a slight moist finish and pervasive aroma of tea tree oil, this is it. However, the sunscreen lacks UVA protection and it's only available in three shades, of which Dark is too rose for anyone's skin. The amount of tea tree oil present is not nearly enough to serve as a disinfectant. **Bronze It SPF 8** *($12.50)* is a sheer, shimmer-laden liquid bronzer whose thin consistency can make even blending a challenge, though the tan color is beautiful. With less than 1% titanium dioxide, UVA protection won't be significant, never mind the low SPF number. **Glow Enhancer** *($12.50)* is an "adapter" product meant to be used alone or mixed with one of The Body Shop's foundations. Either way, this liquid shimmer casts an ethereal pink glow that adds lots of shine.

CONCEALER: ☺ **Concealer Pencil** *($9.50)* is a thick, creamy concealer packaged as a thick pencil that needs regular sharpening. This covers well and blends better than you might expect, but it remains creamy and it creases easily. If you're willing to tolerate the cons, it's OK, but avoid shade 05 (too orange).

☹ **Lightening Touch** *($10.50)* is the same shiny, sheer concealer it always has been, and the two pink and peach shades are still available. You will get a little coverage and soft shine, but that's about it.

☺ <u>POWDER:</u> **Loose Face Powder** *($12.50)* is an average talc-based loose powder that isn't as soft as others, but will work well to keep shine to a minimum, and the three colors that are available are fine, but are best for fair to light skin tones. **Brush-On Bronze** *($16.50)* is an old The Body Shop favorite, but I don't understand why these bronze-colored, very shiny powder beads have maintained such an indispensable status in this line. In any event, this is the same as it ever was, and it works well for a sparkling peachy brown "tan." **Tea Tree Pressed Face Powder** *($12)* is a talc-free, magnesium-based powder that has a sheer, dry texture that can look spotty if it's applied with the enclosed sponge. Brush application produces better results from the three attractive shades, but this isn't as elegant as pressed powders from Clinique or Almay, to name just two other lines.

☺ <u>BLUSH:</u> The **Cheek Color** *($10.50)* is a large traditional powder blush, reminiscent of the size and packaging of M.A.C.'s powder blushes. This has a soft texture and dry, but smooth, application that imparts very sheer color. Most of the shades have a touch of shine, but Golden Pink and Walnut are ultra-shiny and are not recommended for daytime.

<u>EYESHADOW:</u> The collection of 25+ ☺ **Eye Colors** *($8.50)* is not much of an improvement over the previous powder eyeshadows, though the flip-cap compact is attractive. All of these shades, even the dark ones, go on smoothly, but they are frustratingly sheer. Talk about subtle color! And these do not build that well, so you're pretty much stuck with no intensity and a light wash of color that stands a good chance of fading. There are a couple of matte options, but shine is the name of the game here. Jane, Physician's Formula, and Prestige have easier-to-work-with, less expensive shadows that show up nicely on the skin.

☹ **Eye Shimmer Adapter** *($8.50)* has a thick, chunky texture that is heavily iridescent and flakes easily. Even if shine is your thing, this is not the way to get it.

<u>EYE AND BROW SHAPER:</u> ☺ **Eye Definer** *($8.50)* is a routine pencil in terms of the inevitable sharpening, but it does glide on and is minimally creamy, which means there's a low risk of smudging or fading. **Brow & Lash Tint** *($10.50)* is not a tint, but rather a standard clear gel that nicely grooms brows and barely enhances lashes. It isn't sticky and feels exceptionally light.

☺ **Brow Definer** *($8.50)* applies easily and imparts soft, powdery color, but it fades quickly and must be sharpened often in order to use it reliably.

☹ **Liquid Eyeliner** *($10.50)* has a lot going for it—an excellent soft, but firm, brush that is adept at drawing a thin, continuous line and a fast-drying formula that minimizes the risk of smearing—yet this eyeliner breaks down easily so it's all for naught.

<u>LIPSTICK AND LIP PENCIL:</u> ☺ **Lip Color** *($10.50)* has a very slick, but lightweight, creamy texture and soft, glossy finish. Many favorite lipstick colors were carried over from the previous The Body Shop products, and all of them provide semi-opaque coverage. A few shades have a sheer finish, but contrary to claims, none of them are matte. **Liquid Lip Color** *($10.50)* sounds like it's one of those lipstick/lip gloss hybrids,

but it's really just a standard wand gloss with some lightly tinted colors and a Clear option. **Lip Shimmer Adapter** *($10.50)* is a slick, opalescent pink lipstick that is short on color but offers plenty of iridescence. **Lip Liner** *($8.50)* is a standard, but quite workable, lip pencil that features some versatile colors. **Lip Care** *($10.50)* is a very ordinary, but nevertheless emollient, lipstick lip balm that has a particularly glossy finish. It will soothe dry skin quite nicely.

☺ **Lip & Cheek Stain** *($10.50)* is an exceptionally sheer gel-based stain that comes in one pink-berry color. This stays sticky on the skin, and is not preferred to similar versions from Origins or BeneFit.

☹ **Lipscuff** *($9.50)* is an abrasive lip exfoliant that wraps walnut shells in a wax-based lipstick formula along with irritants like mint. It will definitely exfoliate chapped lips, but not without considerable irritation.

☺ <u>MASCARA</u>: **Define and Lengthen, Curling Mascara** and **Volumizing Mascara** *(all $10.50)* don't do much of anything when it comes to adding noticeable impact to lashes. They all perform similarly—building minor length without clumps or smearing—but they are some of the most boring mascaras around. The **Waterproof Mascara** *($10.50)* has two things going for it: it's very waterproof and yet it's easy to remove. On the other hand, you could fall asleep while trying to get anywhere with length or thickness.

<u>BRUSHES</u>: The latest version of The Body Shop's ✔☺ **Brushes** *($8.50–$24.50)* is a huge improvement over the threadbare assortment from a few years back. Each brush is synthetic (animal rights activists, take note) and exquisitely soft and beautifully shaped. What's more, each brush is dense enough to hold and deftly apply color. The best ones to consider are the ✔☺ **Face & Body Brush** *($24.50)*, **Blusher Brush** *($22.50)*, **Eyeshadow Blender Brush** *($16.50)*, and, if you're inclined to use one, the **Foundation Brush** *($22.50)*. The ☺ **Brow & Lash Brush** *($8.50)* is functional, but unremarkable, and the ☺ **Lipstick/Concealer Brush** *($12.50)* would be a sure bet if only it came with a cap.

☺ <u>SPECIALTY</u>: **Matt It Face and Lips** *($12.50)* is a basic silicone serum that contains a tiny amount of aloe and chamomile to reinforce The Body Shop's natural persona. This has a silky finish and will allow for smooth application of foundation, but don't count on it to provide significant shine control or to give a creamy lipstick a matte finish. **Facial Blotting Tissues** *($10 for 130 sheets)* are decent oil-absorbing papers available with or without powder. The powdered versions include the **Rose, Pink**, and **Natural**, while the others use wood pulp (paper) and fragrance. The sheets themselves are half the size of those from most other lines, but they do fit nicely into a small evening bag or your pocket.

BONNE BELL (MAKEUP ONLY)

Bonne Bell was one of the first drugstore lines with products aimed specifically at the teen market. The (now discontinued) skin-care line, though minimal, was tightly linked to "will it ruin my date?" acne anxiety, while the makeup sported a decidedly youthful look, from flavored lip glosses to shine-stopping powders. The line has been revamped more than once, and its current collection represents a return to its roots, with the mantra "We Are Girls." Many of the makeup items that had a more "vanilla wrapper" look have been replaced by a group of products with a more upbeat, kid-oriented look called Gear Bonne Bell.

Anyone who has a sweet spot for all manner of flavored lip balms should look no further than this line—the options seem endless, although from my perspective, it's endlessly repetitive! Whether you crave glittery lip balm or cherry cola–flavored gloss, chances are you'll find it here. For more information about Bonne Bell, call (216) 221-0800 or visit www.bonnebell.com.

☺ **Gel Bronze Face and Body Bronzer** *($3.69)* is a lightweight gel formulation that spreads beautifully over the skin and gives it a rather natural-looking, extremely sheer tan appearance. It has no after-feel, so it works great for someone with normal to oily skin who doesn't want a feeling of makeup on the skin. One major drawback of this product is that it tints the skin, which means once in place it doesn't come off until it sloughs off along with your skin cells, and that can look choppy and uneven—but it does last and will not come off on clothing.

☺ <u>CONCEALER:</u> **2X Stick No Shame Concealer** *($3.49)* is a slightly greasy lipstick-style concealer that has a clear core of salicylic acid and tea tree oil, though neither is present in a high enough concentration to have an impact on blemishes. Plus, this wax-based concealer is the last thing you'd want to place over any blemishes, though it works decently over dark circles with minimal risk of creasing. The four shades are quite good, but restricted to lighter skin tones. Medium is too peach for most skins.

<u>POWDER:</u> ☺ **No Shine Pressed Powder with Tea Tree Oil** *($3.89)* is a soft-textured, talc-based powder that contains a minuscule amount of tea tree oil, which basically just adds fragrance. There are four great shades, all best for fair to light skin. **Powder Bronze** *($3.89)* isn't as nice as others in this price range (including Wet 'n' Wild's bronzing powders), but it's nevertheless a consideration. There are two great shades, both with a matte finish and a dry texture, that go on with more intensity than you may think, so be careful.

☹ **Glimmer Dust Loose Shimmer** *($3.69)* is an assortment of very shiny, talc-based loose powders. Brushing on shiny loose powder can still be a messy undertaking. **Cosmic Cheeks Glitter Gel** *($2.89)* is simply flecks of glitter suspended in a gel base. Because of its texture, it doesn't work well over other makeup colors (the gel would smear or rub off the other products), and if you want to apply other products over it, the glitter can chip off. If you want glitter on the face, there are better ways to do it.

<u>EYESHADOW:</u> ☹ **Eye Shades** *($3.49)* are sheer cream-to-powder eyeshadows that produce a moderate amount of shimmer. These have a bit of a slick finish, which can make them crease easily, but if shine is the goal and duration isn't, then these would work. **Eye Fusion** *($3.79)* is a collection of sheer, shimmery liquid-to-powder eyeshadows. These have a sponge tip, which does not facilitate application, and as such they are more bothersome to apply than similar eyeshadows without that feature.

☺ **Powder Pak** *($2.39 for 2 shadows, $2.39 for compact)* are powdery eyeshadows in a small selection of mostly pastel colors that are sold in sets of two. They are extremely sheer, but have a soft, blendable texture. By the way, if you decide to try these, you will need the sold-separately compact.

EYE AND BROW SHAPER: ✔☺ **Eye Definer** *($2.39)* is a small group of standard pencils. Being standard is not equivalent to being bad—quite the contrary; these are an excellent option if you prefer pencils, with a reasonable color selection that covers the basic shades and a bit beyond.

LIPSTICK AND LIP PENCIL: All manner of lip balms and glosses set Bonne Bell apart from the "adult" side of the cosmetics world. Almost every lip product here has some kind of sweet candy- or berry-flavored taste. ☺ **Lip Lix** *($2.39)* are very emollient, greasy lipstick/glosses that are good for dry lips. **Lip Lites** *($3.49)* are greasy glosses in a tube with flavors ranging from raspberry to chocolate mud pie. Avoid the Clear version, which contains spearmint and wild mint oils. **Lip Burst** *($3.49)* is a very sheer, tinted, oily gloss available in various food flavors. **Lip Rush** *($3.89)* is almost identical in every respect to Lip Burst, but is lighter in feel and application. **Flip Gloss** *($3.69)* and **Flip Gloss Shimmer** *($3.69)* are non-sticky sheer glosses in a unique package that allows you to open the cap and draw up the lip color with one stroke. Very clever, but it's still just gloss! **Flip Shades** *($3.49)* have the same clever packaging as the Flip Gloss, but these are sheer, glossy, flavored lipsticks. **Lip Fashion** *($3.79)* is a flavored, very slippery lip gloss packaged with a roller-ball applicator. **Lip Shox** *($3.79)* is a brush-on iridescent glaze that is similar to Lip Fashion, but offers fuller-coverage colors. **Lip Shake** *($3.69)* is swirled, iridescent lip gloss that has a slick and greasy texture and the fruity/dessert flavors that are a staple at Bonne Bell. **Lip Frosting** *($3.09)* is mineral oil–based, frosted and flavored lip gloss in a squeeze tube. For a thicker, but sheer, gloss this is fine. **Lip Smackers** *($1.49–$4.69)* are standard lip balms that will nicely moisturize dry lips while adding flavor and shine. Included in this mix are **Jewel Lips, Cosmic Lips, Original Flavored, Swirl Gloss,** and **Roll-On Shiner.** All in all, the choices are vast and this is clearly a cornerstone of the Bonne Bell line. **Sun Smackers SPF 24** *($1.89 each, $4.39 for 3)* are the basic Lip Smacker formula, but they have no UVA-protecting ingredients, making them a poor choice for sunscreen. **Lix Treme SPF 24** *($2.89)* has an identical formula to the Sun Smackers above, and the same comments apply. **Cool Shine Creme Lipstick** *($4.39)* products are standard sheer lipsticks that feel slightly greasy and have a soft glossy finish. Although the color range is good, each shade is, of course, flavored.

☹ **Smackers Sponge-On Sparkler** *($2.79)* and **Smackers Sponge-On Glitter Gloss** *($3.49)* are very glossy, utterly shiny, and sticky lip glosses. Any of the regular Lip Smackers have a texture preferable to these, and the glitter portion is overkill. **Smackers Sponge-On Layered Cake** *($3.89)* is so contrived and cutesy that I honestly hope this was designed to appeal exclusively to very young girls who will undoubtedly be impressed with this shimmery layer-cake lip gloss that seems more like a toy than makeup.

☺ <u>MASCARA:</u> **Lash Gloss Clear Mascara** *($3.49)* is simply a great bargain if you need a standard, but effective, clear mascara that doubles as brow gel. As mascara this barely does a thing for lashes and is for a "bare minimum" look only. This comes in two tints (lime green and sky blue), which are both so sheer as to be inconsequential.

☹ <u>BRUSHES:</u> **Brush Up Makeup Brush Kit** *($3.49)* is a collection of five utterly childish brushes that can be considered cute and compact, but also impractical and pretty useless, even in a pinch.

BORGHESE

Under the guidance of President and CEO Georgette Mosbacher, Borghese has had a welcome face-lift. According to Mosbacher, "Over the past several months, we've been restructuring and refocusing the company…. We've streamlined the lines, kept the best, and pared the total skincare and cosmetics collections down to what's essential, what's exciting…. We've also recently introduced innovative new skincare products, just right for today's market place. Like Cura C™ Vitamin C Eye Treatment with its revolutionary new texture and anhydrous water-free formula, a legacy treatment that's sure to build on our Cura C™ formulations. And Retin Intensivo Intensive Retinol Treatment, a gentle Vitamin A refinisher that helps smooth wrinkles." Mosbacher might be a great business-woman, but she should have done more research into exactly what is best in the world of skin care. While some of these products dazzle, the sunscreens are abysmal (they lack UVA-protecting ingredients); the cleansers and toners are lackluster; there are no products for blemish-prone skin; and the vitamin C products contain only vitamin C, while the skin needs a wider blend of ingredients that complement its structure. Where the line excels is with their moisturizers, which are replete with quality antioxidants and water-binding agents. With a little more work this could be an impressive line. Whether or not Borghese's new footing can get this struggling company back as a player in the cosmetics world is yet to be seen. For more information about Borghese, call (866) BORGHESE or visit www.borghesecosmetics.com. **Note:** All Borghese products contain fragrance unless otherwise noted.

BORGHESE SKIN CARE

☺ $$$ **Crema Saponetta Cleansing Creme** *($30 for 7 ounces)* is an extremely standard, detergent-based cleanser that is fairly alkaline and, therefore, drying and irritating for skin. It does contain some good water-binding agents that can help mitigate the irritation, but not by much because they are present in such a tiny amount.

☺ $$$ **Fango Effetto Immediato Spa Comforting Cleanser** *($29.50 for 8.4 ounces)* is a standard cleansing lotion that contains a small amount of detergent cleansing agents. This would work well for someone with normal to dry skin. The water-binding agents are nice, but their benefit for skin would be washed down the drain or wiped away.

☹ **Esfoliante Delicato Gentle Cleanser Exfoliant** *($24.50 for 2.6 ounces)* uses sodium lauryl sulfate as the main cleansing agent and it also contains peppermint and cypress oil, all of which make it too drying and irritating for all skin types.

☹ **Fango Active Mud Soap** *($19.50 for 5.3 ounces)* is a very standard, tallow-based soap that contains a good deal of fragrance, peppermint, and menthol, which makes this too irritating for all skin types.

☺ $$$ **Gel Delicato Gentle Makeup Remover** *($29.50 for 8.4 ounces)* is a very standard, detergent-based, wipe-off makeup remover that would work as well as any.

☺ $$$ **Effetto Immediato Spa Soothing Tonic** *($26.50 for 8.4 ounces)*, with PVP (a film-forming agent) as the third ingredient, has a bit of a sticky application. It also contains some irritating plant extracts. This isn't terrible, but it isn't soothing either. The water-binding agents are very good, but the other problems are hard to ignore.

☹ **Tonico Minerale Stimulating Tonic** *($27.50 for 8.4 ounces)*. Alcohol is the second ingredient, which makes this tonic stimulating to the point of being irritating and drying for all skin types.

✓☺ $$$ **Advanced Spa Lift for Eyes** *($45 for 1 ounce)* is an excellent lightweight moisturizer for any part of the face. It is silicone-based and has an impressive group of antioxidants, water-binding agents, and anti-irritants. It does contain mica, which gives this a slight shine. Reality check: this product won't lift the skin anywhere.

☹ **Botanico Eye Compresses** *($47.50 for 60 pads)*. Witch hazel (that has an alcohol base) is listed as the second ingredient, which means that this can be a skin irritant with repeated use. That's a shame because this product contains some good water-binding agents that would have made it a good lightweight moisturizer.

☺ $$$ **Cura-C Anhydrous Vitamin C Treatment** *($65 for 1.7 ounces)* is just silicone, Vaseline, ascorbic acid, and fragrance. Ascorbic acid is a good form of vitamin C, but it can be irritating. Further, the skin needs more than just vitamin C—there are many elements that help to keep it healthy and functioning optimally. This is a one-note product and for this kind of money your skin deserves an aria.

☺ $$$ **Cura C Vitamin C Eye Treatment** *($42.50 for 0.5 ounce)* contains a form of vitamin C that is less irritating than, though just as effective as, the vitamin C in the Anhydrous version above. The same basic comments about the skin needing a wider array of ingredients pertain to this one as well. This is fragrance-free.

☺ $$$ **CuraForte Moisture Intensifier** *($65 for 1.7 ounces)* contains peppermint oil, which is a skin irritant and has no place in a moisturizer, or in any skin-care product for that matter.

✓☺ $$$ **Cura Notte Night Therapy, for Normal to Dry Skin** *($43.50 for 1.7 ounces)* is an excellent mix of antioxidants, water-binding agents, plant oils, and anti-irritants in an emollient base that would work well for dry skin. This does contain a tiny amount of peppermint oil, but most likely not enough to cause a problem for skin. It also contains a small amount of salicylic acid, but the pH of this product isn't low enough for it to be effective as an exfoliant.

✔☺ **$$$ Cura Notte Night Therapy, for Normal to Oily Skin** *($43.50 for 1.7 ounces)* is similar to the Normal to Dry Skin version above only this one leaves out the emollient thickening agents. That does make it lightweight and better for slightly dry skin (you don't need to apply a moisturizer over oily areas). The comments for the Normal to Dry Skin version above apply to this one as well.

☹ **Cura Vitale Time-Defying Moisturizer, for Normal-to-Dry Skin, SPF 8** *($42.50 for 1.7 ounces)* does not contain the UVA-protecting ingredients of avobenzone, zinc oxide, or titanium dioxide, and the SPF 8 is far below the standard of SPF 15 set by the National Cancer Institute and the American Academy of Dermatology. This is not recommended.

☹ **Cura di Vita Protettivo Protective Moisturizer, SPF 15** *($42.50 for 1.7 ounces)* does not contain the UVA-protecting ingredients of avobenzone, zinc oxide, or titanium dioxide, and is not recommended.

✔☺ **$$$ Dolce Notte ReEnergizing Night Creme** *($50 for 1.85 ounces)* is a very good emollient cream that contains a good amount of antioxidants and water-binding agents.

✔☺ **$$$ Energia Skin Recovery Creme** *($49.50 for 1.7 ounces)* is a very good emollient cream that contains a good amount of antioxidants and water-binding agents. It would be an excellent option for someone with normal to dry skin. The sugarcane in this product cannot function like an AHA and the bilberry extract cannot inhibit melanin production.

✔☺ **$$$ Equilibrio Equalizing Restorative** *($42.50 for 1.7 ounces)* is similar to the Energia Creme above, but has a more matte finish. It is a better option for normal to slightly dry or combination skin.

☺ **$$$ Fluido Protettivo Advanced Spa Lift for Eyes** *($45 for 1 ounce)* is a very good emollient cream that contains a good amount of antioxidants and water-binding agents.

☺ **Hydra-Puro Moisture Renewing Oil Free Fluid** *($35 for 1.7 ounces)* is a very good gel/lotion that contains a good amount of antioxidants and water-binding agents. It would be an excellent option for someone with normal to slightly dry skin.

☹ **Spa Solaire Self Tanning Face Creme SPF 15** *($23.50 for 1.7 ounces)* does not contain the UVA-protecting ingredients of avobenzone, zinc oxide, or titanium dioxide, and is not recommended.

☹ **Spa Solaire Self Tanning Body Creme SPF 15** *($25 for 5 ounces)* does not contain the UVA-protecting ingredients of avobenzone, zinc oxide, or titanium dioxide, and is not recommended.

☺ **Fango Active Mud for Face and Body** *($30 for 7 ounces)* is an extremely standard clay mask that contains bentonite and coloring agents as the primary ingredients. This would work as well as any clay mask. The amount of water-binding agents and antioxidants is so minimal as to be barely present.

BORGHESE MAKEUP

I have a feeling that those behind the reemergence of Borghese's makeup followed the expression "if it ain't broke, don't fix it" as their guiding principle. Most of the comprehensive (but not overwhelming) makeup collection is the same as it was when I last reviewed this line in 1998. One of the positive changes is that the foundations no longer all have the same name; yet, although the textures have improved, every single shade of Borghese makeup has a subtle shine. It is most pronounced in the liquid foundations and less obvious in their powder and liquid-to-powder formulas, but still visible. This is disconcerting, especially since there are some viable shades (especially for dark skin) and excellent textures among the four foundations. Unfortunately, the shine doesn't stop there. The loose and pressed powders, both bronzers, the cream-to-powder blush, and eyeshadow trios are all inherently iridescent—and not in the underplayed, subtle glow way that many other shiny products have. If you have any amount of wrinkling, crepey skin, or less-than-smooth skin texture, all of this shine will only magnify it.

So what's worth shopping for within the Borghese makeup line? Within the accessible, well-organized tester unit, you will find their pencils to be ordinary, but effective; the Brow Milano is still exceptional; and the lipsticks are supremely creamy and richly pigmented. The mascaras have potential, but both also have significant drawbacks that keep them from being superior. Although there are some reputable products, the rather high prices should give you pause before you reach for your credit card.

FOUNDATION: ☺ $$$ **Hydro-Minerali Crème Makeup** *($32.50)* has a luscious light texture that blends beautifully and affords a natural, slightly creamy finish with sheer to light coverage. All of the 13 shades have a soft but noticeable shine, but if that doesn't bother you there are some excellent options for light and dark skin. The following shades are too pink, rose, or peach: No. 2.5 Rose, No. 3 Biscotto, No. 4 Principessa Beige, No. 5 Caramello, No. 7 Sienna, and No. 9 Caffe (slight rose). This formula is best for normal to dry skin. **Hydro-Minerali Natural Makeup** *($31.50)* is similar to the Crème Makeup above, but this has a lighter, fluid texture. You will still achieve a natural, slightly moist finish, but this one does provide a touch more coverage. Each of the 13 shades has a soft but noticeable shine, and the best ones to consider are No. 1 Alabastro, No. 1.5 Lino, No. 2 Latte, No. 8 Amaretto, and, for darker skin, No. 9 Caffe and No. 11 Espresso. No. 10 Terra is OK, but may turn red on dark skin. The shades to avoid are the same as the Crème Makeup above, with the exception of No. 9 Caffe. **Molto Bella Makeup SPF 8** *($35)* is a compact liquid-to-powder makeup that has an initially slick, almost greasy texture that quickly dries to a light matte finish. This blends superbly and provides light to medium coverage. The meager SPF provides inadequate UVA protection, so you will need a separate sunscreen. Otherwise, this is ideal for those with normal to oily skin. Each of the six shades is shiny, though it's a low-key shine. Three shades are too peach or rose for most skin tones: Neutrale 2, Neutrale 3, and Neutrale 4. Oro 3 is slightly peach, but may work for some medium skin tones. For a similar makeup with truly neutral shades, consider Stila Sport Pivotal Skin Foundation ($25).

☺ $$$ **Hydro Minerali Dual Effetto Powder Makeup SPF 8** *($28.50)* is talc-based and contains zinc oxide and titanium dioxide as the sunscreen ingredients, but the SPF misses the mark. Still, this can work nicely for added sun protection over a regular sun-screen or foundation with sunscreen. Given that plus, I wish the texture and application were better. This provides decent coverage, but is too dry and looks that way on the skin. The ten shades all have shine, so this isn't the best choice for oily skin. The dark shades (Sienna, Caffe, Terra, and Espresso) are lovely, but almost all of the others are too peach. No. 2 Latte and No. 4 Principessa Beige are OK, but all in all this can't compete with the fabulous powder foundations from Chanel, Estee Lauder, and Lancome. **Prima Visa** *($25)* is a thick, silicone-based makeup primer that has a finish that is more moist than dry, which is uncharacteristic for this type of product. This works well as a silky finish mois-turizer, but is not essential for getting makeup to last.

⊗ <u>**CONCEALER:**</u> **Impeccabile/Absolute Concealer** *($25)* has a great smooth tex-ture and is easy to blend, but the two colors give you a choice of pink or peachy pink, and that has me seeing red. There are far better concealer shades at the drugstore or depart-ment store.

<u>**POWDER:**</u> ⊗ **Powder Milano Loose Powder** *($38.50)* has a fine texture, but it's exceedingly shiny and each of the three shades leaves a white cast on the skin. This lists titanium dioxide as an active ingredient, but no SPF is indicated—so it cannot be relied on for sun protection. Titanium dioxide is also listed as an active ingredient (sans any SPF number) for the ☺ $$$ **Powder Milano Pressed Powder** *($30)*, which has a sublime texture and two shiny, but good, talc-based colors. With less obvious shine, this would certainly earn a happy face. **Milano Multi-Bronzer** *($29)* offers three colors (sandy pink, tan, and bronze) in one compact. The effect of combining these shades is attractive, but the shine is too strong for it to look natural.

⊗ **Powder Milano Bronzer** *($30)* is a very shiny pressed bronzing powder whose color is too orange to look convincing on most skin tones.

☺ $$$ <u>**BLUSH:**</u> **Blush Milano** *($29)* isn't the same satin-smooth blush I remember. This has taken on more of a waxy texture that nevertheless allows for a smooth, sheer application of blush. The color selection features a good balance of vivids and neutrals, though each shade is shiny. The worst offenders in regard to shine are Puccini Rosegold and Pisa Rosewood. **Milano Illuminare Cheek Color Duo** *($29)* is a cream-to-powder blush and iridescent highlighter in one compact. The blush portion comes in attractive colors, but stays slick on the skin (so it doesn't stay in place), while the highlighter is just shiny with a capital "S." This may be an evening-look option for those with normal to dry skin.

☺ $$$ <u>**EYESHADOW:**</u> **Shadow Milano Trios** *($32)* have the same texture, applica-tion, and sheer qualities as the Blush Milano above. Although there are some great color combinations available, every shade in each trio is too shiny. These aren't worth consider-ing unless you have perfectly taut, unlined eyelids. **Eye Shadow Base** *($16.50)* is essentially a matte finish concealer masquerading as a specialty product. This is only available in one light shade, and works well, but a concealer provides needed coverage and this does not.

<u>EYE AND BROW SHAPER:</u> ☺ $$$ **Eye Accento Pencil** *($18.50)* is a nice, but standard, pencil that features a sponge tip on one end for softening the line. This is less creamy than others are, and therefore less prone to smear. Avoid the plum (purple), navy, and green hues. ✓☺ **Brow Milano** *($20)* is an excellent tinted brow gel that has a terrific brush that allows you to reach every hair. There are only two shades (one for blondes and one for brunettes), but they're both great.

☺ $$$ **Linea Perfetta Brow Pencil** *($18.50)* is a very standard, stiff-textured, hard brow pencil. It works, but you'll get little payoff for the effort.

<u>LIPSTICK AND LIP PENCIL:</u> ✓☺ $$$ **B-Moisture Lipcolour** *($23)* has a strange name. I've heard of B-movies (where would Jayne Mansfield have been without them?), but what are we supposed to think of a "B-Lipstick"? Luckily, this creamy, opaque lipstick makes it to the A-list with its smooth texture and first-rate colors, including some exquisite reds and corals. ✓☺ **Lip Treatment Moisturizer with SPF 15** *($18.50)* is a great find! This has an in-part titanium dioxide–based sunscreen and a slick texture that imparts sheer, iridescent color. Naturale has no color, but it would work well on its own as a lip sunscreen.

☺ $$$ **Perfetta Lip Pencil** *($18)* is, aside from the Italian name, the same basic pencil you'll find for less in dozens of other lines. The small color selection is well-edited.

☹ **B-Gloss** *($17)* is a standard wand lip gloss with a thick, sticky texture. This is unimpressive all around, especially given the price.

<u>MASCARA:</u> ☺ $$$ **Superiore State-of-the-Art Mascara** *($17.50)* takes some serious effort to build satisfactory length and minimal to no thickness, and there will be a few minor clumps along the way. It's not terrible, but is hardly worth this price.

☹ **Superiore State-of-the-Art Mascara, Waterproof** *($17.50)* is an incredible mascara when it comes to lengthening and thickening with ease and without a clump or flake in sight. Yet it fails miserably as waterproof mascara, especially if you want to take a swim or get stuck in a downpour. If you don't intend to use this for its waterproof claim, it earns a happy face.

BURT'S BEES

Almost all the skin-care lines in the world prefer to identify themselves as companies established to create elegant, scientific formulations conceived with an in-depth understanding of the skin's functions and needs. I say almost, because Burt's Bees makes no such claim. Quite the contrary; this line is about as unglamorous and as unscientific as it gets (the picture of Burt on the label made me think I was buying fishing gear). Talk about being an iconoclast!

This is how the company describes its history on its Web site: "I guess you could say it all started because there weren't many jobs up there north of Bangor. Though we found, grew, or traded for most of what we needed, I figure a person's got to have at least 3,000 dollars a year in actual greenbacks to survive in this old world, especially if you've got kids. I'd been let go from my last three part-time waitressing jobs at Dottie's…. Burt was enjoying similar commercial success selling quarts of honey off the tailgate of his Datsun pick-up…. By the end of summer we got around to the heart of the matter, which was the beeswax. Well, how we got started making lip balm … is another story…." This is a skin-care line?

Aside from its humble, amorphous beginning, Burt's Bees is about natural, earth-friendly skin-care products, as well as overly fragranced products. Its philosophy in this respect is fetching and sincere: "We believe that Mother Nature has the answers and She teaches by example [I know they don't mean tornados or earthquakes, right?]. Our ingredients are the best that Mother Nature has to offer."

For those seeking a line of skin-care products with truly natural ingredients, this line is one of the few that steadfastly adheres to its commitment; there is no hypocrisy here. If the ingredient lists are accurate, and there is no reason to assume otherwise, then you will not find preservatives or synthetically derived ingredients of any kind. Just from the all-natural point of view, there will definitely be people who will be excited about these products, but I'm not one of them. Many of the plant extracts and oils used in these products, including orange oil, cinnamon oil, clove oil, lemon oil, orange peel, eucalyptus oil, pine tar, alcohol, lime oil, and balsam peru, are problematic for skin and present a significant risk of irritation or a sensitizing reaction. Ouch! Plus you can't rely on this line for all your skin-care needs because there are no sunscreens of any kind, no products for oily skin, and definitely none for blemish-prone skin. Both the intriguing philosophy and inexpensive products are attractive, but it takes more than that to establish reliable products that are good for skin.

I know that most people are attracted by fragrance and in this regard these products excel. They are also notable for the lack of preservatives, which can be beneficial for those who can't tolerate preservatives. (That lack may be an issue for product stability, although I did not have these products tested for contamination.) But for any other skin-care need, I suggest you use your wisdom and recognize that while Mother Nature is assuredly wise about the Earth, *She* does not have everything the skin needs. In fact, Mother Nature offers up many problematic things for skin, including the sun and poison ivy. For more information about Burt's Bees, call (800) 849-7112 or visit www.burtsbees.com.

BURT'S BEES SKIN CARE

☹ **Bay Rum Exfoliating Soap** *($5 for a 3.25-ounce bar)* is much like all the soaps in this line; its alkaline base with a pH of over 10 makes it very drying and irritating. To make matters worse, this product contains orange, cinnamon, clove, and lemon oils. It smells nice, but for skin it is problematic.

☹ **Burt's Beeswax and Honey Face Soap** *($5 for a 1.9-ounce bar)* doesn't contain the irritating extracts of the Bay Rum soap, but there is still an unspecified wafting fragrance and the pH is still over 10, which makes it very drying and irritating for skin.

☹ **Farmer's Friend Gardener's Soap** (*$5 for a 5.25-ounce bar*) has an alkaline base with a pH of over 10 and it contains eucalyptus oil, which makes it drying and potentially irritating for skin.

☺ **Farmer's Market Orange Essence Cleansing Creme** (*$9 for 4 ounces*) is a fairly standard cold cream, with plant oils, lanolin, and plant extracts. It is still highly fragrant, but for a cold cream it's just fine. It can leave a greasy film behind on the skin.

☹ **Ocean Potion Detox Soap** (*$5 for a 3.5-ounce bar*) is just soap with a pH over 10, which makes it drying and irritating for all skin types. The spruce oil and fir needle oil do make it smell nice. They can't "detox" anything, but they can cause skin sensitivity.

☺ **Farmer's Market Citrus Facial Scrub** (*$7 for 2 ounces*). You would be far better off just buying some ground-up almonds and using that rather than risking the irritation from the orange peel, orange oil, and clove powder this product contains.

☹ **Burt's Complexion Mist, Chamomile** (*$6 for 4 ounces*) is just water and fragrant plant oils. You might as well put perfume on your face.

☹ **Burt's Complexion Mist, Grapefruit** (*$6 for 4 ounces*) is similar to the Chamomile version above, except that this one uses lime, lemon, and grapefruit oils, which are all potential skin irritants.

☹ **Burt's Complexion Mist, Lavender** (*$6 for 4 ounces*) is just water and fragrant plant oils, and the lavender oil is a photosensitizer.

☹ **Farmer's Market Complexion Mist with Carrot Seed Oil** (*$7 for 4 ounces*) is similar to the Chamomile version above and the same comments apply.

☹ **Garden Tomato Toner** (*$9 for 8 ounces*) lists alcohol as the second ingredient, which makes it too irritating for all skin types.

☺ **Baby Bees Skin Creme** (*$11 for 2 ounces*). The clay in this product can be drying and sort of negates the emollients. This is a bit of a confused product that may be problematic for dry skin, but it is completely inappropriate for combination or oily skin.

☺ **Burt's Beeswax Moisturizing Creme** (*$12 for 2 ounces*) is similar to the Skin Creme above and the same comments apply.

☺ **Burt's Jasmine Decollete Creme** (*$18 for 3.5 ounces*) contains nothing special for the neck area. This is similar to the Skin Creme above and the same comments apply. This one does contain a teeny amount of royal jelly, but I have yet to see research of any kind indicating that it is somehow a preferred skin-care ingredient. It is a good water-binding agent, but that's about it.

☺ **Farmer's Market Carrot Nutritive Creme** (*$10 for 1 ounce*) is a very good, basic moisturizer for dry skin.

☺ **Burt's Beeswax & Bee Pollen Night Creme** (*$8.50 for 0.5 ounce*) is a very good, basic moisturizer for dry skin. There is no research to show that bee pollen, especially in meager amounts, has any benefit for skin.

☺ **$$$ Burt's Beeswax & Royal Jelly Eye Creme** (*$11 for 0.25 ounce*). There's clay in this one, but it's present in such a tiny amount that it won't have much, if any, effect on

The Reviews B

skin. Still, it seems strange to put such a drying ingredient in a moisturizer. Aside from that, this is fairly emollient and quite ordinary, though it can be OK for normal to dry skin.

☺ **Wise Woman Comfrey Comfort Salve** *($4 for 0.6 ounce)* is a very emollient, though standard, moisturizer that would be OK for very dry skin. What would really be wise is if one of Burt's products contained a sunscreen with UVA-protecting ingredients.

☺ **Marshmallow Vanishing Crème** *($9.99 for 1.5 ounces)* is very good emollient moisturizer that contains mostly plant oils, thickeners, emollients, antioxidants, and a small amount of water-binding agents.

☹ **Parsley Blemish Stick with Willowbark** *($6.99 for 0.3 ounce).* The first ingredient is alcohol, and if that wasn't bad enough it also contains lemon oil and eucalyptus. The claim that this will normalize skin is disingenuous, as you are much more likely to end up with red, irritated dry skin after using this.

☹ **Herbal Blemish Stick** *($6.99 for 0.3 ounce)* is almost identical to the Parsley version above and the same comments apply.

☹ **Pore Refining Mask** *($5.99 for 1.8 ounces)* contains an assortment of irritating plant extracts inclusing peppermint, comfrey, and eucalyptus! What a terrible product!

☹ **Burt's Beeswax Lip Balm, Lifeguard's Choice** *($2.50 for 0.15 ounce)* has no sunscreen, and without that there is nothing about this appropriate for daytime, much less for use at the beach! It also contains peppermint oil, which can be irritating and drying for the lips in the long run.

☹ **Burt's Beeswax Lip Balm** *($2.50 for a tin or tube)* is almost identical to the version above and the same comments apply.

☺ **Wings of Love Powdered Facial Tissue** *($3 for 65 sheets)* are small pieces of rice paper dusted with cornstarch. This is an option for absorbing oil during the day, but depending on how oily your skin is, these can set down uneven splotches of powder on the face. And though cornstarch is very absorbent and drying, it can also be problematic for breakouts. For those who prefer this way of taking care of shine during the day, these are an option, and they are far cheaper than those sold by Shiseido at three times the price.

BURT'S BEES MAKEUP

Burt has kept his bees busy in the makeup department as well. Although the collection, called Wings of Love, isn't plentiful, there are some flattering colors. Yet, unless you're adamant about using makeup that is as close to 100% natural as you can get, there is little reason to choose this makeup over the far more elegant (and far less irritating) cosmetics from almost every major brand. The majority of Burt's Bees makeup is based on plant oils or nut oils and on beeswax, which means its use is limited to those with dry skin. However, just about all of the cosmetics contain one or more irritating essential oils, with the most notable offender being the All-Natural Lipstick, which contains a significant amount of peppermint oil. The allure of pure, natural products is assuredly a strong pull for many women—yet their use should not come at the expense of causing unnecessary irritation. If you still want to stick your hand into the beehive, beware that none of the color representations on the packaging match the actual color of the product when used on skin.

☺ **FOUNDATION: Tinted Facial Moisturizer** *($11)* comes in a squeeze tube and is as thick as toothpaste, but once you begin blending this it turns into a soft, moist emulsion that smooths over the skin with ease. True to its name, this provides a sheer tint of color and the emollient, oil-based formula is best for dry to very dry skin. Of the four shades, only Ethnic is suspect as being too coppery for dark skin tones. The rest of the colors are fine, though this does have a very strong fragrance.

☹ **CONCEALER: Concealing Crème** *($9)* is honestly 100% natural, but I doubt that will be much consolation if you attempt to use this very thick, greasy concealer that loses even more points because it offers such transparent and short-lived coverage.

☹ **POWDER: Loose Powder** *($16)* is a talc-free loose powder. This has a slightly thick texture and a much drier finish than most other powders because it also contains calcium carbonate (chalk) and clay. Even very oily skin won't want to put up with this powder's unpleasant texture.

☺ **BLUSH: Blushing Creme** *($9)* is for dry skin only, and only then if you don't mind putting up with an almost-too-greasy texture and extraordinarily sheer color. Speaking of color—the only non-iridescent shade available is Clarity. The other shades offer minimal color and maximum shine.

LIPSTICK AND LIP PENCIL: ☹ **All-Natural Lipstick** *($9.50)* has a soft, slightly greasy texture and offers a selection of pretty, medium-coverage colors. Unfortunately, the formula contains enough peppermint oil to cause a tingling, burning sensation as soon as it's applied. **Lip Shimmer** *($6.50)* is heavy on the iridescence and, just like the Lipstick, is hindered by the inclusion of peppermint oil.

☺ **Lip Pencils** *($9)* are standard pencils that go on quite creamy, so don't expect this to be a strong barrier to prevent lipstick from feathering. These also contain peppermint oil, but not nearly as much as the Lipstick and Lip Shimmer products above.

CALVIN KLEIN

Calvin Klein's re-emergence onto the cosmetics scene in 1999 was a pleasant surprise for me, since I am probably one of the few makeup artists who remember that Klein launched a color line back in the late 1970s. In fact, his was the first department-store makeup line I worked for—and what a line it was, with a stellar collection of neutral matte eyeshadows and blushes. Few other lines were dabbling in such practical colors, and women at that time seemed content to spend their cosmetic dollars on varying shades of blue, green, violet, and pink eyeshadows, and that spelled certain doom for the Calvin Klein color line, which primarily espoused neutral taupes, tans, and browns as the way to color and shade your features. Although Klein's original line was shelved shortly after being launched, almost two decades later Klein made a second attempt to establish a makeup (plus skin-care) line. However, it looks as though the second time around isn't turning out much differently from the first. This skin-care and cosmetics collection used to be readily available in Nordstrom and other department stores, but it's now sold almost exclusively online. Only two Nordstrom stores in the United States carry the line, along with a handful of Sephora stores.

Still, thanks to its availability on Sephora.com, including the Calvin Klein products in this book is warranted, and I can't deny my nostalgia for Calvin Klein's makeup. Although it's not the same straightforward, simple line I remember, there are enough positives to make it worthwhile, particularly the concealers, blushes, lipsticks, and foundation shades.

What's difficult to explain is why this enticing line was largely ignored by department-store cosmetics shoppers. It certainly has enough shiny, trendy products to keep makeup mavens busy, and the Klein name is practically synonymous with understated, modern, and casual American elegance. I suspect the oversaturation of designer makeup lines was responsible for Klein's exodus from department stores, just as it was for Tommy Hilfiger's now-defunct makeup line. Perhaps the lesson here is that having an established brand name is not always the hot ticket it seems to be. Inevitably, the more different industries a brand tries to tap into, the higher its chances of getting a cold shoulder from overwhelmed consumers. Even if Calvin Klein's cosmetics line becomes a distant memory (again), his formidable fashion, textile, fragrance, and accessories dominion will be more than enough consolation. For more information about Calvin Klein, call (800) 715-4023 or visit www.sephora.com.

CALVIN KLEIN SKIN CARE

☺ **Balancing Milk Cleanser** *($20 for 6 ounces)* is just a standard creamy cleanser that can leave a slightly emollient feel on skin, which can work well for someone with normal to dry skin, but you would need a washcloth to remove makeup effectively. It contains a mix of plant extracts that are both irritants and anti-irritants, so they cancel each other out.

☹ **Toning Gel Cleanser** *($20 for 6 ounces)* is a standard, detergent-based, water-soluble cleanser that contains both arnica and eucalyptus, which are irritants for skin, and this is not recommended.

☺ $$$ **Micro-Exfoliator** *($22 for 4 ounces).* The buzz on this product is that it contains the same gritty substance used in microdermabrasion machines. Well, it does, but that can be problematic for skin when used on a regular basis because it is so rough on skin (microdermabrasion is done once every other month). It's especially not a good idea for someone with normal to dry or sensitive skin.

☺ $$$ **Makeup Remover** *($16 for 4 ounces)* is as standard a detergent-based makeup remover as it gets. It will work as well as any.

☺ $$$ **Protective Moisture Cream SPF 15** *($30 for 1.7 ounces)* is an overpriced, but good, avobenzone-based moisturizer. It would work well for dry skin, but there is no reason to consider this formulation over other far less expensive avobenzone-based sunscreens. The tiny amount of arnica in this is probably not a problem for skin.

☺ $$$ **Protective Moisture Lotion SPF 15** *($30 for 1.7 ounces)* is a good, in-part avobenzone-based sunscreen. The price is absurd for what you get, which is just sunscreen in a lightweight, standard moisturizing formula, but this silicone-based sunscreen would still be an option for most skin types, although not for someone with dry skin. The tiny amount of arnica is probably not a problem for skin.

☺ $$$ **Oil Control Hydrator** *($30 for 1.7 ounces)* is a standard, silicone-based gel that has a light matte feel (it contains nylon-12, a good absorbent), though it won't control oily skin. It is more just a good lightweight moisturizer for normal to slightly oily skin, leaving it feeling soft and smooth. The tiny amount of arnica is probably not a problem for skin.

CALVIN KLEIN MAKEUP

FOUNDATION: ✓☺ $$$ **Sheer Coverage Foundation SPF 20** *($29)* has an excellent SPF 20 with avobenzone as part of its active sunscreen ingredients, so it does have sufficient UVA protection. That can be good news for someone with oily skin, though the formulation isn't all that matte. The name is actually quite accurate—this is a very sheer foundation that would be excellent as a moisturizing tint with sunscreen for those with normal to dry skin. If you have problems with titanium dioxide as a sunscreen ingredient and want to get sunscreen in your foundation, this is one to try. The eight shades are beautifully neutral, though Walnut is slightly orange for dark skin.

☺ $$$ **Light Coverage Foundation SPF 8** *($29)* comes in 15 mostly neutral shades, each with a disappointing SPF 8. It does have titanium dioxide as part of the sunscreen, but the low SPF number just doesn't swing. The coverage is almost as minimal as the Sheer Coverage version above, but this one has a softer, less dewy finish. The formula is still best for normal to dry skin, but only if you're willing to wear a separate SPF 15 sunscreen underneath. Watch out for Toffee, Almond, Cinnamon, and Nutmeg—each is red or orange enough to be a problem for darker skin. **Medium Coverage Foundation with SPF 8** *($38)* is a cream-to-powder foundation that is more creamy than powdery. Most of the 12 colors pass muster, but the too-low SPF number is disappointing. Almost any stick foundation with an effective SPF 15 sunscreen can beat this average makeup. If you decide to settle for average, avoid Ivory, Linen, Vanilla, Shell, Cinnamon, and Toffee.

☺ $$$ **POWDER:** The **Pressed Powder** *($26)* and **Loose Powder** *($32)* each offer six beautifully neutral colors. Both are standard, talc-based powders that have a silky-smooth texture with a sheer application and incredibly natural finish. **Bronzing** *($24)* is a pressed-powder bronzer that has a superior smooth texture and even application with only a hint of shine. The single color available is a bit on the orange side to look convincing on fair skin, but is otherwise recommended.

✓☺ $$$ **CONCEALER:** **Concealer** *($17)* is an excellent liquid concealer available in four skin-friendly shades. It has a terrific soft-matte finish with minimal risk of creasing, and it remains a favorite.

BLUSH: ☺ **$$$ Blush** *($24)* comes in a beautiful array of muted colors that have a soft, silky finish, although the price is absurd for what you get. It's easily replaced by far less expensive options at the drugstore—but you won't be disappointed if you splurge here.

☺ **$$$ Cheek Color Wash** *($23)* is a fairly standard cream blush with a sheer finish that leaves a good deal of shine on the cheek. For an expensive evening glow, these work well. **Highlighter** *($23)* is described as a "sheer blush that adds color quietly," but on the skin it merely leaves a faint (and I mean really faint) hint of color and a shimmer finish. If you're shine-inclined, Revlon's SkinLights offers the same concept for half the price.

EYESHADOW: ☺ **Eye Shadow** *($15)* has a sheer, suede-smooth texture that blends well and clings to the skin nicely. The colors are attractive, though almost all of them are sparkly, and that can not only be distracting but also play up less-than-perfect eyelids. These can be used wet or dry, and there are some almost matte options that would make good powder eyeliner or brow colors. **Eye Shadow Palette** *($25)* is a sensible assortment of five workable colors in a Lucite compact with an eyeshadow brush. If the color combination appeals to you and the soft shine isn't bothersome, this is almost a bargain!

☺ **Eye Color Wash** *($14)* is a great name for just a very ordinary liquid-to-powder eyeshadow with shine that comes in a squeeze tube. This is a messy way to apply eyeshadow because it's difficult to control color placement, plus it creases easily and needs to be set with powder to get it to stay. If you like this type of eyeshadow, consider the longer-wearing options from BeneFit or Revlon.

EYE AND BROW SHAPER: ☺ **Eye Definer** *($14)* is a standard pencil with a sponge tip at one end. It does have a good smooth application in comparison to many that tend to be more greasy and thick, but it fades quickly and can smear with little provocation.

☺ **$$$ Brow Groomer** *($16)* is a very standard clear brow gel that has a great dual-sided brush for making sure each brow hair is tamed. This is assuredly overpriced, but it works.

☹ **Eye Gloss** *($14)* is, just as the name implies, a gloss for the eyes. This greasy mess is supposed to look good, but I don't understand this trend. It makes everything you've just applied slide around and crease almost immediately. If you want to add a "transparent sheen" to eyelids, consider a clear silicone gel instead.

LIPSTICK: ✔☺ **$$$ Lip Color** *($16)* is a very good nicely creamy lipstick with a smooth, relatively non-greasy finish and opaque coverage. The range of 30+ colors is exquisite, and many have a good stain.

☺ **$$$ Lip Gloss** *($17)* is a very standard, minimally sticky lip gloss with a good amount of iridescence and soft, sheer colors.

☺ **Lip Color Wash** *($15)* is a great name for a standard, semi-sheer glossy-finish lipstick in a great group of can't-go-wrong colors. And if you can't decide between the colors, consider **Lip Color Wash Palette** *($25)*, which features five sheer lip colors in one slim compact with an enclosed lip brush. **Lip Definer** *($14)* is a standard lip pencil with a lip brush on one end. It does have a good creamy finish, but don't expect it to keep lip color from bleeding.

☺ $$$ <u>MASCARA:</u> **Mascara** *($16)* is just OK. This builds minimal length and no real thickness, though it doesn't clump or smear. It's just lackluster all the way around, though the Khaki shade is perfect for naturally blonde lashes.

☹ $$$ <u>BRUSHES:</u> **Brushes** *($16–$38)*. With all the superior brushes available from department-store lines such as M.A.C., Bobbi Brown, Laura Mercier, and Trish McEvoy, there is no reason to consider these. The bristles are soft, but not as lush and densely packed as most, plus the shapes of the **Large Eye Shadow** *($24)* and **Powder Brush** *($38)* are too large—almost clumsy—and not the best for most face shapes. The only brushes to consider are the **Eyeliner Brush** *($16)*, **Blush Brush** *($32)*, and **Small Eye Shadow Brush** *($18)*.

☹ $$$ <u>SPECIALTY:</u> **Liquid Crystals for the Body** *($25)* is a dry-finish, lightweight lotion that's imbued with either fleshy pink or bronze sparkles. Although this is a consideration for evening, the sparkles tend to flake because the base formula is not emollient.

CAMOCARE (SKIN CARE ONLY)

If you feel that chamomile is an important skin-care ingredient then look no further, because this line agrees. Here you'll find the showcased and glorified focal point is chamomile—ergo the name CamoCare. But should you be looking for chamomile in your products? Is this the be-all and end-all for good skin care? Hardly. Chamomile is a good anti-irritant and soothing agent, but it is scarcely the only one—in fact, there are dozens and dozens of other effective ingredients used in cosmetics specifically to reduce irritation and inflammation. Showcasing one ingredient is always a problem for a skin-care line, because when newer research comes along establishing that other options exist—and there is a lot of research out there about a lot of ingredients having benefit for skin—it's hard to explain the benefit of using just chamomile alone. Either it is the best element for skin or it isn't, and if it isn't, why name a product line after just one small aspect of a formulary?

It is interesting to note that while chamomile is a good anti-irritant and has antioxidant properties, it is far from the best one. However, many of the CamoCare products also include plant extracts that are known to cause irritation, including lemon, peppermint, orange extract, lavender, and tangerine. That mixture negates the purpose of concentrating on the chamomile in the first place, which is to counteract the irritation caused by environmental factors (primarily sun damage) and not the irritation from the product itself.

Of course, CamoCare wants you to believe that their chamomile is the best one, and their Web site cites three studies from the University of Bonn, Germany, proving that the CamoCare products are superior to two other options. These three studies are not published or even dated. If you assume that the results are accurate (though they're clearly not unbiased), it is nice to know that these products are soothing when compared to some other cream. However, what the studies failed to look at were other creams that contained equally good or better topical anti-irritants and antioxidants. Not to mention that the studies only looked at a small group of women and only for the issue of irritation. There are a lot of skin-care issues besides irritation.

Aside from chamomile, CamoCare has jumped on other bandwagons (I guess chamomile isn't enough after all). The first one is AHA and BHA, though CamoCare's products only contain plant extracts and not the actual acids, which means these are not really effective for exfoliation (and that's what AHAs and BHA are for!). Several of the products contain alpha lipoic acid, which is the showcase ingredient (along with vitamin C) in Dr. N.V. Perricone's products (reviewed in this edition). Alpha lipoic acid is a good antioxidant, but again, the same comment applies for it as for chamomile—there are lots of good antioxidants, and alpha lipoic acid is neither the best nor the only one. However, for the money, if you are looking for a topical alpha lipoic acid product, this is by far a cheaper way to get it.

The last bandwagon is the addition of vitamin C products. CamoCare's ingredient of choice is Ester-C and, according to CamoCare, it's supposed to be the only stable form of vitamin C. That isn't true, as there is much research showing that magnesium ascorbyl phosphate and ascorbyl palmitate, among others, are more stable and acceptable to skin. Ester-C is a trade name for a combination form of vitamin C that contains mainly calcium ascorbate. The company that sells Ester-C maintains that this form allows for more bioavailability of the vitamin C. However, the company's research has not been published in a peer-reviewed journal (Source: The Bioavailability of Different Forms of Vitamin C, Linus Pauling Institute, Oregon State University, http://www.orst.edu/dept/lpi/ss01/bioavailability.html). There are studies showing Ester-C to have no differences when compared to ascorbic acid (Source: *Biochemical Pharmacology*, June 1996, pages 1719–1725). For more information about CamoCare, call (800) 226-6227 or visit www.camocare.com.

☺ **Camomile Light Foaming Cleanser** (*$9.95 for 4 ounces*) is a standard, detergent-based, water-soluble cleanser that includes some plant extracts that can be anti-irritants, though because they're in a cleanser their effect would just be rinsed down the drain. This would work well for most skin types, except for very dry skin. It does contain fragrance and preservatives.

☺ **Camomile Moisturizing Cleanser** (*$9.95 for 4 ounces*) is a standard, cold cream–type, plant oil–based cleanser that needs to be wiped off. It can work for dry skin.

☹ **Camomile Oil Free Toner** (*$8.95 for 4 ounces*). This product is a mixed bag, with very few strong points aside from the alpha lipoic acid. The fragrant plant extracts in this product negate the effectiveness of the plant extracts that can be anti-irritants.

☹ **Camomile Stimulating Toner** (*$8.95 for 4 ounces*). The fragrant plant extracts in here negate the effectiveness of the plant extracts that can be anti-irritants. Still, this can be an OK toner for most skin types, with one good antioxidant and an anti-irritant.

☹ **Camomile Toning Therapy** (*$10.95 for 8 ounces*) does at least leave out the irritating plant extracts. It is a simple toner of just water, gentle detergent cleansing agent, slip agent, anti-irritant, and preservatives. This is an OK toner for most skin types.

The Reviews C

☹ **12% Alpha + Beta Hydroxy Intense Treatment** *($19.95 for 2 ounces)* does not contain any AHAs or BHA at all. However it does contain some plant extracts that are distantly related to AHAs and BHA (about as distantly related as wheat is too bread—you can't make a sandwich out of wheat); however, even if they worked as exfoliants (which they don't), the pH of 5 is too high for them to be effective. This also contains several plant extracts that can be skin irritants, including peppermint.

☺ **$$$ C-Spot** *($29.95 for 1 ounce)* is a rather ordinary, lightweight lotion. The teeny amount of vitamin C is barely detectable, and the lactic acid is present in too small an amount to function as an exfoliant.

☺ **$$$ Night Skin Firmer** *($40 for 1 ounce).* If you're looking for a vitamin C product this would be an OK option, but it lacks many other elements the skin needs to make it really worth the money or good for the health of your skin.

☺ **$$$ Day Skin Firmer** *($37.50 for 1 ounce)* is similar to the Night Skin Firmer above except that this product contains no plant oils. The plant extracts in here sound like they are related to AHAs, but they are not, and they have no exfoliating properties. Because this does not contain sunscreen, it is not recommended to be worn alone during the day.

☺ **$$$ EPF Daily Facial Moisturizer SPF 15** *($19.95 for 1 ounce)* is a very good, in-part zinc oxide–based sunscreen in a very standard, ordinary moisturizing base. It would work well for someone with normal to dry skin.

☺ **$$$ Eye Lifting Moisture Cream** *($17.59 for 0.5 ounce)* is a product with a minuscule amount of interesting ingredients, but the small quantity of them in here makes it little more than a standard moisturizer for dry skin.

☺ **Facial Therapy** *($20 for 2.4 ounces)* is a very emollient, though ordinary, moisturizer for very dry skin; it contains a trace amount of antioxidants.

☺ **Light Facial Therapy** *($13.39 for 1 ounce)* is almost identical to the Facial Therapy above and the same basic comments apply.

✓☺ **Intense Facial Therapy** *($20.69 for 1 ounce)* is definitely an improvement over the Facial Therapy above. This version contains a good mix of water-binding agents, antioxidants, and anti-irritants. It is a very good option for normal to dry skin.

☹ **Under Eye Therapy** *($14.49 for 0.25 ounce)* contains lemon and witch hazel, which can cause irritation—and that won't reduce puffiness.

☹ **Clear Solution** *($11 for 0.5 ounce)* is supposed to clear up blemishes, but all it contains is chamomile extract, alpha lipoic acid, flavonoids (from lemon), and essential oils—at least, that's what's on the label, but I suspect that the label is not entirely complete, nor does it meet FDA ingredient listing guidelines. Regardless of what CamoCare appears not to be disclosing, even the listed ingredients have no research showing them to be effective against acne.

☺ **Revitalizing Mask** *($13.39 for 2 ounces)* is a very good clay mask with glycerin and a teeny amount of alpha lipoic acid. It would work well for someone with normal to oily skin.

☺ **Soothing Cream** *($6.19 for 0.71 ounce)* is a very ordinary emollient moisturizer that contains mostly water, thickeners, lanolin, plant oil, and preservatives.

CARGO (MAKEUP ONLY)

With all the many makeup artist–driven lines available today; the average cosmetics shopper must no doubt be perplexed as to which one to shop. M.A.C. was at the forefront of these niche lines, and thanks to their runaway success, enough spin-offs have been launched to leave one feeling dizzy. So how does Canadian-bred CARGO fit into this slew of choices? For the most part, the line excels in all arenas. Their philosophy is "uncompromised and unparalleled quality," but I wouldn't go so far as to say this line's products have no equals, because they most certainly do. Almost all of these cookie-cutter makeup lines offer women truly neutral foundations, incredibly soft powders, velvety matte blushes and eyeshadows, and an assortment of professionally designed brushes. CARGO does not rise above this protocol, they follow it—though some of their products do have an edge when it comes to price. One distinct benefit of CARGO's creations is that they are created by working makeup artists servicing both the public and private sectors. That equates to mostly practical products in wearable shades that have enough of an edge to begin as trendy, yet with the potential to become classic. There is every reason to consider CARGO's products the next time you happen upon a display at Sephora or one of the regional specialty boutiques that carry it. Although CARGO does not distinguish itself from its competitors in any major way, you can count on getting what the company refers to as "easy to use, easy to wear makeup … with a collection of current and classic colors." For more information about CARGO, call (905) 760-0705 or visit www.cargocosmetics.com.

☺ **FOUNDATION: Liquid Foundation** *($24)* comes in ten exceptionally neutral shades suitable for light to dark skin tones, all named after planets and one constellation—clever, but not helpful for identifying shades! It has a silicone- and talc-based, soft-matte finish that gives sheer to light coverage. Don't expect this one to work well for very oily skin, though; the amount of silicone can make it feel too oily or slippery, despite the fact it is not technically oil. The talc adds to the matte finish, but it isn't enough to hold back the slippery feel. This works best for someone with normal to slightly oily or slightly dry skin.

☺ **Wet/Dry Powder Foundation** *($24)* is a standard, talc-based powder with a soft shine, and that makes it problematic for reducing shine. Also, the formulation is fairly emollient, which explains the slightly heavy, emollient-feeling coverage, at least in comparison to other pressed powders. It would work well for normal to dry skin, but should be avoided by anyone prone to blemishes or oily skin. The same color names apply to these as for the Liquid Foundation, and the colors are all equally excellent. The feel is silky soft, and the application gives sheer to light coverage.

☺ $$$ <u>CONCEALER:</u> **Concealer** *($16)* is a thick, slightly greasy concealer that provides ample coverage and blends down to a soft powder finish. However, the three shades leave much to be desired, especially compared with the options available from Stila, Lancome, and M.A.C.

<u>POWDER:</u> ✔☺ $$$ **Loose Powder** *($24)* has a very fine, sifted texture that glides over skin and leaves a soft matte finish. This talc-based formula is best for normal to dry skin, especially if you have shied away from powder because it always seems to look too powdery on your skin. The five shades are good, though Powder #2 is definitely on the yellow side, which can add a strange cast to the skin.

☺ $$$ **Pressed Powder** *($24)* is a standard, talc-based powder that has a drier, sheerer finish than the Wet/Dry Powder Foundation above, but it is creamier feeling than the Loose Powder. The five shades are mostly great, with only #02 being a bit too yellow for some light skin tones. Each one has a subtle shine, which is not likely to please someone with oily skin.

☺ $$$ **Bronzer** *($25)* has an incredibly smooth texture and comes in three utterly convincing tan-to-bronze shades, but each one is heavily infused with shine, so attempting to create a natural-looking tan-from-the-sun effect is fruitless.

☹ $$$ **Glitter** *($22)* is aptly described by its name. This is iridescent loose powder that comes in a set of three small vials. In spite of making some beauty editors' "best" lists, this remains messy to use and tends to get all over the place, though it does add a good deal of shine wherever it does stick.

☺ $$$ <u>BLUSH:</u> ✔☺ **Blush** *($20)* is packaged in a large tin, the shades are attractive, and most of them offer a good matte finish. The Topeka, Fresno, and Siena shades have a distracting shine. The pigmentation is dense, so you need a deft hand to apply it evenly. Overall, this is an easy recommendation thanks to the luscious texture and smooth application. ✔☺ **ColorTube** *($24)* is a version of the three-in-one type color sticks from companies such as Bobbi Brown and Almay that are meant to be used for the eyes, cheeks, and lips. ColorTube's difference is that it is a thick, pasty cream that you squeeze out like toothpaste and blend onto the skin. This has a slightly emollient texture and four very good sheer colors, plus one iridescent gold hue for highlighting. If you prefer a dewy finish on the cheeks, this is worth considering and advantageous over the three-in-one pencils because there is nothing to sharpen!

☺ <u>EYESHADOW:</u> **Eyeshadow** *($15)* is a large range of eyeshadows that have a great, silky-smooth application. There are shiny shades to wade through as well as several blue and green tones, but the neutral shades, though slightly iridescent, go on easy and have great color density. The matte shades are great, and stay on well without flaking.

☺ <u>EYE AND BROW SHAPER:</u> **Eye/Brow Pencil** *($14)* is available in only three shades. This sharpening-required pencil goes on creamier than most, which means it can tend to smear, but it can also be easier to line over eyeshadows.

☺ <u>LIPSTICK AND LIP PENCIL:</u> **Lipstick** *($16)* is a standard group of lipsticks with a selection of Sheers that are fairly greasy with minimal color deposit, Creams that are more glossy than creamy but still likable, Frosts that are opaque iridescents, and Mattes that have a nice stain but are more creamy than matte. There is only a limited color selection in each category, but the overall color selection is impressive. **Celebrity Artist Lipstick** *($16)* is a selection of lip colors created by such luminaries as Debra Messing of *Will & Grace* fame and Star Jones from television's *The View*. The concept behind these lipsticks (which share the same formulas as CARGO's regular lipsticks) is that two dollars from the sale of each color is donated to the national efforts of Children's Miracle Network. The range of shades is quite good, and the celebrity tie-in is an easy finesse for many consumers. You can even choose the same lipstick worn by Jennifer Aniston during her wedding to Brad Pitt (shade name: Plume). It's an enticing concept and a worthy cause that can make shopping for lipstick feel like a mini good deed! **Lip Pencil** *($14)* products are standard lip pencils that require sharpening. These are creamier than most, and so are not as helpful in preventing lipstick from feathering. The color palette offers a nice mix of familiar stand-bys and unusual hues. **Lip Gloss** *($17)* has a liquid-cream, minimally sticky texture that feels great on the lips. Each generous tin features two shades and the duos are mostly beautiful. **Lip Gloss/Conditioner** *($17)* is simply half shimmer gloss and half lip balm, and for lovers of both, it is convenient.

☺ $$$ <u>MASCARA:</u> CARGO's **Mascara** *($16)* formulation must have been tweaked since I last reviewed it because now it's adept at building good length and noticeable thickness without a lot of effort. It does not clump and lasts all day without flaking, though you may want to avoid the blue, green, and violet shades.

<u>BRUSHES:</u> The brushes in this line are somewhat overpriced, but for the most part have a soft, smooth feel with good density and thickness and come in very workable shapes and sizes. The following are all worth feeling and checking out to see if they meet your needs: ✔☺ $$$ **Dome Brush** *($68)*, **Flat Lip Brush** *($15)*, **Fluff Brush Large** *($34)*, **Fluff Brush Jumbo** *($28)*, **Pointed Mini Crease Brush** *($28)*, **Super Powder Brush** *($60)*, **Kolinsky Eye Liner** *($12)*, and **Medium Fluff Blush** *($28)* are all great! The ☺ **Angle Liner Brush** *($18)* and **Concealer Brush** *($22)* are synthetic bristles that can feel stiff and scratchy on the face, but they are an option for some makeup applications. Actually, the Concealer Brush works better for eyelining than concealing. The **Small Fluff Blush** *($22)* is OK for soft detail work, but is almost too small to be practical.

CAUDALIE (SKIN CARE ONLY)

The ambience accompanying this product line is intended to evoke the world of grapes. The name Caudalie—are you ready for this—is a wine term describing the length of time the taste of a wine stays in the mouth. It is an actual measurement, defined as one second of finish being equal to one Caudalie, and the more Caudalie the wine has the better the wine is supposed to taste. What does any of that have to do with skin care? Following the model of Lancome's Vinefit and a handful of other lines, it is meant to evoke the importance of the grape for skin. This company's belief in the vine almost makes you want to use Welch's Grape Juice as your toner. But of course that's not what Caudalie has in mind.

Despite the cosmetics industry's hype, there are no published studies indicating that grapes in any form, applied topically, can affect the wrinkling process. However, what is true about grapes (stem, seed, pulp, and all) is that they contain proanthocyanidin, a pigment that is considered a very potent antioxidant, and helpful for reducing the sun's damaging effects (Sources: *Current Pharmaceutical Biotechnology*, June 2001, pages 187–200 and *Toxicology*, August 2000, pages 187–197). Proanthocyanidin has also been shown to have wound-healing properties (Source: *Free Radical Biology and Medicine*, July 2001, pages 38–42). It's helpful to know that there's no difference in the antioxidant potential between different types of grapes (Source: *Journal of Agricultural Food Chemistry*, April 2000, pages 1076–1080). However, there is not an abundance of research in this whole area. There is still little known about the bioavailability, absorption, and full-spectrum activity of grape compounds because this has thus far proven difficult to measure (Sources: *European Journal of Internal Medicine*, December 2001, pages 484–489; and *Free Radical Biology and Medicine*, February 15, 2002, pages 314–318).

What is important to keep in mind is that there are many plant extracts, vitamins, and plants with potent antioxidant, anti-inflammatory, and wound-healing properties. No single ingredient has obtained the coveted status of "best" when it comes to skin (or health) care. Almost all antioxidants appear to have some benefit for the skin. Yet, how much of them the skin needs, and exactly how they work in a cosmetic formulation remains unknown, as all of the research on these types of ingredients has been done on the compounds as standalone ingredients, and not when they are just a small part of a moisturizer.

Although almost all of Caudalie's products contain grapes (in one form or another), they share the same problem that besets most "natural" lines, namely the inclusion of several irritating plant extracts and essential oils. Any positive benefit you could potentially gain from slathering yourself with Caudalie's grape-based elixirs would be negated because of unwelcome irritation caused by other ingredients in these products, such as lemon oil, lavender oil, orange peel oil, and others. As much as Caudalie would like you to believe their botanical cocktails are the sought-after fountain of youth, you would be better off spending your money on fresh grapes, grape juice, or—if you're of age—a vintage bottle of Merlot or Cabernet Sauvignon! For more information about Caudalie, visit www.caudalie.com or www.sephora.com.

☺ **$$$ Grape Seed Gentle Cleanser** (*$25 for 6.7 ounces*) is a standard emollient cleanser with a small amount of detergent cleansing agent. It can be an option for normal to dry skin. This also contains a small amount of lemon, lavender, and coriander oil along with additional fragrance, and may be problematic for use around the eyes.

☺ **$$$ Instant Foaming Cleanser** (*$25 for 5 ounces*) is a very good, though very standard, water-soluble, detergent-based cleanser that would be an option for normal to oily skin. This product uses a nonaerosol pump to convert the liquid to a foam. That's fine, but it's not essential for a cleanser. It does contain fragrance. The benefit of the grape water, if any, would be rinsed down the drain.

☹ **Ultra Mild Wine Soap** *($15 for 5.3 ounces)* is standard-issue fragrant bar soap that does contain grape juice, but it can still leave a film on the skin and be drying for most skin types.

☹ **Grape Seed Buffing Cream** *($34 for 1.6 ounces)* is a thick, plant wax–based scrub using jojoba wax. This also contains a host of irritating plant extracts.

☹ **Grape Water Mist** *($12 for 3.4 ounces)* is an incredibly simple toner that contains only grape water and nitrogen. Ironically, nitrogen can generate free-radical damage and cause cell death (Source: *Mechanisms of Ageing and Development*, April 2002, pages 1007–1019). This product is not recommended. Even without the nitrogen, this still wouldn't be preferred to or different from applying grape juice to your skin.

☺ **$$$ C20 Grape Seed Cream** *($37 for 1.3 ounces)* is a standard moisturizer for dry skin that, save for the addition of grape seed oil, is relatively boring. At this price, you would at least expect some other interesting water-binding agents and "newer" antioxidants. It does contain a tiny amount of vitamin E, but it's listed after the fragrance, so its benefit is negligible.

☺ **$$$ C40 Grape Seed Anti-Wrinkle Cream** *($43 for 1.3 ounces)* is similar to the C20 Grape Seed Cream above, but this is a bit more emollient and includes silicone for a silkier texture. Although it does contain grape seed oil, which is a decent antioxidant, it is commingled here with irritants like coriander, lemon peel oil, and orange peel oil, so the positives associated with grapes are compromised. If you want grapes without the irritants (and effective sun protection to boot), consider Lancome's Vinefit Energizing Cream SPF 15 ($37.50 for 1.7 ounces).

☺ **$$$ C80 Emulsion** *($56 for 1.6 ounces)* has a good base formula of some water-binding agents mixed with emollients, an anti-irritant (oat protein), silicone, film-forming agent, and standard thickeners. This also contains several fragrant plant extracts, but they are present in small amounts so that the risk of irritation is minimal.

☺ **$$$ C80 Grape Seed Rejuvenating Cream** *($56 for 1.6 ounces)* is a standard, rather ordinary moisturizer that would be an OK option for normal to dry skin. However, for this kind of price you would expect at least some amount of unique water-binding agents or anti-irritants, which this product simply does not contain, though it does include additional fragrance.

☺ **$$$ Facial Treatment Oil for Dry Dehydrated Skin** *($51 for 1 ounce)* is a good combination of plant oils for very dry skin. It does contain fragrance. Still, nothing about this product that couldn't easily be replaced with a bottle of grape seed oil, which is available at most health food stores.

☹ **Facial Lotion Beauty Elixir** *($56 for 3.8 ounces)* lists the second ingredient as alcohol, and combining that irritant with peppermint, balm mint, and grapefruit extract is anything but beautiful.

☺ **$$$ Grape Seed Eye Contour Cream** *($43 for 0.5 ounce)* is an OK moisturizer for normal to dry skin. This has a slightly matte finish, which can work well under the eyes if you need to use a lighter moisturizer there but do not want to encourage concealer slipping into lines around the eye. This lacks any state-of-the-art water-binding agents or anti-irritants that you'd want to find to warrant spending this kind of money. It doesn't even contain much grape extract for that matter.

☺ **$$$ Vinolift** *($75 for 1 ounce)* claims it can enhance the renewal of collagen and elastin fibers and match the effectiveness of AHAs and retinol without being aggressive. However, these powerful assertions are not mirrored in the product's ingredient list. This contains mostly water, gel-based thickener, anti-irritant, fragrant plant water, slip agents, silicone, emollient, preservatives, plant extracts, fragrance, film-forming agents, and water-binding agents. There are some intriguing ingredients in this product (such as ceramides, which are great for normal to slightly dry skin), but Elizabeth Arden has ceramides with other water-binding agents in their formulations for far less. Moreover, while this is a good moisturizer, what it can do is completely unrelated to how a well-formulated AHA product works or even how a good retinol product is theoretically supposed to work.

☹ **Vinolift Day Fluid, SPF 12** *($59 for 1 ounce)* is described as a sunscreen, but for this amount of money, when you see the low SPF number (SPF 15 is recommended as the minimum by the American Academy of Dermatology and the National Cancer Institute) you have to wonder whether the executives spent too much time swigging wine and not enough time researching what sunscreen needs to do.

☺ **$$$ Vinolift Total Night Care** *($59 for 1 ounce)* is a straightforward moisturizer for normal to dry skin. The interesting ingredients are listed far after the preservatives, so they are barely detectable and offer little benefit for skin. This does contain fragrance.

☺ **$$$ Purifying Grape Seed Mask** *($40 for 1.6 ounces)* is a standard clay mask wrapped up in one of the longest ingredient lists you're likely to see. The odd mix of absorbents and emollient, oily, or wax-based thickeners is bound to be confusing for your skin. Contrary to the claim, this mask cannot regulate skin functions, mattify the skin, or reduce skin flaws. The "buzz" ingredients (some of which are fragrant plant oils) are listed after the preservatives, so they will have little to no impact on the skin, for better or worse. This mask would work best for normal to slightly oily skin, but it is hardly an essential addition to your skin-care routine.

☹ **Revitalizing Moisture Grape Seed Cream Mask** *($40 for 1.6 ounces)*. What could have been a creamy, grape seed oil–enriched mask for dry skin is corrupted by the unnecessary addition of a slew of potent irritants. The list reads like a "who's who" of offenders, including vetiver, lemon, lime, orange, and sandalwood oils—they're all here. What a shame, because this is otherwise a beneficial, indulgent mask for dry skin.

☺ **Grape Seed Lip Conditioner** *($15 for 0.14 ounce)* is a standard, mineral oil– and wax-based lip balm that contains a nice array of emollients that can help lips feel smooth, soft, and comfortable. The price is steep for what you get, but this will take good care of dry, chapped lips.

CELLEX-C (SKIN CARE ONLY)

Originally, Cellex-C was all about vitamin C, and a very specific form of vitamin C, namely L-ascorbic acid. However, following the pattern of most companies, which often tout a single ingredient as being the be-all and end-all for skin, Cellex-C also has added other products that do not include their showcase ingredient. Aside from that development, is L-ascorbic acid really a better form of vitamin C? According to Cellex-C it is. The information on their Web site states that L-ascorbic acid "is the one vitamin that doctors and dermatologists agree can speed wound healing, protect fatty tissues from oxidation damage, and play an integral role in collagen synthesis." That statement is completely erroneous. Not only isn't there a consensus among any group of physicians regarding which vitamin is the best for skin (there is abundant research about vitamin E and vitamin A, too), but also there's a battle among various physicians who sell vitamin C skin-care products as to which form of that vitamin is the best. In this area, the two most notable doctors are Dr. Sheldon Pinnell, creator of Skinceuticals, who sells his own supposedly stable form of L-ascorbic acid (at least it's more stable than the one Cellex-C uses), and Dr. N.V. Perricone, with a skin-care line bearing his name and who lays claim to the efficacy of Ester-C (calcium ascorbate).

It turns out that there is a great deal of research showing that there are many stable and effective ingredients that can assist in wound healing, collagen formation, and protection from free-radical damage. These ingredients include vitamins, minerals, various plant extract antioxidants, and AHAs, just to name a few. Cellex-C boasts that several of their products contain an extremely high concentration of vitamin C (over 15%). However, there is no research showing how much vitamin C the skin needs, whether or not at any concentration it can affect wrinkling.

Of course Cellex-C wants you to believe that the vitamin C in their products is the miracle answer, and after more than a decade they are still using the exact same before-and-after picture they did in the very beginning. Aside from the lack of more "testimonial" pictures, one might wonder: If the little bottle of Cellex-C is supposed to be so amazing, why is the company also selling AHAs, BHA, and other wrinkle creams that don't contain vitamin C? There is no doubt that vitamin C is a good ingredient for skin, but lots of companies use it and it doesn't have to be this expensive.

Cellex-C's Betaplex line is about AHAs and BHA, and uses willow bark as its source of BHA. Willow bark contains salicin, a substance that when taken orally is converted by the enzymes present in the digestive process to salicylic acid. But what it takes to turn salicin into saligenin, and then into salicylic acid is a complicated digestive process. Further, salicin, much like salicylic acid, is stable only under acidic conditions. The likelihood that willow bark in the tiny amount used in these products can mimic the effectiveness of salicylic acid is at best problematic, and in all likelihood impossible. For AHAs the Cellex-C line is a consideration, but even so it goes without saying that there are far less expensive

The Reviews C

versions of AHAs available. For more information about Cellex-C, call (800) CELLEX-C or visit www.cellex-c.com.

✔☺ $$$ **Advanced-C Eye Firming Cream** *($90 for 1 ounce)* definitely contains vitamin C, along with some thickening agents, silicone, plant oil, antioxidants, anti-irritants, preservatives, and fragrance. This would be a very good moisturizer for someone with normal to dry skin.

✔☺ $$$ **Advanced-C Eye Toning Gel** *($70 for 0.5 ounce)* is similar to the Firming Cream above only in gel form and with better water-binding agents. It would work well for normal to slightly dry skin. But there is nothing about this product that makes it preferred for the eye area, especially if the under-eye skin is very dry.

☹ **Under Eye Toning Gel** *($31 for 0.3 ounce)* contains zinc sulphate, eucalyptus, and peppermint, which won't tone anything, but it will irritate skin and that isn't good for any part of the face.

☺ $$$ **Advanced-C Neck Firming Cream** *($115 for 2 ounces)* is similar to the Eye Firming Cream above and the same basic comments apply.

✔☺ $$$ **Advanced-C Serum** *($115 for 1 ounce)* has a very good mix of antioxidants and water-binding agents. It would work well for someone with normal to slightly dry skin.

☺ $$$ **Advanced-C Skin Hydration Complex** *($79 for 1 ounce)* contains water, water-binding agents, an antioxidant, and preservatives. This simplistic formula leaves out the mix of antioxidants that the other equally expensive products in this line contain. This is still a very good moisturizer for normal to slightly dry skin.

✔☺ $$$ **Advanced-C Skin Tightening Cream** *($135 for 2 ounces)* has a formula almost identical to the Eye Firming Cream above, yet this actually prices out cheaper. So, on the off chance you want to waste money on an unnecessarily expensive moisturizer this would be the one to consider.

✔☺ $$$ **Eye Contour Cream** *($64 for 1 ounce)* is almost identical to the Eye Firming Cream above only with somewhat less vitamin C. Given that no one knows how much vitamin C the skin needs, this product would do just as well and this one is cheaper. It is a very good moisturizer for normal to dry skin.

☹ $$$ **Eye Contour Cream Plus** *($70 for 1 ounce)* omits the vitamin C but adds plant extracts of bilberry, sugarcane, and sugar maple. The sugarcane and sugar maple have no AHA exfoliating benefit for skin. Bilberry has some antioxidant potential, but its reputation for skin lightening has no research showing that to be true. This is far less interesting than many of the other pricey moisturizers in this line.

✔☺ $$$ **Eye Contour Gel** *($51 for 0.5 ounce)* is a good combination of antioxidants and water-binding agents that would be very good for normal to slightly dry skin.

☺ $$$ **Fade-Away Gel** *($55 for 0.84 ounce)* contains no ingredients that can cause anything to fade away. It is similar to the Eye Contour Gel above and the same comments apply.

✔☺ **$$$ High Potency Serum** *($90 for 1 ounce)* is similar to the Advanced-C Serum above and the same basic comments apply.

✔☺ **$$$ Serum for Sensitive Skin** *($90 for 1 ounce)* contains nothing that makes it preferred for sensitive skin. It is similar to the Advanced-C Serum above and the same comments apply.

✔☺ **$$$ Skin Firming Cream** *($105 for 2 ounces)* is almost identical to the Advanced-C Eye Firming Cream above and the same comments apply.

✔☺ **$$$ Skin Firming Cream Plus** *($114 for 2 ounces)* is almost identical to the Advanced-C Eye Firming Cream above and the same comments apply.

☺ **$$$ Sun Care SPF 30** *($35 for 4 ounces)* is a very good, in-part zinc oxide–based sunscreen (along with other synthetic sunscreen ingredients) in an exceedingly ordinary moisturizing base. This would be appropriate for normal to dry skin, but there is nothing about this formula that cannot be replaced with a far less expensive version.

☺ **$$$ Sun Care SPF 30+** *($25 for 3.3 ounces)* is a very good, in-part zinc oxide– and titanium dioxide–based sunscreen (along with other synthetic sunscreen ingredients) in an exceedingly ordinary moisturizing base of mostly Vaseline and mineral oil. This would be appropriate for normal to dry skin, but there is nothing about this formula that cannot be replaced with a far less expensive version.

☺ **$$$ Sun Care SPF 15** *($33 for 4 ounces)* is identical to the Sun Care SPF 30+ above, save for a lower SPF rating. The same comments apply.

☹ **Sun Rescue Gel** *($49 for 3 ounces)* contains some very good antioxidants and water-binding agents, but for some inexplicable reason it also contains a good amount of peppermint and zinc sulphate, which are irritating and will only damage skin more.

☹ **Advanced-C Skin Toning Mask** *($55 for 1 ounce)*. The only thing advanced about this product is the price. It is just cornstarch and egg white with vitamin C and a teeny amount of grape extract. It is a waste of time and won't tone anything, at least not any better than what you can mix up yourself in your kitchen for pennies.

CELLEX-C BETAPLEX

☺ **$$$ Betaplex Gentle Cleansing Milk** *($29 for 6 ounces)* is a standard, plant oil–based cleanser that also includes a small amount of detergent cleansing agent. It would be an option for someone with normal to dry skin. This does contain lactic acid as the third ingredient, but the pH of the product isn't low enough for it to have exfoliating properties.

☺ **$$$ Betaplex Gentle Foaming Cleanser** *($29 for 6 ounces)* is a standard, detergent-based cleanser that also contains a small amount of lactic acid, though the pH of the cleanser isn't low enough for it to be effective as an exfoliant. This can be an option for someone with normal to oily skin.

☹ **Betaplex Facial Firming Water** *($29 for 6 ounces)* lists rice wine, which is alcohol, as the second ingredient and that can be drying and irritating for all skin types.

☹ **Betaplex Fresh Complex Mist** *($29 for 6 ounces)* contains several problematic irritating ingredients, including witch hazel and peppermint oil, and is not recommended.

☺ **\$\$\$ Betaplex Line Smoother** *(\$59 for 1 ounce)* supposedly contains about 15% AHA in a gel base. However, the pH of this product is not low enough for the AHA to be effective as an exfoliant.

☺ **\$\$\$ Betaplex New Complexion Cream** *(\$59 for 2 ounces)* supposedly contains about 10% AHA in a rather standard moisturizing base. The pH of this product is not low enough for the AHA to be effective as an exfoliant.

☺ **\$\$\$ Betaplex Smooth Skin Complex** *(\$59 for 2 ounces)* supposedly contains about 8% AHA in a rather standard moisturizing base of mineral oil and thickeners. The pH of this product is not low enough for the AHA to be effective as an exfoliant.

☹ **Betaplex Clear Complexion Mask** *(\$39.50 for 2 ounces)* contains several problematic plant extracts, including peppermint, menthol, orange, lemon, and eucalyptus, and that makes it too irritating for all skin types. It is not recommended.

CELLEX-C ENHANCERS

☺ **\$\$\$ Bio-Botanical Cream** *(\$54 for 2 ounces)* is a good moisturizer for normal to dry skin but isn't as fully loaded with beneficial ingredients as many of the other moisturizers in the Cellex-C group.

☺ **\$\$\$ G.L.A. Dry Skin Cream** *(\$58 for 2 ounces).* The "G.L.A." in the name stands for gamma linolenic acid, a fatty acid used in cosmetics as an emollient, and considered to promote healthy skin growth, which is great and similar to many effective antioxidants. However, there is no research showing G.L.A. to be effective in the treatment of wrinkles (Sources: *British Journal of Dermatology*, April 1999, pages 685–688 and *Dermatology*, 2000, volume 201, number 3, pages 191–195). G.L.A. has been shown to have some anticancer properties when taken orally, but there is no research showing that effect translates to products applied to the skin. This adds up to being a very good moisturizer for normal to dry skin.

☺ **\$\$\$ G.L.A. Extra Moist Cream** *(\$64 for 2 ounces)* doesn't contain the same interesting mix of antioxidants and plant oils as the Dry Skin Cream above.

☺ **\$\$\$ G.L.A. Eye Balm** *(\$54 for 1 ounce)* is almost identical to the Dry Skin Cream above and the same comments apply.

☺ **\$\$\$ Seline-E Cream** *(\$58 for 2 ounces)* contains a good mix of antioxidants in a rather ordinary moisturizing base that would be OK for someone with normal to dry skin.

☺ **\$\$\$ Sea Silk Oil-Free Moisturizer** *(\$49 for 2 ounces)* is a good, but standard, moisturizer that would work well for someone with normal to dry skin. It does contain fragrance.

☺ **\$\$\$ Hydra 5 B-Complex** *(\$66 for 1 ounce)* contains water, hyaluronic acid, pantothenic acid, and preservatives. This rather one-note product would be a very good, but overpriced, moisturizer for normal to slightly dry skin.

☹ **Skin Perfecting Pen** *(\$20 for 0.3 ounce)* contains peppermint, zinc sulphate, and eucalyptus, which makes it far less than perfect; rather it is irritating and drying for all skin types.

CETAPHIL (SKIN CARE

Galderma is the company that manufactures Cetap
of you who are familiar with my work from the begir
Skin Cleanser is a facial cleanser I have been impressed w
when I first discovered this obscure little cleanser, I was almost ai
because no one else knew about it. Back then there were very few good pro
for women to clean their faces. For decades, and until recently, the only options we.
cream or cold cream–like products, which had to be wiped off and then left the face
greasy, and bar cleansers or soaps, which left the face dried out and irritated. Cetaphil
Gentle Skin Cleanser was one of the only water-soluble cleansers available that cleaned
the face without drying it out or leaving it feeling greasy. Times have changed, of course,
and there are now many more alternatives for cleaning the face, but Cetaphil Gentle Skin
Cleanser remains a primary option for women with dry, sensitive skin who don't wear
much makeup. Unfortunately, Cetaphil Gentle Skin Cleanser is not very good for removing makeup, but it is very good in the morning or if you wear minimal makeup, and
now they have Cetaphil Daily Facial Cleanser that *can* be used to remove makeup no
matter what your skin type may be! For more information about Cetaphil, call (800)
582-8225 or visit www.cetaphil.com.

☺ **Cetaphil Gentle Skin Cleanser** *($8.99 for 16 ounces)* is a very good cleanser for
someone with dry, sensitive skin. It is a simple formulation containing thickeners and a
detergent cleansing agent. One word of warning: It doesn't remove makeup very well, so
it is best for daytime or at night if you wear minimal to no foundation. This does contain
sodium lauryl sulfate, but at a less than 1% concentration and, therefore, it poses minimal to no risk of irritation.

☺ **Cetaphil Daily Facial Cleanser for Normal to Oily Skin** *($5.99 for 8 ounces)* is a
standard, detergent-based cleanser that can work for most skin types except for dry to
very dry skin. It removes makeup nicely, far better than the original Cetaphil Gentle Skin
Cleanser, and doesn't irritate the eyes or dry out the skin. It does contain fragrance.

☺ **Cetaphil Gentle Cleansing Bar for Dry, Sensitive Skin** *($2.99 for 4.5 ounces)* is a
standard bar cleanser that uses a detergent cleansing agent. It does contain tallow, which
can cause breakouts. It is best used from the neck down.

☺ **Cetaphil Gentle Cleansing Bar Antibacterial** *($2.99 for 4.5 ounces)* is similar to
the Cleansing Bar above except that this version contains the disinfectant triclosan. Please
refer to Chapter Seven, *Cosmetics Dictionary* for information regarding the efficacy and
controversy about triclosan.

☺ **Cetaphil Moisturizing Lotion for Dry Sensitive Skin** *($8.99 for 16 ounces)* is a
very standard but effective moisturizer for someone with normal to dry skin.

☺ **Cetaphil Moisturizing Cream, Dry Sensitive Skin Treatment** *($10.99 for 16
ounces)* is a very basic cream moisturizer that would be OK for dry skin.

Cetaphil Daily Facial Moisturizer SPF 15 *($7.99 for 4 ounces)* is a good, zone-based sunscreen in a standard moisturizing base that would be OK for some-with normal to dry skin.

✓☺ **Nighttime Facial Moisturizer with Retinol** *($12.95 for 1.05 ounces)* is a fragrance-free retinol product in a relatively emollient base with additional antioxidants. It is packaged appropriately, in an airtight aluminum tube, which keeps the retinol stable. If you're curious to try a retinol product, this is a great option.

CHANEL

A major change for Chanel occurred in mid-1999, when the company launched a completely reformulated line of skin-care products they call Precision. I found that a very intriguing situation. After all, when you sell some of the more expensive skin-care products around, and make great claims about being the best, it takes a lot to say, "No, those really weren't the best, *now* we're selling you the best." Chanel's chemists seem to have used the "kitchen sink" approach to skin care with this new line, throwing in every ingredient under the sun so it can create a full menu of claims and promises. Some of these products contain more than 75 different ingredients. Is that better for skin? That depends on your point of view. The notion that tiny amounts of antioxidants are better than higher concentrations of one or two effective ones has not been established in the least. Plus, the longer the ingredient list, the higher your chances of irritation or allergic reaction. However, on the positive side, having a large group of ingredients does cover a lot of bases, especially for those looking for a little bit of everything (with the emphasis on *a little bit,* because many of the interesting ingredients are present in negligible amounts). From my perspective, if Chanel was going to go to all the trouble of creating a new line, they could have really set a fresh standard for excellence and let go of the coloring agents and fragrance. Now that would have been really new!

Nevertheless, what is definitely impressive is the inclusion of an SPF 15 sunscreen with UVA protection. Finally! It's ironic to consider that just a few years ago Chanel was sending me letters taking me to task for criticizing its SPF 8 products without UVA protection. How sad that it took Chanel so long, and that in the meantime so many women wasted so much money and put their skin at risk. For more information about Chanel, call (212) 688-5055 or visit www.chanel.com. **Note:** All Chanel products contain fragrance and coloring agents.

CHANEL SKIN CARE

☺ **$$$ Aquamousse Foaming Cream Face Wash** *($30 for 5 ounces)* is a rather standard, detergent-based, water-soluble cleanser that uses myristic acid, sodium methyl cocoyl laurate, and potassium hydroxide as the cleansing agents. That can be drying and irritating for the skin despite the addition of vegetable oil to help counteract the dryness. This standard formulation is wildly overpriced for what you get.

☺ $$$ **Gel Purete Foaming Gel Face Wash** *($30 for 5 ounces)* is an very standard, but good, detergent-based, water-soluble cleanser that would work well for normal to oily skin.

☺ $$$ **Gel Tendre Non-Foaming Makeup Remover Face and Eyes** *($30 for 5 ounces)* is an extremely standard, detergent-based eye-makeup remover. It would work as well as any, and is almost identical to many that cost half the price.

☺ $$$ **Lait Tendre Gentle Makeup Remover Face and Eyes** *($30 for 6.8 ounces)*. What a price tag for mineral oil and a tiny amount of detergent cleansing agents! It works, and it would be gentle, but it would be gentler without the fragrance and preservatives, much as using plain mineral oil would be.

☺ $$$ **Demaquillant Yeux Intense Gentle Biphase Eye Makeup Remover** *($23.50 for 3.4 ounces)* is a standard, silicone-based eye-makeup remover. This is definitely less greasy than the Lait Tendre above, but it's still similar to many other versions available for a lot less money.

☹ **Energizing Radiance Lotion** *($32.50 for 6.8 ounces)* With alcohol as the second ingredient this ends up being energetically irritating and drying for all skin types.

☹ **Gentle Hydrating Lotion** *($32.50 for 6.8 ounces)* also lists alcohol as the second ingredient, which makes it neither gentle nor hydrating.

☹ **Oil-Controlling Purifying Lotion** *($32.50 for 6.8 ounces)*. Another alcohol-based toner? What is Chanel thinking? This won't control oil, but it can add dryness and irritation to an oily skin problem.

☹ **Time Fighting Revitalizing Lotion** *($32.50 for 6.8 ounces)*. This toner lists alcohol as the fourth ingredient, which makes this definitely less problematic than the other toners but contains little else of benefit for skin. The teeny amount of water-binding agent in here and the lack of antioxidants makes this an overpriced, poorly formulated toner.

☺ $$$ **Maximum Radiance Delicate Exfoliator** *($30 for 2.6 ounces)* uses plant fiber as the exfoliant in a lotion base that would be appropriate for someone with normal to dry skin. It works well and is fairly gentle.

✓☺ $$$ **Age Delay Eye Rejuvenation Eye Gel** *($50 for 0.5 ounce)* comes with all sorts of beguiling claims that it can correct, prevent, and rejuvenate eye-area problems such as dark circles, puffiness, and fine lines. According to Chanel, the end result should be a wide-awake, luminous look. According to the ingredient list, this is a good, gel-based moisturizer that contains a sufficient amount of silicone to make the skin feel silky-smooth and also some interesting water-binding agents, though it lacks any significant antioxidants. It will address normal to slightly dry skin, but nothing in this product is capable of lightening dark circles or reducing puffiness. It does showcase tamarind seed polysaccharide as one of its main ingredients. What tamarind can do in a cosmetic application is unclear. It doesn't perform well as an antioxidant (Source: *Phytotherapy Research*, March 1999, pages 128–132), but it does work well for wound healing (Source: *European Journal of Ophthalmology*, January-March 2000, pages 71–76). It can be helpful for skin, but no more so than many other ingredients, from vitamin E to copper, and none of that has to do with puffy eyes or dark circles.

✓☺ **$$$ Age Delay Rejuvenation Serum** *($60 for 1 ounce)* is a very good lightweight, silicone-based moisturizer for normal to slightly dry skin. It contains a good mix of antioxidants and water-binding agents, but none of that will delay one second of aging from your face.

☹ **$$$ Radiance Revealing Serum** *($55 for 1 ounce).* This lightweight lotion offers little in the way of antioxidants or water-binding agents, but it does contain proteases, and that is unique. Proteases are enzymes that are part of a process affecting the breakdown of amino acids and proteins in skin (Source: http://www.chemistry-info.net/). There is research showing that proteases applied topically to skin can reduce the visible scaling associated with dry, flaky skin (Source: *Archives of Dermatological Research*, November 2001, pages 500–507). However, breaking down proteins and amino acids may not necessarily be the best way to deal with getting rid of unwanted skin. Whether or not proteases can be of benefit for wound healing when applied topically is unclear (Source: *Experimental Dermatology*, October 2001, pages 337–348). This is a unique product to consider, but given the lack of research for the use of proteases in skin care, it is likely you will be gaining more of an experimental experience than guaranteed results.

☹ **$$$ Eye Correction Anti-Wrinkle Firming Eye Cream** *($50 for 0.5 ounce)* is a good moisturizer for dry skin, but there is nothing about this product that makes it preferable for the eyes. If anything, the other moisturizers in the Chanel line have better antioxidant concentrations and far more interesting water-binding agents.

✓☺ **$$$ HydraMax Balanced Hydrating Cream** *($40 for 1.7 ounces)* is a very good moisturizer for dry skin that contains an impressive mix of antioxidants, water-binding agents, plant oils, and a small amount of anti-irritants. It does contain balm mint, but the amount is so small that it would pose no irritation risk for skin.

✓☺ **$$$ HydraMax Balanced Hydrating Gel** *($40 for 1.7 ounces)* is a lightweight, silicone-based gel moisturizer that would work well for normal to slightly dry skin. It contains an impressive mix of antioxidants, water-binding agents, plant oils, and a small amount of anti-irritants. It does contain balm mint, but the amount is so small that it would have no irritation risk for skin.

☺ **$$$ HydraMax Oil-Free Hydrating Gel** *($40 for 1.7 ounces)* is basically identical to the Balanced version above, only this one includes clay and aluminum starch octenylsuccinate as the third and fourth ingredients, respectively. These absorbents can definitely leave a matte finish on the skin, which may be an option for someone with normal to oily skin. It does contain a good complement of antioxidants and water-binding agents. The minute amount of balm mint and caffeine is probably not a problem for skin.

☺ **$$$ Fluide Multi-Protection Daily Protection Lotion SPF 25** *($26 for 1 ounce)* is a very good, in-part titanium dioxide–based sunscreen in a lightweight, matte-finish lotion that would work well for someone with normal to slightly dry skin. It does contain a small amount of good water-binding agents.

☺ $$$ **Skin Conscience Total Health Oil-Free Moisture Fluid SPF 15** *($45 for 1.7 ounces)* is a decent sunscreen with avobenzone as one of the active UVA-protecting ingredients and it would be good for someone with normal to oily skin. It has a slight matte finish (thanks to the talc and the aluminum starch octenylsuccinate), and contains some very good antioxidants and water-binding agents. That's all good news and this is indeed an option for daily sun protection if you apply it liberally (which the price tag might prevent you from doing). However, while I don't doubt Chanel's claim that this product has been sensitive-skin tested, allergy tested, and comedogenicity tested, without an opportunity to see any test results, I wouldn't suggest you rely on this product to not cause you problems if you have sensitive skin or if you tend to break out. There are more than 80 ingredients in this product, and that should cause concern for someone with sensitive skin, not to mention the fragrance and synthetic sunscreen agents. It's not that the sunscreen ingredients are bad, it's just that synthetic ones like avobenzone tend to produce more irritation than the mineral sunscreen ingredients titanium dioxide and zinc oxide. In terms of breakouts, there are a few suspect ingredients here that will require testing to see how your skin reacts. One more point: This product does contain a teeny amount of salicylic acid, but neither the amount nor the pH of 5.5 this product sports allows it to have any exfoliating benefit for skin.

☺ $$$ **Skin Conscience Total Health Moisture Cream SPF 15** *($45 for 1.7 ounces)* is almost identical to the Oil-Free version above only minus the talc and aluminum starch octenylsuccinate. That makes this one better for normal to dry skin.

✓☺ $$$ **Rectifiance Day Lift Refining Cream SPF 15** *($60 for 1.7 ounces)* is a very good sunscreen with an in-part avobenzone sunscreen for UVA protection. This formulation would work well for normal to dry skin plus it contains an excellent combination of antioxidants and water-binding agents. It does contain lactic acid (AHA) and a teeny amount of salicylic acid (BHA), but the pH of 5 is too high to allow either the AHA or BHA to be effective as exfoliants.

✓☺ $$$ **Rectifiance Day Lift Refining Lotion SPF 15** *($50 for 1.7 ounces)* is almost identical to the Cream version above, only in lotion form, and the same basic comments apply.

☹ $$$ **Rectifiance Day Lift Refining Oil-Free Lotion SPF 15** *($50 for 1.7 ounces)* is similar to the Refining Lotion version above, only with a far more matte finish. Disappointingly, this contains witch hazel distillate, and that can be drying; it also uses aluminum starch octenylsuccinate, an absorbent, to help create the matte finish, and that can be helpful for oily skin.

✓☺ $$$ **Rectifiance Nuit Night Lift Restoring Cream** *($50 for 1.7 ounces)* has one of the longest ingredient listings I've ever seen. Whether you need all of that is a decision that rests with you, but aside from the incredible redundancy between this and several other Chanel products, it turns out to be a good moisturizer for dry skin with a very good assortment of water-binding agents and antioxidants. The pH of the cream isn't low enough for the AHA or BHA to work as exfoliants.

☺ $$$ **Rectifiance Nuit Night Lift Restoring Lotion** *($60 for 1.7 ounces)* is similar to the Cream above only in lotion form, plus it contains aluminum starch octenylsuccinate, which can leave a matte finish on the skin. This may be an option for normal to oily skin, but you have to ask yourself, why apply a moisturizer with ingredients that absorb moisture? The pH of the cream isn't low enough to allow the AHA or BHA to work as exfoliants.

☺ $$$ **Lift Serum Extreme Anti-Wrinkle Firming Complex** *($70 for 1 ounce)* is another lifting product—what a surprise. If the collagen and elastin in this product were so great for preventing wrinkles, why aren't they present in any of the other products? Collagen and elastin are basically just water-binding agents, and that's good, but it's hardly unique and is neither extreme nor lifting. This does contain some good antioxidants and water-binding agents, but not as many as several other Chanel options. Plus this one lists arnica as the fourth ingredient, and that can be a skin irritant.

☺ $$$ **Hydra Serum Vitamin Moisture Boost** *($50 for 1 ounce)* lists alcohol as the third ingredient. That's confusing for a product claiming to be a moisturizing boost, and the ingredients in this one don't make for as interesting a formulation as many in the Chanel camp.

☺ $$$ **Skin Recovery Cream** *($160 for 1.7 ounces)* is an OK moisturizer for normal to dry skin that contains a good mix of emollient, water-binding agents, and teeny, almost inconsequential amounts of antioxidants. Dollar for dollar, this is a far less impressive moisturizer than many others you could select if you were interested in Chanel products.

☺ $$$ **Skin Recovery Emulsion** *($130 for 1.7 ounces)* is similar to the Recovery Cream version above and the same basic comments apply.

☺ $$$ **Skin Recovery Eye Cream** *($95 for 0.5 ounce)* is an emollient moisturizer that contains mostly water, thickeners, film-forming agent, mineral oil, lanolin, silicone, water-binding agents, plant oil, anti-irritant, and antioxidants. This is a good option for normal to dry skin, though for the money the amount of antioxidants you get is not impressive.

☺ $$$ **Solution Destressante Calming Emulsion** *($30 for 3.4 ounces)* is a silicone-based moisturizer with a good antioxidant and some good water-binding agents. It isn't as impressive as others in this group, but it would be an option for normal to slightly dry skin.

☹ **T-Mat Shine Control** *($25 for 1 ounce)* contains alcohol and witch hazel as the second and third ingredients, respectively, which makes this too drying and potentially irritating for all skin types.

☹ **Ultra Correction Anti-Wrinkle Restructuring Lotion SPF 10** *($65 for 1.7 ounces)*. It is incredibly disappointing to see any modern, expensive product that has only an SPF 10. Every national medical association states that an SPF of at least 15 is desirable. Chanel's Ultra Correction does contain an in-part avobenzone-based sunscreen, but the optimum SPF is as crucial for the skin as the UVA-protecting active ingredients. Apart from the low

SPF, this product claims to have "synergistically powerful" ingredients that firm and resculpt the skin "as if surface skin is bonded to its support system." Here's a news flash: Surface skin already *is* bonded to its support system—the dermis and subcutaneous layer of fat. It is the lower layers of skin (plus facial ligaments, muscles, bone, fat, and collagen) that deteriorate with age or years of unprotected sun exposure, and none of them can be affected in any way by this product. Along with the enticing claims comes Chanel's "unique resculpting massage," which supposedly relaxes facial muscles "contracted by aging." Yet facial muscles do not contract with age, they simply diminish in mass. It is this process, coupled with the fact that the skin continues to grow as the muscles and bone break down, that eventually leads to sagging, which can be corrected with plastic surgery but not by massage of any kind.

☹ **Ultra Correction Anti-Wrinkle Restructuring Cream SPF 10** *($65 for 1.7 ounces)* is almost identical to the Lotion version above, only the Cream version is more emollient.

☺ **$$$ Ultra Correction Anti-Wrinkle Restructuring Night Cream** *($75 for 1.7 ounces)* will not help anyone "rediscover the look of youth" unless their skin is dry—in which case this is an OK moisturizer (though not unique or ultra in any way).

☺ **$$$ Controle Imperfections Blemish Control** *($26 for 0.5 ounce)* comes in the tiniest quantity and is the most expensive BHA product I've seen, not to mention that the concentration of BHA is only 0.5%. The somewhat emollient gel base is fine for normal to dry skin, but the pH isn't low enough for it to be effective as an exfoliant (it has a pH of 5), so why bother?

☺ **$$$ Masque Force Hydratante** *($28.50 for 2.6 ounces)* is a standard emollient mask with a film-forming agent. While this is a very good moisturizer with some good water-binding agents for normal to dry skin, the mask part doesn't really add any benefit.

☺ **$$$ Masque Lift Express** *($32.50 for 2.6 ounces)* won't lift the skin anywhere, but it is an OK moisturizer for normal to dry skin.

☺ **$$$ Masque Purete** *($28.50 for 2.6 ounces)* is an exceptionally standard clay mask that would work as well as any. The pH is too high for the BHA it contains to have any exfoliating properties.

☺ **$$$ Lip Correction Lip Cure** *($27.50 for 0.5 ounce)* includes a group of ingredients that can't cure anything. This is basically just film-forming agent, emollients, and talc, sort of a lightweight spackle mixed with hairspray. It goes on greasy and then dries to a matte finish. That's nice, but it doesn't do much for lips and only minimally helps prevent lipstick from feathering.

CHANEL MAKEUP

Chanel's makeup in its distinctively branded black lacquer packaging with the signature intertwined "C" continues to evoke the promise of elegant affluence, all the while carrying on the same strengths and weaknesses seen over the past several years. Their foundations have some of the most enviable textures around, and their latest powders feel incredible since the shine from the past has been replaced by a velvety matte finish. The mascaras are all stellar and the lipsticks offer some lush textures and rich, opalescent colors. Aside from the illusion of high fashion and designer panache, the fact is that much of what Chanel does well, other lines do just as well (and sometimes better) and with a more realistic price range to boot. Underneath all of the sleek packaging lie some very ordinary and even a few lackluster products, such as most of the eye, lip, and brow pencils and a few of the concealers. Overspending on such items does not make sense, and can end up being disheartening.

FOUNDATION: ☹ **$$$ Teint Fluide Universale Multi-Vitamin Natural Makeup SPF 15** *($37.50)*. How disappointing that this silky-feeling foundation, with its satin-smooth finish, light coverage, and relatively inexpensive price tag (given Chanel's tendency for outlandish price points) wastes a decent SPF by including no UVA-protecting ingredients! Come on, Chanel—I know you know this one because you use avobenzone in your skin-care products and you've used titanium dioxide in other foundations. However, if you as a consumer are already using an effective sunscreen with UVA-protecting ingredients, then this still may be a foundation to consider. The five colors are exceptionally neutral, though there are no options for very light or darker skin tones. Despite the strong points, it's hard to know exactly to whom I should recommend this foundation. The soft matte finish is a bit deceiving because this foundation definitely has shine and the shine does stick around all day. This is supposed to reflect light so as to hide wrinkles. If you believe that bit of cosmetics absurdity, go for it—but it will look like shine in any light, and for wrinkles that's not good news. Those with oily skin won't appreciate the added shine either. All in all, the strong points are somewhat negated by the weak points. Therefore, if you're intrigued, try this one on, wear it all day, and check it in really good light before making the investment. **Teint Naturel SPF 8** *($52.50)* has a gorgeous, lightly creamy texture and an impeccable, natural finish that provides light to medium coverage. If this had an SPF 15 with appropriate UVA-protecting ingredients (it fails on both counts), it would be a great option despite the unwarranted price tag. The eight shades are mostly fine, except Warm Beige and Tawny Beige.

✓☺ **$$$ Teint Cristallin Waterlights Sheer Makeup Stick** *($37.50)* has a soft, flawless, creamy application that dries to a silky, very soft powder finish. This is definitely a sheer to light coverage makeup and the eight shades, though all slightly warm-toned (meaning slightly yellow), are wonderful, with some great colors for very light skin tones but none for darker skin tones. Only Sunlit and Sand are slightly peach, but even they are still worth considering. This would be a suitable stick foundation for normal to slightly oily skin. ✓☺ **$$$ Double Perfection Fluide Matte Reflecting Makeup SPF 15** *($40)* has an amazing silky, light texture that blends incredibly well over the skin, but it dries quickly to a solid matte finish that will unfortunately enhance any dry, flaky skin you may already have. The silicone-in-water emulsion and the in-part titanium dioxide–based sunscreen make this excellent for those with normal to oily skin who want to use as few products on the face as possible. Coverage is in the light to medium range, and despite the foundation's

The Reviews C

matte finish, it does not look or feel thick or heavy on the skin and it has good staying power. There are nine gorgeous shades, with nary an overtone of peach, pink, rose, or ash. The colors offer options for light to dark (but not very dark) skin. If the price doesn't bother you, this foundation is highly recommended. ✓☺ $$$ **Bronze Universal de Chanel** *($40)* is a gorgeous cream-to-powder bronzer housed in a large glass jar. It comes in one color, a medium golden tan, and it meshes well with the skin, leaving a sheer semi-matte finish. ✓☺ $$$ **Sheer Brilliance** *($36.50)* is a generous (for Chanel) sized bottle of liquid shimmer that can be used anywhere, though it's recommended for the face, with or without foundation. It has a definite, though subtle, shine and imparts a soft hint of color.

☺ $$$ **Teint Lift Eclat SPF 8** *($52)* has an unbelievably lovely silken texture and blends beautifully to a natural finish capable of light to medium coverage. It works well for someone with oily to combination skin or normal skin, but isn't emollient enough for someone with dry or sun-damaged skin. Seven shades are available, with options for very light skin tones, but not for very dark skin tones. The following shades are too peach or rose for most skin tones: Warm Bisque, Clear Beige, and Golden Honey. Despite the disappointingly low SPF rating, the sunscreen does include some titanium dioxide, but neither is enough for the kind of protection needed to protect from sun damage. **Double Perfection Matte Reflecting Powder Makeup SPF 10** *($45)* does have UVA-protecting ingredients but the insufficient SPF 10 is disappointing, especially given the price tag. Yet this is still a wonderful pressed-powder foundation, with a silky-smooth, seamless finish and 12 stunning, fairly neutral shades. This is best applied dry, using a sponge or a powder brush. **Vitalumiere Satin Smoothing Fluid Makeup SPF 15** *($50)* almost had everything going for it, but Chanel inexplicably didn't include UVA-protecting ingredients. The liquid texture is irresistibly smooth, and blends with ease to a light to medium coverage satin finish. Yet using words like "vibrant" and "young" to describe this is disingenuous considering the incomplete sunscreen (and Chanel knows better because many of their sunscreens do include UVA-protecting ingredients). Still, for those with normal to dry skin willing to pair this with a good sunscreen, the nine colors present some impressive options. The only shades to avoid due to rose or peach tones are Soft Bisque, Natural Beige, and Sienna Caramel. **Vitalumiere Satin Smoothing Crème Makeup SPF 15** *($55)* is the creamy version of the Fluid makeup above, and it is extremely moist. Those with dry skin and a hefty cosmetics budget will appreciate this foundation's rich feel and finish, and it never veers into heaviness or looks too thick on the skin. If only the sunscreen contained adequate UVA-protecting ingredients, Chanel would have hit a bull's-eye. As it stands, a separate sunscreen is needed underneath. Of the nine mostly beautiful colors, watch out for Soft Bisque, Natural Beige, and Sienna Caramel—these are too pink or peach for most skins.

CONCEALER: ☹ **Visage Parfait Correction Perfection Face Kit** *($58.50)* is a compact with a concealer, a yellow color corrector, a shiny bronze "luminizer," a creamy, very shiny "brightener," an itty-bitty wrinkle-fill-in pencil called Line Perfector, and an equally small nylon brush. It is ridiculously overpriced and all the worse for the creamy, thick texture of the concealer and corrector (both will crease), not to mention the notion that a peach-toned, powder-finish pencil will somehow fill in facial lines. There is only one set of colors and they are suited to fair/light skin tones, in spite of Chanel's "one size fits all" decree. **Line Perfector Face Pencil** *($22.50)* is the same golden peach–colored standard pencil available in the kit above, only this is the full-size version. Don't bother. **Estompe de Chanel Corrective Concealer** *($32.50)* is a creamy, lipstick-style concealer with light coverage and poor colors that can easily crease into lines around the eye. **Extreme Estompe Cover Up** *($28.50)* comes in a tube and has a smooth, creamy texture, but the three shades are noticeably peach, green, or pink, and they tend to easily crease into any lines around the eyes.

☺ $$$ **Estompe Professionelle Professional Concealer Duo SPF 15** *($35)* features two thick, creamy concealers in one compact. There are three duos in all, and although the colors are respectable, these can leave a chalky finish on the skin and have a slight tendency to crease. What's keeping this from earning a sad face is the fact that if you're patient enough you can gain great coverage of dark circles and other discolorations—and the sunscreen is pure titanium dioxide.

✓☺ $$$ **Quick Cover** *($32.50)* has a silky, light texture and offers even, opaque coverage. This one could easily take the place of Chanel's other concealers, although it is only available in two (very good) colors.

POWDER: ☺ $$$ **Natural Finish Pressed Powder** *($40)* has a very smooth texture and a soft, dry finish. This talc-based powder comes in five shades, and only Translucent Sun should be avoided since it is too yellow for most skin tones. **Sunlit Powder** *($45)* is a pressed bronzing powder that features two complementary colors swirled together. There are versions for light and medium skin tones, and this has a smooth texture and very subtle sheen. ✓☺ **Natural Finish Loose Powder** *($45)* has an extremely fine, sifted texture and a soft matte finish that looks beautiful on skin. It is talc-based and comes in the same pleasing array of colors as the Pressed Powder above. The Translucent Sun shade is not as yellow here, and has a greater chance of working for light skin tones.

☹ **Powderlights** *($48.50)* is all about packaging. It comes in an awkward container with a powder brush attached to the base of the container as part of the cap. You have to remove the cap and then get the powder onto the brush, either by shaking the powder onto the brush, which is messy, or shaking some of the powder onto a tissue and then using the brush to pick up some of the powder. Why anyone would want to bother with this contrivance, the four unconventional, slightly shiny colors, and the cost is beyond me.

☺ $$$ **Perfecting Bronzing Powder SPF 8** *($38.50)* is available in one shade, a reddish tan that is best for medium skin tones. It is matte and blends nicely, but don't count on it for sun protection with its measly SPF 8 and no UVA-protecting ingredients.

BLUSH: ☺ $$$ **Powder Blush** *($37.50)* goes on very smoothly and has a dry finish. The selection of 14 rich shades is lovely, though some of them are obviously shiny; still, there are enough matte shades here to merit a look.

☺ **$$$ Aqua Blush Waterlights Sheer Cheeks** *($35)* is a replacement for Chanel's former (and preferred) Face Brights. This version has a creamy, slightly wet texture and a moist, slightly sticky sheer finish. The biggest demerit these now have is that each shade is loaded with iridescence—and for a natural or understated look that doesn't hold water. If the concept sounds appealing, Aveda has their own version of this product, Cooling Calming Color ($18), for half the price. **Face Colour Pencil** *($35)* is one more oversized, double-ended pencil. It is a versatile product that has a soft, creamy texture and blends well enough, but the cheek appeal is only for those with dry skin. Some may find it OK to use as a lipstick (although constantly having to sharpen it is a pain), but as an eyeshadow it easily creases.

☹ **Bronze Perfection Face Palette** *($58.50)* is a compact that just about writes the book on shimmer. If your idea of bronzed perfection involves paying top dollar for tiny pie-shaped wedges of a light and dark shiny powder along with peach and coppery tan shimmer creams then look no further.

EYESHADOW: Chanel unabashedly sells shiny eyeshadows. Whereas many of today's eyeshadows with shine have been toned down, Chanel's nicely pigmented shadows really lay it on thick. ☺ **$$$ Quadra Eyeshadow** *($52.50)* has some very strange, contrasting color groupings alongside some worthwhile but shiny sets. There are a few matte shades, but in order to get a return on your investment, it makes sense to use all of the eyeshadows (if you can figure out how to do so without looking clownish), and that means surrendering to some intense iridescence. What a shame the matte choices just aren't here, because the textures are supremely smooth. Of all the Quadra Eyeshadows, Mysteres and Euphoria have the most difficult combinations of colors to work with. **Shadowlights** *($27)* are single eyeshadow colors, and the small selection of shades offers some beautiful neutral options, though most of them have prominent shine. The texture of these is just marvelous, and if you're in the mood to really splurge, the almost-matte options to note are Daylight Beige and Nightlight Taupe. One caution: Applying these too thickly can cause flaking, so start sheer.

☺ **$$$ Basic Eye Color** *($45)* is a compact of eyeshadows holding three similarly toned shades in varying depths of color, including an eyeliner shade. At least one shade in each is shiny. The color groupings are mostly flattering, but they have a dry, grainy texture that can go on choppy. If Chanel shadows put a twinkle in your eye, choosing from the Quadra compacts above will yield better results.

EYE AND BROW SHAPER: ✔☺ **$$$ Sculpting Brow Pencil** *($26)* is a very good option for a brow pencil, with a smooth powder texture and two good shades that allow for a soft, natural look. This can go on too thick unless some restraint is used. What a shame that the price will assuredly raise some brows! ✔☺ **Precision Brow Definer** *($26)* is a standard pencil that has a texture and application that's a step above most brow pencils. This goes on softly and has a dry, smooth finish. If only the price weren't so high!

☺ **$$$ Liquid Eyelines** *($28.50)* now has a very nice, clean application of intense color that dries in good time, stays on, and doesn't smudge. For the money, I would still consider liquid eyeliners from L'Oreal or Almay before this one.

☺ $$$ **Precision Eye Definer** *($26)* is a very expensive, utterly standard pencil that has a soft texture, a slightly dry finish, and an angled sponge tip for blending. Nothing is extraordinary here except the price. **Eye Liner Duo** *($28.50)* is a double-ended, automatic pencil that can also be retracted. One end is a matte shade, the other is shiny. Both sides have a creamy texture and slight powder finish that can easily smudge and smear unless you're very careful. **Aqua Crayon Eye Colour Stick** *($22.50)* is an automatic, nonretractable eye pencil that has a creamy, slick application. Chanel maintains this is waterproof, and although it does hold up well when wet, the creaminess can lead to smudging and fading.

☹ **Perfect Brows** *($67.50)* is a set of three powdered brow colors (taupe, medium brown, and brownish black), Smurf-sized tweezers, and a grooming brush. The intent is for women to mix and match among the three shades to achieve their "Perfect Brow," but this ends up being useless for anyone with light hair (which means all blondes), who could only use the lightest color, and what are brunettes supposed to do with two dark colors, one of which will undoubtedly make the brows look severe? I could go on, but you get the idea. I admit that the concept has merit, because no one's brows are all one color, but there are dozens upon dozens of suitable brow powders and eyeshadows that perform beautifully and aren't so insultingly expensive. **Brow Shaper** *($28.50)* is a brow gel with a very small color selection: Taupe and Clear. There are no shades for brunettes, light blondes, or redheads, and even though it does keep brows in place, it also tends to glob onto the hairs and flake once it's dried. Origins' Just Browsing ($12) is a far superior option. **On-the-Double Eye Crayon** *($28.50)* is a group of standard, dual-ended pencils, all of them too creamy to last, with plenty of shine to spare.

LIPSTICK AND LIP PENCIL: ☺ $$$ **Infrarouge Whisperlight Lipstick** *($21.50)* has a slick, opaque texture and a slightly greasy feel that quickly dissipates into a fairly weightless, reasonably long-wearing lip color. The extensive color selection features several different finishes, including iridescent, metallic, satin, and a sheer version, which is less intensely pigmented. This is just a good creamy lipstick with a luxury price tag. **Hydrabase Creme Lipstick** *($21.50)* has an excellent creamy, slightly greasy texture and a splendid variety of opaque colors. It's not worth this amount of money, but do women buy Chanel for performance or for the image it evokes? **Hydracaresse Hydra Treatment Lipstick SPF 15** *($22.50)* does not contain any UVA-protecting ingredients but it is a very emollient, thick-textured lipstick with rich, opaque colors that leaves a slight stain. The base formula is nearly identical to the Hydrabase Creme Lipstick above.

☺ $$$ **Precision Lip Definer** *($26)* is shockingly similar to dozens of other lip pencils and absolutely not worth the fee, when everyone from Max Factor to Revlon has their version (with a brush) for so much less. **Lip Liner Duo** *($28.50)* is identical in concept and packaging to the Eye Liner Duo above. There is a matte and a shiny side, and many women will invariably find they favor one color over the other, which makes this all the more frivolous.

☺ $$$ **Hydrasoleil Sheer Lipstick SPF 6** *($21.50)* is a small group of light-coverage, slightly greasy lipsticks with no UVA-protecting ingredients. Even with the right sun protection, SPF 6 is well below the recommended SPF 15. **Hydracaresse Hydra-Treatment Lip Care SPF 15** *($22.50)* does not contain UVA-protecting ingredients and is nothing more than a very sheer, greasy lipstick that is available in one peachy pink tint.

☹ **Protective Lip Color** *($22.50)* is little more than a pink lipstick that is sold as a clear base to use before applying lipstick to prevent the color from changing. It doesn't work. **Glossimer** *($24)* has a sumptuous name and a bevy of sparkling colors but all that does little to make this very standard, thick, and sticky gloss deserve such a jaw-dropping price. **Aqua Crayon Lip Colour Stick** *($22.50)* is an automatic lip pencil that is too creamy and smear-prone on its own, let alone paired with a creamy or glossy lipstick!

☺ $$$ MASCARA: ✓☺ **Instant Lash Mascara** *($21.50)* impressively builds long, thick lashes fairly fast, so the name is apropos, and you'll be able to achieve this with no smudging or smearing! ✓☺ **Sculpting Mascara Extreme Length** *($21.50)* and ✓☺ **Extreme Length Fine Lashes** *($21.50)* consist of a single mascara formula that comes packaged with two different brush options. The Extreme Length Fine Lashes contains a very tiny, thin brush that builds exceptionally long lashes with no clumping. The Sculpting Mascara Extreme Length has a full round brush that is far less impressive at building long lashes, though it's still a good lengthening mascara. ✓☺ **Extreme Cils Drama Lash Mascara** *($21.50)* is primarily a lengthening mascara, and has a much cleaner application than it used to. For the most part you will be amazed at how effortlessly this elongates your lashes.

☺ $$$ **Extreme Wear Waterproof Mascara** *($21.50)* lengthens well and thickens minimally. Although it applies easily enough, it is definitely unimpressive at this price, and did not pass the waterproof test with flying colors. **Super Curl Lengthening Mascara** *($21.50)*. They have to be joking with the "super" part of the name, but it isn't too funny considering the price of this below-average mascara. You will achieve some length and the lashes are cleanly separated, but curl is practically nonexistent, as is any thickness. Chanel (and many other lines) have done better with their other mascaras.

☺ $$$ BRUSHES: Chanel does present an attractive, satiny, and comparably priced collection of brushes *($22.50–$45)*. Many of them are very useful, with excellent shapes and sizes. For your consideration, take a look at the ✓☺ **#2 Eyeshadow** *($22.50)*; the small but good for detailed work ✓☺ **#1 Eyeshadow** *($22.50)*; the versatile ✓☺ **#11 Eyeshadow** *($25)*; as well as the soft and full ✓☺ **Blush** *($38)* and ✓☺ **Powder** *($45)* brushes if you're feeling particularly spendy. The **Foundation Brush** *($32.50)* is also excellent if for some reason you're inclined to use one.

Avoid the **#4 Shadow/Line Brush** *($22)*, which is scratchy, the **#15 Lip Brush** *($22.50)*, which is unrealistically tiny, and the **#10 Contour Face Brush** *($38)*, which is too large and flimsy to allow precise contouring.

The Reviews C

CHANTAL ETHOCYN (SKIN CARE ONLY)

Chantal Ethocyn has had a rocky road since it was first launched as the new miracle answer for wrinkles in the 1990s. Thanks to some clever press releases accompanied by an endorsement from a clinical professor of dermatology at UCLA who tested Ethocyn on 20 people, their sales and stock went through the roof. But by the end of 1998 no other physicians had spoken up, nor was there any published research substantiating the company's claims (Source: *Seminars in Cutaneous Medicine and Surgery*, September 1996, pages 139–144). Their revenues decreased 51%, the Securities and Exchange Commission was looking into the company's recordkeeping, the company was struggling with a lawsuit, and the stock price was less than $10 per share (today the stock price is 3 cents a share). Now, after trying a round of drugstore and infomercial sales (which failed), these products have finally found a home on the Internet (though you have to call to order), with price tags that are just hard to swallow. Ah, the business of beauty!

Chantal is Chantal Burnison, the founder of the company. Ethocyn is the trade name of her patented ingredient, ethoxyheptyl bicyooctanoe. It is supposed to be a natural molecule that improves moisture retention and builds elastin in the skin. If Ethocyn is effective, only the Chantal Ethocyn Corporation and the physician who did the original study know about it. (By the way, the original study, which was not published or peer reviewed, was not done double-blind or with a placebo, nor did it compare the product to an alternative vehicle containing, say, vitamin C or vitamin E for that matter. That isn't much of a study.) There isn't much besides Ethocyn in these products. The lack of both antioxidants and impressive water-binding agents and the absence of a sunscreen in the group means the Chantal Ethocyn line leaves much to be desired in comparison to products in the same pricey neighborhood, not to mention in far less expensive ones. For more information about Ethocyn, call (888) 242-6825 or visit www.ethocyn.com.

☹ **Gel Cleanser** *($23 for 6.7 ounces)* lists alcohol as the second ingredient, so this otherwise standard, astoundingly overpriced cleanser/toner is an irritation waiting to happen.

☺ $$$ **A.M. Eye Rescue Cream** *($30 for 0.5 ounce)* is a fairly standard moisturizer for dry skin that contains some water, slip agents, thickeners, water-binding agents, more thickeners, preservatives, and, of course, Ethocyn. It does contain shine and fragrance.

☺ $$$ **Botanical Booster Cream** *($45 for 2 ounces)* is a fairly emollient, Vaseline-based moisturizer that includes some good water-binding agents, Ethocyn, silicone, several fragrant plant oils, preservatives, and coloring agents.

☺ $$$ **Essence Vials** *($45 for 0.33-ounce vial)* is just silicones, water-binding agents, antioxidants, and plant oil. It is a very expensive way to find out if Ethocyn works, which is the only reason to consider any of these products, so if you're curious, the less expensive versions in this line would work just as well.

☺ $$$ **Vital Zone Serum** *($55 for 1 ounce)* is almost identical in every way to the

Essence Vials above. Can they be thinking the price difference of almost $100 is a marketing ruse the consumer will never notice?

☺ $$$ **Ginseng Nourishing Cream** *($40 for 1.75 ounces)* is a very plain moisturizer for dry skin that contains the teeniest amount of ginseng imaginable, and even less Ethocyn than that.

☺ $$$ **Hydrating Complex** *($40 for 1.75 ounces)* is a good, silicone-based moisturizer that would work well for normal to slightly dry skin. This one has the best assortment of water-binding agents and it contains Ethocyn. It also contains fragrance.

☺ $$$ **Phyto Hydra Complex** *($40 for 1.75 ounces)* is similar to the Hydrating Complex above and the same comments apply.

☺ $$$ **Multi Action Day Cream** *($45 for 1.75 ounces)* is almost entirely water, slip agents, thickeners, silicones, shine, teeny amounts of water-binding agents, preservatives, Ethocyn, and fragrance. The plant extracts it contains are meant to sound like they have AHA benefits, but they have no function for skin, especially not such a minuscule amount.

☺ $$$ **Optimum Neck Cream** *($55 for 1.75 ounces)* is as ordinary a moisturizer as it gets. It contains water, thickeners, Vaseline, silicones, shine, preservatives, fragrance, Ethocyn, coloring agents, and fragrance.

☹ **P.M. Eye Renewal Cream** *($30 for 0.5 ounce)* is mostly witch hazel, some thickeners, and Ethocyn. This is not worth the money for any skin type.

☺ $$$ **Ultra Rich Night Cream** *($55 for 1.75 ounces)* is just water, thickeners, water-binding agents, preservatives, Ethocyn, and fragrance. This adds up to an ultrawaste of money and effort.

☺ $$$ **Revitalizing Masque** *($25 for 2 ounces)* is primarily almond meal and clays. That won't revitalize skin, but it can be an option for normal to oily skin.

CHANTECAILLE

Created by Sylvie Chantecaille, this line of makeup and skin-care products being sold at Neiman Marcus and some salons and spas draws on Chantecaille's 20 years of experience as an employee of the Estee Lauder corporation. The fact that she worked for Lauder and helped to create and launch the Prescriptives line is impressive. Experience alone means a lot in the crowded, complicated cosmetics industry, so it isn't startling that this veteran cosmetics-marketing executive would parlay her background into creating her own line. Unsurprisingly, she claims her products are "based on the purest most natural ingredients possible," though it only takes a cursory look at the ingredient listing to see that isn't true. Commenting on the synthetic agents that form the backbone of almost every cosmetic isn't as enticing to the consumer as talking about botanicals and food ingredients like fragrant plant extracts and oils. However, not one product in the Chantecaille product mix can hold a candle to those from Chantecaille's former employer. Whether they're from any of Lauder's department store lines, from Clinique to Prescriptives, they are far better formulated and cost a lot less money. The fragrance spilleth over from Chantecaille's products, the interesting ingredients are in the most meager amounts, and there isn't a sunscreen in the lot. What an utter disappointment. Chantecaille products are available exclusively at Neiman Marcus and Bergdorf Goodman, and at some salons around the country. For more information about Chantecaille, call (212) 343-3614 or visit www.neimanmarcus.com.

CHANTECAILLE SKIN CARE

☺ $$$ **Flower Infused Cleansing Milk** (*$43 for 3.4 ounces*) is basically a highly fragranced, cold cream–style lotion with a gentle detergent cleansing agent. It would be an option, though overpriced, for someone with normal to dry skin. The teeny amount of antioxidants in this product is immaterial.

☹ $$$ **Rice & Geranium Foaming Cleanser** (*$45 for 2.46 ounces*) is an exceptionally standard, detergent-based cleanser that is more drying than most. It can be an option for oily skin, but the real question is why would you want to spend this kind of money when cleansers from Neutrogena are virtually identical and don't contain the amount of fragrance this one does.

☹ **Pure Rosewater** (*$43 for 3.4 ounces*) is an incredibly appropriate name for an absurd product. For this amount of money all you're buying is rose water, slip agent, and preservatives. This is overpriced, in my estimation, by about $42.

☹ $$$ **Flower Harmonizing Cream** (*$95 for 1.7 ounces*) definitely contains plenty of fragrant plant extracts, but other than that this is just water, thickening agents, plant oils, and the tiniest amount of water-binding agents and antioxidant.

☹ $$$ **Retinol Intense** (*$82 for 1.7 ounces*) is similar to the Harmonizing Cream above only with the addition of retinol. There are far better retinol products to consider from Cetaphil to L'Oreal or Lancome.

☹ $$$ **Water Flower Fluid** (*$65 for 1.7 ounces*) is similar to the Harmonizing Cream above only in lotion form, and the same basic comments apply.

✓☺ $$$ **Vital Essence** (*$78 for 1.7 ounces*) contains mostly water, glycerin, slip agent, water-binding agents, plant oils, thickeners, antioxidants, more thickeners, and preservatives. This is a very well-formulated moisturizer for normal to dry skin. The soybean and kudzu extracts in it have no estrogen activity when applied topically (and especially not in this small amount), though they do have antioxidant properties.

☹ $$$ **Jasmine & Lily Healing Mask** (*$57 for 1.7 ounces*) is a very basic emollient and highly fragrant mask. It contains a minute amount of water-binding agents and antioxidants, and is not worth the money in the least.

CHANTECAILLE MAKEUP

Chantecaille's textures are the most notable aspect of the makeup collection; they are all impressive, with silky smoothness and even application. Sylvie Chantecaille claims she created her products by using technology that allows them to imperceptibly mesh with the skin, and it shows. The shortcoming is the shine. Almost everything shines, and although that can have a nice effect for evening or special occasions, for daytime a full face of shine is sort of like wearing a sequined outfit to the office.

FOUNDATION: ☺ $$$ **Real Skin Foundation SPF 15** *($49 with compact; $31 for refill)* and **Real Skin Foundation SPF 30** *($53 with compact; $31 for refill)* are almost identical to Vincent Longo's Water Canvas ($45). As I mention in my review of Longo's Water Canvas, these types of compact foundations are liquidy powders with a gel-like, wet feel that dry to a satiny-smooth, sheer, slightly matte finish. Chantecaille's works well for most skin types, and both versions have a sheerer finish than Longo's. The disadvantage is that Chantecaille has far fewer color choices, with only four shades of the Real Skin SPF 30 and five of the SPF 15 version, though two of those are color-correcting shades of pink (Cool) and yellow (Soft), which may work in a limited capacity for some skin tones. Although the pickings are slim, all of the flesh-tone colors are quite good, but are appropriate only for light to medium skin. An advantage over Longo's version is that they both contain titanium dioxide as the sunscreen! **New Stick Concealer & Foundation SPF 8** *($40)* is similar to many of the stick foundations on the market, from Lauder's Minute Makeup SPF 15 ($32.50) to Clinique's CityStick SPF 15 ($21) and Prescriptives' Exact Matchstick Foundation SPF 15 ($37)—and these are all titanium dioxide–based, too. Chantecaille's seven colors are great and the application is smooth and even for good medium coverage and they would work well for normal to dry skin. But for the money and the sunscreen factor, the Lauder, Clinique, and Prescriptives versions are definitely preferred (note that these products are all from Chantecaille's alma mater). **Compact Makeup** *($47)* is a standard, talc-based pressed powder with a wonderful silky-soft texture, but an absurd price. The six shades are nice and they can be used wet (like most pressed powders can be). This product claims that it is supposed to be hydrating, but it isn't—no powder can be. By its very nature it absorbs oil and water, and that's not hydrating in the least.

☺ $$$ **Future Skin Foundation** *($55)* has a creamy texture that blends out quite sheer and light. The light-reflecting claim comes from the shiny finish, which is indeed noticeable. The nine shades at first appear to be too pink or peach, but they blend on surprisingly neutral. The only one to consider avoiding (if you can put up with the aforementioned shiny finish) is Sand. By the way, although not labeled on the box or the ingredient list, the jar this comes in claims the makeup has an SPF 10. When I inquired as to why there was no SPF ingredient listed as an active ingredient, the company claimed the sun protection came from the seaweed this contains. Can anyone believe that seaweed offers any significant sun protection?

POWDER: ☺ $$$ **Loose Color Powder** *($45)* makes much ado about the fact that it is talc-free, which seems strange given that the Compact Makeup above contains talc. If there is something wrong with talc, why put it in any of these products? Talc is just fine in makeup. It has as silky and smooth a texture as any other mineral used on the face, and, as

The Reviews C

I've commented in the past, there is no health risk associated with the use of talc in face makeup. The shortcoming with this product is that because mica is used instead of talc, the two shades are shiny, which negates using it to reduce shine on the face. It's fine for a shiny dusting, but it's useless for setting makeup or reducing the shine from oil on the face.

☺ $$$ BLUSH: **Cheek Color Powder** *($21)*. With just six shades there isn't much selection, but these do have great soft, matte, silky textures, and the colors are all quite wearable. For equivalent textures and more down-to-earth prices, consider L'Oreal Feel Naturale Blush ($11.99) or Sonia Kashuk Beautifying Blush Powder ($8.99).

☺ $$$ EYESHADOW: **Lasting Eye Shadow Powder** *($21)* and **Shine Eye Shadow Powder** *($21)*. Trying to find the matte shades in this group of streamlined colors is not an easy task. Only a handful are supposed to have shine, but it turns out that most of them do. Of the supposed mattes, the shine isn't glaring, but if you were hoping for more matte selections this isn't the line to frequent. Aside from that, the textures are luscious and the most impressive part of the line. These can be used wet or dry without fear of creasing.

☺ $$$ LIPSTICK AND LIP PENCIL: **Lipstick** and **Lip Sheer** *($21)*. The Lip Sheer is more like a gloss, while the Lipstick is just a very standard, nice creamy lipstick. The color range is impressive but there is nothing extraordinary to get excited about. These claim to have an SPF between 6 and 8, but not only are those numbers too low for sunscreen, there are also no active sunscreen ingredients listed for this lipstick. **Lip Definer** *($19)* is awfully expensive for what amounts to the same standard pencil with a creamy application that almost every other line has. **Lip Gloss** *($21)* claims it protects "against sun, sea, or city," but other than placing a layer of emollient gloss over the lips (which can keep lips moist and keep air off of them), its protective abilities are slim. This is fine as far as glosses go and the colors are impressive, but not enough to warrant this price.

☺ $$$ BRUSHES: The brushes *($20–$70)* from Chantecaille feature exquisite textures and mostly practical shapes and cuts. The various **Eye Shadow Brushes** *($24–$30)* are pricey but worth a look, while the **Face Brush** *($70)* and **Cheek Brush** *($55)*, though nicely shaped, are too soft and fluffy for much control or ability to hold powders evenly. The **Lip Brush** *($28)* should, at this price, come with a cap or be retractable, but it does not have either feature. The **Eye Liner Brush** *($28)* is better for filling in brows than using with liner because the angled cut makes drawing one continuous line a challenge. Lastly, the **Concealer Brush** *($28)* is nicely sized and firm yet soft; however, it is made with natural hair instead of synthetic (nylon) bristles, and these can absorb concealer (and foundation), which means more product ends up on the brush than on your face.

SPECIALTY: **Sylvie Palette** *($120)* and **Olivia Palette** *($120)* are sleek, slim, metallic cases filled with seven eyeshadows and one blush shade, as well as the Basic Eye Brush. The Sylvie Palette features warm colors, while the Olivia (Sylvie's daughter and business partner) Palette opts for cool tones. Although the price is high, if you love Chantecaille's eyeshadows (and these colors in particular), this is actually a money-saving way to get them. The palettes are refillable, too.

CHRISTIAN DIOR

Dior has launched three skin-care collections since the previous edition of this book. It is a bit shocking to report that not one of these collections is impressive or an improvement from the previous line. It turns out that what was true about Dior in the previous editions of this book is still true today: Dior is a great name when it comes to haute couture. Yet, as often happens when a fashion house trademark expands to makeup and skin care, something inevitably gets lost in the translation. The packaging is really the star attraction here, as is typical of many high-end designer lines, and in this realm you will not be disappointed. Many Dior products are so bejeweled and ornamental that you may want to wear the packaging and forget what's inside! If this type of showmanship appeals to you, just be aware that that is what you end up paying for.

Dior's new lines are aimed at the twenty-something crowd, the forty-plus-something group, and the "I've got money to waste" crowd. Dior has attempted to stay abreast of the latest gimmicks and has added a few unique curves. But none of this ends up being beneficial for skin, because the truly interesting ingredients for most of the products are so far down at the end of the ingredient list they are inconsequential to the formula. One area that still remains a concern for this line, as is true for most European lines, is the fragrance wafting from these products, which is invasive. If you wouldn't put perfume on your face, think twice about applying it in the form of an expensive skin-care product. For more information about Christian Dior, call (800) 929-DIOR or visit www.dior.com.

CHRISTIAN DIOR SKIN CARE

CHRISTIAN DIOR iOD SKIN CARE

According to the Web site for *Cosmetics & Toiletries* magazine (www.thecosmetic site.com), "iOd, by Christian Dior, is aimed at appealing to the 17-25 age group. The key ingredient in the products is marine source water, which is demonstrated by the company to have been taken from a pure water reservoir discovered off the coast of Brittany's Ile Grande, 22 meters below sea level. The company presents it as pure in terms of microbiology—there is no life in it and it is stable. The water's mineral … makeup is reportedly similar to the makeup of the skin, which is able to replenish and restore the skin's equilibrium." Aside from the marketing language, regardless of where you get seawater from, seawater is seawater, and it definitely has similarities to the water content in skin cells. But as exotic as "deep sea" seawater sounds, water can only be absorbed by surface skin cells, and that doesn't balance anything or help skin any differently than water from, say, a faucet.

☺ $$$ **Clear Aqua Foam** *($20 for 5.1 ounces)* is an exceptionally standard, water-soluble cleanser that would work for most skin types. It does contain denatured alcohol, but just a teeny amount, not enough to be drying for skin.

The Reviews C

☺ Double Soap *($18 for 5.3 ounces)* is a dual-phase bar soap that, in spite of its attractive, artwork-like appearance, is just standard bar soap coupled with rather drying detergent cleansing agents. This offers no advantage over many far less expensive bar soaps.

☺ Mineral Aqua Gelee *($20 for 5.1 ounces)* is an extremely standard, silicone-based makeup remover. It would work as well as any.

☹ Duo Discs *($21 for 12 discs)* are nothing more than pads soaked in a standard detergent-cleansing base along with menthol and camphor, which can be irritating to skin. The price and the product are both a burn—and nothing in these discs can purify or exfoliate skin.

☺ $$$ Clear Aqua Lotion *($20 for 5.1 ounces)* is an extremely ordinary spray-on toner that would be OK for most skin types. The seawater sounds exotic, but when it comes to cosmetics water is water.

☹ Mineral Aqua Lotion *($20 for 5.1 ounces)* is similar to the Clear Aqua Lotion above, but is spoiled by the addition of alcohol and witch hazel. This spray-on toner is not recommended.

☺ $$$ Hydra-Sorbet Aquatique *($31 for 1.7 ounces)* is a lightweight, silicone-based moisturizer that also contains aluminum starch octenylsuccinate, which creates a matte, somewhat dry finish. In essence, there is little reason to consider this ho-hum formulation. If you have dry skin it won't be moisturizing enough, and if you have oily skin, it could be a good absorbent, but the silicones may feel too slippery, so you would want to try it first.

☹ Matte Aqua Fluid *($31 for 1.7 ounces)* claims it will "remove excess sebum [oil] and leave skin lastingly matte," but considering the amount of alcohol in here (it's the second ingredient), you can count on skin being irritated and confused, as this product also contains mineral oil.

☺ $$$ Aqua Powder *($23 for 0.36 ounce)* is an interesting option for keeping excess shine at bay—no doubt a concern many 17- to 25-year-olds share (the target market for Dior's iOd line). This applies like a powder, changes to a liquid on the skin, and then dries. The technology is similar to Prescriptives' Magic powders (which go on wet and then dry to a shiny finish), but this also has a subtle shine—which kind of defeats the purpose of powdering to reduce shine, doesn't it?

CHRISTIAN DIOR PRESTIGE SKIN CARE

The brochure from Dior states that the "Prestige line utilizes an extremely rare exclusive ingredient—a native flower nectar endowed with exceptional nourishing, energizing, and anti-oxidizing properties. Organically grown in the south of France, it must be hand-picked at dawn in order to preserve the integrity of its composition until it is incorporated in to the formulas." This mystery ingredient is *Kniphofia uvaria* nectar, from a plant of African origin, and it has some sugar and sorbitol added to it. There isn't a shred of research anywhere showing this to have any special properties for skin. Though you have to wonder, if this plant is so fragile and unstable that it has to be picked at a certain hour

The Reviews C

how could it ever hold up during the process of getting it into a cosmetic formulation? These products are ridiculously overpriced and with formulations that leave you wondering where's the meat?

☺ $$$ **Prestige Cleansing Cream** *($55 for 6.9 ounces)* is a basic lotion-style cleanser that needs a washcloth to remove all the makeup. There are no words for how ordinary this is. Lines from Neutrogena to Olay all have options that surpass this one. The tiny amounts of antioxidants and anti-irritants in this product are barely worth mentioning.

☹ **Prestige Rich Lotion** *($55 for 6.7 ounces)*. The second ingredient in this very fragrant, plain toner is alcohol, which makes it richly irritating and drying.

☺ $$$ **Prestige Cream for Eyes** *($70 for 0.5 ounce)* lists the third ingredient as aluminum starch octenylsuccinate, an absorbent that is about as far from moisturizing as you can get. This contains a small amount of water-binding agents, antioxidants, and anti-irritants, but for this kind of money, that's an insult.

☺ $$$ **Prestige Revitalizing Cream** *($150 for 1.7 ounces)*. I almost decided to give up writing about cosmetics when I saw this product. This rather standard moisturizer is easily replaced with a multitude of options for a fraction of the price. If the industry has women believing this very basic moisturizer is worth the money I have got to get another job! This will work for normal to slightly dry skin, and contains tiny amounts of water-binding agents, plant oils, and even smaller amounts of antioxidants. My only thought is, how sad!

☺ $$$ **Prestige Revitalizing Serum** *($170 for 1 ounce)* is a silicone-based moisturizer with wafting fragrance that contains small amounts of antioxidants and water-binding agents. It's an utter disappointment, because given the price tag it should have been so much more.

☺ $$$ **Prestige Massage Mask** *($110 for 1.7 ounces)* is mostly fragrant water, thickeners, talc, silicone, emollient, fragrance, preservatives, vitamin C, and anti-irritants. It would be an OK mask of sorts for normal to dry skin, but for the most part, even if it cost one-fourth as much, this is a real "Why bother?"

CHRISTIAN DIOR SNOW SKIN CARE

Ignoring proven skin-lightening agents such as hydroquinone and (to a lesser extent) kojic acid, Dior has created a whitening line based around magnesium ascorbyl phosphate, a stable form of vitamin C. This is one of the main ingredients in three of the five Snow products. Research into magnesium ascorbyl phosphate's ability to lighten skin via inhibition of melanin is scientifically promising (Sources: *Skin Research and Technology*, May 2002, page 73 and *Journal of the American Academy of Dermatology*, January 1996, pages 29–33). These studies used 3% and 10% concentrations, respectively. Although Dior does use magnesium ascorbyl phosphate as one of the main ingredients in the Snow moisturizers, they are not forthcoming about the percentage—so it's something of a leap of faith that these do indeed contain enough of a concentration to be effective. A few of these products are worth considering, but the prices are steep when you consider that many other lines offer products with magnesium ascorbyl phosphate for less. If you're curious about using higher levels of magnesium ascorbyl phosphate for skin lightening, consider DHC AntioxC ($32 for 1.4 ounces), to name just one.

☹ **Aqua Powder Whitening Cleanser** *($27.50 for 3.5 ounces)* is a talc-based powdered cleanser that must be mixed with water prior to use. This is more of a gimmick than anything else (were they going for a powdered snow effect?), as it does not clean any better than (and is certainly not preferred to) a gentle, water-soluble cleanser. It does contain polyethylene, a synthetic plastic that works as a mild abrasive. This can make for a rather scratchy cleanser that ends up being way overpriced for what you get. Nothing in this cleanser can whiten even one skin cell.

☹ **Radiance Whitening Lotion** *($42.50 for 6.7 ounces)* is an incredibly overpriced, alcohol-based toner that also contains licorice extract—an anti-irritant whose effect is lost when it's paired with alcohol. There is no reason to consider this product, and this contains nothing that can lighten the skin.

☺ $$$ **Enlightening Whitening Day Essence** *($85 for 1.7 ounces)* calls itself an "essential daytime treatment," but without an effective sunscreen, I would think twice before considering this serum-type moisturizer enlightening or even prudent. This also claims to exfoliate the skin, but with a pH of 7, that's about as likely as a sunny, dry winter in Seattle. Other than the magnesium ascorbyl phosphate, there really is no reason to consider this one over the DHC product mentioned above. It does contain fragrance.

☺ $$$ **Anti-Spot Whitening Night Essence** *($57 for 1 ounce)* appears to contain about as much magnesium ascorbyl phosphate as the Day Essence above, and is in a better moisturizing base, though not one that is worth this price. Again, the DHC product is a similar and less costly option to consider before this one.

☺ $$$ **Whitening Airy Emulsion** *($52 for 1 ounce)* barely differs from the Night Essence above, yet Dior recommends this for night and daytime use to "clarify and even-out skin." Of the three Snow moisturizers, this is the most emollient, though with the inclusion of aluminum starch octenylsuccinate, an absorbent material, it's a problem for dry skin. It does have magnesium ascorbyl phosphate as one of the main ingredients, but without an effective sunscreen you won't see lightening results of any kind. It does contain fragrance.

☺ $$$ **Snow UV SPF 35** *($60 for 1.9 ounces)* is a very good but exceedingly overpriced in-part titanium dioxide–based sunscreen in a lightweight, boring moisturizing base. Please keep in mind that to gain the SPF benefit of this product you need to apply it liberally and at this price that isn't very likely to happen!

MISCELLANEOUS CHRISTIAN DIOR PRODUCTS

☺ $$$ **Purifying Wash-Off Cleansing Foam** *($22.50 for 6.8 ounces)* is a standard detergent cleanser that is potentially too drying and irritating for most skin types, though it could be an option for someone with very oily skin. It does contain fragrance.

☺ $$$ **Purifying Cleansing Gelee for Face and Eyes** *($22.50 for 6.8 ounces)* is a standard, silicone-based makeup remover that would work as well as any.

☹ **Purifying Lotion** *($22.50 for 6.8 ounces)* lists alcohol as the second ingredient, and it also contains menthol.

☹ **Refreshing Wash-Off Cleansing Gel** *($22.50 for 6.8 ounces)* uses sodium C14-16 olefin sulfate as the primary detergent cleansing agent, which makes this too drying and potentially irritating for all skin types.

☺ $$$ **Refreshing Cleansing Water for Face and Eyes** *($22.50 for 6.8 ounces)* is a very standard, boring toner.

☹ **Refreshing Lotion** *($22.50 for 6.8 ounces)* lists alcohol as the second ingredient. That isn't refreshing, but it is irritating and drying for all skin types.

☺ $$$ **Cleansing Milk for Face and Eyes** *($22.50 for 6.8 ounces)* is a good, cold cream–style cleanser that is no different from Neutrogena's Extra Gentle Cleanser, except that the Neutrogena product is one-third the price.

☺ $$$ **Softening Wash-Off Cleansing Creme** *($22.50 for 6.8 ounces)* is virtually identical to the Cleansing Milk above only in cream form, and the same comments apply.

☺ **Softening Lotion—Alcohol Free** *($22.50 for 6.8 ounces)* is alcohol-free, and I'm glad it is, but all the toners in this line should be. It would be an OK (but boring) option for normal to dry skin, and contains minute amounts of two water-binding agents and an antioxidant. There are more preservatives and fragrance in this product than beneficial ingredients for skin.

☺ $$$ **Instant Eye Makeup Remover** *($18.50 for 3.4 ounces)* is a good, standard, detergent-based makeup remover, but there are lots of good makeup removers for far less.

☺ $$$ **Duo-Phase Eye Makeup Remover** *($20 for 3.4 ounces)* is a standard, but good, silicone-based eye-makeup remover that would work as well as any.

☺ $$$ **Deep Radiance Exfoliating Creme** *($25 for 6 ounces)* is a standard, lotion-style scrub that uses polyethylene (ground-up plastic) as the abrasive. This can be an option for someone with normal to dry skin, but it really is about as basic as it gets.

☺ $$$ **Capture Essential Time-Fighting Serum for Eyes** *($48 for 0.5 ounce)* is a fairly standard lightweight moisturizer that is a mediocre option for normal to slightly dry skin. For this kind of money there should be a whole lot more of the good stuff than what you get with this product.

☺ $$$ **Capture Eyes Contour Gel** *($45 for 0.5 ounce)* is similar to the Serum for Eyes above and the same basic comments apply.

☹ **Capture Rides Fluide Multi-Action Wrinkle Lotion SPF 8** *($45 for 1 ounce)* has an SPF 8, but that number is pathetic for good all-day skin care. That would be bad enough, but this also doesn't contain the UVA-protecting ingredients of avobenzone, zinc oxide, or titanium dioxide, and is absolutely not recommended.

✓☺ $$$ **Capture Rides Wrinkle Creme for Eyes** *($45 for 0.5 ounce)* is a good moisturizer for normal to dry skin with a nice mix of water-binding agents and antioxidants.

☺ $$$ **Hydra Move Creme** *($42 for 1.7 ounces)* is an emollient moisturizer that is exceedingly boring and not worth even half the price.

☹ **Hydra Move Fluid SPF 10** *($42 for 1.8 ounces)* is a good, in-part avobenzone-based sunscreen (though with 0.5% avobenzone, it's well below the 2% that would be helpful for UVA protection), but the SPF 10 makes this a waste of time anyway, and it is not recommended. It is actually astounding that Dior has a discussion on their Web site defending why SPF 10 is OK, despite recommendations for SPF 15 from the American Academy of Dermatology and the National Cancer Institute. Dior claims this is because it "…is suitable for city use where sunlight exposure is not strong. Obviously, when exposing yourself to strong direct sunlight, we recommend you use a specially developed sunscreen product on top of Hydra-Move." How inane and offensive! First, SPF is about *length of time*, or how long your skin will be protected from the sun, not how intensively! And in any part of the world except extreme northern latitudes in the winter, your skin will see more sun than what an SPF 10 can protect you from during the day. Lastly, increasing evidence of ozone depletion in cities means UV rays can penetrate even more there, meaning it's reasonable to believe that more, not less, protection would be important in those areas.

☺ **$$$ Icone Regulating Creme Dehydrated Skin** *($70 for 1.7 ounces)* is a good, though absurdly expensive, moisturizer for normal to dry skin. This does contain urea, which can be an exfoliant.

☺ **$$$ Icone for Hyper-Sensitive Skin** *($58 for 1 ounce)* is similar to the Dehydrated Skin version above and the same comments apply. However, nothing in this product makes it more suitable for sensitive skin, and Dior didn't even leave out the fragrance in this one.

☺ **$$$ Icone Regulating Gel Sebum Control Treatment** *($44 for 1 ounce)* would be a good lightweight moisturizer with some good water-binding agents for normal to slightly dry skin. It does have some absorbency, but not much.

☹ **Mati-Star Hydrating Mattifying Lotion** *($42 for 1.7 ounces)* contains mostly alcohol along with other irritating ingredients, specifically menthol and camphor. This is an irritation waiting to happen.

☹ **Model Lift SPF 10** *($70 for 1.7 ounces)*. The SPF 10 and the lack of UVA-protecting ingredients makes this anything but lifting.

☺ **$$$ Model Lift Nuit Enriched Firming Night Cream** *($75 for 1.7 ounces)* is an OK, emollient moisturizer that just isn't worth the money given that it's easily replaced by a multitude of better-formulated products from Avon to Neutrogena.

☺ **$$$ Model Lift Yeux** *($48 for 0.53 ounce)* is as average a moisturizer as it gets and it sure won't lift skin anywhere. It lacks the interesting water-binding agents in the Night Cream above and contains even fewer antioxidants (and it's hard to imagine that could be possible).

☺ **$$$ NoAge Essentiel Age-Defense Renewal Serum** *($50 for 1 ounce)*. Basically this is a standard moisturizer for normal to dry skin in a rather ordinary base of thickeners, slip agent, glycerin, and water-binding agents (though most of these are listed well after the fragrance and preservative, so their content is minuscule). The inclusion of RNA has no effect on skin cells (thankfully). It also contains coloring agents.

Dior's brochure for NoAge states it is supposed to contain "…optitelomerase—it helps to safeguard the youthful appearance of your skin. Two powerful antioxidants join optitelomerase to form the 'Ageproof Moisturizing Complex', a winning combination against the external stresses of daily life, including UV rays…." These "external stresses" are a problem because, according to Dior, "Such factors reduce the natural enzyme telomerase, which optimizes cell life." Further, Dior states that it's "…beyond doubt that the decline in the activity of telomerase … is responsible for premature cellular senescence [meaning cells growing old]." Dior appears to be the only one who thinks that telomerase activity plays an essential role when it comes to skin health.

The buzzword being used here involves the reference to telomerase (which this product does *not* contain), and therein lies the hype and the rub, because it turns out you may not want to increase activity of the enzyme telomerase. Even though telomerase is an enzyme that appears to be responsible for creating what are called immortal cells, and immortality sounds like a good thing. Telomerase appears to be responsible for the unchecked growth of cells seen in human cancers. Telomerase levels appear to be carefully maintained in normal body tissues, but the enzyme is reactivated in cancer, where immortal cells are likely required to maintain tumor growth (Source: *Science,* 1994, volume 266, pages 2011–2015). Further, the authors of an article published in *Nature* (June 15, 2000) have this to add: "…scientists report that using telomerase to extend the life-span of human tissue culture cells … may present some level of cancer risk…." That's not necessarily good news for skin.

As disconcerting as all that sounds, I can say without a shred of hesitation that Dior's NoAge products contain no ingredients that can negatively affect the telomerase enzyme, and whether or not they can have a positive effect is completely unclear. Of the antioxidants in NoAge, one in particular, l-ergothioneine, is considered to be effective (though it is present in less than a 0.1% concentration in these products). But whether any amount of this ingredient, or any antioxidant, can work through the surface of skin to affect telomerase activity is unknown.

☺ $$$ **NoAge Eyes** *($50 for 0.5 ounce)* is almost identical to the NoAge Renewal Serum above and the same comments apply.

☺ $$$ **Nutri-Star Creme for Very Dry Skin** *($55 for 1.7 ounces)* is a good, though ordinary, moisturizer for normal to dry skin that has just a minute amount of water-binding agents and is completely not worth the money.

☺ $$$ **Phenomen-A Double Retinol Wrinkle Treatment** *($50 for 1 ounce)* does contain retinol, but other than for the Dior label there is no reason to choose this retinol product over Neutrogena's, RoC's, or Alpha Hydrox's at the drugstore for far less. The amount of retinol in this product is the same as in most.

☺ $$$ **Phenomen-A Yeux Double Retinol Wrinkle Treatment for Eyes** *($45 for 0.5 ounce)* puts retinol in a formula that is really too matte for dry skin. Besides, this rather basic moisturizer with retinol does not come in the kind of packaging that ensures that the retinol will remain stable. There are minuscule amounts of other interesting water-binding agents and anti-irritants, but all in all, if you're looking for retinol, you would do far better to check Neutrogena's, RoC's, L'Oreal's, Alpha Hydrox's, or Cetaphil's at the drugstore for a fraction of this price.

☺ $$$ **Phenomen-A Day Cream** *($70 for 1.7 ounces)* does list active sunscreen agents, but does not indicate an SPF on the label, so it cannot be relied on for adequate sun protection. Other than that, this is a matte-finish moisturizer with thickeners, absorbent, silicone, preservatives, water-binding agents, fragrance, and antioxidants. The only thing phenomenal about it is the price tag. It is just an OK basic moisturizer for normal to dry skin.

☺ $$$ **Vitalmine Radiance Activator** *($45 for 1 ounce)* is one more vitamin C product for you to swallow (well, not literally). This one does contain magnesium ascorbyl palmitate, considered to be one of the more stable forms of vitamin C in terms of reliable antioxidants, but the notion that this is the best antioxidant or that it can stop or improve wrinkling is not supported by any research. This is a good moisturizer for dry skin.

☺ $$$ **Auto-Bronzant Face Self Tanner SPF 10** *($22.50 for 1.7 ounces)*. If you ignore the measly SPF 10, this is just a very standard self-tanner that uses dihydroxyacetone as the ingredient to affect skin color. It holds no advantage over Coppertone or Bain de Soleil, which are available at the drugstore.

☺ $$$ **Auto-Bronzant Golden Self Tanner for Body** *($25 for 1.7 ounces)* is similar to the Face Self Tanner above and the same comments apply.

☺ $$$ **Auto-Bronzant Instant Glow Tinted Body Self-Tanner** *($25 for 4.2 ounces)* is similar to the Face Self Tanner above and the same comments apply.

☹ **Spray Auto-Bronzant Golden Self Tanner for Body** *($26 for 4.2 ounces)* lists the second ingredient as alcohol, which makes this too drying for skin anywhere.

☹ **Spray Auto-Bronzant Golden Self Tanner** *($26 for 4.2 ounces)* is similar to the Spray Body version above and the same comments apply.

☺ $$$ **Ultra Protection UV 30 Face Coat** *($31 for 1 ounce)* is a good, in-part titanium dioxide–based sunscreen in an exceptionally standard moisturizing base. This is overpriced for what isn't even as well-formulated as drugstore versions from Eucerin to Neutrogena.

☺ $$$ **Masque Cocoon Relaxing Moisture Mask** *($35 for 1.8 ounces)* is just water, plant oils, glycerin, thickeners, fragrance, preservatives, and a dusting of water-binding agents. It is a mediocre moisturizer.

☺ $$$ **Masque Stretch-Firming Energy Mask** *($35 for 1.8 ounces)* is just a simple mixture of water, thickening agents, silicone, slip agent, talc, film-forming agent, preservatives, and fragrance. The minuscule amounts of anything interesting are inconsequential.

☺ $$$ **Clarifying Cleansing Mask** *($25 for 1.9 ounces)* is a standard clay mask that also contains small amounts of camphor and menthol, which aren't the best in any amount and may cause irritation.

CHRISTIAN DIOR MAKEUP

The most exciting happening within the world of Dior makeup is their foundations, which have improved considerably and now rate as having some of the most luxurious, elegant textures at the department store. Add to this the fact that someone at Dior finally woke up and realized that women don't want or need pink, rose, and overly peach foundations and you have even more incentive to check out the neutral to yellow foundation color palette. Of course, since Dior has a couture fashion legacy, these improvements don't come cheap, though the price point is a bit easier to handle than you'll find at the neighboring competitor Chanel. You will also find that Dior now has an excellent concealer, and their powders have supple textures and smooth, airy applications.

Seemingly oblivious to the need for at least some matte eyeshadows, all of Dior's orb-enhancing options are bedecked with shine. Although some shades keep the shine on low, it's still enough to draw attention to less-than-perfect lids or sagging brows. The powder blush presents some wonderful colors, while the lipsticks and pencils are nice, but they don't rise above considerably less expensive options. The mascaras are now a 50/50 proposition. Two rank superior, while two are disappointing options, especially for the money.

☺ $$$ <u>FOUNDATION:</u> ✓☺ **Teint Diorlight SPF 10** *($34.50)* is an extremely sheer, beautifully smooth foundation with an ultra-silky texture, a natural finish, and a part titanium dioxide–based sunscreen (though SPF 15 is the number to be looking for). This blends on easily and would be fine for almost all skin types (except very oily) preferring bare minimum coverage. The nine shades have been improved, and the majority of them are fine for light to medium skin tones. Only Blond and Honey Beige lean toward the peachy side of neutral. ✓☺ **Teint Diorlift SPF 10** *($34.50)* comes with an SPF that is unreliable for UVA protection, but if you're willing to wear an effective sunscreen underneath, this could work. The texture is smooth with a lot of slip, so blending takes a while, but this leaves a natural, silken finish with flawless light to medium coverage. This would be an option for normal to very dry skin. Although there are no colors for very light or very dark skin tones, the nine shades are exceptional for light to medium skin tones. By the way, this won't lift your skin anywhere or adequately conceal wrinkles—it's simply a good foundation. ✓☺ **Teint Dior Poudre Foundation** *($42.50, $29.50 for refills)* is a standard, wet/dry, talc-based powder foundation with a soft, very smooth texture that is best used dry for light coverage. This has to be one of the most expensive pressed powders around, yet there's little reason to consider it with this price tag given that everyone from Clinique to Urban Decay has excellent alternative options. The six available shades are mostly fine, with a few of them having a soft peach hue—but this shouldn't be a problem since the application is so sheer. ✓☺ **Teint Diorlift Compact SPF 10** *($34.50)* is the cream-to-powder version of the Diorlift liquid foundation above. Whereas the liquid version does not have UVA protection, this one uses titanium dioxide as the active ingredient, which is great, although SPF 15 would be perfect. What's strange is that this contains almost 18% titanium dioxide—an amount that should make achieving SPF 15 a slam-dunk. In any event, this compact-style foundation applies well and offers light to medium coverage. The dry, powdery finish makes it an option only for normal to slightly oily skin—any dry patches would look terrible with this foundation's finish. Of the nine shades, the only ones to view suspiciously are Blond and Dark Beige. The remaining colors are remarkably neutral, and show that Dior's foundations are finally offering women the kinds of real-skin shades they need.

CONCEALER: ☹ **Hydrating Concealer** *($19.50)* is a creamy, medium- to full-coverage concealer that has a pervasive sweet fragrance. Of the shades available, only Light Beige looks like real skin color.

✓☺ $$$ **Teint Diorlift Smoothing Anti-Fatigue Concealer** *($22.50)* is one of the most expensive concealers around, but if cost isn't an issue this light-textured product offers smooth, relatively opaque coverage and a soft matte finish that presents minimal risk of creasing. The four shades are mostly beautiful—only #300 is too peach for some skin tones. Dior opted to package this with a brush applicator instead of a sponge tip. I prefer a sponge tip, but the brush is still an OK option for dotting on concealer.

POWDER: ☺ $$$ **Diorlight Loose Powder** *($42.50)* is a standard, talc-based powder with a light silky texture and dry finish. This is recommended for oily skin, but the sheen these three colors leave behind will not be of much help taking down excess shine. This does come with a worthwhile brush instead of the oft-included powder puff. **Diorlight Pressed Powder** *($35)* is a talc-free powder with a drier texture than the Loose Powder, though the aluminum starch in the Pressed Powder may prove to be irritating for some skin types. This does have an unbelievably smooth texture and three very good colors, though Medium is slightly peach. **Teint Poudre** *($35)* is a talc-free pressed powder that has a more slippery, emollient feel, so it could be an option for drier skin types. All of the colors are fine.

☹ **Terra Bella Sun Powder** *($31)* has a dry, grainy texture and three overly orange, shiny colors, each with a strong sparkle that just looks fake.

☺ $$$ BLUSH: You will not be disappointed with the sublime texture and application of ✓☺ **Diorlight Blush Final** *($32)*. In a word, it is superlative, and the available colors are mostly excellent, though there are some shiny shades to watch out for. The ☺ **Effects Blush Powder Blush Trio** *($35)* is an interesting option for blush, though not one worth getting too excited about. Of the three colors in each set, one is shiny (for highlighting), one is a brown tone (for contouring), and one is a typical muted shade of blush. They still have a great texture, and the options for defining are interesting, but unless you allot enough time for a full makeup application, this isn't something you would want to bother with every day. **Multi-Touch** *($27.50)* is a cream-to-powder blush that features blendable sheer colors, each with a hint of iridescence. The price is out of line for what you get, but it wouldn't be Dior without that!

☺ $$$ EYESHADOW: **5-Color Eyeshadow Compact** *($49.50)*. The texture of these is like powdered sugar and, while they do blend on smoothly, there isn't much reason for the expense, largely because of the mostly awkward color combinations and

Dior's consistent penchant for too-shiny eyeshadows. If shine is the reason you use eyeshadow, these are the most workable sets to consider: Basic Chic, Discretion, and The Browns. **Single Eyeshadow** *($22)* is a much more savvy way to choose eyeshadow colors, and the texture is identical to that of the 5-Color Eyeshadow Compact above. However, the shine is even more apparent on almost all the colors, making them hard to recommend for a daily makeup application. What a shame, because the soft texture and saturated colors are a pleasure to use! **Duo Couture Eyeshadow** *($25)* has a fashionable name but seems to have taken the most garish eyeshadow pairings (often seen on models at fashion shows) and unleashed them onto the public. The shine is still predominant here, and these share the same enviable texture as the eyeshadows above. **Ombre Plume Creme Eyeshadow** *($22)* comes in a tube with a wand applicator and all of the colors are iridescent to the extreme. The formula blends well, but laying on this much shine is certainly just as possible with far less expensive products.

EYE AND BROW PRODUCTS: ☺ $$$ **Crayon Kohl Eyeliner** *($21)* is just a standard pencil that is longer than most and has a slight cream-to-powder texture. Don't count on this for long wear—it can smear with minimal effort. **Crayon Eyeliner** *($21)* is also a standard pencil, but this version is quite creamy, making smearing almost a certainty. The seasonal colors for this pencil are usually odd shades that do little to add shape and definition to the lash line. **Duo Styl for Eyes** *($22)* is a new twist on standard eye pencils that seems clever and convenient, yet the performance is not as stellar as the packaging. **Eye Styl** features a creamy eye pencil on one end and a very shiny cream-to-powder eyeshadow on the other. The pencil portion is automatic and retractable, which is a plus, though aside from the packaging it isn't that exciting or better than other automatic eye pencils that do not carry a double-digit price tag. **AquaDior Eyeliner** *($21)* is a standard pencil that has a heavy, waxy texture that barely sets, so it stays sticky. It used to come off easily with water, but now it stays on quite well when exposed to it, so the waterproof claim is valid. Still, smoother pencils abound.

☺ $$$ **Diorliner** *($30)* is a long-lasting liquid liner that comes with a good brush that makes an even application easy. The bottom of the pen houses the liquid and you have to click the base to feed the brush. If Dior sold refills, this would be an option; since they don't this is absurdly overpriced for what you get. **Brow Gel** *($16)* is standard, lightweight brow fixative. The brush is excellent, with both long and very short bristles, so every hair will be tamed, and this has a minimally sticky finish. ✓☺ $$$ **Powder Eyebrow Pencil** *($21)* is a standard needs-sharpening pencil that has an extraordinary smooth texture that glides on, dries to a powder finish, and does not smear or flake. The built-in eyebrow brush is scratchy and stiff, but otherwise, this is a superior, price-is-no-object brow pencil that puts many others to shame.

☹ **Eyebrow Pencil** *($21)* has such a dry, hard texture it actually hurts to apply it.

LIPSTICK AND LIP PENCIL: There are enough colors here to keep a lipstick enthusiast busy for hours, starting with ☺ $$$ **Diorific Long-Wearing True Color Lip-**

stick *($22)*, which has a creamy, opaque texture and luminous finish. For this amount of money, these should have enough stain to last through a morning coffee break, but I doubt they'd make it past the morning commute without needing a touch-up. The **Rouge Hydrating Lipstick** *($21)*, is a very creamy, rich lipstick with full coverage and a glossy, slippery finish. **Rouge Dior Addict Colorplay Lipstick** *($22)* has a soft, creamy texture and a slightly greasy-feeling finish. That may feel great, but it won't help in the longevity department. The majority of the colors are fine, with most having an iridescent finish. By the way, the artfully trendy packaging for this lipstick is the real attraction and, along with advertising, is what the consumer ends up paying for. **Glossy Lipstick** *($19.50)* is exactly that, and sheer to boot, while **Rouge Brilliant Automatic Lip Gloss** *($21)* is about as standard a tube lip gloss as it gets, though it does win points for a smooth application and barely sticky texture. The **Lipliner Pencil** *($21)* is a standard, creamy-finish lipliner that comes in a dwindling array of colors and has a lipstick brush at one end. It's exceptionally overpriced for what you get, but it is still a good basic pencil.

✔☺ **Diorific Plastic Shine Lip Gloss** *($22)* features an opaque, deeply pigmented gloss in a supremely luxurious package. The tenacious texture is slightly sticky and most of the colors are iridescent, but for intensity and evening glamour, this is an option.

☹ $$$ **Duo Styl for Lips** *($22)* is a lip pencil and creamy lipstick in one. This may sound convenient, but for paying top dollar you'll have to contend with a poor automatic-pencil texture and a merely OK lipstick formula.

<u>MASCARA:</u> Here is where Dior excels; its reputation for producing superior mascaras is well deserved, though the newest formulas are not surpassing the tried-and-true favorites. ✔☺ $$$ **Mascara Fascination** *($20)* is uniformly excellent. It builds thick, long lashes with minimal effort and holds up well throughout the day. I suppose that's where the "fascination" part comes into play.

☺ $$$ **Mascara Parfait** *($20)* quickly builds length and lush (but not dramatic) thickness, all without a clump or smear.

☹ $$$ **Long'Optic Mascara** *($20)* is billed as an illuminating (meaning iridescent), lengthening mascara, and although this mascara does build some length, be prepared to work at it, as it takes several applications and reapplications to get there. Thickness is nonexistent. On the plus side, it stays on well, doesn't clump or flake, and removes easily. Still, I wouldn't trade in any of my L'Oreal mascaras for this one. **Mascara AquaDior Waterproof Mascara** *($20)* is a less-than-stellar addition to Dior's usually top-notch mascaras. This one is indeed waterproof, but it takes some effort to get any length and the lashes tend to get stuck together in the process. Need I say there are much better waterproof mascaras than this one?

☹ $$$ <u>BRUSHES:</u> There are indeed brushes here, but they pale in comparison to the excellent options at almost every other counter, from Lancome to M.A.C. to BeneFit. In addition, the Dior brushes feature cumbersome metal handles that no doubt cost much more than the brush hairs used, which is a disadvantage for the user.

CLARINS

Clarins is a distinctively French line whose beginnings go back to the early 1950s. It was then that the founder, Jacques Courtin-Clarins, began formulating plant-based treatments for his clients. He parlayed this into a Beauty Institute, and from there, with an all-natural mantra that was slightly ahead of its time, the business just grew. Fast-forward to today and you will notice upon visiting the Clarins counter that the plant-based, natural-extract rhetoric is still intact, and so thick you may want to bring along some salad tongs to get through it. Never wavering from its original marketing angle, Clarins has steadfastly held on to the belief that whatever grows from the ground and smells nice must be the cure for every skin ailment, from breakouts to the dreaded "sponginess" of cellulite.

This line is enormous. It's absolutely one of the most extensive around, and the assortment of plant extracts ranges from the usual to the exotic and on to the no-one-knows-what-in-the-heck-these-are! Clarins has something for every skin concern imaginable—from keeping pollution off the face (not possible) to lifting a sagging jaw line (not possible without surgery). It would seem there is nothing these supposedly miraculous products can't do! And you'll find a horde of plants here with the promise that this can really all come true. However, once you're armed with even a modicum of ingredient knowledge and a fair helping of myth-busting, you'll realize how ridiculously out of whack all of this hype is. That's not to imply that all of these products are bad—there are good ones—or that all of the plant extracts aren't good—because many are very good anti-irritants, emollients, or antibacterials. However, there are many that are potential allergens or skin irritants. Clarins also has its fair share of ordinary, standard, and completely unnecessary products whose claims are at best misleading and at worst downright false, and overall the products are incredibly overpriced for what you get. What is most startling is the redundancy among the Clarins products. There are few differences, for example, between the moisturizers and the masks, cleansers, and the oil-control products are more reruns than they are new alternatives for skin care.

You will find some good choices here, but be prepared to deflect the same kind of plants-as-salvation claims that so much of the skin-care world goes on and on about! For more information about Clarins, call (212) 980-1800 or visit www.clarins-paris.com. **Note:** All Clarins products contain fragrance.

CLARINS SKIN CARE

☺ **Cleansing Milk with Alpine Herbs Dry or Normal Skin** (*$21 for 7 ounces*) contains mint, arnica, and pine, among other ingredients that can cause skin irritation and that are a concern in any formulation. However, the amounts are probably so small as to have little impact. This ends up being just a very standard cold cream–style cleanser that is a cautious option for normal to dry skin.

☹ **Cleansing Milk with Gentian Oily/Combination Skin** (*$21 for 7 ounces*) is actually quite similar to the Alpine Herbs version above only with different problematic plant extracts. The emollients in this cleanser are not appropriate for oily or combination skin. What were they thinking when they formulated this one?

☺ $$$ **Extra-Comfort Cleansing Cream with Bio-Ecolia Very Dry or Sensitized Skin** (*$30 for 7 ounces*) is a very standard, plant oil–based, cold cream–style cleanser that would be an option for someone with dry skin. While this still contains fragrance, a problem for all skin types (but especially so for sensitive skin), it does leave out all of the irritating and problematic plant extracts found in almost every other Clarins product. You wonder why Clarins couldn't have followed this model of healthy skin care for all skin types.

☺ $$$ **Gentle Foaming Cleanser for All Skin Types** (*$22 for 4.4 ounces*) is a fairly drying, detergent-based cleanser. It can be an option for oily skin, but definitely not for all skin types.

☺ $$$ **Gentle Foaming Cleanser for Dry/Sensitive Skin** (*$22 for 4.4 ounces*) is a standard, detergent-based, water-soluble cleanser that can be drying for some skin types. It does contain some emollients that counteract the drying effect of the cleansing agents, but it also contains sodium lauryl sulfate, which can be a skin irritant.

☺ $$$ **Purifying Cleansing Gel** (*$21 for 4.4 ounces*) is a very standard, detergent-based, water-soluble cleanser that can be an option for someone with normal to oily skin. It also contains salicylic acid, but the pH is too high for it to work as an effective exfoliant.

☺ $$$ **One-Step Facial Cleanser with Orange Extract** (*$26 for 6.8 ounces*) amounts to a standard silicone-based, wipe-off cleanser and little else, and that would work well—but the price is over the top. The claim that the minuscule amount of moringa seed can help neutralize the harmful effects of pollution is implausible. Moringa has a small amount of research showing it to have antioxidant properties, but that is true for many substances. What's the big deal about moringa? That's hard to assess, because there's no definitive research indicating that any antioxidant can neutralize the effect of pollution on skin.

☺ $$$ **Gentle Eye Make-Up Remover Lotion** (*$20 for 4.4 ounces*) is gentle enough, but pretty ordinary, containing mostly fragrant water, thickeners, and preservatives. It is not the most effective choice for removing makeup.

☺ $$$ **Instant Eye Makeup Remover** (*$19 for 4.2 ounces*) is more effective than the Gentle version above, but only barely. This one contains a more effective cleansing agent.

☺ **Gentle Exfoliating Refiner for Face** (*$21 for 1.7 ounces*). The abrasive particles in this product are slightly gritty, but they dissipate quickly and end up being fairly tame. This would work well for someone with normal to dry skin.

☺ **Extra-Comfort Toning Lotion Very Dry or Sensitized Skin** (*$23 for 6.8 ounces*) is a good toner for most skin types. It contains water, aloe, silicone, water-binding agents, plant extracts (antioxidants), film-forming agent, slip agents, fragrance, preservatives, and coloring agents. The fragrance in this product can definitely be a problem for sensitive skin, but overall this is a good toner for normal to dry skin.

☺ **Purifying Toning Lotion** *($15.50 for 6.8 ounces)* lacks any interesting waterbinding agents or antioxidants. This does contain a tiny amount of salicylic acid (less than 1%), but the pH isn't low enough for it to be effective as an exfoliant. It also contains some irritating plant extracts and minerals.

☺ **Toning Lotion for Dry to Normal Skin** *($18.50 for 6.8. ounces)* is just an OK, mundane toner of slip agents with a minute amount of antioxidants. It does contain lactic acid, but the amount is too tiny for it to have any exfoliating properties for skin.

☺ **Toning Lotion for Oily/Combination Skin** *($18.50 for 8.4 ounces)* is a standard, glycerin-based toner with some problematic plant extracts. It lacks any significant waterbinding agents or antioxidants.

☺ $$$ **Aromatic Plant Day Cream** *($38.50 for 1.7 ounces)*. The plant extracts include some skin irritants (pineapple and horsetail), as well as some that have wound-healing benefit, but the mix is confusing, and in the long run not helpful for skin. The interesting ingredients (antioxidants and water-binding agents) are present only in minute amounts. This one may smell nice, but the fragrant plant extracts are far better for your nose than for your skin.

☺ **Beauty Flash Balm** *($36.50 for 1.7 ounces)* is an extremely average moisturizer that contains rice starch, which as an absorbent and can be problematic for dry skin.

☹ **Contouring Facial Lift** *($47 for 1.7 ounces)* lists alcohol as its second ingredient, which isn't a lift, but is a problem for irritation and dryness.

☺ $$$ **Total Double Serum Age-Control Extra-Firming Serum** *($75 for two 0.5 ounce bottles)*. Why the need for a two part product is anyone's guess, especially when neither of the parts includes a sunscreen. Assuming that this is not used during the day since it contains no sunscreen, this is just a good moisturizer for normal to dry skin. There is nothing in here that can control age (not even a second's worth) and it doesn't firm skin, unless you consider a hair spray ingredient firming. The Hydro Serum contains mostly water, film forming agent, water-binding agents, slip agents, plant extracts, preservatives, and coloring agents. The plant extracts (along with the yeast and algae) may have antioxidant properties but are not better than many other forms of antioxidants. The Lipo Serum contains mostly thickeners and mineral oil with a small amount of plant oils added to make the product appear more natural. But, primarily, its mineral oil, which makes this an obscenely overpriced concoction. The tiny amount of vitamin A is barely worth mentioning.

☺ $$$ **Extra Firming Concentrate** *($52.50 for 1 ounce)* is a liquidy lotion that is an OK moisturizer for normal to slightly dry skin. Most of the products in the Extra Firming collection contain the same plant extracts. Some are decent antioxidants and anti-inflammatories, but there isn't much of them in here. Then there are the exotic *Kigelia africana,* and the very American *Sequoia giganteum* (giant sequoia), although those have no research showing benefit for skin. If this contained any significant amounts of antioxidants and water-binding agents it would have garnered a much happier face.

☺ $$$ **Extra-Firming Day Cream All Skin Types** *($50 for 1.7 ounces)* lacks a sunscreen, and without that it isn't appropriate for daytime, though it is a good emollient moisturizer for someone with dry skin. There is nothing in it that will firm skin, and the emollients (several plant oils) and thickeners are not appropriate for all skin types. Some of the plant extracts are good antioxidants and there are some water-binding agents, but there are also plant extracts that can be irritants. This is a mixed bag with strong and weak points.

☺ $$$ **Extra-Firming Night Cream All Skin Types** *($73.50 for 1.7 ounces)* is a very emollient, mineral oil–based moisturizer that would be OK for dry skin. It does contain a good amount of emollients, but only a dusting of water-binding agents and antioxidants. The claims about this being extra-firming stretch the truth about what these standard cosmetic ingredients can really do.

☺ $$$ **Extra-Firming Day Cream for Dry Skin** *($63 for 1.7 ounces)* is, like the Night Cream for All Skin Types above, not great for daytime because it lacks sunscreen, but it is a very good emollient moisturizer for dry skin.

☺ $$$ **Eye Contour Balm All Skin Types** *($38.50 for 0.7 ounce)* is an exceedingly ordinary moisturizer that would be OK for dry skin. However, it lacks any state-of-the-art ingredients for skin.

☺ $$$ **Eye Contour Balm "Special"** *($38.50 for 0.7 ounce)* contains mostly water, mineral oil, thickeners, water-binding agent, silicone, plant oils, antioxidants, mica (adds shine), and preservatives. This is a good moisturizer for dry skin but it isn't special, though it is more special than the version above for All Skin Types.

☺ $$$ **Eye Contour Gel** *($38.50 for 0.7 ounce)* is an extremely do-nothing moisturizer for minimally dry skin.

☹ $$$ **Extra-Firming Eye Contour Cream** *($47.50 for 0.7 ounce)* is an OK moisturizer for normal to slightly dry skin that contains some antioxidants and water-binding agents, but not an impressive amount, and that's especially unimpressive considering the price tag.

☺ $$$ **Energizing Morning Cream** *($52.50 for 1.7 ounces)* has one of the longest ingredient listings in the industry, and long ingredient listings are a problem because they substantially raise the likelihood that there is something in it you are going to be allergic to. Despite the complexity and the handful of potentially irritating plant extracts, this product also contains a good mix of antioxidants, anti-irritants, and water-binding agents, although there is just no way to tell how much of them is present, and it's likely that they are present in very small amounts. Remember, without sunscreen this is a problem for use during the day unless an effective sunscreen is also applied.

☺ $$$ **Extra-Firming Eye Contour Serum** *($47.50 for 0.7 ounce)* is a lightweight lotion that contains a small assortment of water-binding agents and antioxidants. The pineapple extract and papain it contains have no research showing they are effective for exfoliation in a cosmetic formulation.

☺ $$$ **Extra-Firming Day Lotion SPF 15** *($57.50 for 1.7 ounces)* is a good, in-part titanium dioxide–based sunscreen, with a mix of antioxidants and water-binding agents that make it a good option for dry skin. It does contain a handful of potentially irritating plant extracts.

☺ $$$ **Extra Firming Neck Cream** *($63 for 1.7 ounces)* is said to be for the neck and not the face, but there is nothing in it that makes this different from the others in the Extra-Firming group, nor is there anything in it that will lift the neck. It is a good moisturizer for slightly dry skin with a teeny amount of antioxidants.

☺ $$$ **Face Treatment Oil "Blue Orchid" for Dehydrated Skin** *($39 for 1.4 ounces)* is a good, though rather ordinary, mix of plant oils that is basically hazelnut oil and fragrant oils. Skip the fragrance and just use the hazelnut oil you get from the health food store for a fraction of this price. This may smell nice but the basic formulation is as ordinary as it comes.

☹ **Face Treatment Oil "Lotus" for Combination Skin/Prone to Oiliness** *($39 for 1.4 ounces)*. This product is supposed to help "balance" surface oils. What it does is place more oils on the skin. It's actually almost identical to the Blue Orchid above only with different fragrant oils, but it still lists hazelnut oil as the first ingredient. Aside from the absurd expense of this product, it's based on one of the more inane myths of the cosmetics industry: that oily skin is oily because it is dry. In real life, oil production is controlled by hormones and not the condition of skin. If that weren't the case, then women with dry skin would also have oily skin, and they don't!

☺ $$$ **Face Treatment Oil "Santal" Dry or Extra Dry Skin** *($39 for 1.4 ounces)*. The fragrant plant oils in this can be irritating, and you can get hazelnut oil, the primary ingredient, at the health food store for far less and with no risk of allergic reaction.

☹ **Face Treatment Oil "Santal" for Dry or Reddened Skin** *($39 for 1.4 ounces)*. Sandalwood, cardamom, parsley, and lavender oils can all cause skin irritation (which isn't great for someone with reddened skin), and again, the primary ingredient is hazelnut oil, which is easily replaced at the health food store for a fraction of the cost.

☺ $$$ **Gentle Day Cream for Sensitive Skin** *($48.50 for 1.7 ounces)* is a good, but rather ordinary, mineral oil–based moisturizer for dry skin. Because it contains no sunscreen, it isn't best for daytime wear unless your foundation contains sunscreen.

☺ $$$ **Gentle Day Lotion** *($48.50 for 1.7 ounces)* is a decent moisturizer for normal to dry skin that contains an OK amount of water-binding agents and antioxidants. Without sunscreen it is inappropriate for daytime.

☺ $$$ **Gentle Night Cream for Sensitive Skin** *($58.50 for 1.7 ounces)* is almost identical to the Day Cream version above, and the same comments apply. Vitamins are present in this cream, but only in negligible quantities. Why this product is more expensive than the other is a marketing caprice, nothing more.

☹ **Hydra-Matte Day Lotion** *($32 for 1.7 ounces)* contains several potentially skin-irritating ingredients, though it has a dusting of some good water-binding agents and antioxidants. It will have a matte finish due to the talc content (it's the fifth ingredient), but the long ingredient list adds up to confusion more than help for skin.

✔☺ **$$$ Hydration-Plus Moisture Lotion SPF 15 for All Skin Types** *($38.50 for 1.7 ounces)* is a good, in-part titanium dioxide–based moisturizer for someone with normal to dry skin. Now this is a daytime sunscreen your skin can live with! The price isn't warranted for what you get, but it does contain an impressive mix of water-binding agents and antioxidants.

☺ **Instant Shine Control Gel** *($20 for 0.7 ounce)* is just silicone. That can have a matte finish but minimal oil-absorbing potential, so this is one to test drive before you buy.

☺ **$$$ Moisture Quenching Hydra-Balance Cream** *($48.50 for 1.7 ounces)* is a good moisturizer for dry skin, although it is similar to many in the Clarins line. It would be more quenching if the interesting ingredients were present in more than minute quantities.

☺ **$$$ Moisture Quenching Hydra-Balance Lotion** *($48.50 for 1.7 ounces)* is similar to the Hydra-Balance Cream version above and the same comments apply.

☺ **$$$ Moisture Quenching Hydra-Balance Lotion SPF 15** *($48.50 for 1.7 ounces)* is a very good, though overpriced, in-part avobenzone-based sunscreen that would be an option for those with normal to slightly oily skin. There are some irritating plant extracts present, but they fall way after the fragrance on the ingredient list, so their presence is unlikely to have an impact on skin. Other than the reliable SPF and UVA protection, there isn't anything that makes this all that interesting for skin.

☺ **$$$ Multi-Active Day Cream Protection Plus All Skin Types** *($55 for 1.7 ounces)* is a day cream without sunscreen, which makes it the last thing you would want to use during the day. Several Clarins salespeople told me that this is the only daytime moisturizer I would need, as the natural ingredients allow the product to have an SPF 6. Even if that were true (and it isn't in the least), an SPF 6, natural or not, would be substandard protection anyway. Hopefully, this is not something Clarins has in their training manual, and merely a contrivance the sales personnel create to defend the product's lack of sun protection. While there are some interesting antioxidants and anti-irritants in this product, their position on the ingredient list (well after the potent fragrance) means they are barely present and, therefore, have little to no impact on the skin, and some of the plant extracts can be skin irritants. It is just an OK option for someone with normal to dry skin—the emollients make it inappropriate for normal to oily or blemish-prone skin types.

☺ **$$$ Multi-Active Day Cream Protection Plus, Dry Skin** *($55 for 1.7 ounces)* is similar to the All Skin Types version above and the same comments apply.

☺ **$$$ Multi-Active Day Cream-Gel** *($55 for 1.7 ounces)* is similar to the All Skin Types version above only minus some of the thickening agents. It could have been a really great moisturizer for normal to dry skin, but the truly interesting ingredients—antioxi-

The Reviews C

dants, anti-irritants, and water-binding agents—are present in such minuscule amounts they have little to no impact on skin. The claims that this product can regulate variations of moisture and temperature, as well as something Clarins calls "Photo-regulating: neutralizes light-induced free radicals," are a bad joke. There is no sunscreen in this product so it can't reduce sunlight's detrimental effect on skin in any way. And temperature? Standard ingredients like this cannot affect the body's heat regulation, so don't count on hot flashes being a thing of the past. In terms of regulating moisture, that's what all moisturizers do to one degree or another, and this one works as well as any.

☺ $$$ **Multi-Active Day Cream-Gel** *($55 for 1.7 ounces)* is a good lightweight moisturizer for normal to slightly dry skin, but the impressive ingredients are not as abundant as you would expect given the price tag.

☺ $$$ **Multi-Active Night Lotion, All Skin Types** *($62 for 1.7 ounces)* is a basic moisturizer for normal to dry skin. Someone with oily skin would not be happy with many of the ingredients in this lotion.

☹ $$$ **Multi Action Night Lotion, for Very Dry Skin** *($62 for 1.7 ounces)* is almost identical to the All Skin Types version above and the same comments apply.

☹ **Normalizing Night Gel** *($31 for 1.06 ounces)* contains several problematic ingredients, including wintergreen, orris root, and zinc sulfate, all of which can be skin irritants. The teeny amount of water-binding agents and antioxidant are inconsequential for skin.

☹ $$$ **Renew Plus Night Lotion** *($53.50 for 1.7 ounces)* contains mostly water, thickeners, plant oils, silicone, plant extracts, water-binding agent, fragrance, vitamin A, and preservatives, along with sodium salicylate (the salt form of salicylic acid), which is not effective for exfoliation. It also includes papain, and there is a little research showing it to be effective for exfoliation, but the amount of it in this product is so tiny that it is ineffectual. There is little benefit to be gained from using this lotion.

☹ $$$ **Skin Beauty Repair Concentrate** *($51.50 for 0.5 ounce)* contains peppermint, which is a skin irritant. What it lacks are any consequential amounts of water-binding agents or antioxidants—you could easily use pure olive oil and gain better results for your skin for a lot less money!

☹ $$$ **Thirst Quenching Hydra Balance Serum** *($45 for 1 ounce)* is an OK moisturizer for someone with normal to dry skin.

☹ $$$ **Ultra Matte Concentrate, for Oily Skin** *($31.50 for 1.06 ounces)* contains several potentially irritating plant extracts that would not be helpful for any skin type. Though there is a tiny amount of salicylic acid, the pH is too high for it to be effective for exfoliation.

☹ **After Sun Gel, Ultra Soothing** *($23.50 for 5.3 ounces)* is basically just water, silicone, aloe, and preservatives. This does feel nice on the skin, but your skin would be just as happy with pure aloe vera.

☹ **After Sun Moisturizer, with Self Tanning Action** *($23.50 for 5.3 ounces)* is a very ordinary moisturizer for dry skin, but there is nothing about this that would be helpful before or after sun exposure. This is a standard self tanner that uses dihydroxyacetone to affect skin color, and it would work as well as any.

☹ **Oil Free Sun Care Spray SPF 15** *($23.50 for 5.08 ounces)* doesn't contain the UVA-protecting ingredients of titanium dioxide, zinc oxide, or avobenzone, and is absolutely not recommended.

☹ **Self Tanning Face Lotion SPF 15** *($24 for 1.7 ounces)*, as all self tanners do, uses dihydroxyacetone to affect skin color. With less than 1% titanium dioxide as one of the active sunscreen ingredients, this product cannot be relied on for UVA sun protection.

☺ **$$$ Self Tanning Gel without Sunscreen** *($21 for 4.4 ounces)*, as all self tanners do, uses dihydroxyacetone to affect skin color. This one would work as well as any.

☺ **$$$ Radiance Plus Self Tanning Cream Gel** *($45 for 1.7 ounces)*, as all self tanners do, uses dihydroxyacetone to affect skin color. This one would work as well as any.

☹ **Self Tanning Milk SPF 6** *($25 for 4.4 ounces)*, as all self tanners do, uses dihydroxyacetone to affect skin color. Though it does contain avobenzone, the SPF 6 is just a welcome mat for wrinkles and sun damage and this is absolutely not recommended.

☹ **$$$ Self Tanning Instant Spray** *($27 for 4.2 ounces)* lists alcohol as the first ingredient, which makes this too irritating and drying for skin, especially when the goal is a smooth-looking tan.

☺ **$$$ Sun Care Cream SPF 20** *($30 for 7 ounces)* is a very good, in-part titanium dioxide–based, sunscreen in a good, but rather standard, moisturizing base that would be an option for someone with normal to dry skin. Keep in mind that you must apply sunscreen liberally to get any benefit from using it. If an expensive sunscreen discourages you from liberal application it can be a serious problem for the health of your skin.

☺ **$$$ Sun Wrinkle Control Cream SPF 15** *($24 for 2.7 ounces)* is a very good, in-part titanium dioxide–based, sunscreen in a good, but rather standard, moisturizing base that would be an option for someone with normal to dry skin. It is similar to the Sun Care Cream SPF 20 above and the same comments apply.

☺ **$$$ Sun Wrinkle Control Cream SPF 30** *($24 for 2.7 ounces)* is similar to the SPF 15 version above and the same comments apply.

☹ **Sun Care Cream Gel SPF 15** *($23.50 for 4.4 ounces)* doesn't contain the UVA-protecting ingredients of titanium dioxide, zinc oxide, or avobenzone, and is absolutely not recommended.

☹ **Sun Care Lotion SPF 6** *($23.50 for 5.08 ounces)* doesn't contain the UVA-protecting ingredients of titanium dioxide, zinc oxide, or avobenzone, and the SPF 6 is an insult for skin. This product is absolutely not recommended.

☹ **Sun Care Oil Intensive Tanning SPF 4** *($23.50 for 5.08 ounces)* is similar to the Lotion SPF 6 above (except that this is an SPF 4) and the same comments apply.

☹ **Sunblock Stick SPF 30** *($20 for 0.17 ounce)* doesn't contain the UVA-protecting ingredients of titanium dioxide, zinc oxide, or avobenzone, and is absolutely not recommended.

☺ **Shimmer After Sun Moisturizer** *($23.50 for 5.3 ounces).* If you're interested in a shiny moisturizer this very basic version provides it.

☹ **Blemish Control** *($17 for 0.5 ounce)* lists its second ingredient as alcohol, and that is too drying and irritating for all skin types. It does contain a tiny amount of salicylic acid, but the pH is too high for it to be effective for exfoliation.

☹ **Minimizing Blemish Cream** *($17 for 0.53 ounce)* contains several problematic ingredients for skin, including alcohol, wintergreen, orris, and zinc sulfate. It does contain a tiny amount of salicylic acid, but the pH is too high for it to be effective for exfoliation.

☺ **$$$ Extra Firming Facial Mask** *($41 for 2.7 ounces)* can't firm skin in the least, but it is a good emollient mask/moisturizer for dry skin.

☺ **$$$ Gentle Facial Peeling, with Plant Extracts** *($29 for 1.4 ounces)* is just waxes that you rub over the skin and that takes some skin cells off as you rub. This can be a problem for the face, but would work well for elbows, lips, knees, and heels.

☺ **$$$ Aromatic Plant Purifying Mask** *($26 for 1.7 ounces).* The word "aromatic" in the title is clearly there to add a marketing twist to this facial mask that is otherwise virtually identical to the Clarins Purifying Plant Mask. This may attract those who are searching for aromatherapy for their skin. What a shame, because the claims that fragrant plant extracts are good for the skin is incredibly misleading for the consumer. It contains mostly water, talc, mineral oil, thickeners, clay, fragrant plant extracts, film-forming agent, fragrance, vitamins, preservatives, and coloring agents. This is an OK mask for normal to dry skin, but it adds no real benefit, other than a possible emotional one.

☺ **$$$ Gentle Soothing Mask** *($33 for 1.7 ounces)* is a mineral oil–based mask with some good water-binding agents and plant oils. It is gentle, but it is also fairly ordinary.

☺ **$$$ Normalizing Facial Mask** *($22.50 for 1.7 ounces)* is a standard clay mask that can absorb oil, but no better than any other clay mask.

☺ **$$$ Skin-Smoothing Eye Mask, with Plant Extracts** *($39.50 for 1.05 ounces)* is just some thickening agents, rice starch, and film-forming agent. There is nothing in it that makes this product preferred for the eye area, and the ingredient list is unimpressive.

☺ **$$$ Thirst Quenching Hydra-Balance Mask** *($31 for 1.7 ounces)* contains mostly water, glycerin, thickeners, antioxidants, fragrance, and preservatives. It isn't thirst quenching in the least, but it is rather ho-hum and unbalanced when it comes to good water-binding agents and plant oils that would really quench your skin's thirst.

☺ **$$$ Lip Beauty Multi-Treatment** *($20 for 0.11 ounce)* is a very good, but very standard, emollient balm that would work great for dry lips.

☺ **$$$ Extra-Firming Age Control Lip & Contour Care** *($29.50 for 0.7 ounce)* is supposed to visibly smooth fine lines through an immediate "lift action" as well as help produce collagen. These primarily ordinary ingredients are not capable of that in any way.

☺ **$$$ Body Lift Advanced Cellulite Control** *($49 for 7 ounces)* capitalizes on the notoriety of a group of ingredients used earlier in this line, the benefits of which are still unproven. The ingredients are called xanthines, and are contained in caffeine, theophylline, and aminophylline (the latter two showed up in the original cellulite products made infamous by the TV show *Hard Copy* several years ago). In essence the true effect of these therapies is completely unknown. The only studies that exist looked at a small group of women (no more than 12 women) and then for only a brief period of time. These studies weren't done double-blind, and they didn't take into consideration that the massage (rubbing the cream into the thigh on a regular daily basis) could have a temporary effect of its own, and they also ignored the tannin content of the caffeine (which can be a skin irritant). Further, the studies didn't evaluate the changes that take place in the thigh with such factors as menstruation or exercise. The likelihood that the alcohol, silicone, and caffeine (which make up the bulk of this formula) in this product are going to change one iota of fat on your thigh or anything in the structure of skin is little more than fantasy. It is interesting to note that this product includes an ingredient called escin. There are studies showing that escin in a pure concentration can be effective in helping fluid and venous movement (venous stasis) when taken orally. While supplements with the substance may be helpful for those with certain leg problems (such as lymphedema or vein problems), the teeny amount in this product, applied topically, would not be helpful for any health concern of the thigh area (and lymphedema is not related to cellulite problems).

CLARINS MAKEUP

Clarins continues to offer a beautiful selection of lipsticks and blush colors, all nicely arranged on the tester unit, as well as two very good mascaras. Although the foundation textures and finishes are quite pleasant, the available shades still showcase more than their fair share of peach and pink tones that must be selling to someone (or why keep them around?). Plus, many of the eyeshadows and other complexion products are still riding a tidal wave of shine that shows no signs of slowing down.

☺ $$$ **FOUNDATION:** Clarins claims that all of their foundations have an anti-pollution complex to "safeguard skin's beauty" from "environmental aggressors." The ingredients in these foundations can't keep pollution off the face (no cosmetic can). What a shame they emphasize the bogus anti-pollution angle when an effective sunscreen, which really can have an impact on skin's health and appearance, is absent. **Multi-Matte Foundation** *($32.50)* is a replacement for Clarins' former Matte Finish Liquid Foundation, and in contrast to its predecessor this foundation offers a lighter texture and slightly less coverage while upping the ante with a stronger matte finish. You will find most of the ten shades appealing. The colors to consider avoiding are 04, 06, 08, and 13—all of these are too peach or pink for most skin tones. **Hydrating Liquid Foundation** *($32.50)* has a moist, lightly creamy texture and a dewy, luminous finish that blends easily. This would be a good option for someone with normal to dry skin seeking light to medium coverage, and the color range of ten shades offers some great options. There are no shades for very light or very dark skin, but those who fall in between these should be pleased. The following colors are slightly peach, orange, or pink: Sunlit Beige, Praline, Tender Gold, and Mahogany. **Extra Firming Foundation** *($36)* is what Clarins recommends if you "need a lift," yet nothing in this formula can perk up even one skin cell. This is a very good makeup, offering a soft, creamy-light texture with excellent blendability, medium coverage, and a delicate matte finish. It would be fine for normal to dry skin and there are ten shades, with Pale Ivory being a great shade for very light skin. The colors to watch out for due to overtones of rose and peach are Tender Gold, Sunlit Beige, and Mahogany. **Matte Powder Compact Foundation SPF 15** *($32.50)* has a silky, luxurious texture and smooth application. It gives skin a light-coverage, soft matte finish that does not look too dry or powdery, yet it lacks effective UVA protection. If you're willing to wear a separate sunscreen underneath, this talc-based powder foundation is recommended for normal to slightly dry or slightly oily skin. Of the eight shades, watch out for Soft Caramel and Chestnut, which are too peach, although Silk Beige, which is just slightly peach, may work for some skin tones. ✓☺ **Smart Stick Foundation** *($32.50)* starts out feeling thick but blends on well, leaving a slightly creamy-feeling soft matte finish. As is true for most stick foundations, any dry areas will be accentuated by the powder portion of this makeup. It is best for normal skin seeking medium coverage. There are 11 shades available, and the only bad apples in the bunch are Sunlit Beige and Latte. Praline, Tender Gold, and Mahogany are great dark shades.

☺ $$$ **Ultra Satin Finish Foundation** *($32.50)* has a creamy, moist texture, and despite its thickness it blends on quite well, though the finish is not as natural-looking as the finish of other Clarins foundations. The main problem is that half of the eight shades are too peach or rose, and those include Tender Gold, Sunlit Beige, Wheat Beige, and Natural Beige. Pale Ivory is an excellent shade for very light skin. This is still worth a look if you have dry skin. **Colour Veil** *($31)* is essentially a very sheer group of color correctors that have a slick, weightless texture and silky feel on the skin. According to Clarins, the three shades have "specialized auto-focus colour pigments." In real-world testing, you can take that to mean "subtle iridescence." There's really no need to consider these peach-toned veils, but if you're curious, Clarins often has samples available. **Shimmer Veil** *($31)* is identical to the Colour Veils, but the colors are intensely shiny. These will not do a thing to conceal lines—if anything, this much iridescence will only enhance them; though to add glimmer and sparkle, this definitely does the job. **Hydra-Balance Tinted Moisturizer SPF 6** *($32.50)* is an updated version of Clarins' former Moisturizing Tint. Perhaps Clarins missed the countless recommendations for SPF 15 as being the minimum amount recommended for daily protection, because even though this is all titanium dioxide, SPF 6 is embarrassingly low. This is a sheer, silicone-based moisturizer that would be fine for normal to dry skin. Of the four shades, the best ones to consider are Bisque and Gold. Amber is too peach and Copper is too orange, but may work for some darker skin tones.

☹ **Natural Veil** *($31)* has a moist, lotion-like texture and comes in one shade that is very peach. Although it is sheer, the poor color shows enough on the skin to make this a problem.

The Reviews C

☹ <u>**CONCEALER:**</u> **Concealer Plus Corrector** *($18)* offers a peach-toned creamy liquid concealer on one end and an equal portion of mint green color corrector on the other. The concealer colors are marginally acceptable and the green tint is just a waste, which makes this product a real "Why bother?"

<u>**POWDER:**</u> ✓☺ $$$ **Face Powder** *($33)* is a loose powder that comes in a generous tub. It has a silky, feather-light texture and a sheer, dry application that looks beautiful on the skin. The three shades are all fine, and each has a satin finish—meaning this is best for those with normal to dry skin who wish to avoid a true matte finish. ☺ $$$ **Bronzing Powder Duo** *($29)* has an agreeable soft texture and comes in a split-pan compact with two peachy-tan colors. Both shades go on sheer, and the final result is best for fair to light skin tones. This does have a very subtle shine that should not be intrusive.

☺ $$$ **Bronzing Sun Compact SPF 15** *($35)* has a gorgeous creamy texture and blends imperceptibly with skin, imparting a very sheer bronze tone with an in-part titanium dioxide–based sunscreen. This would be a slam dunk for normal to dry skin if only there were not large glitter particles suspended in the moisturizing formula! The randomly dispersed, large pieces of glitter can be blended away or picked off the skin, but unless you want this type of shine, why go to the trouble? **Powder Compact** *($29)* has a very soft, smooth texture and a dry finish, but this pressed powder's three shades present only one (Ivory) that looks like skin. **Jewel Powder Compact** *($35)* is a pressed powder, but the only reason to consider it over a less expensive version is for its elegant gold compact that slips into a red velvet pouch; this is certainly a chic way to "take a powder" in public. The single pale shade is very sheer and leaves a soft shine on the skin. **Jewel Highlights Compact** *($35)* presents four strips of peach to tan colors in one compact. You can use the colors separately or sweep a brush over the powder cake to get a little of each shade for a soft, sheer tan effect with subtle shine. Although this is an attractive package, the price tag for what amounts to a decent bronzing powder is a bit much.

<u>**BLUSH:**</u> ✓☺ $$$ **Powder Blush** *($25)* still has a great velvety texture and excellent application. It is highly recommended if the price tag doesn't faze you. Although the shiny shades have been eliminated, so have some of the matte options. However, what remains is choice and still worth a look. **Multi Blush** *($22)* is an excellent option for cream-to-powder blush. The formula is very easy to blend, and the three colors are beautiful, with Tender Chestnut being a great bronze tone.

☺ $$$ <u>**EYESHADOW:**</u> **Soft Shimmer Eye Colour** *($16.50)* has a soft texture and very smooth application, but every single shade is noticeably shiny. If you decide to try this anyway, consider avoiding Plum, Forest, and Midnight. **Eye Colour Duo** *($26)* also has a great smooth application and includes some very effective color combinations, but almost all of them are shiny. The handful of matte options from the past has been reduced to only one: Natural/Clay. **Jewel Eye Highlights** *($35)* continues the parade of sheer, shiny colors that characterize the Clarins eyeshadows. These are quad sets that do present some attractive color combinations if you crave shimmer.

EYE AND BROW SHAPER: ☹ Eye Liner Pencil *($16.50)* is a standard pencil with substandard attributes. This soft-textured pencil is too creamy for it not to smudge and smear in short order. Eyebrow Pencil *($16.50)* is your basic brow pencil that needs sharpening and has a dry, hard texture that allows you to apply soft color, but not without some pain and wincing.

☺ $$$ Liquid Eye Liner *($18)* is worth considering! This comes with a very fine brush that expertly lays down a thin line that can be thickened if desired. The formula takes a bit longer to dry than some others, but once it does, it stays put nicely.

LIPSTICK AND LIP PENCIL: ✔☺ $$$ Le Rouge Lipstick *($21.50)* has a sumptuous creamy texture, rich, opaque colors, and a satin-smooth finish. There are over 30 colors, arranged in six groups. The Emotion group of colors offers some beautiful pink hues, Illusion offers nude shades, Passion features vivid reds, Inspiration has lovely orange and coral colors, Fusion includes neutral pink and mauve-brown tones, and Sensation showcases earthy browns. All in all, a great lipstick—although for the money this is not superior to Revlon's Absolutely Fabulous Lip Cream SPF 15 ($8.99).

☺ $$$ Sheer Lipstick *($18.50)* is a very slick, greasy lipstick available in just three soft colors. Sheer Shimmer Lipstick *($18.50)* is identical to the Sheer Lipstick, only there are more colors and all are heavily iridescent. Lip Color Glaze *($16.50)* makes good on its claim to "provide the colour density of a classic lipstick with the brilliance of a gloss." The color range is stunning, and these have a smooth, slick texture that is absolutely not sticky. Moonlit, a sheer, shimmery silver, is the only color I would advise against. Lip Liner Pencil *($16.50)* is a standard pencil that has a good, easy-to-apply texture and fine colors. The pencil has a brush at one end, which is convenient.

☹ $$$ Sheer Gloss *($16.50)* is a clear, non-sparkly lip gloss that has a syrupy texture and an uncomfortably sticky finish. Felt Tip Lip Liner *($17)* is more of a lip pen than a pencil. This product features a pointed, sponge-tip applicator that allows you to apply soft, gel-based color. Unfortunately, the three colors are sheer and the sponge tip is not preferred to a pencil tip for precise application.

MASCARA: ✔☺ $$$ Pure Volume Mascara *($19.50)* is a formidable mascara that enables you to lengthen, thicken, and lightly curl lashes with minimal effort. A minor drawback is that this can clump a bit on the ends of lashes, but that can be remedied by lightly wiping down the brush before application, or using a lash comb afterwards. ✔☺ Pure Curl Mascara *($19.50)* is a superior lengthening mascara, but no more so than any other good mascara (and there are many in this book for half the price). However, this does go on rather wet and the brush tends to stick lashes together instead of individually defining them, which creates a more dramatic look. It does not clump or flake and is easily removed with a water-soluble cleanser. ☺ $$$ Lengthening Mascara *($19.50)* is true to its name, as this lengthens easily with no clumps along the way. Thickness is minimal, especially compared to the Pure Volume version above.

☹ $$$ Fix Mascara Waterproofing Seal *($16.50)* claims it is "the first waterproofing gel for lashes," but that's entirely untrue, as Estee Lauder beat them to it several years ago with their Raincoat Waterproofing Top Coat for Lashes. That product is no longer available, and I suspect this one will fall by the wayside soon. The notion is to use this clear, wax-based gel over your regular mascara to make it waterproof. It works, but so do lots of waterproof mascaras all on their own, so why do two steps and weigh down already fragile lashes with this rather heavy, sticky product?

☺ $$$ <u>BRUSHES:</u> The majority of Clarins **Brushes** *($16–$28)* have great shapes and are dense enough to hold and apply powder-based color. Strangely, this collection is lacking in medium to large eyeshadow brushes. The **Blush Brush** *($21)* is nice but would be better if the hair was longer and more tapered. The **Lip Brush** *($16)* comes with a cap and has a thicker, fuller cut—a nice change of pace from most other too-small lip brushes. Lastly, the **Jewel Powder Brush** *($28)* is a lavishly packaged retractable powder brush that is a convenient take-along option for midday touch-ups.

CLE DE PEAU BEAUTE

Shiseido's decision to launch this prestige (read "overly expensive") line of skin-care products was a foray into the world of elitism and superciliousness. A decision to let price speak louder than formulations must have caused much executive amusement at the expense of naive, vulnerable women who unknowingly end up caring more about image than substance. The plan was a good one. While Shiseido's relatively inexpensive 5S line of products has left these shores and is no longer being sold in the United States, Cle de Peau Beaute has expanded and grown. Originally sold only at Bergdorf's in the United States, it has expanded its market and is now sold in several upscale department stores and salons around the country, and in Canada. What a way to build panache.

Cle de Peau Beaute means "key to beautiful skin," but even a cursory overview shows that it is merely the key to the most inane waste of money. I wish there were a way I could imbue the reality of what women were really buying with a swoop of a wand. The reality is, aside from having no sunscreen, which leaves skin completely vulnerable to the very damage this skin-care line touts to repair, these products contain nothing unique or out of the ordinary. While most of the products contain some amount of antioxidants and anti-irritants the amounts are so minuscule they are inconsequential for skin; for this kind of money that's insulting. Moreover, the formulations are repetitive, with little significant bona fide differences among the formulations.

Each product contains an assortment of tocopherol acetate, *Fagus sylvatica* extract, dipotassium glycyrrhizate, retinol, serine, disodium adenosine triphosphate, sodium acetylhyaluronate, *Hypericum perforatum* extract, *Rubus suavissimus* extract, *Rosa roxburgii* extract, and *Uncaria gambir* extract.

Tocopheryl acetate is a form of Vitamin E. There is no question it's a very good antioxidant, but this ingredient shows up in thousands of products, and in larger quantities, and arguably in more potent forms than in this one. Dipotassium glycyrrhizate is a component of licorice that has very good anti-irritant properties, but so do lots of plant extracts, and it usually takes more than the trace amounts used in these products to provide benefit for skin. Retinol is used in a few products and, though the research about its effectiveness is debatable, other lines from L'Oreal, Lancome, Cetaphil, and Neutrogena have versions in good formulations as well for a fraction of the price. Serine is an amino acid that in humans is part of a complicated chemical pathway vital to body functions. Topically on skin, without the presence of these other constituents, this ingredient can't make protein for skin, although it is a good water-binding agent similar to the other 20-plus essential amino acids the body and skin need to function. Disodium adenosine triphosphate (ATP) serves as the major energy source within the cell to drive a number of biological processes, such as the synthesis of proteins. However, for the cell to use ATP it must be broken down by hydrolysis to yield adenosine diphosphate (ADP), which is then further broken down to yield adenosine monophosphate (AMP). Whether or not ATP applied topically on skin can affect cellular energy has not been shown. It is unlikely that this complicated chemical molecular process can be generated from the outside in, and by using such small amounts. Sodium acetylhyaluronate is a form of hyaluronic acid, which is a component of skin that when applied topically is an effective water-binding agent. However, this is used in numerous skin-care products and it isn't the only vital component of skin.

Fagus sylvatica extract is the Latin name for beech tree extract and this ingredient hasn't one shred of research showing it to be beneficial for skin. *Hypericum perforatum* extract is the Latin name for St. John's wort, and it actually contains several components that are toxic on skin in the presence of sunlight (Sources: *Planta Medica*, February 2002, pages 171–173 and *International Journal of Biochemistry and Cell Biology*, March 2002, pages 221–241). The association of St. John's wort with improving depression when taken as an oral supplement is unrelated to its topical impact on skin. While it may be a problem for skin there is research showing it has components that have antioxidant properties (Source: *Journal of Agricultural Food Chemistry*, November 2001, pages 5165–5170). *Rubus suavissimus* extract is Latin for the Chinese blackberry extract. Most likely, as is true for most berries, this fruit may have potent antioxidant properties. However, there is no research proving this to be the case and given the abundance of research showing that everything from raspberries to blueberries and green tea have significant benefit, this addition is interesting but not something to rely on.

Rosa roxburghii extract is from the chestnut rose and can be a source of antioxidants for skin (Source: *International Journal of Clinical Chemistry and Applied Molecular Biology*, November 2001, pages 37–43) and *Uncaria gambir* extract is a leaf extract of a shrub in the madder family. Some forms of *Uncaria* have antioxidant properties, but there is no such supporting research for the *gambir* species. However, *Uncaria gambir*, due to its tannin content, most likely does have antioxidant properties, but the tannin content also makes it a potential skin irritant.

These are the cornerstones of the Cle de Peau Beaute products, interesting and potentially effective, but they can be replaced with more effective or far more established potent extracts or supplements in many products, which are used in far greater concentrations. Even if you have money to burn, this is not an appealing way to go about it. If you're looking to take great care of your skin, there are products just as expensive (and inexpensive) that won't waste your money. For more information about Cle de Peau Beaute, call (212) 805-2300 or visit www.cledepeau.com.

☹ $$$ **Cleansing Cream (Crème Demaquillante)** *($60 for 2.5 ounces)* is a standard detergent-based cleanser that can be more drying than most, though the Vaseline in it can reduce the irritation. It does contain fragrance.

☹ $$$ **Refreshing Cleansing Foam (Mousse Nettoyante Fraiche)** *($50 for 3.3 ounces)* is a standard detergent-based cleanser that can be more drying than most, though it can be an option for normal to oily skin. It does contain fragrance.

☺ $$$ **Gentle Cleansing Foam (Mousse Nettoyante Tendre)** *($50 for 3.3 ounces)* is a standard detergent-based cleanser that can be good for normal to dry skin.

☺ $$$ **Absolute Eye Makeup Remover (Demaquillant Pour Les Yeux)** *($35 for 2.5 ounces)* is an exceptionally standard, but good, silicone-based eye-makeup remover. It works, but the cost of this average product is bizarre.

☹ **Cleansing Lotion (Lotion Demaquillante)** *($60 for 6.7 ounces)* is a ho-hum detergent-based toner except that the second ingredient is alcohol. It is not recommended.

☹ **Refreshing Balancing Lotion (Lotion Fraiche)** *($85 for 5 ounces)* lists alcohol as the second ingredient, which makes it too irritating and drying for all skin types. Without the alcohol this would have been a good toner, but nothing in here is worth this absurd price.

☹ **Gentle Balancing Lotion (Lotion Tendre)** *($85 for 5 ounces)* lists alcohol as the third ingredient, which makes it too irritating and drying for all skin types.

☹ $$$ **Eye Contour Balm (Baume Contour Des Yeux)** *($125 for 0.5 ounce)* contains mostly water, plant oils, thickeners, slip agent, Vaseline, preservatives, fragrance, vitamins, anti-irritants, water-binding agents, antioxidants, and more fragrance. The potentially effective ingredients are present in such minute amounts that they are inconsequential. For this kind of money, that is an insult.

☹ $$$ **Energizing Cream (Crème Energisante)** *($135 for 0.5 ounce)* is similar to the Eye Contour Balm above and the same basic comments apply. This version does contain a minute amount of vitamin C, but hardly enough worth mentioning.

☹ $$$ **Enriched Nourishing Cream (Crème Soyeuse)** *($120 for 1.7 ounces)* is similar to the Energizing Cream above and the same comments apply.

☹ $$$ **Clarifying Emulsion (Emulsion Eclat)** *($100 for 1.7 ounces)* is an OK lightweight moisturizer for normal to dry skin, but the interesting ingredients are so far down the list they are almost insignificant.

☹ **Refreshing Nourishing Emulsion (Emulsion Fraiche)** *($120 for 2.5 ounces)* lists alcohol as the second ingredient. The interesting ingredients come well after the preservative and are barely present anyway.

☹ **Refreshing Protective Emulsion (Emulsion Protectrice Fraiche)** *($95 for 1.7 ounces)* is similar to the Nourishing Emulsion above and the same comments apply.

☹ **Enriched Protective Emulsion (Emulsion Protectrice Soyeuse)** *($95 for 1.7 ounces)* contains sunscreen ingredients, but without an SPF rating this product cannot be relied on for sun protection and is not recommended. Also, this product has the same limitations of minuscule amounts of antioxidants and anti-irritants as the other products described above.

☹ **Gentle Protective Emulsion (Emulsion Protectrice Tendre)** *($95 for 1.7 ounces)* is similar to the Enriched Protective Emulsion above and the same comments apply.

☺ **$$$ Revitalizing Emulsion (Emulsion Revivifiante)** *($135 for 1.2 ounces)* contains mostly water, silicone, glycerin, slip agent, thickeners, silicones, alcohols, preservatives, fragrance, antioxidants, anti-irritants, and water-binding agent. This ordinary moisturizer is OK for normal to dry skin, but the waste of money for this standard formulation is almost painful to consider.

☺ **$$$ Gentle Nourishing Emulsion (Emulsion Tendre)** *($120 for 2.5 ounces)* is similar to the Revitalizing Emulsion above and the same comments apply.

☺ **$$$ Energizing Essence (Essence Energisante)** *($125 for 2.5 ounces)* is similar to the Revitalizing Emulsion above and the same comments apply.

☺ **$$$ The Cream (La Crème)** *($450 for 1 ounce)*. I had to check my notes several times before I could settle on an appropriate comment for this product, and then I thought better of it and decided to leave out the four-letter words that truly represent the insanity this price tag represents. It contains mostly water, glycerin, Vaseline, slip agent, arbutin, plant oils, thickeners, silicone, more thickeners, preservatives, fragrance, and minute amounts of antioxidants and water-binding agents. What does set this offensively priced, Vaseline-based moisturizer apart is the 3% to 4% concentration of arbutin. There is research showing that arbutin at higher concentrations can inhibit melanin and improve skin discolorations. However, arbutin has not been shown to be more effective than hydroquinone or magnesium ascorbyl palmitate among other skin lighteners. However, if you're curious to try arbutin, Shiseido's Whitess Intensive Skin Brightener ($120 for 1.4 ounces) has a higher concentration and is one-fourth the price.

☺ **$$$ Eye Contour Serum (Serum Contour Des Yeux)** *($100 for 0.5 ounce)* is an OK, average moisturizer for normal to dry skin.

☹ **Brightening Serum (Serum Eclaircissant)** *($135 for 1.2 ounces)* contains alcohol as the second ingredient, which is too drying and irritating for all skin types.

☹ **Clarifying Serum (Serum Eclat)** *($100 for 2.5 ounces)* contains alcohol as the third ingredient, which is irritating and drying for all skin types.

☹ **Oil Balancing Essence (Essence Equilibrante)** *($50 for 2.5 ounces)* contains alcohol as the second ingredient, which is too irritating and drying for all skin types. The zinc phenolsulfonate in it can also be a skin irritant.

The Reviews C

☹ **Oil Balancing Gel (Gel Equilibrant)** (*$50 for 1 ounce*) contains alcohol, menthol, and camphor, which won't balance anything, but it is exceedingly drying and irritating.

Intensive Treatment Set (three products) (*$125 for 10 treatments of 3 products*) these "treatments," and I use that term lightly, are a redundancy of other Cle de Peau Beaute products and with all the same disappointments. ☺ $$$ **Intensive Treatment (Essence Intensive)** is an ordinary moisturizer that would be OK for normal to dry skin. ☹ **Intensive Lotion (Lotion Intensive)** lists alcohol as the second ingredient and is not recommended. ☺ $$$ **Intensive Mask (Masque Intensif)** is just film-forming agent and some thickening agents and little else. What a waste.

☺ $$$ **Translucency Mask (Masque Transparence)** (*$110 for 3.3 ounces*) is a standard, plasticizing mask that contains polyvinyl alcohol, an ingredient in hairspray. The interesting ingredients are hidden after the preservatives and fragrance and make this of little use for skin at any price.

☺ $$$ **Massage Cream (Crème de Massage)** (*$110 for 3.3 ounces*). The impressive ingredients are barely detectable in this standard emollient moisturizer for normal to dry skin.

CLE DE PEAU MAKEUP

Without question, this is absolutely one of the most expensive collections of makeup sold today. While the prices defy logic or reason, at least the majority of the products perform reliably well and most have beautiful, soft textures that are easy to work with. Of particular interest are the foundations, concealers, and lipsticks. The mascaras, pencils, blushes, and eyeshadows have their strong points, too; however, when you consider that products costing considerably less share these strengths, the decision to purchase from Cle de Peau comes down to how large your cosmetics budget is and how important the image of ultra-high-end prestige is to you and your makeup bag.

<u>Caution</u>: The cosmetics counter personnel may mention that the foundations contain SPF 18 and the lipstick has an SPF 10, yet none of the makeup products list active sunscreen ingredients, and no SPF claim is made on the box or product itself; therefore, you should absolutely not rely on these for sun protection of any kind.

☺ $$$ <u>FOUNDATION</u>: **Teint Naturel Crème Foundation** (*$100*) has the distinction of being the most expensive foundation I have ever reviewed or in existence. Teint Naturel Crème Foundation gets a fair amount of press in upscale beauty magazines, and I surmise that is why I continue to get so many requests to review this makeup. There is no doubt that the price is out-of-line and nothing in this one makes it exceptional or even remotely worth the money. You will not find your face looking like you found the ultimate foundation answer. Overall, it is just a very good foundation with ten excellent neutral shades. This silicone- and talc-based makeup goes on very smooth and dries to a silky-matte finish. What is unique about the formulation is that it's densely pigmented. That can be good in the sense that a little goes a long way, but can be problematic if you

The Reviews C

want a sheer or light coverage. It can be mixed with a moisturizer to thin out the coverage if desired, and that may be a good idea, since using it at full strength results in such intense camouflage, it isn't what anyone would call "natural."

In addition to the shades mentioned above, there are also **Color Control Foundations** *($85)*, which are white and bronze shades that Cle de Peau recommends using to deepen or lighten any of the foundation colors or for contouring and highlighting the face. These two "extras" are an option (and much better than standard color correctors), but before you drop almost $200 for two jars of foundation, please remember that the existing foundation colors should work just fine on their own and any special shading or highlighting can be achieved with considerably less expensive products. This formula is good for normal to oily skin. Using this over dry skin can be tricky because it tends to accentuate the dryness; however, an emollient sunscreen underneath can help it go on more easily. **Creamy Powder Foundation** *($75 for powder cake; $25 for compact; $10 for sponge; $95 for refills)* is an incredibly standard, but undeniably smooth, talc-based powder foundation. It applies easily and quite sheer, with a soft, dry finish. The ten shades are very good, though B10, B20, B30, and B40 can turn peach if used on oily skin. For the money, this is not as impressive as the powder foundation options from Lancome, L'Oreal, Chanel, Estee Lauder, or Laura Mercier.

CONCEALER: Cle de Peau's famed ✔☺ $$$ **Concealer** *($65)* is exceptional. This twist-up stick concealer has a light, smooth texture that glides over the skin and offers substantial, but (almost) imperceptible, coverage in three excellent shades. The soft matte finish poses little risk of creasing, and the only thing that's disconcerting about this is the prohibitive price.

POWDER: Both the ☺ $$$ **Translucent Loose Powder** *($95; $65 refill)* and **Translucent Pressed Powder** *($70; $65 refill)* are talc-based, have super-fine textures, and come in one shade that is supposedly translucent but can look pink on light skin and ashen on dark skin. If your skin matches these shades, both powders look natural, though the Pressed version has a noticeably drier finish. For comparable texture and more than one shade to choose from, consider the powders from Sonia Kashuk, Clinique, or Laura Mercier.

☺ $$$ **Perfect Enhancing Powder** *($37 for powder cake; $13 for case; $6 for powder puff)* is a pressed powder whose texture and application are similar to the Translucent Pressed Powder above, but this one comes in more than one color. Two shades are for highlighting (pale pink and pale yellow) and two are bronze tones for contouring. Each shade provides a matte finish and goes on sheer, but the bronze tones (numbers 72 and 73) are distinctly preferred.

☺ $$$ BLUSH: **Cheek Color** *($40 for powder cake; $30 for compact; $15 for brush)* ends up costing $85 for something other lines wouldn't dare sell for over $30. This pressed powder blush does have an incredibly smooth texture and sheer, even application in five attractive shades, but so do many other powder blushes that don't cost as much as a new VCR!

☺ **$$$ <u>EYESHADOW</u>:** Each **Eye Shadow** *($15 per shade; $20 for case; $10–$12 for sponge-tip applicators)* has a suede-smooth texture that applies well and doesn't flake. However, each of the 30+ shades has a decent amount of shine, and that can magnify any eye-area flaws, including the ones Cle de Peau's skin-care claims to alleviate but cannot. If the shine and ridiculous price don't stop you, at least consider avoiding the following purple, pink, blue, and green shades: 17, 19, 26, 35, 36, 39, 41, 42, 44, 45, and 50.

<u>EYE AND BROW SHAPER</u>: The automatic, retractable ☺ **$$$ Eye Pencil** *($20 for cartridge; $30 for pencil case)* has a soft cream-wax texture that is eminently easy to work with but applies color too softly and tends to smudge and fade before too long. You can set it with powder eyeshadow for longer wear, but at this price, it should be able to hold its own. **Eyeliner Fluid** *($40)* features an average brush that lays down a thicker than usual liquid line. This formula dries quickly and stays on, but is very difficult to remove, and each shade is iridescent.

☺ **$$$ Eyebrow Liner** *($16 for cartridge; $30 for pencil case)* is a very good automatic brow pencil that has the standard hard texture but goes on well without being greasy or looking thick. This has a powder finish and comes in three workable colors. **Eyebrow Shadow** *($16 per shade; $33 for 2-color palette case; $6 for applicators)* allows you to customize a brow compact by choosing from a selection of four matte brow powders and coordinating brow waxes for setting and grooming the brows. This is a practical (albeit pricey) option for creating well-defined brows and both the powder and brow wax perform nicely and do not look or feel heavy. Although you will be charged for the petite brushes that are necessary to use this product, they are quality tools that should serve you well.

<u>LIPSTICK AND LIP PENCIL</u>: Cle de Peau's ☺ **$$$ Lipstick** *($55)* is available in Cream or Sheer formulas, and although both are commendable, the Cream version is the one to choose if you're willing to part with this much money for lipstick. Both formulas have an impeccably smooth, deceptively light texture that floats over the lips and leaves a soft glossy finish. The Cream versions are opaque and densely pigmented, so they tend to last at least until lunch—and the colors are stunning. Still, I wouldn't pass up Revlon's Absolutely Fabulous Lip Cream SPF 15 for this. **Lip Gloss** *($40)* is a very standard semi-liquid gloss packaged with a wand applicator. Your lips won't be able to tell the difference between this and almost any other slightly sticky gloss, but it's an option. **Lip Liner** *($20 for cartridge; $30 for pencil case)* is an automatic, retractable lip pencil that has a rich, creamy application and a limited selection of mostly vivid colors that don't complement Cle de Peau's lipsticks as well as they should.

☺ **$$$ Lip Duo** *($65)* features a lip color, lip powder, and brushes in one elegant compact. The idea behind this is to "make the most of your lips" by first applying the creamy, medium-coverage lip color and then finishing with the "light-controlling" white lip powder. The powder can make a creamy lipstick look semi-matte, but otherwise it adds a strange white hue to the lips that most women will want to remedy by applying more of the lip color. This contrived product simply does not make sense.

☺ **$$$ <u>MASCARA:</u>** The regular **Mascara** *($40)* applies cleanly and wouldn't clump for the world, but is otherwise truly lackluster mascara that builds average length and no thickness whatsoever. In contrast, the **Volume Mascara** *($40)* has a bit more gusto and ably builds noticeable length and some thickness without clumping or smearing. Still, neither formula is spectacular enough to warrant a happy face, especially given the cost.

CLEAN & CLEAR BY JOHNSON & JOHNSON
(SKIN CARE ONLY)

When it comes to dealing with breakouts, the Clean & Clear line has some great options and some really disappointing shockers. For example, you'll find some wonderfully formulated benzoyl peroxide products and gentle cleansers that contain no irritants. But then there's the cleanser for oily skin that contains Vaseline! What were these people thinking? For more information about Clean & Clear by Johnson & Johnson, call (800) 526-3967 or visit www.cleanandclear.com.

☺ **Foaming Facial Cleanser for Sensitive Skin** *($3.79 for 8 ounces)* is a very good, detergent-based, water-soluble cleanser for someone with normal to oily skin. It is definitely far more gentle than any of the other cleansers in this line. It does contain fragrance.

☺ **Foaming Facial Cleanser** *($3.49 for 8 ounces)* is a standard, detergent-based, water-soluble cleanser. It can be more drying than some, but it would be an option for someone with oily skin. It contains a tiny amount of triclosan, a disinfectant, which could be effective for controlling breakouts—but in a cleanser it would just be washed away. It does contain fragrance.

☺ **Continuous Control Acne Cleanser** *($4.29 for 5 ounces)* contains Vaseline and mineral oil; don't ask me why, I'm confused about that, too. These ingredients can be great for dry skin, but they don't work for oily skin that tends to break out. The small amount of menthol is probably not much of a problem for skin. This does contain 10% benzoyl peroxide, but in a cleanser it would just be wiped or washed away.

☹ **Continuous Control Acne Wash, Oil-Free** *($4.99 for 6 ounces)* uses sodium C14-16 olefin sulfonate as the main cleansing agent, which can be too drying and irritating for most skin types. It does contain salicylic acid, but in a cleanser that would just be washed away before it could be of much benefit, and besides the pH of this product is too high for the BHA to work as an exfoliant.

☺ **Daily Pore Cleansing Cloths** *($4.99 for 25 cloths)* are just some soft wipes soaked with standard detergent cleansing agents and fragrance. It would work, but washing the skin clean with a gentle cleanser is easier on skin than wiping.

☹ **Deep Action Cleansing Wipes, Oil-Free** *($4.99 for 25 wipes)* lists the second ingredient as alcohol, and that is too drying and irritating for all skin types. The alcohol doesn't go deeper into the skin or pore, it just causes deeper problems for skin. This also contains a small amount of menthol, which can also be a skin irritant.

☹ **Deep Action Cream Cleanser** *($3.99 for 6.5 ounces)* would have been a fairly gentle cleanser except that it contains menthol, which doesn't help skin in the least. It also contains salicylic acid, which in a cleanser would be wasted because it would just be rinsed down the drain.

☺ **Oil Free Daily Pore Cleanser** *($3.99 for 5.5 ounces)* is a very good, standard, detergent-based, water-soluble cleanser for someone with normal to oily skin. It does contain fragrance.

☹ **Clarifying Toner** *($4.99 for 6 ounces)* contains alcohol as the second ingredient and that is too drying and irritating for all skin types.

☹ **Oil-Fighting Deep Cleaning Astringent** *($3.99 for 8 ounces)* contains alcohol, eucalyptus, camphor, peppermint, and clove, all of which are irritants and have no benefit for controlling breakouts; rather, they can create red and inflamed skin, making matters worse.

☹ **Sensitive Skin Astringent** *($8.99 for 5 ounces)* is shockingly similar to the Oil-Fighting version above (actually, it contains even more alcohol), and the same comments apply.

☺ **Moisturizing Mist** *($4.99 for 2.1 ounces)* is a very lightweight, OK toner that is an option for normal to oily skin. It does contain about 2% salicylic acid but the pH of 7 makes it completely ineffective for exfoliation.

☺ **Deep Action Cleansing Mask, Oil Free** *($4.99 for 4 ounces)* isn't deep cleaning, but like all mineral masks it does offer some oil absorption.

☹ **Invisible Blemish Treatment** *($4.49 for 0.75 ounce)* is over 28% alcohol and that can be irritating and drying for skin, making matters worse rather than better.

☹ **Overnight Acne Patches** *($4.99 for 30 patches)*. The product's pH of 5 means that the 2% salicylic acid is not all that effective for exfoliation. Plus, the patch concept offers no advantage over just applying a well-formulated lightweight product all over the face. Besides, if you are struggling with blemishes all over, how many patches must you place all over the skin at night? One more point: The film-forming agent in here can be a problem for skin.

✓☺ **Persa-Gel 10, Maximum Strength** *($3.49 for 1 ounce)* is a very good, 10% benzoyl peroxide liquid. The company discontinued their 5% version, but for a stronger benzoyl peroxide product, this one would be just fine. At this strength benzoyl peroxide can be irritating for some skin types, in which case a milder 5% or 2.5% version would be better.

☺ **Clear Touch Oil Absorbing Sheets** *($4.95 for 50 sheets)* are an interesting twist on the standard oil-absorbing papers. These are more like soft plastic sheets with a slight rubbery feel (not the rose-petal texture mentioned in the ads). They do work well enough, but it takes several of them to make a difference, just as it does with any of the more standard oil-absorbing papers.

CLEARASIL (SKIN CARE ONLY)

Clearasil has been around as a teenage acne product for decades! Has it cured anyone's acne? From what I remember, these products didn't work for anyone when I was a kid, and they still don't! Many contain problematic ingredients that can worsen skin irritation and redness, and that's not good news for those with blemish-prone skin. For more information about Clearasil, call (866) 252-5327 or visit www.clearasil.com.

☹ **Antibacterial Bar** *($2.72 for 3.25 ounces)* is a standard, tallow-based cleanser with a detergent cleansing agent. It contains the disinfectant triclosan, which has no research showing it to be effective for breakouts, but even if it did, its effects would be rinsed down the drain with the cleanser. The big problem is that this product contains tallow, which can cause breakouts and blackheads.

☺ **Daily Face Wash** *($3.93 for 6.5 ounces)* is a standard, detergent-based, water-soluble cleanser that may be OK for someone with oily skin, though the detergent cleansing agents in it can be more drying than most. It contains the disinfectant triclosan, but its effects are washed away in a cleanser and there is no research showing it to be effective against blemishes.

☹ **Adult Care Acne Tinted Cream** *($4.52 for 0.65 ounce)* contains resorcinol and sulfur, both potent disinfectants, but they are extremely irritating and problematic for skin. It also contains alcohol! Ouch! Further, one of the thickeners is isopropyl myristate, which can cause breakouts. Aside from being very drying and irritating, this product may also clog pores.

☺ **Tinted Cream Maximum Strength** *($5.18 for 1 ounce)* is a 10% benzoyl peroxide product with a tint. Although the benzoyl peroxide is an effective disinfectant, few people have skin that's this color. You can find similar products with tints that won't look strange on your skin.

☺ **Vanishing Treatment Cream Maximum Strength** *($5.18 for 1 ounce)* is unlikely to cause anything to vanish. It is a 10% benzoyl peroxide product that also contains clay and thickeners. One of the thickeners is isopropyl myristate, which can cause breakouts, but the benzoyl peroxide is an effective disinfectant.

☺ **Stay Clear Acne Defense Cleanser** *($5.32 for 6.78 ounces)* is a standard, detergent-based, water-soluble cleanser that also contains salicylic acid. The problem with having salicylic acid in a cleanser is that it will be rinsed down the drain before it has time to absorb into the skin. Even if that weren't a problem, this one contains a small amount of menthol, and that can be irritating for the skin and eyes.

☹ **Stay Clear Deep Clean Astringent** *($3.49 for 8 ounces)* is a 2% salicylic acid toner steeped in alcohol and menthol, and is not recommended for any skin type.

☹ **Stay Clear Deep Clean Pads** *($3.49 for 65 pads)* is similar to the Deep Clean Astringent above minus the menthol, and the same comments apply.

☹ **Stay Clear Zone Control Clearstick** *($4.99 for 1.2 ounces)* is similar to the Deep Clean Astringent above, only in stick form, and the same comments apply.

The Reviews C

CLIENTELE

Hype and exaggerated claims abound in the Clientele group of skin-care products. Actually, they're poured on so thick you can barely step through them. For example, the information on Clientele's Web site states that "It was Clientele that pioneered the antiaging breakthrough in the 1970's that revolutionized the entire cosmetic industry by first introducing antioxidants. Now Clientele's team of doctors has come up with something even more exciting. It combines enzymes and a rare flower that's been around since Ancient Egypt. It's called the Sacred Lotus Flower."

If Clientele was the first company to "use antioxidants" and "provide research that it slows aging," there is no evidence of that, and not a shred of documentation or studies published anywhere. In fact the original product from their line, dating back to the '70s, Moisture Concentrate, doesn't contain one antioxidant or any other significant skin-care ingredient. As for the use of lotus seed extract, it does have a small amount of research showing it to be a good antioxidant and anti-inflammatory, but suggesting it is some kind of miracle is an assertion without any proof whatsoever. However, other antioxidants that Clientele and many cosmetics companies use, such as superoxide dismutase, vitamin E, vitamin C, and vitamin A, among many others, do have abundant research showing their efficacy when applied topically on skin. What is absolutely undeniable, despite this line's claims of a "50% reduction in wrinkles," is that not one plastic surgeon has gone out of business because of these products.

Each of Clientele's three groups of products—Clientele, Time Therapy, and Elastology—makes escalating antiwrinkle claims. If you believe even a fraction of what is described in their brochures, these products should set your face back 20 years. I won't even start on the cosmetic surgery and photographic air-brushing their spokespeople have had, but there is no way those wrinkle-free visages are an unretouched reality or a result of these products. The notion that Clientele is using patented ingredients is bogus, too, because almost every single ingredient in these products shows up in hundreds of other products throughout the industry. What makes reviewing this line particularly confusing is that Clientele has repackaged and renamed many of their products, placed them in different product groupings, and even priced them differently, which is all incredibly strange and mystifying.

For the most part (except for the Elastology line), these products are just some of many in the world of cosmetics that contain an impressive assortment of antioxidants, water-binding agents, and antioxidants. Some of their sunscreens are well-formulated, too. But be careful—this line also has some poorly formulated sunscreens, several over-the-top irritating formulations, inappropriate products for oily and blemish-prone skin, and packaging that would quickly allow antioxidants or plant extracts to deteriorate. For all of Clientele's research (which isn't available anywhere for review), they overlooked a lot of basic issues about skin care.

It is important to point out that with all the bravado today about the use of antioxidants in skin care and their use for eliminating wrinkles or stopping aging, there isn't any research showing that takes place. That's not to say that antioxidants don't and shouldn't play a significant role in skin care, because they absolutely should, it's just that there is no proof they fight aging or wrinkles the way we'd like to hope they would. So while theoretically antioxidants are a wise addition to any skin-care product, we are still at sea looking for solid answers that only the cosmetics industry purports to have found. For more information about Clientele, call (800) 327-4660 or visit www.clientele.org.

CLIENTELE SKIN CARE

☺ $$$ **Gentle Cleansing Bar for Normal to Dry Skin** *($16 for 4 ounces)* is a standard bar cleanser with minuscule amounts of vitamins. There is no advantage in using this bar cleanser over Cetaphil Bar Cleanser found at the drugstore for a fifth of this price.

☹ $$$ **Gentle Cleansing Bar for Normal to Oily Skin** *($16 for 4 ounces)* is almost identical to the Bar for Normal to Dry Skin above only this contains sulfur, which can be a disinfectant, although it is also extremely irritating and drying.

☺ $$$ **Face Wash** *($25 for 8 ounces)* is a standard, detergent-based cleanser that can be an option for someone with normal to oily skin.

☺ $$$ **Blemish Free Face Wash** *($35 for 8 ounces)* is almost identical to the Face Wash above only with 0.5% salicylic acid and an even smaller amount of glycolic acid. However, the pH of 5 is too high for those to be effective as exfoliants.

☺ $$$ **Eye Makeup Remover** *($14 for 2 ounces)* is a standard, detergent-based makeup remover that would work as well as any.

☹ **Surfacing Refining Lotion 40 Normal to Dry** *($30 for 8 ounces)* is mostly alcohol and some menthol, and that isn't refining in the least. Instead, it is drying and irritating, especially for normal to dry skin. What were they thinking?

☹ **Surfacing Refining Lotion 60 Normal to Oily** *($30 for 8 ounces)* is almost identical to the Normal to Dry version above only with more alcohol, which makes it even worse for skin.

☹ **Blemish & Acne Treatment Roll-On** *($25 for 0.35 ounce)*. The sulfur and resorcinol in here are topical disinfectants, but they are also exceedingly irritating and drying for skin. This is poorly formulated for any skin type, but especially for dry, sensitive skin.

☺ $$$ **Activator Normal/Dry Problem Skin Formula** *($50 for 3.18 ounces or 60 packets)* contains sunscreen ingredients (UVB only) but is not rated with an SPF, which is strange. Other than that, this is a good, though expensive and unnecessary, way to apply what ends up being a very good moisturizer for normal to dry skin with some good plant oils, antioxidants, and a small amount of water-binding agents.

☺ $$$ **Activator Normal/Oily Problem Skin Formula** *($50 for 3.18 ounces or 60 packets)* is similar to the Normal/Dry version above only the sunscreen ingredient is titanium dioxide, which can be a problem for blemish-prone skin. Still, this is a good lightweight moisturizer with good water-binding agents and antioxidants. It would be an option for normal to dry skin, but it should not be relied on for any amount of sun protection.

☺ $$$ **Roll-On Alpha Hydroxy Wrinkle Treatment** *($25 for 0.35 ounce)* contains about 5% glycolic acid in a lightweight lotion that has some good antioxidants as well. The pH of 4 makes it effective for exfoliation. This is a pricey AHA product and there are definitely other well-formulated versions available for far less. The application is clever but adds no benefit and ends up transferring bacteria from your skin to the product.

☹ $$$ **Moisture Concentrate** *($40 for 4 ounces)* is an exceptionally standard moisturizer of water, waxes, glycerin, and preservatives, adding up to a complete waste of time and money. It actually contains no water-binding agents, antioxidants, or any remotely interesting ingredient for skin.

☹ **Oil-Free Daytime Moisture Concentrate SPF 8** *($40 for 4 ounces)* not only has an SPF that falls far short of the standard SPF 15, it also doesn't contain the UVA-protecting ingredients of titanium dioxide, zinc oxide, or avobenzone, and is not recommended.

☹ **Preventive Age Treatment SPF 12 Dry Skin** *($35 for 1.1 ounces)* merits the same comments as the Oil-Free Daytime Moisture Concentrate SPF 8 above, only here the SPF is 12, which is still below the standard of SPF 15.

☺ $$$ **Nourishing Night Oils** *($100 for 10 vials)* contains mostly sunflower and olive oil along with some good antioxidants. The price is absurd for what you get, but it is a good emollient for normal to dry skin.

☹ **Time Shield Natural Oils** *($28 for 2 ounces)* is supposed to be a little bit of everything—a precleanser, eye-makeup remover, and antiwrinkle oil—and it even makes claims of having mild sun protection, which is the same as saying this product will leave your skin subject to sun damage, which it will. But mild sun protection is OK with Clientele because this product is also supposed to be a "fast tanning oil," which is a shocking suggestion from a company making so much ado about the antiaging products they sell. Not only is the sun protection abysmal (not rated, but not enough concentration to be much more than an SPF of 6), but it also doesn't contain UVA-protecting ingredients. This is just coconut, almond, olive, and sunflower oil with a tiny amount of antioxidants. You would do just as well with some plain olive oil and, of course, a well-formulated sunscreen.

☺ $$$ **Time Therapy** *($75 for 1.1 ounces)* is a very good, silicone-based moisturizer for normal to dry skin. It contains a good mix of antioxidants and water-binding agents. Some of the plant extracts can be skin irritants (clove and orange) but there probably isn't enough of them to be a problem for skin.

☹ $$$ **Wrinkle Treatment** *($75 for 1.1 ounces)* is similar to the Time Therapy above only with far fewer antioxidants. It is still an option for normal to dry skin, but if you are really shopping this line, choosing this version is not the best idea.

☹ $$$ **Spot Lightening Roll-On** *($25 for 0.35 ounce)* contains hydroquinone, a melanin-inhibiting ingredient that can lighten skin, but there is no information about how much of it this product contains. It is an option but this type of formulation is not unique in any way. .

☹ **Facial Masque for Normal/Dry Sensitive Skin Formula** *($45 for 6 Facial Masque Packets 0.5 ounce each and 3 ounces of Masque Lotion)* is a standard clay mask that you mix up yourself combining the powder packets with the Masque Lotion. The lotion contains too much alcohol and menthol and it is not recommended.

☹ **Facial Masque for Oily Problem Skin Formula** *($45 for 6 Facial Masque Packets 0.5 ounce each and 3 ounces of Masque Lotion)* is almost identical to the Facial Masque for Normal/Dry Sensitive Skin above, only this Masque Lotion contains acetone—that's nail polish remover—which just leaves me speechless.

CLIENTELE TIME THERAPY SKIN CARE

☺ **$$$ Alpha Hydroxy Face Wash for Normal/Dry, Sensitive Skin** *($25 for 4 ounces)* is a standard, detergent-based cleanser with less than 2% glycolic acid, which isn't enough to have exfoliating properties. The tiny amounts of antioxidants in this product would be rinsed down the drain before they had a chance to have benefit for skin. It is an option for normal to oily skin.

☹ **Alpha Hydroxy Face Wash for Normal/Oily Skin** *($25 for 4 ounces)* is similar to the Face Wash for Normal/Dry Skin above only this version contains sulfur, which makes it too drying and irritating for all skin types. It also contains tiny amounts of glycolic and salicylic acids, but the pH of this highly alkaline cleanser is too high for those to be effective for exfoliation.

☺ **Alpha Hydroxy Roll-On Rinse for Normal/Oily Skin** *($20 for 1 ounce)* contains about 5% glycolic acid in a light lotion base that contains some good antioxidants. You are supposed to apply this and then rinse it off, which would rinse the AHA right down the drain. It is a strange suggestion and not one I would recommend if you are hoping for effective exfoliation.

☺ **Alpha Hydroxy Roll-On Rinse for Normal/Dry Sensitive Skin** *($20 for 1 ounce)* is similar to the Roll-On Rinse for Normal/Oily Skin above and the same comments apply. This is not recommended for sensitive skin.

☺ **Eye Makeup Remover Oils** *($15 for 2 ounces)* does, as the name clearly says, contain plant oils, which are easily replaced by any plant oil you have in your kitchen cupboard. This will wipe off makeup.

☹ **Blemish & Acne Roll-On for Normal/Dry, Sensitive Skin** *($15 for 0.35 ounce).* The sulfur and resorcinol in here are topical disinfectants but are also exceedingly irritating and drying for skin. This is poorly formulated for any skin type, but especially for dry, sensitive skin.

☹ **Blemish & Acne Roll-On for Normal/Oily Skin** *($15 for 0.35 ounce)* is similar to the Roll-On for Normal/Dry skin above, only this one adds alcohol, taking a bad product and making it worse.

✓☺ **$$$ Day Serum SPF 25 for Normal/Dry, Sensitive Skin** *($49 for 1 ounce)* is a very good, in-part titanium dioxide–based sunscreen in an emollient base that, while way overpriced, would be good for normal to dry skin. It contains some very good antioxidants and water-binding agents.

☺ **$$$ Day Serum SPF 25 for Normal/Oily Skin** *($49 for 1 ounce)* is almost identical to the Day Serum SPF 25 above and the same comments apply. This is not recommended for oily skin.

✓☺ **$$$ Night Serum, for Normal/Dry, Sensitive Skin** *($49 for 1 ounce)* is a very good emollient lotion for normal to dry skin that contains an impressive mix of antioxidants and water-binding agents.

✓☺ **$$$ Night Serum, for Normal/Oily Skin** *($49 for 1 ounce)* is almost identical to the Night Serum for Normal/Dry Skin above, though it is less emollient; it is a very good option for normal to slightly oily skin.

☹ **$$$ Instant Age Eraser Duo** *($74 for 0.15 ounce of Wrinkle Eye Cream and 0.15 ounce of Treatment Concealer).* This won't erase a minute of age off your skin. The **Wrinkle Eye Cream** is simply a good emollient moisturizer for normal to dry skin that contains some very good antioxidants and water-binding agents. The **Treatment Concealer** is just a very greasy stick concealer that can easily slip into lines on the face, making them more obvious. There is nothing in here that is a treatment of any kind.

✓☺ **$$$ Sacred Lotus Seed Wrinkle Serum** *($49 for 1 ounce)* is a very good emollient moisturizer that contains a very good mix of plant oils, antioxidants, and water-binding agents. What benefit the lotus seed may have is up to you.

☹ **$$$ Spot Lightening Roll-On** *($15 for 0.35 ounce)* contains hydroquinone, a melanin-inhibiting ingredient, but there is no information about how much of it is in this product. It is an option but it is not unique in any way.

CLIENTELE ELASTOLOGY SKIN CARE

☺ **$$$ Gentle Soy Antioxidant Wash** *($35 for 8 ounces)* is a standard, detergent-based cleanser that is an option for normal to oily skin.

☺ **$$$ Makeup Remover** *($25 for 2 ounces)* contains mostly Vaseline and plant oils. There would be little difference between using this versus plain mineral oil or a plant oil like coconut oil or sunflower oil (the second and third ingredients in here). The antioxidants in this formula are nice, but plain olive oil is a great antioxidant and far cheaper than this.

☹ **$$$ Builder with Triple Alpha Hydroxys** *($65 for 1.1 ounce)* is a slightly sticky lotion with a pH that is too high for the glycolic acid in this product to be effective for exfoliation. This product does contain some good antioxidants and anti-irritants, just not very much of them given the price. Several of the plant extracts can be skin irritants.

✓☺ **$$$ Antiaging Activator Plus** *($50 for 1.3 ounces)* is an emollient moisturizer for normal to dry skin that contains an impressive mix of antioxidants, anti-irritants, and water-binding agents.

✔☺ $$$ **Firming Eye Cream** *($45 for 0.5 ounce)* is similar to the Antiaging Activator plus above and the same comments apply.

✔☺ $$$ **Firming Night Cream** *($75 for 1.1 ounce or kit 3 for $84)* is similar to the Antiaging Activator Plus above and the same comments apply.

✔☺ $$$ **Lotus Firming Serum** *($65 for 1 ounce)* contains an exceptional mix of antioxidants, water-binding agents, and anti-irritants. For the money and formulation this is one of the best of this group.

☺ $$$ **Lotus Vitamin C Serum** *($65 for 1 ounce)* contains ascorbic acid as the chosen form of vitamin C, and it's rather high up on the ingredient listing. Unfortunately, ascorbic acid is also considered to be one of the more irritating forms of vitamin C for the skin. Aside from that, this lightweight lotion contains some very good antioxidants and water-binding agents. The pH of 4 is low enough for the glycolic and salicylic acids in here to be effective as exfoliants.

☹ $$$ **50 Restorative Complex** *($100 for 0.5 ounce)* is a very emollient moisturizer for normal to dry skin that contains an impressive mix of water-binding agents and antioxidants. However this does contain phytosterol, which has research showing it can be a problem when applied to skin and exposed to sunlight. It also has progesterone that can easily absorb into skin and then affect your body systemically, not just your skin (Source: *Journal of Steroid Biochemistry and Molecular Biology*, April 2002, pages 449–455). Applying a hormone topically to skin for the sake of skin care without knowing how much you are using or what the risks may be is unwise. There is also pregnenolone acetate in here, a precursor to other hormones that can affect levels of progesterone and estrogen in the body when taken orally. When applied to skin it may work as a water-binding agent. There is no information if absorption through skin is even possible and there is no research showing it can change skin. Please refer to Chapter Seven, *Cosmetics Dictionary*, for more specifics about these ingredients.

☹ $$$ **Soy Estro-Lift Face Therapy** *($75 for 1 ounce)*. The minuscule amount of soy and wild yam in here can have no impact on skin, or at least there is no research showing that topically applied soy or wild yam can have estrogenic or progesterone-like properties for skin. Of more concern is the amount of progesterone this product contains. Please refer to Chapter Seven, *Cosmetics Dictionary*, for more specifics, and see the comments above for the 50 Restorative Complex. This does contain some good antioxidants and water-binding agents, but this product has risks you may want to check out with your physician or health care provider.

☹ $$$ **Soy Estro-Lift Neck Therapy** *($55 for 2 ounces)* is more emollient than the Estro-Lift Face Therapy above, but the same concerns and comments apply.

☹ $$$ **Youth Elixir Wrinkle Cream** *($29.95 for 1 ounce)* is a silicone-based moisturizer for normal to dry skin that contains far smaller amounts of pregnenolone acetate and progesterone than the Estro-Lift products above, though the same concerns and comments apply.

The Reviews C

✓☺ **$$$ Age Blocker with SPF 25** *($75 for 1.1 ounces)* is a very good, in-part titanium dioxide–based sunscreen in an emollient base that would be good for normal to dry skin. It contains some very good antioxidants and water-binding agents, but if the price prevents you from applying this liberally, then it is a product you should not be using.

✓☺ **$$$ Saving Face Oil Free SPF 30** *($65 for 1 ounce)* is a very good, titanium dioxide–based sunscreen in an emollient base with good antioxidants and water-binding agents, though the price may prevent you from applying it generously enough to obtain the SPF on the label.

☹ **Line Smoother Roll-On** *($30 for 0.35 ounce)* contains cornstarch, and that can be a problem for skin as well as not smoothing out anything. This does have a small amount of some good antioxidants, but given that many of the products in this and other lines also do, there is no reason to bother with this one.

☺ **$$$ Vital Factors** *($115 for 1 ounce)* isn't any more vital than any other moisturizer Clientele sells, and is actually a less impressive formula with smaller amounts of antioxidants. It does contain salicylic acid, but the pH of 5 is too high for it to be effective as an exfoliant. This also contains tiny amounts of progesterone and wild yam extract; see comments about the Soy Estro-Lift above for concerns regarding those two ingredients, as well as Chapter Seven, *Cosmetics Dictionary*, for more specifics.

✓☺ **$$$ Sun Kiss Lip Conditioner SPF 15** *($15 for 0.24 ounces)* is a very good, emollient lip balm with a great SPF that uses only titanium dioxide as the active sunscreen ingredient.

CLIENTELE MAKEUP

Clientele's makeup appears to be an afterthought. The majority of the items have dated formulas, poor textures, and color combinations that give a whole new meaning to the phrase "blast from the past." Perhaps what's most confusing is that several of Clientele's makeup products go by different names, and for some the same formulas are marketed to disparate skin types. For example, their Under Eye Concealer and Treatment Conceal are identical. Both are sold with age-erasing claims, and only the packaging differs. Clientele also offers one foundation with no less than *three* distinctive names, but don't try to dispute this with them or you'll get a run-around the size of a football stadium, and still be no closer to understanding what's going on and why. If you are somehow duped into thinking Clientele is the one and only answer for your skin, they do have a few noteworthy makeup items. If you're a curious bystander wondering whether or not you should keep on walking, I would advise you to do just that, and at a rather quick pace just to be safe.

<u>FOUNDATION:</u> ☹ **Elastology Perfect Coverage Liquid Makeup** *($35)* carries over Elastology's theme of firming the skin, but don't count on anything close to that or a makeup that looks natural. The formula is nearly identical to Clinique's alcohol-based Pore Minimizer Makeup, which is bad enough. Compounding matters further, the three colors are an excellent example of what to avoid when it comes to choosing your ideal

foundation color. Note: This product is also sold under the name **Perfect Coverage Makeup** and **Oil-Free Skin Tone Balancer** *($25)*. **Moisturizing Skin Tone Balancer** *($30)* doesn't balance anything, and the four colors for this emollient foundation are just distantly related to neutral tones.

☺ $$$ **Perfect Coverage Makeup Compact** *($35)* is a pressed-powder foundation that is easily replaced by less expensive, readily available versions from Aveda to M.A.C. The three shades are not as noticeably poor as the Perfect Coverage makeup above, but they're still far from neutral.

<u>CONCEALER:</u> ☹ **Under Eye Concealer** *($30)* is sold with the tag line "there's nothing like it! The finest conceal on earth." P. T. Barnum would be proud of this showmanship, but his cast of circus performers would rightly balk at the prospect of using this overly creamy compact concealer that comes in two of the worst shades imaginable. Note: This product is also known as **Treatment Conceal** *($30)*.

☺ $$$ <u>POWDER:</u> **Oil Control Powder** *($25)* is a talc-free pressed powder with a sheer, flaky texture and two average colors. It's a decent option but disappointing for this price. **Oil Control Loose Powder** *($25)* is almost identical to the Oil Control Powder, except this goes on even sheerer and among other colors offered there is a must-avoid shade called Lavender Lift.

☺ $$$ <u>BLUSH:</u> **Contour Blush** *($25)* is a pigment-rich, pressed-powder blush, and despite the name, most of the colors should not be used for contouring (they're too vibrant or pastel). Of the six shades, four have great smooth textures and even applications. Avoid Plum and Rose—both have unusually dry, grainy textures that tend to grab and stick to the skin. The square sponge on a stick that accompanies this blush is not recommended unless you're trying to create a strange swatch of color.

☹ <u>EYESHADOW:</u> **Eye Color Treatment** *($20)* shares the same smooth or grainy texture as the Contour Blush, but these are sold as duos and the bulk of these are wildly contrasting colors that have no place in a professional makeup wardrobe.

☺ $$$ <u>EYE AND BROW SHAPER:</u> **Calligraphy Eye Pencil** *($15)* is priced about three times higher than it should be for such an ordinary, needs-sharpening pencil. You won't notice a performance or longevity difference between this and just about any pencil from Cover Girl.

☺ <u>LIPSTICK AND LIP PENCIL:</u> **Lipstick** *($15)* is a slightly creamy formula that applies well, if a bit dry, and sets to a semi-matte finish with a minimally moist feel. This would be a good choice for those who find a true matte lipstick too drying, but who need an escape from traditional creamy lipsticks that feather into lines around the mouth. **Lip Pencil** *($15)* is a standard, but good, slightly creamy pencil that is available in five shades that work well with Clientele's lipsticks.

☺ <u>MASCARA:</u> The simply-named **Mascara** *($15)* allows you to create adequate length with a touch of thickness. This tends not to clump but some smearing will occur if you're less than precise. This lasts all day and removes easily with a water-soluble cleanser.

☺ <u>SPECIALTY:</u> **All In 1 Glamour Kit** *($59)* is a fold-out, gold-covered case that holds the best and worst of Clientele. Apparently, all of these shades represent actress and infomercial diva Hunter Tylo's favorite colors. If this is to be believed, then Ms. Tylo should seriously reconsider whom she takes makeup advice from! Ironically, the slipcover picture of Ms. Tylo shows her sporting a classic, understated makeup that emphasizes soft tones, which is pretty much the opposite of what you'll find inside this product.

CLINAC

☺ **Clinac Oil Control Gel** *($19.50 for 90 grams)* is a topical gel that uses a film-forming agent to provide a matte feel on the skin and that has some absorbent properties. This product is not unique among the range of matte gel formulations that make claims of absorbing oil. However, this one is as good an option as any. The study being touted in ads as demonstrating that this product works was carried out by the company selling it, and there is no other substantiating research. For more information about Clinac, visit www.dermstore.com.

CLINIQUE

Clinique was Estee Lauder's first attempt to expand its market with a completely separate line and image. Lauder was clearly a mature woman's line and Clinique became known as the indispensable line for the woman under 30 concerned with breakouts, oily skin, and fragrance-free products (meaning less likely to cause allergic or sensitizing skin reactions). Clinique's tremendous success reshaped the way cosmetics lines identified themselves, sending the concept of line loyalty out to pasture. Today, cosmetics companies expand their market either by buying already established companies or by creating new ones. Of course, cosmetics companies keep this multiple-personality identity hidden from the consumer. If the general buying public realized that these apparently different companies were so intertwined with each other, how could the different lines flaunt their independence and claim that their unparalleled formulations are secret? Unless you think Lauder (or any company) would, even if they could, keep secrets from one branch separate from the others.

The niche Clinique built launched the notion of cosmetics being "allergy-tested," "hypoallergenic," "100% fragrance-free," and "dermatologist tested." Of those marketing claims the only one that has significance is the "100% fragrance free," which, for the most part, Clinique maintains (it does have some fragrant extracts in a few products). But unless you can see the test results, what difference does it make if a product is "allergy-tested"? What if the test showed 20% of the women who used it had a sensitizing reaction, dryness, or irritation? Moreover, "hypoallergenic" is a term that is not regulated by the FDA, so any product can claim it. "Dermatologist tested" is also bogus, because without published test results, the term can easily mean nothing more than that a dermatologist picked up the product, looked at the container, and said, "This looks good."

Clinique's products, particularly the skin-care products, are aimed at oily or combination skin types, which is probably why Clinique attracts a younger clientele, but many of these products are exceptionally irritating. Among these disappointing products are the ones that contain a lot of alcohol, which would be drying, or the emollient moisturizers, recommended for oily, acne-prone skin, which could trigger breakouts. The strong points of Clinique products are the lack of fragrance of any kind in many of the products, some great moisturizer formulas, and excellent sunscreens. One thing you can be sure of at most Clinique counters is service. There always seem to be four to five white-jacketed women dashing around behind those cases. (The white jackets are supposed to look medical—how contrived can you get!) One more plus is that the products are by far more affordable than those of numerous other lines in department stores. For more information about Clinique, call (212) 572-3800 or visit www.clinique.com.

CLINIQUE SKIN CARE

☹ **Facial Soap Extra Mild** *($11 for 6 ounces)* is just soap, which means it is too drying and irritating for all skin types. It's not one iota different from other "soaps" at the drugstore.

☹ **Facial Soap Mild** *($11 for 6 ounces)* is similar to the Facial Soap Extra Mild above and the same comments apply.

☹ **Facial Soap Oily Skin Formula** *($11 for 6 ounces)* is similar to the Facial Soap Extra Mild above and the same comments apply.

☺ **Comforting Cream Cleanser** *($16.50 for 5 ounces)* is an excellent emollient cleanser that would be an option for dry skin. It would work just fine, but it is almost identical to Neutrogena's Gentle Skin Cleanser for half the price.

☺ **Extremely Gentle Cleansing Cream** *($22.50 for 10 ounces)* is an exceedingly standard mineral oil– and Vaseline-based wipe-off cleanser that can leave a greasy film on the skin. It is an option for very dry skin, but there is little reason to use this rather than just plain, fragrance-free mineral oil.

☹ **Rinse-Off Foaming Cleanser** *($16.50 for 5 ounces)* is a detergent-based cleanser that uses more drying cleansing agents than most, plus it adds lemon, eucalyptus, pine, and cardamom, and that makes it an irritation waiting to happen.

☹ **Wash-Away Gel Cleanser** *($16.50 for 5 ounces)* is similar to the Rinse-Off Foaming Cleanser above and the same comments apply.

☺ **Extremely Gentle Eye Makeup Remover** *($10 for 2 ounces)* is a basic lotion that will remove makeup—boring, but effective.

☺ **Naturally Gentle Eye Makeup Remover** *($14.50 for 2.5 ounces)* is supposed to be as "gentle to the eyes as tears." Since when were tears made up of hydrogenated polyisobutene, butylene glycol, ammonium acryloyldimethyltaurate/VP copolymer, or acrylates/C10-30 alkyl acrylate crosspolymer? This is a good eye-makeup remover, but it is very basic and no gentler than others. The second ingredient is sesame oil, and if you happen to have that in your kitchen cabinet, it, too, would really be gentle for removing makeup.

☺ **Rinse-Off Eye Makeup Solvent** *($13.50 for 4.2 ounces)* is a standard detergent-based eye-makeup remover that would work as well as any.

☺ **Take the Day Off Makeup Remover, for Lids, Lashes and Lips** *($15.50 for 4.2 ounces)* is a standard, silicone-based makeup remover that would work as well as any.

☹ **7 Day Scrub Cream** *($15 for 3.5 ounces)* is a mineral oil–based scrub that uses polyethylene (ground-up plastic) as the abrasive. This is a fairly unrinseable, heavy, greasy scrub that would only be an option for dry to very dry skin.

☺ **7 Day Scrub Cream Rinse Off Formula** *($15 for 3.4 ounces)* is a very basic, emollient cleanser that uses polyethylene (ground-up plastic) as the abrasive. As a mechanical exfoliant it would be an option for normal to dry skin.

☹ **Exfoliating Scrub** *($15 for 3.4 ounces)* would have been a good option for a scrub in a rinseable, detergent-based cleanser using polyethylene (ground-up plastic) as the abrasive; however, it contains some menthol, and that adds unnecessary irritation to the skin.

☹ **Clarifying Lotion 1** *($10.50 for 6.7 ounces)* is similar to the Lotion 3 below, and the same comments apply.

☹ **Clarifying Lotion 2** *($10.50 for 6.7 ounces)* contains alcohol and menthol, which makes it too irritating and drying for all skin types.

☹ **Clarifying Lotion 3** *($10.50 for 6.7 ounces)* lists alcohol as the second ingredient, and that is too drying and irritating for all skin types, so instead of clarifying it's just a problem for healthy skin.

☹ **Clarifying Lotion 4** *($10.50 for 6.7 ounces)* is similar to, but even more potent than, the Lotion 3 above and the same comments apply.

☺ **Mild Clarifying Lotion** *($10.50 for 6.7 ounces)*. At least this one doesn't have any irritants! It contains about a 0.5% concentration of BHA, and since the pH of this toner is about 4, that makes it effective for some amount of exfoliation. This can be an option for someone with breakouts, but a pH of 3 to 3.5 would make it more effective.

✔☺ **Advanced Stop Signs Visible Antiaging Serum** *($35 for 1.7 ounces)* isn't all that advanced, but it is a very good, silicone-based moisturizer with an excellent blend of antioxidants, water-binding agents, and anti-irritants. However, you will have to wait a very long, long time if you're hoping it will stop you from aging.

✔☺ **All About Eyes** *($26 for 0.5 ounce)* is similar to the Advanced Stop Signs above only with even more silicone, giving it a somewhat silky, slippery feel. It would be a great option for normal to dry skin.

☺ $$$ **Anti-Gravity Firming Lift Cream** *($35 for 1.7 ounces)*. The more than 50 ingredients in this product aren't lifting your skin anywhere, at least not any more than any other moisturizer in Clinique's moisturizing lineup. This is a good moisturizer for normal to dry skin, with a fair to good mix of antioxidants, anti-irritants, and water-binding agents. All in all, the Advanced Stop Signs above has a more impressive formulation.

☺ $$$ **Anti-Gravity Firming Eye Lift Cream** (*$28.50 for 0.5 ounce*) is a good emollient moisturizer for dry skin, but there is nothing in it that can fight gravity in any way, shape, or form. The product says it: "Helps erase the look of lines and builds cushion back into time-thinned skin." Except for the "builds cushion back," that would be true for any moisturizer, but there simply are no moisturizers that can put "cushion" back into skin. The cushioning of skin is provided by the fat layer of skin, which becomes depleted as we age, and this product can't build fat into skin. This is a more emollient version of the Firming Lift Cream above and the same comments apply.

☺ **Anti-Gravity Firming Lift Lotion** (*$35 for 1.7 ounces*) is indeed a lotion version of the Firming Lift Cream above and the same basic comments apply. This silicone-based version does have a soft matte finish and is good for normal to slightly dry skin.

☺ **Daily Eye Benefits** (*$26 for 0.5 ounce*) contains mostly water, slip agent, glycerin, thickeners, plant oil, plant extracts, water-binding agents, a form of vitamin A, Vaseline, and preservatives. This does contain tannin (a plant component found in tea and coffee) that can have potent antioxidant properties, but tannin can also constrict skin and cause irritation, though the amount in this product is so small it probably isn't a problem for skin. This would be an OK moisturizer for normal to dry skin.

☹ **Dramatically Different Moisturizing Lotion** (*$20.50 for 4.2 ounces*). The only thing dramatic about this moisturizer is how dated a formulation it is. This contains only water, mineral oil, sesame oil, slip agent, thickeners, Vaseline, preservatives, and the famous coloring agents that impart the product's well-known soft yellow color. It doesn't contain even a minute amount of any of today's state-of-the-art moisturizing ingredients.

✓☺ **Exceptionally Soothing Cream for Upset Skin, Anti-Itch Cream** (*$30 for 1.7 ounces*) and **Exceptionally Soothing Lotion for Upset Skin** (*$30 for 1.7 ounces*) both contain hydrocortisone acetate, which can indeed soothe irritated skin. What Clinique doesn't warn about is that continuous use of hydrocortisone over time can actually cause skin damage by thinning the skin and breaking down the skin's support structure. If you are aware of this very serious shortcoming and plan only occasional use, there are many reasons why you may prefer Clinique's products to Lanacort or Cortaid. Even though the active ingredient in these products is the same, the moisturizing base in both Clinique products is a far more elegant one, with soothing agents, silicone, and water-binding agents. However, in the long run, the base shouldn't make that much difference, because you should only be using it short-term.

✓☺ **Moisture In Control** (*$31 for 1.7 ounces*) won't control anything. There is no way a product can put moisturizing ingredients in a dry area on the face, while at the same time holding them off the face in other areas and instead applying ingredients that absorb oil. It is a lightweight moisturizer that would be ideal for someone with normal to slightly dry skin. It contains good water-binding agents and antioxidants.

✓☺ **Moisture On-Call** (*$31 for 1.6 ounces*) is supposed to help skin cells "remember" how to produce their own moisture barrier. This is a physiological impossibility, because you can't change the basic way your skin functions with a moisturizer. Of course, any moisturizer used *daily* will help your skin protect its moisturizer barrier, and this is a very good emollient moisturizer. It contains a very good mix of water-binding agents and antioxidants. The caffeine in it has skin-constricting properties, which can be a skin irritant, but the amount of it is so small that it probably has no effect.

✔☺ **Moisture On Line** *($31 for 1.7 ounces)* is almost identical to Moisture On-Call, and supposedly can "re-educate" the skin. There are no moisturizing ingredients anywhere in the world that can change the nature of skin or make skin remember anything! But skin cells can look better if you faithfully reapply the moisturizer every day, which is exactly what the instructions on this moisturizer tell you to do. Aside from the hype, this is an exceptional moisturizer for someone with normal to dry skin, with excellent water-binding agents and antioxidants.

✔☺ **Moisture Surge Eye Gel** *($26 for 0.5 ounce)* is similar to the Moisture In Control and the same basic comments apply. This would be an option for normal to slightly dry skin.

✔☺ **Moisture Surge Extra Thirsty Skin Relief** *($31 for 1.7 ounces)* is a very good, silicone-based moisturizer that contains a nice complement of antioxidants and water-binding agents. It would work well for normal to slightly dry skin.

☹ **Sheer Matteness T-Zone Shine Control** *($13.50 for 0.5 ounce)* can leave a matte feel on skin, but it offers no other benefit, and with alcohol tops on the list along with clove, this isn't the best option for skin.

☺ **Skin Texture Lotion Oil-Free Formula** *($21 for 1.25 ounces)* is a good, lightweight moisturizer with some good water-binding agents and antioxidants. This would be an option for someone with normal to dry skin.

☺ **Total Turnaround Visible Skin Renewer** *($30 for 1.7 ounces)*. Like all of Clinique's Turnaround products, this one contains a teeny amount of salicylic acid; however, the pH of 5 in these formulations prevents the BHA from being effective as an exfoliant. Other than that, in many ways this product is Clinique's rendition of Lauder's Idealist ($42.50 for 1 ounce). While you're trying to decide what to do with all the other Lauder products you own that claim to return your skin to a more youthful state, or whether or not you want your skin renewed with this product or firmed with the one above, keep in mind that Clinique's versions are almost always cheaper. For example, both Idealist and Total Turnaround contain acetyl glucosamine. The limited research establishing this ingredient as being good for wrinkles comes from the company that sells the raw ingredient and from Lauder. But then Lauder feels that lots of ingredients are good for wrinkles, so why this one more than their others is a mystery! Acetyl glucosamine is an amino acid sugar, the primary constituent of mucopolysaccharides and hyaluronic acid, and it's found in all parts of the skin. It has value as a water-binding agent, and is effective (in large concentrations) for wound healing. There is research (Source: *Cellular Molecular Life Science*, February 1997, pages 131–140 and *Biomaterials*, June 2001, pages 1667–1673) showing that chitins (also known as chitosan, which is composed of acetyl glucosamine) can help in the complex process of wound healing. However, that's at least a few generations away from what acetyl glucosamine may accomplish in teeny amounts in a skin-care product. This product contains mostly water, silicones, slip agent, water-binding agents, plant extracts, acetyl glucosamine, vitamin E, fragrant plant extract, thickeners, film-forming agent, and preservatives. This is a good, silky feeling, lightweight moisturizer for normal to dry skin.

☺ $$$ **Total Turnaround Visible Skin Renewer for Oilier Skins** *($30 for 1.7 ounces)* is nearly identical to the original Total Turnaround Cream, although this lotion does have a lighter texture and more of a matte finish on the skin. Again, the pH of 5 and the tiniest amount of salicylic acid make this a poor choice for an exfoliant, but it's still a lightweight, rather elegant moisturizer, and a good option for normal to slightly oily skins with dry areas. Contrary to the claim, this is not capable of "de-shining" the skin, though it is unlikely to make skin look or feel greasy. It is fragrance-free.

☺ **Turnaround Cream** *($26 for 1.7 ounces)* has a great name! It sounds as if this cream can turn your skin back to a younger time, but it can't (anymore than any of the other products in this line, or in the entire Lauder stable of lines can, for that matter). It contains a small amount of salicylic acid (BHA), but the pH of 5 makes it fairly ineffective as an exfoliant. This is an OK, basic moisturizer for normal to slightly dry skin, with very little to offer over many other Clinique moisturizers.

☺ **Turnaround Cream for Dry Skin** *($26 for 1.7 ounces)* is similar to the Turnaround Cream above, but this one is definitely more emollient and has slightly more water-binding agents. That does make it a better option for normal to dry skin, but it still isn't all that interesting for skin.

☺ **Turnaround Lotion Oil Free** *($26 for 1.7 ounces)* is a silicone-based moisturizer with slightly more salicylic acid than the versions above, but the pH is the same, which means that this one is no more effective as an exfoliant than the others. It does contain a good mix of water-binding agents, anti-irritant, and antioxidants, and is a good option for normal to dry skin.

✓☺ **Weather Everything Environmental Cream SPF 15** *($18.50 for 1 ounce)* is a very good, pure titanium dioxide–based sunscreen in a good moisturizing base that has a nice complement of antioxidants and water-binding agents. It would a great option for someone with normal to dry skin.

☺ **Sun Care Body SPF 15 Sun Block** *($15.50 for 3.4 ounces)* is a very good, in-part titanium dioxide– and zinc oxide–based sunscreen in a rather standard moisturizing base that makes it an option for someone with normal to dry skin. It has a small selection of antioxidants and water-binding agents.

✓☺ **Sun-Care Body SPF 25 Sun Block** *($15.50 for 3.4 ounces)* is a very good, in-part titanium dioxide– and zinc oxide–based sunscreen in an emollient moisturizing base that has some antioxidants and a tiny amount of water-binding agents. This would be very good for someone with normal to dry skin.

✔☺ **Body SPF 30 Sun Block** (*$16.50 for 5 ounces*) is similar to the Sun-Care Body SPF 25 Sun Block above and the same comments apply.

☹ **Body Spray SPF 15 Sun Block** (*$16.50 for 5 ounces*) doesn't contain the UVA-protecting ingredients of titanium dioxide, zinc oxide, or avobenzone, and is not recommended.

☺ **Body Spray SPF 30 Sun Block** (*$16.50 for 5 ounces*) is a good, in-part avobenzone-based sunscreen. Unfortunately, alcohol is the first ingredient, which makes this drying and irritating for skin. That means it's not the best, though the sun protection is excellent.

✔☺ **Face SPF 30 Sun Block** (*$16.50 for 2.5 ounces*) is similar to the Sun-Care Body SPF 25 Sun Block above and the same comments apply.

☺ **Lip/Eye SPF 30 Sun Block** (*$15.50 for 0.21 ounce*) is very good in-part zinc oxide– and titanium dioxide–based sunscreen in a standard though emollient balm form.

✔☺ **City Block Sheer SPF 15** (*$15.50 for 1.4 ounces*) is an excellent, titanium dioxide and zinc oxide–based sunscreen in a good, emollient moisturizing base. It also contains a small amount of high-quality water-binding agents and antioxidants.

✔☺ **Super City Block SPF 25 Oil-Free Daily Face Protector** (*$15.50 for 1.4 ounces*) is an excellent, pure titanium dioxide–based sunscreen in a very good, moisturizing base that includes a great mix of antioxidants and water-binding agents. This is best for someone with normal to dry skin because titanium dioxide can be too occlusive for those with oily or blemish-prone skin.

☺ **City Block Oil-Free Daily Face Protector SPF 15** (*$14.50 for 1.4 ounces*) is similar to the Super City Block above, only with a less impressive moisturizing base. Otherwise, the same basic comments apply.

☺ **Face Quick Bronze Tinted Self Tanner** (*$15.50 for 1.7 ounces*) uses the same ingredient to affect skin color as all self-tanners do, dihydroxyacetone. This one would work as well as any. It essentially does the exact same thing as the Self Tanning Lotion below with the exact same ingredient; the price difference is sheer caprice.

☺ **Self Tanning Lotion** (*$15.50 for 4.2 ounces*) uses the same ingredient to affect skin color as all self-tanners do, dihydroxyacetone. This one would work as well as any.

☺ **Deep Cleansing Emergency Masque** (*$18.50 for 3.4 ounces*) is a standard clay mask with some cleansing agents and a mix of irritating and anti-irritant plant extracts. It also contains cornstarch and that can be a problem for those with blemish-prone skin.

☺ **All About Lips** (*$20 for 0.5 ounce*) is a good, silicone-based moisturizer that has a matte finish on lips.

☺ **Superbalm Lip Treatment** (*$10 for 0.24 ounce*) is a standard, Vaseline-based, emollient lip balm with some antioxidants and water-binding agents. The spearmint is the only thing that gets in the way of this being a very good treatment for dry lips.

☺ **Moisture Stick** (*$13.50 for 0.14 ounce*) is a very standard emollient "lipstick" that contains mostly castor oil, thickeners, lanolin oil, plant oil, and a teeny amount of vitamins. This would work well for dry skin.

CLINIQUE ACNE SOLUTIONS

☺ **Antibacterial Facial Soap** *($9 for 5.2 ounces)* is a standard bar cleanser that contains triclosan, a topical disinfectant. There is no research showing that triclosan is effective against acne bacteria. This also contains menthol, which can be a skin irritant.

☹ **Acne Solutions Body Treatment Spray** *($18.50 for 3.4 ounces)* lists alcohol as the second ingredient, and it also contains peppermint. These add up to irritation and dryness, and that doesn't solve anything when it comes to acne.

☹ **Acne Solutions Night Treatment Gel** *($16 for 1.7 ounces)* is similar to the Body Treatment Spray above and the same comments apply.

☹ **Acne Solutions Daytime Shield** *($16 for 1.7 ounces)* is a lightweight, silicone-based moisturizer that could have been a great soothing option for dry skin, except that it contains peppermint, and that adds unnecessary irritation.

✓☺ **Acne Solutions Emergency Gel Lotion** *($13.50 for 0.5 ounce)* is a very good 5% benzoyl peroxide topical disinfectant for blemishes.

☹ **Acne Solutions Spot Healing Gel** *($12.50 for 0.5 ounce)* lists alcohol as the second ingredient, which is too irritating and drying for all skin types.

CLINIQUE MAKEUP

Other than the addition of even more shine-infused products and a couple of new lipstick formulas and mascaras, Clinique's makeup has largely remained the same since the previous edition of this book. They still offer a vast palette of colors and textures, especially in their huge, almost imposing, selection of foundations. Most skin tones will be well served here, although the blushes and eyeshadows still lack significant depth to show up on darker skin tones. Even the High Impact Eyeshadows, which boast "intense color coverage," are still too soft and sheer to work well on dark skin. Those with very light to medium skin tones will find almost limitless options, though more than a few products (and shade names) are a bit too cloying to appeal to the sophisticated cosmetics consumer.

Clinique has pumped up its makeup workshops using cleverly designed brochures and the lure of free gifts to guide women through the selection, application, and inevitable purchase of their makeup. Although these workshops can be helpful, especially for the makeup novice, the information you're given is more often than not geared toward improving "The Expert's" (Clinique Consultant's) average unit (in dollars) sale, and the emphasis of the workshops is on stressing that multiple products are needed to enhance your appearance, including an excess of skin-care products. Clinique is also one of the few major cosmetics players that has yet to offer its own makeup brushes. That means the Consultant must use cotton swabs, cotton pads, and disposable sponge-tip applicators to apply makeup, which is about as elegant and useful as eating filet mignon with a plastic fork.

<u>FOUNDATION:</u> Clinique's vast stable of foundations runs the gamut from barely there to ultra-coverage, and many of them are wonderful and worth considering. Most skin types will find at least one of these formulas meets their needs.

✓☺ **Dewy Smooth Antiaging Makeup SPF 15** *($19.50)* is definitely smooth, with a silky, silicone-based texture that feels amazing and blends without a hitch. Titanium dioxide is not only the sunscreen agent, it also lends an opacity that allows this makeup to provide medium to full coverage with a natural matte finish that feels slightly moist. This does not make skin look dewy or drenched in moisture—it's best for normal to slightly dry skin, or dry skin that will wear a moisturizer underneath. Beyond the sunscreen, there is nothing antiaging about the formula. Ignore the marketing hype and you'll be left with a superior foundation that comes in ten gorgeous colors for very light to dark skin.

✓☺ **Almost Makeup SPF 15** *($17.50)* is a very sheer foundation with a good, titanium dioxide–based sunscreen with an SPF 15. The colors have expanded from four to six, and what's available is great, including the darker (but not very dark) shades. This would work well for normal to dry skin for minimal coverage and a beautiful natural finish.

✓☺ **City Stick SPF 15** *($21)* is a very good stick foundation to consider and the SPF is excellent, with pure titanium dioxide as the only active ingredient. The coverage is sheer to medium, with a definite silky powder finish. As is true for any cream-to-powder foundation, the powder element can be drying for someone with dry skin, and the cream part can be greasy for someone with combination to oily skin, so that makes this one best for those with normal to slightly dry or slightly oily skin. Of the eight shades, the only one to watch out for is Beige Twist, which can be too peach for most skin tones. ✓☺ **City Base Compact Foundation SPF 15** *($21)* is similar to the City Stick SPF 15 foundation above only in compact form, but this one leaves a slightly heavier, creamier finish. The finish is still powdery, with a slightly silky feel, but not enough to hold back much shine in oilier areas, making this a best bet for normal to slightly dry skin. Except for Porcelain Beige, the ten shades are excellent and would work for a wide range of skin tones, from light to dark, but not for someone with very light or very dark skin. The SPF 15 is great, containing titanium dioxide as the only active ingredient. ✓☺ **SuperFit Makeup** *($19.50)* is an excellent option for those with oily skin who have been displeased with ultra-matte foundations. This is a great, soft-matte finish foundation that features a featherlight texture, and it also has 12 mostly excellent, neutral color options (though it lacks a shade for very light skin tones). The only colors to avoid are Petal, which can be too peach, and Spicy, which can turn copper. Champagne and Vanilla are just slightly peach, which may be a problem for oily skin types. SuperFit blends on easily, has good staying power, and easily washes off, though it isn't as oil-resistant as the ultra-matte finish products. You will get shine sooner than you would with a product like Almay's Amazing Lasting Foundation or Revlon's ColorStay. ✓☺ **Stay-True Makeup Oil-Free Formula** *($16.50)* is a very good foundation for fairly opaque, semi-matte coverage. This has an initial thick texture that blends easily and should work beautifully on very oily or normal to slightly oily skin that is looking for a soft matte (as opposed to an ultra-matte) finish. There are some great colors for both light and dark skin tones, but of the ten shades, avoid Stay Beige, Stay Porcelain, (too pink), Stay Sunny (rose), True Toffee (slightly orange), and True Bronze (too reddish-pink).

☺ **Balanced Makeup Base** *($15.50)* is one of Clinique's oldest foundations, although the number of shades has dwindled. This is best for those with fair to light skin tones who have dry to very dry skin. The mineral oil–based consistency is emollient and creamy, but it blends on well, leaving a natural finish. The coverage is light to medium, and four of the seven colors are excellent; the ones to avoid are: Creamy Peach (too peach), Warmer (too peach), and Honeyed Beige (very pink). **Soft Finish Makeup** *($19.50)* is quite similar to Clinique's Balanced Makeup Base above in terms of consistency and coverage, but this one has a silicone-enhanced slip and is slightly more sheer than the Balanced. This also claims to contain "optical diffusers" to diminish the appearance of wrinkles, but a quick check in daylight while wearing it will quickly disprove that. This is still a good foundation for normal to very dry skin. Of the nine shades, all are beautifully neutral except Soft Cream and Soft Porcelain, which are both too pink.

☺ **Superbalanced Makeup** *($17.50)* is Clinique's top-selling foundation worldwide, in no small part because it claims to provide moisture and absorb oil when and where needed—a skin-care dream many women share. However, this ends up doing neither job very well. There is no way any product can differentiate between the oily parts of your face and the dry parts. The absorbent ingredients in it will soak up any oil they come in contact with (including the moisturizing ingredients in this product or in the one you applied to your skin) and the moisturizing ingredients will get deposited over areas you don't want to be moisturized. What that adds up to is a light to medium coverage, light-matte finish foundation that is best for someone with normal to slightly dry or slightly oily skin. Someone with any amount of excess oil would not be happy with the finish or with how it wears during the day. Even more disappointing are the colors, which include some astonishingly poor options for fair to light skin. Although the darker shades are actually some of the best around, many of the lighter colors are strongly peach to orange! Of the 24 shades, the following colors are best avoided by most skin tones: Petal, Fair, Cream, Ivory, Nude Beige, Linen, Porcelain Beige, Golden, Sunny, Warmer, and Honeyed Beige. Alabaster, Light, and Breeze are the best neutral shades to consider if you have fair skin. **Clarifying Makeup** *($17.50)* is an updated, vastly improved version of Clinique's Pore Minimizer Makeup. While the Clarifying Makeup still contains alcohol as the third ingredient, the foundation application itself is impressive. It has a soft, ultra-light texture, sheer-to-light coverage, and a smooth matte, somewhat transparent, finish. The colors are very nice, with most being neutral to yellow-based. Of the nine shades the only one to avoid is Blushing Buff, although the following three shades are borderline peachy and may turn orange on very oily skin: Perfect Almond, Light Beige, and Neutral Spice. A note of caution: This formula tends to separate, and should be thoroughly shaken before use. **Continuous Coverage SPF 15** *($15.50)* is a very opaque, full-coverage makeup that will certainly not look natural. What it will do is provide substantial camouflage for irregular pigmentation or birthmarks. The sunscreen active ingredient is all titanium dioxide, and this, coupled with the thick, powdery finish, can lend a chalky look to the skin. The four available shades are good, but the pluses and minuses mean that this is definitely a trade-off foundation. **Gentle Light Makeup** *($22.50)* is a sheer liquid foundation that feels light as a feather on the skin and blends wonderfully. It dries to a soft matte finish, but only in feel. The actual appearance on the skin is shiny, almost sparkly, as this makeup contains a good deal of gold iridescence, supposedly to make the skin look luminous. According to Clinique, this makeup contains "mosaic-like mirrored particles equal in size and shape." You can sum up that marketing spin in a one-word translation—glitter—which is exactly what you will see on your face. Perhaps this would work for an evening look or for a special occasion, but for day-to-day wear, an artificially shimmering face is no substitute for the clean, dewy glow you could easily achieve by simply not using any powder. Of the nine shades available, only Cream Light and Beige Glow are a bit too peachy pink, but this product is sheer enough that it's almost not an issue. The remaining (sparkling) colors are all excellent, including options for dark skin. Minus the shine, this would be a superior sheer foundation.

☹ **Workout Makeup All-Day Wear** *($15.50)* is a creamy, water-resistant foundation that provides medium coverage and a rather heavy application. Almost all of the six shades are too peach, orange, pink, or rose to look convincing. **Pore Minimizer Makeup** *($15.50)* is back, apparently by popular demand. I still can't understand the appeal of this watery, alcohol- and talc-based foundation. Yes, it does provide a solid matte finish, but the resulting irritation from the alcohol and the meager, often spotty, coverage are simply not worth the effort. Clearly, there were enough women who liked this makeup to convince Clinique to reinstate it (but only in four shades). However, for the uninitiated, this does not deserve consideration over Clinique's Skin Clarifying or SuperFit Makeups.

CONCEALER: ☺ **Soft Conceal Corrector** *($12.50)* comes in a squeeze tube and offers smooth, even coverage in a great, but small, selection of colors (Light is slightly ash-rose). This has a thick texture and soft powdery finish with only a minimal tendency to crease.

☺ **Advanced Concealer** *($12.50)* comes in a squeeze tube, goes on like a thick cream, but quickly dries to a powder. Coverage is very good without looking heavy. This comes in two shades, Light and Medium, and both are excellent. But beware: This concealer works only if the skin under your eyes is smooth; any dry or rough skin will look worse if you place this over it. **Quick Corrector** *($11.50)* comes in a tube with a wand applicator and has a fluid, slightly moist application. It smooths on easily and covers well with a minimally matte finish, though the unstable matte finish can translate into some creasing around the eyes. Avoid Medium, which is too pink. **City Cover Compact Concealer SPF 15** *($13.50)* is one of the few concealers that has a reliable SPF 15 with UVA protection.

With the exception of City Light Pink, the colors are quite workable and capable of almost full coverage. The problem is that this has a creamy consistency that will crease before you're out the door. If the sun protection appeals to you, make sure you try this at the counter first and see how it wears over a period of time—or, for a greatly reduced tendency to crease, consider Lancome's Photogenic Skin-Illuminating Concealer SPF 15 ($20) instead. **Line Smoothing Concealer** *($13.50)* has a creamy-smooth, slightly slippery texture that blends on decently and dries to a natural finish with a hint of iridescence. The claim for this concealer is that it can be used over lines and wrinkles to "build a bridge" without settling into them, thus making these "flaws" less noticeable. While the risk of creasing is minimal, there is enough visible shine to draw attention to lines—so much for that bridge-building claim. The three shades are all slightly peach-toned, but may work for some skin tones.

☹ **Acne Solutions Concealing Cream** *($12.50)* is terrible in just about every respect. This is one of the driest, thickest, most opaque and difficult-to-blend concealers I have encountered. It does contain 1% BHA (salicylic acid), but the pH is too high for it to be an effective exfoliant, and it also includes alcohol and sulfur, making the whole thing a troublesome irritation for the skin. **Concealing Stick** *($13.50)* is a lipstick-style concealer available in only one color, which is too peach for most skin tones. Even if the color were more neutral, this is a greasy product that easily slips and doesn't have the best coverage. Still, enough people must be buying this to warrant keeping it around.

POWDER: ✓☺ **Blended Face Powder & Brush** *($16.50)* is one of the best talc-based loose powders available, and in an attractive array of colors. This has a light, supple finish that clings well without caking. Of the eight shades, avoid Transparency 1 (almost pure white), Transparency 2 (pale pink), and Transparency Bronze (nice color, but too shiny). ✓☺ **Stay Matte Sheer Pressed Powder Oil-Free** *($16.50)* is an excellent, talc-based powder with a slightly dry, sheer finish that is great for oilier skin types. The eight shades are beautiful and there are some good options for light and dark skin tones.

☺ **Soft Finish Pressed Powder** *($16.50)* is intended by Clinique to be used for drier skin, and that makes sense, as this talc-based formula has a creamier, silky feel and smooth, even coverage. The light-diffusing claims are bogus, but there are five great neutral colors. **Superpowder Double Face Powder** *($16.50)* is a standard, talc-based pressed powder with a smooth, soft texture. It can be used alone or as a regular finishing powder. There are eight very sheer shades, and most of them are excellent. As a reminder, you may be told this can be used wet, but attempting this method of application can result in a streaked, choppy appearance.

☺ $$$ **Gentle Light Pressed Powder** *($20)* supposedly "turns skin radiant" but that's courtesy of the sparkles interspersed throughout this talc-based powder. The can't-miss-it shine is not for those concerned with keeping a shiny appearance down, but for everyone else the five beautiful colors are all options, and this applies smoothly. **Gentle Light Powder and Brush** *($21)* is a talc-based loose powder that is exceptionally light and soft, yet is infused with enough shine to make a chorus of Las Vegas showgirls sparkle with envy. The five shades are beautiful, but this is one shiny, sparkly powder!

BLUSH: The color products (blushes, eyeshadows, and lipsticks) are arranged into four groupings: Nudes/Naturals (which are not all that nude), Tawnies/Corals/Reds, Pinks/Roses/Fuchsias, and Violets/Blues/Berries. This is definitely a helpful way to organize a large color collection!

☺ Sheer Powder Blusher ($16.50) has a great selection of colors, but they are so soft and sheer as to be almost nonexistent on the skin when applied. Even after layering some of the "deeper" colors, it was hard to notice any intensity. Most of the colors also have a slight amount of shine, but it, too, is barely noticeable on the skin. This would be a goof-proof option for the blush-shy! Soft Pressed Powder Blusher ($16.50) does up the ante a bit in terms of depth of color, but these are still quite sheer, and darker skin tones will have a hard time getting these to show up. The colors are all fine, though several have a minimal to moderate amount of shine. Gel Blush ($10.50) has been reintroduced. This traditional gel blush is available in four colors that are lovely and sheer, but—as with all cheek stains—these work best on smooth, flawless skin and must be blended quickly if they are to look convincing. This can also be used on the lips for a sheer stained effect.

☹ Blushwear ($14.50) is Clinique's version of a cream-to-powder blush and it really isn't worth considering. This tends to "grab" on the skin and look spotty, dotting the pores with color and sparkles—each of the shades has a subtle to glaring shine. Clinique has done much better with this type of product in the past. For a superior, non-shiny cream-to-powder blush option, consider Paula Dorf Cheek Color Creme ($18).

☺ $$$ Rich Texture Blush ($18.50) is a pressed powder blush that has a blend of three colors in one compact. These are mixed in a speckled pattern but come off as one slightly shiny color on the skin. I'm not sure what Clinique means by "rich texture" as this is rather dry and unappealing, not to mention almost as sheer as their other blushes.

☺ EYESHADOW: Stay the Day Eyeshadow ($11.50) is supposed to last all day with no fading. You may not notice whether it fades or not because the few colors that are still available are all quite powdery and go on very sheer. The softness of these and their inability to cling well to the skin makes them difficult to recommend. Pair of Shades Eyeshadow Duo ($15.50) features 24 different duos in a formula virtually identical to the Stay the Day Eyeshadows, and, thus, these tend to have the same problems. Most of the duos have one very shiny shade, and for an everyday look that can be more sparkles than one face needs. High Impact Eyeshadow ($11.50) is the latest powder eyeshadow from Clinique, and it seems poised to eclipse Stay the Day Eyeshadow. This formula has slight improvements over the existing powder eyeshadows, but all of the colors are shiny, and many of them are, well, *too* colorful for an understated look. For those who want stronger colors (compared to what Clinique ordinarily offers) with lots of shine, these are one more option in a growing field of eyeshadow colors that "color" the eye, rather than shade it. These do work well when used wet, but once you opt to do this, reverting to dry application is difficult. **High Impact Eyeshadow Duos** *($16.50)* share the same traits as Clinique's High Impact Eyeshadow above—these are equally bold (but still not too intense) colors, all of which are quite shiny—almost glittery. There are some good shade combinations, but this much all-out shine is best reserved for unwrinkled eyes or the under-25 set.

☺ **Touch Base for Eyes** *($12.50)* is one of the better cream-to-powder eyeshadows. This comes in a compact that must be kept closed tightly or the product will dry out and be useless. However, it might dry out even if you follow that guideline, so recommending this is risky. Take a look and try it out first before buying, as there are a couple of matte colors (Canvas and Nude Rose) that would work as an eyeshadow base if your foundation or concealer is not up to the task. **Touch Tint for Eyes** *($13.50)* are tubes of semi-sheer, cream-to-powder eyeshadows. These have a creamy, slightly slick texture that makes controlling the color trickier than usual, but they eventually dry down to a soft powder finish. Each of the five colors are shiny, and not the soft, subtle shine seen in many other products. These are an option if you're seeking a departure from powder eyeshadows, but Revlon's Illuminance Cream Eyeshadow ($6.49) gives you more bang and less glaring shine for your buck. **Smudgesicles** *($12.50)* gets my vote for one of the cutest makeup names ever, but the enthusiasm stops there. These are cream-to-powder eye colors in stick form that go on relatively smoothly and blend out sheer. However, they are tricky to use with other colors, and each shade is iridescent. For a one-color, quick eye design, these can be an option.

EYE AND BROW SHAPERS: ☺ **Brow Shaper** *($14.50)* is a powder brow color that comes in four excellent shades. The texture is slightly heavy, but these blend onto the brow quite well, even though the brush that comes packaged with these is too stiff and scratchy. For the money, a matte, brow-toned eyeshadow would work just as well and could also double as an eyeshadow; this version is too heavy for eyeshadow. **Eye Defining Liquid Liner** *($13.50)* is an excellent choice for liquid liner, provided you don't mind the price. This has a great soft-feeling, but firm, brush and applies an intense line of color that can go from thin to thick with precise ease. It stays on well without smearing or flaking, but equally good, less expensive options are available at the drugstore.

☺ **Quickliner for Eyes** *($14.50)* is a standard automatic pencil that provides a smooth, no-tugging application and is very easy to smudge before it sets. It's nearly identical to several less expensive pencils at the drugstore. **Quick Eyes** *($15.50)* is unique—one end is a creamy pencil and the other end houses a powder eyeshadow in the cap that is dispensed onto a smudge tip. While this may seem convenient, the powder shadows are all very shiny and the pencil is too creamy to last the day. **Eye Shading Pencil** *($11)* is a basic pencil with a smooth, creamy feel and some nice colors. Nothing less, nothing more. **Water-Resistant Eyeliner** *($14.50)* is old-fashioned cake liner that you use with a damp brush. The two matte shades (brown and black) are too softly pigmented to make a dramatic line, but if you prefer this type of product, it's worth a look. Otherwise, a deeply pigmented matte eyeshadow would make a brilliant alternative to this.

The Reviews C

☹ **Touch Liner** *($12.50)* is a poor liquid liner that comes in one shiny color that takes forever and a day to dry. The brush tip is also poor, making this a total washout. **Brow Keeper** *($14.50)* is a brow pencil that comes in three good shades and has a soft, creamy, but slightly sticky, consistency. These tend to stay creamy, and are prone to smudging or fading.

LIPSTICK AND LIP PENCIL: ☺ **Different Lipstick** *($11.50)* is a standard collection of lipsticks with a semi-sheer, glossy finish. Don't count on this one for long wear or being any different from any other sheer lipstick. **Lip Shaping Pencil** *($11)* is a standard pencil with a slightly dry texture. These go on nicely, but the formerly large selection of colors has been reduced to just a handful of shades. **Glosswear for Lips Sheer Shimmers** *($12.50)* is a different formula than the original Glosswear (reviewed below), and this one wins out since it is much lighter, smoother, and less sticky. Equipped with the wand applicator, you can dab iridescent glossy, shine and not have to be concerned with lips feeling too goopy. ✓☺ **Long Last Soft Shine Lipstick** *($12.50)* has a luscious feel and smooth, even application with opaque coverage. The color selection is extensive, with equally impressive pale and deep shades. ✓☺ **Long Last Soft Matte Lipstick** *($12.50)* remains my favorite of Clinique's lipstick choices. This is a creamy, smooth formula with a nice stain and a slightly matte finish that feels great.

☺ **Liquid Lipstick SPF 15** *($12.50)* comes in a tube with a wand applicator and has a glossy, non-sticky finish. These have fairly opaque coverage for a gloss, but the sunscreen offers no UVA protection, making these hard to recommend if sufficient sun protection is your goal. **Moisture Sheer Lipstick SPF 15** *($13.50)* also does not contain adequate UVA protection and remains a sheer, glossy lipstick that comes in a nice selection of "juicy" colors. Continuing this pattern of inadequate UVA-protecting sunscreen is **Moisture Surge Lipstick SPF 15** *($12.50)*. Since we've already seen Clinique's revamped sunscreen formulas that all use avobenzone, titanium dioxide, or zinc oxide, it's obvious that they know better and it's bothersome that two of these lipsticks with inadequate UVA-protecting sunscreens were launched *after* Clinique's retooled sunscreen collection! Moisture Surge is just a standard, slightly greasy lipstick with a pleasant selection of shades and a glossy finish. If your aim is to combine lipstick with sun protection, a far better choice would be Revlon, Cover Girl, or Almay's lipsticks with effective sun protection. **Almost Lipstick** *($13.50)* is a sheer, glossy lipstick that is similar to the Different Lipstick above. Although the formula is nothing special, the colors are beautiful. **Glosswear for Lips** *($12.50)* has a sticky texture and some good colors. This is fine for a standard wand-application gloss, but less expensive options abound. **Quickliner for Lips** *($13.50)* is an automatic, non-retractable pencil that is not preferred over less expensive options, as this one tends to smudge and is quite creamy. **Chubby Stick** *($12.50)* is a collection of short, fat pencils with a creamy lipstick application, but they are so soft they never stay sharp enough to draw a good line, making this just a gimmicky, rather unreliable, choice for lip color.

MASCARA: ✔☺ **Lash Doubling Mascara** *($12.50)* does a very good job of living up to its name, as this quickly builds lots of length and a fair amount of thickness with ease. The formula sweeps on with no clumps or smearing—each lash is well defined—and from my perspective, this is hands down the best mascara in Clinique's lineup! ☺ **Naturally Glossy Mascara** *($12)* is a basic mascara that builds some length and minimal thickness. It's fine for a natural, light look. **Full Potential Mascara** *($12)* goes on very well, with no smudging or clumping, and builds moderately long, thick lashes with minimal effort. **Long Pretty Lashes Mascara** *($12.50)* has an accurate name, as this mascara produces lots of length and does so without clumping, smearing, or flaking. Be warned, though: The clean, quick application does not produce any thickness. Still, if length is what you're after, this is well worth trying! If any of you remember Clinique's problematic Longstemmed Lashes, this is a revised (and much improved) version of that ill-fated mascara. **Gentle Waterproof Mascara** *($12.50)* is a bit of a misnomer, as waterproof mascara in general is hard on lashes for both wear and removal. Still, this is reliable mascara that builds nice length and some thickness, and it's truly waterproof.

☺ **Supermascara** *($12)* is supposedly better for contact lens wearers because it is fiber-free. Well, so are the rest of Clinique's mascaras! In comparison, this one pales when it comes to lengthening and long, non-smudging wear.

CLUB MONACO

Club Monaco has noticeably scaled back its cosmetics distribution since the previous edition of *Don't Go to the Cosmetics Counter Without Me*. Although Sephora wanted to hold on to this still-popular line, Club Monaco opted to pull out of all Sephora stores (and their Web site, too) and offer their cosmetics exclusively through the Club Monaco network of stores. Perhaps the competition in Sephora was too fierce—after all, Club Monaco was often snuggled in between similar lines like Stila and NARS, both of which get more consistent press and far greater nationwide retail exposure. Time will tell if privatizing the Club Monaco line will help or hurt Club Monaco cosmetics.

Club Monaco's skin-care products, on the other hand, appear to be an afterthought, with problematic ingredients, poor separation of skin types, and standard formulations even when the products are good. However, if you want to check out their makeup, and if you live in a city where you can locate a source (Toronto, Seattle, Detroit, Los Angeles, Washington, D.C., San Francisco, New York, or Chicago), it is worth a visit. For more information about Club Monaco, call (800) 513-0707 or visit www.clubmonaco.com.

CLUB MONACO SKIN CARE

☹ **Face Foaming Wash** *($14 for 6.8 ounces)* is a standard, detergent-based, water-soluble cleanser that also contains menthol and peppermint, which are irritating for the skin and the eyes. This cleanser is not recommended.

The Reviews C

☺ **Face Lotion Wash** *($14 for 6.8 ounces)* is more of a cold cream–style cleanser than anything else and it would require a washcloth to get all of your makeup off. But at least they left the menthol out of this version. This is an option for normal to dry skin.

☹ **Face Soap Wash** *($15 for 5.3 ounces)* is a standard, detergent-based bar cleanser that also contains sodium xylenesulfonate and sodium lauryl sulfate, and that adds up to irritation and dryness.

☺ **Face Soothing Wash** *($17 for 6.8 ounces)* is just a detergent-based, water-soluble cleanser that also contains Vaseline. It would work well for dry skin, but the price is high for what is really just a very ordinary formulation that doesn't hold a candle to other gentler products sold at the drugstore.

☺ **Eye Colour Remover** *($12 for 3.4 ounces)* is a standard eye-makeup remover that would work as well as any.

☹ **Face Soother** *($15 for 6.8 ounces)* lists witch hazel distillate as its third ingredient, which means it is part alcohol; that is hardly soothing and is a potential skin irritant.

☹ **Face Freshener** *($15 for 6.8 ounces)* contains mostly alcohol and some menthol, among other irritating plant extracts. This isn't freshening, it's irritating.

☹ **Skin Energizing Mist** *($10 for 3.4 ounces)* contains witch hazel distillate, which is part alcohol and can be irritating and drying for most skin types. It also contains several irritating plant extracts, including peppermint and citrus. It is not recommended.

☹ **Face Exfoliant** *($15 for 3.4 ounces)* contains menthol and peppermint, and is not recommended.

☺ **Face Mild Exfoliant** *($15 for 3.3 ounces)*, because it doesn't have the irritating extracts found in the Exfoliant above, is definitely milder. It's just a standard, detergent-based cleanser that uses polyethylene (ground-up plastic) as the exfoliant. This would work well for normal to oily skin.

☺ **Face Day Hydrating Cream** *($19 for 1.7 ounces)* is a silicone-based, lightweight moisturizer that isn't exciting, but it is an OK option for normal to dry skin.

☺ **Face Day Protection Fluid SPF 15** *($19 for 1.7 ounces)* is a good, avobenzone-based sunscreen for normal to oily skin types. It definitely contains oil-absorbing ingredients that can be helpful for oily skin, mixed in with thickening agents, silicone, vitamins, preservatives, and plant extracts.

☺ **Face Night Relief Cream** *($26 for 1.7 ounces)* is an OK emollient moisturizer for dry skin.

☺ **Face Night Relief Gel Cream** *($26 for 1.7 ounces)* is supposed to be for normal to oily skin, but it contains too many problematic ingredients for these skin types. It's OK for normal to dry skin, but it contains only minute amounts of vitamins and water-binding agents, and that's not a relief, it's unfortunate.

☹ **Eye Treatment Gel Cream** *($25 for 0.5 ounce)* lists aluminum starch (octenyl succinate) as the second ingredient, which is a substance good for absorbing moisture but not for adding anything otherwise beneficial to skin. It also contains peppermint, a skin irritant. This is a confusing formulation that isn't great to use anywhere near the eye area.

☹ **Face Vitamin C Serum** *($30 for 1 ounce)*, with alcohol as the third ingredient and only vitamin C and a tiny amount of plant extract as beneficial ingredients for skin, leaves much to be desired for healthy skin care.

☹ **Face Blemish Control** *($12 for 0.5 ounce)* contains alcohol as the second ingredient, which makes it too irritating for all skin types.

☺ **Face Purifying Clay** *($15 for 3.4 ounces)* is a standard clay mask that also contains a tiny amount of menthol, hopefully not enough to be a problem for skin.

☹ **Lip Protection Stick SPF 15** *($7 for 0.16 ounce)* doesn't contain the UVA-protecting ingredients of titanium dioxide, zinc oxide, or avobenzone, and is not recommended. It does contain spearmint and peppermint oils, which are a burn for lips.

CLUB MONACO MAKEUP

If you happen to live in a city that has a Club Monaco store, there is every reason to check out the makeup, which has largely stayed the same since the previous edition of this book. That's good because, for starters, the color palette for the foundations and concealers is among the best in the industry. The shades are very close to being benchmark neutral tones, and there are options for very light to dark skin. The powders, blushes, and matte eyeshadows are worth auditioning too, especially if you're looking for some less traditional, but still workable, colors. You will also find an all-encompassing collection of lipstick shades, from the sheerest red to oranges, violets, and a slew of classic soft tones. The pencils and mascaras are ordinary, and there are some trendy "works in concept but not in execution" products to watch out for, but overall the makeup is commendable and (for the most part) attractively priced.

FOUNDATION: ☺ **Oil-Free Foundation** *($19)* and **Liquid Foundation** *($19)* are practically indistinguishable from each other, and Sephora used to offer only the Oil-Free Foundation, no doubt to avoid confusion. Both of these foundations have a semi-thick, slightly creamy texture that blends on soft and moist. The Liquid Foundation is a bit more emollient, and offers a dewy finish, while the Oil-Free version has a very slight matte finish. They're both best for normal to slightly dry and dry skin seeking medium coverage. The colors are divided into a Neutral range (these are neutral to soft yellow) and a Beige range (neutral to soft peach), and the combined selection of over 20 shades is stellar, with the Oil-Free Foundation shade Beige 4 being the only one to steer clear of.

☺ **Wet/Dry Powder Makeup** *($23)* is a standard powder foundation with a sheer coverage and a soft, dry finish. The Beige colors are slightly peach, but the finish is almost too sheer to notice. You may find this works better as a pressed powder, so test it out alone and then with foundation if you can.

CONCEALER: This ✔☺ **Concealer** *($11)* is a rare find, with a beautiful selection of neutral shades that go on smoothly, cover well, and do not crease! It is a strong contender for success with those who use concealer, but be wary of shade Neutral 4, which can be too ash for most skin tones. Neutral 5 and Beige 5 are too peach for most skin tones, but may be worth testing if the others prove to be too light.

POWDER: ✓☺ **$$$ Loose Powder** *($19)* has an elegant, silky texture and a very soft, dry application. Shades Finale 1, 2, 3, and 4 are excellent. The other four colors consist of three Enhancers, which are too yellow, peach, or pink to look convincing on most skin tones, and a sheer, sparkly loose powder named Radiance. The formulas for all are talc-based. **Pressed Powder** *($20)* also has a great soft, dry texture and goes on beautifully, leaving a sheer matte finish. The four shades are great for fair to medium skin tones. **Bronzers** *($22)* offer three believable tan shades with only a slight shine. They blend on sheer and would work well for fair to medium-dark skin to mimic "sun-kissed" color on the face or body.

BLUSH: ✓☺ **$$$ Blush** *($16)* has a silky texture that is a breeze to apply and blend. This pressed-powder blush has an interesting mix of standard and unusual shades for both light and dark skin. Spotlight is shiny, but the rest are matte.

☺ **Cheek Dew** *($15)* is a cream blush that comes in a pot and is more greasy and sticky than creamy. If this look (glossy cheeks) appeals to you, try mixing Vaseline over your regular blush and see how you like it before buying this.

EYESHADOW: ☺ **Eyeshadow** *($12)* comes in a large selection of shades and with three distinct finishes. The Mattes are almost matte—there is a subtle shine to many of them, but it's hardly noticeable—and there are some great neutral colors. The Satins offer some stunning colors that have more of a sheen than a straight shine, and they may be an option for evening. The Frosts are ultra-shiny and best avoided. These are also less smooth than the Matte or Satin finishes, and may flake off. All three finishes offer a soft, sheer application that blends and builds well to create a subtle eye design. This is one of the few makeup artistry–themed lines whose eyeshadows don't go on from the first stroke. For a soft look or for the makeup novice, that's a plus.

☺ **Shimmer** *($15)* is provided in small vials of loose, shiny, colored powders. If you want shine, there are plenty of pressed powders around that can provide the same performance without the mess and flaking this product causes.

☹ **Eye Grease** *($14)* is, just as the name implies, a very greasy cream eyeshadow. Apparently this is one of the makeup items Club Monaco is "known" for, but for the life of me I cannot figure out why this overly shiny, slick, crease-prone product tops the sales charts. This can look sexy initially, but unless you're planning to sit still and somehow not blink, the effect is short-lived!

☺ **EYE AND BROW SHAPER: Eye Pencil** *($10)* is a standard, slightly creamy pencil with a decent dry finish. The large selection of colors includes a few best-to-avoid greens and blues, plus shiny gold, and sparkling silver. **Brow Pencil** *($10)* is a very standard, dry-textured brow pencil that is not preferred to a brow powder. Still, if you're a dyed-in-the-wool pencil fan, the colors are quite nice.

LIPSTICK AND LIP PENCIL: You'll find four types of lipsticks here, and whereas Sephora's tester units had an organizational scheme, the latest incarnation at Club Monaco has no rhyme or reason, so you're left to check each lipstick that catches your eye. ✓☺ Matte Lipstick ($14) is more creamy than matte, but this is what typically passes for matte in most makeup collections today. The Matte Lipsticks offer the richest colors, with full coverage and a creamy finish that has enough stain so that it will last at least until lunch. ☺ Cream Lipstick ($14) is a good, standard creamy lipstick with a slightly glossy finish and medium coverage. Cream Frost ($14) is identical to the Cream Lipstick, but with iridescence. Sheer Lipsticks ($14) are similar to the Cream Lipstick, only glossier and not as opaque. The colors are wonderful!

☹ Lip Gloss ($14) is about as boringly standard and overpriced as gloss gets, yet this is another hot commodity for the line. Although the colors are nice, these have an overly thick, sticky texture that's just not as appealing as other glosses. Lip Pencil ($10) has a creamy texture and is not as pigmented as other standard pencils, so don't count on it for longevity. It does apply easily, but there is no reason to consider this over an automatic lip pencil.

MASCARA: ☹ Mascara ($12) provides length and some thickness, but the tiny brush makes application more time consuming than it should.

☺ Waterproof Mascara ($12) wins high marks for being an excellent lengthening mascara that, with effort, also builds some thickness without clumping. It's waterproof and lasts all day, but can be quite difficult to remove.

☺ $$$ BRUSHES: Club Monaco's Brushes ($6–$38) do not disappoint if you are expecting a good selection, and although the bristles are not as soft as some other lines (Stila, Trish McEvoy, and Lancome all have softer ones), the shapes and sizes are nicely matched to a variety of needs and should work well. The Fluff Dusting Brush ($38), Large Angled Contour Brush ($34), Round Blending Brush ($22), Eye Lash Comb ($6), and most of the Eyeshadow Brushes ($15–$30) are worth a closer look to see if they meet your needs. The rest of the brushes are either too soft, too small, or too floppy, or just too downright poorly assembled to allow for precision application, and they can be passed up without a worry.

COMPLEX 15 (SKIN CARE ONLY)

☹ Complex 15 Cream ($5.99 for 2.5 ounces) and Complex 15 Lotion ($5.99 for 8 ounces) are simple, rather ordinary, moisturizers that have been around for a long, long time. Dermatologists recommend them a lot, which is the primary reason they stay on the market, but I wonder if any dermatologist has checked out the ingredient lists recently. They're not bad, just exceedingly outdated formulations lacking anything but the teeniest amount of water-binding agent and with no antioxidants. They are really just thickeners and plant oil. There are far more elegant and skin-interesting formulations out there. Also, without sunscreen, these are only an option for nighttime. For more information about Complex 15, call (800) 842-4090 or visit www.drugstore.com.

COPPERTONE (SUN CARE ONLY)

Coppertone makes one of the most woefully disappointing groups of sunscreen products around. Except for a handful of good avobenzone-based sunscreens, all the other sunscreens in its lineup have no UVA protection—there's no titanium dioxide, zinc oxide, or avobenzone in any of them! Clearly, now that the line does include products containing avobenzone, it's not as if the Coppertone people don't know about the issue. Coppertone also boasts that its sunscreens for kids are the ones recommended most by pediatricians. If that's true, be sure you find another pediatrician right away. It would mean your doctor doesn't know about the damage from UVA rays, and I would worry about what else he or she wasn't up to date on. There is something wanton about a corporation so recognized as a sunscreen manufacturer selling such an abundance of pathetically formulated sunscreens. For more information about Coppertone, call (800) 842-4090 or visit www.coppertone.com.

☺ **Sunblock Lotion SPF 30** *($6.99 for 4 ounces)* is a good, in-part avobenzone-based sunscreen in a very standard lightweight moisturizing base that would be OK for someone with normal to slightly dry skin or slightly oily skin.

☺ **Sunblock Lotion Spray SPF 30** *($8.99 for 7 ounces)* is similar to the Sunblock Lotion above and the same comments apply.

☺ **Shade Sunblock Lotion SPF 45, UVA/UVB Protection** *($7.99 for 4 ounces)* is similar to the Sunblock Lotion above and the same comments apply.

☺ **Oil Free Sunblock Lotion for Faces SPF 30** *($7.99 for 3 ounces)* is similar to the Sunblock Lotion above and the same comments apply.

☹ **Shade Sunblock Spray Mist SPF 30** *($7.99 for 4 ounces)* is a good, in-part avobenzone-based sunscreen. Although you will get UVA protection from this one, it also contains about 80% alcohol, which can be drying and irritating for all skin types.

☹ **Shade Oil-Free Gel SPF 30, UVA/UVB Protection** *($6.99 for 4 ounces)* is similar to the Sunblock Spray Mist above and the same comments apply.

☹ **Sport Sunblock Gel SPF 30** *($8.99 for 6 ounces)* is similar to the Sunblock Spray Mist above and the same comments apply.

☹ **Sport Sunblock Gel SPF 15** *($8.99 for 6 ounces)* is similar to the Sunblock Spray Mist above and the same comments apply.

☺ **Endless Summer Sunless Tanning Lotion, Light/Medium** or **Dark** *($10.99 for 3.7 ounces)* uses the same ingredient to affect skin color as all self-tanners do, dihydroxyacetone. This one would work as well as any.

☺ **Oil-Free Sunless Tanner** *($7.99 for 4 ounces)* is similar to the Sunless Tanning Lotion above, and the same comments apply.

☹ **Cool Gel Aftersun Aloe Light, Summertime Fragrance** *($5.49 for 16 ounces)* is just aloe vera with some slip agents, preservative, fragrance, and coloring agents. There is nothing about this that makes it preferred over pure aloe vera gel from the health food store.

☺ Cool Gel Aloe Aftersun *($5.49 for 16 ounces)* is identical to the version above, only with a different fragrance. The same comments apply, just as neither should contain fragrance.

All of the following products are not recommended, either because they do not contain the UVA-protecting ingredients of titanium dioxide, zinc oxide, or avobenzone, or because they have SPF numbers less than 15, which means that they do not provide sufficient protection from sun damage and the subsequent risk of skin cancer and wrinkles. Many of these also contain irritating plant extracts and alcohol. Some make claims of protecting from UVA/UVB radiation; however, the FDA-regulated, mandatory active ingredient list does not list any ingredients capable of protecting from the entire UVA spectrum.

☹ **Waterproof UVA/UVB Protection 4, PABA Free Moisturizing Suntan Lotion** *($4.79 for 4 ounces)*; **Waterproof UVA/UVB Protection 8, Ultra Moisturizing with Aloe & Vitamin E Sunscreen Lotion** *($4.79 for 4 ounces)*; **Bug & Sun Sunscreen with Insect Repellent, Adult Formula SPF 15** *($6.99 for 4 ounces, $8.59 for 8 ounces)*; **Bug & Sun Sunscreen with Insect Repellent, Kids Formula SPF 30** *($6.99 for 4 ounces, $8.59 for 8 ounces)*; **Dry Oil Tanning Spray SPF 4** *($7.49 for 6 ounces)*; **Dry Oil Tanning Spray SPF 8** *($7.39 for 6 ounces)*; **Aloe & Vitamin Lip Balm with Sunscreen SPF 15** *($1.99 for 0.15 ounce)*; **Waterproof UVA/UVB Protection 15, Sunblock Lotion** *($7.99 for 8 ounces)*; **Kids Colorblock Disappearing Wacky Foam, Sunblock SPF 40** *($8.99 for 6 ounces)*; **Kids Colorblock Disappearing Purple Colored Sunblock SPF 40** *($9.29 for 8 ounces)*; **Kids Glitter Sunblock Lotion SPF 30** *($8.99 for 6 ounces)* **Kids Spray & Splash Sunblock Spray SPF 30** *($8.99 for 8 ounces)*; **Kids Sunblock Lotion Trigger Spray SPF 30** *($8.99 for 6 ounces)*; **Kids Sunblock Stick SPF 30** *($4.79 for 6 ounces)*; **Kids SPF 40, 6 Hour Waterproof Sunblock Lotion** *($8.99 for 8 ounces)*; **Kids Sport Sunblock Lotion SPF 30** *($8.99 for 6 ounces)*; **Natural Fruit Flavor Lip Balm with Sunscreen SPF 15** *($1.99 for 0.15 ounce*; **Oil Free Sunblock Lotion SPF 45** *($8.99 for 8 ounces)*; **Oil-Free Waterproof Sunblock SPF 15** *($6.99 for 4 ounces, $8.59 for 8 ounces)*; **Oil-Free Waterproof Sunblock Lotion SPF 30** *($9.49 for 8 ounces)*; **Oil-Free Waterproof Sunscreen Lotion, SPF 8** *($8.99 for 8 ounces)*; **Rub-Free Sunblock Spray SPF 15** *($8.99 for 7 ounces)*; **Shade Sunblock Stick SPF 30** *($4.79 for 0.6 ounce)*; **Sport Stick SPF 30** *($4.79 for 0.6 ounce)*; **Sport Ultra Sweatproof Sunblock SPF 15** *($7.99 for 8 ounces)*; **Sport Ultra Sweatproof Sunblock SPF 30** *($7.99 for 8 ounces)*; **Sport Ultra Sweatproof UVA/UVB Sunblock SPF 15** *($9.19 for 8 ounces)*; **Sport Ultra Sweatproof Sunscreen Spray SPF 4** *($8.99 for 7 ounces)*; **Sport All Day Protection SPF 48, UVA/UVB Sunblock** *($8.99 for 8 ounces)*; **Sport Sunblock Spray SPF 15** *($10.99 for 7 ounces)*; **Sport Sunblock Spray SPF 30** *($8.99 for 7 ounces)*; **Sunblock Gel SPF 30** *($8.99 for 6 ounces)*; **Sunblock Lotion SPF 15** *($6.99 for 4 ounces)*; **Sunscreen Lotion SPF 4** *($7.39 for 8 ounces)*; **To Go Sunblock Spray SPF 15** *($9.99 for 7 ounces)*; **To Go Sunblock Spray SPF 30** *($9.99 for 7 ounces)*; **Tropical Blend Dark Tanning Lotion Spray Sunscreen SPF 2** *($5.99 for 8 ounces)*; **Tropical Blend Dark Tanning Oil Spray Sunscreen SPF 4** *($5.99 for 8 ounces)*; **Water Babies Lotion Spray SPF**

30 *($10.99 for 8 ounces)*; **Water Babies Lotion Spray SPF 45** *($8.99 for 8 ounces)*; **Water Babies UVA/UVB Sunblock Lotion SPF 30** *($10.99 for 8 ounces)*; **Water Babies UVA/ UVB Sunblock Lotion SPF 45** *($8.99 for 8 ounces)*; **Water Babies Sunblock Lotion Single Use Packets SPF 45** *($8.99 for 12 each)*; **Water Babies Sunblock Stick SPF 30** *($4.79 for 0.6 ounce)*; **Waterproof Ultra-Moisturizing SPF 15, with Aloe & Vitamin E** *($10.99 for 8 ounces)*; **Waterproof Ultra-Moisturizing SPF 30, with Aloe & Vitamin E** *($9.99 for 8 ounces)*; and **Waterproof Ultra-Moisturizing SPF 45, with Aloe & Vitamin E** *($10.99 for 8 ounces)*.

CORN SILK (MAKEUP ONLY)

Throughout its existence, Corn Silk has been synonymous with not having to worry about looking like an oil slick by midday. Corn Silk powder was supposed to be the oil-absorbing powder to end all powders. I recall buying it at several different junctures years ago, hoping it would work miracles on my sludge-laden skin. Sad to say, it didn't work wonders back then and it still can't today. Corn Silk is owned and distributed by the Sally Hansen Company. The mainstay loose and pressed powders are still the centerpiece of this line, but the latest products make a mockery of Corn Silk's anti-shine reputation. Not wanting to exclude themselves from the shimmer craze, Corn Silk now sells powders labeled as "Shine Control" that are loaded with sparkling shimmer. I doubt anyone concerned with tempering excess shine will jump at the opportunity to add more, but the choice is there nonetheless. Ultimately, there is little reason to rely on these powders regardless of how oily your skin is. Most companies offer luxurious powders that best Corn Silk's texture, color selection, and unusually dry finish. Still, if you're on a tight budget, there are some decent inexpensive products to try. For information about Corn Silk, call (800) 954-5080 or visit www. sallyhansen.com.

FOUNDATION: The Zero Shine products all claim to be noncomedogenic—a disingenuous term at best and simply untrue when it comes to the waxes used in Corn Silk's stick foundation. The foundations also feature salicylic acid, which can be an exfoliant, but it appears in amounts too small (and with pH levels too high) to have any positive impact on blemishes.

☺ **Zero Shine Liquid Makeup** *($4.96)* has a limited number of shades, and clearly Corn Silk thinks only fair- to light-skinned women have problems with oiliness. For those women, this can be an option for a decent matte finish foundation that offers light to medium coverage and a powdery finish. It blends well but you must be quick, because once this dries into place it's difficult to soften. Avoid Fair Beige and Natural Beige— both are too pink or peach for most skin tones. **Zero Shine Powderstick Makeup** *($6.99)* is a decently smooth stick foundation that comes in four OK colors and applies sheer and light. However, anyone with oily skin will cringe at the amount of waxes, which can exacerbate breakouts and do nothing to help with shine control in the least. Still, for a stick foundation, it does have a soft, matte finish and decent colors, and can be an option for someone with normal to slightly dry or slightly oily skin. Be careful with Natural Beige, which can turn orange on some skin tones.

☺ **Zero Shine Powder Makeup** *($6.99)* is a powder-based foundation with a soft, matte, dry finish. The zero shine won't last all day, but it can make it through the morning. The limited colors are only appropriate for very white skin. **Shine Control Mattifying Loose Powder Makeup** *($5.96)* is a loose powder foundation whose concept and packaging are similar to Origins' As Good As It Gets ($20). This is a soft, slightly thick-textured, talc-based powder that has a soft application and a satin finish. Of the three shades, No Color (which does have a slight yellow tint) and Creamy Natural are fine, but only if you have fair skin. Natural Beige is too orange for most skin tones.

<u>CONCEALER:</u> ☺ **Liquid Powder Concealer** *($3.76)* is a tube concealer with a wand applicator. It has a light, minimally creamy texture and dries quickly into place, leaving a soft matte finish. It's available in three shades, two of which are appropriate for light skin tones; the Yellow shade is fine if your goal is a jaundiced look. Due to the powdery finish, it can appear a bit chalky if you are too heavy-handed with your application or if you use it over dry skin.

☺ **Powder Finish Cover Stick** *($3.76)* is a concealer in a lipstick tube that has a rather thick, somewhat heavy, application. The four colors are good, but the opaque coverage does not look natural. For heavy coverage, this may be an option.

<u>POWDER:</u> ☹ **Classic Translucent Shineless Loose Powder** *($4.56)* and **Classic Translucent Shineless Pressed Powder** *($4.56)* are Corn Silk's original powders, and both have a semi-soft, dry texture courtesy of the walnut shell powder they contain. The talc-free Loose Powder is not as smooth as the talc-based Pressed Powder. Each offers four shades, appropriate for fair to medium skin only. Avoid Mid, which is slightly peach and can deepen to orange once your oil breaks through and mixes with the pigments. **Natural Matte Loose Powder** *($4.56)* and **Natural Matte Pressed Powder** *($4.56)* are both talc-based and have similar soft, dry textures. Both provide a good matte finish. The Pressed Powder has a drier texture courtesy of the clay it contains. For both versions, avoid Mid, which is too peach. These supposedly give more coverage than the Shineless powders above, but the difference is negligible. **Shine Control Invisible Mattifying Powder** *($4.76)* comes in only one shade, which goes on transparent but with a slight yellow cast. This is almost identical in texture and application to the powders above, and is more or less an extraneous product. Corn Silk recommends using this to cover dark circles, but it is too dry and sheer to make a positive difference under the eyes.

☺ **Oil-Absorbing Powder Papers** *($2.76 for 60 sheets)* are standard powdered papers that will take down excess shine, and also leave a powdery finish on the skin, which can look uneven over very oily areas. I prefer oil-absorbing sheets not dusted with powder, but these are an option if you have fair to light skin.

☹ **Shine Control Skin Brightening Loose Powder** *($5.96)* and **Shine Control Skin Brightening Pressed Powder** *($5.96)* are both very soft, talc-based powders that stray from the dry-as-the-desert finish the other Corn Silk powders have. What's maddening about these powders is that they claim to be about shine control, but leave a glistening finish on the skin that is anything but subtle. In fact, these powders outshine most other powders that do not bear such deceiving names. **Bronzers** *($4.56)* are available as pressed or loose powders. Both are slightly shiny and come in an awful orange color that will look artificial on most skin tones.

COVER GIRL (MAKEUP ONLY)

Cover Girl has retained its role as a major contender in the makeup world by continuing to put on a whole new look—and it's an impressive face-lift. They have been busily eliminating most (though not all) of the overly fragranced (meaning malodorous) foundations, blushes, eyeshadows, and pressed powders. Even more significant is the elimination of all of the poor foundation textures, chalky powders, and flaky eyeshadows! Their newest additions are a breath of fresh air, and some of the best prices you will find at the drugstore. Before I get too carried away, I should state that some of the powders still have a wafting, sweet fragrance that is, at best, overpowering. Yet these are now the exception to the rule and are forgivable given the noteworthy improvements Cover Girl has made just over the past few years.

Cover Girl's Web site is extremely easy to navigate, and presents a wealth of product information, along with praiseworthy tips and tricks for successful makeup application and for finding the shades that work best for you. Its consumer relations number is consistently helpful if you have any questions or concerns. For example, if some favorite item was among the many products that were discontinued, you may be wondering what new (and pleasantly improved) item has replaced it, and they will let you know. It is clear that Cover Girl is carrying on with the best intentions and an eagerness to provide not only superior products but also superior service. For more information about Cover Girl, call (800) 543-1745 or visit www.covergirl.com.

FOUNDATION: Cover Girl would win even higher marks if they would provide adequate testers for all of their products. While some stores do sell mini samples of specific formulas, those are few and far between. For now, and even though the colors have gotten remarkably better, without testers the chance of buying the wrong color is fairly high.

☺ **Fresh Complexion Oil Control Makeup** *($6.49)* maintains that it will provide "beautiful coverage that lasts," but they should have inserted the adjective "sheer," as this talc-based pressed-powder foundation barely registers on the skin in terms of coverage. It does have a velvety texture that never looks dry or powdery, but the finish almost leaves a glow on the skin—not something those with oily skin have on their makeup checklist. It's best for normal to dry skin, but you won't net any lasting shine control with this product. The eight shades present some visibly pink and peach colors, but the sheerness makes the color almost irrelevant. The ones to use with caution are Buff Beige, Natural Beige, and Classic Beige. Fair to light skin tones have the best chance of finding a perfect shade, but dark skin tones should look elsewhere. **Fresh Look Clear Up Tinted Acne Treatment Cream** *($5.79 for 0.65 ounce)* is a very good, 10% benzoyl peroxide product in a nonirritating, matte finish gel base. It is also supposed to be a slightly tinted concealer, but it does a poor job of concealing anything and it's available in only one very sheer shade. What it does a good job of is disinfecting, and that is an important step in the treatment of breakouts. However, 10% benzoyl peroxide is quite strong and not the best place to start for all skin types. It would be far better to start with a lower concentration of this active ingredient and move up gradually if your acne does not respond to the lower concentrations. **CG Smoothers All Day Hydrating Makeup** *($7.59)* actually has mostly great colors (15 in all)—what a shame the color on the container doesn't even vaguely resemble the color inside! Still, of all the Cover Girl foundations, this formula is the one I most often see in mini-sizes, so it's inexpensive to experiment with the shades. The talc content gives this sheer-to-medium coverage foundation a soft matte, slightly powdery finish, which is anything but hydrating (and definitely not for 11 hours, as the package states). It would work well for someone with normal to oily or combination skin. The following colors are too pink, rose, or peach for most skin tones: Natural Ivory (just slightly pink), Natural Beige, Medium Light, Warm Beige, Creamy Beige, and Toasted Almond. Soft Sable is a beautiful color for dark skin tones. This is fragrance-free.

✔☺ **AquaSmooth Makeup SPF 15** *($8.50)* is an ultra-light, water-to-powder compact makeup that smooths easily onto the skin and dries to a soft, powdery matte finish. As with similar foundations, quick, deft blending is key—these formulas dry fast, and are not easy to move once they do. The sunscreen is all titanium dioxide, so even sensitive skin should be able to wear this, though the formula and finish are best for normal to slightly oily skin—dry skin will only look more noticeable with this type of foundation. There are 15 shades, offering light to medium coverage. The ones to avoid due to overtones of pink or peach are Natural Ivory, Medium Light, Warm Beige, Natural Beige, Creamy Beige, and Toasted Almond. The remaining shades feature some excellent options for light and dark skin tones. ✔☺ **Fresh Look Makeup Oil-Free for Combination to Oily Skin SPF 15** *($7.59)* has an incredibly reasonable price, the SPF 15 sunscreen is all titanium dioxide, the finish is nicely matte (though not as matte as Revlon's Shine Control Mattifying Makeup SPF 15), and there is a streamlined assortment of nine colors. This really is a great formula with a smooth, even application and no noticeable fragrance. There are shades for very light skin tones, but nothing suitable for darker skin tones. The following colors are too peach, pink, or rose for most skin tones: Natural Ivory (just slightly pink), Creamy Beige, Natural Beige (very pink), and Tawny. ✔☺ **CG Smoothers SPF 15 Tinted Moisture** *($7.59)*. These are exceptionally sheer moisturizers that impart the smallest amount of color to the skin. The four shades are all worth considering, although if you need significant coverage you will want to use concealer along with it. The reformulated product is completely fragrance-free, the base formula is oil-free and less emollient than before, and the sunscreen is in-part zinc oxide, making this product appropriate for normal to slightly dry or slightly oily skin. **Continuous Wear Makeup** *($7.79)* has 15 mostly excellent shades (including colors for darker skin tones) that blend on smoothly and would work well for someone with normal to dry skin seeking sheer to light coverage. Unfortunately, the container is opaque, which makes it next to impossible to identify your possible color—a serious shortcoming I hope will be corrected soon. The following shades are too peach, pink, or rose for most skin tones: Medium Light, Natural Beige, Warm Beige, Creamy Beige, and Toasted Almond.

☺ **Clean Makeup Fragrance Free** *($5.49)* mercifully omits the sickly sweet scent that is present in the Clean Makeup below, as well as the irritating extracts. Unfortunately, almost all of the 15 shades are just too strongly peach, pink, or rose for most skin tones. The only four shades worth considering are Ivory, Classic Ivory, Soft Honey, and Classic Tan. **Ultimate Finish Liquid Powder Makeup** *($7.29)* features a nice smooth texture, although the aluminum starch (second ingredient) is a skin irritant and the isopropyl myristate in it can aggravate breakouts. It may be OK for normal skin types not prone to blemishes, but drier skin will find that it just exaggerates every dry skin cell. The 15 shades are a mixed bag; most are too glaringly peach, pink, or rose for most skin tones; avoid Natural Ivory, Creamy Natural, Classic Beige, Medium Light, Warm Beige, Creamy Beige, Natural Beige, and Toasted Almond. Soft Sable and Tawny are worthwhile shades for darker skin tones.

☹ **Clean Makeup** *($5.49)* is one of the original Cover Girl foundations (launched in 1961) that hasn't yet been discontinued—and I doubt it ever will be, because according to Cover Girl, they sell just over 23 million bottles per year! Yet this dated, basic formula contains clove, menthol, camphor, and eucalyptus, which are extremely irritating for skin, plus the colors are largely unusable for any skin tone and the fragrance is intrusive. **Simply Powder Foundation** *($7.99)* goes on thick and heavy, and easily cakes on the skin. It's a lot more than powder; it's a messy layer over the skin and ranks way below the newest excellent products from Cover Girl.

CONCEALER: ✔☺ **Invisible Concealer** *($4.69)* is a surprisingly excellent, affordable concealer. The five colors are mostly great for lighter to medium skin tones, but the Medium shade can be too rose. This applies smoothly and evenly without creasing, and is one to try! ✔☺ **Fresh Complexion Undereye Concealer** *($4.99)* has a wonderful, lightly creamy texture and a soft application that provides almost too much slip. Although blending this concealer takes a bit more time, the natural matte finish and smooth coverage are worth it. This wouldn't be my top choice if your optimum concern is great coverage, but those with minor imperfections should check it out. Of the four colors, only Natural Beige is too pink to purchase.

☺ **CG Smoothers Concealer** *($5.79)* is a standard, lipstick-style concealer that doesn't go on as greasy as it appears and provides good coverage with minimal creasing. However, four of the six shades are on the peach side, and the coverage is opaque enough for that to be a problem for some skin tones. Neutralizer is OK, but Illuminator is too whitish pink for even very light skin. Whitish pink is not a shade to use over blemishes.

POWDER: ☺ CG Smoothers Fresh Look Pressed Powder Combination to Oily Skin *($5.79)*, CG Smoothers Fresh Look Pressed Powder Normal to Dry Skin *($5.79)*, and Clean Pressed Powder Fragrance-Free Normal Skin *($5.49)* are all talc-based powders that have a similar sheer, smooth, almost invisible finish despite the different names and formulations. The colors are all decent, with only a few having slightly pink or peach tones, but the tones are so slight it's barely worth mentioning. The packaging has been updated for all of these powders, and now the enclosed puff, which used to almost completely hide the powder color, is behind the compact—so the colors are in full view! Though I rarely comment on a product's smell, the scent for the Fresh Look Pressed Powder Normal to Dry Skin is awfully obtrusive. In contrast, the others are mercifully fragrance-free.

☹ Clean Pressed Powder for Normal Skin *($5.49)* is almost identical to its fragrance-free counterpart, but this one includes eucalyptus oil and camphor, both of which are very irritating even in small amounts. Do I need to mention the overpowering fragrance this has? Professional Loose Powder *($5.69)* comes in six mostly well-conceived shades and a fine texture, but that is cancelled out by the pointless inclusion of eucalyptus, camphor, clove oil, and menthol—four potent irritants—and the sickly sweet fragrance.

☹ BLUSH: All of Cover Girl's powder blushes contain menthol, camphor, eucalyptus oil, and clove oil—irritants that have no business being in makeup and serve no positive purpose for the skin. Instant Cheekbones *($5.69)* has three colors in one compact—a blush tone, a contour color, and a shiny highlighter. The colors for these and for the single blush version, Cheekers *($3.79)*, still haven't been updated, which is strange because most of Cover Girl's drugstore contemporaries have more modern blush hues, while these remain rather pastel and intense. That may be OK for darker skin tones, but anyone looking for subtle colors will be left out of the running. Most of the colors are slightly shiny. Classic Color Blush *($5.69)* is a larger-sized powder blush that comes in four single shades that are vivid, but blend on sheer. These are fairly powdery, and the color intensity is too soft for darker skin tones.

EYESHADOW: ☺ Professional Eye Enhancers *($4.69 "4 kit"; $4.69 "3 kit"; $2.99 "1 kit")* are labeled as matte or "perle," but most are very shiny to slightly shiny. Some of the matte shades, however, are indeed matte (but be careful) and are worth checking out. The texture and application of these is much better than in years past. Some of the 3-kit and 4-kit compacts have practical color combinations, so you can really use all of the shades!

The following Quads and Trios offer all matte shades: Chilled Grape, Slates, Shades of Suede, and Tranquil Browns. The following Singles are neutral and matte: Toasted Almond, Snow Blossom, Dewy Pink, Grey Suede, Midnight Jazz, and Hazelnut.

☺ CG Smoothers Gel Eye Color *($5.79)* are chubby pencils that go on somewhat wet, which means they glide on easily, and then the color dries to a matte finish that doesn't budge or smear all day. By the way, though I love the way these pencils go on, trying to keep a point on the pencil isn't easy, and that makes it difficult to create a thin, controlled line. There are several shades, and many of them are very shiny.

EYE AND BROW SHAPER: ✔☺ **Perfect Blend Eye Pencil** *($4.69)* is a fairly standard, but good, pencil that goes on slightly drier than most others and has decent staying power. There are six shades, all come with a sponge tip to ease blending. Avoid Cobalt Blue. ✔☺ **Liquid Pencil Felt Tip Eyeliner** *($5.69)* is an excellent, gel-based liquid eyeliner that applies easily and stays on without fading or chipping off. It is also very easy to wash off, so if you're a fan of this type of eyeliner, this is a strong contender—and the four shades are all contenders, too. ✔☺ **Perfect Point Plus** *($5.39)* is an automatic eye pencil that glides on easily without being greasy and maintains a consistent, sharp point. Chestnut is a great shade for an auburn eyeliner, but Dusky Blue and Midnight Blue are best avoided.

☺ **CG Smoothers Natural Brow and Lash Mascara** *($5.49)* is an acceptably priced, extremely standard, clear brow gel that leaves a minimal sticky feel. This brush isn't ideal, but it works—just take care that you coat the brows evenly, because any clumps will dry and flake off, an unpleasant side effect of this particular gel formula. **Brow and Eye Makers** *($2.89)* feature two short pencils that are the same color. It seems you're supposed to use one for eyes and one for brows, but the dry, waxy texture of these makes them best suited for brow pencil, and then only if you insist on using pencil over powder. Soft Blonde is a good light beige hue, and Henna Brown is an option for redheads.

LIPSTICK AND LIP PENCIL: Cover Girl has an excellent lipstick collection, and continues to offer impressive textures and a vast array of muted and bright colors. ☺ **CG Smoothers Hydrating Lipstick** *($7.59)* claims to provide just as much moisture for your lips as "the leading lip balm," but the fact is that most creamy, slightly greasy lipsticks (like this one) will do just that. This lipstick wears well and has enough stain to keep the color around for part of the day, which would be a better basis for a catchy claim. **Continuous Color Lipstick** *($5.79)* is available in Cremes, Shimmers, and Sheers. All of these are accurately named and have a smooth, slightly greasy texture. The Sheers are more fleeting, but the Cremes and Shimmers (which aren't too iridescent) have enough stain to go the distance, at least until lunch! **LipSlicks Lip Gloss** *($3.69)* is a basic, emollient gloss with some very shiny shades in packaging that makes getting it on the lips very tricky for anyone with thin lips. **Triple Lipstick SPF 15** *($5.89)* is one of the few lipsticks that offer UVA protection, with an in-part titanium dioxide base. This is a creamy, semi-opaque formula with a slightly greasy finish and minimal stain. The color range is impressive. **CG Smoothers Lip Liner** *($5.79)* is as standard a lipliner as they come, in a nice, though limited, range of colors. These do need sharpening, and will work as well as any other pencil.

✔☺ **Outlast All Day Lipcolor** *($10.99)* pretty much lives up to its claim about staying on without coming off on anything. In some cases, you may even find that this has lasted all day, all night, and into the next morning. Other than the price, the only difference between this and Max Factor (Cover Girl's sister company) is that Outlast has slightly more colors (30+ colors!).

MASCARA: ☺ **Super Thick Lash** *($5.49)* is a great mascara, building long, thick lashes with only the slightest tendency to clump. This lasts well without smearing or flaking, and is arguably Cover Girl's most "dramatic" mascara. **Triple Mascara** *($6.29)* is a single mascara that does a good job of lengthening and thickening lashes, plus it doesn't smear or flake and can last all day. While this isn't the cream of the crop of the lengthening and thickening mascaras out there, it is certainly worth a try!

✔☺ **Professional Waterproof Mascara** *($5.49)* has a formula that applies easily and with some effort builds nice length and minimal thickness. Best of all, it really does hold up when wet and it's easy to remove!

☺ **Remarkable Washable Waterproof Mascara** *($5.49)*. Washable, yet waterproof, isn't that an oxymoron? Nonetheless, this applies evenly and builds good length and thickness. It isn't as waterproof as others, withstanding only a little water (such as a light rain) and breaking down underwater—so swimmers and criers will have to look elsewhere. As a plus, this does come off easily without taking your lashes with it!

☹ **Professional Smudgeproof Mascara Classic Look Curved Brush** *($5.49)* builds good length and some thickness, but tends to go on unevenly, an effect that seems to be a hallmark of these awkward curved-brush mascaras. **Professional Smudgeproof Mascara Classic Look Straight Brush** *($5.49)* has an easier-to-wield wand than the curved version above, but this builds lengthy lashes unevenly and needs more fine-tuning than a mediocre mascara should. **Marathon Waterproof Mascara** *($5.49)* is back and just as poor as it was in the past. No matter how this is applied, it tends to clump and somehow manages to make lashes seem shorter. You won't see a modicum of thickness, and to top it off it's extremely difficult to remove.

BRUSHES: ☹ **Large Blush Brush** *($5.29)* is a poor option because the bristles are too soft and too sparse to provide much control. The **Powder Brush** *($6.39)* has a flat-cut top, which tends to work against the natural contours of the face and makes it easy to over-powder. The ☺ **Eyeshadow Brush** *($4.69)* is nicely shaped but quite thick. Some women may prefer that, but I find it tends to apply eyeshadow in stripes and is hard to use for blending.

CRABTREE & EVELYN (FACIAL SKIN CARE ONLY)

Before there was The Body Shop, Bath and Body Works, or even Garden Botanika there was Crabtree & Evelyn. About 25 years ago, this Northeast emporium was a homey mix of Martha Stewart, aromatherapy, and gourmet tidbits. A profusion of potpourri and scented candles, intermingled with maple syrup and knickknacks, kept company with fragrant body lotions in an atmosphere that was New England quaint. Now, with over 130 stores in the United States alone and hundreds more that carry Crabtree & Evelyn products, the name is a mainstay of Americana.

In recent years, Crabtree & Evelyn decided to give their stores a face-lift. The down-home image is being replaced with a slick, contemporary look—lofty ceilings, large storefront windows, and light wood accents—that feels miles away from its New En-

The Reviews C

gland roots. Not only are the stores being renovated, but the traditional product line is being repackaged and new products are being developed. Fragrance is still the main focus of this company, with wafting scents radiating from every product imaginable. While Crabtree & Evelyn excel as an impressive part of the $1.5 billion scent business, their foray into facial skin care is, well, abysmal. No sunscreens, too much fragrance, dated formulations, no variety for different skin-care needs, and a lack of antioxidants all add up to a disappointment. Please do consider a candle or potpourri, but for your face and body, think again. For more information about Crabtree & Evelyn, call (800) 272-2873 or visit www.crabtree-evelyn.com.

☺ **Swiss Skin Care Cleansing Bar** *($8 for 3.5 ounces)* is a standard, detergent-based overly fragrant cleansing bar.

☹ **Swiss Skin Care Cleansing Milk** *($17 for 6.7 ounces)* is an overpriced, mineral oil–based, wipe-off cleanser that also contains an irritating mix of plant extracts, including arnica, sage, and balm mint.

☹ **Swiss Skin Care Herbal Tonifier** *($17 for 6.7 ounces)* is a pricey mix of irritating plant extracts of arnica, sage, balm mint, and menthol. What is somewhat unique is the ingredient listed fourth—urea—which can work as an exfoliant and water-binding agent.

☺ **Swiss Skin Care 24-Hour Emulsion** *($18 for 3.3 ounces)*. The only thing Swiss about this product is the name. It is an exceptionally ordinary mix of water, slip agents, thickeners, silicone, urea, preservatives, plant oil, and a teeny amount of water-binding agents. It is an option for dry skin, but not a very good one.

☺ **Swiss Skin Care Enriched Night Cream** *($22 for 1.7 ounces)* is an OK, mineral oil–based moisturizer for normal to dry skin. It does contain retinol, but the jar-type packaging ensures that this ingredient will not be stable shortly after it's opened. It does contain some good plant oils and water-binding agents, but the addition of spleen and placenta enzymes does not give this product special properties. These two ingredients, much like any part of a human or animal body, are sources of proteins and amino acids that have water-binding and antioxidant properties (Sources: *Placenta*, July 2002, pages 497–502 and *Bioscience, Biotechnology, and Biochemistry*, November 2000, pages 2478–2481). That's helpful for skin but no more so than hundreds of other ingredients with similar or superior attributes.

☺ **Swiss Skin Care Moisturizing Day Cream** *($20 for 1.7 ounces)* does not have an SPF, and, therefore, is a moisturizer to avoid for daytime, although the ordinary formulation of water, thickeners, mineral oil, and preservatives leaves much to be desired at any hour. The teeny amount of water-binding agents is barely detectable.

DARPHIN

I don't know quite how to present this shockingly flawed, inferior, and overpriced line. Not only are the prices unwarranted for what you get, the formulations are some of the most dated, mundane concoctions I've encountered in a long time. For those who think that buying a line that speaks with a French accent is somehow going to net them better skin, I can almost guarantee that the purchase of a group of Darphin products will just bring them problems. Several of the products contain a range of irritating ingredients, including alcohol, camphor, lemon, and menthol. The supposed "AHA products" do not contain AHAs. The basic water-binding agents, anti-irritants, and antioxidants are not unique in the least and almost always are only present in the minutest amounts. And the (missing) icing on the cake is that there are no sunscreens recommended as part of a daily skin-care routine. I imagine that there may be some emotionally pleasant sensation that accompanies the purchase of these products perhaps the act of actually purchasing a $175 moisturizer or a $50 cleanser feels good but, regrettably, none of that will help your skin. If you're going to spend this kind of money for skin care, though it's anyone's guess why you would, I'd suggest you look to lines that are at least well-formulated, with state-of-the-art water-binding agents, sunscreens, AHA or BHA products, topical disinfectants, and antioxidants. For more information about Darphin, call (888) 611-3003 or visit www.darphin.fr. **Note:** All Darphin products are highly fragranced.

DARPHIN SKIN CARE

☹ **Purifying Cleansing Milk** *($48 for 6.7 ounces)* is a basic, plant oil– and cold cream–style cleanser that contains some very problematic ingredients, including menthol, coltsfoot, and camphor.

☺ $$$ **Purifying Foam Gel** *($40 for 4.2 ounces)* is an exceptionally standard, detergent-based cleanser that would be an option for someone with normal to oily skin. The teeny amount of plant extracts and lactic acid have no effect on skin.

☹ **Purifying Toner** *($48 for 6.7 ounces).* With alcohol as the second ingredient and camphor on the ingredient list as well, this ends up being irritating rather than purifying.

☺ $$$ **Oil Free Exfoliating Foam Gel** *($40 for 4.2 ounces)* is a standard, detergent-based cleanser that includes ground-up plastic (polyethylene) as the scrub. It is an option for a topical scrub for normal to oily skin.

☹ **Purifying Vitaserum** *($55 for 0.5 ounce)* contains mostly water, slip agent, pH-balancing ingredient, thickener, zinc oxide, plant extracts, menthol, and coloring agents. What a truly useless product. Menthol is irritating and the aluminum potassium is an absorbent, but that won't purify anything.

☹ **Intensive Purifying Complex** *($85 for 1 ounce)* lists alcohol as the second ingredient. Add to that a number of irritating plant oils and this ends up being a potentially intense problem for skin.

☺ $$$ **Purifying Aromatic Clay Mask** *($45 for 1.7 ounces)* actually contains very little clay. Rather, this is mostly water, thickeners, talc, and preservatives. It will absorb oil, but the thickening agents are fairly emollient and can clog pores.

☹ **Sebomask** *($65 for 1.7 ounces)* is a standard clay mask that also contains camphor, menthol, and lemon. These won't help oily skin, but they can cause irritation and redness.

☺ $$$ **Vitalskin Aromatic Cleansing Milk** *($40 for 6.7 ounces)* is a lotion-style cleanser that could be an option for someone with normal to dry skin. It does contain some irritating plant extracts, but the amounts are so small that they probably will have no effect on skin.

☺ $$$ **Vitalskin Aromatic Toner** *($40 for 6.7 ounces)* is a basic toner with detergent cleansing agents and a water-binding agent. It also contains some plant extracts that are potential skin irritants. Even without the problems this isn't worth the money.

☹ **Vitalskin Concentrate** *($80 for 1 ounce)* contains plant extracts that are mostly skin irritants, and while the water-binding agent is a good one, the teeny amount of antioxidants in this product makes it anything but vital.

☺ $$$ **Vitalskin Creme** *($75 for 1.7 ounces)* is an exceptionally basic moisturizer for dry skin. It is an option, but given the cost this formula is scandalously mundane.

☺ $$$ **Vitalbalm Lip Care** *($20 for 0.12 ounce)* is a basic lip balm, virtually identical to Chap Stick.

☺ $$$ **Intral Cleansing Milk** *($50 for 6.7 ounces)* is a mineral oil–based cleanser that is as exceptionally ordinary as it is overpriced. It is an option for someone with dry skin.

☺ $$$ **Intral Toner** *($50 for 6.7 ounces)* is an extremely simple toner of slip agents and detergent cleansing agents. It's OK, but just barely.

☺ $$$ **Intral Complex** *($95 for 1 ounce)* contains mostly water, slip agent, glycerin, film-forming agent, plant oil, water-binding agents, thickeners, preservatives, antioxidants, and coloring agents. The teeny amount of antioxidants is barely worth mentioning. It does contains horse chestnut, which does have anti-inflammatory properties for skin, but that isn't unique to this product.

☺ $$$ **Intral Balm** *($85 for 1.7 ounces)* is as standard a lip balm as it gets. The price is best described as laughable, although the unsuspecting consumer who thinks they're buying something truly great for skin won't be laughing.

☺ $$$ **Intral Mask** *($50 for 1.7 ounces)* is a basic emollient mask with a good water-binding agent, but only teeny amounts of anti-irritants and absolutely nothing else.

☹ **Cleansing Aromatic Emulsion** *($40 for 4.2 ounces)* lists sodium lauryl sulfate relatively high on the ingredient list, which makes it a potential skin irritant for all skin types. Other than that, this is a confused product. It has mineral oil as the second ingredient (which can leave a greasy film on the face) and also detergent cleansing agents (which can dry the skin).

☺ $$$ **Aromatic Eye Make-Up Remover** *($35 for 3.3 ounces)* is a standard eye-makeup remover with detergent cleansing agents. It would work as well as any. It does contain a small amount of irritating plant extract, which is problematic for the face, but especially problematic for the eye area.

☺ $$$ **Aromatic Balancing Day Cream** *($75 for 0.7 ounce)* is a good, though exceptionally standard, moisturizer that could be easily replaced with just about any moisturizer from Clinique or L'Oreal (except those product lines have better-formulated products).

This is mostly just thickening agents and trace amounts of antioxidants and water-binding agents.

☺ $$$ **Aromatic Soothing Cream** *($60 for 1.7 ounces)*. The amount of "good" ingredients in this one is negated by the many the fragrant oils it also contains, which are significant potential irritants.

☺ $$$ **Aromatic Night Support** *($60 for 1.6 ounces)* is an ordinary moisturizer for dry skin that's hardly supportive.

☺ $$$ **Aromatic Purifying Balm** *($59 for 0.5 ounce)* is a mix of nonfragrant plant oils, wax, and fragrant plant oils. Skip the fragrance, which can be irritating and sensitizing for skin, and simply buy the primary ingredients—hazelnut oil and vegetable oil—from the grocery store and use them instead. They're better for skin and astoundingly less expensive.

☹ **Camomile Aromatic Care** *($59 for 0.5 ounce)* is a mix of nonfragrant plant oils and fragrant plant oils (including camphor oil, which is a significant skin irritant). Skip the fragrances, and consider buying the primary ingredient—almond oil—from the grocery store and use that instead. As I mentioned for the Purifying Balm above, it's better for skin and astoundingly less expensive.

☺ $$$ **Stimulskin Cream** *($175 for 1.7 ounces)*. The only thing stimulating about this moisturizer is the price. I can't find words to describe how basic and unimpressive this formulation is. It contains mostly water, slip agents, thickeners, plant oil, a minuscule amount of water-binding agents, and even less antioxidants. The soy extracts have no estrogen-like properties for skin. It does contain a fractional amount of retinol, but the jar-type packaging ensures that it won't remain stable once it is opened.

☹ **Stimulskin Complex** *($325 for 10 doses—total 1 ounce)* is somewhat similar to the Stimulskin Cream above only this version has more of a serum consistency and some potentially irritating plant extracts. Shockingly, it even lacks some of the antioxidants the Cream contains. Overall, this is a complete waste of money.

☺ $$$ **Arovita C** *($125 for 1.6 ounces)*. If the price doesn't shock you, this ordinary formulation should. The interesting ingredients are barely present, and the minute amount of retinol present will not remain stable in the jar-style packaging.

☺ $$$ **Arovita Eye and Lip Contour Gel** *($65 for 1 ounce)* is similar to the Soothing Eye Contour Gel below except that this one contains more plant oil and is better for normal to dry skin.

☺ $$$ **Predermine Cream** *($140 for 1.7 ounces)* is an OK moisturizer for dry skin. But from Avon to Clinique there are far better-formulated moisturizers out there with far more interesting ingredients than this one, and for a fraction of the price.

☺ $$$ **Predermine Complex** *($295 for 10 uses)*. The fourth ingredient is alcohol along with a scattering of antioxidants and water-binding agents. The alcohol is a problem for skin, but the good ingredients are not unique to this product and are readily found in myriad other products for a fraction of the cost.

☺ $$$ **Predermine Mask** *($75 for 1.6 ounces)* is an extremely basic clay mask that also contains a good deal of zinc oxide. Clay can be an absorbent, but zinc oxide, as a thick emollient, can clog pores, which makes this a confusing product.

☹ **Firming Vitaserum 70** *($125 for 1 ounce)* contains no vitamins. What it does have are arnica and ginseng, both irritating plant extracts, in a very ordinary serum base of water, water-binding agents, preservatives, and fragrance. This is a huge "Why bother?" unless you are interested in acquiring potential skin problems at what works out to about $2,000 a pound.

☹ **Vitaserum 50 Oil Free** *($95 for 1 ounce)* contains urea, which can exfoliate skin, but it can also be found in far less expensive products that don't contain the irritating plant extracts this one does. The lactic acid is in too minute a concentration to be effective as an exfoliant.

☹ **Vitaserum Eye Contour 40** *($55 for 0.5 ounce)* offers no benefit for skin, at least no more than water and some salt with a little hairspray thrown in would. The plant extracts are a mix of irritants and anti-irritants.

☹ **Instant Radiance Vitaserum Intense** *($80 for 1 ounce)* is void of any water-binding agents or antioxidants, but it is filled with irritating plant extracts.

☺ $$$ **Fibrogene Cream** *($135 for 1.6 ounces)* is an exceedingly basic moisturizer for dry skin with teeny amounts of water-binding agents and antioxidants, and I mean really teeny. The price is a burn.

☺ $$$ **Fibrogene Complex** *($145 for 1 ounce)* is a simple, lightweight lotion with some good water-binding agents, but they are overshadowed by some potentially irritating plant extracts.

☹ **Fibrogene Intensive Eye Contour** *($55 for 0.5 ounce)* is void of any water-binding agents, antioxidants, or anti-irritants, but it does contain a tiny amount of irritating plant extracts. It also contains yeast, but there is scant research showing that to be of any benefit for skin. This moisturizer is best summed up as an intensive waste of money.

☺ $$$ **Fibrogene Mask** *($75 for 1.7 ounces)* is a standard clay mask with a tiny amount of antioxidants. It would work as well as any if you don't choke on the price.

☺ $$$ **Hydraskin Light** *($70 for 1.7 ounces)* is a simple, silicone-based moisturizer that would be an OK option for normal to dry skin.

☺ $$$ **Hydraskin Rich** *($70 for 1.7 ounces)* is a basic, though emollient, moisturizer for normal to dry skin. It has slightly more water-binding agents than the Hydraskin Light version above, but overall is just ho-hum and not of much interest for skin, especially not at this price.

☺ $$$ **Hydraskin Night** *($75 for 1.7 ounces)* is similar to the Hydraskin Rich above and the same basic comments apply. The soy flour does not have estrogen-like properties for skin, and this contains more fragrance than it does interesting ingredients.

☺ $$$ **Natural Regulating Fluid** *($65 for 1.6 ounces)* is a lightweight moisturizer for normal to dry skin. The water-binding agents are barely detectable. The urea can exfoliate skin, but for that kind of benefit there are far less expensive products that will work just as well or better.

☺ $$$ **Creme Energique** *($90 for 1.7 ounces)* lacks even a single state-of-the-art ingredient for skin and is nothing more than water and thickening agents! The price is shocking for what is a truly embarrassing formulation that isn't even as interesting as Vaseline Intensive Care.

☺ $$$ **Soothing Eye Contour Gel** *($65 for 0.5 ounce)* is a decent, but overpriced, lightweight moisturizer for normal to slightly dry skin.

☹ **Desincrustant Lotion** *($40 for 1.7 ounces)* lists the third ingredient as sulfur, and that's followed by lemon and arnica extract. As if that weren't irritating enough, this lotion also contains menthol and camphor. All of these are extremely problematic for skin and this product is absolutely not recommended.

☺ $$$ **Rose Aromatic Care** *($59 for 0.5 ounce)* is a mix of plant oils along with a small amount of extremely fragrant oils. The primary plant oils are hazelnut, sweet almond, and sunflower seed, which are easily purchased at any health food store.

☹ **Niaouli Aromatic Care** *($59 for 0.5 ounce)* is just apricot kernel oil and sunflower seed oil mixed with a horde of potentially irritating fragrant oils.

☺ $$$ **Mild Aroma Peeling** *($45 for 1.6 ounces)* is just wax that you rub over your skin that will remove some skin cells. The minute amount of papaya has no exfoliating properties.

DARPHIN SUN PRODUCTS

☺ $$$ **Ecran Soleil SPF 30** *($50 for 1.7 ounces)* is a good in-part titanium dioxide– and avobenzone-based sunscreen. This formula is technically not legal in the United States, where the combination of avobenzone and titanium dioxide is not approved in sunscreen formulations. However, it is a fine option everywhere else in the world. Nevertheless, there is nothing about this product that warrants the price tag. If anything, using an expensive sunscreen may discourage the liberal application that is essential to obtain basic sun protection.

☺ $$$ **Soleil Filtrant SPF 25** *($48 for 5 ounces)* is similar to the Ecran version above and the same comments apply.

☺ $$$ **Vital Protection Day Fluid SPF 15** *($75 for 1 ounce)* is similar to the Ecran version above and the same comments apply.

☹ **Maximal Sun Protection Milk SPF 12** *($48 for 5 ounces)* is similar to the Ecran version above except that this one has only an SPF 12, which falls far short of being "maximal" and makes this closer to "minimal" protection.

☺ $$$ **Self Tanning Face and Body Cream** *($45 for 4.2 ounces)* is a standard self-tanner that uses dihydroxyacetone to affect skin color, the same ingredient every other self-tanner uses. It would work as well as any.

☺ $$$ **Soleil Douceur** *($48 for 5 ounces)* is a good basic moisturizer for dry skin, but that's about it. There is nothing in it that can alleviate or undo the effects of sun exposure.

DARPHIN CLEAR WHITE

☺ $$$ **Clear White Clarifying Milk** *($50 for 6.7 ounces)* is an ordinary wipe-off cleanser; it doesn't get any more standard and boring than this. It does contain a teeny amount of mulberry extract (from a plant that contains arbutin, which has been shown to inhibit melanin), but the concentration in this product is so insignificant as to have no hope of affecting skin color.

☺ $$$ **Clear White Clarifying Toner** *($50 for 6.7 ounces)* is a very good toner that contains a good amount of water-binding agents and antioxidants. The mulberry extract may have an effect on melanin production, but the research supporting this is scant. It does contain some potentially irritating plant extracts.

☺ $$$ **Clear White Clarifying Essential Cream with Fruit Acids** *($95 for 1.7 ounces)* is a good moisturizer that contains a decent amount of water-binding agents and antioxidants. It does contain vitamin C (magnesium ascorbyl phosphate) and mulberry extract (which may have some effectiveness for skin lightening), though the small amounts of these ingredients make it doubtful whether they would be effective. The lemon and pineapple extracts are also barely present, plus they are unrelated to the effectiveness of "real" AHAs.

☺ $$$ **Clear White Clarifying Complex Intense** *($110 for 1 ounce)* is actually no more intense than the Essential Cream with Fruit Acids above, and ends up being almost identical, except for the price.

☺ $$$ **Clear White Clarifying Mask** *($65 for 1.7 ounces)* lists zinc oxide as the second ingredient, so this emollient mask will go on looking white, but that won't change melanin production in skin! The same comments about the skin-lightening properties for the Essential Cream with Fruit Acids above apply here. This version does contain lactic acid, but only about 0.1%, which is eons away from having any effect on skin exfoliation.

DARPHIN MAKEUP

When it comes to their makeup, Darphin is content to offer the same lackluster, borderline embarrassing products it has been selling since the previous edition of this book. While other lines have improved in many respects, Darphin's only redeeming qualities are an excellent mascara, decent brushes, and one overpriced foundation. Actually, overpriced is an understatement for this makeup. Anyone spending this much money deserves products of the nonpareil variety, not the shockingly poor assortment represented here. There is little reason to consider any of the Darphin makeup when there are so many superior, but less expensive, products at the drugstore and at just about every other cosmetics counter at the department store.

☺ $$$ <u>FOUNDATION:</u> **Teint de Rose Foundation** *($45)* has a moist, liquidy texture and is sheer enough to remind you of a tinted moisturizer, not foundation. If you have normal to dry skin and money to spare, this dewy-finish makeup is an option. The six shades offer choices for lighter skin only; darker skin tones would do well to avoid Sublime and Gold, both of which are too peach and rose.

☹ <u>CONCEALER:</u> **Concealer Pencil** *($30)* is a thick pencil that is greasy, crease-prone, and hard to blend without pulling the skin. In addition, the two colors are, in a word, appalling.

<u>POWDER:</u> ☹ **Pastel Loose Powder** *($40)* is talc-based and has an enviable texture and soft application, but the colors are truly misguided.

☺ $$$ **Harmony Compact Powder** *($35)* is talc-based and has a soft texture with noticeable shine. The colors are a mixed bag, with Reflet Harmonie and Ideale Harmonie being the best of the four.

☺ $$$ <u>BLUSH:</u> **Satin Blush** *($30)* has a soft texture that goes on well. The two colors are very sheer, and only show up on fair to light skin. Both shades are shiny, and this is incredibly overpriced considering the beautiful powder blush options from L'Oreal, Sonia Kashuk, and Jane, just for starters.

☹ <u>EYESHADOW:</u> **Aquarelle Eye Shadows** *($25)* are eyeshadow singles that feel silky and apply incredibly sheer. The colors are a hodgepodge of shiny pastels and a range of matte brown shades. The brown shades have a thicker, dry texture that is not the easiest to blend. At this price, you should expect perfection and these don't even come close.

☺ $$$ <u>EYE AND BROW SHAPER:</u> The **Eye Pencil** *($20)* and **Brow Pencil** *($20)* both have standard textures and applications similar to pencils from L'Oreal to Revlon for a quarter of the price. The Brow Pencil tends to chip off as it's applied—not a pretty sight.

<u>LIPSTICK AND LIP PENCIL:</u> ☺ $$$ **Perfect Lipstick** *($22)* is perfect in name only. The reality behind this greasy, slippery lipstick is that its plant-wax texture won't last until lunch, bleeds into lines around the mouth, and offers some truly unattractive colors. If you're in the mood to overspend on lipstick, visit Chanel or Lancome instead. **Lip Contour Pencil** *($20)* is a standard pencil with a smooth texture and slightly dry finish. There is a brush at one end to help with blending, but that extra touch doesn't justify the high price. The three colors are average.

☹ **Perfect Gloss** *($20)* is a very thick, very sticky gloss that would be a foolish investment considering the number of drugstore lip glosses that have preferable textures and prices.

<u>MASCARA:</u> The ✔☺ $$$ **Mascara** *($20)* is a joy to use because it adeptly makes lashes long and well-defined without clumping or smearing, plus it holds up all day. This one isn't much for thickness, but for fail-safe lengthening mascara, it excels.

☺ $$$ <u>BRUSHES:</u> There are three **Brushes** *($30 and $50)* that are soft and workable. In fact, the brushes and mascara are the only justifiable reasons to shop Darphin's makeup line and only then if you have a sizable cosmetics budget.

DDF (SEE DOCTOR'S DERMATOLOGIC FORMULA)

DECLEOR PARIS

To say that not one of the products in this line is nearly as impressive or as current as, say, any from Estee Lauder, L'Oreal/Lancome, Alpha Hydrox, Neutrogena, Eucerin, Avon, or many, many others is an understatement. So what can I tell you about a line whose average product costs about $50 and whose typical recommended skin-care routine costs from $250 to $400 (and that doesn't include sunscreen), for what adds up to nothing more than oil and waxes and a ton of fragrance? If you are someone who feels that spending excessive amounts of money on skin care is worth it, there are far better-formulated lines to consider than this one, which lacks so many excellent contemporary ingredients. Decleor is replete with an implausibly redundant multitude of moisturizers that, for the most part, lack any unique or state-of-the-art water-binding agents, or have more than trace amounts of antioxidants or anti-irritants. The AHA products are abysmal, and the products for oily or blemish-prone skin are so problematic there's a strong likelihood that they will make matters worse, not better. All of that is second-rate, but what is inexcusable is the pathetic, offensive display of sun protection that has appalling SPF ratings and no UVA-protecting ingredients.

Of course, Decleor's brochure tries hard to convince you that every product they sell will give you wrinkle-free, flawless skin, but these formulations fall far short of the ad copy. If anything, the quality of the sunscreens alone ensures that you'll be more likely to end up with wrinkles and damaged skin than anything else. For more information about Decleor, call (888) 414-4471 or visit www.decleor.com. **Note:** All Decleor products are highly fragranced.

DECLEOR PARIS WHITENING

☺ **$$$ Whitening Cleanser** *($34 for 8.4 ounces)* is merely thickeners, almond oil, fragrance, and coloring agents. It is an option for normal to dry skin but there is nothing in this overpriced, exceedingly basic makeup remover that a bottle of almond oil from the grocery store wouldn't replace. As is true for all of the Decleor Whitening products it contains a small amount of mulberry extract. There is a small amount of research showing mulberry extract to inhibit melanin production, but this research has not been carried out on people, only in vitro.

☺ **$$$ Whitening Toner** *($34 for 8.4 ounces)* contains mostly water, slip agents, water-binding agent, fragrance, and preservatives. It does contain mulberry extract.

☹ **Whitening Day Cream SPF 12** *($49 for 1.69 ounces)* does not contain the UVA-protecting ingredients of titanium dioxide, zinc oxide, or avobenzone, plus the SPF 12 is below the SPF 15 minimum standard. This is not recommended.

☺ **Whitening Day Emulsion** *($42 for 1.69 ounces)* is an OK moisturizer for dry skin. It does contain mulberry extract.

☺ **$$$ Whitening Night Cream** *($53.50 for 1.7 ounces)* is an OK moisturizer for dry skin. It does contain mulberry extract.

☺ $$$ **Whitening Aromessence** *($75 for 0.5 ounce)* is primarily hazelnut oil with some fragrant oils. There is nothing in it that can affect the color of skin, other than turning red with embarrassment for wasting this kind of money on such a useless product that is easily replaced with hazelnut oil from the grocery store.

☺ $$$ **Whitening Powder Complex** *($75 for three 3-ounce vials)* is a powder form of ascorbic acid (vitamin C) that is mixed with a lotion of slip agents, mulberry extract, film-forming agent, and preservatives. Even on the off chance that mulberry extract can lighten skin discolorations, all the other Decleor Whitening products contain it, too, so why would you need this if they would help? This is about as unnecessary an extra step as it gets.

DECLEOR PARIS SKIN CARE

☺ **Nutrivital Cleansing Cream** *($29 for 8.4 ounces)* is a standard, cold cream–style cleanser that can be an option for dry skin. Other than the fragrance there is nothing about this formulation that is preferable to Neutrogena's Extra Gentle Cleanser ($7.29 for 6.7 ounces).

☺ $$$ **Eye Make Up Remover with Plant Extracts** *($21.50 for 4 ounces)* is an exceptionally standard, detergent-based eye-makeup remover, but it would work as well as any.

☺ $$$ **Cleansing Oil for the Face and Eyes, with Sweet Almond Oil** *($35 for 8.4 ounces)* is an option for normal to dry skin but there is nothing in this overpriced, exceedingly basic, makeup remover that a bottle of almond oil from the grocery store wouldn't replace.

☺ $$$ **Velvet Cleansing Milk, with Plant Extracts** *($27.50 for 8.4 ounces)* is similar to the Cleansing Oil above and the same basic comments apply.

☺ $$$ **Gentle Cleansing Wash with Plant Extracts** *($33.50 for 8.4 ounces)* is primarily water, mineral oil, thickeners, detergent cleansing agents, plant oils, fragrance, and preservatives. This adds up to an overly expensive, basic cleanser for normal to dry skin.

☹ **Regulating Cleansing Gel, with Plant Extracts** *($33 for 8.4 ounces)* lists sodium C14-16 olefin sulfonate, a detergent cleansing agent, as the second ingredient, which makes it too drying and potentially irritating for all skin types.

☹ **Soothing Cleansing Water** *($35 for 8.4 ounces)* would have been a decent, though ordinary, cleanser for normal to dry skin except that the plant extracts in it are potential skin irritants.

☹ **Prolagene Gel for Face and Body, for All Skin Types** *($31 for 1.69 ounces)*. The third ingredient on the list is fragrant oil, osmanthus oil, which can be a skin irritant.

☹ **Regulating Tonic Lotion, with Plant Extracts, for Combination and Oily Skins** *($27.50 for 8.4 ounces)* lists the second ingredient as orris root, and the fourth is alcohol; together that makes this potentially too drying and irritating for all skin types.

☹ **Phytopeel Natural Exfoliating Cream with Plant Extracts and Essential Oils, for All Skin Types** *($35 for 1.69 ounces)* is a standard waxy scrub that contains several potentially irritating plant extracts, including lemon, lavender, and thyme.

The Reviews D

☺ **Micro Exfoliating Face Gel** (*$28 for 1.69 ounces*) is a very standard mix of thickening agents and ground-up apricot pits.

☺ **$$$ Contour Firming Serum for the Eyes, with Plant Extracts, for All Skin Types** (*$39 for 0.5 ounce*) is as ordinary a moisturizer as it gets. How embarrassing.

☹ **Day Alpha Hydrating Cream, with Plant Extracts and Alpha-Hydroxy Acids, SPF 12, for All Skin Types** (*$45.50 for 1.69 ounces*). The SPF 12 is below the minimum SPF 15 recommended by the National Cancer Institute and the American Academy of Dermatology. This does contain glycolic and lactic acids (AHAs), but the pH isn't low enough for them to have any exfoliating properties.

☺ **$$$ Essential Harmony** (*$61.50 for 1.69 ounces*) is a decent, overly fragrant moisturizer of water, thickeners, plant oils, and preservatives.

☺ **$$$ Essential Harmony, with Plant Extracts and Essential Oils, for All Skin Types** (*$61.50 for 1.69 ounces*) is a blend of emollient oils and fragrant oils, but primarily this is just hazelnut oil, and absurdly overpriced.

☺ **$$$ Anti Fatigue Eye Contour Gel, with Plant Extracts, for All Skin Types** (*$32 for 0.5 ounce*) contains mostly water, slip agent, plant extracts (mostly fragrant), thickener, and preservatives. What a waste of money, as this is completely lacking in any water-binding agents or antioxidants.

☺ **Dermo Floral Tonic Lotion** (*$27.50 for 8.4 ounces*) is an ordinary toner for normal to slightly dry skin. The plant extracts are a mix of irritants and anti-irritants and negate each other.

☺ **$$$ Floral Moisturizer Spray, with Plant Extracts** (*$21.50 for 5 ounces*) is an OK toner of water, slip agent, aloe, water-binding agent, and preservatives.

☺ **$$$ Firming Neck Gel, with Plant Extract, for Mature Skins** (*$53 for 1.69 ounces*) is an OK, though ordinary, moisturizer for normal to slightly dry skin. The soy flour has no estrogen-type properties for skin.

☹ **Hydra Floral Hydrating Fresh Emulsion** (*$48 for 1.69 ounces*) contains peppermint as the third ingredient, and that makes this too irritating for all skin types.

☹ **Aromessence Rose d'Orient Smoothing Concentrate** (*$59 for 0.5 ounce*) is an overpriced mixture of basic oils. This contains mostly water, sweet almond oil, black currant oil, corn oil, and fragrant oils. It's easily replaced with plain almond oil or olive oil, which has great antioxidant properties.

☹ **Aromessence Iris Time Care Concentrate** (*$79 for 0.5 ounce*) is more like applying fragrance than providing skin care, and the price is absurd for what you're getting. The oils are primarily fragrant and that can cause problems for skin. The first two ingredients are hazelnut oil and sunflower oil, which your grocery can easily supply without the fragrance for far less.

☹ **Nourishing Balm Stick** (*$14.50 for 0.14 ounce*) isn't nourishing in the least, at least not any more nourishing than Chap Stick, which is almost identical to this standard mix of waxes and fragrance.

☹ **Hydra Floral Hydrating Comforting Cream** *($48 for 1.69 ounces)* contains peppermint as the third ingredient, which makes this too irritating for all skin types.

☺ **Hydra Matte Regulating Fluid** *($29 for 1.7 ounces)* is a very basic, silicone-based moisturizer that also contains a teeny amount of tea tree oil. Tea tree oil can have antibacterial properties, but not when it's present in such a minute quantity.

☺ **$$$ Radiant Lifting Fluid with Plant Extracts, for All Skin Types** *($45 for 1.69 ounces)* is a good, though ordinary, moisturizer for normal to dry skin. The plant oils in this product are not appropriate for oily or combination skin.

☺ **$$$ Soin Climatique Moisturising Face Cream, with Plant Extracts and Essential Waxes for Dry Skins** *($56 for 1.69 ounces)* is a good, though ordinary, moisturizer for dry skin.

☺ **$$$ Soothing Anti Redness Day Cream for Sensitive Skin** *($61 for 1.7 ounces)* is an OK, though astoundingly basic, moisturizer of waxes and plant oil. This can actually make skin redder because the fragrant oils present a risk of irritation and sensitizing reactions.

☺ **Night Repair Cream with Plant Extracts and Essential Oils, for Normal Skins** *($41 for 1.69 ounces)* is an OK, tedious moisturizer of mostly waxes and plant oil.

☺ **$$$ Stimulating Concentrate, with Plant Extracts and Essential Oils, for Mature Skins** *($76 for 0.5 ounce)*. The only thing stimulating about this is the price. It is merely a blend of emollient and fragrant oils. Skip the fragrant oils, which are serious skin irritants, and mix this up yourself with pure hazelnut and jojoba oil from your grocery store.

☺ **$$$ Timecare Serum, with Plant Extracts, Fruit Acids, and Aromatic Essences, for Mature Skins** *($76 for 1 ounce)* does contain a tiny quantity of antioxidants, but overall this is just an OK moisturizer for dry skin. The soy flour provides no estrogen-like benefits for skin.

☺ **$$$ Vitalite Nourishing and Firming Face Cream, with Plant Extracts and Essential Oils** *($62 for 1.69 ounces)* is a good blend of emollients, plant oils, water-binding agents, and a small amount of antioxidant. This would be a good option for normal to dry skin.

☺ **$$$ Vitaroma Re-Sourcing Emulsion Lift Contour** *($56 for 1.69 ounces)* does contain a tiny amount of retinol in appropriate packaging, but it is also loaded with fragrant oils and little else of benefit for skin. If you are interested in a retinol product, L'Oreal, RoC, and Cetaphil all have similar versions for far less and with less fragrance.

☺ **$$$ Vitaroma Re-Sourcing Creme Contouring Eye Lift** *($37 for 0.5 ounce)* is similar to the Emulsion Lift Contour above and the same comments apply.

☺ **$$$ Vitaroma Extremely Nourishing Cream, with Plant Extracts and Essential Oils, for Dry Skins** *($39 for 1 ounce)* is a blend of waxes, emollient oils, and fragrant oils. The amount of antioxidants is so tiny as to be barely detectable. This is an OK option for normal to dry skin.

☹ **Vitaroma Lift Total Resculpting Cream** *($78 for 1.69 ounces)*. The only thing this product can resculpt is your wallet. The fourth ingredient, aluminum starch octenylsuccinate (an absorbent), makes this a poor choice for dry skin, and the oil and emollients make it a poor choice for oily skin. What a shame, because this is one of the only products in Decleor's lineup that includes state-of-the-art antioxidants and water-binding agents.

☺ $$$ S.O.S. Regulating Tinted Gel *($27 for 0.5 ounce)* contains rice starch, and that can be a problem for blemish-prone skin. It does contain a teeny amount of glycolic and lactic acids, but the high pH makes them ineffective as exfoliants. The minuscule amount of tea tree oil is too small for it to be effective as a disinfectant.

☺ $$$ S.O.S. Blemish Correcting Tinted Gel *($27 for 0.5 ounce)* is almost identical to the S.O.S. Regulating Tinted version above and the same comments apply.

☺ $$$ Corrective Care *($20 for 0.5 ounce)* is just water and mineral oil and a teeny amount of plant extracts that can be antioxidants. This is easily replaced by plain old mineral oil.

☺ $$$ Contour Mask for Eyes and Lips, with Plant Extracts, for All Skin Types *($31 for 1 ounce)* is an OK blend of water-binding agent, plant oils, and film-forming agents. It won't change skin in the least, but it can feel good on normal to dry skin.

☺ $$$ Intensive Eye and Lip Cream Mask *($36 for 1 ounce)* is not intensive in the least. It is actually rather boring, and similar to the Contour Mask above.

☺ $$$ Hydravital Face Mask with Plant Extracts for All Skin Types *($34 for 1.69 ounces)* is a good mix of water-binding agents and plant oils. It would feel good for dry skin, but there is nothing vital or impressive about this in the least.

☺ $$$ Regulating Purifying Mask with Plant Extracts and Natural Aromatic Essences, for Combination Skins *($34 for 1.69 ounces)* is as standard a clay mask as it gets. This would be an option for someone with oily skin. The teeny amount of tea tree oil is not enough to have any disinfecting properties for skin.

☺ Timecare Mask, with Plant Extracts and Aromatic Essences *($38 for 1.69 ounces)* is a silicone-based moisturizer with some emollients, water-binding agents, film-forming agent, fragrant plant oils, and minute amounts of antioxidants. Essentially this is a waste of time for skin.

☺ $$$ Intensive Anti-Shine Care *($31 for 1 ounce)* is mostly silicone and film-forming agent. Although the tea tree oil in it may have some antibacterial properties, the orris root can be a skin irritant.

☺ Calming and Restoring After Sun Face Mask *($22 for 2.5 ounces)* is mostly water, aloe, hazelnut oil, film-forming agent, silicone, and some fragrance. It is a good basic moisturizer for normal to dry skin, but it won't restore anything. Keep in mind that your skin would do just as well, if not better, with just some pure aloe vera you can buy at the health food store. Of course, you should not be tanning or exposing your skin to sun without the benefit of a well-formulated, liberally applied sunscreen, something Decleor doesn't offer.

☺ $$$ Aromessence Solaire Defense Against Sun Damage *($59 for 0.5 ounce)* is just sunflower seed, rice bran, and wheat germ oils with some fragrant oils added as well. Given that Decleor's sun products guarantee sun damage, it is ironic to offer a product under the guise of defending against it, especially as nothing in this product can undo the damage that results from unprotected sun exposure. This is just plant oils that are easily replaced by any of the same emollient oils found at the grocery store.

☹ **Tan Accelerator, Sun Tan Care with Plant Extracts** *($22 for 2.5 ounces)* contains nothing that will enhance a tan. But over and above that, the notion of encouraging tanning in the first place is unconscionable and dangerous for skin. This product does contain a form of tyrosine, an amino acid that can stimulate melanin production. However, according to information on the FDA's Web site (www.fda.gov), tyrosine's "use is based on the assumption that it penetrates the skin, increases the tyrosine content of the melanocytes, and thus enhances melanin formation. This effect has not been documented in the scientific literature. In fact, an animal study reported a few years ago demonstrated that ingestion or topical application of tyrosine has no effect on melanogenesis [the creation of melanin]."

☹ **Tan Enhancing After Sun Moisturizer** *($26.50 for 4.2 ounces)* includes nothing that will enhance a tan. However, the notion of encouraging tanning in the first place is unconscionable and dangerous for skin.

☹ **High Tolerance Protection Sun Cream for Sensitive Skins, SPF 10** *($43.50 for 1.69 ounces)* does contain zinc oxide and titanium dioxide as the active sunscreen ingredients, but the SPF 10 is below the standard set by the National Cancer Institute and the American Academy of Dermatology.

☹ **High Protection Sun Stick Long Lasting Care SPF 25** *($18 for 0.26 ounce)* does not contain the UVA-protecting ingredients of titanium dioxide, zinc oxide, or avobenzone, and is absolutely not recommended.

☹ **High Protection Sun Cream Water Resistant SPF 30** *($26.50 for 2.5 ounces)* is similar to the Sun Stick above and the same comments apply.

☹ **Moderate Protection Soothing Hydrating Cream Water Resistant SPF 15** *($26.50 for 4.2 ounces)* is similar to the Sun Stick above and the same comments apply.

☹ **Very High Protection Comfort Hydrating Cream, SPF 40** *($26.50 for 2.5 ounces)* is similar to the Sun Stick above and the same comments apply.

☹ **Satin Bronzing Gel SPF 2** *($26.50 for 4.2 ounces)* is an insult for skin, and an offensive product for any skin-care company claiming to be concerned about the health of skin, much less to claim that it has the ability to reduce wrinkles. Wearing a product with this low an SPF number is like laying out a welcome matte for wrinkles, skin discoloration, and a risk of cancer.

☹ **Self Tanning Age Prevention Cream SPF 6** *($36 for 1.69 ounces)*. The comments for the Satin Bronzing Gel SPF 2 above apply here as well.

☹ **Wrinkle Defense Protective Sun Cream SPF 8** *($26.50 for 1.69 ounces)*. The comments for the Satin Bronzing Gel SPF 2 above apply here as well.

☹ **Protective Sun Oil Water Resistant SPF 8** *($26.50 for 5 ounces)*. The comments for the Satin Bronzing Gel SPF 2 above apply here as well.

☹ **Self Tanning Hydrating Emulsion SPF 4** *($26.50 for 6.7 ounces)*. The comments for the Satin Bronzing Gel SPF 2 above apply here as well. However, this does contain dihydroxyacetone, the same ingredient all self-tanners use to affect the color of skin. For indoor self-tanning it would work as well as any.

☹ **Self Tanning Hydrating Satin Gel SPF 2** *($26.50 for 4.2 ounces)*. The comments for the Self Tanning Hydrating Emulsion SPF 4 above apply here as well.

☹ **Self Tanning Hydrating Emulsion SPF 4** *($26.50 for 4.2 ounces)*. The comments for the Self Tanning Hydrating Emulsion SPF 4 above apply here as well.

☹ **Express Self Tan Hydrating Spray SPF 6** *($26.50 for 6.7 ounces)*. The comments for the Self Tanning Hydrating Emulsion SPF 4 above apply here as well.

☺ **$$$ Wrinkle Prevention Eye and Lip Care** *($36 for 0.5 ounce)* is mostly water, plant oils, aloe, anti-irritants, film-forming agent, and fragrance. This is a mediocre moisturizer for normal to dry skin that has no ability to prevent or change wrinkles.

☺ **$$$ Natural Face Oil Neroli** *($59 for 0.5 ounce)* is just hazelnut oil with fragrant oils. What a waste! It's easily replaced with plain hazelnut oil, and then you would be sparing your skin from the potential irritants in this product.

☺ **$$$ Natural Face Oil Ylang Ylang, with 100% Natural Aromatic Essences, for Combination Skins** *($59 for 0.5 ounce)* is, except for a change in fragrance, identical to the Neroli version above, and the same comments apply.

☺ **$$$ Arommessence Essential Balm, for All Skin Types** *($57 for 1 ounce)*, except for a change in fragrance, is identical to the Neroli version above, and the same comments apply.

☺ **$$$ Angelique Night Balm** *($57 for 1 ounce)* is a good emollient balm of plant oils and thickeners, along with fragrance. It's basic and greasy, and not very different from just using a plant oil like hazelnut oil on your skin. The tiny amount of vitamin E is barely detectable.

☹ **Natural Face Oil Angelique, with 100% Natural Aromatic Essences, for Dry Skins** *($55 for 0.5 ounce)* contains too many potentially irritating and sensitizing plant oils. This is far more of a problem for skin than a help.

DERMABLEND

Dermablend is one of the original opaque makeup products designed to cover serious skin discolorations. For years Dermablend's main group of products was known as the Corrective Cosmetics System, and consisted of the original Cover Creme and Setting Powder. This cream foundation and pure talc powder provided serious, opaque coverage, but in exchange for hiding your flaws, the thick texture looked obvious and greasy on the skin. It came down to deciding whether that finished total-coverage look was preferable to the considerably more natural look attainable from most other foundations or concealers. Dermablend does not disappoint if you have something to hide, but in public (especially in daylight), it will be no secret to others that you're wearing heavy-duty makeup. The formulas are waterproof, but can still rub off on clothing and furniture, even when set with powder.

In recent years, Dermablend launched a more traditional group of foundations called Reflections. Reflections contains the patented ingredient Melasyn, which claims to provide a healthy, even skin tone and to self-adjust in any light. The compound was invented by Dr. John Pawelek from the Yale School of Medicine. Essentially, it is a synthetic, melanin-colored ingredient derived from the aloe plant. All that means is that Melasyn is a coloring agent being used, in this case, in Dermablend's foundation. Unlike the popular self-tanning ingredient dihydroxyacetone (DHA), Melasyn washes right off and does not affect the color of the skin cells. It produces a more yellow or ashy brown color, which can be advantageous for those whose skin tone is uneven due to loss of pigmentation. Dr. Pawelek believes Melasyn will protect skin from UV radiation much the same way our own melanin does, but thus far the research into this theory has only come from Dr. Pawelek himself, and this research is lacking any substantiated proof or approval from the FDA. Beyond this history, Melasyn's inclusion in some of Dermablend's products does not change the other drawbacks inherent to the formulas.

Whether or not to use makeup to camouflage rather than enhance skin is a personal decision. The need for this type of makeup is intertwined with potentially delicate self-esteem issues, which made me hesitant to assign face ratings to the products. In the end I decided the ratings were needed for women who want to comparison shop the various full-coverage makeups out there. Dermablend is worth exploring if you can tolerate the unavoidable trade-offs in exchange for concealing what's bothersome about your skin. For more information about Dermablend, call (877) 900-6700 or visit www.dermablend.com.

DERMABLEND SKIN CARE

Primarily a makeup line, Dermablend has only a handful of mostly unimpressive and poorly formulated skin-care products. The majority of them are easily overlooked and several are best avoided at all costs.

☻ **Facial Cleanser** *($14.50 for 6.3 ounces)* is a standard, detergent-based, water-soluble cleanser that could work well for someone with normal to oily skin, but the lemon, lime, grapefruit, and orange oils make this an irritation waiting to happen. It does contain coloring agents.

☻ **Remover** *($14.50 for 6.3 ounces)* lists the second ingredient as TEA-lauryl sulfate, and its potential to cause irritation and sensitizing reactions makes this remover a problem.

☻ **Facial Toner Normal to Dry** *($15.50 for 8.75 ounces)* contains witch hazel distillate, which is mostly alcohol, and that is potentially too drying and irritating for most skin types. That's a shame, because overall the other water-binding agents and anti-irritants are quite good. This does contain retinol, but the packaging does not ensure that it will remain stable.

☹ **Facial Toner Normal to Oily** *($15.50 for 8.75 ounces)* is almost identical to the version above for Normal to Dry skin and the same comments apply, which is strange given that these are recommended for use by very different skin types.

☺ **$$$ Advanced Enzyme Moisturizer with Photosomes SPF 15** *($35 for 1.7 ounces)* is a very good sunscreen that uses only titanium dioxide and zinc oxide as the active sunscreen ingredients. It comes in a good moisturizing base that would work well for someone with normal to dry skin.

☺ **$$$ Advanced Enzyme Moisturizer with Ultrasomes** *($35 for 1 ounce)* is a good moisturizer for someone with dry skin. It contains mostly water, plant oil, thickeners, water-binding agents, antioxidants, and preservatives.

☺ **Fade Creme with Sunscreen and AHA** *($17.50 for 1.7 ounces)* doesn't contain titanium dioxide, zinc oxide, or avobenzone to protect skin from UVA damage and doesn't list an SPF number, so it is not recommended for sun protection. However, as a 1% hydroquinone-based skin-lightening product to fade brown spots or patching, it is very good for someone with normal to dry skin. It does contain fragrance. Also, the small amount of lactic acid (AHA) and the pH over 6 means it will not be effective for exfoliation.

☺ **Advanced Chromatone Plus with Alpha Hydroxy Fade Cream with Sunscreen** *($18.25 for 3.75 ounces)* doesn't contain titanium dioxide, zinc oxide, or avobenzone to protect skin from UVA damage and doesn't list an SPF number, so it is not recommended for sun protection. However, as a 2% hydroquinone-based skin-lightening product to fade brown spots or patching it is very good for someone with normal to dry skin. It does contain fragrance.

☺ **$$$ Eye Revitalizing Complex** *($20 for 0.5 ounce)* is a good emollient moisturizer that contains an interesting blend of emollient, water-binding agents, and antioxidants. The emu oil is a good emollient, but it has no other special properties for skin.

☺ **Hydrating Complex Cream** *($30 for 3.75 ounces)* is a very basic, but good, Vaseline-based moisturizer that would work well for normal to dry skin. It also contains a good mix of antioxidants and water-binding agents.

☺ **$$$ Vitamin C Serum** *($25 for 0.5 ounce)* is a silicone-based moisturizer that uses a good amount of ascorbic acid, a form of vitamin C. This is a fairly irritating form of the vitamin, but it is effective as an antioxidant. It lacks any other interesting components for skin, but for those looking for vitamin C, this is an option.

☹ **Self Tanner with Melasyn SPF 14** *($22 for 3.5 ounces)* does not contain the UVA-protecting ingredients of titanium dioxide, zinc oxide, or avobenzone, and is absolutely not recommended.

☺ **$$$ Wrinkle Fix Line Smoother for Lips and Eyes** *($14.50 for 0.12 ounce)* is little more than a lip gloss—it would be hard to get more greasy and ordinary than this, and I would never recommend it for the eye area.

DERMABLEND MAKEUP

FOUNDATION: ☺ **Cover Creme** *($25)* is Dermablend's original foundation. It offers completely opaque coverage via a thick-textured, slightly greasy cream. This claims to have an SPF 30, but with no active ingredients listed, do not rely on it for your sole source of sun protection. There are over 20 shades, though many of them have decidedly unnatural overtones of peach, pink, rose, orange, and copper. The best neutral shades to consider are Pale Ivory, Warm Ivory, Almond Beige, Yellow Beige, Sand Beige, Natural Beige, Saffron Beige, Golden Beige, Caramel Beige, Olive Brown, Toasted Brown, and Chocolate Brown. Cover Creme is also available as **Compact Cover Creme** *($18)*, which features 13 shades, of which most are decent. This also claims an SPF 30, but it, too, lists no active sunscreen ingredients.

☺ **Cover Creme Smooth** *($17.50)* is a creamy, emollient compact makeup that offers a split pan of foundation and concealer. Both have the same slick, slightly greasy texture and moist application. In contrast to the regular Cover Creme, this offers medium coverage and only six OK to poor shades. If you have dry to very dry skin and need good coverage, consider Medium, Tan, and Deep as good bets.

☺ **Leg and Body Cover** *($16.50)* provides the most significant coverage of any foundation I have ever seen, but the result is a dry, ashen finish that does not look natural or skinlike in the least. The SPF 14 claim comes without a listing of active ingredients, so do not rely on this for sun protection. **Quick Fix** *($16)* is an emollient, lipstick-style concealer that provides intense coverage and can definitely crease into lines around the eyes. Dermablend recommends this as an ace in the hole for blemishes, but using this thick, wax-based concoction over a blemish only proves that misery loves company. There are ten shades, and most are a far cry from realistic skin tones. Beige, Ivory, Caramel, and Deep are the only shades worth considering. **Concealer with Melasyn** *($18)* has a light, moist texture that smooths on well enough but then nosedives into a sticky, almost stiff finish. The five shades are a disappointment, with Ivory being the only one that resembles skin.

☺ **Setting Powder** *($18)* is nothing more than talc and a preservative—not the critical product it's made out to be if you're considering Dermablend. The instructions for Cover Creme indicate this is "the key to the wearability and smudge-resistance of Dermablend," but any talc-based powder will do the same thing, and then you can ignore the mediocre colors offered here.

☺ **Matte & Shimmer Bronzer** *($18)* is a pressed-powder bronzer duo, featuring three very good matte, tan shades, each paired with a complementary ultra-shiny color. There are better and less expensive bronzing powders to consider before this one.

☹ **Reflections Waterbased Face Foundation with Melasyn** *($20)* is noticeably lighter in weight than the ones above, with a somewhat moist texture that has good initial slip. However, this quickly dries to a solid, sticky matte finish that looks too obvious on skin.

Because this cannot provide intense coverage, it should have little appeal to those with serious discolorations, and is not worth considering if you want a good, medium-coverage foundation.

DERMALOGICA

Dermalogica's name implies a relationship to dermatology, which makes it sound as if you are getting serious skin care. The subtitle on Dermalogica's products is even more commanding: "A Skin Care System Researched and Developed by the International Dermal Institute." But what is the International Dermal Institute? Are there any dermatologists there? Apparently not: the International Dermal Institute is a school for facialists who want an education beyond what is required for their cosmetology license, and the classes are taught by facialists. (If you're going to get a facial, although I would not suggest you spend your hard-earned money on one, it is best to go to someone who has training from somewhere other than just a cosmetology licensing school. In that regard, the International Dermal Institute provides a good, albeit expensive, service.)

Does the professional atmosphere of the school associated with Dermalogica mean better products? The proof is in the pudding, and this pudding is, for the most part, just Jell-O, not chocolate mousse. The company's literature expounds at length on the ingredients the products *don't* contain. Nevertheless, there are still many plant extracts in these products that are potentially serious irritants and problems for skin. In fact, most of these products are marred by the presence of unnecessary, irritating plant extracts. Aside from rather standard, though overpriced, cleansers, toners, and moisturizers, what is most disturbing is the number of poorly formulated sunscreens. A skin-care company that aligns itself with a medical image should know better. For more information about Dermalogica, call (800) 831-5150 or visit www.dermalogica.com.

☹ **Anti-Bac Skin Wash** *($37.50 for 16 ounces)* is a standard, detergent-based cleanser that also contains mint, menthol, and camphor, none of which serve any purpose for skin other than to cause irritation and inflammation. This does contain triclosan, an antibacterial ingredient that has no research showing it to be effective for acne, even though there is controversy as to whether or not daily use may be problematic in regard to generating bacterial resistance.

☺ **The Bar** *($16 for 5 ounces)* is a detergent-based bar cleanser that contains a small amount of tea tree oil, but not enough to be effective as a disinfectant. The plant extracts are a mix of anti-irritants (antioxidants) and irritants. It also contains fragrance.

☺ $$$ **Essential Cleansing Solution** *($37.50 for 16 ounces)*. This cold cream–type, wipe-off makeup remover would work for someone with very dry skin.

☹ **Skin Purifying Wipes** *($14 for 20 wipes)* contains mint, menthol, and camphor, and that isn't purifying in the least, just irritating. It does contain triclosan as well as a small amount of salicylic acid, though the pH is too high for it to be effective as an exfoliant.

☹ **Dermal Clay Cleanser** *($37.50 for 16 ounces)* contains menthol, mint, lemon, and arnica, all of which are too irritating for any skin types.

☺ **Special Cleansing Gel** *($37.50 for 16 ounces)* is a standard, detergent-based, water-soluble cleanser that can be OK for someone with oily or combination skin. It contains a tiny amount of balm mint, which can be irritating for some skin types.

☺ **Ultracalming Cleanser for Face and Eyes** *($24.50 for 8 ounces)* contains a mix of irritating and anti-irritant plant extracts, which is confusing, not calming. Aside from the plants, it is just a standard, detergent-based cleanser.

☺ $$$ **Soothing Eye Makeup Remover** *($21 for 4 ounces)* is a standard, detergent-based eye-makeup remover that would work as well as any. At least this one doesn't contain fragrance of any kind.

☺ $$$ **Daily Microfoliant** *($40 for 2.6 ounces)* is a good, though standard, detergent-based mechanical scrub that uses both silicates and oatmeal as the exfoliants. It also contains salicylic acid, but the pH is too high for it to be effective as an exfoliant. The papain it contains has no research showing it to be effective in cosmetic formulations for exfoliation. It also contains a mix of plant extracts that are anti-irritants and potential irritants.

☹ **Gentle Cream Exfoliant** *($30 for 2.5 ounces)* contains several potentially irritating ingredients, including sulfur and lemon. The abrasive is a type of ground-up rock, and that is anything but gentle. It also contains papain and salicylic acid, similar to the Daily Microfoliant above, and the same comments apply.

☺ $$$ **Skin Prep Scrub** *($25 for 2.5 ounces)* is a detergent-based, water-soluble cleanser that uses cornmeal as the scrub. It would probably be better to just use cornmeal from the grocery store if you want a cornmeal scrub, because then at least you wouldn't be applying some of the irritating plant extracts that are present in this product, including arnica and ivy. However, these ingredients are probably present in such small amounts that they don't have much effect on skin, but why are they in here at all?

☹ **Multi-Active Toner** *($21.50 for 8 ounces)* contains mint and lavender, which makes this too irritating for all skin types.

☹ **Soothing Protection Spray** *($26 for 8 ounces)* contains lavender, lemon, sage, and clover, all of which are potential irritants, and that isn't protecting for skin in the least.

☺ $$$ **Gentle Soothing Booster** *($41 for 1 ounce)* contains plant extracts that can have antioxidant and anti-irritant properties along with slip agents and preservatives. That can be beneficial for skin, but water-binding agents would have made this a really great formula for skin.

☺ **Active Moist** *($42 for 3.5 ounces)*. If it weren't for the potentially irritating plant extracts in this one, it could have been an OK emollient moisturizer for someone with dry skin.

☹ **Active Firming Booster** *($41 for 1 ounce)* contains too many irritating plant extracts for all skin types, including lemon, arnica, pine, pellitory, and orange. This won't firm anything, but it could cause irritation.

☺ **Barrier Repair** *($33 for 1.25 ounces)* is a silicone-based moisturizer that also contains some vitamin E, plant oils, vitamin C, and anti-irritants. The silicone feels silky on skin and this would be an option for someone with normal to dry skin.

☺ $$$ **Intensive Eye Repair** *($37 for 0.5 ounce)* is a very good emollient moisturizer for dry skin. It contains some great emollients, water-binding agents, antioxidants, and vitamins. One word of warning: There is a small amount of arnica in here, a substance that can cause irritation, especially around the eyes, for some sensitive skin types. It also contains wild yam extract; for more explanation about why this extract has no effect on skin, please refer to Chapter Seven, *Cosmetics Dictionary*. It does contain fragrance.

☺ **Intensive Moisture Balance** *($37 for 1.75 ounces)* is similar to the Intensive Eye Repair product above only with fewer emollients, and the same basic comments apply. It would be good for someone with normal to dry skin.

☺ $$$ **Intensive Moisture Concentrate** *($45 for 1 ounce)*, like many moisturizers, contains a film-forming agent as the main ingredient. This places an imperceptible layer of plastic over the skin that makes the skin temporarily look smoother. It also contains some good antioxidants and a tiny amount of water-binding agents. It is just a good lightweight moisturizer for slightly dry skin and isn't as well formulated as the other two Intensive products above. It does contain fragrance.

☺ $$$ **Specific Skin Concentrate** *($45 for 1 ounce)* is similar to the Intensive Moisture Concentrate above, and the same comments apply. This one does contain some potentially irritating plant extracts, but it's likely that the amounts are too small to be a problem for skin.

☺ **Skin Smoothing Cream** *($46 for 3.5 ounces)* is a good emollient moisturizer for someone with dry skin. It contains all the appropriate emollients, plant oils, antioxidants, and water-binding agents. It also contains some irritating plant extracts, but not very much of them, so it probably won't be a problem for most skin types.

☺ $$$ **Total Eye Care SPF 15** *($33 for 0.75 ounce)* is a good lightweight moisturizer for normal to dry skin that has a titanium dioxide–based sunscreen and some good water-binding agents. It also contains lactic acid, though the product doesn't have a low enough pH for it to work as an exfoliant.

☹ **Oil Control Lotion** *($30 for 1.7 ounces)*. This salicylic acid lotion also contains mint, camphor, and menthol, which won't control oil in the least, but will cause redness, dryness, and irritation.

✓☺ $$$ **Special Clearing Booster** *($37 for 1 ounce)* is an absurdly expensive, standard 5% benzoyl peroxide–based product. There are far cheaper benzoyl peroxide products available at the drugstore or by prescription than this one.

☹ **Skin Renewal Booster** *($41 for 1 ounce)* is a 10% AHA and 0.5% BHA product that also contains sulfur. The pH of this product isn't low enough for the AHA or BHA to be effective exfoliants, and the sulfur is unnecessarily irritating.

☹ **Solar Defense Booster SPF 30** *($30 for 1 ounce)* does contain avobenzone, so this one has good UVA protection! Sadly, this is negated by the pointless inclusion of mint and lemon.

☹ **Waterproof Solar Spray SPF 25** *($26 for 4 ounces)* is similar to the Solar Defense Booster above and the same comments apply.

☹ **Solar Shield SPF 15 (stick)** *($8.95 for 0.28 ounce)* doesn't contain the UVA-protecting ingredients of avobenzone, zinc oxide, or titanium dioxide, and is not recommended.

☹ **Full Spectrum Sunswipes SPF 15** *($20 for 15 wipes)* doesn't contain the UVA-protecting ingredients of avobenzone, zinc oxide, or titanium dioxide, and is not recommended.

☹ **Full Spectrum Block SPF 15** *($24 for 4 ounces)* doesn't contain the UVA-protecting ingredients of avobenzone, zinc oxide, or titanium dioxide, and is not recommended.

☹ **Protective Self-Tan SPF 15** *($24 for 4 ounces)* doesn't contain the UVA-protecting ingredients of avobenzone, zinc oxide, or titanium dioxide, and is not recommended.

☹ **Ultra Sensitive Bodyblock SPF 15** *($22 for 4 ounces)* is a pure titanium dioxide–based sunscreen in a good moisturizing base for normal to dry skin. Unfortunately, this also contains mint, lemon, and grapefruit extracts, which makes it a problem for any skin type, but especially for someone with sensitive skin.

☹ **Ultra Sensitive Face Block SPF 25** *($22 for 1.75 ounces)* is similar to the Ultra-Sensitive Bodyblock above and the same comments apply.

☹ **Pigment Relief SPF 15** *($45 for 1.7 ounces)* doesn't contain avobenzone, zinc oxide, or titanium dioxide for UVA protection, and is not recommended. Mulberry extract and vitamin C are present in such minute amounts that they can have minimal to no effect on inhibiting melanin production.

☹ **After Sun Repair** *($28 for 3.5 ounces)*. After using most of Dermalogica's sunscreens, you will need after-sun repair, because most of the sunscreens won't protect you from the damage caused by the sun's UVA rays. However, this moisturizer won't repair the skin. It contains several potentially irritating plant extracts, including Szechuan pepper and clove flower. The other ingredients can make a good moisturizer for normal to dry skin, but for the most part this is just a "Why bother?" product.

☹ **Medicated Clearing Gel** *($31 for 2 ounces)* contains tea tree oil, but not enough to be effective as a disinfectant. It also contains salicylic acid, but the pH is too high for it to be effective as an exfoliant. And besides that, it contains a range of potentially irritating plant extracts including thyme, rosemary, sage, and citronella.

☹ **Anti-Bac Cooling Masque** *($31 for 2 ounces)* contains a host of irritating plant extracts, including balm mint, menthol, camphor, sage, and orange. It does contain triclosan, but there is no research showing it to be effective against acne.

☺ **$$$ Intensive Moisture Masque** *($34 for 2 ounces)* is an OK moisturizing mask that contains thickeners, plant oils, a small amount of antioxidants, fragrance, and preservatives. This is really just a thick moisturizer for normal to dry skin.

☺ **$$$ MultiVitamin Power Concentrate** *($42.50 for 45 capsules)*. The plant oils in this product are from a variety of citrus and they can be potential irritants. The form of vitamin C is ascorbic acid and in this silicone-based, encapsulated packaging it would be stable. If you want vitamin C and vitamin E, too, this is a fine option, but there are better formulations that include impressive water-binding agents as well.

☺ **$$$ Multivitamin Power Firm for Eye and Lip Area** *($42 for 0.5 ounce)* is similar to the Power Concentrate above except that this one leaves out the irritating fragrance and adds some good anti-irritants and additional antioxidants to the mix.

☺ **$$$ MultiVitamin Power Recovery Masque** *($36 for 2.5 ounces)* is a standard peel-off mask. This won't change a wrinkle on your face but it can be a good mask for normal to dry skin. It contains a very good mix of antioxidants, plant oils, water-binding agents, and anti-irritants. All in all, it would be great if all Dermalogica's moisturizers were as well formulated as this mask, which can only provide a limited amount of benefit given that it's used infrequently and worn for only a short period of time.

☹ **Skin Hydrating Masque** *($31 for 2.5 ounces)* contains vitamin K, which has no effect on surfaced capillaries. The form of vitamin C, ascorbic acid, is not stable in a water-based product such as this, and several of the plant extracts are skin irritants.

☹ **Skin Refining Masque** *($30 for 2.5 ounces)* is a standard clay mask that also contains some plant oil and water-binding agents. Unfortunately, it also contains a large number of potentially irritating plant extracts.

☺ **$$$ Treatment Foundation** *($30)* is a sheer makeup that has a soft, moist texture. It feels surprisingly light on the skin, and the coverage is similar to what most tinted moisturizers provide. The eight shades include some fairly neutral options, with the only poor choices being shades 1 and 2, which are both too pink. This really doesn't have any treatment benefits beyond moisturizing the skin, though thankfully it is free of the irritants present in many other Dermalogica products.

☹ **Colour Correctors** *($15)* are similar in texture and application to the Treatment Foundation above. The idea is to use the white shade to highlight or lighten a too-dark color and use the coppery red shade to deepen your foundation shade or add contour. Since both shades are so sheer, and most women won't want to bother with this extra step, this product is relatively useless.

DHC

DHC is a Japanese cosmetics company that was launched in the United States in the mid-1990s. At that time, the highlight of the line was a single bar of soap. The brochure stated, "For more than 15 years women in Japan have relied on this clear, pure, gentle bar of soap." That has all changed as the line has grown to include lots of other cleansers, and this bar soap has taken a back seat to a broad and varied array of other cleansers.

The strong points for this line are that most of the products do not contain coloring agents, and the formulations are rather basic and straightforward, which is best considering the way skin uses good water-binding agents and emollient oils. While DHC boasts that it doesn't use fragrance, that simply is not the case across the board. Some of these products absolutely contain fragrance in the form of fragrant extracts, and there are a handful of other irritating ingredients to look out for too, including alcohol, lemon, and ginseng (though this line does make far less use of these ingredients than many other lines).

There are lots of good DHC moisturizers to consider, but you can ignore the claims about firming and getting rid of wrinkles; these products can't live up to those claims any more than any other cosmetics company's products can. While the latest ingredients are present—from vitamin C (the good one) to retinol (though not in packaging that will keep it stable)—they also want you to believe that olive oil will keep your skin young. Olive oil is an emollient plant oil similar to all nonfragrant plant oils. The concept of it having antiaging properties stems from some evidence that diets high in olive oil may help prevent heart disease (Sources: *European Journal of Clinical Nutrition*, January 2002, pages 72–81 and *Lipids*, November 2001, Supplemental pages S49–S52 and pages 1195–1202). There are also a small number of studies using animal tests showing that topically applied olive oil can protect against UVB damage (Sources: *Carcinogenesis*, November 2000, pages 2085–2090 and *Journal of Dermatological Science*, March 2000, Supplemental pages S45–S50). It does seem that olive oil is a good antioxidant. Assuredly, it's a good moisturizing ingredient, and research shows similar results for other oils as well. Just keep in mind that DHC products aren't the exclusive source for those ingredients.

For more information about DHC, call 1-800-DHC-CARE or visit www.dhccare.com.

DHC SKIN CARE

☺ **Deep Cleansing Oil** *($22 for 6.7 ounces)* actually doesn't contain much oil at all. This is just an emollient, wipe-off cleanser with a tiny bit of vitamin E for effect and rosemary oil for scent (even though it can be a skin irritant). The recommendation is to use this product with another cleanser in the line, though for dry skin it would work just fine.

☺ **Facial Wash for Oilier Skin** *($18 for 6.7 ounces)* is a standard, detergent-based, water-soluble cleanser. This typical formulation is definitely an option for normal to oily skin. It does contain fragrance.

☹ **Gentle Cleansing Foam for Normal Skin** *($14 for 4.9 ounces)* is a fairly alkaline cleanser that contains myristic acid and potassium hydroxide as the cleansing agents, and that can be too drying for most skin types. The little bit of olive oil won't undo the dryness of the cleansing agents.

☺ **Make Off Sheet** *($6 for 50 sheets)* is similar to almost all of the wipe-off makeup removers that supply the wiper for you. This one contains a detergent cleansing agent with some slip agents. It would work as well as any.

☺ **Mild Cleansing Cream for Drier Skin** *($14 for 4.9 ounces)* is an exceptionally standard, mineral oil–based, wipe-off cleanser. This is just pricey cold cream with lots of ordinary thickening agents and it doesn't rinse easily off the face. It can be a good option for someone with dry skin.

☹ **Mild Soap** *($12 for 3.1 ounces)* is a standard, tallow-based bar soap that can be too drying for most skin types.

☹ **Pure Soap** *($12 for three 1.4-ounce bars)* is almost identical to the Mild Soap above and the same comments apply.

☺ **Oil-Free Makeup Remover** *($15 for 3.3 ounces)* is a very standard, typical, detergent-based makeup remover that can work as well as any.

☺ **Facial Scrub** *($14 for 4.9 ounces)* uses ground-up apricot seeds as the exfoliant, and also contains some thickeners and fairly drying detergent cleansing agents. That makes this a standard, OK exfoliant for someone with normal to oily skin.

☺ **Acerola Lotion** *($15 for 3.3 ounces)* does contain a minute amount of acerola, which is a source of vitamin C; however, acerola is unlikely to be a good source of vitamin C because much of the vitamin is destroyed during the drying and processing (Source: *Natural Medicines Comprehensive Database*, www.naturaldatabase.com). This is just an OK toner for normal to dry skin.

☺ **Balancing Lotion for Normal Skin** *($12 for 6 ounces)* is a rather ordinary toner that contains mostly water, slip agent, glycerin, water-binding agents, AHA, and preservatives. There isn't enough AHA for it to act as anything other than a water-binding agent. That's not bad, just maybe not what you were expecting. One of the water-binding agents is placental protein; it's a good water-binding agent, but there are other sources of plant protein that work as well, and given that skin can't tell the difference, why use placenta?

☺ **Soothing Lotion for Drier Skin** *($15 for 6 ounces)* is similar to the Balancing Lotion above and the same comments apply. At least this one doesn't contain placenta.

☹ **Clean Finish Lotion for Oilier Skin** *($14 for 6 ounces)* is mostly alcohol, along with ginseng, sage, and resorcinol, and that makes it extremely irritating and sensitizing for all skin types.

☺ **$$$ Mild Lotion** *($34 for 6 ounces)* is merely water, glycerin, slip agent, cucumber juice, and preservatives. The price is insulting for what is nothing more than an exceedingly ordinary toner.

☺ **$$$ Nourishing Mist** *($35 for 6 ounces)* is virtually identical to the Mild Lotion above and the same comments apply.

☹ **Blotting Lotion** *($9 for 2 ounces)* lists the second ingredient as alcohol. That, along with the irritating plant extracts, makes this too irritating and drying for all skin types.

☺ **White Cream** *($34 for 1.4 ounces)* contains a good amount of magnesium ascorbyl phosphate, a form of vitamin C that does have research showing it to have some effect on inhibiting melanin production. Other than that, this is a good moisturizer for normal to dry skin with a nice mix of some plant oils and anti-irritants. It does contain fragrance.

☺ **White Lotion** *($29 for 1.3 ounces)* contains a tiny amount of mulberry extract, but so little it's unlikely to have any effect on inhibiting melanin production. This product is not preferred to the White Cream above. The placental extract in this product has no skin-lightening properties; if anything, there is research showing that it can encourage melanin production (Source: *International Journal of Dermatology*, January 1995, pages 61–66), which is counterproductive to reducing brown skin discolorations.

☹ **Renewing AHA Cream** *($34 for 1.5 ounces)* contains 10% lactic acid (AHA), although the pH of 4.5 is not the best for effective exfoliation. This is a standard moisturizer for normal to dry skin, but not much else.

☹ **Acerola Gel** *($12.50 for 1.4 ounces)* contains a fractional amount of acerola and little else. This is a mediocre gel moisturizer for normal skin. See the comments about acerola for the Acerola Lotion above.

☹ $$$ **Advanced Collagen Treatment** *($40 for 1 ounce)* is not advanced in the least; it just contains some water, slip agent, water-binding agents, preservative, and fragrance. The water-binding agents are great, but this lacks the antioxidants and anti-irritants that would have made it really advanced.

☺ **AntioxC** *($32 for 1.4 ounces)*. The vitamin C in this product is magnesium ascorbyl phosphate and that's considered a good, stable, and effective form, but it won't change a wrinkle; nor is this vitamin better than other antioxidants. It also contains some good plant oils and water-binding agents. This is a very good, lightweight moisturizer for someone with normal to slightly dry skin.

☹ **Ceramide Quick** *($28 for 4 ounces)* actually doesn't contain any ceramides. It's just a simple "toner" that contains mostly water, slip agent, soybean germ extract, glycerin, and preservative. It's OK, but there is little about this product that can restore ceramide levels to your skin, at least not any more than any other simple moisturizer can.

☹ $$$ **Collagen Eye Stick** *($29 for 0.12 ounce)* is a very emollient, clear, lip gloss–type moisturizer for very dry skin. Don't expect the collagen to do anything special because it's just a water-binding agent, nothing more, so it can't help shore up your own collagen. This does contain some good plant oils, but would have been really special if it contained some interesting antioxidants. The teeny amount of mulberry extract can't affect melanin production.

☹ $$$ **Concentrated Eye Cream** *($29 for 0.7 ounce)* is a good lightweight moisturizer for someone with normal to slightly dry skin. The teeny amount of royal jelly in it can have emollient properties, but it's not an antiwrinkle cure, while the rosemary and ginseng extract can be skin irritants. It does contain some good plant oils and water-binding agents, though the teeny amount of vitamin E is barely detectable.

☺ **Dual Defense SPF 25** *($24 for 3.5 ounces)* is a good, partly titanium dioxide–based sunscreen for someone with dry skin in a very basic moisturizing base.

☺ **Emollient Balm** *($30 for 3.3 ounces)* contains mostly water, antioxidant, olive oil, slip agent, water-binding agents, preservatives, vitamin E, soy extract, anti-irritants, and plant extracts. Some of the plant extracts can be skin irritants, but for the most part this is a decent moisturizer for dry skin. The placental protein in this product has no special properties over many other water-binding agents or antioxidants. The soy and vitamin E are present in such minute amounts that they have no real effect on skin.

☺ **Rich Moisture for Normal to Drier Skin** *($24 for 3.3 ounces)* is a good emollient moisturizer for dry skin. The ginseng can be a skin irritant, though the amount is probably too scant to be of real concern. There's a minuscule amount of royal jelly, which sounds good and can be an emollient, but it serves no great purpose for skin care.

☺ **Extra Nighttime Moisture** *($30 for 1.5 ounces)* is similar to the Rich Moisture above and the same basic comments apply. This version does contain a minuscule amount of retinol, but the clear packaging will allow light to decompose this little amount very quickly.

☺ **Hydrating Nighttime Moisture** *($28 for 1 ounce)* is a very good, lightweight moisturizer for someone with slightly dry skin.

☺ **Light Moisture for Normal to Oilier Skin** *($24 for 3.3 ounces)* lists olive oil as the second ingredient, and some of the water-binding agents, like collagen, which is good for dry skin, aren't the best for oily skin. This is a good moisturizer for normal to dry skin; just don't use it over oily areas. It also contains retinol, but the clear packaging allows for decomposition of this highly unstable ingredient.

☹ **$$$ Milk Protein** *($35 for 0.84 ounce)* is a "toner" that contains water, slip agent, yogurt, alcohol, lactoferrin, and preservatives. Yogurt is a relatively useless ingredient for skin care, but lactoferrin is just the opposite. It is a protein, usually derived from milk (particularly breast milk), that can also be found in saliva. Lactoferrin can have antiviral, antibacterial, and anti-inflammatory effects on skin (Sources: *Biochemistry and Cell Biology*, 2002, volume 80, number 1, pages 103–107 and *British Journal of Dermatology*, April 2001, pages 715–725). That's great, but this would have really come highly recommended if it also contained some interesting antioxidants and water-binding agents.

☺ **Moisturizer** *($28 for 3.3 ounces)* contains mostly water, slip agent, olive oil, water-binding agents, glycolic acid, preservatives, and anti-irritants. The amount of glycolic acid, less than 2%, makes this ineffective as an exfoliant. Other than that, this can be a good moisturizer for someone with dry skin. The placental protein is similar to other proteins that have good water-binding and antioxidant properties, but it isn't a miracle ingredient.

☺ **Oil-Free Hydrator for Oilier Skin** *($22 for 3.3 ounces)* could be a good, very lightweight moisturizer for slightly dry skin. It contains mostly water, slip agent, glycerin, water-binding agents, preservatives, and anti-irritants. The placental protein in it is similar to other proteins that have good water-binding and antioxidant properties, but it isn't a miracle ingredient.

☺ **Olive Virgin Oil** *($36 for 1 ounce)*. At first I thought this was a joke, but it isn't. This is pure virgin olive oil. Even if virgin olive oil was a great skin-care ingredient, why would you bother buying this from a cosmetics company for such an absurd amount of money as opposed to getting the exact same thing from a grocery store for a fraction of the price? Olive oil is a good antioxidant moisturizing oil, but that's about it.

☺ **Skin Conditioning Oil** *($30 for 1 ounce)* is just olive oil and some fragrance oils of lavender and rosemary. You don't need the fragrance, so all that counts is the olive oil. You can find much better olive oil than this at your grocery store for a lot less money and forgo the potentially skin-irritating fragrances.

☺ **Pure Squalane** *($25 for 1 ounce)* is, as the name states, pure squalane, an oil derived from shark liver, plants, or human and animal sebum. It is a natural component of skin and is considered a good emollient that has antioxidant and immune-stimulating properties (Sources: *Lancet Oncology*, October 2000, pages 107–112 and *Free Radical Research*, April 2002, pages 471–477). That's great, but there are lots of oils in the world you can use that cost far less than this one and that would work well on dry skin, including pure olive oil; only use the one from your kitchen, not the one DHC sells (see above) with an inflated price tag.

☺ $$$ **Retino A Essence** *($36 for 0.17 ounce)* is a good moisturizer for dry skin, but it is not as interesting as many other moisturizers DHC has to offer.

☹ **Soothing Eye Gel** *($24 for 0.7 ounce)* would just be a pretty do-nothing eye gel except that this one contains orange peel and lemon, which can irritate the skin around the eyes.

☺ **Tocophero E Cream** *($26 for 1.2 ounces)* is a very good emollient moisturizer for dry skin. It does contain a good amount of vitamin E (scientific name tocopherol, even though the name of the product is Tocophero), as well as some plant oils and water-binding agents.

☺ **Water Base Moisture** *($12 for 2 ounces)* has a strange name, given that all DHC's moisturizers are "water-bases." Nonetheless, this is a good, lightweight moisturizer that contains some very good water-binding agents, and the placental extract does have antioxidant properties.

☺ $$$ **Wrinkle Relief** *($28 for 0.7 ounce)* won't relieve you of wrinkles any more than any other antiwrinkling moisturizer. This version contains mostly plant oils, silicone, royal jelly, water-binding agent, vitamin E, and preservatives. The royal jelly has no research showing it to be effective for wrinkles. This is just a good moisturizer for dry skin.

☹ **B Mix Cream** *($29 for 1.7 ounces)* is supposed to reduce shine and help oily skin, but its ingredient list shows that it's impossible for it to have such an effect. First of all, the claim that any form of topically applied vitamin B can have any effect at all on oily skin is not substantiated. Second, the amounts of B vitamins in this moisturizer are minuscule. Third, the emollients in this cream, including caprylic/capric triglyceride, castor oil, and olive oil, are a serious problem for oily skin.

☺ $$$ **Hydrating Facial Mask** *($16 for 3.5 ounces)* is a standard clay mask with some film-forming agent that allows it to be peeled off the skin. It is exceptionally ordi-

The Reviews D

nary, but can help absorb oil. There's a small amount of water-binding agents in this mask, but the clay prevents them from having the intended effect on skin.

☺ $$$ **Mineral Mask** *($31 for 3.5 ounces)* is similar to the Hydrating Facial Mask above and the same comments apply. This does contain a small amount of menthol, which can be a skin irritant, but there probably isn't enough of it to have much of an impact.

☹ $$$ **Firming Kelp Facial Mask** *($30 for 0.6-ounce liquid and 3.5 ounces gel)* is used in steps. Step 1 is a toner that you place on the skin before you apply the mask, which is Step 2. The toner is just water and some water-binding agents. The DNA in this product won't affect your own DNA, and you wouldn't want it to! The mask is mostly film-forming agent (hairspray), so you peel this one off. That can help skin feel smooth and soft, just as any peel-off mask does.

☹ **Peel-Off Pack** *($9 for 2.1 ounces)* is just water, polyvinyl alcohol (film-forming agent), alcohol, water-binding agents, and preservatives. This is like placing a layer of hairspray and alcohol on the face and then peeling it off. What a waste of time for skin.

☹ **Retino-A Pack** *($27 for 1 ounce).* The minuscule amount of retinol and other vitamins in this product is a bit shocking. It's just a peel-off mask with polyvinyl alcohol as the film-forming agent. It also contains clay and some water-binding agents, but the whole combination negates their function on skin.

☺ $$$ **Lip Conditioner** *($11 for 0.12 ounce)* is a very emollient, very basic "lipstick" for dry lips. It contains mostly lanolin, thickeners, plant oils, preservatives, and a minute amount of vitamin E.

DHC MAKEUP

DHC is clearly a skin care–driven line, but their small selection of makeup has some products for light to medium skin tones that are normal to oily. The price differences between these makeup products and the skin-care products are puzzling, since they have similar formulas and contain the same buzz ingredients this line espouses. Basically, the color line is for DHC devotees only. There is nothing extraordinary in this line that cannot be found in other lines, and many of them offer a broader color palette than DHC.

FOUNDATION: ☺ $$$ **Liquid Makeup** *($27)* has a smooth silicone base that dries down to a soft matte finish and provides light to medium seamless coverage. This is a simple, but effective, formula with a weightless feel those with oily skin will enjoy. Of the five shades, Ivory, Beige, and Ocher are decent (though slightly peach), while Pink and Tawny are musts to avoid. **Water Base Face Color** *($19)* is extremely watery, and is actually a very light formula that contains talc for a dry finish. This can feel slightly sticky, but it is matte and an option for those with normal to oily skin who prefer sheer coverage. The five shades go on much lighter than they appear. Only Pink (an accurate name) is too pink for all skin tones. There are no shades for darker skin tones.

☺ **Velvet Skin Coat** *($20)* is a simple, ultra-silky silicone gel that is supposed to fill in pores and fine lines before you apply foundation. This will smooth out the skin's texture and, to a minor, but short-lived, extent, will fill in pores and lines, but putting this Coat on is not an essential step.

POWDER: ☺ $$$ **Face Powder** *($12)* is talc-based and has a very soft texture and sheer satin finish that would be best for normal to dry skin. There are three shades, and while Medium and Deep (which are really quite light) are good, Light is pure white and is not recommended.

☹ $$$ **2 Way Compact** *($31 with compact; $23 for refill)* is a wet/dry pressed powder that has a smooth, dry texture. It lays down a very sheer application of powder whether you use a damp or dry sponge. The formula contains talc, but not as the main ingredient. Instead, this powder contains sericite (a form of mica) and barium sulfate, a metal-based salt that is known to cause skin reactions when used topically. The five colors are decent, except for Tawny and Pink.

LIPSTICK AND LIP GLOSS: ☺ **Fresh Lip Color** *($12)* is a lightly emollient, medium-coverage lipstick that feels great on the lips and comes in a small but enticing group of colors. **Lip Gloss Color** *($10)* is a very good, but typical, lip gloss with a pleasant texture that's not distractingly sticky.

☹ $$$ **Perfect Lipcolor** *($20)* is an ultra-matte lipstick that is intensely pigmented and barely felt on the lips. Used alone, this tends to wear unevenly and can look "cracked," while still managing to come off on coffee cups or your significant other. It fares much better (and is more comfortable) when paired with a lip gloss.

☹ **MASCARA:** The **Mascara** *($15)* has one of the smallest, shortest brushes I've ever seen, but manages to build reasonable length and thickness if you're patient. Regrettably, this tends to smear easily and streak, and is simply not on a par with most mascaras.

DIANE YOUNG

Diane Young is a New York City facialist and aesthetician whose appearances on QVC have made her line of products an infomercial curiosity. Her credentials as a skin-care expert seem to have garnered her some attention in fashion magazines, and the name of her salon, Diane Young Antiaging Salon, definitely gets attention. Her product line offers a host of products promising nothing less than returned youth. Young's Coneflower (echinacea) Neckline Firmer is supposed to be "clinically proven to decrease lines up to 36% in 4 weeks and to increase skin firmness up to 21% in 4 weeks." Just add that to an endless list of other unpublished skin-care studies with miraculous promises. It seems that it only takes a promise of youth to catch the attention of consumers.

Young's niche in the world of skin care is her use of plants that are relatively unique. An extract called mahanimba, from the Asian neem tree, is one of these. Yet this isn't quite as exotically appealing as it sounds. The neem extract, even though it has been shown to have antimicrobial properties, can also have potential toxic effects (Sources: *Life*

Sciences, January 2001, pages 1153–1160; *Journal of Ethnopharmacology*, August 2000, pages 377–382; *Phytotherapy Research*, February 1999, pages 81–83; and *Mutation Research*, June 1998, pages 247–258.)

Another plant is *long xu cai*, a very exotic name for a form of algae that may have antioxidant properties. There's also malkagni, a shrub native to India that may also have antioxidant properties. Then there are the standard plants used in any product line that wants you to think natural thoughts, including cucumber, chamomile, aloe, and horsetail. What any of that can do for the skin is more folklore than established knowledge, but there is no way around it—plants look good on a label. Keep in mind that even if a plant does have known beneficial properties, that information is often derived from research done using a pure concentration in a tincture form or a specific individual "tea" product. There are few, if any, published studies that establish what happens once a plant is added to a cosmetic. In minute amounts, mixed with 10 to 50 other ingredients, and preserved and packaged in a range of containers (most plant concentrates require dark packaging to maintain stability), it's hard to tell if it retains any of its original properties. There are exceptions, but they are few and far between. What you are relying on with the addition of all these plants is the hope that they will have an effect, and what you get is merely the feel-good emotional reaction from thinking you are putting something "natural" on your skin.

There are some very nicely formulated moisturizers in this small product group, and aside from the prices and some fairly extravagant claims, it isn't a line to be dismissed outright. For more information about Diane Young, call the Diane Young Antiaging Salon at (212) 753-1200, or call QVC at (800) 455-6685, or visit www.dianeyoung.com or www.qvc.com.

DIANE YOUNG SKIN CARE

☺ $$$ **Age Lift Hydrating Cleansing Milk** *($28.50 for 2.5 ounces)* is an overpriced, lotion-style cleanser that can be an option for normal to dry skin. It does contain fragrance.

☺ $$$ **Age Lift Intensive Hydration Cream** *($58 for 1.3 ounces)* is an OK moisturizer for normal to dry skin that has some good plant oils, but that lacks antioxidants other than algae. Including some state-of-the-art water-binding agents would have added some credibility to this incredible price tag. This does contain fragrance.

☺ $$$ **Awaken Younger Night Cream** *($58 for 1.5 ounces)* is my favorite name for a skin-care product, but what can this overnight miracle really do? It's complicated to explain. First, it contains heavy water, which is used in nuclear reactor coolant systems, but there is no information on what that can do for skin. It also contains banana extract, which has antioxidant properties. The lactic acid in this product has no exfoliating properties because the pH is too high for it to be effective. It also contains phytosterols, cholesterol-like components of plants, which, while they may lower cholesterol when eaten (Source: *Annual Reviews of Nutrition*, 2002, volume 22, pages 533–549), may be potentially phototoxic when applied to skin (Source: *Photochemistry and Photobiology*, September 1997, pages 316–325). All in all, this is a confusing moisturizer for normal to dry skin that does have some antioxidants and a small amount of water-binding agents, but it is anyone's guess if it's worthwhile for skin, or if you will wake up looking one iota different.

☺ $$$ **Coneflower Eyeline Firmer** *($30 for 0.5 ounce)* contains some good antioxidants and water-binding agents in a lightweight lotion that would be an option for normal to dry skin. But there are also some irritating plant extracts that are problematic for the skin, especially the eye area, including clove and citruses. It does contain retinol, but the packaging ensures that it won't remain stable in the formulation.

☹ $$$ **Coneflower Facialine Firmer** *($40.92 for 1.5 ounces)* contains a mix of plant extracts that can be anti-irritants and irritants, and it lacks any state-of-the-art water-binding agents or antioxidants. It does contain fragrance.

☺ $$$ **Coneflower Neckline Firmer** *($37.50 for 1 ounce)* is an OK, emollient, gel-like moisturizer for normal to dry skin. It lacks any state-of-the-art water-binding agents or antioxidants. It does contain fragrance.

☺ $$$ **De-Aging Sunscreen Oil Free Firming Moisturizer SPF 15** *($38.50 for 1.5 ounces)* is a good, in-part avobenzone-based sunscreen. The moisturizing base is nice, but not worth the exorbitant price tag. This does contain glycolic acid and salicylic acid, but the pH is too high for them to have exfoliating properties.

☺ $$$ **Immediate Appeal Gel Exfoliant** *($38.50 for 0.5 ounce)*. This blue gel can be rubbed over the skin, and that will roll off dead skin cells. That can make skin feel soft, but the ingredients in this product don't amount to much and the price is hardly appealing for what you get.

☺ $$$ **Coneflower Lipline Firmer** *($41 for 0.5 ounce)* is to be rubbed over skin for exfoliation. BeautiControl and Mary Kay have identical versions for a fraction of the cost.

☺ $$$ **Years Younger Skin Lightening and Brightening System** *($68 for 3-piece kit)*. The first piece of this kit includes **Years Younger Skin Brightening Serum** *(1 ounce)*, which contains two ingredients: magnesium ascorbyl phosphate (a form of vitamin C) and calcium d-pantetheine s-sulfonate. There is some research showing that both of these ingredients have the ability to inhibit melanin production. It also contains bearberry, which may also have some melanin-inhibiting properties. It is an interesting option for skin lightening, albeit a very pricey one. The second piece, **Years Younger Age Spot Lightening Serum** *(0.5 ounce)*, is similar to the Brightening Serum only minus the vitamin C and bearberry. Instead, this contains plant extracts that sound like they are related to AHAs, although they have no ability to exfoliate skin. The **De-Aging Sunscreen SPF 15** *(0.25 ounce)* is the third piece, but in this tiny amount you would not be able to use this sunscreen liberally and, therefore, you would not be getting the benefit of the SPF on the label. This is not good news, because liberal sunscreen application is crucial to preventing

The Reviews D

skin discolorations. The third piece of the kit is sold separately, but what a shame the Brightening Serum isn't, because it would be an interesting product to try.

☹ $$$ **Wrinkle Firming Finish** *($68.75 for 0.5 ounce)* contains dimethyl sulfoxide (DMSO) as the second ingredient, which can be a potent skin irritant. For more information about DMSO, please refer to Chapter Seven, *Cosmetics Dictionary*.

☺ $$$ **Years Younger Eye Serum** *($49.50 for 0.5 ounce)* contains a mix of plant extracts (arnica, pellitory, and lime) that can be skin irritants and also some anti-irritants. It lacks interesting antioxidants and water-binding agents.

☺ $$$ **Years Younger Serum** *($45.50 for 1 ounce)* is a very good, lightweight moisturizer for normal to slightly dry skin that contains a great mix of water-binding agents, anti-irritants, and a small amount of antioxidants. The name is enticing, but these ingredients won't net you younger skin anymore than any other well-formulated moisturizer will.

☺ $$$ **Years Younger Soothing Serum** *($50 for 1 ounce)* is almost identical in every way to the Years Younger Serum above and the same comments apply.

☺ $$$ **Dry Parts Moisture Mask Salon Treatment** *($56.50 for 1.5 ounces)* is a very good, emollient moisturizer that contains a good mix of plant oils, water-binding agents, anti-irritants, and a tiny amount of antioxidants. The small amount of grapefruit oil in this is unlikely to cause irritation.

☺ $$$ **Intensive Enzyme Appeal Salon Treatment Mask** *($69 for 1.5 ounces)* lists the second ingredient as papain, an enzyme that in its pure form can exfoliate skin. However, there is little research showing it can do that in a cosmetic formulation. If you were curious to give it a try this is one to consider, but AHA and BHA products can exfoliate as well or better and many of them are a lot less expensive than this. This mask also contains some irritating plant extracts, including clove and cinnamon.

☺ $$$ **Line Lifting Salon Treatment Skincare System** *($125 for 4 treatments)*. You're supposed to mix the **Line Lifting Powder**, which contains mostly egg white, cornstarch, and oatmeal, with the **Line Lifting Activator**, which is mostly, aloe, thickener, and some good water-binding agents. This ordinary group of ingredients is almost laughable given the price tag.

DIANE YOUNG MAKEUP

Diane Young's makeup philosophy is that women need to add lots of artificial shine to their faces because, as we age, our skin loses its subtle color and brightness. To that end, Young's makeup offers several options to replace what time takes away. However, any woman seriously hoping to recapture her "youthful glow" is advised to look elsewhere. Not only is adding layers of iridescence the wrong way to look younger, these are some of the most expensive, poorly formulated, and remarkably disappointing makeup products available. There is nothing in this color line that cannot be found in a better version elsewhere, including products at your local drugstore, and with them you won't have to put up with makeup that sounds like it's a face-lift in a bottle that can treat, cover up, diffuse light from, or lighten wrinkles. If your goal is to downplay wrinkles, your best bet is to apply a moisturizing sunscreen (for daytime) followed by a natural-finish concealer over discolored or dark areas. A sheer veil of non-shiny powder will add a polished look and still allow the dewiness of the moisturizer to show through, and your wrinkles will appear softer.

FOUNDATION AND BLUSH: ☺ $$$ Young Glow! Pearlized Underbase *($35)* is a sheer, lightly creamy moisturizer with a soft golden shimmer that is subtle but still too sparkly for daytime wear. For evening, this can add a glow to the skin, but the same effect can be achieved with considerably less expensive products. **Young Glow! Pearlized Bronzer** *($35)* is nearly identical to the Underbase above, only this has a sheer peachy tan color that does little to create a bronzed look. **Young Glow! Pearlized Blush** *($24.50)* is a light liquid-cream blush that comes in a jar and provides a sheer wash of shiny color that does light up the face, but not in the understated, lit-from-within way you're hoping for.

☹ **Foundation of Youth Liquid Makeup** *($45)* is a sheer, slightly moist liquid foundation that has a shiny finish and an unattractive peach tint that is supposed to be a "one shade fits all" color. If you really want a shiny foundation, there are considerably less expensive options in wonderfully neutral tones from Revlon, Ultima II, Prescriptives, and Clinique.

☹ **CONCEALER: Look Younger Perfecting Pencils** *($22.50)* are standard pencils that have a creamy consistency and a decidedly unnatural peach hue. They're described as "an incredible beauty tool," but I suspect most women will find this as useless as I did, and the effect, while not too convincing, is short-lived. **Wrinkle Treatment Concealer** *($39.50)* is a pen-style liquid concealer dispensed onto a brush tip when you click the base of the product. Although this is sold as a wrinkle filler, this silicone concealer has an inordinately dry, almost grainy, texture that accentuates, rather than hides, every wrinkle, line, crack, or crevice on your face. The price is insulting for even a superior concealer, which this assuredly is not. **Red Neutralizer** *($19.75)* is an incredibly thick-textured, full-coverage concealer whose ashen tone is neither flattering nor natural looking on most skin tones. This greasy product contains only petrolatum, lanolin, preservatives, and pigment, and given Young's authoritative antiaging approach this seems quite dated and inelegant. **Cover All Undereye Concealer** *($22.50)* is a very greasy cream concealer that initially covers well but shamelessly creases and moves throughout the day, so don't expect long-lasting, worry-free results from this one. **C-Circles Vanish** *($47.25)* has an awful, thick, dry texture, and although it will camouflage dark circles, the unattractive finish essentially substitutes one problem for another, not to mention the problem of the outlandish price!

☹ **POWDER: Young Glow! Pearlized Powder** *($45)* is a shiny, very overpriced talc- and mica-based powder that will make you look younger much the same way chewing food with your mouth open makes you look well mannered. **Young Glow! Pearl Powder in a Puff** *($46)* is nothing more than a fluffy powder puff infused with white and opalescent glitter. I am almost speechless that women are paying such a premium price for something as simple as glitter.

__EYE AND BROW SHAPER:__ ☹ __Eye Lift Silky Eye Liner__ *($24.50)* is a creamy eyeliner packaged in a small pot. This stays creamy on the skin, and smears with the slightest provocation. ☺ $$$ __Brow Lift Coloring & Sculpting Wax__ *($22.75)* is supposed to be "the solution for fading, thinning, drooping, aging brows." Regardless of how old your brows look, this product, which is simply tinted wax, is no substitute for a long-wearing matte brow powder, brow mascara, or even a standard brow pencil. It works to add definition to brows, just not as well as lots of other brow-enhancing options.

__LIPSTICK AND LIP GLOSS:__ ☹ __Young Glow! Enduring Lip Color__ *($24.77)* is supposed to "give you back the natural lip color that you had as a youthful twenty-something." Funny, I've yet to see someone in his or her 20s (or any age, for that matter) whose lips were naturally opaque, iridescent pink! This silicone-based liquid lipstick comes with a built-in brush that you click color into from the base of the container. Although this applies smoothly and the brush is easy to work with, the formula stays uncomfortably sticky and eventually cracks and peels off the lips, which is hardly the picture of youth. Further, what remains on the lips is extremely difficult to remove. The "universal rose" color is actually a soft, but bright, pink that certainly won't appeal to everyone.

☺ $$$ __Young Glow! Pearlized Lip Gloss__ *($22.50)* is a very standard, sticky gloss that has more than its fair share of iridescence and an outrageous price.

☹ __BRUSHES:__ __Set of 4 Brushes in a Bag__ *($39)* includes a decent __Powder Brush__ with a 1-inch handle, a stiff, scratchy __Brow Brush__, a sparse __Eyeliner Brush__, and an excellent __Eyelid Crease Brush__. The bag is on the small side and aside from the one good brush, this set has little going for it. __Sponge on a Stick Trio__ *($36.50)* features three different sizes of makeup sponges, each fastened to a plastic stick that resembles a thermometer. One sponge is recommended for the eye area, one for the cheek, and one for all over the face. These makeup contrivances are not preferred to considerably less expensive synthetic makeup sponges.

☹ __SPECIALTY:__ __Diane Young Ultimate 12-piece Color Collection__ *($139)* encompasses almost every product above that earned a frown. This is ultimately a disappointing collection of mostly inferior products whose look-young-now premise is poorly executed.

DIFFERIN

In the world of prescription acne treatments, the vitamin A derivatives called tretinoin (basic to such products as Retin-A and Renova) have been in a class by themselves for many years, backed by a great deal of research proving their efficacy for treating acne as well as skin discolorations and also for improving cell production. Adapalene, another vitamin A derivative (trade name Differin), was patented by Galderma and joins this group with similar impressive results. Differin is a prescription-only, topical acne medication that contains the active ingredient adapalene.

Remember, if abnormal skin cells in the layers of skin and in the pores are left to do their own thing, they just accumulate there, creating an environment in which blemishes can flourish. Aside from topical and oral antibiotics that primarily address the issue of killing off the bacteria responsible for producing pimples, tretinoin was for a while the only prescription product available that could help exfoliate skin cells (especially inside the pores), literally changing the way the skin cells are produced. It works for more than half of the people who can tolerate the treatment, but therein lies the rub—tolerance—because tretinoin can irritate the skin, too. Even Dr. James Leyden, an associate of Dr. Albert Kligman, the original patent holder for Retin-A, said, "Retinoid [Retin-A] therapy ... due to the side effects, has always been a double-edged sword, limiting its use in many patients."

Where does Differin fit into this picture? Differin has been shown in clinical studies to be significantly less irritating than tretinoin. According to a study published in the *Journal of the American Academy of Dermatology* (March 1996), Differin was significantly more effective in reducing blemishes and also better tolerated than tretinoin gel. Other more recent studies have come to the same conclusion, which is that, by several measures, adapalene cream and gel were less irritating after multiple dosing than various tretinoin creams and gels (Sources: *International Journal of Dermatology*, October 2000, pages 784–788 and *Journal of Cutaneous Medical Surgery*, October 1999, pages 298–301).

It seems that Differin has a radarlike ability to positively affect the skin-cell lining of the pores, substantially improving exfoliation and helping to prevent blockage. Moreover, for those with oily skin, the original Differin comes in a lightweight gel formula that is barely felt on the skin. It contains little more than water and cellulose, a sheer thickening agent. Differin is also available in a cream base for those with dry skin and blemishes.

DOCTOR'S DERMATOLOGIC FORMULA (DDF)
(SKIN CARE ONLY)

DDF is an acronym for Doctor's Dermatologic Formula. Can there be any doubt what this line is supposed to represent to the consumer? Getting right to the point, this is one of many cosmetic product lines headed up by a physician. The physician in this case is Dr. Howard Sobel, a real, live, credential-loaded dermatologist and plastic surgeon. According to Sobel, "Having an active full-time dermatology practice in Manhattan keeps me on top of skin care issues. I care about the quality and effectiveness of the products I use in my practice and dispense to my patients." As great as that sounds, there is no way these formulations substantiate the notion that this doctor is "on top of skin care issues." Many of the products contain fragrances (all of them well-known and researched skin irritants and sensitizers), several products contain alcohol and menthol (which are unnecessary skin irritants), the claims about getting rid of wrinkles are completely without substantiation, and many of the ingredient lists on the products do not meet FDA regulations regarding the appropriate names of ingredients (which means you don't really know what you are putting on your skin).

Yet there will be lots of consumers who will believe these products are superior because they carry a physician's endorsement. Highlighting the concern about just how serious the issue of doctors selling skin-care products is (and how prevalent), an article in the August 1999 issue of the *Tufts University Health & Nutrition Letter* stated that the "American Medical Association has issued guidelines advising physicians not to sell health-related products for profit. When a doctor stands to gain from something a patient buys, it creates a conflict of interest." The American College of Physicians–American Society of Internal Medicine has also issued ethical guidelines for physicians selling products, which were in turn reported in the *Annals of Internal Medicine* (December 7, 1999). That paper stated that sales of cosmetics and vitamins by physicians are "ethically suspect."

Aside from the "medical" hype, the strength of the DDF line is that there are some well-formulated sunscreens, AHA exfoliants, skin-lightening products, and an array, actually an overabundant and redundant assortment of, moisturizers containing state-of-the-art water-binding agents and antioxidants. And not all of the prices are hard to swallow. If you pick and choose carefully, there are some great products to consider, but be wary and proceed with caution. For more information about DDF, call (800) HDS-SKIN or visit www.ddfskin.com.

☺ $$$ **Antioxidant Cleansing Bar** *($20 for 4.3 ounces)* has an ingredient list that completely disregards FDA regulations. I suspect this is just a standard bar cleanser, but without a legitimate ingredient list there is no way for you to know what you are really putting on your face.

☺ $$$ **Skin Brightening Soap** *($20 for 4.3 ounces)* is a standard bar cleanser that can be potentially drying for most skin types. It does contain some plant extracts that are known to inhibit melanin production, but in a cleanser their effectiveness would just be rinsed down the drain.

☹ **10% Glycolic Cleansing Pads** *($24 for 60 pads)* no doubt contains 10% glycolic acid, but it also contains alcohol and menthol, which are unnecessarily irritating and problematic for skin.

☹ **Daily Cleansing Pads Glycolic 5%** *($25 for 60 pads)* is similar to the 10% Glycolic Cleansing Pads above only minus the alcohol, which is a plus. However, it does contain witch hazel distillate (which is mostly alcohol), so it still may be a problem for skin, and it also contains menthol.

☹ **Blemish Foaming Cleanser** *($23 for 6.7 ounces)* is a standard, detergent-based cleanser that contains about 2% salicylic acid, though the pH of the product is too high for it to be effective as an exfoliant. It also contains eucalyptus, which can be a skin irritant.

☺ $$$ **Earthy Herbal Foaming Cleanser** *($20 for 6.7 ounces)* isn't herbal in the least. Instead, this is an exceptionally standard, detergent-based cleanser that contains minuscule amounts of plant extracts. It also contains fragrance. It is an option for normal to oily skin.

☺ $$$ **Laid Back Lavender Foaming Cleanser** *($20 for 6.7 ounces)* is virtually identical to the Earthy Herbal version above except for the lavender fragrance in this one. The same basic comments apply.

☺ $$$ **Pick-Me-Up Pink Grapefruit Foaming Cleanser** *($20 for 6.7 ounces)* is virtually identical to the Earthy Herbal version above except for the grapefruit fragrance. The same basic comments apply.

☹ **Glycolic Exfoliating Wash 7%** *($31.25 for 8.45 ounces)* is a standard, detergent-based, water-soluble cleanser that contains no more than 2% glycolic acid, which is not enough to be effective for exfoliation. The claim of 7% does not agree with the position of the glycolic acid on the ingredient list. Even if it were effective, the glycolic acid would be quickly rinsed away in a wash, although what might get left behind is the irritation of the mint oil in here.

☺ $$$ **Non-Drying Gentle Cleanser** *($25 for 8.45 ounces)* is an exceptionally standard, detergent-based cleanser that would be good for most skin types except dry skin. It does contain a coloring agent.

☺ $$$ **Salicylic Wash 2%** *($28 for 8 ounces)* is a standard, detergent-based, water-soluble cleanser that contains salicylic acid (BHA). The effectiveness of the BHA would be rinsed away, however, and the pH of the product is too high for it to be effective as an exfoliant.

☺ $$$ **Sensitive Skin Cleansing Gel** *($27.50 for 8.45 ounces)* is an exceptionally standard detergent-based cleanser that would be good for most skin types except dry skin.

☺ $$$ **Wash Off Cleanser** *($24 for 8.45 ounces)* is an exceptionally standard, detergent-based, water-soluble cleanser that would be good for most skin types except dry skin. This also contains lemon oil, which can be a skin irritant, though it is present in such a small amount that it most likely would not be a problem for skin.

☺ $$$ **Eye Make-Up Remover Pads** *($15 for 60 pads)* is actually a better toner formulation than an eye-makeup remover. It will take off makeup well enough and will leave some good ingredients behind as well.

☺ $$$ **Almond, Bergamot, Herbal, Strawberry;** and **Coconut Face & Body Polish** *($23 for 8 ounces)* are exceptionally standard, but good, detergent-based scrubs that use almond meal and ground-up plastic (polyethylene) as the scrub particles. The only real differences between these are the fragrances.

☺ $$$ **Face & Body Scrub** *($23 for 8 ounces)* is similar to the assorted fragranced Face & Body Polish versions above only minus the fragrance and almond meal. That makes this one far preferred as a scrub for all skin types.

☺ $$$ **Pumice Acne Scrub** *($26 for 8 ounces)* thankfully doesn't really contain pumice! Rather, it uses polyethylene (ground-up plastic), which is far easier on skin, in a standard, detergent-based, water-soluble cleanser. It also contains 2.5% benzoyl peroxide, an effective topical disinfectant, but in a scrub it will be rinsed away before it has much of a chance to make a difference.

✔☺ $$$ **Aloe Toning Complex** (*$22 for 8 ounces*) is a very good toner that contains an impressive array of water-binding agents and antioxidants.

☹ **Glycolic Toner 5%** (*$23 for 8 ounces*) contains alcohol and menthol, which makes it too irritating for all skin types.

☹ **Glycolic Toner 10%** (*$27 for 8 ounces*) contains alcohol and menthol, which makes it too irritating for all skin types.

☺ $$$ **Skin Purifying Tonic** (*$15 for 6 ounces*) contains a good combination of antioxidants, but lacks water-binding agents. It also contains a small amount of plant extracts that may be skin irritants.

☺ $$$ **Rosacea Relief** (*$47 for 1 ounce*) is a lightweight gel lotion that contains mostly water, slip agents, thickener, yeast, plant extracts, and preservatives. The plant extracts for the most part have either anti-irritant properties (a form of licorice extract and horse chestnut) or antioxidant properties (barley and cocoa). That can be nice for skin but this also contains lemon extract, which can be a skin irritant, and the showcased ingredient, trade name Gatuline (also known as pilewort; scientific name *Ranunculus ficaria*, which isn't the best option for treating rosacea. Actually, the only information indicating that pilewort has any benefit with regard to rosacea comes from the company selling the ingredient; there is no other research demonstrating that to be the case. However, there is a small amount of research showing that pilewort extract possibly has antibacterial and antifungal properties, and it is used homeopathically in the treatment of hemorrhoids. However, topically, it can cause skin irritation and may cause photodermatitis (Source: *Natural Medicines Comprehensive Database*, http://www.naturaldatabase.com). Given the abundant research regarding the efficacy of topically applied MetroGel, MetroCream, MetroLotion, and Noritate (all prescription-only pharmaceuticals) in the treatment of rosacea, and the fact that they are actually cheaper then this cosmetic, you could easily bypass this and your skin wouldn't be missing much.

☹ **Faux-Tox** (*$75 for 0.5 ounce*). I knew it was just a matter of time before a cosmetics company would decide to capitalize on the popularity of Botox by boasting that their product's ability to get rid of wrinkles was equal to that of Botox. (Refer to Chapter Seven, *Cosmetics Dictionary*, for details about the Botox medical procedure for wrinkles). There are companies in this book claiming to have myriad products that can mimic just about any procedure a plastic surgeon can perform, from lasers to chemical peels and even face-lifts. However, there isn't a single product that can come remotely close to creating results that in any way, shape, or form, resemble the results of a cosmetic corrective medical procedure. If they could, why would anyone bother with the costly and relatively risky treatments offered by plastic surgeons or dermatologists?

DDF's Botox wannabe is Faux-Tox. This pricey product, which over a years' time wouldn't cost that much less than an actual Botox treatment, claims to contain a "... non-toxic, antiaging peptide, chemically combined from naturally derived amino acids, [that] helps prevent fine lines induced by repeated facial movements without the loss of facial expression." And the results are supposed to be visible within two weeks. The miracle ingredient in this lightweight lotion is Argireline, which is the tradename for the synthetically derived peptide called acetyl hexapeptide-3. The company selling acetyl hexapeptide-3, Centerchem (www.centerchem.com), is from Spain and, according to their Web site, "Argireline works through a unique mechanism which relaxes facial tension leading to a reduction in superficial facial lines and wrinkles with regular use. Argireline has been shown to moderate excessive catecholamines release."

I strongly doubt that any of that is true because there isn't a shred of research substantiating any part of it. However, even if it were vaguely true, that would not be good news for your body because you wouldn't want any cosmetic without any safety data, efficacy documentation, or independent research messing around with your catecholamines. Catecholamines, such as epinephrine, adrenaline, and dopamine, are compounds in the body that serve as neurotransmitters. Epinephrine is a substance that prepares the body to handle emergencies such as cold, fatigue, and shock. A deficiency of dopamine in the brain is responsible for the symptoms of Parkinson's disease. None of that sounds like something you want a cosmetic to inhibit or reduce. What if you accidentally overuse the product and apply too much? What is excessive for your body? The entire notion is more worrisome than almost anything I've encountered in my research for this book.

✔☺ $$$ **Cellular Revitalization Age Renewal** *($125 for 1.7 ounces)* is a very good, though very overpriced, moisturizer for dry skin. It contains emollients, silicone, water-binding agents, plant oils, antioxidants, preservatives, and fragrance.

☺ $$$ **Dramatic Radiance TRF Cream** *($95 for 1.7 ounces)* isn't dramatic in the least, but it is a very good moisturizer for normal to dry skin. It contains some very good plant oils, yet it has only a small amount of water-binding agents and antioxidants. For this price tag, you would definitely expect more.

✔☺ $$$ **EPF Eye Serum C3** *($39 for 0.5 ounce)* is a very good lightweight moisturizer that contains a good mix of water-binding agent, anti-irritants, and antioxidants.

✔☺ $$$ **EPF Serum C3 Environmental Protection** *($60 for 1 ounce)* is similar to the EPF Eye Serum C3 above and the same basic comments apply.

☹ **EPF Moisturizer C3 SPF 15** *($72 for 1.7 ounces)* does not contain the UVA-protecting ingredients of titanium dioxide, zinc oxide, or avobenzone, and is not recommended.

☺ $$$ **Glycolic Moisturizer 10%** *($32.50 for 2 ounces)* is a good 10% AHA exfoliant in a very standard moisturizing base. There are teeny amounts of some good antioxidants in here that do minimally help skin, though they don't help exfoliation.

☹ **Glycolic Gel 10% for Oily Skin** *($34 for 1.67 ounces)* contains alcohol as the second ingredient, which makes it too drying and irritating for all skin types.

☺ $$$ **Glycolic Eye Gel** *($37 for 1 ounce)* contains about 7% glycolic acid, but the pH of the gel is too high for it to be an effective exfoliant. Although that does make it better for the eye area, why put it on at all? Other than that, it does contain some very good water-binding agents and antioxidants in a lightweight gel base. This is a very good lightweight moisturizer for normal to slightly dry skin; just ignore the AHA part of the name.

☺ **Luminous Moisture Shelter SPF 15** *($36 for 1.67 ounces)* is an in-part avobenzone-based sunscreen, though the amount of avobenzone isn't all that much, and more is better than less for UVA-protecting ingredients. There are some good antioxidants and water-binding agents in this moisturizer, but a better sunscreen would have been more impressive. The luminous part comes from the mica, which adds shine to the skin.

☺ **Matte Finish Photo-Age Protection SPF 30** *($22 for 4 ounces)* is a very good, in-part avobenzone-based sunscreen. However, the second ingredient is alcohol and that isn't helpful for skin.

✓☺ **Moisturizing Photo-Age Protection SPF 15** *($22 for 4 ounces)* is a very good, in-part avobenzone-based sunscreen in a silicone-based moisturizer lotion that contains some very good antioxidants.

☺ $$$ **Retinol Energizing Moisturizer** *($85 for 2 ounces)* does contain retinol, along with other antioxidants, and a small amount of water-binding agents. This is a very good moisturizer for normal to dry skin. It does contain fragrance.

✓☺ $$$ **Retinol Energizing Serum with Protein Complex** *($70 for 1 ounce)* is a very good, lightweight moisturizer that would be an option for someone with normal to slightly dry skin. Along with a small amount of retinol it includes some very good antioxidants and water-binding agents.

✓☺ $$$ **Retinol Eye Renewal** *($49 for 0.5 ounce)* is similar to the Energizing Serum above and the same comments apply.

✓☺ $$$ **Silky-C Serum** *($65 for 1 ounce)* is indeed silky, as the primary ingredients are forms of silicone. It also contains vitamin C, retinol, water-binding agents, and antioxidants. This would be a very good moisturizer for normal to dry skin.

✓☺ **Ultra Lite Oil Free Moisturizing Dew** *($28 for 1.67 ounces)* is a very good, lightweight moisturizer for someone with normal to slightly dry skin. It contains an impressive mix of water-binding agents and antioxidants.

✓☺ $$$ **Vitamin K Cream** *($47 for 1 ounce)*. The only research establishing vitamin K as effective for reducing the presence of capillaries on the surface of skin was performed by the company that manufactures the ingredient and by the patent holder. Otherwise, this is a very good moisturizer for normal to dry skin with some very good water-binding agents and antioxidants. There is probably not enough vitamin C in this product to affect skin color, though this also contains kojic acid, which may have some effectiveness for inhibiting melanin production.

✓☺ $$$ **Erase Eye Gel** *($39 for 0.5 ounce)* contains a good amount of vitamin C along with other good antioxidants. The vitamin C and kojic acid may inhibit melanin production. For the effectiveness of the vitamin K in this product see the comments on the Vitamin K Cream above. This would be a very good lightweight moisturizer for normal to slightly dry skin.

✓☺ **$$$ Bio-Molecular Firming Eye Serum** *($75 for 0.5 ounce)* is a very good lightweight moisturizer for normal to slightly dry skin that contains a good amount of antioxidants and water-binding agents.

✓☺ **$$$ Nourishing Eye Cream** *($37 for 1 ounce)* is a very good emollient moisturizer for normal to dry skin that contains a good amount of antioxidants and water-binding agents.

✓☺ **$$$ Soothing Eye Gel** *($37 for 1 ounce)* is similar to the Bio-Molecular Firming Eye Serum above and the same comments apply.

☺ **Sun Gel SPF 30** *($22 for 4 ounces)* is a very good, in-part avobenzone-based sunscreen. However, the primary ingredient is alcohol, and that isn't helpful for skin.

☺ **Sun Mist SPF 30** *($22 for 4 ounces)* is almost identical to the Sun Gel SPF 30 above and the same comments apply.

☺ **Moisturizing Photo-Age Sunscreen SPF 30** *($22 for 4 ounces)* is a very good, in-part avobenzone-based sunscreen in an emollient, moisturizing base that would be an option for normal to dry skin. It also contains some very good antioxidants, but only a teeny amount of water-binding agents.

✓☺ **Organic Sunblock SPF 30** *($22 for 4 ounces)* is a very good sunscreen that uses only titanium dioxide and zinc oxide as the active ingredients, making it an excellent option for sensitive skin. It also contains some very good antioxidants.

✓☺ **Sport Proof SPF 30** *($22 for 4 ounces)* is similar to the Moisturizing Photo-Age Sunscreen SPF 30 version above except that this one is a water-resistant formula.

☺ **After Sun Security** *($22 for 8 ounces)*. There is nothing in this product that can change the negative effect sun exposure has on skin. However, it is a very good emollient moisturizer with some very good plant oils, emollients, water-binding agents, and a small amount of antioxidant. It does contain fragrance.

☺ **Sun Free Self Tanner** *($22 for 4 ounces)* is a standard self-tanner that uses dihydroxyacetone to affect skin color. This would work as well as any.

✓☺ **Aloe Cort Cream** *($25 for 2 ounces)* is a basic hydrocortisone cream identical in effectiveness to Lanacort and Cortaid, which are sold at the drugstore for less than $5 per ounce. The continuous use of hydrocortisone over time can actually cause skin damage by thinning the skin and breaking down the skin's support structure. If you are aware of this very serious shortcoming and plan only occasional use, it can be effective for reducing skin irritation, but there is no reason to use this one rather than the drugstore versions.

☺ **Collagen Dry Skin Mask** *($18 for 2 ounces)* is more of an emollient moisturizer than anything else. It isn't as interesting as most of DDF's moisturizers, but for a mask it will do well enough.

☺ **Detoxification Mud Mask** *($23 for 2 ounces)* is mostly just clay and water. That makes it a decent absorbent for oily skin, although it won't detoxify anything.

☹ **Clay Mint Mask** *($24 for 4 ounces)* is a standard clay mask, although the mint oil can cause skin irritation.

☹ **Sulfur Therapeutic Mask** *($26 for 4 ounces)* is a standard clay mask that also contains 1% sulfur. Sulfur is a topical disinfectant that is very irritating and highly alkaline, and that can cause problems for skin. It also contains eucalyptus oil, which adds even more irritation to the mix.

☹ **Medicated Skin Cleanser 5% Benzoyl Peroxide** *($22 for 8.54 ounces)* is a standard, detergent-based cleanser that contains sodium C14-16 olefin sulfate as the cleansing agent, which makes it too irritating and potentially sensitizing for all skin types. The benzoyl peroxide is a good topical disinfectant, but in a cleanser its benefits would be washed down the drain before they could do the job. Besides, this should not get in the eyes and splashing the face makes that a potential risk.

☹ **Medicated Skin Cleanser 10% Benzoyl Peroxide & Tea Tree Oil** *($24 for 8.45 ounces)* is similar to the 5% version above and the same basic comments apply. This version does contain a tiny amount of tea tree oil, but not enough to work as an effective disinfectant for acne.

✓☺ **5% Benzoyl Peroxide Gel with Tea Tree Oil** *($18 for 2 ounces)* contains 5% benzoyl peroxide in a simple gel base and is a good topical disinfectant for blemishes. It also contains a teeny amount of tea tree oil, but not enough for it to work as an effective disinfectant.

☹ **10% Benzoyl Peroxide and 3% Sulfur** *($19 for 2 ounces)*. The 10% benzoyl peroxide in this product is effective as a disinfectant, but the sulfur, despite its disinfecting properties, is too irritating and alkaline for skin.

☹ **Infusia Blemish Patches** *($19.99 for 48 large round patches and two 0.5-ounce bottles of Activator Mist)*. The patches are coated with a mixture of 1.5% salicylic acid, film-forming agent (a hairspray-like ingredient to stick the patches to skin when they are sprayed with the Activator Mist), and a teeny amount of antioxidants and water-binding agents. There is also an array of plant extracts that are a mix of irritants and anti-irritants. The Activator Mist is little more than water with a tiny amount of antioxidants and a minute additional amount of salicylic acid. Salicylic acid is a good exfoliant, but there is no benefit to applying it to skin via this method, and the hairspray ingredient can be a problem for skin.

☺ **$$$ Fade Cream SPF 30** *($27.50 for 1.67 ounces)* contains almost too small an amount of avobenzone (for UVA protection) to be all that effective as a sunscreen, but it does contain 2% hydroquinone, which is effective for inhibiting melanin production. It also includes some good antioxidants.

☺ **$$$ Fade Gel 4** *($45 for 1 ounce)* contains an interesting mix of 2% hydroquinone and 2% kojic acid, both of which can inhibit melanin production. It also contains 10% glycolic acid and 2% salicylic acid, which help exfoliate skin. Unfortunately, this is all in an alcohol base, and that isn't the best for any skin type, although for skin lightening it is an option.

☺ **$$$ Holistic Skin Lightener** *($39 for 2 ounces)* contains minuscule amounts of alternative herbal skin-lightening agents, including mulberry and bearberry extracts, as well as a teeny amount of kojic acid, but not enough of them to affect melanin production. It does contain about 10% glycolic acid, but the pH is too high for this to be effective for exfoliation.

✓☺ $$$ **Intensive Holistic Lightener** *($45 for 1 ounce)* contains some convincing amounts of alternative melanin-inhibiting ingredients, including arbutin, bearberry extract, and a teeny amount of kojic acid. It also has a good assortment of antioxidants, which are overall beneficial for skin. As an alternative to hydroquinone, this is an option to consider.

☹ $$$ **Surface Peel Creme** *($25 for 2 ounces)* is just wax and plastic scrub particles (polyethylene) that you rub over skin. It does help exfoliate skin, although this type of mechanical exfoliant formula is really best for knees, elbows, and lips, but not the face.

☹ $$$ **Glossy Lip Therapy SPF 15** *($15 for 0.25 ounce)* is a very good emollient lip balm that contains an in-part avobenzone-based sunscreen. The peppermint in it, however, can cause some irritation to lips.

☹ **Stress Relief Eye Pads** *($15 for 12 pads)*. Balm mint is listed as the second ingredient. Although that may feel temporarily soothing, in the long run it can be irritating for skin.

DOVE (SKIN CARE ONLY)

For more information about Dove, call (800) 451-6679 or visit www.dovespa.com.

☺ **Beauty Bar, Nutrium** *($3.29 for two 4.75-ounce bars)* is a standard, tallow-based bar cleanser with detergent cleansing agents and a small amount of plant oil. It is milder than typical "soap," but it can still be drying for skin, and tallow is not great for blemish-prone skin. It does contain fragrance and coloring agents.

☺ **Beauty Bar, Pink** *($2.45 for two 4.75-ounce bars)* is almost identical to the Beauty Bar, Nutrium above only minus the plant oil, and the same basic comments apply.

☺ **Beauty Bar, Sensitive** *(2.45 for two 4.75-ounce bars)* is identical to the Beauty Bar, Pink above, and the same comments apply. It doesn't contain coloring agents, but it does contain fragrance. There is nothing about this bar cleanser that makes it better for sensitive skin.

☺ **Beauty Bar, Unscented** *(2.45 for two 4.75-ounce bars)* is unscented, but not fragrance free! It is basically identical to the Beauty Bar, Sensitive above and the same comments apply.

☺ **Beauty Bar, White** *($2.45 for two 4.75-ounce bars)* is virtually identical to the Beauty Bar, Sensitive above and the same comments apply.

☺ **Daily Hydrating Cleansing Cloths, Sensitive Skin** *($6.99 for 30 cloths)* contains mostly standard detergent cleansing agents soaked on to some fairly soft cloths. It will remove makeup. This also contains a teeny amount of vitamins and anti-irritants, though it also contains fragrance, which isn't the best for sensitive skin (or any skin type for that matter). It isn't hydrating, but it is an option for removing makeup.

☺ **Daily Hydrating Cleansing Cloths, Regular** *($6.99 for 30 cloths)* is similar to the Hydrating Cleansing Cloths, Sensitive Skin above and the same comments apply. This version does contain a teeny amount of water-binding agents, but that doesn't make it hydrating in the least.

DR. DENNIS GROSS, M.D. SKIN CARE

Dr. Dennis Gross is another dermatologist with a skin-care line. He specializes in corrective cosmetic procedures and his line is meant to be an adjunct to the services he provides in his office. The claim that his products use "state-of-the-art technology" is greatly exaggerated. When it comes to state-of-the-art antioxidants, water-binding agents, and anti-irritants, all of the Gross products come up short. Dozens and dozens of lines in all price ranges have better options for up-to-date formulations than this one. And one of the sunscreens is only an SPF 10, rather shocking given Gross's status as a dermatologist.

Several of the products in this line contain emu oil. While there is research showing it to be a good emollient that can help heal skin, it is not different from the same benefit other plant oils offer, from grape to olive or even mineral oil for that matter (Source: *Australasian Journal of Dermatology*, August 1996, pages 159–161). All in all, there is nothing outstanding or even particularly interesting about this small line of products and it is best overlooked in favor of better options. For more information about Dr. Dennis Gross, M.D. Skin Care, call (888) 830-SKIN or visit www.mdskincare.com.

☹ $$$ **Dr. Dennis Gross M.D. Skin Care Alpha-Beta Peel** *($65 for 30 Peel Pads and 30 Neutralizing Pads)* is an at-home peel that won't do much peeling, which is a good thing for your skin because you would not want to do serious skin exfoliation on a regular basis or accidentally leave it on for too long; you wouldn't have much skin left. The 2% salicylic acid content and the alpha hydroxy acid content of the Peel Pads are good, but the product's pH of 4 makes this no better than a number of less expensive products from Neutrogena or Alpha Hydrox. There is no reason to go through this procedure and expense for what ends up being a standard AHA/BHA product. What is actually more problematic is the Neutralizing System. This silicone-based toner has a pH of 9! That is incredibly alkaline, and there is a good deal of research showing that to be a significant problem for skin.

☺ $$$ **All-in-One Facial Cleanser with Toner** *($25 for 8 ounces)* is a very good detergent-based cleanser that would be an option for someone with normal to oily skin. The teeny amount of emu oil provides no emollient benefit for skin.

☹ $$$ **Antiaging Vitamin-C Gel** *($45 for 1 ounce)* is a silicone-based moisturizer that also contains a teeny amount of salicylic acid, although the pH is too high for it to be effective as an exfoliant. There is no research showing that vitamin C of any kind can prevent skin from aging, even if it is a good antioxidant (among many other good antioxidants). What this lacks are any state-of-the-art water-binding agents or effective anti-irritants.

☹ **Auto Balancing Moisture with Sunscreen SPF 10** *($30 for 2 ounces)*. A dermatologist selling a sunscreen with an SPF 10! What will we see next, oncologists selling cigarettes? This sunscreen does contain avobenzone, but the gold standard for sunscreens today is SPF 15 (Source: American Academy of Dermatology, http://www.aad.org).

☺ **$$$ Firming Eye Gel with Vitamin-C** *($30 for 1 ounce)* is an OK emollient moisturizer for normal to dry skin that contains a small amount of vitamins E and C and a teeny amount of water-binding agents.

☺ **$$$ Lift & Lighten Eye Cream** *($28 for 0.5 ounce)* is an OK, basic, emollient moisturizer for normal to dry skin, but there is nothing in it that will lift skin. The teeny amount of kojic acid won't have much effect on skin discoloration, and the vitamin K has no independent research showing it to be effective for reducing the appearance of spider veins. It also contains salicylic and lactic acids, but the small amounts (less than 1%) and the pH (too high) make them ineffective for exfoliation.

☺ **$$$ Maximum Moisture Treatment** *($34 for 1 ounce)* is an OK emollient moisturizer with small amounts of vitamins E, C, and A and a water-binding agent.

☺ **Waterproof Sunscreen SPF 15** *($28 for 7 ounces)* is a very good, in-part avobenzone-based sunscreen in a lightweight silicone base. However, there is nothing in it that makes it preferable to other avobenzone-based sunscreens available at drugstores for less than half the price.

☺ **Waterproof Sunscreen SPF 30** *($28 for 7 ounces)* is similar to the Sunscreen SPF 15 above and the same comments apply.

☺ **$$$ All-in-One Tinted Moisturizer SPF 15** *($32)* is a very good, lightweight, tinted moisturizer with an in-part avobenzone-based sunscreen. This elegant, silky formula has a moist but nongreasy, sheer-coverage finish that those with normal to dry skin will appreciate. The three shades are fine and can work for all but very light or very dark skin tones.

DR. HAUSCHKA

Dr. Rudolf Hauschka is no longer around, although the cosmetics company bearing his name definitely is. Sold primarily at health food stores, the products are a standout for their high prices alone. A cleansing cream at $18 for less than 2 ounces is literally one of the most expensive around.

If plants are your thing, these formulations, according to the ingredient lists, are some of the most "pure" (although not 100% because some still contain animal-derived ingredients, as well as Vaseline). However, the products don't appear to contain what is listed on the labels because the consistency of the formulations indicates other ingredients must be present. Also, the ingredient list does not comply with FDA regulations so it is difficult to know exactly what you would be putting on your skin.

What about the effectiveness of the products in this line? These products are loaded with fragrant oils and plant extracts that have the potential for a good deal of irritation on

The Reviews D

skin. However, there are also plenty of benign nut and vegetable oils that can be quite good for dry skin. While they can be beneficial, current research demonstrates that they aren't enough. Given what is now known about the need for antioxidants and water-binding agents, this line comes up astoundingly short on both fronts.

I am also skeptical about the disclosure of the ingredients in the products because preservatives are not listed on the label. If that is truly the case, the risk of contamination after just a couple of weeks of use is fairly significant, especially considering all the plant extracts these contain. The company insists that the ingredient lists are accurate; if its claim is true, I'd be concerned about keeping the products around for more than two weeks after opening.

Another problem with Hauschka products is that the ingredients are essentially identical product to product to product, with very few exceptions. What makes that strange are the widely varying claims, which range from getting rid of acne to firming skin—all from the same ingredients. Much of the information the company espouses about its ingredients defies published research (even from alternative medical sources), but will those faithful to the image of "natural" be likely to care? For more information about Dr. Hauschka, call (800) 247-9907 or visit www.drhauschka.com.

DR. HAUSCHKA SKIN CARE

☺ $$$ **Cleansing Cream** *($18 for 1.7 ounces)*. This cream would be a good scrub. It contains almond meal, and would work for someone with normal to dry skin.

☹ **Cleansing Milk** *($26 for 4.9 ounces)*. The alcohol in this product (the second ingredient) makes it inappropriate for most skin types. For "a gentle cleanser," that much alcohol just doesn't make sense.

☹ **Facial Toner for Normal to Dry, Sensitive Skin** *($27 for 3.4 ounces)* contains mostly water, alcohol, and witch hazel, and is an irritation waiting to happen.

☹ **Clarifying Toner for Oily, Impure Skin** *($27 for 3.4 ounces)* has similar ingredients to the Facial Toner above and the same comments apply.

☺ $$$ **Eye Contour Day Cream for All Skin Conditions** *($28.50 for 0.34 ounce)* is an OK emollient moisturizer with some good plant oils, but it lacks water-binding agents and antioxidants, and that makes it less than stellar for any skin condition.

☹ **Eye Solace** *($21 for 1.7 ounces)* contains too much alcohol to be used around the eye area, plus it lacks water-binding agents and antioxidants, making this a completely outdated formulation.

☺ $$$ **Moisturizing Day Cream** *($42.50 for 3.4 ounces)*. Without sunscreen, this moisturizer is absolutely not recommended for daytime. The alcohol and witch hazel are a problem in a moisturizer, although the plant oils could make up for that. But without antioxidants and water-binding agents, it is just ho-hum and lacks any state-of-the-art benefits for skin.

☺ **Normalizing Day Oil for Oily, Troubled Skin** *($27 for 1 ounce)* contains mostly water, plant oils, plant extract, and fragrance. The oils found in a kitchen cabinet (almond, wheat germ, peanut, and jojoba) are just as good for dry skin. What is strange is that this product is recommended "for oily, impure skins . . . [to] remove signs of blemishes and large pores." I can't imagine anything less helpful for oily skin or blemishes than more oil.

☺ **Quince Day Cream** *($21.50 for 1 ounce)*. Without sunscreen, this moisturizer is absolutely not recommended for daytime. This is an OK emollient moisturizer for dry skin, but it lacks antioxidants and water-binding agents. The quince seed has skin-constricting properties, which makes it a potential skin irritant, but there is only a tiny amount of it in here so it probably has little to no impact on skin.

☹ **Rhythmic Night Conditioner for All Skin Conditions** *($22.95 for 10 0.34-ounce ampoules)* contains mostly water, rose oil, witch hazel, royal jelly, and silver. Silver can be a skin irritant with long-term use, as can the rose oil and witch hazel. As for the royal jelly, it keeps showing up in products, even though the claims for this ingredient have never been substantiated.

☹ **Rhythmic Conditioner for Sensitive Skin** *($26 for ten 0.34-ounce ampoules)* is mostly fragrance with some plant extracts that are a mix of anti-irritants and irritants. Fragrance is a serious problem for sensitive skin and given the concentration of it in this product, this is more like putting expensive cologne on your face. What this lacks overall to provide any real skin care are any antioxidants and water-binding agents.

☺ **Rose Day Cream for Dry, Sensitive Skin** *($26 for 1 ounce)* doesn't contain sunscreen, so it should not be used during the day. It is an OK emollient moisturizer but that's it. There are no antioxidants, and there's only a teeny amount of one water-binding agent, making this an extremely ho-hum formulation.

☺ **$$$ Toned Day Cream for Normal, Dry, Sensitive Skin** *($27 for 1 ounce)* is a very standard moisturizer for dry skin.

☺ **After Sun Lotion** *($16.50 for 3.4 ounces)* is an OK moisturizer for dry skin, though the amount of alcohol in it can be problematic for some skin types.

☺ **Sunscreen Lotion SPF 15** *($18.50 for 3.4 ounces)* is a very good, titanium dioxide–based sunscreen that would be good for someone with dry skin. It can leave a white cast on the skin.

☺ **Sunscreen Lotion SPF 20** *($21 for 3.4 ounces)* is similar to the Lotion above except that this one has a higher SPF.

☺ **Sunscreen Cream for Children SPF 22** *($21.95 for 3.4 ounces)* doesn't contain anything different to make it better for children, but it is a good titanium dioxide–based sunscreen and the plant oils make it good for dry skin.

☹ **Sunscreen Lotion SPF 8** *($21.95 for 3.4 ounces)* has too low an SPF to be recommended. The company is honest about this product allowing tanning to happen, it just forgot to mention how detrimental that is for skin.

☺ **$$$ Water Resistant Sun-Block Stick SPF 30** *($11 for 0.17 ounce)* doesn't list any active ingredients, so it cannot be relied on for sun protection.

☹ **Translucent Bronze Concentrate** *($27.95 for 1 ounce)* is supposed to soften the appearance of small red blood vessels, but with alcohol as the third ingredient, I strongly doubt that claim because alcohol can cause surface capillaries to look worse. It's expensive for a rather unimpressive tinted moisturizer.

☺ **$$$ Cleansing Clay Mask** *($27.95 for 3.06 ounces)* is a standard clay mask that has some benefit for absorbing oil.

☺ **$$$ Moisturizing Mask** *($38 for 1.1 ounces)* contains mostly water, plant extract, plant oils, glycerin, Vaseline, lanolin, thickeners, water-binding agent, and fragrance. It is a decent moisturizer for dry skin.

☺ **$$$ Rejuvenating Mask** *($34.50 for 1 ounce)* is similar to most of the moisturizers in this line, and contains mostly water, plant extracts, alcohol, glycerin, plant oils, and thickeners. It is an option for dry skin.

☺ **$$$ Firming Mask** *($34.50 for 1 ounce)* contains nothing that can firm skin, but it is an emollient moisturizer that can be good for dry skin. Too bad it still lacks any significant antioxidants or water-binding agents, which could have made it great.

☹ **Facial Steam Bath** *($26.50 for 3.4 ounces)* is supposed to be used with steam heat. That's not recommended, because repeated use of steam heat can cause surfacing of capillaries, increase the severity of rosacea, and damage skin. As much as I love soaking in a Jacuzzi, I don't fool myself into thinking it's helping my skin.

☺ **$$$ Lip Balm** *($10 for 0.15 ounce)* is a good, basic emollient balm for dry lips.

☺ **$$$ Lip Care Stick** *($7.50 for 0.16 ounce)* is similar to the Lip Balm above except in stick form.

Dr. Hauschka Makeup

In line with the same transcendental vibe as the skin-care line, Dr. Hauschka's makeup is a small collection of products that asks you to "compose and conduct the symphony within you—colorfully, beautifully, and uniquely." Termed Decorative Cosmetics, the makeup line purports to "work in harmony with the true nature of your skin, fine-tuning those thoughts and feelings that are reflected in your face." If I were wearing Dr. Hauschka makeup right now, I wonder if it would tune into the fact that I am simultaneously perplexed and amused by this statement. Although it is true that makeup can enhance facial expression by defining the features, there is no way any cosmetic can somehow sense and aid in the communication of facial emotions and movement. That's about as ridiculous as the notion that exercising facial muscles will prevent skin from sagging. There isn't much reason to give this makeup more than a passing glance, as the products are downright ordinary to inadequate, and the prices should snap even the most meditative soul back to reality.

☺ **$$$ <u>FOUNDATION</u>: Translucent Make-up** *($25.50)* has a smooth, creamy texture that feels quite light on the skin and blends very well to a natural, sheer coverage finish. What's problematic are the overpowering fragrance and the fact that only one shade (Intrada) looks like skin. The other two shades are too rosy peach for most skin tones.

☹ <u>CONCEALER:</u> **Cover Stick** *($12.50)* has an awful, thick texture, heavy application, and two of the worst colors you're likely to encounter while shopping for concealers.

☺ $$$ <u>POWDER:</u> **Translucent Face Powder, Loose** *($25.50)* is a talc-free sheer powder that has a soft, but overly dry, texture that can feel grainy. This is the first powder I have seen that uses tapioca starch in place of talc, and the texture difference is telling. Only one shade is available, and it is fine for fair to light skin. **Translucent Face Powder, Compact** *($23.50)* is talc-based and has a smoother, softer texture and application than the Loose Powder above. Again, there is only one color, and it is suitable for fair to light skin.

☺ $$$ <u>BLUSH:</u> **Rouge Powder** *($23.50)* claims to contain nourishing ingredients to balance the skin, but is just a soft, sheer, matte-finish blush that comes in three warm-toned colors. If you believe the all-natural rhetoric, you'll likely not mind paying top dollar for standard powder blush.

☹ <u>EYESHADOW:</u> **Eyeshadow Duo** *($25.50)* features five duos, all of which are shiny and have a fairly soft texture, but a dry, grainy finish and sheer application. Even fans of shiny eyeshadow would balk at this underachieving formula, especially at this price.

☺ <u>EYE AND BROW SHAPER:</u> **Kajal Eyeliner** *($14.50)* is a standard eye pencil that has a soft texture and smooth application. This has a drier finish, so smudging and smearing should be minimal. Avoid Espressivo (blue) and Grazioso (green) if you're going for an elegant, understated look. By the way, I have no idea why this German-bred line has chosen Italian names for all of its colors!

☺ $$$ <u>LIPSTICK AND LIP PENCIL:</u> Dr. Hauschka's **Lipstick** *($21.50)* has a smooth, creamy, rose-scented texture and a pleasant range of 12 semi-transparent colors. It's fine as far as creamy lipsticks go, but numerous less expensive options are available at the drugstore. **Lipliner** *($14.50)* is routine fare. This needs-sharpening pencil has a soft, but not too creamy, texture and a soft, dry finish to help keep lipstick in place.

☹ <u>MASCARA:</u> The **Mascara** *($19.95)* lengthens nicely without clumping, but it also breaks down easily and flakes, making this a must to avoid.

☺ $$$ <u>BRUSHES:</u> Both the **Face Powder Brush** *($56.50)* and the **Blush Brush** *($38.95)* are nicely shaped and dense enough for a controlled application of powder. They're not quite as elegant or versatile as the brushes from M.A.C. or Shu Uemura, but if these appeal to you, they do perform nicely.

DR. JEANNETTE GRAF, M.D. (SKIN CARE ONLY)

According to the mini-brochure that accompanies these skin-care products, "Fighting aging is the mission of Dr. Jeannette Graf. Her particular focus is in the area of cosmetic dermatology, where her strong clinical background in research, development, and product formulation has led to her being recognized as a leading American skin care expert." One point they left out of her background is that Graf is listed as an advisory board member for the NuSkin line of skin-care products. Graf appears to be open-minded about what products you use.

Dr. Graf's forte in the field of science was in connective tissue (ligaments and tendons) and peptide chemistry. Peptides are any group of organic compounds derived from two or more amino acids linked by peptide bonds, and they are found in all living tissues. As far as the topical effects of using peptides on skin are concerned, they are hardly the fountain of youth, although they are good water-binding agents, just like all amino acids and proteins. Put that all together, and you'll notice that the hooks in this line are Graf's Vita-Peptide complex, along with yeast, minerals, copper, and retinol. Vita-Peptide supposedly enhances the penetration of ingredients into the skin, although only two of Graf's products contains it. The glycopolypeptide ends up being just a very good water-binding agent for skin. In terms of helping ingredients penetrate into the skin, lots of standard ingredients that show up in hundreds of products can do that very well, from glycerin to propylene glycol, so Graf's clinical claims end up being more marketing hype than help for skin. The yeast and minerals can be good water-binding agents, too, but they are not unique to this line. Retinol is readily available in products from drugstore lines for far less, and copper, which can be effective for wound healing, is also available at the drugstore in Neutrogena's Active Copper products.

The Graf product lineup does present some worthwhile options, although the assortment of mostly well-formulated moisturizers dressed up as specialty treatment products really starts to get repetitive, with the major distinctions between the various formulas boiling down to texture differences, such as serums versus creams or lotions. All the claims for these products focus on baby-boomer buzzword favorites, such as "firms the skin," "reduces the appearance of wrinkles," and "addresses the visible signs of aging."

Graf's line falls short in several areas. The first is the lack of products for breakouts (because even those fighting aging can struggle with that problem). It also lacks an effective sunscreen. Finally, the cleansers aren't the best and there are no skin-lightening products, so you'll need to look elsewhere for those basic "antiaging" skin-care staples. Thankfully, Graf left the fragrance and coloring agents out of most of her products. For more information about Jeannette Graf, M.D., call Home Shopping Network at (800) 284-3100 or visit www.hsn.com. **Note:** The prices below reflect advertised prices on the Home Shopping Network as this book goes to press. The actual retail prices for Jeannette Graf products are typically 30 to 50 percent higher.

☹ **Protein Action Cleanser** *($18.50 for 7 ounces)*. This otherwise gentle, water-soluble cleanser is flawed by the inclusion of potent skin and eye irritants like cinnamon and eucalyptus oil. This cleanser is not recommended.

☺ $$$ **Retinol Facial Cleanser** *($17.50 for 4 ounces)* is an extremely standard, lotion-style cleanser that would be an option for normal to dry skin—but don't expect this one to rinse easily from the skin. The tiny amount of rosemary extract in this cleanser should not be a problem for irritation. However, the minute amount of retinol would be wiped away during the cleansing process, so even if it could make a difference it wouldn't have the chance.

☹ $$$ **Copper Collagen Infusion** (*$24.50 for 4 ounces*) is a thick, glycerin-based gel moisturizer that contains an interesting assortment of water-binding agents and antioxidants, including sea salt. The sea salt can be a potential skin irritant and can increase skin sensitivity to UVB radiation (Source: *Der Hautarzt*, June 1998, pages 482–486). Copper can have an impact on wound healing, but wrinkles aren't wounds, and there is no published research establishing copper as being effective for wrinkles. The notion that it may be effective for wrinkles or for any amount of skin firming is strictly theory. If you are interested in copper, keep in mind that Neutrogena has a line of copper products that you can try, and they omit the salt that this product contains.

☺ **Deep Wrinkle Treatment Gel** (*$24.50 for 2 ounces*) claims it helps to reduce the appearance of medium and deep wrinkles, but if your wrinkles are from the sun as opposed to just dry skin, you're in for a rude awakening. This strictly glycerin and silicone-based moisturizer can indeed make dry skin feel softer and smoother, but its effect on non-dry-skin-induced wrinkles is superficial, like that of any other moisturizer. Strangely, the array of interesting antioxidants and anti-irritants found in most of Graf's other moisturizers is absent here except for the pentapeptide-3, although there is no independent research showing that to be beneficial for skin.

☺ $$$ **Deep Wrinkle Eye Cream** (*$18.50 for 0.5 ounce*) is a rather standard emollient moisturizer that would work fine for someone with dry skin.

☺ **Moisture Release Treatment** (*$22.50 for 2 ounces*) is quite similar to the Deep Wrinkle Eye Cream above, only this one has a teeny amount of minerals and slightly more antioxidants, which makes it a somewhat more interesting moisturizer for normal to dry skin. There is no reason this cannot be used around the eye area. This does contain butyloctyl salicylate, a derivative of salicylic acid, but the pH of this moisturizer is too high for any exfoliation to occur. The teeny bit of ginseng present will most likely not cause irritation.

☺ **Moisturizing Face Cream** (*$22.50 for 2.25 ounces*) is strikingly similar to the Deep Wrinkle Treatment Gel above, yet this one avoids antiwrinkle claims and instead talks about transforming dry, adult skin back to its baby-soft texture. Your skin will assuredly feel soft after using this silicone-based moisturizer, but the effect, as with all moisturizers, is temporary. This is slightly richer than the Deep Wrinkle Treatment Gel, and would be best for dry to very dry skin.

☹ **Normalizing Face Lotion** (*$22.50 for 2 ounces*) is a standard moisturizer that is not as elegant as some of the other moisturizers in this line. The milk protein is neither unique nor particularly helpful for skin, even as a water-binding agent, because it is present in such a minute quantity.

✓☺ **Overnight Recovery Treatment** (*$24.50 for 2 ounces*) is almost identical to the Deep Wrinkle Eye Cream above, save for the addition of a longer list of antioxidants as well as a broader assortment of water-binding agents. For these reasons, it is preferred to and a better value than the Eye Cream. This does contain ginseng extract, but the amount is too small to be a problem for most skin types.

☺ **Retinol Moisture Barrier Face Cream** (*$21.50 for 1.1 ounces*) is a very ho-hum moisturizer that contains a tiny amount of retinol, about the same as every other retinol product on the market, from Cetaphil to L'Oreal, Lancome, Estee Lauder, and just about everyone else. It is packaged in a container that will help keep the retinol stable, but there is no reason to consider this basic formulation over the ones from Cetaphil or L'Oreal for half the price.

☹ **Retinol Rejuvenator Facial Serum** (*$24.50 for 1 ounce*) is a lightweight, silicone-based fluid that features retinol, but the retinol is listed after the rosemary leaf extract, which is a considerable skin irritant when present in this amount.

✓☺ **Skin Energizing Booster AM/PM** (*$24.50 for 1 ounce*) is one of the more elegant formulas in Graf's line, and is one of two that contains polypeptide. This is a lightweight serum that would work well for normal to slightly dry skin.

☹ **Facial Sunscreen Lotion SPF 15** (*$19.50 for 1.7 ounces*) does not contain the UVA-protecting ingredients of avobenzone, titanium dioxide, or zinc oxide, and is not recommended. And this is supposed to be an antiaging line from a physician?

☹ **Psor-Ease Lotion** (*$19.95 for 3 ounces*) is a 2% salicylic acid lotion that has a pH of 4.5, which makes it minimally effective as an exfoliant (Source: *Cosmetic Dermatology*, July 1998, pages 27–29). This is supposed to be helpful for psoriasis to "help reduce the itching, irritation, flaking, and scaling" that are often the bane of a psoriasis sufferer's existence. Salicylic acid can be effective at reducing the thick scaling of psoriatic skin, but it does little to prevent or ease the severe itching. If you have psoriasis and want to test out a 2% salicylic acid product, there are other products to consider, especially if you are looking for reliable exfoliants that are less expensive and that have a lower pH, which will make the exfoliant more effective.

☹ **Brightening Peel** (*$24.50 for 2 ounces*) is an extremely thick, emollient product that is designed as a gentle foaming peel, but it leaves much to be desired on all counts. For one thing, it uses willow bark extract as the main exfoliant, which is not the same as salicylic acid and does not have the same exfoliating or peeling properties. Salicylic acid does show up toward the end of the ingredient list, but the product's overall pH of 5 makes this minimally to not at all effective for exfoliating skin. It also contains sugarcane and sugar maple extracts, but these distantly related AHA knockoffs won't exfoliate skin either. To top it all off, this contains detergent cleansing agents and citrus extracts that can be irritating if left on the skin for five minutes (as the directions indicate) and the petrolatum (Vaseline) base not only makes it difficult to rinse off but also tends to leave a greasy film on the skin.

☺ **Calm Down Anti-Itch Cream** (*$24.50 for 2 ounces*) is a completely standard, but effective, 0.5% hydrocortisone cream that is easily replaced by significantly less expensive options at the drugstore, such as Lanacort or Cortaid. Please keep in mind that repeated long-term use of any topical cortisone can cause the skin to thin and become more fragile.

☺ **Soothe & Hide** *($24.5 for 1.6 ounces)* is just a tinted average moisturizer that has minimal coverage. The oatmeal is a good anti-irritant, but that doesn't add up to a great moisturizer overall.

DR. LeWINN'S PRIVATE FORMULA
(AUSTRALIA AND UNITED KINGDOM ONLY)

In Australia the hype behind this line has reached almost mythic proportions. The products come with a medical ambience thanks to the claims of being formulated by a distinguished "Plastic Surgeon to the Stars," Dr. Laurence LeWinn, although he is no longer around to add any insight to his products. Considering the hype of the cosmetics industry overall, whether or not he ever was a Hollywood plastic surgeon is anyone's guess. Mentioning to almost any Australian that Americans have never heard of these products or a plastic surgeon named LeWinn brings stares of amazement!

As you would expect, all the attention is based on claims ranging from wrinkle elimination to protecting skin from environmental abuses. Yet this line contains no sunscreen and not one original or unique formulation. What the consumer is left with is a great deal of cosmetic drama with Beverly Hills prices.

If there is extensive research behind these products, as claimed, it is hard to tell what kind of research it was. Retinyl palmitate is the showcase ingredient in several products, backed by claims that it's similar to tretinoin, the active ingredient in Renova and Retin-A. However, retinyl palmitate is as far removed from tretinoin as a tree is from paper. Several of the products also contain skin irritants. An ingredient the company calls "Actifirm" is simply a combination of echinacea and hydrocotyl extracts, and though both have good antibacterial and anti-irritant potential for skin, neither has any firming action on skin. Overall there ends up being little substance behind the hype and you would be far better off with a real plastic surgeon or simply better formulated, less expensive products. For more information about Dr. LeWinn's Private Formula, visit www.privateformula.com.au. **Note:** All prices listed are in Australian dollars.

☺ **$$$ Creamy Facial Cleanser** *($32.50 for 178 ml)* is just plant oils, a minuscule amount of vitamin A, thickeners, and fragrance. Your face and budget would do just as well using plain almond oil or apricot oil to wipe off your makeup.

☹ **Derma-Wash Facial Cleanser** *($32.50 for 178 ml)* contains sodium lauryl sulfate as the detergent cleansing agent, which is potentially too irritating and drying for all skin types.

☺ **$$$ Mega-C Facial Polishing Gel** *($39.50 for 178 ml)* is a decent, though ordinary, topical exfoliant that uses jojoba beads (a waxy, hard extract from the jojoba plant) as the scrub. It is an option for normal to dry skin.

The Reviews D

☹ **Derma-Tone Mild Astringent** *($32.50 for 178 ml)* contains alcohol as a significant part of the formula, making it hardly mild and too drying and irritating for all skin types.

☹ **Nutri-Zone Skin Freshener** *($32.50 for 178 ml)*. With lemon as the third ingredient this may feel temporarily refreshing, but it ends up being more irritating and drying if used day after day.

☹ **Fruits of Youth AHA Concentrate** *($69.50 for 50 ml)* doesn't contain any AHAs. This includes sugarcane, orange, sugar maple, and lemon, which are intended to sound like AHAs, but they have no exfoliating properties, plus the lemon and orange can be skin irritants.

☺ **$$$ A+ Revita-Cell** *($49.50 for 56 grams)* is a decent, plant oil–based moisturizer, but for the money it lacks any interesting or significant water-binding agents or antioxidants (the teeny amount of vitamin A and vitamin E is barely detectable).

✓☺ **$$$ Advanced Night Cream** *($54.50 for 56 grams)* is a very good emollient moisturizer for dry skin that contains a good assortment of antioxidants and water-binding agents.

☹ **Day Cream Moisturiser** *($64 for 113 grams)* makes claims about protecting from the sun, but has no SPF number and, therefore, should not be used for sun protection. It is a decent emollient moisturizer, but wearing it during the day is a serious risk to your skin.

☺ **$$$ Firming Eye Cream** *($44.50 for 28 grams)* is an OK moisturizer for normal to dry skin. The collagen and elastin in this cream have no ability to firm skin in the least, although they are good water-binding agents. The teeny amounts of vitamins (antioxidants) are barely detectable.

☺ **$$$ Mega-B Super-Boost Hydrator** *($75 for 30 ml)*. This is just water, water-binding agent, and vitamin B5. Vitamin B5 has good hydration benefit for skin, but so do lots of other ingredients, and it doesn't have to cost this much to gain that benefit. What this product lacks are antioxidants—now that would have really given the skin a boost.

☺ **$$$ Mega-C Bio-Deliverant Serum** *($95 for 30 ml)* is a good lightweight lotion that contains antioxidants, water-binding agents, and anti-irritants. The price is bizarre for what you get, but overall it is a well-formulated product.

☺ **$$$ Mega-C Cell-Structure Cream** *($125 for 60 ml)* is similar to the Mega-C Bio-Deliverant Serum above, only this version contains L-tyrosine. Tyrosine can theoretically stimulate melanin production, but for someone with skin discolorations that is not necessarily a good thing. The type of packaging used for this product means that the vitamin C won't remain stable.

☹ **Mega Moist Oil-Free Moisture Cream** *($69.50 for 56 grams)* contains some good antioxidants and water-binding agents, but the showcase ingredients, retinol and L-ascorbic acid, will not remain stable because the product comes in a jar container that allows them to be easily exposed to air.

☹ **Tissue Firming Serum** *($54.50 for 30 ml)* lists arnica as the third ingredient and rosemary as the fourth, both bothersome skin irritants and a problem when used repeatedly.

☺ **Sunless Tanning Lotion** *($34.50 for 227 ml)* uses dihydroxyacetone to affect the color of skin, as is true for all self-tanners. This will work as well as any.

☺ **$$$ Mega-C Lip Plump** *($49.50 for 15 ml)* contains nothing that will plump lips, although it does contain vitamin C, some good water-binding agents, and antioxidants. It's a good moisturizer for normal to slightly dry skin but that's about it.

DR. MARY LUPO SKIN CARE SYSTEM
(SKIN CARE ONLY)

Dr. Lupo is a dermatologist with an impressive list of credentials who has created her own skin-care line. You'll find some interesting AHA products, but also a handful of overblown claims. Her sunscreens claim to have UVA protection, yet one clearly doesn't contain any UVA-protecting ingredients, and her Conditioning Cleanser contains sodium lauryl sulfate (SLS), which is known to be one of the most irritating detergent cleansing ingredients around. Surely as a dermatologist, Lupo should know about these issues? I always find it disappointing to see a line from a medical professional that ignores such fundamentals.

Still, some of Lupo's AHA products are good, particularly the lightweight ones. They're pricey for what you get, but they are well-formulated. For more information about Dr. Mary Lupo Skin Care System, call (800) 419-2002 or visit www.drmarylupo.com.

☹ **$$$ Conditioning Cleanser** *($22 for 6 ounces)* is an OK, standard, detergent-based, water-soluble cleanser, though one of the cleansing agents is sodium lauryl sulfate, which can be a skin irritant. There probably isn't much of it in here, but I am always concerned when I see ingredients like that listed in a product designated as "conditioning," and it is particularly disappointing in a line formulated by a dermatologist.

☺ **$$$ Gentle Purifying Cleanser** *($22 for 7 ounces)* is a fairly standard, detergent-based, water-soluble cleanser that is in many respects quite good for most skin types, except dry skin. It does contain fragrance.

☺ **AHA Renewal Gel I** *($25 for 3.5 ounces)* is a good 2.5% AHA gel containing lactic acid. However, the 2.5% concentration is at the low end of being able to exfoliate skin. Still, it contains no other irritants and is an option if you have sensitive skin.

☺ **AHA Renewal Gel II** *($25 for 3.5 ounces)* is similar to the Renewal Gel I above only with a 5% concentration of AHA. The same basic comments apply, though this version will be better for exfoliation.

☺ **AHA Renewal Lotion I** *($25 for 3.5 ounces)* is similar to the AHA Renewal Gel I above only in an ordinary lotion base. The same basic comments apply.

✔☺ **AHA Renewal Lotion II** *($25 for 3.5 ounces)* is similar to the Renewal Lotion I above only with a 5% concentration of AHA. The same basic review applies, though the higher concentration of AHA makes this far better for exfoliation,

☹ **Daily Age Management Moisturizer SPF 15** *($23 for 2 ounces)* does not contain avobenzone, titanium dioxide, or zinc oxide for UVA protection, and it is not recommended.

The Reviews D

☺ **Daily Age Management Oil Free Moisturizer SPF 15** *($23 for 2 ounces)* is a titanium dioxide–based sunscreen with a great SPF in a very standard lotion base that would be best for someone with normal to dry skin.

☺ **Full Spectrum Sunscreen UVA/UVB SPF 27** *($17.50 for 3 ounces)* is a good in-part avobenzone-based sunscreen that would work well for someone with normal to slightly dry skin. This very standard formulation holds no advantage over Neutrogena's avobenzone-based sunscreen at a fraction of the price.

☺ **$$$ Intensive Target Moisturizer** *($39.70 for 1 ounce)* is a very good, silicone-based moisturizer that also contains good amounts of vitamin E and vitamin C as well as a small amount of water-binding agent and other antioxidants. It is an option for someone with normal to dry skin.

☺ **$$$ Vivifying Serum C** *($39.95 for 1 ounce)* uses the stable version (magnesium ascorbyl palmitate) of vitamin C, so if you want vitamin C in a lightweight gel this one is definitely an option, although the addition of some interesting water-binding agents would have made this more than a one-note product. This also contains human leukocyte (white blood cell) extract. White blood cells are the colorless cells in blood that help protect the body from infection and disease. However, there is no research showing that applying white blood cells topically can have any effect on skin whatsoever.

DR. OBAGI NU-DERM (SEE OBAGI)

DR. PERRICONE (SEE N.V. PERRICONE, M.D.)

ELIZABETH ARDEN

Elizabeth Arden was a pioneer in the beauty industry. At the turn of the 20th century, Arden began her legacy when she opened her first salon, with the now familiar red door. Over the next several years she introduced new products and services to women unaccustomed to such choices, and almost single-handedly made it acceptable for modern women to wear makeup. And while Arden understood and met these beauty needs, she was also adept at self-promotion and packaging, helping to solidify the idea that what holds the product should be as beautiful as the woman who uses it. She was the front-runner in the cosmetics industry for quite some time, until another young go-getter by the name of Estee Lauder began her own empire—one that would eventually lead to the Elizabeth Arden line being almost an afterthought in the mind of many consumers.

Perhaps what's most intriguing today is Arden's scaled-back presence in upscale department stores and heavy expansion into the mass market. It is becoming increasingly common to see Arden's vast stable of fragrances (including the Halston and Elizabeth Taylor brands) carried in stores like Wal-Mart, Target, and Kohl's. This "mid-tier" positioning has been a financial boon to this struggling line. In fact, because of this refocused distribution, Arden's net losses were cut by half between 2001 and 2002 (Source: *The Rose Sheet*, June 10, 2002). Although Arden's facial and cosmetic products are still sold almost exclusively in department stores, I can't imagine that the whole line won't eventually show up in these mainstream stores, especially if the cash registers keep ringing.

When it comes to skin care, Arden's products are a strange mix of unique and some fairly standard formulations. A major improvement is that most of the sunscreen products contain UVA-protecting ingredients. What is impressive about the line is Arden's patented use of ceramides, which are a significant component of the skin's intercellular matrix and are at the forefront of what we now know to be significant options for dealing with skin. However, they aren't the only significant option. Many lines now use other versions of ceramides as well as a great many other just as impressive ingredients that are also components of the skin's intercellular matrix, ranging from phospholipids to hyaluronic acid. None of them will change a wrinkle, but they do help the skin behave and look better. For more information about Elizabeth Arden, call (212) 261-1000 or visit www.elizabetharden.com. **Note:** Arden skin-care products contain fragrance unless otherwise noted.

ELIZABETH ARDEN SKIN CARE

☺ **$$$ 2-in-1 Cleanser** *($15 for 5 ounces)* is a standard, detergent-based cleanser that is more drying (meaning alkaline) than most. It also contains some plant extracts that can be skin irritants.

☺ **$$$ Millennium Hydrating Cleanser** *($27 for 4.4 ounces)* is a mineral oil–based cleanser that also contains some detergent cleansing agents, which makes it an option for normal to dry skin.

☺ **$$$ Ceramide Purifying Cream Cleanser** *($21 for 4.2 ounces)* is similar to the Millennium cleanser above and the same comments apply.

☺ **Hydra-Gentle Cream Cleanser** *($15 for 5 ounces)* is a silicone-based, cold cream–style cleanser that is very basic, but still an option for dry skin.

☹ **Oil Control Refining Cleanser** *($15 for 6.8 ounces)* contains several problematic ingredients that can cause skin irritation, including sodium lauryl sulfate, lemon, and rosemary. None of that will help control oil in the least and no other ingredients in this standard, detergent-based cleanser can do so either.

☹ **Sensitive Skin Calming Foaming Cleanser** *($15 for 6.8 ounces)* lists the fifth ingredient as sodium lauryl sulfate, a detergent cleansing agent that is a significant skin irritant. It also contains lemon and orange oil, and altogether that makes this decidedly inappropriate for sensitive skin.

☺ **Visible Difference Deep Cleansing Lotion** *($15 for 6.8 ounces)* is a standard, detergent-based cleanser that can be more drying than most, which doesn't deep-clean, though it can be irritating.

☹ **Modern Skincare One Great Soap** *($15 for 5.3 ounces)* is a standard bar cleanser that can be fairly drying for most skin types.

☺ $$$ **All Gone Eye and Lip Make-up Remover** *($16 for 3.4 ounces)* is a standard, silicone-based wipe-off makeup remover that would work as well as any, and without leaving a greasy film on the skin. It doesn't contain fragrance, but it does contain coloring agents.

☺ **Smooth the Way Cleansing Scrub for Face and Body** *($16.50 for 6.8 ounces)* is a standard, detergent-based cleanser that uses plastic beads as the exfoliant. It is an option for normal to oily skin. It does contain a small amount of plant extracts that may be skin irritants, but probably not enough to have much impact on skin.

☹ **Ceramide Purifying Toner** *($21 for 6.7 ounces)*. Alcohol is the second ingredient and there are several potentially irritating plant extracts, which makes this toner one to avoid.

☺ **Hydra Splash Alcohol Free Toner** *($15 for 6.8 ounces)* is indeed alcohol-free and is an OK toner for most skin types. It contains some good water-binding agents.

☹ **Millennium Revitalizing Tonic** *($26 for 5 ounces)* contains alcohol as the third ingredient, as well as some menthol. That isn't revitalizing, but it is potentially irritating and drying.

☹ **Oil Control Clarifying Toner** *($15 for 6.8 ounces)*. Alcohol is the second ingredient, making this too drying and irritating for any skin type.

☹ **Refining Toner** *($15 for 6.8 ounces)* is similar to the Oil Control Clarifying Toner above and the same comments apply.

☺ **Sensitive Skin Calming Skin Toner** *($15 for 6.8 ounces)* is similar to the Hydra Splash Toner above and the same comments apply.

☺ $$$ **Bye Lines Anti-Wrinkle Serum** *($40 for 1 ounce)* contains coriander oil, which can be a skin irritant, rather high up on the ingredient list, and that's disappointing, because otherwise this is a rather elegant silicone serum with good water-binding agents and a small amount of antioxidants.

☺ $$$ **Ceramide Advanced Time Complex Capsules** *($59 for 60 capsules)*. Each capsule contains mostly silicones, plant oil, water-binding agents, and antioxidants. This is an expensive way to obtain what amounts to a good moisturizer for normal to dry skin, but it will feel nice on the skin.

☺ $$$ **Ceramide Defining Eye Brightener** *($42.50 for 0.5 ounce)* is a silicone-based moisturizer with a good amount of plant oils, water-binding agents, and antioxidants. The balm mint in it can be a skin irritant, not an eye brightener, but there probably isn't enough of it to have much impact on skin.

✓☺ $$$ **Ceramide Defining Skin Brightener** *($49.50 for 1.7 ounces)* is similar to the Eye Brightener version above only minus the balm mint.

☺ $$$ **Ceramide Eyes Time Complex Capsules** *($40 for 60 capsules)* isn't as impressive a formulation as the other Ceramide products and isn't worth the trouble.

✓☺ $$$ **Ceramide Firm Lift, Intensive Lotion for Face and Throat** *($46 for 1 ounce)* won't lift skin anywhere, but it is a good silicone-based moisturizer for normal to dry skin with some good water-binding agents and antioxidants.

✓☺ **$$$ Ceramide Night Intensive Repair Cream** *($46 for 1 ounce)* is similar to the Ceramide Firm Lift above and the same basic comments apply.

✓☺ **$$$ Ceramide Time Complex Moisture Cream** *($46 for 1.7 ounces)* is similar to the Ceramide Firm Lift above and the same basic comments apply.

☹ **Ceramide Time Complex Moisture Cream SPF 15** *($46 for 1.7 ounces)* does not contain the UVA-protecting ingredients of titanium dioxide, zinc oxide, or avobenzone, and is not recommended.

☹ **Ceramide Eye Wish SPF 10** *($40 for 0.5 ounce)*. My only wish for this product is that it was an SPF 15 with UVA-protecting ingredients of titanium dioxide, zinc oxide, or avobenzone. Without them, this is not recommended.

☺ **Eight Hour Cream** *($14 for 1.7 ounces)* is an ordinary emollient moisturizer for dry skin that contains mostly Vaseline (over 55%), lanolin, mineral oil, fragrance, salicylic acid, plant oil, and vitamin E. The teeny amount of salicylic acid is ineffective as an exfoliant.

☺ **$$$ Extreme Conditioning Cream SPF 15** *($35 for 1.7 ounces)* is a very good, in-part avobenzone-based sunscreen in a silicone-based moisturizer. It contains only small amounts of water-binding agents and antioxidants, but they are present and can be helpful for skin.

☺ **$$$ Eye Care Concentrate** *($31 for 0.5 ounce)* is a very standard moisturizer for dry skin that contains mostly water, mineral oil, silicone, thickeners, plant oils, and preservatives.

☹ **Good Morning Eye Treatment** *($21.50 for 0.33 ounce)* lists alcohol as its fourth ingredient, which makes it a poor treat for the eye area.

☺ **$$$ Good Morning Skin Serum** *($29.50 for 0.5 ounce)* is a silicone-based lotion that contains several plant extracts, some of which can have antioxidant properties for skin and some that can be skin irritants. The teeny amount of mulberry is not enough to inhibit melanin production. What this product lacks is a significant quantity of water-binding agents; that would have made this a far better way to say good morning for skin.

☺ **Good Night's Sleep Restoring Cream** *($35 for 1.7 ounces)* is an OK emollient moisturizer that contains a small amount of antioxidants and water-binding agents.

☺ **$$$ Let There Be Light Lotion SPF 15** *($25 for 1.7 ounces)* is a good, in-part titanium dioxide–based sunscreen in a silicone base that would work well for someone with normal to dry skin. It also contains some good antioxidants and water-binding agents along with a generous amount of shine (it contains mica rather high up on the ingredient list). Your skin would be better off if the beneficial ingredients were more prominent than the shine.

☹ **Matte Moisture Lotion** *($30 for 1.7 ounces)* lists alcohol as its second ingredient, and there are also several potentially irritating plant extracts. That is disappointing, because many of the other ingredients make for a very good, matte finish moisturizer for normal to combination skin.

The Reviews E

☺ $$$ **Millennium Day Renewal Emulsion** *($56 for 2.6 ounces)* is a very standard moisturizer that contains mostly water, plant oil, thickeners, lanolin, more thickeners, and preservatives. Your skin would benefit more if the formulation of this product was renewed.

☺ $$$ **Millennium Eye Renewal Creme** *($40.50 for 0.5 ounce)* is similar to the Millennium Day Renewal Emulsion above and the same comments apply.

☺ $$$ **Millennium Night Renewal Creme** *($84.50 for 1.7 ounces)* is similar to the Millennium Day Renewal Emulsion above and the same comments apply.

✓☺ $$$ **Millennium Energist Revitalizing Emulsion** *($60 for 1.7 ounces)* is a silicone-based, emollient moisturizer with a good blend of water-binding agents and antioxidants.

☹ **Modern Skin Care Daily Moisture SPF 15** *($30 for 1.7 ounces)* does not contain the UVA-protecting ingredients of titanium dioxide, zinc oxide, or avobenzone, and is not recommended.

☺ **Sensitive Skin Calming Moisture Lotion** *($30 for 1.7 ounces)* includes a generous amount of fragrant plant extracts, but that does not add up to being a good thing for sensitive skin. This is not as well-formulated as many other moisturizers in the Arden lineup for normal to dry skin.

☺ $$$ **Skin Illuminating Complex** *($45 for 1.7 ounces)* is an OK, silicone-based moisturizer with a small amount of water-binding agents and antioxidants. It is an option for normal to dry skin.

☺ $$$ **Velva Moisture Film** *($38.50 for 6.7 ounces)* is an exceptionally ordinary moisturizer for dry skin that contains water, thickeners, lanolin, and preservatives.

☺ **Visible Difference Perpetual Moisture** *($30 for 1.7 ounces)* will not provide any more moisture for skin than other Arden moisturizers. This is a just a very good, silicone-based moisturizer for normal to dry skin with a good blend of water-binding agents and antioxidants.

☺ $$$ **Visible Difference Refining Moisture Cream Complex** *($49 for 2.5 ounces)* is an average, though emollient, moisturizer for dry skin that contains minuscule amounts of antioxidants and water-binding agent.

☺ $$$ **Visible Whitening Pure Intensive Capsules** *($59 for 50 capsules).* The capsules contain mostly silicones, vitamin C, and plant extracts. Vitamin C and the mulberry extract both have some research showing they can inhibit melanin production, but this is not the most effective (or cost-effective) way to apply these two rather standard skin-lightening agents.

✓☺ $$$ **Visible Whitening Block SPF 20** *($42.50 for 1.7 ounces)* contains a very good, in-part avobenzone-based sunscreen along with a good amount of vitamin C, in a form that has been shown to have some effect in inhibiting melanin production. This two-in-one product is a great option because no skin-lightening product can work without an effective sunscreen. It also contains some good water-binding agents. All in all, this a far better option for skin and skin lightening than the Capsules above.

☺ **Daily Bronzer Self Tanning Boost for the Face** *($18.50 for 1.7 ounces)* is a standard self-tanner that uses dihydroxyacetone to affect the color of skin. It would work as well as any.

☺ **Modern Skin Care Oil Free Self Tanning Lotion for Face & Body** *($21 for 4.2 ounces)* is similar to the Daily Bronzer above and the same comments apply.

☺ **Quick Spray Oil-Free Spray Self Tanner** *($21 for 4.2 ounces).* Alcohol is listed as the first ingredient, which means that this standard self-tanner will dry more quickly than most, but it can also be drying for skin, and that will not make the tan look pretty. This is a trade-off between efficiency versus texture. And basically, because you don't apply self-tanner all the time, the alcohol is probably not a problem, especially if you moisturize well after the tanner has set.

☺ **Triple Protection Oil Free Sunblock SPF 15** *($18.50 for 4.2 ounces)* is a very good, in-part avobenzone-based sunscreen in a standard moisturizing base that would be an option for someone with normal to slightly dry or oily skin.

✓☺ **Triple Protection Face Block SPF 30** *($19.50 for 4.2 ounces)* is similar to the Oil Free Sunblock SPF 15 above and the same basic comments apply. This version is better formulated because it contains some good water-binding agents and antioxidants, and is preferred for all skin types.

☺ **Triple Protection Sunblock Spray SPF 15** *($18.50 for 4.2 ounces)* is similar to the Triple Protection Oil Free Sunblock SPF 15 above and the same comments apply.

☹ **Clear the Way Mask** *($15 for 3.4 ounces)* won't clear anything. It is just a standard, plastic, peel off–style mask that contains some absorbents. But it also contains peppermint and menthol, which are skin irritants, and that clearly isn't great for skin.

☹ **$$$ Deep Cleansing Mask** *($15 for 3.4 ounces)* is a standard clay mask with some token plant extracts thrown in that are a mix of anti-irritants and irritants. This is an option for someone with normal to oily skin, but it won't deep clean, it can only absorb some excess oil.

☹ **Hydrating Mask** *($15 for 3.4 ounces)* is an emollient mask that also contains an absorbent that absorbs moisture, which undoes hydration. This mask is a bit confused, but it may be an option for someone with normal to slightly dry or slightly oily skin.

☹ **Peel & Reveal Revitalizing Treatment** *($30 for 1.7 ounces)* lists alcohol as the second ingredient and plastic as the third. This peel-off mask is not the best way to exfoliate skin. Although peeling off the plastic will make skin feel temporarily smooth, the alcohol can cause irritation and dryness. None of that is revitalizing for skin, rather it's depressing.

☹ **$$$ Visible Difference Eight Hour Lip Protectant Stick** *($13 for 0.13 ounce)* is a good basic, emollient, clear lipstick that is mostly Vaseline, thickeners, and lanolin oil.

ELIZABETH ARDEN MAKEUP

Arden's makeup collection has seen few additions since it was last reviewed, save for some exquisite new foundations and an awesome concealer. If anything, quite a few products have been eliminated, from their innovative Lip Talkers and Semi-Matte Lipstick to their waterproof mascara. It seems that the focus of today's Elizabeth Arden makeup is foundations, and here the line does offer some superlative options, though none of them contain adequate UVA-protecting ingredients or high enough SPF protection. Yet the fact that the majority of the makeup has remained unchanged is hardly a detriment, but more a compliment, since several of the products are outstanding as is.

FOUNDATION: ☺ $$$ **Flawless Finish Skin Balancing Makeup** *($25)* is a natural matte finish makeup with a beautifully smooth, lightweight texture that blends easily and provides light to medium coverage. It is worth a try if you have normal to oily skin, though those with very oily skin will likely want a more solid matte finish. Among the 17 shades are some excellent options for very light skin tones, but darker skin tones are left with unattractive orange-toned colors. The following shades are too ash, orange, or pink for most skin tones: Buff, Honey, Fawn, Mocha II, Cappuccino, and Java (this one may work for some dark skin tones). **Flawless Finish Radiant Moisture Makeup SPF 8** *($25)* is an elegant, moisturizing foundation for those with normal to very dry skin. What a shame the sunscreen lacks adequate UVA protection and is woefully low. This wonderfully creamy makeup provides light to medium coverage and a natural, dewy finish, just be sure to pair it with an effective sunscreen. The 17 shades include plenty of neutral options, and the ones to avoid due to peach or pink tones are Bisque, Cameo, Honey, Mocha II, Fawn, Cappuccino, and Java. **Flawless Finish Mousse Makeup** *($28)* is a foundation that comes in a metal can that uses a propellant to distribute an airy, bubbly, flesh-toned foam that blends on better than you might expect, though you might waste some product until you get used to the dispensing method. The coverage is sheer and the texture has enough slip to allow for adequate blending. This dries to a soft matte finish and should work well for normal to slightly oily or dry skin. If you're prone to breakouts, you will appreciate the absence of potentially pore-clogging thickening agents in this formula. There are 16 shades, including some great colors for very light skin tones, but avoid the following shades: Melba, Cameo, Summer 3, Mocha II, and Natural. **Flawless Finish Bare Perfection Makeup SPF 8** *($25)* is, save for a too-low SPF without adequate UVA protection, an impressive foundation suitable for normal to dry skin. With a smooth, moist texture and satin finish capable of delivering sheer to light coverage, it's worth a look. Just remember that you must wear an SPF 15 with proper UVA protection underneath this and you'll be all set. There are 17 shades to consider, but most of the darker colors are too peach or orange. The shades that should be avoided due to overtones of peach, orange, or pink are Bisque, Cameo, Honey, Mocha II, Cappuccino, and Bronze II.

✓☺ **Flawless Finish Dual Perfection Makeup SPF 8** *($28)* is a pressed powder meant to be used wet or dry as a foundation, though wet can be really choppy and streaky. It is a standard, talc-based powder that has a silky feel and very smooth finish. The SPF is too low, but it is part titanium dioxide, so it's worth using this with an effective SPF 15 sunscreen or foundation. This formula works best for someone with normal to slightly dry or slightly oily skin, and most of the 16 colors are excellent. The only ones that should be viewed suspiciously are Ivory, Cameo, Cream, Buff, and Cappuccino. ✓☺ **Flawless Finish Makeup Stick SPF 15** *($18)* is a superlative stick foundation that has an incredibly smooth, silky texture and a very soft, demi-matte finish that is not at all dry or too powdery. That makes this best for someone with normal to slightly dry skin because any oily areas will show shine quickly given the minimal powder finish of this makeup. In fact, it almost leaves a sheen on the skin, which can be attractive. There are ten shades, with no options for very dark skin. A few of the lighter shades are slightly peach or pink, but the sheer to light coverage you net from this makes this almost a non-issue. The only colors to consider avoiding are Cameo and Bisque—both are too pink for most skin tones. Last, but not least, is the pure titanium dioxide sunscreen—a brilliant icing on the cake.

☺ $$$ **Flawless Finish Sponge-On Cream Makeup** *($28)* is a fairly thick and somewhat greasy mineral oil– and petrolatum-based compact makeup, making it an option only for someone with dry skin. This one starts out very thick and moist, providing medium to full coverage with a creamy, opaque finish. It blends well enough, but most women will not require this much coverage, and the fragrance is quite strong. Of the 16 shades, the following are too pink, orange, or peach to recommend: Honey, Cappuccino, Porcelain Beige, Toasty Beige, Warm Beige, Gentle Beige, and Toasty Rose. **Let There Be Light Radiant Skin Compact SPF 15** *($20)* is a cream-to-powder shimmery highlighter with an in-part titanium dioxide–based sunscreen. It adds luminescence (shine) to the skin. If this type of product is of interest, Revlon's SkinLights is the place to turn for less expensive options, including shimmer with sunscreen.

CONCEALER: ✓☺ Flawless Finish Concealer *($14)* is an excellent concealer that has a lightweight, smooth texture and an opaque, soft matte finish that poses almost no risk of creasing. The four available colors are superbly neutral, although Deep can be slightly peach for some skin tones. This is one to try if you happen upon an Arden counter!

☺ **Visible Difference Eye-Fix Primer** *($15.50 for 0.25 ounce)* is supposed to be a sheer cream for the eyelid to prevent makeup creasing, and it's basically silicone, talc, and wax. Forget this boring formula, and just use the Flawless Finish Concealer above, which would work as well, if not better, than this product.

POWDER: ☺ $$$ **Flawless Finish Loose Powder** *($20)* is a fine-milled powder that has a sheer, very soft texture that's almost invisible on the skin. This talc-based formula doesn't have the best colors, but each of the five shades applies so sheer it doesn't matter. ☺ $$$ **Flawless Finish Pressed Powder** *($20)* has a standard, smooth texture and dry finish that can take on a chalky appearance on the skin. The five shades are OK, and they tend to go on lighter than they appear. Test this one carefully before making a purchase. **Bronzing Powder Duo** *($22.50)* is a talc-based pressed-powder bronzer that features two shiny colors in one compact. For some reason, Arden overlooked the fact that bronzed skin should have a golden brown to red-brown cast, as the two colors here are too peachy rose to resemble a tan.

☺ $$$ <u>BLUSH:</u> **Cheekcolor** *($20)* features a velvety smooth texture and a soft, sheer finish that is a pleasure to apply. There are some beautiful, primarily warm-toned matte shades and almost as many shiny pastel options. What's helpful in this product is that the blushes are divided into three color families that correspond well with the line's eye and lip colors.

☺ <u>EYESHADOW:</u> The lovely selections of **Eyeshadow Singles** *($10 for eyeshadow pan, $3 for duo compact)* are divided into four color groups, from neutrals and browns to plums and purples. This is a welcome separation that makes coordinating colors a breeze. The shadows all have a wonderful satin-matte, nonpowdery finish and a texture similar to Arden's blushes: like velvet. These go from sheer to moderate in intensity, and there are enough matte shades to make this well-organized collection a must-see.

<u>EYE AND BROW SHAPER:</u> ☹ **Smoky Eyes Powder Pencil** *($15)* has a powdery texture and a finish that is meant to be smudged, but this applies unevenly and tends to clump and flake off. ☺ **Smooth Lining Eye Pencil** *($14)* is a creamier standard pencil that goes on well and offers some deep and a few iridescent colors, but the finish also makes it prone to smearing. For a soft look, these do blend out well. ☺ $$$ **Dual Perfection Brow Shaper and Eyeliner** *($16)* has a dry, grainy texture and is meant to be used wet, but the colors are shiny and that just doesn't fly for the brow and the eye. ☺ **Eye Defining Liquid Liner** *($13.50)* has an improved brush that allows you to glide on this quick-drying liquid in one stroke. The formula lasts well, and the two colors are suitably black and brown.

<u>LIPSTICK AND LIP PENCIL:</u> ☺ $$$ **Exceptional Lipstick** *($16.50)* is a great name for just a standard, creamy lipstick. These all tend to have a slight to strong glossy finish and enough stain to allow for longer wear. The color range is what's really exceptional! **High Shine Lip Gloss** *($13.50)* is a fine, slightly sticky lip gloss, but standard is the name of the game here, and budget-conscious cosmetics shoppers will want to look elsewhere. ☺ **Lip Definer** *($13.50)* is an automatic, nonretractable pencil that goes on smoothly and has a creamy consistency that won't do much to keep lipstick from bleeding. **Crystal Clear Lip Gloss** *($12.50)* is a very thick, sticky gloss that is flavored with spearmint, which tastes nice but can be irritating for the lips. ☺ $$$ **Visible Difference Lip Fix Creme** *($17.50)* is supposed to prevent lipstick from feathering. It works well for some lipsticks, but I don't care for the squeeze-tube applicator. It goes on like a moisturizer and must dry before you put on your lipstick, which is less than convenient for touch-ups during the day. I prefer anti-feathering products that come in lipstick or lipliner forms so there's no waiting between applications, and you don't need to remove what you have on to reapply more.

☺ $$$ <u>MASCARA:</u> It is almost shocking that Arden has not launched any new mascaras in over four years. What's available is worthwhile, though you would be wise to explore the numerous A-list drugstore mascaras before these. **Defining Mascara** *($16)* is great for lengthening, though it takes a while to build the lashes. Clumping is minimal, and if thickness isn't your major goal, it's worth a try. **Two-Brush Mascara** *($16.50)* is seemingly for those who can't decide what type of mascara brush they prefer. This dual-ended mascara features a regular-size spiral brush that allows for some average lengthening but little else, and a small, short-bristled brush that allows you to reach every lash while building considerable length and some thickness. Most women will prefer one side to the other, which means you're paying top dollar for half a mascara—and who wants to do that? **Natural Volume Mascara** *($16)* is capable of building lots of length and moderate thickness, but it takes several strokes to reach that point, and it tends to smear as it wears, unless you apply it sparingly—but that can be done with any number of less expensive mascaras.

☺ $$$ <u>BRUSHES:</u> A small but reliable assortment of brushes *($20–$40)* is sold at most Arden counters. There are five brushes, and you will find the **Face Brush** *($40)* is dense and soft, but not too full or floppy for controlled application, while the **Blush Brush** *($35)* has a great shape and is also dense yet soft. The sable **Eye Brushes 1, 2,** and **3** *($20–$35)* are fine, but are overpriced for what you get, although each brush comes with its own case, which is great for traveling.

ELIZABETH GRANT (SKIN CARE ONLY)

Elizabeth Grant launched her skin-care line in London back in 1958. The good news is that these products have evolved over time and are relatively up to date with some good water-binding agents, antioxidants, and anti-irritants. The bad news is there isn't very much of the impressive ingredients in any of these overly expensive products.

Over the years this mail order/Internet company has gained a following of some measure, which is reflected in the number of e-mails I receive asking why I haven't reviewed these products before. Now that I have, I am stunned by some of the most over-the-top claims (and prices asked) I've heard for what turn out to be some good, but definitely not remarkable, skin-care products. This line offers nothing that products from many companies, from Lauder to Clinique, Neutrogena, and Olay, can't outdo and for a lot less money.

For all the claims of superior formulations, this line doesn't even have a sunscreen with UVA-protecting ingredients. Likewise, if you have oily or blemish-prone skin there are no products to address that concern. Yet the line does have a Torricelumn Pur Antiaging Time Retardant Night Cream that sells for $279.99 for 1.76 ounces. First, there is no such thing as "torricelumn." It is merely a marketing term the company uses to represent an assortment of plant extracts and vitamins that it claims can make Barbara Bush look like Elizabeth Grant (check out Grant's picture on the Internet). None of the ingredients in these products is unique to Grant's line and none of them has a shred of evidence showing they can get rid of wrinkles. For more information about Elizabeth Grant, call (877) 751-1999 or visit www.elizabethgrant.com.

☺ $$$ **Gentle Cleansing Milk** *($16.99 for 4 ounces)* is a good, though basic, emollient cleanser that is an option for normal to dry skin. It does contain fragrance and coloring agents.

The Reviews E

☺ $$$ **Hydrating Cleanser with Torricelumn** *($15.99 for 4 ounces)* is just a good, very standard, detergent-based cleanser that would work well for normal to oily skin. There is nothing hydrating about it, though it is cleansing and that's a good thing for a cleanser to do.

☺ $$$ **Torricelumn Pur Cleanser** *($34.99 for 4 ounces)* is a lotion cleanser with some plant oils, water-binding agents, and a small amount of antioxidants. It is a good option for someone with normal to dry skin, but there is nothing in this product that warrants the price tag.

☺ $$$ **Gentle Eye Make Up Remover** *($13.99 for 4 ounces)* is an OK eye-makeup remover, but the tangerine extract in it isn't good for the eye area. Otherwise, this is just plant water, detergent cleansing agents, and preservatives.

☺ $$$ **Apricot Face Scrub** *($17.99 for 1 ounce)* is a lotion-style scrub that uses pumice and walnut shell as the abrasive, and it contains a small amount of menthol, which makes it less than gentle on skin. The plant extracts are meant to sound like they are related to AHAs, but they have no exfoliating properties or any real benefit for skin.

☹ **Pore Closing Lotion** *($13.99 for 4 ounces)*. There isn't anything in this product that will close even one pore on your face, and the lemon oil can be a skin irritant.

☺ $$$ **Toning Lotion** *($29.99 for 4 ounces)* is an OK toner with some plant extracts that can be good antioxidants and anti-irritants, plus a small amount of water-binding agents. This is an option for most skin types. It does contain fragrance.

☺ $$$ **Complete Renewal Treatment** *($54.99 for 1 ounce)* is a very ordinary moisturizer that contains mostly water, thickeners, and preservatives. The antioxidants and water-binding agents are present in such teeny amounts they're barely worth mentioning. This does contain urea, and in this concentration it is a good exfoliant, but there are far cheaper urea-based moisturizers at the drugstore that would work just as well, such as Eucerin's Dry Skin Therapy Plus Intensive Repair Cream ($7.99 for 4 ounces).

☺ $$$ **Enriched Featherlight Moisturizer** *($49.99 for 1 ounce)* is similar to the Complete Renewal Treatment above and the same basic comments apply.

☹ **Featherlight Day Protection SPF 15** *($49.99 for 1 ounce)* does not contain the UVA-protecting ingredients of titanium dioxide, zinc oxide, or avobenzone, and is not recommended.

☹ **Diminu-X Skin Firming Cream** *($59.99 for 1 ounce)* is just water, witch hazel, film-forming agent, and preservatives. The plant extracts are a mix of irritants and anti-irritants, and though there are some good antioxidants and water-binding agents, they are present in such small amounts as to be undetectable. This does contain fragrance.

☺ $$$ **Firming Throat Cream** *($27.99 for 1 ounce)* is an exceptionally standard moisturizer for dry skin that contains mostly water, thickeners, Vaseline, preservatives, and minuscule amounts of antioxidants and anti-irritants. This won't firm any part of your body.

☺ $$$ **Gentle Eye Serum** *($37.95 for 0.5 ounce)* is a simple mix of water, glycerin, water-binding agent, and a tiny amount of antioxidants. It would be an OK option for someone with normal to slightly dry skin.

☺ $$$ **Intensive Eye Cream** *($29.99 for 0.5 ounce)* is a very good moisturizer for normal to dry skin.

☹ $$$ **Rejuvenating Serum AM** and **Rejuvenating Serum PM** *(Sold as set, two containers for $79.99 for 1 ounce each)*. Neither of these are rejuvenating in the least, and the two products are practically identical. These are OK, lightweight moisturizers for normal to slightly dry skin. The arnica in them can be a skin irritant with repeated use.

☹ $$$ **Torricelumn Pur Antiaging Time Retardant Night Cream** *($279.99 for 1.76 ounces)*. I had to check out this price and formulation for a long time before I could believe my eyes. I still have no words to express how offensive a price this is for what amounts to an extremely basic, and I mean really, really basic, moisturizer for normal to dry skin. Are you ready for this? All it contains is mostly water, glycerin, thickeners, water-binding agent, film-forming agent, preservatives, emollient, silicones, more preservatives, teeny amounts of vitamin E, algae, plant oil, and coloring agents. Shocking! It isn't completely without merit, but it's easily replaced with moisturizers from Lauder to Clinique, Olay, and Neutrogena that are far better formulated and a fraction of the price.

☹ $$$ **Torricelumn Pur Instant Hydration Boost** *($189.99 for 1.76 ounces)* is similar to the Retardant Night Cream above and the same comments apply.

☹ $$$ **Torricelumn Pur Antiaging Eye Refiner** *($79.99 for 0.5 ounce)* is similar to the Retardant Night Cream above and the same comments apply.

☹ $$$ **Revitalizing Treatment** *($69.99 for both Revitalizer 1 and Revitalizer 2)* is a two-part skin treatment you are supposed to use for seven days every month. Revitalizer 1 ends up being just a very ordinary 7% glycolic acid lotion-like toner in a base with a pH of 4.5 that gives it some, but not great, exfoliating properties. However, this isn't an improvement over Alpha Hydrox's glycolic acid products at the drugstore for a lot less money. You then apply the Revitalizer 2 moisturizer over it, which has a formula similar to the Complete Renewal Treatment above.

☹ $$$ **Cucumber Mask** *($23.99 for 1 ounce)* is a standard clay mask with the teeniest amount of cucumber thrown in. It would work as well as any clay mask to absorb oil. It does contain fragrance and coloring agents.

☹ $$$ **Torricelumn Pur Moisture Replenishing Mask** *($149.99 for 1.76 ounces)* is similar to many of the moisturizers in the Grant line, with some good water-binding agents, some plant oils, and a tiny amount of antioxidants. This also contains PVP, a plastic that you peel off the face. I'm sure the price tag will be very seductive for a lot of women who will believe it must contain something remarkable for skin, but it is almost laughable how unremarkable this mask is. It isn't bad, it just isn't worth this price by any stretch of the imagination.

☹ $$$ **Lip Contour Cream** *($29.99 for 0.5 ounce)* is a very basic moisturizer that is overpriced for what ends up being just a simple emollient for dry skin.

The Reviews E

☺ $$$ **At Last Lipstain Kit** *($19.99)* consists of three containers of lip stain and one lip balm. The concept and application are similar to Lip Ink, in that each color is essentially pigment suspended in an alcohol and film-forming agent base. These go on decently, but tend to sting the lips, and the color needs to be applied several times to build intensity and coverage. You wind up with a slightly sticky matte finish that tends to flake and chip off on its own. However, you will get more mileage out of each shade when the Moisturizing Stick is used. This mineral oil–based clear lipstick allows for comfortable wear without disturbing the color beneath it, just like the Moisturizing Top Coat sold with Max Factor's Lipfinity, but Grant's lip stains don't hold a candle to that long-wearing lipstick juggernaut. Moreover, this is a kit whose colors are of limited appeal, and the repetitive irritation from the alcohol makes it problematic.

ELLA BACHE (SKIN CARE ONLY)

Ella Bache was born in Hungary at the turn of the 20th century. She eventually became a pharmacist, an unusual feat for women of her day, and along the way developed her own skin-care line. Her long-established heritage is being kept strong as family members continue to operate the company. Regrettably, the heritage she left behind is now dated technology from more than 30 years ago. The claims that these products have state-of-the-art formulations, thanks to "ongoing scientific research, new product development, [and] the use of high quality ingredients" are at best painfully overstated, and in reality just not true. One after the other, these products are burdened with formulations that are really more like those of Vaseline Intensive Care or Jergens, which are available at the drugstore. Almost every Ella Bache moisturizer is a redundant mix of Vaseline, mineral oil, lanolin, waxes, and zinc oxide. What is especially appalling is that these same emollient, waxy ingredients even show up in products for oily and blemish-prone skin. Astoundingly, there are no sunscreens of any kind—not a one!—the cleansers are little more than cold creams; and the toners contain alcohol, even the ones for dry skin! Perhaps most glaringly absent from almost all of these fairly pricey products are any significant water-binding agents, antioxidants, or anti-irritants. And (almost without exception) there isn't a unique or particularly interesting ingredient in the lot. Ella Bache skin-care products were probably once really impressive in the 1950s, 1960s, and maybe even the 1970s. However, given the prodigious amount of readily available research regarding all aspects of skin care, wrinkles, aging, and acne that has taken place over the past 25 years, these products were already out of date by the mid-1980s. For more information about Ella Bache, call (800) 922-2430 or visit www.ellabache.com.

ELLA BACHE CLASSICS

☺ $$$ **Cleansing Milk, for Dry and Sensitive Skin** *($26 for 6.7 ounces)* is a very basic, overpriced, cold cream–style cleanser that is little more than mineral oil, thickening agents, and fragrance. It is an option for normal to dry skin, although plain mineral oil would work as well.

☹ **Mild Cleansing Soap, for All Skin Types** *($10 for 4.40 ounces)* is a very standard bar soap that can be drying and irritating for most skin types.

☺ **$$$ Rinse-Off Cleansing Cream for Sensitive Skin** *($21 for 2.50 ounces)* doesn't rinse very well, at least not without the aid of a washcloth. It is similar to the Cleansing Milk above only this one contains a good amount of lanolin and is only appropriate for dry to very dry skin.

☺ **$$$ Lash Conditioning Cleanser for All Mascara Types** *($25 for 1.58 ounces)* is just coconut oil, Vaseline, water, lanolin, preservatives, and fragrance. There is nothing in this product that warrants the price and you would do just as well with plain Vaseline or just some olive oil from your kitchen cabinet.

☹ **Toning Lotion, for Normal and Sensitive Skin** *($25 for 6.76 ounces)*. With alcohol as the second ingredient, and menthol present, too, this is a serious problem for all skin types, but especially for sensitive skin. Then there's the addition of phthalate, a potential toxin that can be absorbed through skin, which makes this actually a little scary.

☺ **$$$ Complexion Diffusing Cream, for Reactive Skin** *($37 for 1.58 ounces)* is simply water, thickeners, silicone, tomato extract, preservatives, fragrance, and coloring agents. Tomato extract has weak antioxidant properties, though it can also be a skin irritant. All in all, it doesn't get much more ordinary than this as a moisturizer for normal to dry skin.

☹ **Exfoliating Cream for Dry and Sensitive Skin** *($25 for 1.72 ounces)* has a pH of 6, and that makes the salicylic acid in this product ineffective for exfoliation. Add alcohol as the second ingredient, and this becomes a problem for all skin types for any reason.

☺ **$$$ Hydrating Softening Cream for Dry and Sensitive Skin** *($37 for 1.58 ounces)* is very basic and very boring for very dry skin.

☺ **$$$ Hydrating Toning Cream for Dry and Dehydrated Skin** *($41 for 1.58 ounces)* is similar to the Hydrating Softening Cream above and the same basic comments apply. This does contain a very tiny amount of vitamin C and a water-binding agent, but that doesn't change much about what is nothing more than a mundane moisturizer for dry skin.

☺ **$$$ Moisturizing Base for All Skin Types** *($28 for 16.90 ounces)*. This weightless moisturizer is OK for normal to oily skin, but lacks water-binding agents and antioxidants and holds no real benefit for skin.

☺ **$$$ Skin Softening Lotion for Sensitive Skin** *($32 for 4.22 ounces)* is shockingly mundane and completely not worth the effort, because any drugstore moisturizer would do better things for your skin than this formulation.

☺ **$$$ Surfacing Balancing Cream, for Sensitive Skin** *($31 for 1.62 ounces)* is an option for dry skin, but calling this standard and uninteresting is an understatement.

☹ **Surface Regulating Cream, for Combination and Oily Skin** *($34 for 1.74 ounces)* is a standard moisturizer for dry skin that contains mostly water, Vaseline, lanolin, thickeners, preservatives, and fragrance. Recommending this for oily skin is all wrong, not to mention a humiliation.

☺ $$$ **Ultra-Rich Cream, for Dry and Dehydrated Skin** *($30 for 1.58 ounces)* is a standard moisturizer for dry skin that contains mostly Vaseline, water, plant oil, lanolin, fish oil, fragrance, and preservatives.

☹ $$$ **Ultra-Rich Special Eye Cream** *($31 for 1.02 ounces)* isn't all that rich. It's just an overpriced emollient moisturizer lacking antioxidants and any amount of water-binding agents.

☺ $$$ **Beautifying Mask** *($30 for 2.99 ounces)* is just water, plant oil, clay, zinc oxide, thickener, preservatives, and coloring agents, so it can't do anything particularly beautifying. As an exceptionally standard mask for normal to slightly dry or slightly oily skin, it is an option, but the question is really, "Why bother?"

☺ $$$ **Balancing Mask, for Sensitive Skin** *($30 for 2.64 ounces)* is just clay, thickener, talc, rice starch, fragrance, and preservatives. There is nothing in this product helpful for sensitive skin, though as a standard clay mask for absorbing oil, it's an option.

☺ $$$ **Firming Mask, for Tired Skin** *($28 for 2.64 ounces)* is similar to the Balancing Mask above and the same basic comments apply.

☹ **Softening Mask, for Sensitive Skin** *($28 for 2.82 ounces)* is similar to the Balancing Mask above and the same basic comments apply. This also contains menthol, which is a skin irritant and a problem for all skin types, and even more so for someone with sensitive skin.

ELLA BACHE ANTI-WRINKLE

☺ $$$ **Age-Defense Day Cream** *($64 for 1.7 ounces)* contains mostly thickening agents, plant oils, and a trace amount of vitamin E. It is just a standard moisturizer for dry skin, and there is nothing in it that can prevent even one minute of aging. Because this doesn't contain sunscreen, it should not be used during the day.

☺ $$$ **Age-Defense Night Cream** *($70 for 1.67 ounces)* is similar to the Age-Defense Day Cream above only with slightly more emollients. The same basic comments apply.

☺ $$$ **Eye Lift Gel** *($45 for 0.53 ounce)* is one of the better-formulated moisturizers Bache sells. It contains some good water-binding agents and a small amount of antioxidants in a lightweight gel formulation. It is an option for someone with normal to slightly dry skin.

☺ $$$ **Intensive Anti-Wrinkle Serum** *($90 for 1.07 ounces)* is similar to the Eye Lift Gel above and the same basic comments apply.

ELLA BACHE MOISTURIZING FOR YOUNG SKIN

☺ $$$ **Rinse-Off Cream Cleanser, for Face and Eyes** *($26 for 4.19 ounces)* is a basic moisturizer of thickening agents, Vaseline, mineral oil, lanolin, preservatives, and fragrance. That's OK for dry skin but that's about it.

☹ **Refreshing Alcohol-Free Toner** *($26 for 4.76 ounces)* is actually just water, preservative, trace amounts of aluminum sulfate (an ingredient used in deodorants), more preservative, and fragrance. I have no words for how completely useless this is for skin, except this one: Unbelievable.

☺ $$$ Rich Moisturizing Cream, for Dry and Very Dry Skin *($36 for 1.58 ounces)* is a very basic moisturizer for dry skin. The black currant extract can have antioxidant properties, but this product contains so little of it that it can't offer much benefit for skin.

☺ $$$ Moisturizing Matt Finish Cream, for Normal to Oily Skin *($36 for 1.58 ounces)* is a fairly lightweight, silicone-based moisturizer that contains a small amount of antioxidant and even less water-binding agent. It's OK for someone with normal to slightly dry skin.

☺ $$$ Moisturizing Cream Mask *($30 for 2.57 ounces)* is a ho-hum formulation that includes just thickeners and some fragrant plant extracts.

ELLA BACHE MOISTURIZING FOR MATURE SKIN

☺ $$$ Moisturizing Cream Special for Eyes and Lips *($32 for 1.01 ounces)* is a standard emollient moisturizer for dry skin, similar to just about every other Bache moisturizer. The only difference is that this one contains a tiny amount of water-binding agents and colostrum. Colostrum is the cloudy-clear "pre-milk" that female mammals secrete prior to producing milk, and that contains immunoglobulins (disease resistance factors). While there is a small body of evidence indicating that adult consumption of colostrum may have disease-fighting potential, this is hardly substantiated and there is no known benefit when colostrum is applied topically to skin. The only study that does exist showed colostrum to have no wound-healing function on skin (Source: *Journal of Dermatologic Surgery and Oncology,* June 1985, pages 617–622).

☺ $$$ Moisturizing Cream Special for Face *($39 for 1.71 ounces)* is almost identical to the Moisturizing Cream Special for Eye and Lips above and the same comments apply.

☺ $$$ Moisturizing Cream Special for Neck *($32 for 1.01 ounces)* is almost identical to the Moisturizing Cream Special for Eye and Lips above and the same comments apply.

ELLA BACHE ANTI-AGING

☺ $$$ Cream Emulsion *($52 for 1.71 ounces)* is a basic moisturizer for dry skin, and the soybean protein in it has no estrogenic properties for skin.

☺ $$$ Intensive Concentrate Emulsion *($65 for 1.05 ounces)* is similar to the Cream Emulsion above and the same comments apply.

☺ $$$ Ultra-Rich Cream *($52 for 1.6 ounces)* is emollient, but incredibly basic. It contains mostly Vaseline, water, mineral oil, waxes, lanolin, thickeners, fragrance, preservatives, and fragrant plant oils.

☺ $$$ Cream Mask *($47 for 2.46 ounces)* is similar to the Ultra-Rich Cream above and the same comments apply.

ELLA BACHE CLEARING FOR BROWN SPOTS

☺ $$$ Intensive Clearing Serum Special for Brown Spots *($63 for 1.05 ounces)* does contain vitamin C and bearberry, which both have some evidence showing they can inhibit melanin production. However, without the diligent and daily use of an effective sunscreen, it will have no effect whatsoever.

The Reviews E

☺ $$$ **Moisturizing Clearing Cream** (*$45 for 1.58 ounces*) is a standard moisturizing formula with trace amounts of vitamin C and bearberry (bearberry contains arbutin; for more details about bearberry and arbutin, refer to Chapter Seven, *Cosmetics Dictionary*). In this minute amount it is unlikely that these ingredients can have any effect on melanin production.

ELLA BACHE OILY SKIN

☹ **Cleansing Milk, for Normal to Combination Skin** (*$25 for 6.67 ounces*) is a standard, mineral oil–based, cold cream–style cleanser that is completely inappropriate for anyone with any amount of oily skin. The menthol in here is a skin irritant.

☺ $$$ **Deep Cleansing Scrub, for Combination to Oily Skin** (*$21 for 6.17 ounces*) is a lotion scrub that uses silica (sand) as the abrasive. It is an option, but is easily replaced with a gentle cleanser and plain baking soda.

☹ **Exfoliating Lotion, for Combination to Oily Skin** (*$32 for 4.22 ounces*) lists the second ingredient as alcohol, which makes it too irritating and drying for all skin types. The potato starch can also be a problem because it can encourage the growth of bacteria.

☺ $$$ **Matt Finish Solution, for Oily to Problem Prone Skin** (*$24 for 4.22 ounces*) is a basic clay mask that also contains some tea tree oil, but not enough for it to be effective as a topical disinfectant.

☺ $$$ **Purifying Solution, for Oily Skin** (*$70 for 20 ampoules*) contains just water, vitamin C, thickeners, preservatives, and fragrance. Vitamin C has no effect on oil production or oily skin, it is just a good antioxidant. This lacks water-binding agents and anti-irritants, which, given the price tag, would have been far more purifying for oily skin.

☹ **Refining Toning Lotion, for Combination to Oily Skin** (*$27 for 6.76 ounces*). This lists alcohol as the first ingredient and that makes it a problem for all skin types. It also contains phthalate, a toxin that can be absorbed through skin, and is not recommended.

☹ **Refining Toning Lotion, for Oily and Problem-Prone Skin** (*$27 for 6.67 ounces*) is a product that would be a serious problem for problem skin. It contains only alcohol, water, camphor, and coloring agents. None of that is helpful for skin, but it is extremely irritating and drying.

☹ **Absorbing Cream, for Oily Skin** (*$30 for 2.11 ounces*). Add up the Vaseline, mineral oil, fish oil, lanolin, and zinc oxide this product contains, and it's clear this is an oily skin nightmare. My goodness, what were they thinking!

☺ $$$ **Equalizing Emulsion, for Combination to Oily Skin** (*$37 for 4.22 ounces*). With mineral oil as the second ingredient (and also containing thickening agents and waxes), this is only appropriate for normal to dry skin. It does contain a small amount of water-binding agents and vitamin C, but overall it's just a very ordinary moisturizer.

☹ **Tinted Correction Cream, for Oily Skin** (*$30 for 1.46 ounces*) has the same confounding problems as the Absorbing Cream above, and is absolutely not recommended for oily skin.

☺ **$$$ Absorbing Mask, for Oily Skin** (*$30 for 2.99 ounces*) contains mostly clay, plant oil, alcohol, and fragrance. This is a confused product for someone with oily skin but can be an option for someone with normal to slightly dry or slightly oily skin.

☺ **$$$ Equalizing Mask, for Combination to Oily Skin** (*$28 for 6.17 ounces*) is just a very standard, but OK, clay mask for absorbing oil. It would work as well as any.

ELLEN LANGE SKIN CARE

Ellen Lange is an aesthetician based in New Jersey who began her own skin-care line back in 1996. The main outlets for her namesake product line are Sephora stores and Sephora's Web site, www.sephora.com. For the consumer, what makes Lange's line so captivating seems to be the skin-care background of its creator. Her aesthetician's license and her family's medical background may lead people to believe that these products are somehow superior, but a closer look shows that's just not the case. In this instance, the array of products is a mixed bag. On the downside, the cleansers and toners are average, and the sunscreens do not have adequate UVA protection—that fact alone should make anyone instantly leery of a company's claims. However, Lange does excel with her moisturizers, as most of them contain a very good, though far from unique, assortment of antioxidants and water-binding agents such as ceramide and sodium PCA.

The other attention-getting aspect of this line is Lange's Retexturizing Peel Kit, which is supposed to be a do-it-yourself AHA peel. This kit does contain about 5% glycolic acid, but because it has a base with a pH close to 5, that renders it ineffective for exfoliating the skin. Keep in mind that the kind of peel done at most salons usually uses 15% to 20% glycolic acid and that the amount in many typical AHA products is about 8%, with a pH of 3 to 4. That means that Lange's kit cannot be as effective as many other AHA products being sold these days.

One interesting claim Lange makes for her moisturizers concerns the size of the molecules in them, and the way that affects the skin. The MicroThera products claim to contain molecules "1/10th the size of traditional cosmetic product molecules. The small size allows it to absorb quickly into your skin and rapidly release its nourishing ingredients." In contrast, the MacroThera products "use … molecules four times the size of those found in traditional cosmetics." Is this an important feature or merely a marketing ploy? From my perspective, it's a little of both. The MicroThera products contain standard cosmetic ingredients, and many of these do indeed have a smaller molecular size, which increases their ability to enhance the penetration of other ingredients (glycerin is a prime example of such an ingredient). The MacroThera line contains ingredients that have a larger molecular structure (such as collagen) that cannot penetrate into the skin—so they stay on the surface and work to smooth skin and prevent moisture loss. They all work fine at what they do, and the product names are intriguing enough, but the ingredients in Lange's products are not new discoveries or unique to this line in any way.

For more information about Ellen Lange Skin Care, call (800) 652-6438 or visit www.ellenlange.com.

☺ $$$ **Daily Maintenance Cleanser** *($24 for 6 ounces)* is similar in many ways to Cetaphil Daily Facial Cleanser ($8.99 for 16 ounces). Lange's version does contain minerals that have some antioxidant properties, but in a cleanser they would just be rinsed away. This contains coloring agents, though it is fragrance free.

☺ $$$ **Daily Maintenance Singles** *($20 for 36 packets)* contain a cleanser that is identical to the Daily Maintenance Cleanser above, except that these come in single-use packets, and the same comments apply.

☺ $$$ **Daily Maintenance Eye Makeup Remover** *($12 for 2.8 ounces)* is a standard, detergent-based eye-makeup remover that contains a long list of minerals. Although these can work as antioxidants, they are best in a product that is designed to be left on the skin, not wiped away like this one. This contains coloring agents, but is fragrance free.

☹ **Daily Maintenance Refresher** *($20 for 6 ounces)* contains witch hazel as the second ingredient, which makes this otherwise gentle toner too irritating for all skin types.

☹ **MicroThera A.M. SPF 15** *($35 for 2 ounces)* does not contain the UVA-protecting ingredients of titanium dioxide, zinc oxide, or avobenzone, and is absolutely not recommended.

☺ $$$ **MicroThera P.M.** *($40 for 1.5 ounces)* is a very good, though overpriced, moisturizer for dry to very dry skin. The sugarcane extract is not the same as an AHA, though even if it were both the amount of it present and the pH of the product would make it ineffective for exfoliation. This does contain minute amounts of citrus extracts, but probably not enough to cause irritation.

✓☺ $$$ **MicroThera Eye Care** *($32 for 0.5 ounce)* is a very good moisturizer for dry skin with a good assortment of water-binding agents, antioxidants, and moisturizing agents.

☹ **MacroThera A.M. SPF 15** *($36 for 1.4 ounces)* does not contain the UVA-protecting ingredients of titanium dioxide, zinc oxide, or avobenzone, and is absolutely not recommended.

☺ $$$ **MacroThera P.M.** *($42 for 1.4 ounces)* contains mostly water, thickeners, film-forming agents, slip agent, anti-irritant, emollient, water-binding agents, vitamin E, and preservatives. The really good ingredients are tucked in way at the end of the ingredient list and so are in short supply, but the basic ingredients make this an OK option for someone with normal to dry skin.

☺ $$$ **MacroThera Eye Care** *($34 for 0.35 ounce)* is a very emollient, plant oil–based moisturizer that will address dry skin around the eyes or elsewhere. The antioxidants are not as plentiful as in the MicroThera Eye Care, but this will take very good care of dry skin.

✓☺ $$$ **MultiDose Serum Therapy** *($36 for 1 ounce)* is a lightweight serum (primarily a synthetic fluid or mineral-like ester called trimethylolpropane) that does contain some vitamins, water-binding agent, thickeners, and preservatives. The vitamins are good antioxidants, but this doesn't "dose" the skin in the least, as no one knows how much of any vitamin the skin needs topically. It would be a very good moisturizer for normal to dry skin.

☺ $$$ **Velvet Vinyl** *($45)* is a "dynamic duo" featuring a bottle of Velvet (for a "luminous" finish) and one of Vinyl (for a "glossy" finish, of course). Both are silicone-based serums, with the Velvet being reminiscent of M.A.C.'s Creme Matifiance, except that this one has a slight shimmer. The Vinyl product is less slippery-smooth and more emollient, leaving a dewy sheen on the skin. Both are options for use with normal to slightly dry skin by those who don't mind the expense and the small amount of shine left on the skin.

☹ **Retexturizing Peel Kit** *($65)* is the product that put Ellen Lange on the map and is the line's best seller. The kit contains four products: First, a **Peel Prep**, which uses papaya extract in a gel base. This is presumably the start of the exfoliation process, but papaya's exfoliating effects on the skin are minimal, at best, and it's also unstable, especially in comparison to a well-formulated AHA or BHA product. After the Prep come the **Peel Accelerator Pads**, which use glycolic acid along with irritants like witch hazel and menthol. These pads feel somewhat abrasive, and the pH of 5 makes them ineffective for exfoliation. The menthol and witch hazel, though, can cause irritation, especially if used every day as directed. After the Pads, the next step is to brush on the **Glycolic Peel Solution** and leave it on the skin for ten minutes. Although the foaming action (it foams right before your eyes) is kind of cool, the pH of the Solution is 4.5—again too high to allow it to be effective as an exfoliant. This also contains menthol, most likely to give users the impression that the peel is "working" because their skin is tingling. Finally, after washing off the Solution, you apply the **Post Peel Cream**, which is perhaps the saving grace of this whole kit. It is a basic moisturizer that feels light and silky on the skin and contains a nice assortment of water-binding agents, emollients, and antioxidants. There is a tiny amount of witch hazel and sodium lauryl sulfate in the cream, but in these tiny amounts they are extremely unlikely to be a problem for skin. All in all, the money spent on this peel would be better spent on the real deal—an AHA (or BHA) peel using a concentration of between 10% and 20%, and with a pH of 3.

☹ **Blemish Controlling Peel** *($65)* also has four parts. The **Purifying Peel Prep** is just a standard, detergent-based cleanser. The **Oil Reducing Pads** are mostly water, alcohol, and glycolic acid. The pH of 4 is in the ballpark for effective exfoliation (but so are Alpha Hydrox's glycolic acid products at the drugstore without the alcohol). The Pads are soaked with the **Alpha/Beta Peel Solution** that comes next, but the Solution has a pH of 5, which means there will be minimal to no exfoliation. After all, it turns out this Solution doesn't contain any AHAs or BHA, but instead contains several irritating plant extracts including camphor, eucalyptus, lemon, and cinnamon, none of which have any positive effect on skin. Last is the **Moisture Control Gel**, which is a ho-hum moisturizer with no antioxidants or significant water-binding agents. To control blemishes an effective exfoliant and topical disinfectant are essential, and this kit falls short on both counts.

ENGLISH IDEAS & LIP LAST (MAKEUP ONLY)

English Ideas is a small cosmetics company whose founders believe "cosmetics needed to go beyond makeup artistry and towards science." With the goal of designing "solutions to unresolved cosmetic problems," English Ideas features a wide assortment of products that masquerade as unique scientific breakthroughs, while remaining hopelessly ordinary, outdated, or just plain ineffective. Even the products that do work do so at a price, such as skin or lip irritation. The line's first claim to fame was their Lip Last Lipstick Sealant, which does indeed work to help lipstick last longer, but also burns the lips, and for some may give credence to the phrase "beauty is pain, pain beauty"! Besides, with the advent of PermaTone color technology, used in Max Factor Lipfinity and Cover Girl Outlast lipsticks, products like Lip Last seem almost archaic.

The rest of the line is composed of all sorts of sealants, enhancers, primers, and treatments for common cosmetic woes. Yet there is truly nothing groundbreaking here, and several products have an unpleasant texture or finish that just doesn't live up to the English Ideas "Innovation in Cosmetics" theme. There are some decent foundations with effective sunscreens to consider, but why pay top dollar for less-than-remarkable products? If elegance and current cosmetics technology are what you're seeking, shopping this line is not the best idea, English or otherwise.

For more information about English Idéas & Lip Last, call 1-800-LIP-LAST or visit www.englishideas.com.

FOUNDATION: ☺ $$$ **Perfect Powder SPF 15 Pressed Powder Foundation** *($28)* is a sheer, slightly shiny, talc-free powder foundation with titanium dioxide as the active sunscreen. There are eight respectable shades available, with options for darker skin tones, and the texture is dry but smooth. Keep in mind that it takes a liberal coverage of sunscreen to get the SPF on the label, so a sheer-finish application will not protect you from sun damage. As an adjunct to foundation with sunscreen, this is an expensive option.

☺ $$$ **Perfect Liquid SPF 15 Foundation** *($30)* comes in a pump bottle and has titanium dioxide as its active sunscreen agent. This has a slick, smooth application and dries quickly to an opaque, matte finish, which would be great for very oily skin. Four of the six shades are too peach or pink for most skin tones, but the two winning shades are LF4 and LF5 (for medium to dark skin tones). **Perfect Primer** *($28)* is a thick, viscous, pure-silicone primer, with added antioxidants, that has an incredibly slippery texture (that's the nature of silicones) and leaves a soft, slick feel on the skin. This can make the skin look smoother, but the claim about keeping foundation perfect for 8 to 12 hours is debatable.

EYESHADOW AND EYE PRODUCTS: ☺ **Kolour Shadow SPF 15 Eye Shadow** *($15)* uses zinc oxide as its sunscreen and although that is a reliable ingredient for UVA protection, it lends a dry, chalky texture to these powder eyeshadows. They blend decently and are pigment-rich, but the trade-off in texture for these mostly shiny shadows is undesirable.

☹ **Eye Perfection Color Corrector and SPF 15 Eyelid Foundation** *($35)* features three powdery colors in one compact: flesh tone, pale yellow, and mint green. The SPF is zinc oxide–based and has the same texture issues as the Kolour Shadow SPF 15 Eye Shadow above, only this product tends to flake off easily. **Eye Solution Hydrating Eye Gel with Vitamin C** *($45 for 0.5 ounce)* would have been a great, lightweight gel for the eye area, but the formula contains witch hazel as one of the main ingredients, which, along with bitter orange and balm mint, should not be used anywhere near the eyes. **Eye Refine** *($55 for 0.5 ounce)* is an AHA and retinol cream recommended for use around the eyes and on eyelids. This creamy emulsion contains far too many irritants to even think of putting it near the eyes, and AHAs should never be used on the eyelids anyway; in any case, the pH is too high to allow exfoliation. **Eye Potion Eye Firming Treatment** *($18)* is a very pale pink, iridescent liquid that you apply with a wand to give a visual "lift" to the eye area. It is quite drying and the witch hazel present isn't good for the eye area—not to mention that the shimmer enhances wrinkles.

EYE AND BROW SHAPER: ☺ **Kolour Liner Eye Pencil with Vitamin E** *($12)* is a completely standard, creamy pencil with a slightly powdery finish that smears easily. ☹ **$$$ Brow Last Brow Sealant** *($18)* is nothing more (literally) than alcohol and cellulose (a thickening agent), and even with two brushes it's not worth the high-end price tag.

☺ **Brow Enhance** *($15)* is a standard pencil with an unusually pleasant texture that applies easily and evenly without streaking or looking heavy. If you prefer pencil to powder for brows, this is one to consider, but only one shade is available and it's best for brunettes.

☹ **Liner Last Eye Liner Sealant** *($18)* is nothing but alcohol with thickeners and a hairspray-type fixative, and that is too potentially irritating for the eye area. **Brow Hi-Lites Eye Brow Gel** *($22)* is an absurdly overpriced brow gel whose colors all have a strong metallic tint and a sticky texture.

LIPSTICK AND LIP PENCIL: ☺ **Kolour Creme SPF 15 Lipstick** *($15)* is a very creamy, opaque lipstick with an unreliable sunscreen and a slightly glossy finish. The color range is impressive. ✓☺ **Kolour Crayon** *($13.50)* is a great lip pencil (similar to many but still good) that applies smoothly and offers a slight powder finish with an impressive stain.

☺ **$$$ Lip Hi-Lites** *($22.50)* have a slight cream-to-powder texture and are applied with a sponge tip. Each shade has a slightly greasy feel and an ultra-shiny finish. For the money, any iridescent drugstore gloss from Wet 'n' Wild to Maybelline would work just as well if not better.

☺ **$$$ Lip Last Transparent Lipstick Sealant** *($17.50)*. All this very tiny bottle contains is alcohol, fragrance, flavor, and a film-forming agent (like hairspray) that burns when you apply it to the lips—there is even a warning on the bottle. If you apply an even layer, you definitely get a great covering over your lip that creates a matte seal and can prevent feathering and bleeding, though not any better than most ultra-matte lipsticks (Revlon ColorStay comes to mind). This does last for a good length of time but tends to roll and chip off the lips, taking your lipstick with it. Your lipstick will still stay on, but only slightly longer than usual. Given the trade-off of the irritation factor compared to far more innovative products such as Max Factor's Lipfinity, there are better ways to keep lipstick on lips than this pricey liquid. **Lip Enhance** *($15)* bills itself as lipliner and foundation in one, but is really just a standard, pink-toned pencil with an overly thick texture. **Lip Solution Hydrating Lip Gel** *($24 for 0.5 ounce)* is supposed to "moisturize lips under any circumstances," but this concoction lacks any emollients, oils, or waxes that could form a barrier to protect the lips from moisture loss and the environment. It's not a bad product, just a senseless one that will leave your lips wanting more.

☹ **Lip Works Lip Balm SPF 18** *($9)* is just a very sheer gloss that leaves your lips out to dry when it comes to UVA-protecting ingredients. The **Grapefruit** version contains irritating grapefruit oil, and the **Tea Tree** version also contains camphor and menthol. The **Concealer** shade of Lip Works Lip Balm is reputed to hide cold sores, which is far beyond the reach of this product (and most any concealer, for that matter). **Professional Lip Brush** *($20)* is a decent brush, but the overly long, inconvenient handle does not come with a cap—meaning that once this is used, traces of lipstick will be all over whatever the brush touches. **Lip Refine AHA Exfoliating Cream** *($32 for 0.5 ounce)* is a lotion that contains AHAs and is supposed to exfoliate the lips. I would be concerned about AHAs on the lips because of the delicate nature of the skin in that area, but this product doesn't have a low enough pH to allow any exfoliation. Even if it did, there are far less expensive and far more effective AHA products available.

☺ **Lip Makeup Remover** *($10)* uses plant oil to cut through Lip Last. It works, but any oil would do the same thing. This product makes much ado about not containing mineral oil, as if this were somehow bad for skin; it isn't. In fact, because mineral oil doesn't go rancid like plant oils, it is better for the skin in many ways.

☹ <u>MASCARA:</u> **Mega Mascara All Weather Mascara** *($24)* is an absolute mess. This builds negligible length, no thickness, and makes lashes feel dry and stick together; it also tends to flake throughout the day. This is an extremely stubborn mascara that comes with warnings about how difficult it is to remove—and these should be taken seriously, as few mascaras are as maddeningly tenacious as this one. **Mega Primer** *($16)* is a sticky lash primer that forms a white coating to bulk up the eyelashes. It's completely unnecessary given the prevalence of superior mascaras that can achieve long, lush lashes without the help of an additional product. **Duo Lash Treatment Mascara** *($28)* is a double-sided mascara with one end being the Mega Primer reviewed above and the other a standard mascara that will eventually lengthen lashes with no clumping. The primer makes no discernible difference and is a complete waste of money.

EPICUREN (SKIN CARE ONLY)

Figuring out a way to describe how truly unbelievable I found the claims espoused by Epicuren took me awhile. They rank up there with some of the worst. (Although, to my chagrin, I must admit that the number of companies on my "overblown offenders" list gets longer and longer by the day.) Epicuren's marketing nonsense (though an expletive I can't use would have been far better than the word "nonsense") is just infuriating because I'm certain there are lots of consumers who will want to believe what this company professes. First, let's take the natural air out of this overinflated balloon of claims. Epicuren claims that its products are hypoallergenic, noncomedogenic, and absolutely free of chemical preservatives or fragrances. According to the FDA, "hypoallergenic" and "noncomedogenic" are not regulated terms, and cosmetics companies can use them however they like. There are plenty of ingredients in these products that can trigger skin reactions, and these products absolutely contain fragrance. *All* ingredients are chemicals, and fragrant oils and fragrant extracts are chemicals with preservatives to keep them stable. Grapefruit might sound wonderful but get a bit of it into an open cuticle and you will have definite proof that what's natural is not automatically the best for skin.

Epicuren's claims about natural versus chemical are meaningless, especially as their products contain plenty of synthetic ingredients—didn't the marketing people read their own ingredient listings? Further, many of these products contain exceptionally "chemical" ingredients that range from polyacrylamide to triethanolamine, tetrasodium EDTA, butylene glycol, benzoyl peroxide, cetyl alcohol, diazolidinyl urea, carbomer, propylparaben, and on and on. The notion that these are natural-based products is just ludicrous.

While some of the unnatural ingredients on the Epicuren label are easy to spot, others are disguised with names like P.C.M.X., the trade name for chloroxylenol, a preservative, or Plantaren 2000, a detergent cleansing agent. That's not bad, but it is definitely not natural either.

It is important to point out that almost none of the items on the Epicuren ingredient labels meet FDA regulations for accurate ingredient identification, leaving you in the dark as to what you are really putting on your skin. Given how few regulations exist for cosmetics companies to follow, it is inexcusable when a company can't even comply with the one thing legally required of them.

Epicuren's collection of other erroneous or misleading information is extensive. Just as an example, Epicuren states that its zinc oxide sunscreen "is truly a new millennium product; especially, in the wake of all the medical publications such as the *New England Journal of Medicine*, etc. on the dangers caused [by] using chemical sunscreen ingredients that irritate the skin, such as octyl methoxycinnamate, benzophenone-3, benzophenone-4 and octyl dimethyl and PABA." What is really incredible is that Epicuren didn't notice that some of its own sunscreens contain some of the very ingredients it criticizes, including octyl methoxycinnamate and benzophenone-3, and at levels ranging from 5% to 7.5%. Epicuren also claims that its products are free from petrochemicals, although some of the products contain isoparaffin and Vaseline, both decidedly petrochemical-based ingredients.

I won't even get started on the prices for these products. For more information about Epicuren, call (800) 235-1217 or visit www.epicuren.com. **Note:** All Epicuren products are highly fragranced.

The Reviews E

☺ $$$ **Herbal Cleanser** *($48 for 4 ounces)* is a standard, detergent-based cleanser (which isn't natural in the least) that would work well for normal to oily skin.

☹ **Citrus Herbal Cleanser** *($41 for 4 ounces)* contains lemon oil (and it does smell like lemon oil) and that can be irritating to the eyes. Even if I thought its claim that this product contains "natural surfactants" was true, all surfactants are potentially drying.

☺ **Gelle Cleanser** *($17 for 4 ounces)* uses a standard, detergent-based cleanser with some water-binding agents, making it an option for normal to oily skin.

☺ $$$ **Apricot Cream Cleanser** *($31 for 4 ounces)* is a good, emollient plant oil–based cleanser that contains mostly plant oil, though it does need to be wiped off and can leave a slight greasy feel on the skin.

☹ **Milk Cleanser** *($34 for 8 ounces)* contains several potentially irritating plant extracts, including grapefruit, rosemary, and camphor. Aside from that, this would have been a good emollient cleanser for dry skin.

☹ **Medicated Acne Cleanser** *($54 for 8 ounces)* is a standard, detergent-based cleanser that contains triclosan. Triclosan is a good disinfectant but it has not been shown to be effective against the bacterium that causes blemishes. This also contains some potentially irritating plant extracts.

☺ $$$ **Medicated Acne Gel** *($49 for 4 ounces)* contains 10% benzoyl peroxide, a concentration that makes it effective for disinfecting the bacterium in skin that can cause acne. The gimmick in this product is that it is supposed to contain 5% asymmetric oxygen, something that is supposed to "make it the most effective acne treatment known." It is true that oxygen can kill bacteria, but the notion that this can penetrate skin and help is at best minimally possible, not to mention that oxygen is a problem for generating free-radical damage.

☺ $$$ **Crystal Clear Makeup Remover** *($27 for 4 ounces)* is a standard, but good, silicone-based eye-makeup remover that also contains trace amounts of vitamins and a mix of plant extracts that, for the most part, can be good anti-irritants.

☺ $$$ **Apricot Facial Scrub** *($34 for 4 ounces)* is supposed to be "a surgical scrub." Run for your life if your doctor is scrubbing with finely ground apricot and walnut shells, which is what this product contains, along with thickeners, fragrance, and preservatives. It is a decent scrub, but there is no reason to use this over other far less expensive scrubs or just plain baking soda for that matter.

☺ $$$ **Fine Herbal Scrub** *($51 for 4 ounces)* is almost identical to the Apricot Facial Scrub above only with a smaller amount of abrasive, and the same basic comments apply.

☺ $$$ **Extra Fine Citrus Herbal Scrub** *($37 for 8 ounces)* is similar to the Fine Herbal Scrub above and the same comments apply. Of course, given the simple formulation, it begs the question to ask why not just use crushed almond or walnut shells for a lot less money and identical results?

☺ $$$ **Citrus Herbal Polisher** *($41 for 8 ounces)* is just baking soda and detergent cleansing agents. Can you imagine charging this amount of money for baking soda and a cleansing agent! Unbelievable!

☺ **$$$ Benzoyl Peroxide Scrub** *($27 for 4 ounces)* contains 2% benzoyl peroxide along with crushed nuts and detergent cleansing agents. None of that is a problem for skin, though the benzoyl peroxide is better in a leave-on product than in a rinse-off-the-skin cleanser. This also contains plant oils that can be a problem for oily skin types. All in all, there are far less expensive ways to gain the benefit of an exfoliant scrub (baking soda) or benzoyl peroxide (from products at the drugstore).

☹ **Acne Conditioning Astringent** *($16 for 4 ounces)* lists alcohol as its second ingredient, which makes this astringent too irritating and drying for all skin types.

☺ **$$$ Enzyme Conditioner** *($22 for 2 ounces)* is a good toner with water-binding agents and a small amount of antioxidants. The lemon and sage extracts can be skin irritants. Whatever claims Epicuren makes about the benefit of "enzymes" in their products, none of them have even one shred of research supporting them. Actually, this product doesn't even contain enzymes!

☺ **$$$ Protein Mist** *($20 for 4 ounces)* is similar to the Enzyme Conditioner above and the same comments apply.

☺ **$$$ Acidophilus Probiotic Emulsion** *($60 for 4 ounces)*. If you want acidophilus, there are yogurts and supplements that are a far better source than this cosmetic formulation; in fact, it's unlikely the acidophilus in this product is still active. Besides, there is no known benefit for skin when it's applied topically. Other than that, this is just an OK moisturizer with some plant oil and a teeny amount of vitamin E, very average and boring.

☺ **$$$ Botanical Elixir** *($48 for 1 ounce)* claims to contain "33 highly beneficial botanical substances." That's a lot of plants to put on one face! There is no way to tackle the claims surrounding each of the substances appearing in this lotion (though you can look them up in Chapter Seven, *Cosmetics Dictionary*), but the amount of each ingredient is minuscule, and a few are relatively irritating to skin, including arnica, lemon, and the fragrant oils. This turns out to be a good emollient moisturizer with some excellent antioxidants and water-binding agents, but the anti-irritants are negated by the presence of the irritating plant extracts.

☺ **$$$ Colostrum Serum** *($80 for 2 ounces)*. Colostrum is a fluid secreted in animal and human breast milk at the start of milk production. The source of the colostrum used in cosmetics or supplements is animal. While there is absolutely no question that human colostrum transfers many important active immunological compounds to a newborn, that is where the benefits start and stop, at least for nourishing the body. When it comes to topical application of colostrum, there have been no studies monitoring its effect on human skin. The only study that does exist showed colostrum to have no wound-healing function on skin (Source: *Journal of Dermatologic Surgery and Oncology,* June 1985, pages 617–622).

☺ **$$$ Custom Blended Aromatherapy Aloe Vera Gel** *($14 for 4 ounces)* is just what the name implies. Your skin would be far better off if you just picked up some plain aloe vera gel from the health food store and skipped this fragranced version.

The Reviews E

☺ $$$ **CXc Stabilized Vitamin C Topical** *($172 for 2 ounces)* is supposed to contain a 15% concentration of ascorbyl glucosamine, although whether or not that is helpful for skin isn't supported by research. In fact, ascorbyl glucosamine, a form of vitamin C, has little to no research showing it to have the antioxidant or skin-lightening properties of other forms of vitamin C. The only study that does exist showed it to be ineffective for skin lightening (Source: *Dermatology*, 2002, volume 204, number 4, pages 281–286). Most likely it is a good antioxidant and the other ingredients, which include a small amount of water-binding agents, a teeny amount of vitamins E and A, and fragrance, make it a good moisturizer for normal to dry skin. But for that price you could soak in a tubful of orange juice!

☺ $$$ **Enzyme Concentrate** *($56 for 1 ounce)* actually doesn't contain any enzymes of any kind on the ingredient list. So much for product names and claims. What you do get is a lightweight moisturizer for normal to slightly dry skin that contains some good water-binding agents and antioxidants.

☺ $$$ **Live Enzyme Gel Plus** *($68 for 2 ounces)* is similar to the Enzyme Concentrate above and the same comments apply.

☺ **Epicuren Emulsion** *($26 for 2 ounces)* is similar to all of Epicuren's enzyme products, so this one doesn't contain any enzymes either. What it does contain are some good water-binding agents in an emollient base of plant oils and thickeners. It's OK but lacks antioxidants and anti-irritants.

☺ **Evening Emulsion** *($32 for 2 ounces)* is similar to the Epicuren Emulsion above and the same comments apply.

☺ $$$ **Eye Brightener** *($44 for 0.5 ounce)* is a fairly ordinary, lightweight lotion. The plant extracts are a mix of irritants and anti-irritants. The teeny amount of vitamin E is barely noticeable. It can be an option for normal to slightly dry skin.

☺ $$$ **Eye Cream** *($56 for 0.5 ounce)* is a good emollient moisturizer for normal to dry skin that contains a good blend of antioxidants and water-binding agents.

☺ $$$ **HydroPlus** *($48 for 2 ounces)* is an average emollient moisturizer for normal to dry skin.

☺ $$$ **Instant Lift** *($89 for 2 ounces)* won't lift skin anywhere and the price is a real letdown for what amounts to just an OK moisturizer.

☺ **Moisture Surge Gel** *($28 for 1 ounce)* is just water-binding agent, thickener, and grapefruit extract. It's OK as a very lightweight moisturizer for normal to slightly dry skin.

☹ **Pigment Balancer** *($38 for 0.5 ounce)* contains an unknown amount of hydroquinone, but in the long run the quantity doesn't matter because the jar-type packaging ensures that this highly unstable ingredient, which is easily affected by air and light, will deteriorate shortly after it's opened.

☹ **Glycolic Polymer Solution 5% or 10% Gel or Lotion** *($20 for 2 ounces)*. Both of these glycolic acid–based lotions have a pH of 5.5 to 6, and that is too high to allow either one to be effective as an exfoliant.

☺ $$$ **Pro-Collagen III** *($30 for 0.33 ounce)* supposedly "selectively amplifies the biosynthesis of Collagen III in human skin.… The phenomenal results are typically visible within 48 hours." If that were possible, how would the skin know when to stop making collagen? Would your skin just plump up forever? After all, this is merely a good moisturizer for normal to dry skin with some good water-binding agents and vitamins, and there is absolutely nothing special in this product that would even begin to warrant the exaggerated claims.

☺ $$$ **Retinol Concentrate** *($48 for 0.5 ounce)* is basically a good moisturizer for normal to dry skin, with antioxidants and plant oil. Even though there is a small amount of research suggesting that what retinol does is related to the effects of Retin-A or Renova, it isn't conclusive. What is conclusive is that retinol is an unstable ingredient and requires packaging that doesn't let air or light in. This product's jar packaging ensures that the retinol will be gone shortly after you open it. If you are interested in retinol, many lines, from L'Oreal to Cetaphil, have versions that are packaged to ensure its stability.

☹ $$$ **Rose Otto** *($48 for 0.5 ounce)* is just fragrant oils and plant oil. Using plain apricot or avocado oil (you can get those at any health food store) would be far better for your skin.

☹ $$$ **Skin Rejuvenation Therapy (SRT)** (available in **SRT #1**: Bulgarian Rose Otto, Jasmine, Neroli, Lavender, and Vetiver; or **SRT #2**: Melisse, Clarysage, Myrrh, and Frankincense) *($60 for 1 ounce)*. According to the Epicuren brochure, "This is the ultimate treatment for cell rejuvenation to help reverse the signs of aging." But if this is the ultimate then what are all the other vitamin, enzyme, AHA, herbal, and colostrum products in this line for? The protein derived from DNA is just a water-binding agent and (thankfully) cannot affect the genetic material in your skin cells. The fragrance in these SRT products can be irritating for skin, but aside from that they can be good moisturizers for normal to dry skin. Just don't expect one wrinkle to change, because it won't.

☺ $$$ **Ultra Rose Treat Emulsion** *($71 for 4 ounces)* contains some good antioxidants and water-binding agents in an emollient base, and it would be an option for normal to dry skin. The teeny amount of lactic acid in this product has no exfoliating properties for skin.

☺ $$$ **Youth Teen Anti-Oxidant Serum Moisturizer** *($48 for 1 ounce)* is a good lightweight moisturizer with good antioxidants. It lacks water-binding agents and anti-irritants. There is nothing about this product that makes it better for skin of any age.

✓☺ $$$ **Zinc Oxide Sunblock Sunscreen SPF 20** *($28 for 2 ounces)* is a very good, zinc oxide–based sunscreen in an emollient base that contains some very good antioxidants.

✓☺ $$$ **YouthTeen SPF 30 Sun Protection** *($34 for 4 ounces)* is a very good, in-part avobenzone-based sunscreen in a lightweight gel that contains some very good antioxidants. It is a great option for normal to oily skin.

☺ $$$ **YouthTeen SPF 20 Lip Balm** *($8 for 0.33 ounce)* is a very good, in-part avobenzone-based sunscreen. The emollient base would be good for dry lips.

The Reviews E

☹ **Invisible Spray Sunscreen SPF 20** *($18 for 4 ounces)*; **Skin Treat Sunscreen SPF 15** *($20 for 4 ounces)*; **Sport Treat Sunblock SPF 30** *($34 for 4 ounces)*; and **Enzyme Lip Balm SPF 15** *($8 for 0.33 ounce)* do not contain the UVA-protecting ingredients of titanium dioxide, zinc oxide, or avobenzone, and are not recommended.

☺ **$$$ Bulgaricum Home Mask** *(64 for 4.5 ounces)* is a very fancy way to sell yogurt for the skin. You're supposed to mix the *Lactobacillus bulgaricus* powder in this product with Epicuren's Pure Aloe, and you get a mixture that is supposed to detoxify and oxygenate skin. However, in general, skin doesn't like oxygen (oxygen triggers free-radical damage), ergo the need for *anti*oxidants. If you like yogurt for your skin, there are far cheaper versions than this, like pure yogurt and pure aloe vera from a health food store, for a fraction of the cost.

ERA FACE FOUNDATION

☺ **$$$ ERA Face Foundation** *($65)* is an aerosol spray that mists a light layer of foundation onto the skin. The effect is supposed to be akin to airbrushing (as in photographs), but this just doesn't hold true in real life. The main problem with this type of foundation is that it's difficult to keep the mist from getting to places where you don't want it—namely, your lips, eyelashes, eyebrows, hairline, clothing, countertops, or someone else passing by you at the wrong moment. The mist is propelled out forcibly enough to be a messy proposition, which may be all some women need to steer clear of products like this. In all fairness, ERA Face Foundation does come with a cloth headband to protect the hairline, as well as blending tools to aid in application, but that's a lot of trouble for what ends up being just a foundation.

ERA Face Foundation is available in ten shades, and the majority are quite good. Shades R4 and R9 are a bit too peach for most skin tones, but the final look depends on how much is sprayed on—the less you use the more natural each color looks. The texture is neither too oily nor too watery, and it blends easily into the skin with the included puff. You can also use a regular makeup sponge or, if you prefer, your fingers. The formula and finish are best for normal to very oily skin—normal to dry skin would fare best using a moisturizer beforehand. The fine mist produced with this makeup allows for medium to full, yet very fine-textured, natural-looking coverage. The pigments in ERA Face Foundation are suspended in a water bubble that essentially bursts upon contact with the skin, and dries down in ten seconds to a solid matte finish. You can layer for more coverage, or you can use the included sponge to buff the product to a more solid matte finish.

Are there benefits to using an aerosol foundation like ERA? Mostly, no. It may have use for the body, but it isn't exactly body-style makeup, since traces of it can rub off on clothing. This spray-on method of application takes experimentation to create the desired effect and not look like you've used too much product. There are other foundations available that can boast natural coverage, silky textures, and real-skin colors that do not come with the drawbacks inherent with spray-on foundations. I suggest approaching this type of makeup with caution, and try to experience it at a salon or spa before purchasing. Call (310) 456-9700 or visit www.classifiedcosmetics.com to find a location near you that carries the ERA Face Foundation.

One more word of warning: Although ERA sprays on a light veil of foundation, the silicone- and talc-based formula is water and transfer resistant. That's yet another reason to approach this with caution, as something this tenacious will not be easy to remove when it lands where it is not supposed to be. Removing ERA Face Foundation will require more than a standard, water-soluble cleanser! An oil- or silicone-based makeup remover works well, but still takes some effort, as the makeup tends to "stain" the skin.

ERNO LASZLO

Throughout its history, the Erno Laszlo line has had more owners than Elizabeth Taylor has had husbands. The company changed hands yet again in 2002, when Cradle Holdings, a new cosmetics entity created under the private equity firm Fox Paine, purchased it. At the helm of this operation is Robert Nielson, the former Group President of Estee Lauder Companies. Considering his pedigree and 40+ years of experience, one would think he would jump right in and begin overhauling the antiquated aspects of this line. However, although some outdated skin-care products have been discontinued, it appears as though the standard principles of Dr. Laszlo's skin-care routine and history are still intact. What has been given the proverbial axe are almost all of the makeup products—and what remains is hardly worth mentioning, especially at these prices. At press time, it was still not clear whether or not Laszlo's makeup line will continue to fade into obscurity or will revive itself. Meanwhile, the various counter personnel I interviewed felt strongly that the "new" focus of Laszlo would be on its skin-care heritage.

According to the company's brochure, Dr. Erno Laszlo, a Hungarian dermatologist, was "the first to combine the exact science of his profession with the art of cosmetology" using "precisely diagnosed treatments dispensed with a doctor's touch." Great copy, except that Erno Laszlo was never licensed to practice medicine in this country, and some say he was never even a medical doctor in Eastern Europe.

In his time, Laszlo's claim to fame was prescribing skin-care regimens for wealthy women who could afford to "succumb to the 'Laszlo Ritual' of daily skincare." His ritual included washing with old-fashioned bar soap (he had women with dry skin cover their face in oil before using the soap), then splashing the face 30 times with a basin full of the soapy rinse water, and then splashing the face 30 times with scalding hot water. When that was done, his patients would finish by soaking their skin with apple cider vinegar. Dr. Laszlo proclaimed that nothing cleaned better than hot water and soap, but because soap's alkaline content changed the skin's pH level, apple cider vinegar was needed to restore it.

One of the problems with legendary or ancient skin-care routines is that new research more often than not negates what we once thought to be true. After all, the good doctor couldn't have known about sun damage or the need for exfoliation, or that hot water can hurt skin and cause surfaced capillaries. He clearly didn't know that soap is too irritating and that irritation is a problem for skin (it's one of the major causes of collagen destruction). Plus, alkaline substances (that's what soap is) have studies showing they can increase bacteria content in skin and damage the skin's healing process. With today's gentle cleansing techniques, you leave the pH of the skin alone, so there is no reason to worry about bringing it back to the right pH.

In 1966 Laszlo sold the right to use his name and retail his products to Chesebrough-Pond's. Now, some 30 years after Laszlo's death (and, as mentioned above, a slew of other owners), most of the skin-care routines still include using bar soap and all of that soapy and hot-water splashing, but the rest of the regimen is just loosely based on the "doctor's" concepts. For more information about Erno Laszlo, call (800) 865-3222 or visit www.ernolaszlo.com.

ERNO LASZLO SKIN CARE

☹ **Active pHelityl Cleansing Lotion** (*$30 for 6.8 ounces*) is a relatively standard, detergent-based, water-soluble cleanser that also contains some emollients, which can make it better for normal to dry skin; however, it also contains some fairly irritating plant extracts, and that's disappointing.

☺ $$$ **Active pHelityl Oil Pre-Cleansing Oil for Dry to Slightly Oily Skin** (*$32 for 6.8 ounces*) is supposed to be used before you use the soaps (reviewed below) to protect the skin and help remove makeup. But your skin wouldn't need protection if you weren't using such a drying product to wash your face. Given that this is mostly mineral oil and fragrance, skip the fragrance and just use plain mineral oil for far less; that's what Dr. Laszlo used to do.

☹ **Active pHelityl Soap for Dry and Slightly Dry Skin** (*$23 for 6 ounces*) is a standard, tallow-based bar of soap with the same ingredients found in all soaps. This one does contain some plant oil, but that won't help the dryness caused by the other ingredients.

☹ **Beta Wash** (*$32 for 6.8 ounces*) uses sodium C14-16 olefin sulfate as the main cleansing agent, along with sodium lauryl sulfate, which makes it too drying and potentially irritating for all skin types.

☹ **HydrapHel Cleansing Bar for Extremely Dry Skin** (*$27 for 6 ounces*) is a standard bar cleanser with a tiny amount of emollients, but it can still be quite drying, which isn't good for dry skin.

☹ **HydrapHel Cleansing Milk for Extremely Dry Skin** (*$28 for 6.8 ounces*) contains several potentially irritating plant extracts, including lemongrass, pine needle, arnica, and kiwi. They can be a problem for any skin type, but especially for dry skin.

☺ $$$ **HydrapHel Cleansing Treatment Liquid Cleanser for Extremely Dry Skin** (*$25 for 4.3 ounces*) is little more than an expensive, standard cold cream, and not very different from just using mineral oil or Vaseline by itself (the two primary ingredients in this product). It can be an option for dry skin, but it can leave a greasy film.

☹ **Sea Mud Cleanser** *($22 for 4.4 ounces)* contains fairly drying detergent cleansing agents as well as some fairly irritating plant extracts, including arnica and pine needle. There is sea mud in it, but that just adds to the dryness.

☹ **Sea Mud Soap for Normal, Slightly Oily, and Oily Skin** *($27 for 6 ounces)* is as standard a bar of soap as it gets, containing tallow and sodium cocoate with a little sea mud thrown in. This is too drying and irritating for all skin types.

☹ **Special Skin Soap for Oily and Extremely Oily Skin** *($27 for 6 ounces)* contains the standard soap ingredients of tallow and sodium cocoate, along with the detergent cleanser sodium lauryl sulfate, which is very drying and irritating.

☹ **Multi-pHase Eye Makeup Remover for All Skin Types** *($28 for 4 ounces)* is basically just silicone and plant extracts. The plant extracts include some that can cause irritation and that should not be used repeatedly on skin, particularly not around the eyes.

☺ **$$$ pHelitone Gentle Eye Makeup Remover** *($18 for 3 ounces)* is far more gentle than most of the above cleansers because there are no irritating plant extracts or drying cleansing agents in it. This is just a basic makeup remover that uses a gentler detergent cleansing agent and some slip agents, with no fragrance or coloring agents. If they could figure out a "gentle" formulation for this product, why not be gentle with all skin types?

☹ **Conditioning Preparation for Oily to Extremely Oily Skin** *($28 for 6.8 ounces)* is almost pure alcohol, and very irritating to the skin, plus it contains resorcinol, which makes this product a serious skin irritant.

☹ **Heavy Controlling Lotion PM Oil Control for Slightly Oily to Extremely Oily Skin** *($28 for 6.8 ounces)* won't control anything, and the alcohol makes it too drying and irritating for all skin types.

☺ **$$$ HydrapHel Skin Supplement Freshener for Extremely Dry and Dry Skin** *($28 for 6.8 ounces)*. At least this one doesn't contain any alcohol. This would be an OK, basic toner for most skin types.

☹ **Light Controlling Lotion Toner for Slightly Dry to Oily Skin** *($28 for 6.8 ounces)*. The amount of alcohol this contains makes it too irritating for all skin types.

☹ **Regular Controlling Lotion PM Oil Control for Slightly Dry and Normal Skin** *($30 for 6.8 ounces)* is alcohol-based, which makes it too irritating and drying for all skin types, but that is particularly inexcusable in a product for dry skin.

☹ **AHA Revitalizing Complex** *($65 for 1 ounce)* contains about 3% to 4% AHAs and BHA combined, but the pH is too high for it to be an effective exfoliant, not to mention that far more effective and less expensive AHA and BHA products are widely available.

☺ **Active pHelityl Cream PM Moisturizer for Slightly Dry Skin** *($32 for 2 ounces)* is a standard, emollient, Vaseline-based moisturizer. This is easily replaced by a number of moisturizers at the drugstore, from Lubriderm to Cetaphil, for a fraction of the price.

☺ **$$$ Retinol Reparative Therapy** *($87 for 1 ounce)* is just another retinol product, and an exceptionally overpriced one at that. Given this formulation, there is no reason to consider it over L'Oreal's, Neutrogena's, or Cetaphil's, all of which are just as good for one-eighth the price, and their products are contained in more airtight packaging (which keeps the retinol stable).

☺ $$$ **Retinol Reparative Therapy for Eyes** *($69 for 0.5 ounce)* is virtually identical to the Retinol Reparative Therapy above and the same basic comments apply. The price difference between these is a marketing contrivance if I've ever seen one!

✓☺ $$$ **Antioxidant Complex for Eyes, Lightening, Firming, Protective Eye Treatment for All Skin Types** *($42 for 0.5 ounce)* is a lightweight lotion that contains some very good antioxidants and water-binding agents. It also contains mulberry extract and magnesium ascorbyl phosphate (a stable form of vitamin C), both of which can have a melanin-inhibiting effect on skin, but the amounts present in this product are minuscule and not enough to have any effect. The tiny amount of lemon has little risk of causing irritation.

✓☺ $$$ **Antioxidant Concentrate for Eyes, Intensive Therapy for the Eye Area** *($48 for 0.5 ounce)* is a very good emollient moisturizer with an array of very good water-binding agents and antioxidants.

☹ $$$ **Antioxidant Mattifying Complex** *($55 for 2 ounces)* is more of a lightweight moisturizer for normal to oily skin than something that will provide much oil-absorbing properties. The film-forming agents can leave a matte feeling, though it won't last long, while the witch hazel (mainly alcohol) can be an irritant. This contains only a tiny amount of antioxidants.

☹ **Antioxidant Moisture Complex SPF 15 Oil-Free Moisturizer for All Skin Types** *($55 for 2 ounces)* doesn't contain the UVA-protecting ingredients of avobenzone, zinc oxide, or titanium dioxide, and is not recommended.

✓☺ $$$ **Antioxidant Moisture Complex Cream for Extremely Dry to Normal Skin** *($67 for 2 ounces)* is a very good emollient moisturizer for someone with dry skin. It contains a good mix of antioxidants and water-binding agents.

☹ **Daily Moisture Protection Lotion SPF 15 AM Moisturizer with Sunscreen for All Skin Types** *($50 for 2.5 ounces)* doesn't contain the UVA-protecting ingredients of avobenzone, zinc oxide, or titanium dioxide, and is not recommended.

☹ **Cellular Exchange Therapy SPF 15** *($97 for 2.5 ounces)* doesn't contain the UVA-protecting ingredients of titanium dioxide, zinc oxide, or avobenzone, and is not recommended. The price is shocking for such a poorly formulated sunscreen.

✓☺ $$$ **Retexturizing SAP Complex** *($67 for 1 ounce)* is a good, silicone-based moisturizer that also contains some very good antioxidants, anti-irritants, and water-binding agents.

☺ $$$ **HydrapHel Emulsion AM Moisturizer for Extremely Dry and Dry Skin** *($50 for 2 ounces)* is a very good emollient moisturizer with an impressive group of antioxidants, water-binding agents, and anti-irritants. Do not wear this during the day unless you are also wearing an additional moisturizer or foundation with effective sun protection.

☺ $$$ **HydrapHel Complex PM Moisturizer for Extremely Dry and Dry Skin** *($57 for 2 ounces)* is a fairly standard, mineral oil–based moisturizer with a tiny amount of antioxidants and water-binding agents. The HydrapHel Emulsion AM version above is a far better formulation than this one.

☹ $$$ **Moisture-Firming Throat Cream for All Skin Types** *($42 for 2 ounces)* would be a good emollient moisturizer for dry skin, but it contains some fairly irritating plant extracts, including ginseng and arnica.

☹ $$$ **pHelitone Replenishing Eye Cream for All Skin Types** *($42 for 0.5 ounce)*. This is pricey for what amounts to little more than water, thickeners, Vaseline, and a teeny amount of vitamin E.

☹ $$$ **pHelityl Cream PM Moisturizer for Normal Skin** *($57 for 2.1 ounces)* is an exceptionally ordinary emollient moisturizer for normal to dry skin.

☺ $$$ **pHelityl Lotion AM Moisturizer for Slightly Dry to Slightly Oily Skin** *($50 for 3 ounces)* is an OK emollient moisturizer for someone with dry skin. But someone with even slightly oily skin is not going to be happy with this much oil in a product of any kind, and without sunscreen it's useless to anyone for daytime. This does contain small amounts of antioxidants, but for the money this leaves much to be desired.

☹ $$$ **R.E.M. Intensive Night Therapy** *($85 for 2 ounces)*, with emollients, waxes, and plant oil, is intensely emollient and would work for dry skin. What isn't so intense is the small amount of water-binding agents and antioxidants it contains.

☺ $$$ **R.E.M. SPF 30** *($68 for 2.5 ounces)* is a very good, avobenzone-based sunscreen that also contains some good water-binding agents and antioxidants. It's interesting to point out that the third ingredient is *Taraktogenos kurzii* seed oil, also known as chaulmoogra oil. This oil was once the treatment for leprosy worldwide due to its antimicrobial properties (Source: *Proceedings of the National Academy of Sciences USA*, February 2000, pages 1433–1437). It can be a skin irritant.

☹ $$$ **Total Skin Revitalizer Facial Hydration Enhancer for All Skin Types** *($56 for 1 ounce)* is just a totally ordinary, lightweight, emollient moisturizer for normal to dry skin. There is nothing enhanced about it and it definitely is not for all skin types.

☹ $$$ **Total Skin Revitalizer for Eyes Hydration Enhancer for the Eye Area** *($48 for 0.5 ounce)* is an OK moisturizer for normal to dry skin with tiny amounts of antioxidants and water-binding agents.

✓☺ $$$ **C10 Radiance Cream** *($62 for 1.05 ounces)* is a silicone- and Vaseline-based moisturizer that includes a good mix of antioxidants and a water-binding agent.

☹ **Beta Wash** *($32 for 6.8 ounces)* uses sodium C14-16 olefin sulfate and sodium lauryl sulfate as the main cleansing agents, which would be irritating enough for any skin type, but then this product throws more fuel on the fire by including camphor, menthol, and peppermint.

☹ $$$ **Beta Complex Acne Treatment** *($65 for 2 ounces)* contains a 1% salicylic acid concentration, but the price is mind-boggling, especially given that the pH is too high for this to be an effective exfoliant.

☹ **Beta Target Blemish Treatment** *($18 for 0.5 ounce)* contains too much alcohol, eucalyptus, peppermint, menthol, and camphor for any skin type, much less blemish-prone skin.

☹ **Beta Mask** *($36)* has the same problems as the Beta Target Blemish Treatment above and the same comments apply.

☹ **Oil-Free Sunblock SPF 25 for All Skin Types** *($22 for 4.3 ounces)* doesn't contain the UVA-protecting ingredients of avobenzone, zinc oxide, or titanium dioxide, and is not recommended.

☺ **Self-Tanning Lotion SPF 8** *($22 for 4.2 ounces)* doesn't contain the UVA-protecting ingredients of avobenzone, zinc oxide, or titanium dioxide, and the low SPF 8 makes this absolutely not recommended for sun protection. However, it works fine as a self tanner.

☹ **Sun Control Mist SPF 15** *($22 for 3.5 ounces)* doesn't contain the UVA-protecting ingredients of avobenzone, zinc oxide, or titanium dioxide, and is not recommended.

☺ **$$$ Salve Extreme** *($65 for 2 ounces)* isn't particularly extreme, but it is a good emollient moisturizer with an interesting blend of water-binding agents. What it lacks, especially for this price, is an equally interesting mix of antioxidants.

☹ **Intensive Decollete Cream SPF 20** *($82 for 1.75 ounces)*. The only thing intense about this poorly formulated sunscreen (it doesn't contain the UVA-protecting ingredients of titanium dioxide, zinc oxide, or avobenzone) and moisturizer is the inane price. It is not recommended.

☺ **$$$ Hydra-Therapy Skin Vitality Treatment, Two Phase Moisture Mask for All Skin Types** *($38 for four applications of each phase)* is a two-part system that is so amazingly ordinary it is almost embarrassing. You mix an ordinary liquid of water, film-forming agent, water-binding agent, slip agent, and preservatives with a simple powder that is mostly algae and some salts, apply it to your face, let it set, and then rinse. What a waste of time and money!

☹ **Sea Mud Mask** *($38 for 7 ounces)* is basically a standard clay mask, but it also contains alcohol and peppermint, which makes it too irritating for all skin types.

☺ **$$$ pHelitone Firming Eye Gel Mask for All Skin Types** *($30 for 0.5 ounce)* is an absurdly standard, lightweight gel for minimally dry skin. It lacks any interesting water-binding agents or antioxidants.

☺ **$$$ Lip Therapy** *($42 for 0.5 ounce)* is a very good emollient moisturizer.

ERNO LASZLO MAKEUP

☹ **FOUNDATION: Regular Normalizer Shake-It** *($34)* is Laszlo's worst foundation—why this one is still being sold is perplexing, as there is little to extol in this watery, alcohol-laden makeup. It's difficult to apply, can streak, provides minimal coverage, and can dry out the skin.

☹ <u>CONCEALER:</u> **Conceal Correcteur** *($29)* is another click-pen concealer whose delivery system feeds concealer onto a built-in synthetic brush tip. This formula starts out creamy, then dries quickly to a powdery finish that is quite smooth. However, the price is ridiculous for what you get, and the two poor shades will be problematic for most skin tones.

☺ $$$ <u>POWDER:</u> **Controlling Face Powder** *($30)* and **Controlling Pressed Powder** *($27)* are both talc-based and have a supremely soft texture and a natural finish on the skin. The two shades are decent, though Translucent Shell can be too pink for fair skin. Laszlo recommends this for oily skin, but normal to dry skin will fare best with this powder. **Duo-pHase Face Powder** *($30)* and **Duo-pHase Pressed Powder** *($27)* are recommended by Laszlo for normal to dry skin. However, with a lighter, drier, talc-based texture and stronger matte finish than the Controlling powders above, these are preferred for normal to oily skin. The two colors are identical to those of the powders above.

☺ $$$ <u>EYE PENCIL:</u> **Multi-pHase Eye Pencil** *($16)* is a standard pencil that is neither noteworthy nor worth this price.

<u>MASCARA:</u> ☺ $$$ **Multi-pHase Mascara** *($19)* easily defines lashes without clumping or smearing, and lengthens well while providing a touch of thickness. This is a fine mascara, but there are several less expensive options in other lines that can outperform it.

☺ $$$ **Multi-pHase Advanced Mascara** *($19)* is hardly exciting, especially at this price. As a lengthening mascara, it succeeds, though it never goes beyond average, even with lots of effort. This is about as advanced as sending a telegram instead of an e-mail.

ESOTERICA

Owned by the Medicis Pharmaceutical Corporation, Esoterica is probably one of the most long-enduring cosmetics lines being sold in drugstores around the world. This is the original skin-lightener line, using hydroquinone as the active ingredient in its fade creams. There is a great deal of research showing hydroquinone to be effective for inhibiting melanin production, but hydroquinone is also an exceptionally unstable ingredient susceptible to deterioration with exposure to light or air. The traditional jar packaging Esoterica uses ensures that the hydroquinone won't last until the product is used up. What's even more disappointing are the poorly formulated sunscreens. Effective sunscreens, meaning they have an SPF 15 or greater and contain UVA-protecting ingredients, are a crucial element for avoiding skin discolorations. For more information about Esoterica, visit www.drugstore.com or www.medicis.com.

☹ **Skin Discoloration Fade Cream SPF 10** *($7.96 for 3 ounces)* does not contain the UVA-protecting ingredients of titanium dioxide, zinc oxide, or avobenzone, and is not recommended.

☹ **Skin Discoloration Cream Facial With Sunscreen** *($7.69 for 3 ounces)* does not contain the UVA-protecting ingredients of titanium dioxide, zinc oxide, or avobenzone, and is not recommended.

☺ **Skin Discoloration Fade Cream Regular** *($7.69 for 3 ounces)* contains 2% hydro-quinone, which is effective for inhibiting melanin production; however, the jar packaging means that the product's stability is not well-protected.

☺ **Skin Discoloration Fade Cream, Sensitive Skin, Unscented** *($7.69 for 3 ounces)* is similar to the Fade Cream Regular above only with 1.5% hydroquinone, and the same basic comments apply.

ESTEE LAUDER

What sets the venerable Estee Lauder company apart from its rivals is that it owns most of the cosmetics lines it competes with. Lauder's formidable reach includes Clinique, Origins, Prescriptives, M.A.C., Bobbi Brown, Stila, Aveda, Jane (a drugstore line aimed at teenagers), and La Mer, among others. That sort of takes the notion of cosmetic secrets and throws it to the winds, doesn't it? Would Estee Lauder keep so-called secrets from its own companies?

Of course, Estee Lauder is still the grande dame of makeup lines, with a loyal follow-ing and a plethora, if not endless redundancy, of products. Ask any of the salespeople who work for this seasoned cosmetics company and they will tell you that the products sell themselves. A few years ago, Night Repair and Eyezone were jumping off the shelves; then Estee Lauder's AHA product, Fruition (discontinued in favor of the far better formulated Fruition Extra), caught fire; and now Idealist and LightSource are the flavor du jour. It only takes a cursory look at the stable of Estee Lauder products, from the line itself to its protégés, to notice that there is an overwhelming number of antiwrinkle products (over 300 in all). But the question to ask is this: If just 10 of its products could live up to their claims to get rid of wrinkles, why would you need an additional 290 products claiming to do the same thing? The Estee Lauder lineup boasts some wonderful moisturizers, but also some absurd prices for products that can't live up to their more glorious claims. For more information about Estee Lauder, call (212) 572-4200 or visit www.esteelauder.com. **Note:** All Lauder skin-care products contain fragrance unless otherwise noted.

ESTEE LAUDER SKIN CARE

☺ **Perfectly Clean Solid Cleanser Normal to Dry** *($16.50 for 4.2 ounces)* is a pricey bar cleanser that is almost identical to Cetaphil's Bar Cleanser but at five times the price. This contains fragrance and coloring agents. Despite the Vaseline content, it can still be fairly drying for all skin types, but especially for dry skin.

☺ **Perfectly Clean Solid Cleanser Normal to Oily** *($16.50 for 4.2 ounces)* is simi-lar to the Normal to Dry version above only minus the Vaseline. The same basic comments apply.

☺ **Perfectly Clean Foaming Lotion Cleanser, Normal/Dry and Dry Skin** *($16.50 for 4.2 ounces)* is a standard, detergent-based cleanser that also contains a good amount of plant oil, making it a good option for someone with normal to dry skin.

☺ **Perfectly Clean Foaming Gel Cleanser, Normal/Oily and Oily Skin** (*$16.50 for 4.2 ounces*) is an exceptionally standard, detergent-based, water-soluble cleanser for normal to oily skin.

☺ **Soft Clean Milky Lotion Cleanser** (*$16.50 for 6.7 ounces*) is a lotion-style cleanser that doesn't contain any detergent cleansing agents, making it an option for normal to dry skin. It doesn't remove makeup very well and may require using a washcloth to get everything off.

☹ **Rich Results Hydrating Cleanser** (*$18.50 for 4.2 ounces*) contains menthol, coriander, and sage, which can all be skin irritants.

☹ **Splash Away Foaming Cleanser** (*$18.50 for 3.4 ounces*) is a fairly drying, detergent-based, water-soluble cleanser. It can be an option for normal to oily skin.

☺ **Tender Creme Cleanser** (*$26 for 8 ounces*) is a standard, lotion-style cleanser with no detergent cleansing agents that can be an option for normal to dry skin. For the money, Neutrogena's Extra Gentle Cleanser is almost identical for a third the price.

☺ **Gentle Eye Makeup Remover** (*$13.50 for 3.4 ounces*) is an exceptionally standard, detergent cleanser–based eye-makeup remover and it works the same as most, though this one does not contain fragrance.

☺ **Take It Away Makeup Remover** (*$18 for 6.7 ounces*) is a fairly standard, wipe-off makeup remover that would work for most skin types.

☹ **$$$ So Polished Exfoliating Scrub** (*$19.50 for 1.7 ounces*) is a detergent-based cleanser that uses pumice as the abrasive. This can be an option for normal to oily skin, but it isn't preferred over using plain baking soda with a gentle cleanser.

☹ **Clear Finish Purifying Toner N/D** (*$16.50 for 6.7 ounces*). This extremely standard toner contains menthol, which can be a skin irritant for most skin types.

☹ **Clean Finish Purifying Toner N/O** (*$16.50 for 6.7 ounces*) is similar to the version above, only this one adds grapefruit to the menthol irritation factor.

☹ **$$$ Re-Nutriv Extremely Delicate Skin Cleanser** (*$32.50 for 7.5 ounces*) is a very standard, mineral oil–based, cold cream–style cleanser. There is very little reason to spend this amount of money for what is essentially Pond's Cold Cream. This can be an option for very dry skin, though the price is not warranted. The teeny amount of royal jelly in this product has no benefit for skin.

☹ **$$$ Re-Nutriv Moisture-Rich Creme Cleanser** (*$27.50 for 3.4 ounces*) is similar to the Delicate Skin Cleanser above, only less greasy, and the same basic comments apply.

☺ **$$$ Re-Nutriv Intensive Hydrating Cream Cleanser** (*$35 for 4.2 ounces*) is an emollient, cold cream–style cleanser that is an option for someone with normal to dry skin, but it holds no advantage over far less expensive versions at the drugstore or even other versions in this line!

☹ **Re-Nutriv Gentle Skin Toner** (*$30 for 6.7 ounces*) is an exceptionally standard toner whose second ingredient is cetrimonium chloride, a cleansing agent and disinfectant. It isn't bad for the skin, it just isn't all that gentle. It also contains arnica, which is a problem when used repeatedly on skin.

☺ $$$ **Re-Nutriv Creme** *($78 for 1.75 ounces)* is a very emollient, mineral oil–based moisturizer for dry skin. It does contain some good water-binding agents and antioxidants.

☹ $$$ **Re-Nutriv Firming Eye Creme** *($47.50 for 0.5 ounce)*. This won't firm the eye area, and the amino acids, elastin, and collagen cannot get rid of wrinkles, though they are good water-binding agents. What this lacks is the assortment of antioxidants that many of the other Lauder products contain.

☺ $$$ **Re-Nutriv Firming Throat Creme** *($55 for 1.7 ounces)* is a good emollient moisturizer for dry skin that contains a good mix of water-binding agents and a small amount of antioxidants. There is nothing in this formulation that makes it better for the throat than the face.

☹ $$$ **Re-Nutriv Intensive Firming Plus** *($95 for 1.7 ounces)* is a very overpriced, basic moisturizer for dry skin that doesn't begin to compare to lots of other far better formulated Lauder moisturizers. It does contain a small amount of AHAs, but the pH is too high for them to be effective for exfoliation.

✓☺ $$$ **Re-Nutriv Intensive Lifting Creme** *($150 for 1.7 ounces)*. While this is a good moisturizer with lots of good water-binding agents, antioxidants, and anti-irritants, there is nothing in it that will lift skin anywhere, and the price is nothing less than obscene given the ingredient list. Estee Lauder charges a lot less for other moisturizers that have a similar ingredient list.

✓☺ $$$ **Re-Nutriv Intensive Lifting Serum** *($170 for 1 ounce)* contains an impressive array of water-binding agents, anti-irritants, and antioxidants in an emollient, Vaseline-based moisturizing lotion. Everything from retinol to grape extract, mulberry, and a bevy of plant extracts make an appearance here. The concentration of each isn't much and this won't lift skin anywhere, but it is definitely an excellent moisturizer for normal to dry skin.

☺ $$$ **Re-Nutriv Intensive Lifting Series** *($250 for 14 vials, total 0.95 ounce)*. Do women really believe that there is anything in this product worth $4,000 for 16 ounces? Actually, this isn't even as impressive as the Intensive Lifting Serum above, as it lacks many of the unique plant extracts and water-binding agents its sister contains. This one is good for normal to dry skin, but for the money, this just doesn't add up.

✓☺ $$$ **Re-Nutriv Ultimate Lifting Cream** *($250 for 1.7 ounces)*. If this is the ultimate cream, it makes you wonder why Lauder needs to sell the other 300 antiwrinkle, antiaging products in their line. Ultimately, this Cream uses the kitchen-sink approach to skin, meaning it contains a little bit of everything. But what if skin needs more than just fractional amounts of a lot of ingredients? No one knows, but here you are playing for a great deal of money, and it's an expensive guessing game. There are lots of water-binding agents, antioxidants, anti-irritants, and emollients in here that are great for skin, but many Lauder products contain similar assortments for a lot less.

☺ $$$ **Re-Nutriv Replenishing Creme** *($78 for 1.7 ounces)* is an emollient moisturizer that contains some good water-binding agents, though it lacks any of the interesting antioxidants typical of many less expensive Lauder moisturizers. This one also contains several plant extracts that are potential skin irritants, including lemon, clove, and cinnamon.

☺ $$$ **Re-Nutriv Lightweight Creme** *($75 for 1.75 ounces)* isn't all that light. It contains lots of thickening agents, plant oils, and a small amount of water-binding agents and antioxidants. It is an OK, though exceedingly overpriced, moisturizer for dry skin.

☺ $$$ **Re-Nutriv Intensive Lifting Mask** *($70 for 1.7 ounces)* is mostly an emollient moisturizer that adds nothing in the way of extra benefit over many of the other Lauder moisturizers. It does contain some very good plant oils, anti-irritants, and some antioxidants.

☹ $$$ **Resilience Elastin Refirming Creme** *($60 for 1.7 ounces)* is a good, but extremely ordinary, moisturizer for someone with normal to dry skin. It does contain some good water-binding agents, but lacks many of the interesting antioxidants found in other Lauder products. Elastin is merely a good water-binding agent; there is no research showing it can affect the quality of elastin in skin.

☹ $$$ **Resilience Elastin Refirming Lotion** *($62.50 for 1.7 ounces)* is similar to the Elastin Refirming Creme above, only in lotion form, and the same review applies.

☹ $$$ **Resilience Eye Creme Elastin Refirming Complex** *($42.50 for 0.5 ounce)* is an OK moisturizer for normal to dry skin, with several state-of-the-art water-binding agents and emollients like Vaseline and shea butter, but only a teeny amount of vitamin E. However, it won't lift the skin anywhere and there is nothing about it that makes it better for the eye area than the face. There are also minute amounts of plankton, caffeine, and barley, among other extracts. If these ingredients are the answer for wrinkles, then why aren't they in the other products for wrinkles that Lauder sells? Or does everything get rid of wrinkles? Must be, because there is no uniformity among these myriad antiwrinkle products.

☹ $$$ **Resilience Eye Creme** *($42.50 for 0.5 ounce)* is an OK, silicone- and film-forming agent–based moisturizer for normal to dry skin. It does contain a decent assortment of water-binding agents, but lacks the antioxidants and anti-irritants found in many other Lauder products.

☹ $$$ **Resilience Lift Eye Creme** *($42.50 for 0.5 ounce)* is similar to the Resilience Eye Creme above only with more emollient, and the same comments apply.

✓☺ $$$ **Resilience Lift Overnight** *($70 for 1.7 ounces)* is an emollient, Vaseline-based moisturizer that contains a very good assortment of water-binding agents and antioxidants.

✓☺ $$$ **Resilience Lift Face and Throat Cream SPF 15** *($65 for 1.7 ounce)* and **Resilience Lift Face and Throat Lotion SPF 15** *($45 for 1 ounce)* are two good sunscreens with part titanium dioxide to help provide UVA protection. But no one is spending this much money on these two products just for sun protection! Clearly, the word "lift" is meant to imply that these can make a serious difference in the appearance of skin. They can't. They are simply standard sunscreens in good moisturizing bases that contain an array of water-binding agents and antioxidants, and that isn't going to lift the skin anywhere.

☺ $$$ **Verite Light Lotion Cleanser** *($22.50 for 6.7 ounces)* is an emollient, cold cream–style cleanser that is an option for someone with dry skin.

☹ $$$ **Verite Soft Foam Cleanser** *($22.50 for 4.2 ounces)*. One of the detergent cleansing agents in this product, sodium C14-16 olefin sulfonate, is not the best for any skin type, but especially not for sensitive skin. Though the Vaseline does help soften the effect, in the long run it just ends up being confusing for skin.

☺ $$$ **Verite Soothing Spray Toner** *($22.50 for 6.7 ounces)* is an OK toner for normal to dry skin that contains mostly water, slip agent, water-binding agents, plant extracts, fragrance, and preservatives.

✓☺ $$$ **Verite Calming Fluid** *($60 for 1.7 ounces)* won't calm anything, but it is a very good moisturizer with great water-binding agents and antioxidants for someone with normal to dry skin.

☺ $$$ **Verite Moisture Relief Creme** *($50 for 1.75 ounces)* is an OK moisturizer for someone with normal to dry skin.

✓☺ $$$ **Verite Special Eye Care** *($50 for 1.7 ounces)* is a very emollient, Vaseline-based moisturizer that contains a good mix of water-binding agents and antioxidants.

☺ $$$ **100% Time Release Moisturizer Creme** *($35 for 1.7 ounces)* is a moisturizer with a small amount of water-binding agents and antioxidant that is OK for someone with normal to dry skin. It is one of the more ordinary offerings in the Estee Lauder lineup.

☺ $$$ **100% Time Release Moisture Lotion** *($35 for 1.7 ounces)* is similar to the Creme version above and the same basic comments apply.

✓☺ $$$ **Advanced Night Repair Protective Recovery Complex** *($70 for 1.7 ounces)* isn't all that advanced, but it is a very good moisturizer with a first-rate mix of antioxidants, water-binding agents, and anti-irritants. One strange twist: It also contains a good amount of sunscreen, which doesn't make sense in a product that's meant to be used at night, although the sunscreen is not rated with an SPF.

✓☺ $$$ **Advanced Night Repair Eye Recovery Complex** *($45 for 0.5 ounce)* claims to address pretty much every eye-skin-care woe you can think of, from puffiness to dark circles, wrinkles, and tired skin. It sounds like the ultimate choice for eyes, but we've all heard this song before with countless other Lauder eye products, from Uncircle to Unline to Eyezone, along with a vast selection from the ten other lines under Lauder's ownership. Still, skin-repairing claims aside, this is undeniably a very good, silicone-based moisturizer that would take good care of dry skin anywhere on the face.

☺ $$$ **Age Controlling Creme** *($60 for 1.7 ounces)* is a good, lanolin-based, emollient moisturizer for someone with very dry skin that also contains some plant oils, Vaseline, mineral oil, and a small amount of water-binding agents and antioxidants. There is nothing in this product that can control even one minute of aging.

☺ **Clear Difference Oil-Control Hydrator for Oily Normal/Oily and Blemish-Prone Skin** *($27 for 1.7 ounces)* is a silicone-based moisturizer that contains some good water-binding agents and an antioxidant. It also contains salicylic acid, but the pH of the product is about 4, and that is just borderline for allowing it to be effective for exfoliation. There is nothing in it that can control oil production.

✔☺ **Estoderme Emulsion** *($27.50 for 4 ounces)* is a good emollient moisturizer for dry skin that contains some good water-binding agents and antioxidants.

☹ $$$ **Eyezone Repair Gel** *($35 for 0.5 ounce)* contains mostly water, film-forming agents, algae, slip agent, water-binding agent, vitamin A, and preservatives. The tiny amount of algae and even smaller amount of vitamin A here won't do anything for skin, much less repair it, but this is an OK, ordinary moisturizer for slightly dry skin.

☹ $$$ **Time Zone Eyes Ultra-Hydrating Complex** *($40 for 0.5 ounce)* is a lightweight, ordinary moisturizer for normal to slightly dry skin.

☹ $$$ **Time Zone Moisture Recharging Complex** *($55 for 1.7 ounces)* is similar to the Eyes Ultra-Hydrating Complex above, only with more emollients. It would be good for dry skin.

✔☺ $$$ **Fruition Extra Multi-Action Complex** *($70 for 1.7 ounces)*. The original Fruition was discontinued, and the Extra is now the only version available. The original was supposed to be an exfoliating AHA product, but it didn't contain enough AHA to have any effect; basically it was just a good lightweight moisturizer. Fruition Extra adds salicylic acid to the mix, so this is a BHA product now. It does work well as an exfoliant, but is incredibly overpriced for what you get, which is a good, lightweight moisturizing base with silicones, film-forming agents, water-binding agents, antioxidants, fragrance, coloring agents, and preservatives.

✔☺ $$$ **Future Perfect Micro-Targeted Skin Gel** *($45 for 1.75 ounces)* is not more perfect than any other moisturizer in the Lauder group. It is just a good, silicone-based, emollient moisturizer for normal to dry skin that contains a good mix of water-binding agents and antioxidants.

✔☺ $$$ **Idealist** *($42.50 for 1 ounce)*. The spin on this product is that it's a non-retinol and non-AHA wrinkle remover; it claims to be the best option around for skin. If that's the case, does that mean Estee Lauder's Fruition Extra and Diminish are now history, along with all the other AHA, BHA, and retinol products the other Estee Lauder–owned lines sell? That would never happen, of course, despite Estee Lauder's claim that Idealist is now the answer for your less-than-youthful visage. The two standout ingredients, according to Estee Lauder "… are acetyl glucosamine and sodium lactobionate." For some reason, if these two ingredients can banish wrinkles, the only company that knows about it is Estee Lauder.

What we do know about N-acetyl glucosamine is that it's an amino acid sugar, the primary constituent of mucopolysaccharides and hyaluronic acid, and is found in all parts of the skin. It has value as a water-binding agent and is effective (in high concentrations) for wound healing. There is also research (*Cellular-Molecular-Life-Science*, 53(2), February 1997, pages 131–140) showing that chitins (also known as chitosan—which is composed of acetyl glucosamine) can help in the complex process of wound healing.

However, that is a few generations removed from the acetyl glucosamine being included in a skin-care product. Besides, you have to wonder what any of that has to do with exfoliation, especially in the tiny concentration this product contains. And please understand that wound healing isn't related to wrinkles because wrinkles aren't wounds. What about the sodium lactobionate? It seems to be used in solutions as a preservative, but I wasn't able to find any research confirming Estee Lauder's contentions for it. It's a mystery. All told, this is a good, lightweight moisturizer for normal to dry skin—the silicone will leave a silky feel on the skin—and it does have plenty of anti-irritants and antioxidants. Whether or not the acetyl glucosamine and sodium lactobionate do something different is yet to be seen.

☺ $$$ **LightSource Transforming Moisture Creme SPF 15** (*$45 for 1.7 ounces*) is a very good emollient moisturizer, containing a reliable SPF 15 using avobenzone as one of the active ingredients. This would work well for someone with normal to dry skin. Now to the claims! Lauder's brochure for this product states that it contains "Millions of micro-crystals [emeralds that] convert light into positive energy, giving your skin an amazing brightness and freshness—even without makeup. Skin experiences an upsurge of energy—and is empowered to remain active … [to do] all the things it's always done, but now with dramatically enhanced levels of performance." Wow! Actually, I'm speechless. I don't know what to say about any of this. Can minuscule amounts of crushed "reflective" stones give skin energy? Not that I've seen. Is there a shred of clinical published research proving any of this to be true (other than what the Lauder company asserts)? Not a one. But at least Lauder had the good sense to add an effective sunscreen, because there will no doubt be women who will believe that sunlight's negative effects can somehow be tamed or converted by this product, and they can't. By the way, about the "millions of micro-crystals"—the amount of emerald in this product is at best described as a trace.

☺ $$$ **LightSource Transforming Lotion SPF 15** (*$45 for 1.7 ounces*) is similar to the LightSource Creme version above only without the Vaseline, which makes it better for normal to slightly dry skin, and the same basic comments apply.

☺ $$$ **Skin Perfecting Creme Firming Nourisher** (*$35 for 1.75 ounces*) is a good, lightweight, emollient moisturizer for dry skin. This product does contain arnica, a possible skin irritant with repeated use, but the amount is so small that it probably won't have any impact on skin.

☺ **Skin Perfecting Lotion Lightweight Moisturizer** (*$27.50 for 1.7 ounces*) is indeed lightweight, but it's also boring. The Creme version above is far better formulated because it has both more interesting water-binding agents and less fragrance.

✓☺ **Swiss Performing Extract Moisturizer** (*$25 for 1.7 ounces*) is a very emollient and very good moisturizer for someone with dry skin. It contains a good mix of antioxidants, plant oils, and water-binding agents. The minor concern about arnica for the Skin Perfecting Creme above applies here as well.

☺ $$$ **Uncircle** *($37.50 for 0.5 ounce).* There is nothing in this product that will have any greater effect on circles than would any other moisturizer in this line. Vaseline and film-forming agent are not what I or anyone else would call an exotic or excitingly new formulation, and fish cartilage can't affect anything around the eyes. It does contain some good water-binding agents and a small amount of antioxidants, and that's good, just not great.

☹ **Unline Total Eye Care** *($35 for 0.5 ounce).* Although many aspects of this one make it a good moisturizer, the mint and wintergreen oil are irritants and a particular problem for the eye area.

✓☺ $$$ **Nutritious Bio Protein** *($45 for 1.7 ounces)* is a very good moisturizer for normal to dry skin. However, despite the clever name, you can't feed the skin from the outside in. Still, it does contain some very good antioxidants and water-binding agents.

✓☺ $$$ **Diminish Retinol Treatment** *($70 for 1.7 ounces)* came on the scene with a fanfare of claims about getting rid of lines, evening-out skin tone, improving skin texture, and on and on, much like the claims about several of the other products in this line. It definitely contains retinol, but only about 0.1% or 0.2%. Other than that, the rest of the ingredients are an impressive mix of water-binding agents and antioxidants.

✓☺ $$$ **Day Wear Super Anti-Oxidant Complex SPF 15** *($37.50 for 1.7 ounces).* The antioxidants are not exactly at the top of the ingredient list, nor are they any more special than those in hundreds of other products, so none of that is all that super. What is good about this day cream is that it contains an SPF 15 sunscreen that is in-part titanium dioxide, one of the better ways to protect against sun damage. In that regard, this product is right on, as are most of Estee Lauder's sunscreens.

☺ **Spotlight Skin Tone Perfector** *($30 for 1.7 ounces)* is a good, silicone-based moisturizer for normal to slightly dry skin. This product is meant to improve skin color, thanks to the presence of some vitamin C and plant extracts that include mulberry root and licorice. There is some research that indicates these ingredients in pure form can inhibit melanin formation, but probably not in the tiny amount present in this product. It also contains shine.

☺ **Enriched Under-Makeup Creme** *($25 for 4 ounces)* is definitely emollient, but also boring. This is a very ordinary moisturizer for someone with very dry skin.

☹ **Counter Blemish Lotion** *($14 for 0.45 ounce).* Alcohol is listed as the second ingredient, and it also contains zinc phenolsulfonate and cinnamon, which means this ends up causing irritation and dryness, effects that don't counter blemishes in the least.

☺ **Go Bronze Tinted Self Tanner for Face** *($18.50 for 1.7 ounces)* and **Go Bronze Tinted Self Tanner for Body** *($25 for 5 ounces)* are like all other self-tanners in that they use the active ingredient dihydroxyacetone to turn the skin brown. The advantage to the tint is that it lets you see where you've applied it, helping to achieve a more even tan look.

☺ **Stay Bronze Moisturizing Tan Extender for Face** *($19.50 for 1.7 ounces)* is just a self-tanner that uses dihydroxyacetone, the same ingredient in all self-tanners, to affect the color of skin. It would work as well as any other.

☺ **$$$ So Clean Deep Pore Mask** *($19.50 for 3.4 ounces)* is a standard clay mask that also contains some good water-binding agents, though their effectiveness would be negated by the absorbing properties of the clay. This would work as well as any for absorbing oil.

☺ **$$$ So Moist Hydrating Mask** *($19.50 for 3.4 ounces)* is indeed hydrating, but no more so than any other moisturizer in the Estee Lauder family.

☺ **$$$ Stress Relief Eye Mask** *($27.50 for ten 0.4-ounce packets)* is a somewhat sticky mask that doesn't feel great on the skin, although it is a good lightweight moisturizer. Still, there is nothing in it that will give the skin relief from anything.

☺ **$$$ Triple Creme Hydrating Mask** *($27.50 for 2.5 ounces)* contains good moisturizing ingredients, so it would feel good on dry skin, but no more so than any other moisturizer in the Estee Lauder lineup.

✓☺ **Sunblock for Body SPF 25** *($18.50 for 5 ounces)* is a good, in-part titanium dioxide– and zinc oxide–based sunscreen in a good emollient moisturizing base with a small amount of water-binding agents and antioxidants. It would be a good option for normal to dry skin.

✓☺ **Sun Block for Face SPF 15** *($18.50 for 1.7 ounces)* is similar to the Sunblock for Body SPF 25 above and the same basic comments apply.

✓☺ **Sun Block for Face SPF 30** *($18.50 for 1.7 ounces)* is similar to the Sunblock for Body SPF 25 above and the same comments apply.

☹ **Oil Free Sun Spray SPF 15** *($18.50 for 4.2 ounces)* doesn't contain the UVA-protecting ingredients of titanium dioxide, zinc oxide, or avobenzone, and is not recommended.

ESTEE LAUDER WHITELIGHT BRIGHTENING SYSTEM

☺ **$$$ WhiteLight Brightening Cleansing Foam** *($26 for 4.2 ounces)* is a standard, rather gentle, water-soluble cleanser that has a mild foaming action. It contains a nice assortment of anti-irritants and water-binding agents, which can be helpful for skin, though they would be rinsed off before they had much chance to have any benefit. Like all the WhiteLight products, it does contain fragrance. If left on the skin, the vitamin C, along with the mulberry extract in this product, may inhibit melanin production, but in a cleanser that benefit would be rinsed down the drain.

☹ **$$$ WhiteLight Brightening Cleansing Powder** *($26 for 4.2 ounces)* is a wax- and talc-based cleansing powder that forms a soaplike lather when used with water. This can feel mildly abrasive on the skin as well as be overly drying. It can also leave a soapy film on the skin (the fourth ingredient is sodium hydrogenated tallow glutamate). The comments about the vitamin C and mulberry ingredients in the Cleansing Foam above apply here, too.

☺ **$$$ WhiteLight Brightening Treatment Lotion** *($30 for 4.2 ounces)* claims it is "far more than a toner," but based on the ingredient list this is much closer to a toner than anything else. It contains mostly water, slip agents, vitamin C, antioxidants, tourmaline (a gemstone), clay, fragrance, preservatives, and mica (a shiny earth mineral). This is good, but not great. The vitamin C and mulberry extract can help inhibit melanin production.

☹ **WhiteLight Concentrated Brightening Stick** *($30 for 0.22 ounce)* is essentially a silicone-based cream-to-powder stick concealer that has a strange mauve tint. This does little to conceal brown or tan discolorations, except for giving a somewhat ashen appearance when applied. Even if you are all for the use of color correctors, mauve is traditionally used to neutralize yellow or sallow undertones, not brown ones. It does contain a small amount of mulberry extract, which may help inhibit melanin production.

☺ $$$ **WhiteLight Brightening Moisture Creme** *($37.50 for 1 ounce)* is a good moisturizer for normal to dry skin that contains mostly water, emollient, slip agent, thickeners, silicone, antioxidants, water-binding agents, anti-irritants, fragrance, and preservatives. It does contain a small amount of mulberry extract, which may help inhibit melanin production.

☺ $$$ **WhiteLight Brightening Protective Base SPF 30** *($30 for 1.7 ounces)*. Diligent use of sunscreen with UVA-protecting ingredients is the most important element for reducing skin discolorations, and this moisturizer covers that need nicely. Featuring one of the longest ingredient lists you'll likely ever see for a sunscreen, it contains an impressive group of antioxidants and water-binding agents and includes zinc oxide as one of the active sunscreen ingredients. It is worth considering if you have normal to dry skin that's not prone to breakouts.

☺ $$$ **WhiteLight Concentrated Brightening Serum** *($65 for 1.3 ounces)* promises to make "the look of porcelain-perfect skin a reality," but the effect is entirely cosmetic, thanks to the lavender opalescent powder it contains, which lends an ethereal soft blue glow to the skin. This silicone-based serum has a good assortment of antioxidants and anti-irritants. But if what you're paying for is the promise of perfect skin and no skin discolorations, this product is incapable of delivering that, despite its otherwise state-of-the-art formula. It is best for normal to slightly dry or slightly oily skin.

ESTEE LAUDER MAKEUP

If any line has a golden touch when it comes to launching new makeup products, it's Estee Lauder. Season to season, they seem to have a divining rod on the pulse of what women want—or maybe the women who frequent the Lauder counter have simply come to expect their choices to be dictated by this well-heeled company. The cosmetics collection is nothing short of exhaustive, at least when it comes to the sheer number of products available. The tester units have become more accessible, but if you're hoping to compare different foundations, concealers, or powders, you'll need a salesperson's assistance, because it is almost impossible to navigate this line alone.

It is interesting to note that other Lauder-owned companies, from Clinique to Prescriptives, often launch similar, if not identical, products. For example, several months after Lauder's Equalizer foundation debuted, Lauder-owned Origins came out with Stay Tuned Balancing Face Makeup, a nearly identical formula (sans sunscreen) that costs less than half of Lauder's Equalizer. The same thing happened with Lauder's Fresh Air Continuous Moisture Tint SPF 15. Again, a nearly identical Origins product, Nude & Improved Bare-Face Makeup SPF 15, came on the scene, boasting effective sun protection and a significantly smaller price tag. The only real difference among many of these products is the marketing angle and the targeted consumer demographic.

Lauder's selection of makeup excels in their foundation textures and colors (including improved options for darker skin) and their eyeshadows, which are superior to those from most other department-store lines. Other strong points include some reliable concealers and blushes, and an ever-imposing selection of lipsticks. The makeup loses momentum with its uninspired collection of mascaras and merely OK brushes. Given that other lines under the Lauder umbrella (such as Clinique and Stila) are ably producing superior versions of these makeup must-haves, there's no reason to remain loyal to Lauder's namesake line.

FOUNDATION: Estee Lauder's foundations offer something for everyone in terms of texture and formulation. However, several of the formulas are without the recommended UVA-protecting ingredients, and while a couple have the benchmark SPF 15 rating, there are still those that miss the mark. It's even more important to take great care in finding the right shade, as Estee Lauder still likes to sneak in the occasional rosy pink and peach colors. However, foundation samples are readily available for almost all of the formulas reviewed below—so don't hesitate to ask for these if you're uncertain about shade or formula.

✓☺ **$$$ So Ingenious Multi-Dimension Makeup SPF 8** *($32.50)* is a truly silky liquid makeup. This airy foundation establishes a new benchmark when it comes to an ultra-smooth feel, great application, and a natural, non-drying matte finish. If only the titanium dioxide sunscreen was boosted to a higher number; the SPF 8 is an embarrassment! As is, you'll have to pair this with an effective sunscreen to net a full day's worth of protection. There are 16 shades available, with options for very light and darker skin tones. Although most of them are admirable, they aren't as across-the-board brilliant as those from Lauder's So Ingenious Powder Makeup are. The following shades are too gray, peach, or pink for most skin tones: Fresco, Auburn, Outdoor Beige, Pebble, and Linen. If you have normal to slightly dry skin and prefer sheer to medium coverage, this one should be on your short list! ✓☺ **So Ingenious Multi-Dimension Powder Makeup** *($32.50)* offers an ultra-smooth, suede-like texture that does not have an overly dry finish. This provides a clean, quick application and blends extraordinarily well over the skin, leaving a soft matte finish. As is typical with powder foundations, coverage is light to medium, and this type of foundation is best suited to all except very oily or very dry skin types. Essentially, talc-based powder foundations like this are middle-of-the-road options for those whose skin is neither too greasy nor too parched. Lauder has set a precedent by introducing 16 beautiful skin-realistic shades. There are suitable options for light and dark skin tones, and the only colors to view with caution are Cool Champagne (slightly pink) and Cool Praline (very slightly peach), but even these shades may work for some skin tones and should not be altogether ignored. By the way, this product features Lauder's

QuadraColor technology, which supposedly allows pigments to self-adjust depending on what type of light you're in. You won't see this powder magically fine-tune itself as you go from sunny outdoors to the fluorescent lighting of your office, but it's natural finish and seamless coverage do keep it from looking too thick or chalky on the skin, regardless of the lighting. This comes with a dual-sided sponge, with one side porous and the other smooth. The smooth side affords a nicer finish and more even coverage, but test both sides to see which one you prefer. ✔☺ **Equalizer Smart Makeup SPF 10** *($32.50)* is similar in concept (and number of shades) to Lauder-owned Origins Stay Tuned Makeup ($15). Both of these foundations make the same improbable claim of being able to moisturize dry areas while absorbing oil from oily areas. How a product could hold back its moisturizing ingredient from one area while absorbing oil or moisture from another is a mystery, and in fact it doesn't work—which you will be able to tell immediately from the first application. All claims aside, Equalizer leapfrogs over Stay Tuned by adding an all titanium dioxide–based sunscreen. (What would have really been smart would have been an SPF 15; an SPF 10 is cheating skin for no good reason.) It also has a very silky, light texture, offering sheer to medium coverage with a soft, slightly powdery finish that would be great for those with normal to slightly oily skin. If you have any dryness, it can feel tight and look flaky soon after it's blended. There are 20 shades, and the majority of them are wonderful. Several colors do shy toward being a bit too peach, but not nearly enough to warrant avoiding them. However, there are two colors that you should steer clear of, Vanilla and Copper, because they are just too peach or pink to come across as natural on almost any skin tone. There are a couple of options for very light skin tones, but darker skin tones have the edge here, as almost all of the deep colors are gorgeous.

☺ $$$ **Futurist Age-Resisting Makeup SPF 15** *($32.50)* leaves out the most important antiaging weapon anyone can have: a sunscreen with UVA-protecting ingredients! How disappointing that a foundation with such a superlative texture and luminous finish has this as its major flaw. If you have normal to dry skin and are prepared to wear a sunscreen underneath, you will get a great medium-coverage foundation, but be careful of the following colors, all of which can be too rose, orange, or copper for most skin tones: Fawn, Pale Almond (slightly pink), Tender Cream, Cool Sand, Golden Petal, Cameo, Sunlit Topaz, and Bare Beige. **Lucidity Light-Diffusing Makeup SPF 8** *($29.50)* claims it has "special light-diffusing pigments" that "actually reflect light away from fine lines and wrinkles so they seem to disappear," but this is just a standard, silicone-based moisturizing foundation with a smooth texture and medium coverage. Any wrinkles will still be plainly visible, if not magnified—but that's true of any foundation. Lucidity's SPF 8 is not only too low for daily protection, it does not contain UVA-protecting ingredients. It's an option if you have normal to dry skin and are willing to wear a separate sunscreen underneath. Of the 13 shades, the following can be too peach or pink for most skin tones: Outdoor Beige, Cool Beige, Neutral Beige, Sun Beige, Rich Ginger, and Vanilla Beige. Porcelain and Ivory Beige are slightly pink, but still worth considering if you have light skin. **Minute Makeup Creme Stick Foundation SPF 15** *($29.50)* has a light, creamy texture that applies smoothly and dries to a soft, powder finish. But don't let the name fool you—it takes as long to apply as any other makeup, unless you're going for spot application. Consider this one if you have normal to dry skin and prefer sheer to medium adjustable coverage. There are eight mostly excellent shades, and only Maize and Golden tend toward the peachy side, though not irreparably so. One word of warning: Estee Lauder claims this is non-acnegenic. I disagree. Several ingredients in it could trigger breakouts, not the least of which is the active sunscreen ingredient, titanium dioxide, which is great for UVA protection but can be problematic for acne-prone skin. **Double Wear Stay-in-Place Makeup SPF 10** *($29.50)* is great—at least when it comes to a terrific matte texture that doesn't move. Someone with normal to oily skin will be impressed with the application and the way it holds up over a long day, though it can provide too much coverage—this is pretty thick stuff—and, as is true for most ultra-matte foundations, it's hard to remove. Of course, the SPF should be a 15 even though it does have a pure titanium dioxide base. As the formula stands, you would require another sunscreen underneath, which can add an oily or layered feel on oily skin. Still, this is one of the last strong contenders in a diminishing selection of ultra-matte, long-wearing makeup. Of the 12 shades available, four can be too peach, pink, or rose for most skin tones: Pebble, Bronze, Spice, and Soft Tan. **Enlighten Skin-Enhancing Makeup SPF 10** *($29.50)* has a wonderful texture, and uses titanium dioxide as the sunscreen agent; what a shame it only has an SPF 10, which leaves the skin in need of more sun protection. The application is smooth and sheer, leaving a beautiful, slightly matte finish. It is best for someone with normal to combination or slightly dry skin. The eight-shade color selection isn't as strong as the selections of Lauder's newer foundations, though there are some options for very light skin tones. The following colors are too pink or peach for most skin tones: Neutral Beige, Gentle Ivory, Outdoor Beige, and Vanilla Beige. **Re-Nutriv Intensive Lifting Makeup** *($65)* is elegantly packaged in a frosted-glass jar complete with golden cap and trim. This is billed as Lauder's ultra-luxurious makeup, perfect for dry to very dry skin. Yet this silky, silicone-based formula blends down to a natural matte finish that is not at all emollient or something those with dry skin would enjoy. It's best for those with normal to slightly dry or slightly oily skin seeking medium coverage and a whatever-it-may-cost makeup. The seven shades are impressively neutral, with the exception of the peach-tinged Radiant Wheat and Radiant Tan. Do I need to mention that this won't lift the skin even one centimeter?

☺ $$$ **Maximum Cover Camouflage Makeup for Face & Body SPF 15** *($26)* goes on creamy-smooth and tends to stick to the skin, which can feel uncomfortable. It doesn't provide as much coverage as the name implies (this isn't Dermablend), but it does cover well, provides a titanium dioxide sunscreen, and blends to a solid matte finish. The range of seven shades is commendable, with only Creamy Tan being a bit too peach. There are no options for darker skin tones.

☺ **$$$ Impeccable Protective Compact Makeup SPF 20** *($29.50)* has a texture similar to the Minute Makeup SPF 15 above, only this is slightly creamier and offers heavier coverage and has inadequate UVA protection. If you are willing to wear an adequate sunscreen underneath, this could work well, but there are better options out there, such as Clinique's City Base Compact Foundation SPF 15 ($21). Of the eight shades, Vanilla and True Beige can be too pink or rose. **Fresh Air Continuous Moisture Tint SPF 15** *($34)* is an impressive tinted moisturizer in terms of its silky, easy-to-blend texture, radiant finish, and four wonderful shades that offer a sheer veil of color. What's disappointing, not to mention shocking, is the lack of adequate UVA protection from the sunscreen. This would have been an easy one to recommend for normal to dry skin, but with the insufficient sunscreen, there is no reason to consider this over Origins Nude and Improved Bare-Face Makeup SPF 15 ($15).

☹ **Double Matte Oil Control Makeup SPF 15** *($29.50)* was launched after the winning Double Wear Makeup, and one would have thought the reliable SPF would carry over since this foundation has a similar theme. Well, the SPF is higher, but it doesn't contain UVA protection. In addition, the texture is thick, five of the nine colors are poor, and the finish is slightly sticky and chalky, making this a bona fide "Why bother?" Oilier skin looking for a foundation with reliable sun protection would do well to consider Revlon's Shine Control Mattifying Makeup SPF 15 instead. **Maximum Cover Color Corrector** *($26)* is the exact same formula as the Maximum Cover Makeup above, but this is a mint green shade. Not only is green an odd color to use on the face, this is too opaque to look anything but obvious. **Polished Performance Liquid Makeup** *($26)* and **Country Mist Liquid Makeup** *($21)* are holdovers from several years ago, and they're both standard, no-frills, emollient foundations for normal to dry skin that come in disappointing colors and are not worth considering over Lucidity. **Fresh Air Makeup Base** *($21)* is equally disappointing, though it has a lighter texture and a clay-based matte finish that would only please someone with oily skin. If that's you, consider Clinique's superior Stay True Makeup over this one.

<u>CONCEALER:</u> ☺ **$$$ Double Wear Stay in Place Concealer SPF 10** *($17)* is a liquidy, ultra-matte concealer that provides intense coverage and includes a titanium dioxide sunscreen. You must be exact in your blending, as this dries very quickly to a matte finish that won't budge. There are six shades, and the two darkest colors are a bit peach, but they may work for some skin tones. For dark circles, this is preferred to Estee Lauder's **Smoothing Creme Concealer** *($17)*. The Smoothing Creme comes in a squeeze tube, so be cautious of pressing out too much. However, it does have a pleasant, creamy texture and a natural finish that allows for semi-opaque coverage with minimal chance of creasing. The three colors are all worthy of consideration, but there is nothing for very light or dark skin tones. **Lucidity Light-Diffusing Concealer SPF 8** *($18)* features a fountain pen–style applicator. You need to turn the base of the concealer to feed the product onto a sponge tip, and then apply. The typical problem with this method is that it often gives

you too much concealer, and thus you end up wasting or over-applying product. Still, the texture of this is exceptionally smooth, with a soft matte finish, and the six shades are mostly excellent and provide even coverage. The only color to be cautious with is Light, which is too peach for most fair skin tones. The titanium dioxide–based sunscreen has an SPF 8, which is too low to rely on for significant sun protection, though it's a nice adjunct to a foundation with SPF 15.

☺ $$$ **Uncircle Concealer SPF 20** ($17) is a thick cream concealer in a pot that offers an excellent sunscreen, but despite this and the one very good color, it can crease into lines, so test it carefully before making the investment.

☹ **Automatic Creme Concealer** ($15) comes in only two colors and a mauve tint. The mauve is unnecessary and the other shades are too rosy peach to recommend.

POWDER: ☺ $$$ **So Ingenious Multi-Dimension Loose Powder** ($30) is impressive for the sizable packaging alone! The powder looks like it's suspended in air as you gaze upon the clear container, an entirely impressive presentation from every angle. What's inside is just as impressive—a silky, imperceptibly light talc-based powder. The six colors become peachier as you go from light to dark, but the sheer application prevents that from having any effect on the skin. This powder is so smooth you may not even notice the shiny particles on hand to add a glistening finish, though I did. They're not too intrusive, but still noticeable and diminish this as an option for anyone looking to use powder for a polished matte finish. **Equalizer Smart Loose Powder** ($28) provides a comparatively small amount of loose powder in a container that is covered with a built-in screen. You take the enclosed thin powder puff and press down, and a sheer veil of powder is forced up onto the sponge. This is supposedly an innovation for those on the go who wish to use loose powder as if it were pressed, but it's still a messy proposition, and you'll end up with excess powder on your fingers no matter how careful you are. This talc-free formula uses nylon-12 as the absorbent, and each of the five peachy, but sheer, shades contains "thirsty micro-sponges" to intercept oil for all-day shine control." Even if these so-called sponges worked, they would be too exhausted trying to mop up the emollients and lavender wax already in the formula, let alone your skin's oil. Consider this an overpriced, but fine-textured, light-coverage powder that's ideal for normal to dry skin. Anyone seeking serious shine control would fare better with Lauder's Double-Matte powders. **Lucidity Translucent Loose Powder** ($27) and **Lucidity Translucent Pressed Powder** ($22) are standard, but good, talc-based powders. Both have six great colors (though Medium Intensity 3 can be too peach) and a wonderful soft, silky finish with a faint hint of shine. Lucidity is supposed to change the way light focuses on your face. It doesn't. Though they feel nice and smooth, neither of these looks any different from dozens and dozens of other powders. **Enlighten Skin-Enhancing Powder** ($22) is a standard, talc-based powder, available as a pressed powder only. It has a light, dry texture and applies extremely sheer. It is sold with a brush rather than a puff and that makes sense, given the concept of this "no powder" powder, whose four shades are all excellent. **Double-Matte**

Oil-Control Loose Powder *($22)* and Double-Matte Oil-Control Pressed Powder *($22)* are talc- and silica-based powders. They both have a great texture, with a dry, slightly chalky finish, which can be a problem for some skin tones; however, someone with very oily skin will appreciate how well these absorb. The pressed version has a thicker texture, but it still provides light coverage. All the colors are good options for very light to medium-dark skin tones. Bronze Goddess Soft Matte Bronzer *($27)*, which has a much smoother texture, downplayed (but still visible) shine, and a beautiful tan color.

☺ $$$ Re-Nutriv Intensive Smoothing Powder *($50)* is a very smooth, talc-based loose powder with an outrageous price tag! The "radiant finish" attributed to this silky powder is simply shine—and lots of it. The four colors are mostly excellent, though Medium is just too peach to look natural on the skin. If you fall for the notion that shiny powders will minimize wrinkles, consider the considerably less expensive options from Revlon SkinLights first. Instant Sun All-Over Bronzing Duo *($27)* is a dual-sided powder bronzer that applies unevenly and is quite shiny. It's not worth considering, especially over Lauder's Bronze Goddess Soft Matte Bronzer reviewed above.

☺ $$$ BLUSH: Blush All Day Natural CheekColor *($21.50)* has a soft, dry texture that feels slightly grainy and doesn't apply as smoothly as it could. Still, it does the job, goes on color-true, and the varied shade selection has options for very light to medium skin tones. Each blush color has some amount of shine, with the most obvious being Potpourri, Raspberry, Rose Marble, and Pink Sand. Minute Blush Creme Stick for Cheeks *($26)* has a light, creamy, slippery texture that dries to a sheer, minimal powder finish. The six colors are gorgeous, with a couple of options for deeper skin tones (Russet and Spice). This type of product works best for normal to dry skin types. Note: Each shade tends to go on warmer than it looks from the stick. BlushLights Creamy CheekColor *($25)* is a silky-smooth cream-to-powder blush that offers eight sheer, attractive colors, but must be applied with a deft hand because it dries almost immediately to a soft powder finish. Although each shade has a hint of shine, only Honey Shimmer and Pink Shimmer are too shiny for daytime wear.

EYESHADOW: ✓☺ Color Intensity Microfine Powder Eyeshadow *($13.50)* has an ultra-smooth texture and applies exceptionally well without being too powdery. These are pressed quite softly, so be cautious of the powder cake breaking apart. As for the color intensity, these are somewhat bolder than what Lauder has offered in the past, but not by much. What's really great is the selection of matte shades. Sand Dollar, Fawn, Brown Sugar, Hazelnut, Dusk, Twilight, and Chocolate are the ones to check out the next time you're near a Lauder counter. Equally impressive are the ✓☺ $$$ Color Intensity Duos *($25)* and Color Intensity Quads *($35)*. The Duos feature some sensible (though mostly shiny) pairings, with Truffle the sole matte option. The Quads actually provide five colors—three well-coordinated eyeshadows that vary set to set, and two cake eyeliner/brow filler shades that are the same in each set. Although these are predominantly shiny, Vintage, Tulip, and Brunette are great combinations. ✓☺ Pure Color Eyeshadow *($20)* are single eyeshadows packaged in weighty, Lucite cubes with a crystal flip cap. The product inside lives up to the ostentatious container, as each shade has a satin-smooth texture and beautiful application that blends well. There are a few matte options to consider, such as Tea Box, Espresso Cup, Plum Pop, and Caramel Square. Each shade is sheer compared to Lauder's Color Intensity Microfine eyeshadows.

☺ $$$ **Go Wink Liquid** and **Go Wink Powder Eyeshadows** *($16)* offer more choices for adding glitz and gleam to your eyes. The liquid version is actually a cream-to-powder formula that comes with a wand applicator. It dries quickly to a reasonably solid powder finish, and the iridescence is visible from across the room. The powder version is a multitextured eyeshadow that is pretty to look at, but it's really just another shiny eyeshadow to embrace or ignore, depending on your preferences.

☹ **Shadow Stay Eyelid Foundation** *($15)* is a silicone- and wax-based stick that has a sheer mauve tint. This goes on a bit thick, does not prevent eyeshadows from creasing, and is absolutely not needed if you have a reliable matte-finish concealer on hand.

EYE AND BROW SHAPER: ☺ $$$ **Automatic Pencil for Eyes** *($22.50, $10 for refill)* is a standard, twist-up, retractable pencil in an elegant container. It is among the more pricey pencils on the market, but the refills are a bargain and then you have the sexy container, if you're into that kind of thing. Some of the colors are too shiny and fairly greasy, so be careful; this can smear under the eye. **Automatic Brow Pencil Duo** *($22.50, $10 for refill)* comes in the same elegant, refillable packaging as the Automatic Pencil for Eyes above. This has a soft, slightly creamy texture that applies evenly without being too thick or greasy. The price is steep, but if you're a dyed-in-the-wool brow pencil fan, it's worth an audition and there are options for blondes and redheads.

☺ **Brow Gel** *($15)* is a standard brow groomer with a good brush and minimal sticky after-feel.

☺ **Eye Defining Pencil/Smudger** *($15)* is a basic pencil that needs sharpening and has a creamy texture that glides on. These claim to have a "non-smudge" formula, but they are creamy enough so they can definitely smudge by midday. ☺ $$$ **Two-in-One Eyeliner/Browcolor** *($25)* goes on wet or dry, but works best when used wet. It comes in one compact with two colors: Brown and Black. Although it does work to fill in brows or line the eye, the color selection is limited and almost any matte eyeshadow can perform the identical function. These two colors are also represented in Lauder's Color Intensity Quad Eyeshadows.

☹ **Liquid Eyeliner** *($15)* comes in two shades and features a thin brush that applies an even line. As nice as that is, this tends to dry so slowly as to seriously try your patience and risk smearing. **Natural Brow Filler** *($15)* is a fat, one-color eyebrow pencil that isn't by any means a one-size-fits-all product. The broad tip makes it hard to control the color through the brow, and the color isn't in the least natural if you have very light or dark brows.

LIPSTICK AND LIP PENCIL: ☺ $$$ **Pure Color Long-Lasting Lipstick** *($22)* is being called "the most technologically advanced color line on the market" by Lauder executives, but I assume none of them have experimented with as many lipsticks as I have. Although this lavishly packaged lipstick is a comfortable, creamy formula with a smooth texture and opaque coverage, the finish is glossy enough to slip into any lines around the mouth. The mostly splendid colors also have minimal to no stain, which means they won't wear nearly as well as other options from Lauder, such as their True or Go Pout lipsticks. **Pure Color Crystal Lipstick** *($22)* promises "sheer electricity, daring shine," but the only thing that will get a charge out of this slick, glossy lipstick is your credit card. The colors are fine, but fleeting. **Sumptuous Lipstick** *($18)* claims it has a "never-before-seen gel-based formula that glides on, stays on," but after one test drive you'll be ready to dispute the claim for yourself. This creamy, opaque lipstick is silicone-based, so it does glide on with ease and feels light on the lips. Yet aside from having a small amount of stain, these won't redefine anyone's expectations for a long-wearing lipstick (well, except for perhaps Lauder's). **Go Pout Lip Color** *($16)* presumably adds dimension and fullness to the lower lip and shadows the contour of the upper lip. Quite a feat for a standard lipstick! However, all this adds up to is a good creamy lipstick with a fair amount of iridescence. That can indeed affect the way light is reflected off the lips (or anywhere else), just not in the way the marketing language wants to make you think it does. **True Lipstick** *($17.50)* comes in Satin or Matte. Both have a slick feel and are opaque. The Satins have a glossy finish, whereas the Mattes (which are not matte in the least) have a creamy finish. There is enough stain in the products to let these colors go the distance, but the number of shades is dwindling to make room for Lauder's newer formulas.

☺ $$$ **Futurist Lipstick SPF 15** *($17.50)* is a rather standard, creamy lipstick that has enough of a greasy feel to make those with bleeding-lipstick problems cringe. The SPF 15 sounds impressive, but alas, without UVA protection there is no reason to consider this part of your or anyone else's future plans. **All Day Lipstick** *($15)* is extremely creamy, bordering on greasy, with medium coverage and no stain to speak of. Consider yourself lucky if you can get this to last past mid-morning! **Lip Blush SPF 15** *($16)* does not have adequate UVA protection, so count on this being nothing more than a very standard, sheer, glossy lipstick. **High Shine Lip Lacquer SPF 15** *($16)* also does not have reliable UVA-protecting ingredients, making this just a sticky, semi-opaque "wet" gloss. **Automatic Pencil for Lips** *($22.50; $10 for refill)* is a standard, twist-up, retractable lipliner, but the tip of the pencil comes out of a wider than normal opening, which makes it too thick to be capable of drawing a thin outline around the mouth.

☺ $$$ **Pure Color Gloss** *($20)* carries over the opulent packaging of its lipstick predecessor, but this costly gloss offers little innovation when it comes to feel, performance, or finish. It's just minimally sticky lip gloss with sheer, iridescent colors. **Go Pout Sheer Lip Glaze** *($16)* is for those who couldn't get enough pouting from the original Go Pout lipstick. This smooth, non-sticky iridescent lip gloss offers sheer colors that leave an alluring, iridescent glossy finish. If packaging isn't your paramount interest, you'll find that this lasts longer and is richer than the Pure Color Gloss above.

The Reviews E

☺ **Lip Defining Pencil/Brush** *($15)* is a standard pencil with a creamy feel and enough stain to help lip color cling a little longer. The pencil includes a brush at one end, which is a convenient feature.

MASCARA: ☹ **$$$ More Than Mascara** *($18)* is just mascara, plain and simple. It does little to impress, especially at this price. For decent length without clumps, this remains an effective, but boring, option. **Illusionist Maximum Curling Mascara** *($19.50)* is a rather disappointing mascara, especially when you consider the grandiose claims attached to it. Illusionist begs you to "give your lashes dramatic curl and unprecedented lift in one sweep," but it takes several sweeps to build average length, minimal thickness, and no discernible curl. This doesn't clump, smear, or flake and is an option if you need lengthening mascara, but it's no match for less expensive options such as L'Oreal's Le Grand Curl ($7.49).

☹ **Pure Velvet Dramatic Volume Mascara** *($18)*. If length, thickness, and volume are your goals, this mascara may send you over the edge trying to achieve them. You will get a clean, sheer application, but it's incredibly slow going. **Lash Primer Plus Full Treatment Formula** *($16)* is sold as a pre-mascara conditioning base for lashes. It is an unwarranted step, given the industry-wide availability of superlative one-step mascaras. The formula itself is no more conditioning than most mascaras, so that promised benefit is easy to dispel.

☺ **$$$ Futurist Lash-Extending Mascara** *($18)* is a distinct improvement over the other Estee Lauder mascaras, building nice length and thickness with no clumps or smudges. This tends to go on wetter than most, so be extra-cautious of smearing.

☺ **BRUSHES:** Estee Lauder's **Brushes** *($15–$35)* were mildly retooled, though the improvement is still not enough to make these worth considering over the excellent brushes from Lauder's vast portfolio of brushes from other lines, from Aveda to Stila. Both the **Powder Brush** *($25)* and **Blush Brush** *($20)* are options, but they're almost too soft and are not dense enough to control application. There is only one **Eyeshadow Shading Brush** *($15)* and it remains a fine option for a smaller, flat shadow brush. The **Eyelining Brush** *($15)* is the same nylon "push" eyeliner brush made popular by Trish McEvoy. The synthetic **Concealing Brush** *($15)* is versatile, and can double as an eyeshadow brush, while the retractable **Golden Lip Brush** *($15)* and oversized, but stout, **All Over Face and Body Brush** *($35)* are easily passed up in favor of more practical options from other lines.

EUCERIN (SKIN CARE ONLY)

For more information about Eucerin, call Beirsdorf Inc., at (800) 227-4703 or visit www.eucerin.com.

☺ **Gentle Hydrating Cleanser** *($7.99 for 8 ounces)* isn't hydrating, though it is a very good, very standard, detergent-based, water-soluble cleanser for normal to slightly dry or slightly oily skin. It is fragrance and color-agent free.

☺ **Aquaphor Healing Ointment** (*$5.69 for 1.75 ounces*) is a basic, ordinary moisturizer for dry skin that contains mostly Vaseline, thickeners, and mineral oil.

☺ **Daily Sun Defense Sensitive Skin Lotion SPF 15** (*$7.99 for 6 ounces*) is a good avobenzone-based sunscreen in an ordinary, though emollient, moisturizing base.

☺ **Facial Moisturizing Lotion SPF 25** (*$8 for 4 ounces*) is a very good in-part titanium dioxide– and zinc oxide–based sunscreen in a fairly emollient, though standard, moisturizing base for someone with normal to dry skin.

☹ **Face Renewal Alpha Hydroxy Moisturizing Lotion SPF 15** (*$6.99 for 4 ounces*) does not contain the UVA-protecting ingredients of titanium dioxide, zinc oxide, or avobenzone, and is not recommended.

☺ **Dry Skin Therapy Plus Intensive Repair Cream** (*$7.99 for 4 ounces*) is not intensive in the least; it is just a very ordinary, urea-based moisturizer with some mineral oil and thickening agents. Urea is a good exfoliant that can be helpful for skin, but this cream lacks good water-binding ingredients and antioxidants.

☹ **Itch Relief Moisturizing Spray** (*$7.89 for 6.8 ounces*) contains menthol, a counter-irritant, but that means it is also irritating for skin and not recommended for regular use.

☺ **Original Moisturizing Creme** (*$4.99 for 2 ounces*) is an extremely heavy, ordinary moisturizer. It would be best for someone with extremely dry, parched skin, but there are many more elegant and interesting formulas readily available.

☺ **Original Moisturizing Lotion** (*$6.89 for 8 ounces*) is basically just thickeners and mineral oil, which makes it a mediocre moisturizer for very dry skin.

☺ **Daily Replenishing Lotion** (*$6.99 for 12 ounces*) is a very standard, though emollient, moisturizer for dry skin.

☺ **Plus Alpha Hydroxy Moisturizing Lotion** (*$7.49 for 6 ounces*) contains urea as the ingredient to exfoliate skin, and that's a possibility. This would work for exfoliation, but there are many more elegant formulations to consider.

☺ **Plus Alpha Hydroxy Moisturizing Creme** (*$7.99 for 6 ounces*) is similar to the Lotion above, and the same comments apply.

☺ **Q10 Anti-Wrinkle Sensitive Skin Creme** (*$10.59 for 1.7 ounces*) does contain coenzyme Q10, and while that's a good antioxidant there is no evidence that it has any effect on wrinkles. This is an OK basic moisturizer for someone with normal to dry skin, but that's about it.

☹ **Q10 Anti-Wrinkle Sensitive Skin Lotion SPF 15** (*$10.59 for 1.7 ounces*) does not contain the UVA-protecting ingredients of titanium dioxide, zinc oxide, or avobenzone, and is not recommended.

EXUVIANCE BY NEOSTRATA

Exuviance is a line of skin care products owned by another line of skin care products called NeoStrata (reviewed in this book). Both were created by Dr. Eugene Van Scott and Dr. Ruey Yu, two researchers who own the original patent for the use of glycolic acid

The Reviews E

(AHA) in relation to its ability to diminish wrinkles. Both the Exvuiance and NeoStrata lines contain glycolic acid (AHA) but some also contain a polyhydroxy acid (PHA) called gluconolactone (which is also patented by Scott and Yu) with similar claims. Gluconolactone is supposed to be gentler and longer acting than glycolic acid. However, according to an article in *Cosmetic Dermatology* (July 1998), skin can't tell the difference between the various effective AHAs and gluconolactone, and the possibility of gluconolactone staying on the surface of skin longer than other AHAs did not prove out. So PHA ends up being as good as AHA.

Aside from the type of AHA or PHA these products contain, in terms of efficacy, they don't hold a candle to the NeoStrata line of products. Most of the Exuviance options have pH levels that are too high for the AHA or PHA to be effective for exfoliation. If you are looking for AHA products, this is not the best line out there. There are some good cleansers and decent sunscreens to consider, but the toners and skin lightening products contain alcohol, as does the blemish product, and the moisturizers are good but not great. Overall, this isn't an exciting line. For more information about Exuviance, call (800) 225-9411 or visit www.neostrata.com.

☺ **Gentle Cleansing Creme Sensitive Formula** ($19 for 6.8 ounces) is a lotion-style cleanser that is an option for normal to dry skin. There is nothing about this formula that makes it preferred for sensitive skin.

☺ **Purifying Cleansing Gel** *($19 for 8 ounces)* is a standard, but good, detergent-based, water-soluble cleanser for normal to oily skin. It does contain about 4% AHAs, but the pH of 5 isn't low enough to make it effective as an exfoliant.

☹ **Moisture Balance Toner** *($18 for 6.8 ounces)* lists alcohol as the second ingredient, and that makes it unacceptable for any aspect of skin care. It isn't moisturizing in the least, but it is drying and irritating.

☺ **Soothing Toning Lotion Sensitive Formula** *($18 for 8 ounces)* is a disappointing formulation that is mostly water, preservatives, slip agent, silicone, plant extracts, and coloring agents. There is less than a 1% concentration of PHA (polyhydroxy acid) in this product, so it has no exfoliating properties.

☹ **Skin Rise Morning Bionic Tonic** *($32 for 1 ounce)* contains several potentially irritating plant extracts, including peppermint, grapefruit, menthol, and eucalyptus, and is not recommended.

☺ **Essential Multi-Defense Day Creme SPF 15** *($25 for 1.75 ounces)* is a good, in-part titanium dioxide–based sunscreen. The moisturizing base is just thickeners with some silicone; it's nothing very interesting. This has a pH of 4.5 which makes the AHA minimally effective for exfoliation, though it is still an option for sun protection.

☺ **Essential Multi-Defense Day Fluid SPF 15** *($23 for 2 ounces)* is similar to the Day Creme SPF 15 above, only in lotion form. The primary and rather significant difference between the two is this version has a pH of 3, which makes the approximately 7% concentration of AHA effective for exfoliation. This is one of the few sunscreens that include an effective concentration of AHA and an effective pH level as well.

☺ **Fundamental Multi-Protective Day Creme SPF 15 Sensitive Formula** *($25 for 1.75 ounces)*. Aside from containing slightly less AHA than the Day Creme SPF 15 above, it also has a pH of 5 that makes it even less effective for exfoliation. However, it is an option for a sunscreen.

☺ **Fundamental Multi-Protective Day Fluid SPF 15 Sensitive Formula** *($23 for 2 ounces)* is similar to the Day Creme SPF 15 Sensitive Formula above, and the same comments apply.

☹ **Essential Skin Lightener Gel** *($14.50 for 1.6 ounces)* would be a good 2% hydroquinone and glycolic acid skin-lightening product if it weren't for the alcohol it contains, which is unnecessarily irritating and drying for skin.

☺ **Evening Restorative Complex** *($27.50 for 1.75 ounces)* is a very good, silicone-based moisturizer for normal to dry skin that contains some good water-binding agents and antioxidants. The pH of 4.5 makes the AHA minimally effective for exfoliation.

☺ **$$$ Hydrating Lift Eye Complex** *($24.50 for 0.5 ounce)* isn't very different from the Evening Restorative Complex above; for all intents and purposes they both work well for normal to dry skin. The comments about AHA effectiveness are the same.

✓☺ **$$$ Vespera Bionic Serum** *($55 for 1 ounce)* is a good, lightweight gel moisturizer for normal to slightly dry skin that contains some good antioxidants and water-binding agents, along with effective AHAs for exfoliation. The price is out of line for what is essentially the same product as the Evening Restorative Complex and Hydrating Lift Eye Complex above.

☹ **Blemish Treatment Gel** *($13.50 for 0.5 ounce)* lists alcohol as the first ingredient, which makes this product too irritating for all skin types, much less blemish-prone skin. The pH of 6 makes the salicylic acid it contains ineffective for exfoliation.

☹ **Rejuvenating Treatment Masque** *($16.50 for 2.5 ounces)* is basically alcohol and film-forming agent. This is an irritation waiting to happen.

☺ **Essential Multi-Protective Lip Balm SPF 15** *($8.50 for 0.14 ounce)* is a very good emollient lip balm with an effective, in-part titanium dioxide– and zinc oxide–based sunscreen.

EXUVIANCE MAKEUP

The small assortment of Exuviance makeup products takes the "makeup as skincare" approach by including gluconolactone in all the makeup products. Although Exuviance makes much ado about gluconolactone being a superior moisturizing and gentler AHA, information presented in *Cosmetic Dermatology* (July 1998) doesn't bear this out. That is, it's hard to see any better possibilities for gluconolactone than for the older, mainstay AHAs such as glycolic acid and lactic acid. What each makeup item does include is an effective sunscreen, and that's good news, because as far as antiaging goes, that feature is far more essential than any buzz ingredient. Exuviance's three foundations

The Reviews E

do not offer a middle-of-the-road option when it comes to coverage. You're left to choose between the opaque CoverBlend or the sheer Skin Caring option. The CoverBlend Concealing Treatment Makeup SPF 20 is truly in a class by itself when it comes to traditional full-coverage makeup, and it's highly recommended if you need significant coverage for discolored areas on the face or body. The tube concealer also offers full coverage (though the colors are not the most neutral around), and the loose powder is a fine, albeit overpriced, option.

FOUNDATION: ✔☺ **CoverBlend Concealing Treatment Makeup SPF 20** *($22)* is a remarkable full-coverage foundation that effectively conceals minor and major discolorations without looking heavy or feeling thick and greasy on the skin. Since this is a rather opaque makeup, I don't agree with Exuviance's claim that it provides "natural" coverage, but this is certainly more attractive on the skin and easier to work with than DermaBlend or almost any other heavy-duty foundation you may have tried. The silicone-based formula features an excellent titanium dioxide– and zinc oxide–based sunscreen, and although it appears thick in the jar, it has a soft, light texture that is surprisingly easy to blend. Concealing Treatment Makeup dries to a solid matte finish, which may not be to everyone's liking, but you will certainly get more longevity out of it than you will with traditional creamy or greasepaint-type foundations. Those with normal to dry skin will definitely need to apply moisturizer before using this makeup, and you're not likely to need any setting powder, unless you want to further enhance the matte effect. Almost complete coverage is achieved with one application, and this layers well for areas that need more camouflage. There are 14 shades, but not all of them are praiseworthy. The following colors are too pink, peach, or rose for most skin tones: Neutral Beige, True Beige, Blush Beige, and Palest Mahogany. Bisque and Ivory are slightly peachy pink, but may work for some fair skin tones since the dry-down result is lighter than the color you see in the container. True Mahogany, Blush Mahogany, and Deep Mahogany are beautiful for dark skin tones, though the titanium dioxide and zinc oxide sunscreen can cause a slightly ashen finish.

☺ **$$$ Skin Caring Foundation SPF 15** *($26)* has a titanium dioxide sunscreen and a strong silicone base that starts out feeling light and silky but blends down to an ultra-matte, dry finish that only those with very oily skin will appreciate. Coverage is sheer to light and it does maintain its solid matte finish for most of the day. As with most ultra-matte foundations, it will exaggerate any dry spots. There are 14 shades available, and though some of them appear too pink, peach, or rose in the bottle, they dry down to a soft, sheer color. The following colors are noticeably peach, pink, or rose on the skin: True Beige, Neutral Beige, Palest Mahogany, and Blush Mahogany.

☹ **CoverBlend Corrective Leg & Body Makeup SPF 18** *($16)* is more akin to traditional full-coverage makeup when compared to the Concealing Treatment Makeup above. Although this silicone- and talc-based makeup with a titanium dioxide– and zinc oxide–based sunscreen does indeed provide substantial, water-resistant coverage, three of the four shades are simply too peach or pink to look convincing on most skin tones. If you're going to wear opaque makeup on the body, you don't want to use colors that stand out against the skin and draw attention to what you're trying to hide. If you have dark skin and need this type of makeup, Mahogany is a worthwhile deep tan shade to consider.

☺ $$$ <u>CONCEALER:</u> **CoverBlend Multi-Function Concealer SPF 15** *($16)* is a slightly creamy, full-coverage concealer that includes a titanium dioxide– and zinc oxide–based sunscreen. This applies quite well, and has only a slight tendency to crease—though the complete coverage may only be of interest to those with severe dark circles or other skin flaws that are not effectively covered by traditional concealers. If you need serious coverage and don't mind the trade-off of a less-than-natural finish, this is worth a try. There are four shades available, and only Mahogany is a must-avoid due its too strong peachy gold overtones.

☺ $$$ <u>POWDER:</u> **CoverBlend Antiaging Finishing Powder** *($18)* is a fine-textured, satin-finish loose powder that contains only talc, gluconolactone, pigments, and preservatives. The gluconolactone is supposed to provide an antiaging benefit, but don't count on startling results from a powder containing this ingredient. This simple formula works well with the CoverBlend foundations, and the two shades are equally good options.

FACE STOCKHOLM

This boutique line of makeup has great personality and style. The two Swedish owners, mother and daughter Gum Nowak and Martina Arfwidson, have a passion for what they do and have created an interesting niche in the cosmetics world for women who want makeup to be fun and casual. However, many of their skin-care products are lackluster and have major problems, especially their sunscreens and with the presence of irritating ingredients. The prices are another factor: they are unreasonable for what you get. For more information about FACE Stockholm, call (888) 334-FACE or visit www.facestockholm.com or www.beauty.com.

FACE STOCKHOLM SKIN CARE

☺ $$$ **Aloe Vera Cleansing Cream** *($18 for 4 ounces)* is an emollient, wipe-off, cold cream–style makeup remover that can be an option for dry skin, but this product has no advantage over Pond's Cold Cream.

☺ $$$ **Aloe Vera Cleansing Lotion** *($18 for 4 ounces)* is similar to the Cleansing Cream above only in lotion form, and the same basic comments apply.

☺ $$$ **Foaming Facial Cleanser Normal to Oily Skin** *($18 for 4 ounces)* is a standard, detergent-based, water-soluble cleanser that works quite well, both for removing makeup and for not drying out the skin.

☹ **Eye Makeup Remover** *($22 for 8 ounces)* is a standard, detergent-based makeup remover, but this one contains sodium lauryl sulfate, making it an exceptionally irritating one.

☺ **$$$ Apricot Gel Scrub Normal to Oily** *($16 for 2 ounces)* is a completely over-priced scrub of gel, thickening agents, and ground-up apricot seeds. Baking soda mixed with Cetaphil Gentle Skin Cleanser would work as well and be far less expensive.

☺ **$$$ Honey Almond Scrub** *($16 for 2 ounces)* is virtually identical to the Apricot Gel version above except that this one uses almonds instead of apricot seeds.

☹ **Aloe Vera Toner All Skin Types** *($18 for 8 ounces)* is just aloe vera gel, some plant extracts that are a mix of irritants and anti-irritants, fragrance, and preservatives. Your skin would do just as well with plain aloe vera from the health food store without the fragrance and the confusing mix of plant extracts.

☺ **Vegetable Toner All Skin Types** *($18 for 8 ounces)* contains water and plant extracts. The vegetable extracts can have antioxidant properties when eaten, but there is no research showing that to be the case when applied topically on skin. This lacks any water-binding agents or anti-irritants and isn't of much interest for skin.

☺ **Aloe Vera Gel** *($18 for 8 ounces)* contains mostly aloe vera gel, along with some plant extracts and preservatives. The plant extracts don't add much to this basic formulation, and you would do just as well with plain aloe vera from the health food store for a lot less.

☺ **Aloe Vera Moisture Cream All Skin Types** *($24 for 2 ounces)* is an ordinary emollient moisturizer for dry skin. This is absolutely not suited for all skin types, especially oily skin.

☺ **Aloe Vera Facial Lotion All Skin Types** *($14 for 4 ounces)* is an extremely emollient, ordinary moisturizer. It would be very good for someone with dry skin. As with the Moisture Cream All Skin Types above, this one is absolutely not suited for all skin types.

☺ **Daily Eye Care** *($26 for 1 ounce)* is just an average moisturizer for dry skin.

☺ **Eye Gel** *($24 for 1 ounce)* is a lightweight gel that does contain some good water-binding agents, but it also contains some plant extracts that can be skin irritants.

☺ **Orchid Oil Moisturizer All Skin Types** *($28 for 2 ounces)* is a very basic moisturizer for dry skin that contains mostly water, thickeners, plant oils, and fragrance.

☺ **Vitamin A Cream All Skin Types** *($26 for 2 ounces)* is similar to the Orchid Oil Moisturizer above and the same basic comments apply. The teeny amount of vitamin A in this product is barely detectable.

☺ **Vitamin Cream All Skin Types** *($29 for 2 ounces)* doesn't contain any vitamins and is just a basic, very mundane moisturizer for dry skin.

☹ **Moisture Cream SPF 15 All Skin Types** *($25 for 2 ounces)* doesn't contain the UVA-protecting ingredients of titanium dioxide, zinc oxide, or avobenzone, and is not recommended.

☺ **$$$ Detoxifying Green Clay Masque** *($32 for 2.6 ounces)* is a standard clay mask that also contains some plant oils, plant extracts (mostly anti-irritants), water-binding agents, and antioxidants. Ironically, this contains by far some of the most interesting ingredients of any other product in this line. Unfortunately, any benefits from these ingredients are lost in a mask because they are "absorbed" by the clay.

☺ $$$ **Hydrating Rose Petal Antioxidant Face Masque** *($32 for 2 ounces)* is a very good moisturizer with an impressive mix of plant oils, water-binding agents, antioxidants, and anti-irritant.

☹ $$$ **Sage and Aloe Mask All Skin Types** *($18 for 2 ounces)* is just a bunch of thickeners and emollients; it would be good for dry skin (not for all skin types as the name implies). Someone with oily or blemish-prone skin would not appreciate the avocado oil this mask contains.

FACE STOCKHOLM MAKEUP

In many ways, FACE Stockholm is the Swedish-bred version of M.A.C., though FACE Stockholm actually debuted four years before M.A.C. came on the scene. This makeup artistry–themed line was truly ahead of its time back then, and has expanded quite a bit over the past two decades, offering a veritable smorgasbord of color products. Best of all, FACE's makeup line has a wonderfully balanced selection of matte and shiny finishes along with mostly reliable textures, plus one of the most extensive lineups of shades you're likely to see. Any look is possible using these products, from barely there naturalism to flamboyant diva. Of course, in a line of this size, not everything is spectacular. Some of the products are well-intentioned but impractical to use, even downright unnecessary, but the tried-and-true products are commendable and the choices abundant. With only a handful of boutiques in the United States (all but one in New York) and its scarcity in department stores, few people are likely to happen upon it.

FOUNDATION: ☺ **Liquid Foundation** *($24)* is a standard moisturizing foundation with an even, light-to-medium coverage application and 13 mostly great colors. This would be best for those with normal to dry skin that is not prone to breakouts. The only colors to avoid are Sno, which can be too pink, Parlemo 2, which is shiny, and Sommar, which can be too peach. **Matte Foundation** *($24)* is a decent, though basic, option for a light-textured, light-to-medium coverage, soft matte finish foundation. The lack of modern silicones and an emollient fairly high on the ingredient list means this won't stay matte for long, so it is ideally for those with normal to slightly oily skin. There are 17 colors available, including four color correctors, which should be avoided along with the shades Sno, Sommar, and Parlemo 2. $$$ **Powder Foundation** *($27)* is talc-based and has excellent shades (15 in all) and a wonderfully soft, dry finish. These work best as powders rather than as foundation and are definitely preferred over the regular Pressed Powders in this line, which are all shiny. The only shades to avoid are July, March, and November, which are fairly peach to overly yellow.

☹ $$$ **Picture Perfect Foundation** *($28)* comes in a jar and is a very thick, emollient formula that is meant for full coverage. The mineral oil–based texture is greasy enough that the product's directions emphasize the need to use powder to get any longevity from the makeup, and they're right—you would need to powder all day long to keep this from slip-sliding away, especially if you plan to use it for television or theatrical makeup. The 15 shades have some worthwhile colors, but this formula has enough draw-backs to pass it up entirely, including a far from natural look and a far too heavy application for most skin types. Its one redeeming quality is that its moist finish would definitely appeal to those with very dry skin.

☹ <u>CONCEALER:</u> **Corrective Concealer** *($16)* doesn't correct, it just places strange shades of yellow or peach on the skin, though Neutralizer is a consideration for light skin tones. The **Concealer Wheel** *($18)* and **Skin Wheel** *($18)* present five flesh-tone or color-correcting cream concealers in one pan. Each shade gets its own pie-wedge shape, but none of the colors blend well or look convincing on the skin, plus they tend to move too easily on the skin. **Concealer Wand** *($12)* is a wand-applicator type concealer that has an extremely poor range of colors; all of them are either too pink, peach, ash, or green to recommend. **Concealer Stick** *($13)* is a standard, lipstick-style creamy concealer. Two of the five colors are poor—only Light Amber, Amber, and Dark Amber resemble skin tones—and this tends to crease and fade, too.

<u>POWDER:</u> ☺ $$$ **Loose Powder** *($21)* has a lovely soft texture that feels great on the skin, though the kaolin (clay) present provides a dry, matte finish that is best for normal to oily skin. The best shades to consider are 1 through 4, 7, and 8. Shades 5 and 6 are a bit too peach, while shades 9 through 15 are either unconventional colors or too shiny for daytime wear.

☺ $$$ **Bronzer** *($20)* is a standard, pressed-powder bronzer that comes in an excellent group of five colors. Three shades omit the iridescence, but the oils do leave a sheen, which is a boon for those with normal to dry skin. Ibiza and Cancun are workable colors, but they are too sparkly to look like the real thing.

☺ $$$ **Pressed Powder** *($20)* offers some beautifully neutral shades and a sheer, satin texture that applies well, though each shade leaves a shiny finish. For normal to dry skin that doesn't need shine control, this will work well. $$$ **Pressat Puder** *($18)* (yes, that's the correct spelling) is a collection of sheer, shiny, pastel pressed powders. These are supposed to add a glow, but along with the shine, the strange assortment of colors, such as lilac, blue, and purple, end up creating a strange hue on the skin. **Galaxy** *($15)* is just large flecks of loose glitter, much like what you'd find at an arts-and-crafts store. It's fairly messy to apply because it doesn't cling well, but for all-out shine, this is as glitzy as it gets.

<u>BLUSH:</u> ☺ **Blush** *($15)* is a group of standard, single-tin blushes that have a great soft texture and smooth, soft application. The enormous color selection has some excellent matte-finish options for all skin tones. These tend to be less grainy than M.A.C.'s Matte Powder Blush ($16). Still, you'll find comparable blush textures and, to a lesser extent, colors from such lines as Stila, Lorac, Trish McEvoy, and Bobbi Brown. **Blush Shimmer** *($15)* has a texture identical to the Blush above, but each of the four shades is shiny.

☺ $$$ **Creme Blush** *($18)* is standard cream blush that has an old-fashioned, slightly greasy texture, so be cautious unless you have dry skin. It goes on sheerer than the color in the pot would lead you to think. This can't compete with the more current cream-to-powder blush textures from other lines that have a more even and less slippery application. **Highlighters for Face and Body** *($18)* are tins of greasy, iridescent color that can be used anyplace you want to add slippery shine. **Glitter Stick for Face and Body** *($22)* are more shimmery than glittery, and these have a smooth, creamy texture that makes them easy to blend—though don't count on the formula staying put. For overpriced shimmer, these do the job. **Trinity** *($18)* eyeshadows are pots of creamy, rather slick eyeshadows that are also meant to work for blush or lip color. They're heavy on the shimmer and can make the face, lips, and eye area look greasy. **High Lighter Quad for Face and Body** *($22)* presents four coordinated, shiny colors in one container. The emollient, waxy formula goes on well, but tends to migrate and isn't as modern a way to gleam up as the less expensive options from Revlon SkinLights.

EYESHADOW: ✔☺ **Pearl Shadow** and **Matte Shadow** *($15)* are a find. The smooth matte texture and application are excellent and there are dozens of colors—over 65 with oodles of neutral options available! For shine-lovers, the Pearl formula includes over 30 choices. Each formula has its share of blue, green, purple, and fuchsia hues to wade through, but their inclusion is forgivable given the overall color selection.

☹ $$$ **Eyedust** *($17)* are tins of extremely shiny powder. They are messy to use and hard to control, but they do create shine all over and work as well as any. **Upstage Collection, Theatrical Shades** *($16)* is aptly named, as these greasy, bold colors are strictly for theatrical and exaggerated makeup only. If you're a member of the Cirque du Soleil troupe, this may be of interest!

EYE AND BROW SHAPER: ☺ **Eye Liner** *($12)* is an extremely standard, soft-finish pencil that comes in a wide range of colors. Avoid the green Gron and blue Greco. $$$ **Brow Shadow** *($18)* is a group of six matte eyeshadows that match most brow colors rather nicely. This is a great way to apply brow color. **Cake Eyeliner** *($12)* is a traditional (and worthwhile) cake eyeliner that's used wet to create a dramatic line along the lashes. **Brow Fix** *($13)* comes in two shades, clear and a medium brown. They work well to make brows look fuller and keep them in place without feeling sticky, but more shades would have been nice.

☺ **Eye-Lip Liner Pencil** *($12)* is a standard pencil whose two shades of peach and brown are of little use for the lips, though they can work as creamy eye pencils.

☹ **Liquid Eyeliner** *($12)* is hard to apply evenly and tends to go on choppy. The brush is too long and soft to rely on for effective control.

LIPSTICK AND LIP PENCIL: ☺ $$$ **Lipstick** *($17)* is exceptionally creamy without being greasy, and there is a superlative selection of 114 full-coverage shades. Looking for that just-right red? How about iridescent silver or a soft taupe? Chances are, it's here! ✔☺ **Matte Lipstick** *($17)* has the distinction of being one of the few truly matte lipsticks available. This has a smooth, not-too-thick texture that provides lush coverage and long wear. There are over 30 exceptional shades available for fair to dark skin tones. **Lipstick Veil** *($17)* is a fine sheer, glossy finish lipstick in a small but winning selection of shades.

☺ **Lipgloss Wand** *($14)* is just an emollient, sticky lip gloss with a great range of colors. **Pot Lipgloss** *($14)* is a slightly sticky, but very glossy, pot of gloss with a remarkably vivid application of color. **Lip Pencils** *($12)* are modestly priced standard creamy pencils whose colors run from understated to over the top. These apply nicely, too!

☺ **MASCARA: Mascara** *($14)* isn't what I would consider impressive, but it's nevertheless a reliable mascara that provides some length and a smidgen of thickness. If you want a basic mascara that doesn't clump or flake, here it is!

☺ **BRUSHES:** FACE Stockholm offers over 25 **Brushes** *($6–$30)*. The sable hair eyeshadow brushes are excellent and there are many reasons to check these out, especially for size options. The powder and blush brushes tend to be too floppy for controlled application, and not as dense as what you'll find in brushes from similar lines—then again, they cost about half as much as those other lines charge! There are some workable nylon brushes as well, though they aren't as luxurious as the sable options. The only superfluous brushes to avoid are the **Fan Duster #19** *($14)*, **Spooly Brush #20** *($6)*, and **Sponge Applicator #23** *($5)*.

☺ **SPECIALTY:** Makeup artists and neat-niks take note: there are all kinds of great makeup bags, cases, organizers, palettes, and boxes to consider from FACE Stockholm. They range in price from $6 for the **Pro Palette 4-Pan Compact** to $220 for the **Pro-Traveler Makeup Box**, and offer some intriguing, practical ways to organize, store, and travel with only a few or many cosmetics!

FASHION FAIR

It has always struck me as somewhat sad and ironic that women of color, who on average buy cosmetics at three times the rate of other ethnic groups, have such a limited number of options. One would think a cosmetics line like Fashion Fair would be a welcome oasis in a desert of limited choices, but in fact the opposite is true. Although Fashion Fair distinctly prides itself as a line for women of color, the textures and color choices of many of its products leave much to be desired and can't hold a candle to other lines such as M.A.C. and Prescriptives, which have recognized the oversight in makeup shortages for women of color and have offered some successful corrections. Also, there are now much better lines specifically devoted to African-American women, particularly Iman (available at J.C. Penney) and Black Opal (a small but good drugstore line).

I can only surmise that this 30-year-old line is still around because of the powerful "this line is especially for you" branding statement it makes to the African-American community. Fashion Fair is a division of Johnson Publishing, Inc., the company that publishes the popular *Ebony* and *Jet* magazines, where Fashion Fair gains regular exposure. Yet glossy magazine spreads can't compensate for the poorly organized, inadequately staffed Fashion Fair counters where the mostly uninspired products present few satisfying options.

Of utter disappointment are the skin-care products. They are mostly greasy, cold cream–like cleansers, water-soluble cleansers with strongly irritating cleansing agents, alcohol-based toners, and greasy, mediocre moisturizers. Layering greasy moisturizers on darker skin tones can cause a buildup of dead skin cells, making skin look dull and uneven. Almost all of the toners are exceedingly drying and irritating, which is another cause of dull, uneven skin tones, not to mention breakouts. An even more glaring defect is the lack of effective sunscreens. Surely by now Fashion Fair knows that darker skin tones also run the risk of sun damage, and that a major cause of ashen discoloration on dark skin tones is damage caused by the sun. For more information about Fashion Fair, call (312) 322-9444 or visit www.fashionfair.com.

FASHION FAIR SKIN CARE

☺ **Botanical Cleansing Gel** *($12.50 for 6.7 ounces)* is a good, but standard, detergent-based, water-soluble cleanser for someone with normal to oily skin. It does contain fragrance, but the minuscule amounts of the plant extracts in here hardly make this botanical.

☺ **Cleansing Creme with Aloe Vera** *($14.25 for 4 ounces)* is a standard, mineral oil–based, wipe-off cleanser that can leave a greasy film, although it can be an option for someone with dry skin.

☺ **Deep Cleansing Lotion Balanced for All Skin Types** *($15 for 8 ounces)* is almost identical to the Cleansing Creme above, except this version contains more mineral oil, lanolin, and some very emollient thickening agents. This is a fairly greasy cleanser that needs to be wiped off and isn't very different from using just plain mineral oil. Calling this suitable for all skin types is absurd, though for someone with very dry skin it is an option.

☹ **Facial Shampoo Original Formula for Normal or Oily Skin** *($11 for 3 ounces)* is a standard, detergent-based, water-soluble cleanser that uses sodium lauryl sulfate as the main cleansing agent, which makes it potentially too drying and irritating for all skin types.

☹ **Foaming Facial Cleanser** *($17.50 for 5.5 ounces)* is similar to the Facial Shampoo above and the same comments apply.

☺ **Gentle Facial Shampoo Mild for Dry Sensitive Skin** *($11 for 3 ounces)* is a standard, detergent-based, water soluble cleanser that could be good for someone with normal to oily skin, but it is completely inappropriate for someone with dry sensitive skin. It does contain fragrance.

☹ **Gentle Facial Polisher for All Skin Types** *($13.25 for 3 ounces)* is a detergent cleanser that also contains synthetic scrub particles (polyethylene). It does contain menthol, which can be irritating for many skin types.

☺ **Botanical Skin Purifier I for Normal to Oily Skin** *($11.50 for 6.7 ounces)* won't purify anything; it is just about as ordinary a toner as you can get, containing mostly water and glycerin. The lemongrass that's present can be a skin irritant.

☺ **Botanical Skin Purifier II for Normal to Dry Skin** *($11.50 for 6.7 ounces)* can't balance skin, but it is an OK, ordinary toner for the skin type indicated. The small amount of plant extracts in this one may have antioxidant properties.

☹ **Deep Pore Astringent Regular for Normal to Oily Skin** *($13.25 for 8 ounces)* is primarily alcohol and fragrance, and that makes it too drying and irritating for all skin types.

☹ **Skin Freshener I Normal to Oily Skin** *($11.50 for 6 ounces)* is similar to the Deep Pore Astringent above and the same comments apply.

☹ **Skin Freshener II Dry or Sensitive Skin** *($11.50 for 6 ounces)* has basically the same ingredients as Skin Freshener I above and can be just as drying. Alcohol isn't appropriate for any skin type, but it's even less so for someone with dry or sensitive skin.

☹ **Toning Lotion Mild for Dry Sensitive Skin** *($13.25 for 8 ounces)* is similar to the Freshener II above and the same comments apply.

☹ **Daytime Moisturizer SPF 15** *($25 for 2 ounces)* doesn't contain the UVA-protecting ingredients of titanium dioxide, zinc oxide, or avobenzone, and is not recommended.

☺ **Dry Skin Emollient for Excessively Dry Skin** *($21 for 2 ounces)* is an extremely basic and rather greasy moisturizer that contains mostly mineral oil, water, wax, and Vaseline.

☺ **$$$ Eye Cream** *($19 for 0.5 ounce)* is a very basic, thick, emollient moisturizer that would be OK for dry skin. The minuscule amounts of water-binding agents and antioxidants are barely detectable.

☺ **Hidden Beauty Skin Enhancing Creme** *($25 for 1.9 ounces)* is supposed to be a blend of antioxidant vitamins and beta hydroxy acid. However, the amount of vitamins is minuscule, and though this does contain BHA, the high pH makes it ineffective for exfoliation.

☺ **Moisturizing Creme with Aloe Vera for Dry Skin** *($18.50 for 4 ounces)* is a very emollient, very standard moisturizer that would be OK for very dry skin. The tiny amount of water-binding agents and antioxidants it contains is hardly worth mentioning.

☺ **Moisture Lotion for All Day Beauty** *($14.75 for 4 ounces)* is a standard, mineral oil–based, emollient moisturizer for someone with dry skin, but it's rather unimpressive, and without sunscreen it's not good for all-day protection.

☺ **Moisturizing Lotion for Normal to Oily Skin** *($18.50 for 4 ounces)* is a very standard moisturizer, but what can Vaseline and lanolin be doing in a product for oily skin?

☹ **Oil-Free Moisturizer** *($21 for 4 ounces)* is indeed an oil-free moisturizer, but it also contains isopropyl myristate and isopropyl palmitate high up on the ingredient list, and both of those thickening agents are problematic for causing blackheads and breakouts.

☹ **Oil-Control Lotion** *($16.50 for 3 ounces)* contains mostly alcohol and some minerals that have some ability to absorb oil. The alcohol causes more problems than the minerals can help.

☺ **Special Beauty Creme with Collagen** *($19.50 for 2 ounces)* is an extremely basic moisturizer for someone with very dry skin. Collagen is a good water-binding agent, but it doesn't affect the collagen in your skin one little bit, and this product offers no other interesting or beneficial ingredients for skin.

☹ **Deep Pore Cleansing Masque for Normal to Oily Skin** (*$15.25 for 2 ounces*) is just some absorbents and a layer of plastic that you apply and then peel off the face. There is little reason to consider this for any skin type.

☺ **Vantex Skin Bleaching Creme with Sunscreens** (*$17.50 for 2 ounces*) doesn't contain enough sunscreen or UVA-protecting ingredients to protect skin from any amount of sun damage, but it is a good 2% hydroquinone (for skin lightening) product in a slightly moisturizing base. You would still need a reliable sunscreen for this product to be effective.

FASHION FAIR MAKEUP

What you will find among the Fashion Fair makeup are merely average foundations with few great shades to extol, poor concealers, exceedingly shiny blushes and eyeshadows, standard pencils, and overly greasy lipsticks. Beyond that, the few odds and ends worth considering are certainly not exceptional enough to seek out, but if you happen upon a counter and want to peek for yourself, at least you will have a good idea of what to avoid.

FOUNDATION: ☺ **Oil-Free Perfect Finish Souffle** (*$20*) goes on thick and creamy but dries to a medium matte finish. It can be tricky to blend, but the color selection and coverage are excellent for someone with normal to oily skin (it may look somewhat pasty on normal to dry skin). The only colors to avoid are Copper Glo, Brown Blaze Glo, and Bronze Glo. **Perfect Finish Creme Makeup** (*$18.50*) is a thick-textured, creamy makeup that blends well and offers sheer to medium coverage and a natural finish. This non-powdery makeup is best for normal to dry skin. There are 15 shades, but the following are too orange for most skin tones: Brown Blaze Glo, Honey Glo, Copper Glo, Beige Glo, and Amber Glo. Fawn Glo, Topaz Glo, Pure Brown, and Ebony are OK, but you'll find M.A.C. offers better versions of these colors. Brown is a beautiful shade for very dark skin tones. **Oil-Free Perfect Finish Creme to Powder Makeup** (*$21*) may be oil-free, but this contains enough emollients and waxes to give it a slightly greasy texture and minimal powder finish that won't prevent oil from breaking through. Still, this does blend quite well and offers soft, sheer-to-light coverage. If you have normal skin (no oily areas, no dry patches) this is worth testing, and the 15 shades (which go on lighter than they appear) are mostly very good. Only Amber, Honey, Topaz, Bronze, Tawny, and Copper are unlikely to work for most medium to dark skin tones.

☺ **Fast Finish Foundation** (*$22.50*) is no faster than other makeups, but this stick foundation does have a smooth texture and powder-dry finish going for it. For those with normal to oily skin looking for medium coverage and a tenacious matte finish, there are some contenders among the 12 shades. The following colors are too orange, golden, or copper for most dark skin tones: Honey, Copper, Tender, and Bronze. Note: This formula is very difficult to remove, and almost stains the skin.

☹ **Oil-Free Liquid** (*$19.50*) used to pass as a good matte foundation, but compared to the far more elegant, silky textures now available from lines such as Lancome, Chanel, and Almay, this has a terribly sticky finish and is difficult to spread over the skin. There are some worthwhile colors among the ten shades, but the application and finish make this tough to recommend. **Sheer Foundation** *($15.50)* does provide a light, sheer coverage and has an emollient feel that dry skin will enjoy. However, seven of the eight shades are simply too peach, pink, orange, or rose for all skin tones. There are many more modern foundations to consider ahead of this one.

CONCEALER: ☺ **Cover Tone Concealing Creme** *($18)* is for use on dark circles or over blemishes and scars. It has a very dry, thick consistency and provides heavy coverage with a slightly sticky finish. The six shades are passable, with the best ones being Tender Glo and Pure Brown Glo—but think twice before using such an unnatural-looking, difficult-to-blend concealer.

☹ **Coverstick** *($12)* quickly slips into lines around the eye, provides substandard coverage, and the two shades are awful.

☺ POWDER: **Transglo Face Powder** *($17.50)* is a talc-based loose powder that has a superb lightweight texture and finish, though each sheer shade has an obvious shine. This is not recommended for daytime wear, but is an option for evening. **Transglo Pressed Powder** *($16)* has a soft, sheer texture that applies easily and looks natural. The four slightly shiny shades are decent and this formula is best for normal to dry skin.

☺ $$$ **Fragrance-Free Pressed Powder** *($16)* is identical to the Transglo Pressed Powder above except that this does not contain fragrance.

☺ $$$ **Oil Control Loose Powder** *($18.50)* has an incredibly silky texture, but disappointingly peach to cantaloupe orange colors. However, each of the five shades goes on very sheer, almost translucent. This may be worth a test-run because the non-chalky finish works so well on dark skin tones.

☹ **Oil Control Pressed Powder** *($17.50)* is fragrance-free, talc-based, and has a drier texture than the Oil Control Loose Powder above. The application is still soft and coverage is good, but this tends to apply unevenly and is hard to pick up with a powder brush.

☺ BLUSH: **Beauty Blush** *($15)* comes in an interesting variety of colors, all fragranced. They go on dry, but smooth, and include both vivid and subtle shades, although most of the shades scream shine. Golden Lights is classified as a **Beauty Highlighter** *($15)* and is simply an ultra-shiny gold pressed powder. M.A.C., Lorac, and NARS have far better blush textures and colors for dark skin tones.

☹ EYESHADOW: Fashion Fair has done away with its mostly garish trio and quad eyeshadow sets, and now offers only single ones in their **Eyeshadow** *($10)*. Lamentably, every color is very shiny, and although these blend well, the shine can flake off.

EYE AND BROW SHAPER: ☺ **Eye Liner Pencils** *($10)* are creamy pencils with a sponge tip on one end. This needs-sharpening pencil lasts longer than you might expect, but if you want to avoid the potential for smearing, use a matte powder eyeshadow for lining.

☹ **Liquid Eye Liner** *($13)* has three very shiny shades, and because the brush is hard to control, application tends to be wildly uneven. **Brow Pencil** *($9)* is an automatic pencil with a very dry, heavy texture and only one shade. **Brush-On Brow** *($13)* has two shades of matte powders that are rather waxy and apply too heavily to look natural.

LIPSTICK AND LIP PENCIL: There are three types of lipsticks available: Cremes, Frosts, and Forever Matte. The ☺ **Cremes** *($12.50)* have a thick texture and slightly greasy consistency with a nice selection of opaque colors. The **Frosts** *($12.50)* are identical in texture to the Cremes except they are unmistakably iridescent.

☺ **Forever Matte** *($13)* isn't really matte; it's actually quite creamy with a nice stain for longer wear and a shiny finish. There aren't many color options for this lipstick, but most of them are rich shades that complement dark skin. **Automatic Lip Color** *($12.50)* is just iridescent lip gloss with a wand applicator and a nice, non-sticky feel. **Lip Liner Pencils** *($10)* are standard, creamy pencils with a small, but good, selection of colors. **Lip Moisturizer** *($12.50)* is an emollient, colorless lipstick that will nicely remedy dry, chapped lips.

☹ **Lip Highlighter** *($12)* is an opalescent, semi-opaque white lipstick meant to create a highlight when used with other lip colors. It's hardly subtle and such an effect can be achieved without such a contrived product. **Sheer Crystal Lip Gloss** *($12)* is an extremely thick, syrupy gloss that has a stringy texture akin to melted cheese. Elizabeth Arden and M.A.C. clear gloss options are unequivocally preferred.

☹ **MASCARA:** Fashion Fair's **Sensitive Eyes Mascara** *($11)* is an incredibly do-nothing product that builds negligible length and definition, even with considerable effort. Unless you like minimum payback with maximum effort, this is one to ignore.

FLORI ROBERTS

Flori Roberts is a cosmetics line aimed at African American women that seems to be satisfied with staying exactly the same, never improving or reformulating its products, even as the industry's style changes and as improved formulations come along. Unfortunately that means it leaves much to be desired in the skin-care arena. It has more than its share of greasy moisturizers and drying toners (containing lots of irritating ingredients), which can create problems that weren't there before for darker skin tones. Irritation on darker skin tones can make skin look flaky and ashen, and none of that is good. This line needs an overhaul, but it doesn't look like it's coming anytime soon. For more information about Flori Roberts, call (877) 57FLORI or visit www.floriroberts.com.

FLORI ROBERTS SKIN CARE

☹ **My Everything Double O Soap Gold for Normal to Oily Skin** *($13 for 4 ounces)* is a standard bar soap that is drying and irritating, but to add insult to injury this product also contains peppermint oil, eucalyptus oil, and camphor. My, oh my!

☺ **My Everything Treatment Foaming Gel Cleanser** *($12 for 6 ounces)* is a standard, detergent-based, water-soluble cleanser that can be an option for normal to oily skin. It does contain fragrance.

☺ My Everything Treatment Fresh Foaming Cleanser Normal to Oily *($15 for 6 ounces)* is a detergent-based, water-soluble cleanser that also contains several plant oils, making it inappropriate for someone with normal to oily skin. It also contains spearmint, which can be a skin irritant.

☹ My Everything Treatment Gentle Creamy Cleanser Normal to Dry *($15 for 6 ounces)* is a standard lotion cleanser that for some inexplicable reason also contains peppermint, sage, and rosemary oils, which can all be skin irritants.

☹ My Everything Gentle Eye Makeup Remover *($9 for 3 ounces)* isn't gentle. Putting peppermint, sage, and rosemary, which are strong irritants, especially for the eye area, in an eye-makeup remover is a cruel joke.

☹ My Everything Treatment Double O Complex Normal to Oily *($15 for 8 ounces)* contains alcohol and a host of irritating ingredients, such as peppermint oil, eucalyptus oil, clove oil, and camphor. This toner does nothing for the skin other than irritate and dry it, making it a problem for skin of all types and colors.

☹ My Everything Treatment Gentle Refining Toner Normal to Dry *($15 for 8 ounces)*. The second ingredient listed is witch hazel distillate, which contains mostly alcohol, and that makes this a problem for all skin types.

☹ My Everything Treatment Skin Balancing Astringent/Toner *($15 for 8 ounces)* contains mostly water, witch hazel, slip agent, lactic acid, anti-irritant, and preservatives. This is about a 5% AHA product, and it will exfoliate, but the witch hazel and orange oil in it make it more irritating than necessary.

☹ My Everything Treatment Exfoliating Facial Scrub and Primer *($12.50 for 4 ounces)* is mostly corn syrup, ground-up peanuts, water, ground-up plastic, and thickeners. This is a strange scrub combination that offers little advantage over using a clean washcloth.

☺ My Everything Treatment Advanced Formula Creme *($28.50 for 3.25 ounces)* makes claims about sun protection, but it doesn't contain enough sunscreen to protect skin from sun damage, nor does it contain any UVA-protecting ingredients. It is just a very ordinary moisturizer containing mostly thickeners and silicones and the tiniest amount of water-binding agent and antioxidants.

☺ My Everything Treatment Chromatone Plus Fade Creme *($15 for 3.75)* is a standard 2% hydroquinone fade cream in an emollient base.

☹ My Everything Treatment Eye Treatment Complex *($18.50 for 1 ounce)* is just a combination of a long list of thickeners, and is one of the more poorly formulated moisturizers I've ever reviewed.

☺ My Everything Hydrophilic Moisture Complex Normal to Dry *($20 for 2 ounces)* is an OK, but very boring, moisturizer for normal to dry skin. The teeny amount of lactic acid it contains is not effective as an exfoliant.

☺ My Everything Creme *($25 for 3.25 ounces)* is an ordinary moisturizer of thickeners and a small amount of plant oils.

☺ **My Everything Treatment Oil Control Serum Normal to Oily** *($14 for 1 ounce)* is a simple, lightweight gel moisturizer that won't control a drop of oil. It contains mostly water, aloe, thickeners, glycerin, water-binding agent, and preservatives.

☹ **My Everything Treatment Oil Free Moisturizer** *($16.50 for 3 ounces)* is a do-nothing product of slip agents and preservatives that won't help any skin type. This does contain sunscreen ingredients, but the protection isn't rated and it doesn't have any UVA-protecting ingredients, so that part is also disappointing.

☹ **My Everything Treatment Revitalized Protection Moisturizer** *($16.50 for 4 ounces)* doesn't contain enough sunscreen to protect skin from sun damage, nor does it contain any UVA-protecting ingredients, and it is not recommended. In addition, the AHA is present in a concentration of less than 1%, which makes it ineffective for exfoliation.

FLORI ROBERTS MAKEUP

When it comes to makeup, Flori Roberts seems content to offer African-American women poor foundation colors, blushes that are shiny and dry, and several eyeshadow color combinations that were popular (who knows why?) back when everyone was wondering, "Who shot J. R.?"

Women of color do require stronger colors (and stronger colors can tend to have a grainy texture), but that doesn't mean the blushes can't be silky-smooth and have stronger pigment at the same time; a feat that many other lines have accomplished. There is no logical reason to choose Flori Roberts over the superior choices from Iman (often positioned right next to Roberts at J.C. Penney) or from diverse lines such as Prescriptives and M.A.C. The tester units are not user-friendly in the least, nor does anyone who services them seem to care how they look or whether testers are even available. When you add everything up, stopping by this counter shouldn't be on anyone's cosmetics "to do" list, unless you like the challenge, which is on par with fitting a square into a circle!

FOUNDATION: ☹ **Touche Satin Foundation** *($17)* is a thick, cream-to-powder compact makeup that is decidedly creamy. It does blend on well, offering medium to full coverage, but most of the colors are just awful. The only possible considerations may be Walnut, Mahogany, or Mocha; the rest are too peach, pink, or red.

☺ **Oil-Free Hydrophilic Foundation** *($21)* is a liquid foundation that offers sheer to light coverage and a slightly sticky matte finish. This can be an option for normal to oily skin, but it takes a long time to set, so be prepared to blend. The eight revised shades are somewhat of an improvement over the previous pitiful lot. Still, shades B, C, D, and E are must-avoid colors.

☹ **Hydrophilic Demi Creme to Powder** *($18.50)* is a creamy foundation with light to medium coverage and barely a hint of a powdery finish. Those with normal to dry dark skin may want to consider Demi Sable or Demi Tan, but these are merely the passable shades among some otherwise incredibly deficient colors.

The Reviews F

POWDER: ☹ **Chromatic Loose Powder** *($17.50)* has a smooth, soft, talc-based texture and a lovely dry finish, but all of the three colors are too peach or pink.

☺ **Pressed Powder** *($13)* is a talc-based powder with a beautiful texture and finish, but the colors are not the best. However, No. 6 and No. 7 could work on medium skin tones as rosy bronzing powders. **Compact Face Powder** *($16.50)* has a nice, dry talc-based texture that meshes well with the skin and will assuredly absorb excess oil, but five of the seven colors are too peach to recommend. Only Dark and Brown are worth (careful) consideration.

☺ **BLUSH: Radiance Blush** *($13)* comes in a large assortment of colors, all with slight to glaring shine. Even without the shine, the grainy, sandpaper-like texture of these leaves much to be desired. The intensity of these colors is great for ebony skin, but good luck getting them to apply evenly.

☹ **EYESHADOW: Signature Eyeshadow Trios** *($15)* have some of the most unusual and shiny color combinations you are ever likely to see in the world of makeup. No one needs this much shine and definitely not as their only eyeshadow option.

☺ **EYE AND BROW SHAPER: Eye Contour Pencils** *($8.50)* are standard pencils, but a bit drier than most on the market. There are only three shades, black, brown, and navy blue, which is, to say the least, limited. The dry texture means they don't apply very easily, but they also don't smear as fast.

☺ **LIPSTICK AND LIP PENCIL:** Flori Roberts lipsticks used to pass with flying colors (pun intended), but compared with today's creamy, lightweight textures, these almost feel like a step backward on the lips. **Lipstick** *($11)* has a thick, rather unpleasant greasy texture and a bevy of intense, saturated colors, most with strong iridescence. This lipstick will easily creep into any lines around the mouth. **Liqui-Lip Gloss** *($11)* is a wand applicator–type standard gloss with a liquidy, non-sticky texture and striking, full-coverage colors. **Lip Polish** *($9)* offers two shades of ultra-shiny, sticky gloss in a pot. Better glosses abound at the drugstore. **Lip Contour Pencil** *($8.50)* is completely ordinary in every respect, though the texture is nicely creamy without being greasy. **Lip Base Coat** *($10.50)* is a chocolate-brown lipstick that is supposed to balance one's natural lip color. Although women of color may find that their natural lip color does not match top to bottom, any color balancing is best done with a lip pencil, not with a greasy lipstick such as this. **Lip Oil Stick** *($10.50)* is an emollient clear lip balm packaged as a lipstick, and is a good, albeit oily, option for dry lips.

☹ **MASCARA: Lash Set 2000 Mascara** *($12)* is a boring mascara that builds meager length while somehow making lashes look sparse and stunted. If you are in the unique position of wanting to use mascara to downplay your lashes, look no further.

GALDERMA (SEE CETAPHIL)

GATINEAU

Gatineau, a French line of skin-care products, has been around for years. Created originally by Jeanne Gatineau in 1937, it has grown into a well-established European skin-care line. More recently this line has found its way to the United States and is being sold on QVC. Aside from their allure as French imports, these products claim to be suited for sensitive skin, and particularly for those with rosacea. Alas, these highly aromatic products simply can't live up to that claim. The fragrance alone is enough to knock those with sensitive skin for a loop. Yet if the fragrance doesn't bother you, the good news is that there aren't many other offending ingredients. Very few problematic plant extracts grace these products, and when they do there isn't very much of them. On the other hand, there is a regrettably short supply of water-binding agents, antioxidants, and anti-irritants, though there are a few notable exceptions. That's especially disappointing given the price tags, which range from $15 to $65, and that's U.S. dollars, not Euros.

Adding an oddly innovative twist to what would otherwise just be another selection of antiaging potions aimed at the over-50 crowd is a group of products claiming to be the first laser treatment packaged in a cosmetic. You're expected to believe that these are equivalent to a real laser treatment, only gentler. Ingredients in these products are supposed to capture the positive energy of light and transform it into mini-beams that smooth the appearance of the skin's surface, erasing wrinkles, fine lines, and minor imperfections. Honestly, I am not making this up! (Wait, I need to stop laughing if I'm going to finish writing this review.... OK, I'm better now.) This tops the list as one of the most far-fetched marketing claims to come out of the cosmetics industry, and in an industry filled with over-the-top claims that's really saying something. It is a major understatement to suggest that there isn't a single ingredient in these so-called laser products that can in any way, shape, or form have that effect or any significant effect on skin. Not one wrinkle on your face will change, but you may blush from embarrassment for getting sucked into such nonsense. For more information about Gatineau, call (888) 345-5788 or visit www.qvc.com.

☺ **Soothing Cleanser** *($28 for 13.5 ounces)* is little more than water, mineral oil, thickeners, and fragrance. It's soothing for dry skin, but Pond's Cold Cream is just about identical for a fraction of the price.

☹ **Gentle Cleansing Toner** *($28 for 13.5 ounces)* contains mostly water, slip agents, preservatives, fragrance, and coloring agents. This exceptionally ordinary toner has a minuscule amount of sericin, which is a protein substance derived from silk spun by silk worms, that can have water-binding properties for skin. Despite the association with silk, the skin can't tell the difference between one form of protein and another.

☺ $$$ **Gentle Eye Make-Up Remover** *($15 for 1.6 ounces)* is an exceptionally standard and overpriced eye-makeup remover that uses a basic detergent cleansing agent.

☺ $$$ **Oxygenating Exfoliating Treatment** *($34 for 3.3 ounces)* is an exceptionally standard, detergent-based cleanser that contains jojoba wax particles as the scrub. There are some emollients in it that make it better for normal to dry skin. However, there is absolutely nothing oxygenating in here. That's actually good news, because oxygen can generate free-radical damage, something almost every other skin-care product in the world is trying to prevent.

☹ $$$ **Antiaging Eye Compresses Pack** *($39 for 6 packets)* contains mostly water, collagen, glycerin, thickeners, and preservatives. Does anyone still believe that collagen is the answer for their wrinkles? Gatineau seems to. Yet, there is not one shred of research showing that topical application of collagen has any benefit for skin other than being a good water-binding agent, period. The collagen craze ended in the early '90s when this once-popular ingredient left many women disappointed, and this overpriced treatment will prove the same.

☹ $$$ **Anti-Wrinkle Serum** *($42 for 0.51 ounce)*. While this does contain some beneficial water-binding agents and an antioxidant, the amounts are so minuscule as to be almost nonexistent. All in all, this contains far more preservatives and fragrance than it does any of the good stuff.

☹ $$$ **Anti-Aging Day Moisturizer** *($39 for 1.6 ounces)* does contain avobenzone for UVA protection, but because it doesn't list the sunscreen ingredients as active ingredients (required by the FDA for sunscreens), and has no SPF rating it cannot be relied on for sun protection. That isn't terribly disappointing, as this is just an OK emollient moisturizer with some good plant oils for dry skin. The tiny amount of lactic acid is ineffective as an exfoliant.

☹ $$$ **Anti-Aging Night Moisturizer** *($46 for 1.6 ounces)* is an OK moisturizer for dry skin, but the price is over the top for such a basic formulation. The grapeseed oil is a good emollient and antioxidant, but that can be said for a lot of plant oils, including the olive oil that's sitting right in your kitchen cabinet. The minute amounts of antioxidants and a water-binding agent in this product are insignificant for skin.

☹ $$$ **Anti-Aging Firming Throat Gel** *($49 for 1.6 ounces)* contains menthol, but it is probably present in such a small amount that it wouldn't cause irritation. The teeny amount of antioxidants present isn't firming at all, but deflating.

☹ **Anti-Fatigue Skin Care Concentrate** *($59 for 1 ounce)* lists alcohol as the third ingredient, and for skin that is just exhaustingly drying and irritating.

☹ $$$ **Hydrating Eye Contour Gel** *($28 for 0.5 ounce)* is an OK moisturizer for dry skin. The plant extracts are a mix of anti-irritants and irritants, but the worthwhile water-binding agents are in minute supply.

☺ $$$ **Melatogenine Eye-Care Cream** *($45 for 0.5 ounce)* is a good moisturizer for normal to dry skin, but there is nothing in it that will stop aging or change a wrinkle.

☹ $$$ **Hydrating Creamy Mask** *($30 for 2.5 ounces)* lists clay as the third ingredient, which is hardly hydrating. Rather this is just a very basic clay mask that has some oil-absorbing benefit for skin.

☺ $$$ **Lip Care Balm** *($26 for 0.5 ounce)* is a mineral oil– and plastic-based lip balm that is definitely emollient. It does contain very small amounts of some very good water-binding agents and antioxidants.

☺ $$$ **Laser Radiance Contour Serum** *($45 for 0.5 ounce)* contains mostly water, slip agent, mineral oil, glycerin, water-binding agent, silicones, thickeners, film-forming agent, preservatives, more thickeners, anti-irritant, antioxidants, and more water-binding agents. For the most part this is a good moisturizer for normal to dry skin, but the really interesting ingredients are there in barely detectable amounts. It goes without saying, but I just have to say it, that there is nothing in any of the Laser-named products that could have any laser-like effect on skin.

☺ $$$ **Laser Radiance Day Moisturizer** *($55 for 0.8 ounce)* is similar to the Contour Serum above and the same basic comments apply.

☺ $$$ **Laser Radiance Night Moisturizer** *($65 for 1.6 ounces)* is similar to the Contour Serum above and the same basic comments apply.

☺ $$$ **Laser Radiance Energizing Mask** *($35 for 2.5 ounces)* is an exceptionally standard clay mask that has a mere dusting of water-binding agents and antioxidants hiding behind the fragrance and preservatives.

GIORGIO ARMANI (MAKEUP ONLY)

Anyone with even a passing interest in today's fashion scene is no doubt familiar with the Armani name. Giorgio Armani is credited with giving tailored elegance, power, and sex appeal to forgotten standbys like men's suits, and turning Hollywood's A-list stars into fashion icons as they parade through countless awards ceremonies adorned in his elegance-laden creations. According to Armani, "The goal I seek is to have people refine their style through my clothing without having them become victims of fashion." Since Armani has always been passionate about textures, it's no surprise that his makeup presents an impressive collection that features some of the smoothst, lightest textures you're likely to find. From foundations to blushes, eyeshadows, and mascaras—even pencils—the makeup selection includes some truly stellar products. According to the brochure for Armani's makeup, the supreme textures and silky application are the result of Micro-fil technology. This supposedly allows for a precise way of blending and layering select ingredients, offering a heightened sense of color that fits like a second skin. Regardless of how that technology is labeled, almost all of the makeup uses standard silicone polymers along with ordinary ingredients like nylon-12. Of course, many cosmetics companies have their equivalent version of Micro-fil, but somehow Armani's is just a step above the rest.

The color collection was designed in part by fashion makeup artist Pat McGrath—and let me forewarn you that Ms. McGrath's use of color (at least for eyeshadow and eye pencil) is not what I would describe as classic or understated makeup. Nestled among the taupes, browns, grays, and soft blacks you will find a fair amount of pastel blues, greens, and lavenders that might catch your eye, yet may not be what's most flattering on or around them, especially since most of these shades are vibrantly shiny. On the subtle side, the shade range for foundations and powders is remarkably neutral, and caters beautifully to both very light and dark skin tones. Although the Armani makeup line is not widely available, it will become more accessible as more Armani stores (and select department stores) introduce it throughout 2003. In the meantime, if you live in or are visiting New York City, San Francisco, or Las Vegas this line is well worth perusing, if for nothing else than to experience some truly neutral foundations and play with an extremely user-friendly tester unit. For more information about Giorgio Armani makeup, call (212) 988-9191 or visit www.giorgioarmani.com.

FOUNDATION: ✔☺ $$$ **Luminous Silk Foundation** *($42)* has a fluid, ultra-smooth texture that floats over the skin and dries to a natural finish with a faint hint of shine. For light coverage and an unbelievably skin-like result that comes in 14 gorgeous colors for fair to dark skin, this foundation is tough to beat. It is best for normal to slightly dry or slightly oily skin. ✔☺ $$$ **Silk Foundation Powder** *($40)* is a wet/dry talc-based powder foundation that has a buttercream-smooth texture, excellent application, and soft matte finish. The 14 brilliant shades feature options for all skin tones (except very dark) and do not look ashen or chalky. This provides light to medium coverage and is worth the splurge if you prefer powder foundations. ✔☺ $$$ **Fluid Sheer** *($42)* is similar to the Luminous Silk Foundation, but is meant to "polish, sculpt, and illuminate facial contours." There are seven translucent "enhancers," each with a soft shimmer that looks great in photographs, but can be distracting in daylight. For a touch of shine or to softly highlight your features in the evening, these are fine, and they blend well with foundation or moisturizer. The only shades to avoid are numbers 5 and 6—two color-correcting shades that are well-intentioned but too peach or yellow to recommend.

☺ $$$ **CONCEALER: Skin Retouch** *($26)* is described as "a cream graft of color" but is a bit too creamy for its own good. The initially thick texture melts into skin and blends well, but it's also crease-prone unless a generous amount of powder accompanies it. The seven shades coordinate well with most skin colors, though 0 is almost white and 4 is too peach for those with a medium skin tone. For the money, a soft matte concealer such as Elizabeth Arden's Flawless Finish ($14) is preferable to this.

POWDER: ✔☺ $$$ **Sheer Powder** *($38)* is a very smooth, talc-based pressed powder that has a soft, almost imperceptible finish on the skin and comes in seven stunning neutral colors. ✔☺ $$$ **Micro-fil Loose Powder** *($42)* has an equally wonderful texture and a seamless finish that is seemingly incapable of looking too dry or powdery on skin. The five colors are excellent, though each one leaves a very soft shine—something those with oily skin will not be thrilled with, but those with dry skin will find attractive. ✔☺ $$$ **Sheer Bronzer** *($33)* was bound to be great, as Giorgio Armani himself is a huge proponent of bronzing powder (and being perpetually tan, but that's another story) and was actively involved in choosing these four sun-kissed colors.

Although all of them have a subtle shine, each shade has a good balance of red, brown, and orange pigment that allows for the illusion of a real tan—though it would have been even more convincing had the shine been nixed.

☺ $$$ **Sheer Shimmer** *($33)* is indeed shimmery, but the effect is sheer and not too intrusive. Billed as "special effects for the face," these can nicely enhance a taut brow bone, aquiline nose, or delicate collarbone, without announcing their presence when they're used sparingly.

BLUSH: ☺ $$$ **Sheer Blush** *($33)* does have an incredibly smooth, powder-based texture and flawless application, but each shade is shiny and too distracting for subtle daytime wear. The shades are quite soft, but would have been better with a matte finish that you could then add shine to if desired.

✓☺ $$$ **Color Retouch** *($35)* is a velvety cream blush that offers sheer, dewy colors and an easy application. There are not as many shades of the Color Retouch as for the Sheer Blush above, but if you're a fan of cream blush (and not on a cosmetics budget) this is worth a test run.

☺ $$$ **EYESHADOW:** The large selection of pressed powder **Eyeshadow** *($22)* features an impressive smooth texture that is a pleasure to work with. The shades start sheer but easily allow you to build intensity, and they cling well to skin. Disappointingly, most of the 25+ colors have some amount of shine, though there are some subdued options to consider. Numbers 1, 13, 14, 15, 24, 25, and 27 are too blue, green, or lilac (purple) to recommend.

EYE AND BROW SHAPER: ✓☺ $$$ **Smooth Silk Eye Pencil** *($22)* is a standard pencil in that it needs regular sharpening, but otherwise it has a wonderfully silky application that sets to a reasonably solid finish. Finally, an overpriced eye pencil that has more going for it than the cache of a designer logo! Unless you're interested in using eye pencil for shock value, avoid numbers 3, 5, and 6.

LIPSTICK AND LIP PENCIL: ✓☺ $$$ **Smooth Lipstick** *($21)* is billed as being "beyond matte" but ends up going right past matte so that you're left with a semi-opaque, light-textured creamy lipstick with a soft glossy finish. The colors are exquisite.

☺ $$$ **Sheer Lipstick** *($21)* is "the lipstick of the future" and although that sounds promising, this silicone-based lipstick is merely one more glossy lipstick to consider if price isn't an issue, and if transparent, fleeting color is what you're after. **Shine Lipstick** *($21)* is even more glossy (and more slippery) than the Sheer Lipstick and has a short life-span on the lips—yet the colors, particularly No. 8 Armani Red, are an intriguing blend of classic and fashion-forward hues. **Smooth Silk Lip Pencil** *($22)* is a standard creamy lip pencil that glides over the lips and comes in great colors—but so do many other pencils that cost far less and are as close as your neighborhood drugstore.

☺ $$$ **Shine Lip Gloss** *($16)* is a thick, viscous tube gloss that is similar to M.A.C.'s LipGlass ($11.50) and, given the price difference and wide availability of M.A.C. (and countless other lip gloss–toting lines), this is one you can safely pass up.

The Reviews G

MASCARA: ✓☺ $$$ **Soft Lash Mascara** *($20)* is an admirable lengthening mascara that does not clump or flake and allows you to define lashes quickly. Thickness is harder to come by, but for clean, long-lasting length this does the job.

☺ $$$ BRUSHES: Consulting makeup artist Pat McGrath has put together a useful and elegant selection of **Brushes** *($20–$54)*, although the salesperson confided that the **Face Brush** *($54)* and **Blush Brush** *($38)* needed to be retooled due to hair breakage (I noticed this as well). The best brushes to consider are the **Blender** *($34)*, **Eye Contour Brush** *($38)*, **Eyeshader Brush** *($38)*, **Eyebrow Brush** *($20)*, and **Eyeliner Brush** *($20)*. The **Combing Brow and Lash Brush** *($20)* is not necessary when an old, clean mascara wand does the same thing, and the **Lip Brush** *($20)* is sans cap and nonretractable, which means it's for at-home use only. At this price, it should be completely versatile!

GIVENCHY

The name Givenchy rolls off the tongue like an infusion of French wine and haute couture fashion. Yet as eloquent and refined as it sounds, image doesn't equal substance when it comes to cosmetics, and it turns out the Givenchy products have more packaging accent than product quality. Skin care is the most disappointing aspect of this line, and it has been pared down to almost nothing since the previous edition of this book. Ordinary formulations abound, and despite the presence of some exotic-sounding ingredients, these are mostly waxy bases with few to no current formulations and not even one sunscreen to be found. For more information about Givenchy, call (212) 931-2600 or visit www.sephora.com. **Note:** All Givenchy products contain fragrance.

GIVENCHY SKIN CARE

☹ $$$ **Creamy Cleansing Foam** *($28 for 4.2 ounces)* is a standard, detergent-based, water-soluble cleanser that uses cleansing agents (myristic acid and potassium hydroxide) that are considered more drying and irritating than most.

☺ $$$ **Regulating Cleansing Gel, Purifying Care for Radiant Skin Combination and Oily Skin** *($22 for 4.5 ounces)* is a standard, detergent-based, water-soluble cleanser that would work well for someone with normal to oily skin. The plant extracts are a mix of anti-irritants and irritants. It does contain coloring agents.

☺ $$$ **Make-off Emulsion** *($28 for 6.7 ounces)* is merely a mineral oil–based, wipe-off cleanser that includes slip agents, fragrance, and preservatives. It will take off makeup and can leave a greasy film on the skin. This is virtually identical to using plain mineral oil, which is available for about $2 for 16 ounces.

☺ $$$ **Gentle Exfoliating Massage** *($45 for 1.7 ounces)* is a standard, synthetic-based scrub (ground-up plastic is the abrasive) mixed with thickening agents and mineral oil. It can be an option for dry skin, but can leave a film on the skin.

☹ **Bain des Soin Toner for Combination/Oily Skin** *($28 for 6.7 ounces)* lists alcohol as the second ingredient, which would be drying and irritating enough for any skin type, but this one also includes camphor, menthol, and coltsfoot, and is absolutely not recommended.

☺ $$$ **Bain des Soin Toner for Normal/Dry Skin** ($28 for 6.7 ounces) would work for normal to dry skin, but it is exceptionally ordinary and utterly undistinguished.

☺ $$$ **Balancing Mist** ($30 for 5 ounces) contains mostly water, ginseng, silicone, water-binding agent, fragrance, and preservatives. The coltsfoot here can be a problem for skin, but all in all this is just a very basic toner for normal to dry skin. There's also a small amount of lactic acid, but due to the product's high pH it has no exfoliating properties for skin.

☹ $$$ **Regulating Mist** ($30 for 5 ounces) contains urea, which can exfoliate skin, but there are several plant extracts that can be skin irritants.

☺ $$$ **Double Sequence Eye Contour Firming Balm** ($75 for 60 doses) is a two-step process that comes in medical-looking vials. As therapeutic as this appears to be, the ingredients are less than remarkable. This is a combination that may make for a good moisturizer, but it won't firm anything. Dose 1 contains several thickeners, water-binding agents, plant oils, emollients, preservatives, and plant extracts. Dose 2 is almost identical except for the addition of urea, which can have exfoliating properties. There are some antioxidants, interesting water-binding agents, and anti-irritants, but in such teeny amounts it makes them practically insignificant.

☺ $$$ **Lifting Double Sequence** ($100 for 0.5 ounce total, 30 treatments) is a lighter-weight, silicone-based version of the Eye Contour Firming Balm above. The two Doses are OK moisturizing formulations with some interesting water-binding agents, but this is by far more image than substance. You are actually spending $3,200 for a pound of this stuff, and all you get is a moisturizer for normal to slightly dry skin. For this kind of money you would have enough for a great face-lift in less than a year or two.

☺ $$$ **Firm Profile** ($55 for 1.7 ounces) is a shockingly standard moisturizer for normal to dry skin. Some of the plant extracts can be skin irritants.

☺ $$$ **Firm Profile Eye** ($45 for 0.5 ounce) is similar to the Firm Profile above and the same basic comments apply.

☺ $$$ **Firm Profile Serum** ($50 for 0.26 ounce) is similar to the Firm Profile above. This one does contain more film-forming agent, and lists the fourth ingredient as alcohol, but none of this makes it any more firming than the other Profile formulas.

☺ $$$ **Hydra-Tricellia Evolution Fluide** ($47 for 1.7 ounces) contains mostly water, thickeners, sunscreen agents (though this is not rated with an SPF and there are no UVA-protecting ingredients), fragrance, preservatives, film-forming agents, vitamin E, silicone, water-binding agents, more preservatives, plant extracts, and coloring agents. The teeny amount of beneficial ingredients for skin makes this an exceedingly over-fragrant and overpriced moisturizer for normal to dry skin.

☺ $$$ **Hydra-Tricellia Mask** ($42 for 10 treatments, 0.25 ounce each) could be an OK mask for someone with normal to slightly dry skin, but this is mostly a "Why bother?" because there are far better moisturizers available than this one.

☹ **Essential Matte Long Lasting Shine Control Fluid** *($39 for 1.7 ounces)* lists alcohol as the second ingredient, and the only thing long lasting about this will be the irritation and dryness it will cause if you use it regularly.

☹ **Gentle Exfoliating Massage** *($45 for 1.5 ounces)* is little more than mineral oil and plastic (polyethylene) that you apply and then peel off the face. Period. This is incredibly overpriced for what ends up being a mediocre, do-nothing formulation.

☹ **Regulating Purifying Mask for Oily Skin** *($38 for 2.8 ounces)* is a standard clay mask that also contains a lot of alcohol, which makes it too irritating and drying for any skin type.

GIVENCHY MAKEUP

The entire Givenchy color line was phased out of department stores in 1999. I doubt that anyone seriously missed it, however, since there was little to notice and the colors (particularly for foundations) were some of the worst around. It turned out a revamping was in the works as well as a streamlined, niche-driven distribution process. The image-is-everything line is now available in select Sephora stores (they have the same parent company, Louis Vuitton Moet-Hennessey) as well as on www.sephora.com. Department stores are now nowhere in the Givenchy makeup picture. But is there any reason to seek out Givenchy for makeup? If futuristic, cosmetics-as-art packaging intrigues you, yes. Each piece of Givenchy makeup comes in elegantly sculpted, decadently angled containers, each equipped with a built-in mirror. One cannot help but feel indulgent simply holding a Givenchy compact—even the powders are pressed into unusual shapes and embossed with beveled edges. Yet for all of this elegant posturing, the line remains mostly unexciting when it comes to performance. There are a few standouts, but overall the experience of Givenchy makeup is akin to mistaking your cubic zirconia for a diamond.

☺ **$$$ FOUNDATION:** **Teint Miroir Lift ConFort Foundation SPF 10** *($38)* is a liquid foundation that has a smooth silicone base that blends very well, drying to a natural matte finish. This provides medium coverage and would be an option for normal to oily skin, but the sunscreen lacks UVA-protecting ingredients and four of the six shades are just too peach to look convincing in daylight. Only Ivory 1 and Spice 6 are realistic colors. **Teint Miroir Satine Foundation SPF 15** *($38)* is a sumptuous creamy foundation for normal to dry skin that blends easily, offering sheer to light coverage and an appropriate satin finish. The sunscreen is in-part titanium dioxide. Again, the poor colors are this otherwise stellar foundation's undoing. Only Ivory 61 is an option among the five shades. **Teint Miroir Mat Foundation SPF 15** *($38)* has a fluid, sheer texture that feels amazingly light and blends with just a bit too much slip. The natural matte finish has a dimensional quality to it, which looks more skin-like. What's not skin-like in the least are the majority of the six colors. Used over oily skin, the peachy hues will only look increasingly orange throughout the day. Ivory 81 and Spice 86 are the best choices. The sunscreen is in-part titanium dioxide. **Teint Miroir Soleil Bronzing Foundation** *($30)* is a liquid bronzing lotion that comes in two utterly believable tan colors. What a shame that these sheer colors are overpowered with iridescence.

☹ <u>CONCEALER:</u> **Corrective Concealer** *($22)* is a horribly greasy stick concealer that comes in three hideously obvious colors and is not recommended.

☺ $$$ <u>POWDER:</u> **Flawless Effects Pressed Powder & Brush** *($36)* is a collection of talc-based pressed powders in which the powder cake is divided into four separate colors that can be used separately or as one. However, the majority of these powder quads feature odd or unbecoming colors that do little to flatter the complexion. For pricey bronzing powder, Warmth 4 and Sun 5 are possibilities. The included powder brush is retractable and quite soft and workable. **Semi-Loose Face Powder** *($40)* is called semi-loose because it is very softly pressed. Don't drop this compact, as even a light impact will cause the powder to break. The shades share the same comments as the Pressed Powder above, except that these have noticeable shine.

<u>BLUSH:</u> ☺ $$$ **Powder Blush** *($36)* is a pressed-powder blush with dual-toned colors. One half is barely shiny, the other blindingly so. This does have a smooth, soft texture and nonpowdery application; but think twice about adorning your cheeks with this much shine.

☹ **Powder & Cream for Cheeks & Eyes** *($35)* features a split pan of powder and cream colors in one compact. The powder portion is fine, but the cream tends to blend unevenly and comes off in chunks. What seems like a versatile timesaver quickly turns into a middling frustration.

☺ $$$ <u>EYESHADOW:</u> **Mono Eyeshadow Powder** *($20)* are actually duos, though the colors are so close it's really like getting one shade per compact. These all have an OK but slightly stiff application and a texture that feels nicer than it applies. Each of the sheer shades is shine-laden *and* there are lots of greens, blues, and violets to avoid.

<u>EYE AND BROW SHAPER:</u> ☺ $$$ **Miroir Eyebrow Definition Pencil** *($19)* rises above the fact that it needs regular sharpening by having a great, effortless application and a soft powder finish that isn't heavy in the least. It's unfortunate there are only two colors.

☺ $$$ **Precision Liquid Eyeliner** *($30)* is a very good liquid eyeliner that is dispensed from a click-pen applicator. Although this is only capable of drawing a thick line, the formula dries in place and stays on—which is what you should expect, especially at this price!

☹ **Eyeliner Pencil Miroir** *($18)* is a completely below-standard creamy pencil that leaves a slightly tacky finish. This will smudge easily, too, though the colors are surprisingly tame.

<u>LIPSTICK AND LIP PENCIL:</u> ☺ $$$ **Rouge Miroir Lipstick SPF 8** *($21)* does not contain adequate UVA protection, and the SPF 8 is almost laughable. This has a thick, emollient texture with a greasy finish and colors with light to medium opacity. For the money, I wouldn't choose this over the creamy lipstick choices from Revlon, Almay, or L'Oreal. **Transparent Miroir** *($21)* is a simple, sheer-and-glossy lipstick that comes in great colors, but it's overpriced for such a basic formulation! **Lacque Miroir Crystal Lipgloss**

($24) is an uncomfortably sticky gloss that you apply with a brush. The sheer, metallic colors somehow fit with the space-age mirrored packaging.

☺ $$$ **Eau de Rouge Semi-Matte Liquid Lipstick** *($24)* stays slick and moist as it imparts intense color and a high-gloss finish that is as far from matte as you can get! The brush applicator is easy to work with, and this is overall a pleasant product. **Lacque Miroir Lip Shine** *($24)* is a moderately sticky, wand-type lip gloss that also features highly pigmented, exquisite colors, each with a glass-like shine. **Lip Liner Miroir** *($19)* is a standard, creamy-smooth lip pencil whose colors have an appreciable stain.

☺ $$$ <u>MASCARA:</u> **Thickening Lash by Lash Mascara** *($19)* is not the best of its kind, but it does unquestionably produce ample length and slight thickness without a lot of effort. It has a small tendency to smear, but is otherwise excellent. **Lengthening and Curling Lashes Mascara** *($19)* directs you to "sweep away the competition with this glamorous, state-of-the-art mascara," but Givenchy is apparently unaware of the vast selection of outstanding mascaras that easily improve on this good, but not spectacular, formula. This builds nice, non-overdone length without clumping and leaves a soft curl, making it an option for an enhanced but still natural look.

GLYMED PLUS (SKIN CARE ONLY)

Glymed Plus is one of many skin-care lines being sold by dermatologists and spas. Of course there is nothing particularly medical about these products. As far as spa lines are concerned, I've yet to see anything particularly special about any of them in comparison to similar lines sold at department stores or drugstores, other than the price tag, that is. Glymed claims its products are naturally manufactured (who doesn't?), but they aren't, though I imagine you could argue that there's no such thing as "unnatural" manufactured cosmetics. The ingredients in Glymed products aren't any more natural than those in any other cosmetics line, and that means they include plenty of synthetics and a share of plant-extract ingredients. There are some good AHA moisturizers here, but the Acne Management line contains several unnecessary irritants, and similar and gentler formulations with the same active ingredients are available for less at the drugstore. The new Cell Science line is a revamp of Glymed's Oxy Radical Anti-Oxidant Therapy. The new version has a few more interesting water-binding agents and antioxidants, but these aren't particularly unique and means these products would work the same as hundreds of others containing antioxidants. For more information about Glymed Plus, call (800) 676-9667 or visit www.glymedplus.com.

GLYMED AGE MANAGEMENT SYSTEM

☺ $$$ **Gentle Facial Wash** *($29 for 8 ounces)* isn't all that gentle, but it is a good, albeit exceptionally overpriced, detergent-based, water-soluble cleanser that would work well for normal to oily skin. It does contain about 2% to 3% AHA, which isn't much, but the pH is too high for it to be effective as an exfoliant anyway.

☺ $$$ **Skin Recovery Mist** *($28.75 for 4 ounces)* is an OK toner for normal to dry skin.

☺ $$$ **AHA Accelerator** *($59.95 for 4 ounces)*. It goes without saying that there are less expensive AHA products available with similar or better formulations than this one (Alpha Hydrox at the drugstore is one that comes to mind). This does have a good concentration of AHA and a pH that makes it effective as an exfoliant. It does contain fragrance.

☹ **Facial Hydrator** *($47.75 for 4 ounces)* lists alcohol as the second ingredient, and that is too irritating for most skin types. It also contains lemon, citrus, and balm mint oils, which add irritation without bringing any benefit to the skin.

✓☺ $$$ **Treatment Cream** *($69.55 for 2 ounces)* is a very good emollient, glycolic acid–based AHA moisturizer with about 7% AHA and a pH of 3.5, which makes it an effective exfoliant for dry skin. It does contain fragrance.

☺ $$$ **Eye and Lip Renewal Complex** *($36.75 for 0.75 ounce)* contains mostly water, thickeners, silicone, plant oil, AHA (about 3%), vitamins, water-binding agents, plant extracts, fragrant oils, film-forming agent, and preservatives. The amount of AHA isn't enough for it to be effective as an exfoliant, and that's good, because it would be a problem for the lips, which can be irritated far more easily than other skin. It's a good moisturizer for normal to slightly dry skin, but there is nothing about it that makes it especially suited to the eyes or lips. The DNA and RNA in this product cannot affect skin cells. It does contain fragrance.

☺ $$$ **Vital-A Retinyl Cream** *($36.25 for 1.5 ounces)* contains retinyl palmitate, a form of vitamin A. There is research showing it can improve the thickness of skin, and that's good. This also contains lactic acid (about 7%), but the pH is too high for it to be effective as an exfoliant. Overall, this is a good basic moisturizer for dry skin with minimal water-binding agents.

☺ $$$ **Photo-Age Environmental Protection Gel SPF 20** *($47.25 for 7 ounces)* is a very good, titanium dioxide–based sunscreen. It works well but it can leave a white film on the skin. The gel feel is a great option for some skin types that like gels and want titanium dioxide–based sun protection to prevent irritation to skin and eyes. Only the price is a problem, because concern about the cost can affect how liberally you are likely to apply it and liberal application is essential to get the full benefit of the SPF.

☹ **Photo-Age Protection Cream SPF 15** *($27.50 for 2 ounces)* doesn't contain UVA-protecting ingredients and is not recommended.

☺ **Tan-In Self-Activating Tanning Cream** *($21 for 7 ounces)* uses dihydroxyacetone, just as all self-tanners do, to affect the color of skin. This one would work as well as any.

☹ **Alpha-Hydrox Exfoliant Masque** *($39.40 for 4 ounces)* is a waxy mask that contains mostly paraffin and scrub particles. The wax does help roll off the outer layer of skin cells, but it can be pore clogging for some skin types. It also contains small amounts of AHA and BHA, but they aren't effective as exfoliants because the pH is too high for them to work.

✓☺ $$$ **Derma Pigment Bleaching Fluid** *($33.60 for 2 ounces)* is a good, 2% concentration, hydroquinone-based moisturizer. It contains mostly water, slip agents, aloe, thickeners, and preservatives. Less expensive versions of skin-lightening products like this are available, of course, but this is definitely an option to consider.

☺ $$$ **Derma Pigment Skin Brightener** *($33.60 for 2 ounces)* contains mostly water, AHA (about 8%); glycerin, plant oil, aloe, antioxidants, kojic acid, thickeners, water-binding agents, and preservatives. This is a good glycolic acid–based moisturizer for normal to slightly dry skin. Kojic acid has some ability to inhibit melanin production, but it suffers from poor stability and is a relatively unreliable ingredient. This is a good AHA product with some good elements for normal to dry skin.

✓☺ $$$ **Living Cell Clarifier** *($33.60 for 2 ounces)* contains live yeast cells, sort of like the stuff that makes bread dough rise. There is no known benefit for using these on skin, but it won't hurt skin either. This product also contains bearberry, licorice, a form of vitamin C that can be helpful for inhibiting melanin production, other antioxidants, water-binding agents, and anti-irritants. The yeast part is hokey, but overall this is a well-formulated lightweight moisturizer for normal to slightly dry skin.

GLYMED CELL SCIENCE

☹ $$$ **Cell Science High Purification Skin Cleanser** *($29 for 8 ounces)* is a basic lotion cleanser that is an option for someone with normal to dry skin. It contains a tiny amount of antioxidants, but that still doesn't warrant this price tag. It does contain fragrance.

✓☺ $$$ **Cell Science Daily Skin Repair Cream** *($68.25 for 2 ounces)* contains some very good antioxidants and water-binding agents in an emollient base that would be good for someone with dry skin, although this won't repair skin any better than any other well-formulated moisturizer. It does contain fragrance.

✓☺ $$$ **Cell Science Daily Cell Repair Serum** *($68.25 for 0.5 ounce)* is similar to the Repair Cream above only in lotion form, and the same basic comments apply.

✓☺ $$$ **Cell Science Photo-Sunscreen SPF 35** *($40.95 for 2 ounces)* is a good in-part titanium dioxide–based sunscreen in an emollient base that contains some good water-binding agents and a tiny amount of antioxidants. This is an option for normal to dry skin.

☹ $$$ **Cell Science Skin Repair Fruit Enzyme Masque** *($41.80 for 2 ounces)* lists cornstarch as the fourth ingredient, and that can be a problem for skin. It does contain papain and pineapple, but those have limited, if any, ability to exfoliate skin. The water-binding agents in it are great for skin, but the cornstarch pretty much undoes their benefit. It does contain antioxidants.

GLYMED VITAMIN C PRODUCTS

✓☺ $$$ **Vitamin C Cream** *($82.95 for 2 ounces)* definitely contains magnesium ascorbyl phosphate, a good, stable form of vitamin C, as well as some other very good antioxidants, but it has only a small amount of water-binding agents. Fortunately, the RNA and DNA in this cream cannot do anything to affect the genetic makeup of your skin cells. Though it's very overpriced, if you are looking for vitamin C this is a product to consider. It does contain fragrance.

☺ **$$$ Vitamin C Serum** *($67.95 for 0.5 ounce)* is not as well formulated with a variety of ingredients as the Vitamin C Cream above, though this does contain more vitamin C. Vitamin C is a good, skin-friendly ingredient, but it is not the be-all and end-all of antioxidants. This does contain fragrance.

GLYMED SERIOUS ACTION

☹ **$$$ Serious Action Skin Wash** *($28.60 for 8 ounces)* is a standard, detergent-based, water-soluble cleanser that contains 2.5% benzoyl peroxide. That can be an option for disinfecting blemish-prone skin, but in a cleanser the benefit would be mostly washed down the drain.

☹ **$$$ Serious Action Exfoliant Scrub** *($28.60 for 8 ounces)* is similar to the Skin Wash above, with similar issues, only this version contains plastic scrub particles.

☹ **Serious Action Skin Astringent No. 5** *($26.95 for 8 ounces)* contains alcohol and menthol, which are problematic ingredients for irritation and dryness and have no positive effect on any skin type.

☹ **Serious Action Skin Astringent No. 10** *($28.05 for 8 ounces)* is similar to Astringent No. 5 above and the same comments apply.

☹ **Serious Action Masque** *($39.50 for 4 ounces)* is a standard clay mask that also contains eucalyptus and camphor, which makes it unnecessarily irritating for all skin types.

☹ **Serious Action Skin Gel** *($58.85 for 4 ounces)* is aimed at controlling breakouts, but this is a lot of money for some fairly irritating ingredients, including alcohol (second on the ingredient list), camphor oil, and eucalyptus oil. There are far better products for breakouts than this, not to mention for far less money.

✓☺ **Serious Action Skin Medication No. 5** *($26.95 for 4 ounces)* is a good 5% benzoyl peroxide gel that also contains a teeny amount of tea tree oil. It is a very good option for blemish-prone skin.

✓☺ **Serious Skin Medication No. 10** *($26.40 for 4 ounces)* is similar to the No. 5 version above, except that this one contains 10% benzoyl peroxide.

☹ **Serious Skin Peeling Lotion** *($28.05 for 2 ounces)* contains sulfur, salicylic acid, resorcinol, and alcohol, so I would absolutely call this seriously irritating. There are far better ways to exfoliate skin and disinfect it at the same time without using these three ingredients.

G.M. COLLIN

This French line of skin-care products was launched in 1957. Since then, G.M. Collin has become an international spa/salon line with a complex group of products asserting lofty claims and promising nothing less than perfect skin. Despite fervent assurances from the brochure that this line is technologically advanced, product after product poses a conundrum. For example, many of the products do contain some very impressive water-binding agents, anti-irritants, and antioxidants, and yet many of them also contain an assortment of irritating plant extracts such as menthol, lemon, grapefruit, eucalyptus, and arnica. Several of the products also contain alcohol and a few contain sodium lauryl sulfate, a cleansing agent and emulsifier known as a potent skin sensitizer.

Even more puzzling are some basic formulation issues. As a rule, throughout this book, I have not gone into detail about the issue of preservatives and their varying pros and cons. I do explain, at the beginning of Chapter Three, some of the questions surrounding formaldehyde-releasing preservatives, and the problem with some of the parabens having estrogenic properties. These technicalities are difficult to assess and overall I agree with most of the cosmetics chemists I interviewed for this book. And that means I believe that a well-preserved cosmetic is better than one subject to contamination by bacteria, molds, and fungus. While there is much disagreement over the issue of preservatives, there are two preservatives—methylchloroisothiazolinone and methylisothiazolinone (together they go by the trade name Kathon CG)—that are universally recognized as being acceptable for use only in rinse-off products (Sources: *Contact Dermatitis,* November 2001, pages 257–264 and *European Journal of Dermatology,* March 1999, pages 144–160). Even the manufacturers of these two ingredients concur (Source: Rohm and Haas, http://www.rohmhaas.com). It is therefore a bit shocking that G.M. Collin would use Kathon CG in several of their leave-on skin-care products, and those products are not recommended.

The G.M. Collin line has some excellent moisturizers and its sunscreens are well-formulated, but overall there are far more letdowns than satisfactions, and that's disappointing. In essence, it seems that for every brilliant ingredient used there is an equally abysmal ingredient in the mix. For more information about G.M. Collin, call (800) 341-1531 or visit www.gm-collin.com. **Note:** All G.M. Collin products contain fragrance.

☹ **Royal Jelly Cleansing Milk** *($22.50 for 6.75 ounces).* There is no research showing royal jelly to have benefit for skin, which makes this just a basic detergent-based cleanser. The menthol it contains makes it a problem for all skin types.

☹ **Hydramucine Cleansing Milk** *($22.50 for 6.75 ounces)* is a standard, detergent-based cleanser that also contains lemon, eucalyptus, and grapefruit, which makes it too potentially irritating for all skin types.

☹ **Biovegetal Floral Cleansing Milk All Skin Types** *($22.50 for 6.75 ounces).* The mint, lemon, and rosemary in this product can be skin irritants. Other than that, this is just a very standard lotion cleanser.

☹ **Mild Cleansing Gel Oily Normal or Sensitive Skin** *($22.50 for 6.75 ounces)* isn't mild in the least, though it is a standard, detergent-based, water-soluble cleanser. The citronella, grapefruit, lemon, and mint can be skin irritants.

☹ **Biovegetal Phytoaromatic Gommage** *($22.90 for 1.7 ounces).* The main detergent cleansing agent is sodium lauryl sulfate, which makes this too potentially irritating and drying for all skin types.

☹ **Hydramucine Lotion** *($23 for 6.75 ounces)* contains several irritating plant extracts, including lemon and eucalyptus.

☹ **Isotonic Lotion** *($23 for 6.75 ounces)* contains Kathon CG, which should not be used in leave-on skin-care products. This toner is not recommended.

☹ **Biovegetal Floral Water Lotion** *($23 for 6.75 ounces)* contains a mix of irritating plant extracts and anti-irritants along with a great deal of fragrance. It also contains Kathon CG, which should not be used in leave-on skin-care products. This is more like wearing eau de cologne than applying a lotion for skin care.

☹ **Puractive Lotion Normal to Oily Skin** *($23 for 6.75 ounces)* contains several irritating plant extracts including arnica, sage, lemon, citronella, and cornmint. It also contains Kathon CG, which should not be used in leave-on skin-care products. This toner is not recommended.

☺ **Desincrustant Lotion Oily Skin** *($23.50 for 6.75 ounces)* contains mostly water, detergent cleansing agent, disinfectant, fragrance, and coloring agents. This has no benefit for oily skin other than as an extra cleansing step.

☺ **$$$ AHA + Ceramide Skin Care Normal to Oily Skin** *($37.50 for 1.7 ounces)* doesn't contain any AHAs. The sugarcane, citrus, and apple extract may sound like AHAs but they have no exfoliating properties and are night-and-day different from such true AHAs as lactic, glycolic, malic, and citric acids.

☺ **$$$ AHA + Ceramide Skin Care Phase I** *($31.50 for 1.7 ounces)* is similar to the AHA + Ceramide Normal to Oily Skin above, and the same comments apply.

☺ **$$$ AHA + Ceramides Skincare Mature Fatigued Skin** *($37.50 for 1.7 ounces)* is similar to the AHA + Ceramide Normal to Oily Skin above, and the same comments apply.

☹ **AHA Gel Oily Skin** *($38 for 1.7 ounces)* lists alcohol as the second ingredient and also contains irritating plant extracts, which makes this too irritating and drying for all skin types. Regrettably, this one really does contain glycolic acid and salicylic acid in a pH that would make it effective for exfoliation.

☹ **Biovegetal "Hydration Cream"** *($30 for 1.7 ounces)* contains Kathon CG, which should not be used in leave-on skin-care products. This product is not recommended.

☺ **$$$ Biovegetal Eyelid Relaxing Gel** *($24 for 0.5 ounce)* is an OK gel moisturizer with a teeny amount of antioxidants, but only a minuscule amount of water-binding agents.

☹ **Biovegetal Eyelid "Sculpture" Cream** *($24 for 0.5 ounce)* contains Kathon CG, which should not be used in leave-on skin-care products. This product is not recommended.

☹ **Biovegetal Equilibrium Gel** *($30 for 1.7 ounces)* contains Kathon CG, which should not be used in leave-on skin-care products. This product is not recommended.

☹ **Biovegetal "Vitality" Cream** *($31 for 1.7 ounces)* contains sodium lauryl sulfate high up on the ingredient list, which makes this too irritating and sensitizing for all skin types. What sodium lauryl sulfate is doing in a moisturizer is anyone's guess.

✓☺ **$$$ Retinol Action + Q10 Vitamin A Skin Care** ($56 for 1.7 ounces) contains an excellent group of water-binding agents, antioxidants, plant oils, and retinol. This would be a very good moisturizer for someone with normal to dry skin.

☺ **$$$ Vitamin C Concentrate** ($56 for 1 ounce) contains a great deal of fragrance (it has more orange fragrance than it does vitamin C), but it does contain some good water-binding agents and antioxidants and would be an option for someone with normal to slightly dry skin. The RNA it contains cannot affect the genetic component of skin cells.

☺ **$$$ Daily Ceramide Comfort** ($66 for 75 capsules for a total of 0.84 ounce) is a silicone-based lotion placed in capsules for no other reason than to make it look more medicinal and extraordinary. It isn't. Aside from the silicone this just contains some good plant oils, water-binding agents, and a tiny amount of antioxidants. It actually does not contain ceramides, but that isn't a shortcoming because there are other equally good water-binding agents in this product; it's just that the name is misleading.

☹ **Royal Jelly Cream** ($30 for 1.7 ounces) contains Kathon CG, which should not be used in leave-on skin-care products. This product is not recommended.

☹ **Ultraderm Hydro-Restructuring Complex** ($54 for 0.8 ounce) contains Kathon CG, which should not be used in leave-on skin-care products. This product is not recommended.

✓☺ **$$$ Ultraderm Native Collagene Gel** ($49.90 for 1.7 ounces) is a lightweight gel with a very good mix of water-binding agents and antioxidants. The gimmicky claims this makes about the DNA and RNA in it are nonsense; they can't affect cell function but they can function as good water-binding agents.

✓☺ **$$$ Ultraderm Hydro Nutritive Cream** ($52.50 for 1.7 ounces) is similar to the Native Collagene Gel above only in cream form, and the same basic comments apply.

✓☺ **$$$ Ultraderm Hydro Restorative Cream** ($69 for 1.7 ounces) is similar to the Native Collagene Gel above only in cream form, and the same basic comments apply.

✓☺ **$$$ Time Corrector Eyelid Gel-Cream** ($43 for 0.8 ounce) is similar to the Native Collagene Gel above only in cream form, and the same basic comments apply.

☺ **$$$ Vitalift Cream** ($46.50 for 1.7 ounces). There are a few good water-binding agents and plant oils in this moisturizer, but it is not as impressively formulated as others in this line. It contains a small amount of arnica, which can be a skin irritant.

☺ **$$$ Vitalift Concentrate** ($41 for 0.8 ounce) is similar to the Vitalift Cream above and the same basic comments apply.

✓☺ **$$$ Sensiderm Cream** ($34 for 1.7 ounces) is a good emollient moisturizer for normal to dry skin with some interesting anti-irritants, water-binding agents, antioxidants, and plant oils. Omitting the fragrant plant oil would really have made this one good for sensitive skin.

☺ **$$$ Hydramucine Cream** ($30 for 1.7 ounces) contains some irritating plant extracts, though it also contains some very good water-binding agents, antioxidants, and emollients.

☹ **Hydramucine Concentrate** *($36 for 0.8 ounce)* contains Kathon CG, which should not be used in leave-on skin-care products. This product is not recommended.

✓☺ $$$ **Nutrivital Cream** *($33.50 for 1.7 ounces)* is an emollient moisturizer for normal to dry skin that contains an impressive group of plant oils, water-binding agents, and antioxidants.

✓☺ $$$ **Phyto-Lipidic Complex** *($35 for 0.8 ounce)* is mostly emollient oils with some excellent water-binding agents and antioxidants. This would be a very good option for someone with dry skin.

☺ $$$ **Vasco-Tonic Concentrate** *($37 for 0.8 ounce).* There is nothing in here that can affect the (vascular) blood flow to skin, but it is a good basic moisturizer for dry skin with a few good anti-irritants and water-binding agents.

☺ $$$ **Puractive Gel Cream Oily Skin** *($30 for 1.7 ounces)* is a moisturizer that contains several problematic plant extracts that can be skin irritants, while it lacks any significant water-binding agents or antioxidants. There is absolutely nothing in this cream that is beneficial for oily skin; if anything, it's too emollient for oily skin.

☹ $$$ **Puractive Concentrate Oily Skin** *($35 for 0.8 ounce)* is a mix of good water-binding agents along with some irritating plant extracts. This is just a lightweight moisturizer for normal to slightly dry skin, but be cautious of the potential for irritation. There is nothing in this product that can control oil.

☺ **SPF 30 Total Sunblock** *($27 for 5 ounces)* is a very good, titanium dioxide–based sunscreen with a matte finish that would be good for normal to slightly dry skin. It does contain a small amount of water-binding agents and a teeny amount of an antioxidant.

☺ **SPF 15 Sun Protection** *($25 for 5 ounces)* is similar to the SPF 30 above and the same comments apply.

☺ **SPF 14 Spray Lotion** *($25 for 5 ounces)* is similar to the SPF 30 above and the same comments apply. This would be better if it had a rating of SPF 15, but the difference isn't enough to leave this out as a sunscreen option.

☺ $$$ **After Sun Restoring Skin Care** *($23 for 5 ounces)* contains nothing that can restore skin after exposure to sun. It is simply a basic moisturizer that does contain some good water-binding agents, and a teeny amount of antioxidant, but none of that can undo sun damage.

☹ **Bronze Control Self Tanning Skin Tan Without Sun** *($24 for 6.75 ounces)* contains Kathon CG, which should not be used in leave-on skin-care products. This product is not recommended.

☹ **Luminance Concentrate** *($49 for 1.7 ounces)* lists alcohol as the third ingredient and also contains eucalyptus, which makes it too irritating and drying for all skin types.

☹ **Stilligel** *($24.90 for 0.5 ounce)* is a lightweight gel with a list of plant extracts that creates a strange combination of anti-irritants (butcher broom and licorice) and irritants (arnica and sage). Overall, it lacks water-binding agents and antioxidants, which might have made up for the plant confusion.

☹ **Puractive Mask** *($28 for 2.7 ounces)* contains sodium lauryl sulfate high up on the ingredient list, which makes it too irritating and sensitizing for all skin types.

☹ **Biovegetal Acne Complex with Essential Oils** *($34 for 1.7 ounces)*. The teeny amount of salicylic acid in this product can't help exfoliate skin. This ends up being more fragrance than skin care.

☹ **Biovegetal Phytoaromatic Mask** *($23 for 1.7 ounces)* contains sodium lauryl sulfate high up on the ingredient list, which makes it too irritating and sensitizing for all skin types.

☺ $$$ **Kerato-Peel Gommage** *($27.90 for 2.7 ounces)* is just wax and clay that you rub over your skin to help remove skin cells. It can feel great on lips, knees, and elbows, but it is best not to use it on the face.

☺ $$$ **Exfozyme Exfoliant** *($27.90 for 2.7 ounces)* is an exceptionally standard clay mask that can absorb some amount of oil. It would work as well as any.

☺ $$$ **Vitalift Mask-Gel** *($25 for 1.7 ounces)* is a mask that is a good option for normal to slightly dry or slightly oily skin, but there is nothing in it that will lift skin anywhere.

☹ **Hydramucine Mask-Cream** *($28 for 2.7 ounces)* contains Kathon CG, which should not be used in leave-on skin. This product is not recommended.

GUERLAIN

Guerlain is steeped not only in its own rich history, but also in an over-inflated sense of self-importance. Visiting their counters is almost like shopping for fine jewelry—the skin-care and makeup packaging is the epitome of bejeweled artifice, and the counter personnel treat it as such. Nevertheless, it's what's inside these baubles that really counts, because beautiful packaging can't help your skin. If it could Guerlain would be *the* line to set your sights on. To fashion your skin in all things Guerlain would take hundreds and hundreds of dollars. Guerlain's Paris pedigree, having evolved from a centuries-old fragrance house to a "lifestyle" line that prides itself on luxurious indulgences that promise to beautify (and perfume) almost every inch of you, still manages to hook plenty of unsuspecting women. Yet behind all of the beguiling names and extraordinary claims lie some of the most unremarkable, overpriced skin-care products available. It may sound luxurious to find gold is included in some of their formulations, unless you happen to know that applied topically gold is simply a potent allergen; there is no research showing it to have any effect on wrinkles or aging.

Guerlain's skin-care products contain a preponderance of ordinary cosmetic ingredients, with only a smattering of antioxidants, water-binding agents, and anti-irritants. If you are looking to spend money on skin care, there are many other pricey lines with formulations that are far better and more thoughtfully formulated than these. For example, there are dozens and dozens of moisturizers in this line that are at best described as mediocre and out of date, while the sunscreens are poorly formulated! And despite the specialty claims they make for each product grouping, repetitive formulations are the hallmark of the Guerlain line. For more information about Guerlain, call (800) 815-7720 or visit www.guerlain.com. **Note:** All Guerlain products contain fragrance.

GUERLAIN SKIN CARE

GUERLAIN BLUE VOYAGE

☺ $$$ **Issima Blue Voyage Ready to Go Cleanser** *($72 for three 0.33-ounce packets)* is an extremely standard, wipe-off makeup remover, and I mean really standard. The extreme cost (it would be over $432 for 6 ounces, which is the basic quantity you get with most cleansers) is a joke. This is easily replaced by almost any other makeup remover.

☹ **Issima Blue Voyage Recovery Creme SPF 15** *($72 for three 0.33-ounce packets)* doesn't contain the UVA-protecting ingredients of titanium dioxide, zinc oxide, or avobenzone, and is not recommended. Even more disconcerting is the fact that the amount in each packet isn't enough to provide even a modicum of the liberal application necessary to net the benefit of the SPF.

☺ $$$ **Issima Blue Voyage In-Flight Serum** *($72 for three 0.33-ounce packets)* adds up to a good, though very standard, moisturizer for normal to dry skin for a bizarre amount of money. This does contain some antioxidants and water-binding agents, but in such minuscule amounts as to be of almost no consequence.

GUERLAIN ISSIMA

☺ $$$ **Pure Veil Cleansing Milk** *($32.50 for 8 ounces)* is an exceptionally standard and astoundingly overpriced mineral oil–based cleanser that would be an option for someone with dry skin. The fractional amounts of antioxidants and plant extracts in here are barely detectable.

☹ **Issima Pure Dew Cleansing Foaming Gel** *($32.50 for 5.4 ounces)* contains sodium lauryl sulfate as one of the main cleansing agents, which makes it potentially too irritating and sensitizing for all skin types.

☺ $$$ **Issima Flower Cleansing Cream** *($42 for 6.8 ounces)* is a very basic, cream-style cleanser that is astoundingly similar to Neutrogena's Extra Gentle Cleanser ($5.49 for 6.7 ounces).

☺ $$$ **Perfect Eye and Lip Makeup Remover** *($28 for 3.3 ounces)* is an ordinary, silicone-based makeup remover that would work as well as any.

☺ $$$ **Issima Smoothing Gentle Exfoliator** *($37 for 2.5 ounces)* is a mineral oil–based cleanser with ground-up plastic as the abrasive. This can be an option for dry skin. The teeny amounts of lemon and papaya have no benefit for skin.

☹ **Issima Fresh Purifying Iris Toner** *($32.50 for 6.8 ounces)* lists alcohol as the second ingredient, which makes this too drying and irritating for all skin types.

☹ **Issima Success Smoothing Toner** *($42 for 6.8 ounces)* is similar to the Fresh Purifying Iris Toner above, and the same comments apply.

The Reviews G

☺ $$$ **Moisturizing Mallow Toner** (*$32.50 for 6.8 ounces*) is as ordinary a toner as it gets. This contains mostly water, slip agents, preservatives, and fragrance. The tiny amount of water-binding agents and anti-irritants means they are practically nonexistent.

☹ $$$ **Issima Eye Mythic Creme** (*$50 for 0.5 ounce*). The only thing mythic about this product is the claims it makes. This lacks any substantial interest, containing the teeniest amount of water-binding agents and antioxidants imaginable from an unimaginably overpriced moisturizer.

☹ **Issima Hydramythic Fluid SPF 15** (*$58 for 1 ounce*) doesn't contain the UVA-protecting ingredients of titanium dioxide, zinc oxide, or avobenzone, and is not recommended.

☺ $$$ **Issima Serum Mythic Radiant Youth Secret** (*$75 for 1 ounce*) does contain some very good antioxidants and water-binding agents, but for the money you would expect the concentrations to make up more than just a fractional amount of the formulation.

☺ $$$ **Hydramythic Fresh Moisturizing Stick** (*$58 for 0.35 ounce*) is a pathetically boring formulation of just water, glycerin, slip agents, film-forming agent, thickeners, silicone, and fragrance.

☺ $$$ **Issima Substantific High Density Nourishing Day Lotion SPF 15** (*$145 for 1 ounce*) does contain a tiny amount of avobenzone (0.5%), but it may not be enough to protect your skin from the sun's UVA radiation. Nonetheless, the high cost of this rather basic moisturizer ensures that you won't apply it liberally and, therefore, won't obtain the SPF benefit. This does contain some good antioxidants and water-binding agents, but the amounts are barely detectable.

☹ **Issima Substantific High Density Nourishing Day Cream SPF 10** (*$145 for 1.7 ounces*) doesn't contain the UVA-protecting ingredients of titanium dioxide, zinc oxide, or avobenzone and the SPF 10 is brazenly low. Even if that were not the case, this is an exceptionally mundane moisturizer with minuscule amounts of beneficial ingredients.

☺ $$$ **Substantific High Density Nourishing Decongesting Night Care** (*$155 for 1.6 ounces*) is an exceptionally mundane moisturizer with minuscule amounts of beneficial ingredients.

☺ $$$ **Issima Midnight Secret Late Night Special Treatment** (*$95 for 1 ounce*) is an extremely ordinary moisturizer for normal to dry skin, but nothing more. The secret must be that there's nothing interesting inside the bottle, because the impressive ingredients are present in less than minute concentrations.

☺ $$$ **Issima Success Day Smoothing Anti-Wrinkle Day Care** (*$125 for 1.7 ounces*) does not have an SPF rating and, though it does contain sunscreen ingredients, it does not contain the UVA-protecting ingredients of titanium dioxide, zinc oxide, or avobenzone; therefore, it cannot be relied on for sun protection. There are some good water-binding agents and antioxidants, but the amounts are almost embarrassingly minute given the cost.

☺ $$$ **Issima Success Night Firming Anti-Wrinkle Night Care** *($145 for 1.7 ounces)* is similar to the Issima Success Day version above only minus the sunscreen agents. The same basic comments apply.

☺ $$$ **Issima Success Eye** *($85 for 0.5 ounce)* is a lackluster moisturizer for normal to dry skin. The only success visible is that Guerlain can get away with charging such inflated prices for such standard products.

☺ $$$ **Issima Successlaser Resting Phase Treatment** *($75 for 1 ounce)* is a shockingly standard moisturizer with an infinitesimal amount of water-binding agents.

☺ $$$ **Issima Successlaser Wrinkle Minimizer SPF 15** *($95 for 1 ounce)* is similar to the Substantific High Density Nourishing Day Lotion SPF 15 above, and the same comments apply.

☹ $$$ **Issima Success Lift Radiant Lifting Serum** *($95 for 1 ounce)* is primarily just thickeners, slip agents, and minuscule amounts of antioxidants and water-binding agents. The only thing lifted up with this product is the price.

☹ $$$ **Issima Serenissime Restructuring Treatment with Active Genesium** *($190 for 1 ounce)* ends up costing $3,040 a pound for extremely standard ingredients and something called "genesium," which supposedly can tackle all the things that cause the skin to age. However, there is no such thing as "genesium"—it is just a marketing term. The ingredients in this product are the same ones found in product after product in this line. It does have some good water-binding agents and some antioxidants, but they are overwhelmed by the waxy thickening agents and mineral oil, of the same kind you can find in a thousand other products. Even the interesting ingredients are listed well after the fragrance and preservatives, meaning they are barely present.

☹ $$$ **Issima Super Aquaserum Optimum Hydrating Revitalizer** *($135 for 1.7 ounces)* is about a 3% AHA product, though that low concentration and the product's pH of 5 prevent this from having any exfoliating properties. The urea in this product can be an exfoliant, too, but not when it is present in such a tiny amount. I can't even comment about the price; I am just flabbergasted at how preposterous it is for what is just an OK moisturizer.

☹ $$$ **Serum SOS, Sensitive and Intolerant Skins** *($75 for 1 ounce)*. The main thing that's intolerable about this product is the price. It is just a very average moisturizer for dry skin with minimal amounts of water-binding agents and antioxidants.

☹ $$$ **Midnight Star, Extraordinary Radiance Treatment** *($58 for ten 0.03-ounce vials)* is an extraordinarily basic and another redundant unimpressive moisturizing formulation making claims that are not possible with the minute amounts of helpful ingredients.

☹ $$$ **Beautyissme A, Face and Eyes Anti Wrinkle Treatment** *($375 for three 0.51-ounce bottles and 28 eye patches)*. This product contains three separate bottles of ingredients that you are supposed to apply consecutively along with the eye patches over an eight-week period, under the theory that each bottle contains subsequently stronger formulations, a spurious assertion. Each one is in fact little more than an OK moisturizer similar to many in the Guerlain array of products. **Phase One** contains mostly water, plant oil, thickeners, glycerin, absorbent, preservatives, water-binding agents, vitamin E, silicone, more preservatives, more water-binding agents, gold, and coloring agents. **Phase Two** is similar only minus the absorbent, which makes it a better moisturizer, but that's about the only difference. **Phase Three** is almost identical to Phase Two. The **Hydrogel Eye Contour Patches** contain more preservative than any interesting ingredients. All told, these are actually abysmal formulations for the money.

☺ $$$ **Issima Eyeserum Eye Contour Treatment** *($72 for 0.5 ounce)* is a standard formulation for normal to dry skin that contains several plant extracts that can be irritants and others that are anti-irritants. The remaining ingredients are completely ordinary and average, with only minuscule amounts of antioxidants and water-binding agents (even less than what show up in the other Guerlain moisturizers).

☺ $$$ **Issima Intenserum Beauty Treatment** *($185 for 14 0.08-ounce ampoules)* is, to say the least, inanely overpriced, though it is an OK lightweight moisturizer for someone with normal to dry skin. However, these ingredients do not warrant a price tag that's even one-fifth of this one.

☺ $$$ **Issima Neck Firming Creme** *($89 for 1.7 ounces)*. There is nothing in this moisturizer that makes it better for the neck. It is just an average moisturizer, the same old, same old product, like most of those that Guerlain sells.

☺ $$$ **Issima Moisturizing Revitalizing Mask** *($47 for 1.7 ounces)* lists talc as the fourth ingredient, which makes this hardly what anyone would call moisturizing. The negligible amounts of antioxidants and water-binding agents this contains are barely worth mentioning.

☹ **Issima Matiday Oil-Control Hydrating Fluid** *($52 for 1 ounce)* is primarily silicones and aluminum starch octenylsuccinate, which can absorb oil, but so can most pressed powders. The zinc sulfate and orris root it contains can be skin irritants.

☹ **Issima Creme Camphrea, Anti-Blemish Care** *($25 for 0.56 ounce)*. Mineral oil and beeswax for blemish care? They've got to be kidding! On top of that, it also contains camphor. Irritation and grease, now there's an original combination. Do not put this on blemish-prone skin.

☹ **Issimat T-Zone Matifying Secret** *($40 for 0.5 ounce)* lists alcohol as the second ingredient, which makes this too drying and irritating for all skin types, and that isn't exactly secret, just something many cosmetics companies choose to ignore.

GUERLAIN MAKEUP

Guerlain's has arranged its makeup in three categories: Terracotta encompasses the original bronzing powder and all of its spin-offs; Meteorites follows suit with its multicolored powder beads and accompanying "light-reflecting" products; and Divinora features makeup essentials such as foundation, blush, eyeshadow, and mascara, all packaged in textured gold tubes and compacts. There are some impressive foundations to consider in terms of texture and finish, and reliable sunscreen, but Guerlain needs to take a look at how well other counters like Stila, Chanel, and Lancome are doing with their impressively neutral shades. A beautiful application and even coverage mean nothing if the color is too peach or pink to work on most skin tones. If you find the elitist trappings of Guerlain get the better of you, the products to focus on are the blushes, powder eyeshadows, liquid eyeliners, the Terracotta Compact foundation, and lipsticks. If you're willing to spend this much on makeup, knowing what to pay attention to and what to ignore can help prevent some costly and, in some cases, unattractive mistakes.

FOUNDATION: ☺ $$$ **Divinora Silky Smooth Foundation SPF 12** *($37)* is a liquidy foundation that has a very smooth texture that blends expertly into the skin, leaving a soft matte finish. This also features an in-part titanium dioxide sunscreen and provides light to medium coverage. The seven shades offer some decent colors, though each has a soft to strong peach or rose tint. Shades No. 540 and No. 770 are the worst offenders—the rest are options for normal to slightly oily skin. **Divinora Ultra-Fluid Foundation SPF 15** *($36)* is an admirable ultra-matte foundation with an excellent in-part titanium dioxide sunscreen and a better SPF rating than the one above. This has a very soft, fluid texture that feels quite silky. Since this is a true ultra-matte makeup, it dries quickly and tends to stay put, so blending must be meticulous. If you have oily skin and prefer light to medium coverage, this is worth trying—though the only two shades to consider seriously are Rose Clair and Dore Fonce. The other five shades are disappointingly peach or pink. **Issima Foundation** *($55)* is a thick, creamy foundation that applies well and leaves a moist finish that dry skin will love. Of the seven shades, the only ones that resemble skin are Almondine No. 6, Noisette No. 9, and Coconut No. 8. The price is exorbitant and this has none of the antiaging benefits it brags about (especially since this is sans sunscreen), but it's one of the few truly emollient foundations available.

✔☺ **Terracotta Ultimate Bronze Compact Foundation SPF 15** *($32.50)* is a soft-textured cream-to-powder makeup whose finish is more creamy than powdery. The sunscreen is in-part titanium dioxide, and this comes in four gorgeous colors, each with a soft bronze tint. This can be used as a light-coverage all-over foundation, or you can choose a deeper shade to use as a natural-looking bronzer with added sunscreen.

☺ $$$ **Issima Antiaging Creme Foundation SPF 12** *($48)* has a light, but moist, texture and a soft creamy finish suitable for normal to dry skin. Unfortunately, this sheer to light coverage makeup has only one shade that looks like skin, and that's Beige Creme No. 52. All the other shades are embarrassingly peach, pink, or rose.

☹ **Terracotta Tinted Day Cream SPF 8** *($32)* does not contain adequate UVA protection and the SPF is too low. The moist, sheer texture is fine for normal to dry skin, but the colors are just too peachy orange to look convincing on most skin tones. **Terracotta Refreshing Tinted Gel** *($32.50)* is a sheer iridescent bronzer that lays on lots of shine, and is just inappropriate unless glittery bronzed cheeks are what you had in mind.

Terracotta Refreshing Stick Bronzer *($32.50)* has a cool, wet feel and glides over the skin, but it's blindingly shiny and not nearly as attractive as the natural finish bronzing sticks from Bobbi Brown.

☺ $$$ <u>CONCEALER:</u> **Divinora Concealer SPF 12** *($26)* is a cream-to-powder stick concealer that does not list active sunscreen ingredients but that does contain a fair amount of titanium dioxide. Even so, without an active ingredient list this cannot be relied on for sun protection. And you may want to skip this crease-prone concealer altogether because the three colors are a bit too peach or pink to pass for neutral. **Palette Touch** *($35)* has five creamy colors in one compact. Three of them are sheer, iridescent shades for lips and cheeks, while the other two are color-correcting concealers in mint green and pale yellow. It's nicely packaged, but I doubt anyone would get much use from it. **Meteorites Highlighter** *($29)* is a collection of sheer, softly iridescent creams whose shades are appropriate for highlighting facial features. But you do realize that you can easily achieve this same effect for less, right? **Terracotta Duo Matte & Shine** *($26)* is not really a concealer, but more of a creamy bronzer along with a cream-to-powder iridescent highlighter in one compact. It's OK, but more or less a superfluous spin-off product.

☺ $$$ <u>POWDER:</u> **Meteorites Voyage Compact Powder** *($145, $42.50 for refill)* is a prismatic rainbow of pastel and muted colors in a breathtaking compact accompanied by a price that should leave you all choked up. This soft, dry-finish powder can also be purchased in a standard compact for the price of the refill. **Meteorites Powder for the Face** *($42.50)* is delicately described as "a shower of heavenly light." Celestial language aside, these are multicolored powder beads that all have a slight to moderately intense shine. There are much less expensive ways to gleam yourself up than this, and you'll have no trouble finding facsimiles of this product at The Body Shop, the drugstore, or less expensive cosmetics counters. This is Guerlain's top-selling product, but I honestly (and literally) do not see what all the fuss is about—and the price is outlandish. **Les Voilettes Loose Powder** *($43)* is a talc-based powder with a sumptuous silky texture that looks beautiful on the skin, though the four sheer shades are just too peachy pink to earn a smiling face. **Les Voilettes Pressed Powder** *($39.50)* is almost identical to the Loose Powder above, only this is the pressed version, and the same comments apply. **Terracotta Bronzing Powder** *($32.50)* presents four believable, tan-looking colors, although three of them have noticeable shine that negates the natural look (real tanning does not yield iridescence), while Shade No. 4 (designed as the Men's Bronzer) is perfectly matte. So women's tans are supposed to shine but not men's? Go figure. These may have been worth the splurge if the shine were absent, but until then there are much better options for bronzing powder, such as Bobbi Brown and even Bonne Bell! If you decide to splurge on Guerlain, you will find Terracotta has a smooth texture and applies evenly—though a little goes a long way. **Radiant Compact Powder Finish** *($32)* is yet another pressed powder that has a silky texture, sheer finish, and talc-based formula. The pastel, opalescent colors are odd and don't resemble real skin tones.

☺ $$$ <u>BLUSH:</u> **Divinora Radiant Blush** *($34)* is an attractive group of dry-finish powder blushes that sweep on easily and feel quite silky. The sheer colors are almost all matte, though they lack the intensity to show up on darker skin. These are worth a look if you have fair to medium skin and want to spare no expense when it comes to blush.

<u>EYESHADOW:</u> ☺ $$$ **Divinora Radiant Color Single Eyeshadow** *($22)* has an exceptionally silky texture that applies evenly, blends easily, and lasts. However, each shade has a touch of shine, so choose carefully and avoid the blue and green hues if your goal is to shape and shade the eye, not "color" it.

☺ $$$ **Meteorites Eyeshadow Pen** *($20)* is a cream-to-powder eyeshadow applied with a built-in sponge-tip applicator. Neither the pastel, iridescent colors nor the manner in which this dispenses the color make for a subtle or sophisticated eye design. **Protective Base for the Eyelids** *($25)* is essentially a cream-to-powder concealer that is supposed to prime the eyelids for eyeshadow application. Although this blends down to a soft matte finish, the colors are peachy pink! There is no reason to consider this over a neutral-toned matte finish concealer.

<u>EYE AND BROW SHAPER:</u> ☺ $$$ **Divinora Eye Pencil** *($20)* is a very standard, creamy pencil that tends to smudge unless it's set with powder. This comes in lots of colors, with an emphasis on iridescence. **Divinora Brow Pencil** *($20)* is also a standard pencil that is quite easy to apply and is not too thick or greasy. It does stay creamy on the skin, so some smearing may be apparent at the end of the day.

✓☺ $$$ **Eye-Liner** *($26)* is a very good liquid eyeliner that applies smoothly, dries quickly, and stays put. Avoid the unattractive iridescent colors.

☹ **Loose Powder Kohl** *($25)* is a rather senseless product. The packaging resembles the inkwell-type container used for liquid eyeliner, but housed inside is pigmented shiny loose powder. The applicator is just a stick—no wand, sponge tip, or brush—and so the messy powder goes on unevenly and flakes everywhere.

<u>LIPSTICK AND LIP PENCIL:</u> ☺ $$$ **Kiss Kiss Pure Comfort Lipstick** *($22)* is fine as a standard creamy lipstick with a smooth texture and full coverage colors. The price is indulgent, but once you see the container this lipstick is housed in, you'll know why.

☺ $$$ **Divinora Sheer & Shine Lipstick SPF 10** *($22)* does not contain adequate UVA protection and is otherwise an overpriced sheer, glossy lipstick with some pretty colors. **Divinora Color & Shine Lipstick SPF 12** *($22)* is also without sufficient UVA protection, but it does have an elegant creamy-slick texture that feels great on the lips and provides rich, glossy color. **Lip Liner Pencil** *($20)* is a very standard creamy pencil that offers rich colors and a nice stain—though any of the liners from Almay, L'Oreal, or Revlon can compete with or surpass it.

☺ $$$ **Meteorites Lip Gloss** *($19)* is a standard wand-application gloss with a sticky texture and some truly peculiar colors. **Terracotta Gloss & Shine** *($19)* has an identical texture to the Meteorites Lip Gloss, but features more realistic, bronze-tinged shades.

<u>MASCARA:</u> ☹ $$$ **Divinora Enticing Eyes Mascara** *($22)* is not as spectacular as the lavish gold container that holds it. This mascara produces OK length and a smidgen of thickness without clumps, but, simply put, the performance does not justify the price.

☺ $$$ **Super-Cils Mascara Waterproof** *($22)* builds excellent length and appreciable thickness, all without clumps or smearing. It's indeed waterproof, but so are many other waterproof mascaras that cost less than half of this one.

☺ $$$ <u>BRUSHES:</u> Guerlain sells a **Terracotta Brush** *($28.50)* to complement their Terracotta Bronzing Powder, as well as a **Meteorites Brush** *($28.50)* to use with their pastel powder beads. Both brushes are soft and well-shaped, though the Meteorites Brush is preferred for its density.

GUINOT (SKIN CARE ONLY)

What's in a name? If it's French, usually a high price tag and the promise of "European" skin care. Of course, in Europe the women praise American know-how when it comes to skin care—but I guess the grass is always greener in someone else's lawn. As it turns out, French products are no different from American products. All the gimmicky plant extracts and vitamins, standard thickening agents, basic detergent cleansing agents, preservatives, slip agents, emollients, lightweight silicone moisturizing gels, and problematic ingredients are virtually identical, it's just that the claims have a French accent.

Guinot is a long-established salon/spa line of skin-care products with a reputation for being an elegant, elite, serious, and intricately designed way to take care of skin. Their price tags definitely make these products elite, and the packaging can be described as elegant, but in terms of formulation these products are rather ho-hum, with some downright inferior and old-fashioned formulations.

Despite the extravagant-sounding product names, this line seems unusually overpriced for what you get, and in need of revamping. I could go on at length about the claims, which range from "remodels your silhouette" to "blackheads disappear," "transforms the appearance of oily skin," "diffuses the water needed to keep skin moist all day," and (this one's my favorite) "dynamizes the complexion, smoothing away signs of fatigue." It would take another entire book to do justice to this kind of obtuse profundity. That's not to say there aren't some good products mixed in here, but they just can't deliver what the claims may lead you to believe they can. Guinot's name turns out to be the most impressive part of this skin-care line, which means its elite, serious image is just that: image. For more information about Guinot, call (800) 444-6621 or visit www.guinotusa.com. **Note:** All Guinot products are highly fragranced.

☺ $$$ **Moisture Rich Cleansing Milk** *($25 for 6.7 ounces)* is a standard plant oil– and mineral oil–based wipe-off cleanser that can leave a greasy film on the skin, though it can be an option for someone with dry skin. It does contain coloring agents.

☹ **Purifying Cleansing Gel** *($25 for 6.7 ounces)* contains sulfur and sodium lauryl sulfate, which makes it irritating and drying for all skin types, and that's not purifying in the least.

☺ $$$ **Wash-Off Cleansing Cream** *($28.50 for 5 ounces)* is similar to Neutrogena's Extra Gentle Cleanser ($5.49 for 6.7 ounces), which makes it an option for dry skin, though neither product removes makeup very well.

☺ $$$ **Refreshing Cleansing Milk** *($25 for 6.7 ounces)* is virtually identical to the Moisture Rich Cleansing Milk above and the same comments apply.

☺ $$$ **Gentle Eye Cleansing Gel** *($19.50 for 4.2 ounces)* is a standard, detergent-based makeup remover that would work as well as any. This does contain coloring agents.

☹ **Purifying Toning Lotion** *($25 for 6.7 ounces)* contains lemon and sulfur, which are too irritating and drying for all skin types, and there isn't one redeeming ingredient in the entire formulation.

☺ $$$ **Moisture-Rich Toning Lotion** *($25 for 6.7 ounces)* is a rather standard toner. The plant extract is cornflower, which can have anti-inflammatory properties, and the urea can be an exfoliant, but there are far more interesting toners around than this one.

☺ $$$ **Gentle Face Exfoliating Cream** *($36 for 1.7 ounces)* isn't the best way to exfoliate skin because the cream is hard to rinse off and can leave a greasy film on skin.

☺ $$$ **Longue Vie Cellulaire, Vital Face Care** *($67 for 1.6 ounces)* is an OK moisturizer for normal to dry skin, but the vital water-binding agents are so far at the end of the ingredient list that they don't end up amounting to much that's vital for skin.

☺ $$$ **Continuous Nourishing and Protecting Cream** *($36 for 1.6 ounces)* is a simple moisturizer of thickener, plant oils, fragrance, and preservatives.

☺ $$$ **Skin Revitalizing Concentrate** *($52 for 1 ounce)* is a silicone-based moisturizer for normal to slightly dry skin, but this is one of the more ho-hum, do-nothing formulations in this line, and that's saying a lot given how mediocre most of the Guinot products are.

☺ $$$ **Desensitizing Serum** *($41 for 1.7 ounces)* is an OK moisturizer for dry skin, but rather basic and uninteresting. The negligible amounts of vitamin C and anti-irritants this includes make them barely detectable.

☺ $$$ **Newlight Lightening Starter Lotion** *($27 for 6.7 ounces)* is an exceptionally ordinary toner of mostly water, slip agents, preservatives, yeast, and minute amounts of vitamin C and bilberry. Yeast has no effect on skin, though vitamin C and bilberry can have melanin-inhibiting properties, although not when they are present in such a tiny amount.

✓☺ $$$ **Newlight Deep Action Lightening Serum** *($64 for 1.07 ounces)* contains a good amount of vitamin C (magnesium ascorbyl phosphate) and there is research showing that it can inhibit melanin production. It also contains a small amount of some very good water-binding agents.

☺ $$$ **Newlight Lightening Cream** *($65 for 1.7 ounces)* is a basic moisturizer with a tiny amount of vitamin C and even smaller amounts of water-binding agents. The amount of vitamin C in this product is not enough to affect the color of skin in any way.

☺ $$$ **Newlight Lightening Mask** *($33 for 1.7 ounces)* is similar to the Lightening Cream above except that this one also contains clay so you can apply it as a mask.

✓☺ $$$ **Pigmentation Mark Prevention SPF 15** *($25 for 1.7 ounces)* is a good, in-part titanium dioxide–based sunscreen in a moisturizing base that contains small amounts of some very good water-binding agents and antioxidants. Used long-term, this will help prevent skin discolorations, but no more than other well-formulated sunscreens will.

✓☺ $$$ **Skin Defense SPF 15** *($48 for 1.6 ounces)* is similar to the Pigmentation Mark Prevention above and the same basic comments apply.

☺ $$$ **Pure Balance Serum** *($36.50 for 1.7 ounces)* can't balance skin and is just a very mediocre, matte-finish moisturizer. The zinc sulfate in here can be a skin irritant.

☹ **Pure Balance Cream** *($29 for 1.7 ounces)* is supposed to reduce the size of pores and disinfect skin. It can't. If anything, this product contains thickening agents that can cause problems for oily or blemish-prone skin. The teeny amounts of zinc sulfate and clay won't balance skin. Clay can absorb oil, but zinc sulfate can be a skin irritant.

☺ $$$ **Pure Balance Mask** *($33 for 2.1 ounces)* is mostly chalk and clay. That will indeed absorb oil and would be an option for oily skin types, except that this product contains alcohol and camphor, which can be skin irritants.

☹ **Pure Balance Concealer** *($22 for 0.5 ounce)* is a strange color and it contains camphor, which can be a skin irritant.

☺ $$$ **Youth Replenishing Skin Cream** *($70 for 1.6 ounces)* is an OK moisturizer with minuscule amounts of water-binding agents and antioxidants. This won't restore one second of youth to your skin.

☺ $$$ **Hydrazone Moisturizing Cream Dehydrated Skin** *($67 for 1.6 ounces)* is just water, wax, preservatives, and fragrance. The minute amount of vitamin A is almost nonexistent.

☺ $$$ **Liftosome Lifting Cream** *($72 for 1.6 ounces)* is just a very ordinary moisturizer for dry skin that contains the same boring ingredients as most Guinot products. This does contain tiny amounts of two decent water-binding agents, but that doesn't warrant the price tag for this otherwise run-of-the-mill product.

☺ $$$ **Eye Lifting Creme** *($39 for 0.5 ounce)* is an OK moisturizer for normal to slightly dry skin. As usual in this line, the interesting ingredients are present in such small amounts that they can have little to no impact on skin.

☺ $$$ **Anti-Wrinkle Cream for the Eyes** *($34 for 0.5 ounce)* is a simple emollient moisturizer for dry skin, but it lacks even a light representation of worthwhile ingredients for skin.

☹ **Anti-Wrinkle Rich Night Cream** *($48.50 for 1.5 ounces)* is a Vaseline-based moisturizer with a small amount of water-binding agents. Though boring, it could be an option for dry skin, except that it contains sulfur, which makes this too potentially irritating for skin.

☺ $$$ **Firming Neck Cream** *($40 for 1 ounce)*. Not only won't this firm skin anywhere on the face or body, it is just an extremely average moisturizer for dry skin.

☺ **$$$ Lifting Day Cream** *($48.50 for 1.6 ounces)*. This ordinary, lanolin-based moisturizer for dry skin contains a minuscule amount of some very good water-binding agents. Given the price tag, it is only minimally passable as a moisturizer for dry skin, and because it doesn't contain sunscreen it should not be used for daytime.

☺ **$$$ Long Lasting Moisturizing Cream** *($41 for 1.7 ounces)* is an OK moisturizer for dry skin, but it's very ordinary, and nothing in this product will make it last any longer than any other Guinot moisturizer.

☺ **$$$ Intense Protection Cream** *($35 for 1.7 ounces)*. There is nothing intense about this product except that it is intensely boring. It is just water, thickeners, fragrance, and preservatives. What a waste.

☺ **$$$ Radiance Renewal Cream** *($52 for 1.7 ounces)* is similar to the Intense Protection Cream above and the same comments apply. It has a few more bells and whistles (a form of vitamin A, vitamin E, and water-binding agents), but they are present in such microscopic amounts as to be useless for skin.

☹ **Anti-Fatigue Eye Gel** *($29.50 for 0.5 ounce)* is a basic gel with no water-binding agents or antioxidants, while the plant extracts are a mix of irritants (ivy) and anti-irritants (horse chestnut), which makes it a rather fatiguing formulation.

☺ **$$$ Huile Fine Nutri Comfort** *($40 for 1 ounce)* contains mostly fragrant oils and wheat germ oil plus a minute quantity of vitamin A. This may be comforting to smell, but it can be irritating when applied to skin. Skip the fragrance and just buy some wheat germ oil at the health food store; it would be cheaper and you would net better results for dry skin, too.

☺ **$$$ Moisture Supplying Radiance Mask** *($32 for 1.7 ounces)* is just an emollient moisturizer with microscopic amounts of water-binding agents and antioxidants.

☹ **$$$ Radiance Mask** *($32 for 1.6 ounces)* contains menthol and camphor in a Vaseline- and lanolin-based moisturizer. Irritating and ordinary, that's not exactly radiant, is it?

☺ **$$$ Anti-Redness Treatment** *($28 for 1 ounce)*. There is nothing in this product that can reduce redness, and it's about as ordinary a moisturizer as it gets. The plant extract is a good anti-irritant, but the amount is barely detectable.

☺ **$$$ Instant Eye Mask** *($31 for 1 ounce)* is hardly worth the effort to put this on the face, as there are far better moisturizers for skin than this.

☺ **Self Tanning Cream** *($25 for 5.5 ounces)*. Like all self-tanners, this uses dihydroxyacetone to affect the color of skin, and it would work as well as any.

☺ **$$$ Sun Screen SPF 30** *($27 for 2.6 ounces)* is a good, in-part avobenzone–based sunscreen in a silicone-based, lightweight moisturizer. There is not one thing in this sunscreen that makes it preferred over many other avobenzone-based sunscreens found at the drugstore, such as those from Ombrelle or Coppertone.

☺ **$$$ Moisturizing Sun Spray SPF 15** *($27.50 for 5.4 ounces)* is a good, in-part titanium dioxide–based sunscreen in an ordinary moisturizing base.

☺ **After Sun Recovery** (*$22 for 7.03 ounces*) is an exceedingly dull moisturizer that features the smallest amount of vitamin C imaginable.

H₂O+ SKIN CARE

Boutique-oriented cosmetics lines have had their problems over the past few years as they've faced decreasing sales and high overhead. H₂O+ is one such company, and it began closing its doors in the late '90s. New direction and an influx of money helped turn the company around, however, and they are opening new stores with a sleek, steely look that is more upscale and elegant than before. Along with the new look are new, relatively upscale formulations, accompanied by fairly upscale prices.

As was true with the original product line, H₂O+ is "focused solely on the benefits of water-based, oil-free skin care." It is the exception to the rule for any company to make products that are not water-based, but stating that they are water-based does sound good. However, that doesn't mean that nonaqueous products (that is, products that are not water-based) are problematic. Quite the contrary, because there is research showing that water-based formulations cause the breakdown of plant extracts and antioxidants, and many formulators are experimenting with new ingredient technology that involves non-water-based formulations. Even H₂O+ knows this, since one of their retinol products is in a decidedly non-water-base formulation.

What is unique to H₂O+ is the cornucopia of plant extracts their products contain, such as *Crithmum maritimum, Undaria pinnatifida, Coffea arabica* (coffee), *Viola tricolor* (pansy), *Pfaffia paniculata, Frangula alnus,* and *Veronica officinalis,* along with a number of other seaweeds and algae extracts. All of these extracts are reviewed in Chapter Seven, *Cosmetics Dictionary,* but suffice it to say that many of these extracts do have a small amount of research showing them to have antiinflammatory and/or antioxidant properties. Their exotic identities and seaworthy origins, however, do not make them better or more significant for skin than other ingredients from other sources that can provide the same benefits.

For the most part the H₂O+ product renovations are well-done, including some impressive ingredients that can be of benefit to a variety of skin types. Where the line falls down is with its products for oily or blemish-prone skin, which are void of ingredients that can exfoliate or disinfect. There are also some sunscreens that don't have UVA-protecting ingredients, which is surprising given that so many of the other products contain state-of-the-art water-binding agents and anti-irritants. Of course, you still have to get past the claims, but that is no different for this line than for most others. Thankfully, you won't have to swim against the current to get to the interesting stuff, because there's more good than bad to be found on these shelves. For more information about H₂O+ Skin Care, call (800) 242-BATH or visit www.h2oplus.com. **Note:** All H₂O+ products contain fragrance unless indicated otherwise.

☺ **Marine Cleansing Gel** (*$18.50 for 5.7 ounces*) is a standard, detergent-based, water-soluble cleanser that would work well for someone with normal to oily skin. The sea minerals are a mix of anti-irritants and irritants. The marine plant extracts can have some antioxidant properties, but in a cleanser the benefits of these would be washed down the drain.

☺ **Moisturizing Marine Cleansing Cream** (*$21 for 8 ounces*) is mostly mineral oil and wax, which makes it a very basic, cold cream–style cleanser and overpriced for what you get. The token addition of marine plant extracts doesn't have an impact on skin.

☺ **Oil Control Cleansing Mousse** (*$17.50 for 7.5 ounces*) is an exceptionally standard, detergent-based cleanser for normal to oily skin with a minuscule amount of marine plant extracts and Dead Sea salts. None of that can affect oily skin in any way, shape, or form.

☺ **Sea Mineral Cleanser** (*$14.50 for 5.7 ounces*) is a lotion-style cleanser that definitely contains some Dead Sea salts, but the amount is minuscule and the research for these minerals is that they are effective for dermatitis, not for general skin care. This can be an option for someone with normal to dry skin.

☺ **Smoothing Facial Cleanser** (*$19.50 for 5.7 ounces*). The plant extracts in here sound like they are related to AHAs, but they have no exfoliating properties for skin. This lotion cleanser is extremely basic and can be an option for normal to dry skin.

☺ **Dual Action Eye Makeup Remover** (*$16 for 4.5 ounces*) is a very standard, silicone-based eye-makeup remover that would work as well as any. This does not contain fragrance.

☺ **Water-Activated Eye Makeup Remover** (*$14.50 for 4 ounces*) is a standard, detergent-based, water soluble cleanser that would work well for someone with normal to oily skin.

☺ **$$$ Oil-Controlling Exfoliator** (*$17.50 for 4 ounces*) is a standard, detergent-based cleanser that uses ground-up plastic (polyethylene) and pumice as the topical abrasives. It would work as well as any for someone with normal to oily skin. The plant extracts sound as if they are related to AHAs, but they have no exfoliating properties for skin.

☺ **$$$ Sea Mineral Scrub** (*$17.50 for 4 ounces*). The abrasives in this product aren't sea minerals, just ground-up plastic. This is a standard, detergent-based cleanser with minimal amounts of plant extracts and Dead Sea salts. This can be a decent option for someone with normal to oily skin.

☺ **Marine Toner** (*$16 for 8 ounces*) contains mostly water, slip agent, plant extracts, salts, fragrance, preservatives, and coloring agents. The plant extracts have minimal antioxidant properties.

☺ **$$$ Oasis Mist** (*$15 for 6 ounces*) is similar to the Marine Toner above only this version contains a good water-binding agent, making it a better formulation for all skin types.

☹ **Toner Plus** (*$16.50 for 8 ounces*) lists alcohol as the second ingredient, which makes it too irritating and drying for all skin types.

✓☺ **Eye Mender Restorative Firming Treatment** (*$25 for 0.5 ounce*) is a good, silicone-based moisturizer for someone with normal to dry skin. It contains an impressive assortment of water-binding agents and antioxidants. It does contain coloring agents.

✓☺ **Eye Oasis Moisture Replenishing Treatment** *($22.50 for 0.5 ounce)* is similar to the Eye Mender above and the same comments apply.

✓☺ **Face Oasis Hydrating Treatment** *($32 for 1.7 ounces)* is similar to the Eye Mender and Eye Oasis above and the same comments apply.

✓☺ **Green Tea Antioxidant Face Complex** *($32 for 1.7 ounces)* is an emollient moisturizer for normal to dry skin that contains some very good antioxidants and water-binding agents.

✓☺ **Instant Lift Eye Serum** *($28 for 0.95 ounce)* is a good, silicone-based moisturizer with an impressive mix of water-binding agents and antioxidants.

☹ **Intensive Moisture Complex SPF 15** *($28 for 1.7 ounces)* doesn't contain the UVA-protecting ingredients of titanium dioxide, zinc oxide, or avobenzone, and is not recommended.

✓☺ **Intensive Night Recovery Complex** *($30 for 1.7 ounces)* is a very good emollient moisturizer for normal to dry skin that contains some very good water-binding agents, antioxidants, and emollients.

☺ **Intensive Night Repair Supplement** *($24 for 1 ounce)* is similar to the Night Recovery Complex above except that it contains a small amount of salicylic acid. However, the pH of this product is too high for the BHA to be effective as an exfoliant. This is still a good moisturizer for normal to dry skin, though the Night Recovery Complex above has a more impressive combination and concentration of ingredients.

☺ **Line Defense Retinol Complex** *($38 for 1 ounce)* is mostly silicone, retinol, film-forming agent, thickeners, and fragrance. If you're looking for a retinol product, this one is as good as any and the formulation and packaging help ensure that it remains stable.

☺ **Marine Daily Hydrator** *($23 for 4 ounces)*. This does not contain sunscreen and would not be a wise choice for daytime, though it is an OK moisturizer for normal to dry skin. It does contain a tiny amount of water-binding agents and antioxidants, but it is not up to the standards of other moisturizers in this line.

☺ **Marine Daily Moisture Cream** *($22 for 1.7 ounces)* is similar to the Marine Daily Hydrator above and the same basic comments apply.

☺ **Marine Enzyme Serum** *($22.50 for 1 ounce)* is a very good lightweight lotion moisturizer for normal to slightly dry skin. It contains a good assortment of water-binding agents, antioxidants, and anti-irritants.

☹ **Oil Controlling Hydrator** *($25 for 1.6 ounces)* lists alcohol as the second ingredient and will help generate dry, irritated skin, but it won't control anything.

☺ **Smoothing Hydrocomplex** *($22.50 for 1 ounce)*. Both the plant extracts (touted as exfoliants, which they are not) and the product's high pH mean that it does not have exfoliating properties for skin. As a moisturizer there are better formulated versions to choose from in this line.

☺ **Express Bronzer Medium Tan** or **Deep Tan** *($16.50 for 4 ounces)*, just like all self-tanners, use dihydroxyacetone to affect the color of skin. They would work as well as any. The plant extracts in these have no exfoliating properties.

☹ **Lip & Eye Stick SPF 15** *($12.50 for 0.25 ounce)* doesn't contain the UVA-protecting ingredients of titanium dioxide, zinc oxide, or avobenzone, and is not recommended.

✓☺ **Solar Block SPF 30** *($15 for 1.7 ounces)* is a good, in-part titanium dioxide–based sunscreen in an emollient base that would work well for normal to dry skin. The plant extracts have some anti-inflammatory properties, but there's not very much of them in here.

☺ **Solar Defense Spray SPF 15** *($16.50 for 4 ounces)* is a good, in-part avobenzone-based sunscreen in a silicone base that also contains a large amount of alcohol, which isn't the best for skin, so it is only a consideration for the neck down and only if you are not worried about dry skin.

☹ **Solar Shield SPF 15** *($15 for 1.7 ounces)* doesn't contain the UVA-protecting ingredients of titanium dioxide, zinc oxide, or avobenzone, and is not recommended.

☺ **Solar Relief** *($15 for 4 ounces)* is an ordinary moisturizer with a small amount of some interesting plant extracts that have some anti-irritant and antioxidant properties. Overall this is just an average moisturizer that offers no recovery whatsoever from sun damage.

☹ **Acne Spot Treatment** *($12 for 0.5 ounce)* lists alcohol as the second ingredient, which won't help acne, but will help generate dry, irritated skin.

☺ **$$$ Hydrating Marine Moisture Mask** *($24 for 4 ounces)* is a good emollient moisturizer similar to many H₂0+ moisturizers. This mask version doesn't add anything special, but it will feel nice on skin.

☹ **Pore Refining Peel-Off Mask** *($22 for 3 ounces)* lists alcohol as the second ingredient, which won't help acne, but will help generate dry, irritated skin.

☺ **$$$ Purifying Exfoliation Mask** *($18 for 3 ounces)* is a standard clay mask with some ground-up plastic as the abrasive. The clay has some oil-absorbing properties and the abrasive can exfoliate, but so can a washcloth.

☺ **$$$ Sea Mineral Mud Mask** *($24 for 4 ounces)* is a standard clay mask that can absorb oil.

☺ **Line Defense Lip Plumper** *($20 for 0.5 ounce)* contains nothing that will prevent or change lines around the mouth, especially as this is just water and silicones with tiny amounts of emollients and plant extracts. It's OK, but not exciting.

☹ **Lip Mender** *($10 for 0.5 ounce)* is mostly just Vaseline and wax, but it also contains peppermint and clay, which can irritate skin and burn lips.

H₂0+ WATERWHITE LINE

☺ **Waterwhite Brightening Cleansing Mousse** *($25 for 7.5 ounces)* is a standard, detergent-based cleanser that would work well for most skin types.

✓☺ **Waterwhite Brightening Tonic** *($22.50 for 6 ounces)* is a very good, irritant-free toner that contains some excellent water-binding agents, anti-irritants, and antioxidants. The plant extracts and vitamin C in this product may have melanin-inhibiting properties for skin.

✓☺ $$$ **Waterwhite Brightening Essence** (*$45 for 0.85 ounce*) contains some very good water-binding agents, antioxidants, and anti-irritants in a lightweight lotion that would be good for someone with normal to slightly dry skin. The extracts and vitamin C that can inhibit melanin production are present in such small concentrations that they are unlikely to have much impact on skin.

✓☺ $$$ **Waterwhite Brightening Lotion SPF 15** (*$35 for 1.5 ounces*) is a good, in-part avobenzone-based sunscreen in a silicone base that contains a good concentration of vitamin C that may help inhibit melanin production. It also contains some good anti-irritants. This would be an option for normal to slightly dry skin.

✓☺ $$$ **Waterwhite Brightening Night Cream** (*$40 for 1.7 ounces*). There are over 65 ingredients in this formulation. It ends up being a very good, emollient moisturizer with an impressive mix of water-binding agents, anti-irritants, and antioxidants. The tiny amount of peppermint probably won't have a negative impact on skin. As far as skin lightening, it doesn't contain high enough concentrations of the skin-lightening ingredients to have that effect.

☺ $$$ **Waterwhite Brightening Mask** (*$30 for 3.5 ounces*) contains mostly water, rice starch, thickeners, vitamin C, water-binding agents, fragrance, plant extracts, and preservatives. The rice starch negates the benefits of the water-binding agents. As far as skin lightening, it doesn't contain high enough concentrations of the skin-lightening ingredients to have that effect.

HARD CANDY (MAKEUP ONLY)

Hard Candy is a modern-day success story. Founder Dineh Mohajer was a pre-med student in Southern California who had an eye for fashion. Frustrated that she couldn't find a blue pastel nail polish that matched her blue sandals (don't you just hate that?), she decided to create her own at home. Soon after adding blue dye to a standard white nail polish, she found herself back on campus getting an extraordinary amount of attention from the female students, who flipped over the color. And not long after trademarking the name "Hard Candy" in 1995, Mohajer stepped into the ultra-trendy Fred Segal boutique and presented her new colors (four in all), which were snatched up immediately. From there the line exploded to a broad range of flashy, glittery, brash colors and products, including a brief stint with men's nail polish.

In May 1999, Hard Candy was purchased by Sephora, which features the line in many of its stores. Interestingly, Sephora also purchased Hard Candy's chief competitor, Urban Decay, and the two former nail polish rivals are now under the same corporate umbrella.

Although the story of Hard Candy is intriguing, its products and displays are strictly image. This is a teen-oriented color line that relishes the chance to provide sparkly, glittery *everything,* from polish to pencils. Yet even though Hard Candy appears to be your one-stop shimmer shop, the formulations are either exceptionally standard or leave much to be desired, which proves the old adage, "all that glitters is not gold." If glitter appeals to you, most other lines (including the aforementioned Urban Decay) best Hard Candy when it comes to product performance, though there are a few sleeper products here that you may want to examine. For more information about Hard Candy, call Sephora at (877) SEPHORA, or visit www.hardcandy.com.

☺ $$$ <u>FOUNDATION:</u> There is only one foundation-type product in the Hard Candy lineup, called **Hint Tint SPF 15** *($29.50)*, which has been reformulated and re-packaged, with both changes making improvements over the original. This product now contains an in-part avobenzone sunscreen and a cushiony, moist texture that is a pleasure to use. The sheer coverage and finish is typical of a tinted moisturizer, and the formula is best for those with normal to dry skin. All of the five shades are commendable, with Angel being excellent for very light skin and Luscious serving as a beautiful color for dark skin.

<u>POWDER:</u> ☺ $$$ **Peace Powder** *($26)* is a talc-based pressed powder with a silky, yet waxy, texture that feels almost creamy and applies sheer. Each shade has a touch of shine and a slightly powdery finish, and all of them are beautiful neutral tones. **Bronze-n-Brush** *($22.50)* is a pressed-powder bronzer that has a great tan color and (believe it or not) a rather subdued shine. The brush that accompanies it is retractable, but not the best choice for an even, controlled application of powder.

☹ **Sonic Sparkle Dust** *($15)* is loose glitter powder that has a terribly rough texture and does not adhere well to skin.

<u>BLUSH:</u> ✔☺ $$$ **Stain for Lip & Cheek** *($18)* is an exceptional gel-based stain that comes in a squeeze tube and has three excellent colors that (and this is the best part) blend easily over the skin. Most gel blushes tend to dry almost immediately and can look uneven, but this provides enough slip and "play time" for you to get the color on evenly. The effect is a long-lasting, sheer wash of color that works best on small-pored, even-textured skin.

☹ $$$ **Blush-n-Brush** *($22.50)* is a standard pressed-powder blush that has a soft, dry texture and decent application; there are three shades, each with a soft shine. The included blush brush is mediocre and no match for a professional brush.

☹ **Blush Highlight Duet** *($28)* comes in a compact with one-half cream blush and the other a cream-to-powder highlighter. The blush part has a heavy, thick texture that blends on sticky (though it's sheer), while the highlighter is too shiny for anything but an evening look. **Roller Girl Face Shimmer** *($18)* looks like a mini bottle of roll-on deodorant, but instead is glitter suspended in a clear gel base that you stroke on anywhere you want shine. This does not blend well at all, so the effect can look more like glitter war paint than anything else. **Sonic Stick** *($18)* is more sheer shine; it just dispenses the glitter in stick form.

☹ <u>EYESHADOW:</u> The **Eye Shadow Quartets** *($35)* are absurdly overpriced and have an opaque, dry, powdery texture. The color combinations are mostly unworkable and all of the shades are either eye-glaringly shiny or blend poorly. **Eye Shadow Loners** *($15)* have a powdery application and a widely varying texture that goes from sheer and smooth (the lighter colors) to grainy and thick (the darker, glittery colors). Every shade is very shiny and these tend to cling unevenly. **Eye Lacquer** *($15)* is intensely shiny cream-to-powder eyeshadow that comes in a click-pen dispenser that puts the colors onto an angled sponge-tip applicator. These eyeshadows dry quickly and stay put, but this much glitter is incredibly distracting.

<u>EYE AND BROW SHAPER:</u> ✓☺ $$$ **Training Brow Pencil** *($16)* is recommended if the price (and regular sharpening) doesn't bother you. The texture is light and powdery, with a good sheer application that builds nicely.

☺ $$$ **Eye Glider** *($17)* is just a standard pencil with a creamy application and shiny colors. **Glitter Shadow Pencil** *($18)* has a smooth, powdery texture and glides well, but be prepared for the glitter to fly everywhere, even when the pencil is being sharpened. **Eye Base Pencil** *($15)* is a standard, but thick, pencil with a soft, creamy texture. This is supposed to provide a base for the Sonic Sparkle Dust to cling to, but the pale, shiny gold color can crease and the glitter powder tends to grab unevenly, which ends up being more comical than attractive. **Training Brow Kit** *($28)* is cute but overpriced for what you get: two shades of almost matte eyeshadow in a compact with an itty-bitty pair of tweezers and a minuscule brow brush. There are scads of inexpensive true-matte brow colors and far better tweezers to use that negate the need for this kit, though some will probably find it appealing.

☹ **Super Sonic Pencil** *($19)* is a standard chunky pencil with a waxy, sticky texture that is truly awful, with or without the flecks of glitter. **Training Brow Gel** *($14)* is exceedingly standard, sticky, and not worth the price tag. Use hairspray on an old toothbrush instead and treat yourself to a bottle or two of nail polish.

<u>LIPSTICK AND LIP PENCIL:</u> ☺ $$$ **Super Good Lipstick** *($16)* is more like "super standard." This is a slick, creamy lipstick with a glittery finish and unbecoming colors. **Super Plump Lipstick** *($18)* does not plump anything, but it does have a pleasantly lightweight texture and sheer, semi-glossy finish—what a shame the color selection is so limited. **Caffeine Lipstick** *($17)* is supposedly enriched with caffeine for a quick lift every time you lick your lips. Please ignore this gimmick, because the notion of encouraging consumers to lick their lips and consume lipstick to get a hit of caffeine is not good for anyone's health.

☺ **Lip Stix SPF 12 Lip Gloss** *($15)* lacks UVA protection, so this remains just a sheer, glittery gloss dispensed in the same manner as the Eye Lacquer above.

☹ **Glitter Dip Lipstick** *($17)* is a creamy lipstick speckled with chunks of glitter. As the color wears off, the glitter remains. If you like shiny lips that feel like sandpaper, check this out. **Lip Gloss Cubes** *($12)*, **Super Shine Lip Gloss** *($12, $30 for Mini Super Shine Gloss Set)*, and **Super Clear Lip Gloss** *($12)* are standard lip glosses that come in various types of packaging and a wide assortment of pastel, iridescent hues along with a few traditional shades. What's problematic, and especially unappealing, is that all of these have a sticky, goopy texture that lacks any elegance or sophistication. In fact, this gloss is kid's stuff. **Lip Sync Quartet** *($35)* features three lip colors and one gloss in a compact.

The space-age iridescent colors have a sticky, hot-caramel texture that is just awful, and the included lip brush is a joke. **Super Good Lip Pencil** *($12)* is below standard, needs sharpening, and the color choices are depressing, and that isn't super in the least.

☹ MASCARA: Hard Candy's **Mascara** *($15)* has some truly strange colors, and though it is a reliable lengthening mascara that defines lashes and adds a soft curl without clumping it tends to smear throughout the day. The **Glitter Mascara** *($16)* is a mess when it comes to application and figuring out a way to keep the glitter particles from flaking (painfully) into your eye.

SPECIALTY: As the backbone of this line's business, the $$$ ☺ **Nail Polish** *($12)* features a wild assortment of colors and textures, from the chip-prone glittery shades to the palest pastels. These are quite ordinary except for the colors. Still, if one of these somehow fits into your wardrobe or color scheme, why not?

☺ $$$ **Palm Palette** *($35)* is an on-the-go arsenal of shine in one difficult-to-open compact. There are several kits that include eyeshadow, blush, and lip colors, plus mini applicators. This would be *the* cool item to have and share at a teen slumber party, but will elicit "what was I thinking" reactions in the light of day. Great name, though!

HELENA RUBINSTEIN

Entrepreneur, philanthropist, international businesswoman, and author—the legendary Helena Rubinstein was a multifaceted woman. Raised in Poland, Rubinstein immigrated to Australia while still in her twenties and opened up the country's first beauty salon in 1902. Her initial claim to fame in the cosmetics arena was a family recipe for face cream. That isn't surprising, because family recipes for moisturizers were all that women had in those days given that the cosmetics industry wasn't yet born. That fabled face cream, whose content remains a mystery, gave birth to an entire skin-care line. Rubinstein eventually opened salons in Europe and New York, the forerunners of what are now known as day spas. With the line's growing popularity, department stores were soon selling Rubinstein's products alongside the products of two other cosmetics divas of the era, Estee Lauder and Elizabeth Arden. In her day, Rubinstein was a household name as the guru of beautiful skin.

When Rubinstein passed away in 1965 the line's confidence and flair seemed to disappear, and it finally stopped being sold in the United States in 1985. L'Oreal bought Helena Rubinstein in 1988 and relaunched it stateside in 1996 in a number of Saks Fifth Avenue and Bergdorf Goodman stores. There is also a Helena Rubinstein Gallery in New York City.

Despite the L'Oreal-backed revival, it is doubtful that Rubinstein would think the present-day version of her namesake line lived up to her philosophy that "creation must be bold—it must surpass what has been done before." In this case, a good deal of it is the same old, same old. For more information about Helena Rubinstein, call (212) 343-9966 or visit www.helenarubinstein.com. **Note:** All Rubinstein products contain fragrance unless otherwise noted.

HELENA RUBINSTEIN SKIN CARE

☺ $$$ **Mat Specialist Deep Clarifying Cleansing Foam** *($21.50 for 4.4 ounces)* is a detergent-based cleanser that also contains clay. It can leave a matte feel on the skin. The menthol in it can be a skin irritant.

☺ **Fresh Foaming Gel Gentle Water Dissolve Cleanser** *($21.50 for 6.7 ounces)* is a very simple, but good, detergent-based cleanser that would work well for most skin types.

☺ $$$ **Glycolic Exfoliating Cleanser** *($23.50 for 4.2 ounces)* does contain about a 5% concentration of glycolic acid, but the pH of the product isn't low enough for it to be effective as an exfoliant.

☺ **Pure Cleansing Water Toning Face and Eye Cleanser** *($23.50 for 6.7 ounces)* is supposed to be a cleanser, eye-makeup remover, and toner. All it ends up being is a very ordinary, boring toner composed of water, glycerin, slip agents, and preservatives with little benefit for skin in any arena.

☺ **Fresh Cleansing Fluid Express Face and Eye Cleanser** *($23.50 for 6.7 ounces)* is an option for normal to dry skin.

☺ $$$ **All Mascaras! Complete Eye Make Up Remover** *($22 for 4.2 ounces)* is an exceptionally standard, silicone-based makeup remover that would work as well as any.

☹ **Mat Specialist Clarifying Treatment Tonic** *($21.50 for 6.7 ounces)* lists alcohol as the second ingredient, and along with menthol that means the only thing clear about this toner is the irritation and dryness it can cause.

☺ **Glycolic Exfoliating Lotion** *($24 for 6.7 ounces)* could have been a very good 8% glycolic acid–based, toner-style exfoliant, but the product's pH of 5 means it doesn't have exfoliating properties.

☹ **Fresh Honey Stimulating Hydrating Tonic** *($21.50 for 6.7 ounces)* lists alcohol as the fourth ingredient, which means that the freshness and stimulating effect will be short-lived and soon replaced by irritation and dryness.

☺ **Delicate Aromatic Lotion** *($21.50 for 6.7 ounces)* is just water, glycerin, slip agent, fragrance, preservatives, and coloring agents. It is an ordinary, obsolete toner.

☺ $$$ **Prodigy Skin Life Treatment** *($125 for 1.76 ounces)* lists aluminum starch octenylsuccinate, an absorbent, as the third ingredient, which will negate any hydrating or moisturizing benefits that might result from the other ingredients. It contains a modicum of water-binding agents and antioxidants and is incredibly overpriced for what is a poorly formulated lotion.

☹ **Hydro Urgency Intense Moisture Replenishing Lotion SPF 15** *($46.50 for 1.7 ounces)* does not contain the UVA-protecting ingredients of titanium dioxide, zinc oxide, or avobenzone, and is not recommended. The only thing urgent about this product is the need to find a better formulated sunscreen.

☺ $$$ **Hydro Urgency Intense Moisture Replenishing Cream** *($46.50 for 1.7 ounces)* is a basic emollient moisturizer for normal to dry skin with a small amount of water-binding agents and a minute amount of vitamin E.

☺ **$$$ Hydro Urgency Intense Moisture Replenishing Cream Gel** *($46.50 for 1.7 ounces)* is similar to the Replenishing Cream above and the same comments apply.

☺ **$$$ Face Sculptor Line Lift Cream** *($75 for 1.7 ounces)* is an emollient moisturizer that contains mostly water, silicone, glycerin, thickeners, sunscreen, emollient, water-binding agents, antioxidants, and preservatives. This is a good moisturizer for normal to dry skin, but given the price you would expect an exceptional one and it doesn't fall into that category. It is strange for a product to have this amount of sunscreen but no SPF rating.

☺ **$$$ Throat Sculptor Lift Up Cream** *($65 for 1.7 ounces)* is similar to the Face Sculptor Line Lift Cream above and the same comments apply. There is nothing in this moisturizer that can sculpt or that makes it better for the throat.

☺ **$$$ Eye Sculptor with Pro Phosphor** *($52 for 0.5 ounce)* is similar to the Face Sculptor Line Lift Cream above and the same comments apply.

☺ **$$$ Face Sculptor Concentrated Line Lift Serum** *($78 for 1 ounce)* is similar to the Face Sculptor Line Lift Cream above and the same comments apply. There is nothing concentrated about this product in the least.

☹ **$$$ Night Sculptor Anti Puffiness Face and Eye Line Lift** *($75 for 1.7 ounces)* is similar to the Face Sculptor Line Lift Cream above only this version lacks antioxidants. There is nothing in this product that will eliminate or reduce puffiness around the eyes or lines for that matter.

☺ **$$$ Power A for Eyes Pure Retinol Repair System** *($55 for 0.5 ounce)* does contain retinol and some good water-binding agents, but it is essentially identical to L'Oreal's (L'Oreal owns Rubinstein) Line Eraser Pure Retinol Concentrate ($14.99 for 1 ounce). It even has the same packaging. This doesn't contain fragrance.

☹ **$$$ Power A Pure Retinol System** *($80 for 1.7 ounces)* doesn't contain retinol, though it does contain retinyl palmitate, which is a whole other generation removed from the active component of vitamin A. Overall this is just an average moisturizer for dry skin.

☹ **$$$ Power A Essence** *($80 for 1 ounce)* lists alcohol as the third ingredient, which means that this lotion ends up being more problematic for skin than anything else.

☹ **$$$ Collagenist Plumping Treatment Anti-Wrinkle Firmness** *($72 for 1.6 ounces)* does contain collagen, but collagen has no ability to firm skin or fight wrinkles. Collagen has shown up in skin-care products since the 1980s, and there still isn't a shred of research showing it to be the answer for wrinkles. There are other good water-binding agents in here, but at such minimal concentrations that they just don't add up to this price tag. It also contains a form of salicylic acid, but the pH is too high for it to be effective as an exfoliant. This is an OK emollient moisturizer for dry skin.

☹ **$$$ Collagenist Intensive Plumping Serum** *($72 for 1.6 ounces)* is similar to the Power A Essence above and the same comments apply.

☺ **$$$ Force C Premium Super Anti Fatigue Eye Care** *($42 for 0.5 ounce)* is a very good, silicone-based moisturizer for normal to dry skin that contains a good amount of antioxidants (vitamin C), plant oils, and anti-irritants. If you are looking for a vitamin C product, this would be an option.

☺ $$$ **Force C Premium Super Energizing Cream** *($56 for 1.7 ounces)* is similar to the Anti-Fatigue Eye Care above only in cream form, and the same basic comments apply. This does contain a form of salicylic acid, but the pH of the product is too high for it to be effective as an exfoliant.

☺ $$$ **Force C Premium Super Energizing Fluid Vitamin C Time Release SPF 15** *($56 for 4.2 ounces)* is a good titanium dioxide–based sunscreen in a matte-finish lotion. It contains minimal amounts of vitamin C. The plant extracts are meant to sound like they are similar to AHAs, but they have no exfoliating properties.

☹ **Force C with Pure Vitamin C Exfoliating Radiance Disks** *($30 for 10 discs)*. They're kidding, right? This is just aluminum starch octenylsuccinate (an absorbent), detergent cleansing agents (one is tallow-based), a teeny amount of vitamin C, and film-forming agent. Unbelievable! This is a drying cleanser that's soaked onto a sponge disk that swells when you add water. Not only is it a waste of money, it's one of the most absolutely poorly formulated vitamin C products I've ever seen. This is nothing more than a gimmick that some women will fall for.

☺ $$$ **Urban Active Age Defense System Fluid SPF 15** *($50 for 1.76 ounces)* is a good titanium dioxide–based sunscreen in a rather ordinary emollient moisturizing lotion that has minimal amounts of water-binding agents and antioxidants, which makes it outrageously overpriced. This is easily replaced with similar or far better formulations available at the drugstore for far less money.

✓☺ $$$ **Urban Active Age Defense System Cream SPF 15** *($50 for 1 ounce)* is similar to the System Fluid above only in cream form. This one does contain a larger assortment of water-binding agents and antioxidants and is preferred to the version above.

☺ $$$ **Golden Beauty Sun Tan Express Crystal Self Tanning Gel** *($25 for 1.7 ounces)* contains dihydroxyacetone, the same ingredient all self-tanners use to affect the color of skin. This would work as well as any.

☺ **Golden Defense SPF 15 Moisturizing Sun Lotion** *($26.50 for 5.07 ounces)* is a very good avobenzone-based sunscreen in a standard silicone-based moisturizer that is an option for normal to slightly dry skin. However, there is nothing in this formulation to make it preferred over Ombrelle, which can be found at the drugstore and is also made by L'Oreal.

☹ **Mat Specialist 2 Way Shine Control Fluid Oil Free** *($36.50 for 1.7 ounces)* lists alcohol as the fourth ingredient, which may be too potentially drying and irritating for all skin types.

☹ **Mat Specialist Instant Purifying Mask** *($27 for 2.08 ounces)* is similar to the 2 Way Shine Control above and the same comments apply.

☹ $$$ **Hydro Urgency Instant Moisture Mask** *($27 for 1.76 ounces)*. There is nothing urgent about this average emollient mask. It does contain a tiny amount of water-binding agents, which is nice, but it's completely ordinary.

☺ **$$$ Lip Sculptor Smoothing Effect Balm** *($30 for 0.5 ounce)* is just an ordinary silicone-based lip gloss with a teeny amount of vitamin E. This won't smooth one line around your lips.

HELENA RUBINSTEIN FUTURE WHITE LINE (CANADA ONLY)

☺ **$$$ Future White Whitening Fluid SPF 40** *($60 for 1.11 ounces)* is a good in-part titanium dioxide-based sunscreen in an OK emollient moisturizing base that can be an option for normal to dry skin. However, other then the sunscreen, which can be extremely helpful for preventing skin discolorations caused by sun damage, there are no other melanin-inhibiting ingredients in this product. It is a rather basic sunscreen that is easily replaced by far less expensive options.

☹ **$$$ Future White Whitening Eye Care** *($68 for 0.5 ounce)* contains about 3% glycolic and lactic acid, which isn't enough to be effective for exfoliation. This adds up to a rather basic moisturizer for normal to dry skin, with little to offer for any skin type, and absolutely nothing to inhibit or reduce skin discolorations.

☺ **$$$ Future White High Precision Whitening Essence** *($90 for 1.01 ounces)* contains about 7% AHAs in a pH of 4.5, which makes it somewhat effective for exfoliation. It also contains kojic acid, which can be effective for inhibiting melanin production, though it is considered a fairly unstable ingredient. This is an option for most skin types.

HELENA RUBINSTEIN MAKEUP

Very few Rubenstein makeup items can be called bold, groundbreaking, or even uniquely intriguing. The foundations feature some admirable textures, but those with sunscreen lack UVA protection. The concealer is abysmal, the majority of the blushes and eyeshadows are layered with shine, and the pencils are ordinary. The one saving grace of this sprawling collection is its truly remarkable mascaras. Knowing this line is owned by L'Oreal, it's not surprising that the mascaras are stellar. Other than that, the makeup, though lavishly packaged, is unexciting.

<u>FOUNDATION:</u> ☺ **$$$ Illumination Natural Radiance Reviving Makeup SPF 15** *($40)* is a liquid foundation with a smooth texture that blends well and dries to a natural matte finish. The sunscreen lacks UVA protection, but this is an option for normal to slightly dry or slightly oily skin when paired with an effective sunscreen. Most of the eight shades (for light to medium skin tones) are acceptable—only G202 and 103 are too peach to consider. **Double Agent Skin Adjusting Makeup** *($38.50)* is an ultra-matte makeup that contains multiple silicones and denatured alcohol for a featherlight, silky texture and a dry, almost powdery finish. This provides light to medium coverage and has enough playtime to allow for adept blending, but it still must be blended quickly and precisely because this does not budge once it has dried. The eight shades have a soft peach or golden cast, but not enough to warrant avoiding them, though G02 is too yellow for most skin. **Face Sculptor Makeup Rich Lifting Foundation** *($44)* sounds like the perfect tool to mold your visage into the shape you want. While it would be nice if all it took was

a foundation to lift a sagging jawline and eliminate crow's-feet, this one doesn't even come close to fulfilling its alluded-to promises. Face Sculptor is a good, creamy foundation for normal to dry skin that provides light coverage and slips elegantly onto the skin, leaving a radiant finish, but that's the extent of it. Of the eight shades, avoid the pink-tinged 12 and peachy 104. **Color Fitness Energizing Tinted Moisturizer SPF 12** *($30)* lacks significant UVA protection and has an SPF that is marginal for daytime wear. Otherwise, this well-formulated, emollient tint would work best for normal to dry skin. The three shades are appropriately sheer and workable. However, I wouldn't choose this over a tinted moisturizer with an effective sunscreen.

☺ $$$ **Illumination Natural Radiance Reviving Compact Makeup SPF 15** *($42)* does not list any active sunscreen ingredients, so the SPF claim is bogus. This is a standard, overpriced cream-to-powder makeup with a smooth application and satin finish that feels dry. The six shades provide sheer to light coverage, but steer clear of P103 and P104, as both are too peach. **Illumination Natural Radiance Reviving Compact Makeup SPF 14** *($42)* is a talc-based, pressed-powder foundation that includes noticeable shine and excludes any effective UVA protection. This is pricey for what amounts to a subtle shimmering powder that has a creamy feel and sheer application that can build to medium coverage. The six shades are mostly neutral, with only 06 being too orange.

☹ **CONCEALER:** **Touch It Up Cover Cream Concealer** *($22.50)* is a too-creamy compact concealer that not only emphasizes lines around the eye but also tends to slip into them and crease. The four shades include a yellow color corrector, but this is not an easy concealer to live with.

POWDER: ☺ $$$ **Softwear Loose Powder with Micro Fibres** *($35)* is a very sheer, talc-based loose powder that feels light and airy on the skin and comes in three OK shades. This holds no advantage over less expensive loose powders from Clinique or Sonia Kashuk, to name but two. **Double Agent Mattifying Pressed Powder** *($30)* is talc-based and has a light application and suitably dry finish. This is best for normal to oily skin, and (thankfully) the shiny particles were left out. The six colors are not the most neutral around, and 03 is too pink for most skin tones. Nothing about this formula will "smooth dryness," but it will assuredly accentuate it!

☺ $$$ **Compact Bronzer SPF 30** *($30)* contains titanium dioxide as part of the active sunscreens and is a fine option for a sheer, creamy bronzer with a non-greasy finish. This builds well so you can create anything from a soft glow to a bold Tahitian tan. ☺ $$$ **Compact Bronzer** *($32)* is a decent pressed bronzing powder that can initially go on strong, but it blends well to a shiny sateen finish. If not for the shine, this would be perfect for a sun-kissed look.

☹ **Opalescence Pressed Loose Powder** *($35)* is a talc-based pressed powder that's just loosely pressed, so the pickup on the brush and application is more akin to traditional loose powder. This is not preferred over either regular pressed powder or loose powder.

☺ **$$$ <u>BLUSH</u>: Color Statement for Cheeks Radiant Blush** *($30)* has a soft, blendable texture and features nine mostly shiny shades of varying intensity. Redbrown, Fight for Chocolate, and Think Pink as deeper tones, while the remaining shades are decidedly sheer. The only matte option is Cherish Cherry—don't even ask about the perplexing shade names!

☺ **$$$ <u>EYESHADOW:</u>** The **Color Statement for Eyes Radiant Eyeshadow** *($18.50)* is sold as singles and comes in an extensive range of shades that offer something for every taste and skin tone, including women of color. These have a standard powder eyeshadow texture and apply easily. The matte shades tend to be sheer and the shiny shades (which outnumber the mattes) apply heavier, so watch out for flaking. The darker shades have great pigmentation and should be used sparingly.

<u>**EYE AND BROW SHAPER:**</u> ☺ **$$$ Two On Line Bicolor Eye Pencil** *($16)* is a dual-sided standard pencil that glides on with relative ease, but it is creamy enough to eventually smear unless it is set with a powder eyeshadow.

☺ **$$$ Silky Eyes Smooth Glide Eye Pencil** *($16)* is also a standard pencil that has an impressive color range, but otherwise it's no different from the best smooth-applying pencils available at the drugstore (L'Oreal and Cover Girl come to mind). **Spectacular Liner Ultra Precise Liquid Eyeliner** *($25)* is a suitable liquid liner that applies easily but sheer, and lasts, but you will not notice a tremendous difference between this and the outstanding liquid liners sold by L'Oreal.

☹ **Eyebrow Pencil** *($16)* needs sharpening, has a hard texture, and yet smudges easily even with deft application. Don't bother with this one.

<u>**LIPSTICK AND LIP PENCIL:**</u> ☺ **$$$ Ritual Rouge Intense Color Long Lasting Lipstick** *($21)* is a beautifully creamy, but elegantly light, lipstick that features full-coverage iridescent and cream-finish colors. **Ritual Rouge Brilliant** *($21)* has a texture and application almost identical to the one above, but comes in sheer, glossier colors that have subtle impact and a short life span on the lips. **Rouge Pulse High Impact Color** *($21.50)* extends the range of Rubinstein's lip colors. This creamy, slightly greasy lipstick feels smooth and moist, but is too emollient to last until lunch. **Forever Gloss** *($18.50)* is a smooth-textured wand gloss with mostly iridescent pigmented colors. For some reason, the Clear shade is sticky, while the others are not. **Lip Pencil** *($16)* is a standard creamy pencil that is a pleasure to use and does not feel too thick or waxy. The large color range favors pinks, plums, and nudes, which is smart given the popularity of those colors.

☹ **Liquid MetalLacquer for Lips** *($21)* is a liquidy lip color that is applied with a sponge-tip wand and goes on sheer. Its high concentration of alcohol allows the formula to evaporate quickly, leaving a weightless veil of relatively budgeproof color. What's disappointing about this is how it wears—within hours you will find this has flaked or chipped off, leaving an unsightly ring of color on the outside of the lips. For this price, you should expect more.

MASCARA: Rubinstein offers no less than eight mascaras, and almost all of them are excellent and wear beautifully. ✔☺ $$$ **Spectacular Mascara** *($22)* is a superior lengthening mascara that goes on wetter than most, but produces copiously long lashes that last all day without smearing. This does tend to stick the lash tips together for a more dramatic finish. ✔☺ $$$ **Crescendo Mascara** *($22)* is the perfect all-purpose mascara. Length, thickness, and definition are achieved in equal parts for striking lash enhancement rather than lash overkill. ✔☺ $$$ **Extravagant Mascara** *($22)* is tremendous. This is an expert lengthening mascara that allows you to get to each and every lash, plus it builds subtle thickness.

☺ $$$ **Generous Mascara** *($22)* takes a while to get going but eventually shows you what a good, clump-free lengthening and minor thickening mascara it is. The application is slightly wet, but clean. **Long Lash Mascara** *($22)*, launched in 1958, became one of the first mascaras to usher out the era of cake mascaras. This features a threaded metal rod rather than a brush. Although it looks strange, the rod allows you to build length and thickness and to adeptly define every lash with ease. It's waterproof and a bit stubborn to remove. Since this contains silk fibers, it is not recommended for contact lens wearers.

☺ $$$ **Vertiginous Mascara** *($22)* has a name that means "causing or tending to cause dizziness or vertigo," but thankfully you or your lashes won't experience any of that with this average formula that builds OK length and a bit of thickness. It wears well without flaking, but simply isn't as impressive as the ones above. **Vertiginous Mascara Base** *($20)* is a lash primer that's basically a mascara minus pigment. It does a good job adding an undercoat of oomph and soft curl to lashes, but no more so than a single, excellent mascara—of which Rubinstein indeed has a few! **Vertiginous Mascara Waterproof** *($22)* builds quick, impressive length with some minor smearing and OK lash separation. This is waterproof and requires an oil- or silicone-based product for complete removal.

☹ **Spectacular Mascara Waterproof** *($22)* is waterproof, but it's less than spectacular when it comes to length and thickness, plus it tends to smear, which makes it the weakest of all the Rubinstein mascaras.

☺ $$$ **BRUSHES:** Considering the sheer scope of Rubinstein's makeup, it is a bit shocking that they offer only a few **Brushes** *($20–$35)*. What's available is pretty much a rank-and-file selection, and none of them are top-notch. So much for Rubinstein's credo, "Creation must be bold! It must surpass what has been done before."

HYDRON

Hydron is sold on QVC, and it is simply captivating to watch the host of the show swear by it while enthusiastic callers echo the sentiment. The presentation is *very* convincing, but before you pick up your phone and order, you need more information than just what the company wants you to know.

The Best Defense Collection by Hydron supposedly can restore your skin's natural moisture balance by creating a water-insoluble film over the surface of your skin. According to the company, "Hydron is a polymer, which is an extremely high-molecular- weight compound." What Hydron really is, is polyhydroxyethyl-methacrylate. That makes it basically a film-forming agent, like most of the other acrylates that show up in skin-care products. The other aspect of Hydron is that, like any polymer, its molecules are too large to penetrate the skin, so it sits on top and covers the surface. That water-insoluble film also has water-binding properties, which are nice and can benefit dry skin, but the film is hardly miraculous or rare, nor the only way to keep water in the skin; and it's not unique in terms of function compared to other film-forming agents used in lots and lots of skin-care products. There are some very good moisturizers and cleansers to consider in this line, but you will wait a lifetime if you're expecting to see wrinkles disappear. For more information about Hydron, call (800) 4-HYDRON or visit www.iqvc.com or www.hydron.com. **Note:** All Hydron products contain fragrance unless indicated otherwise.

☺ **Best Defense Gentle Cleansing Creme** *($16.50 for 6 ounces)* is a standard lotion cleanser that would be an option for someone with normal to dry skin. It offers no advantage over using Neutrogena's Extra Gentle Cleanser ($5.49 for 6.7 ounces), which is almost identical.

☺ **Oil Control Facial Cleansing Gel** *($15.75 for 4 ounces)*. There is nothing in this product that will control oily skin. This is just a good, standard, detergent-based cleanser that would work well for normal to oily skin. It does contain triclosan, a disinfectant, but there is no research showing that to be effective against the bacterium that causes blemishes.

☺ $$$ **Best Defense Gentle Eye Make Up Remover** *($17 for 4 ounces)* is a standard, silicone-based makeup remover that would work as well as any. This doesn't contain fragrance.

☺ $$$ **Best Defense Micro-Exfoliating Creme** *($16.75 for 3.6 ounces)* is similar to the Gentle Cleansing Creme above only this contains ground-up plastic (polyethylene) as the abrasive. It is an option for normal to dry skin, but is overpriced for a standard scrub.

✓☺ **Best Defense Botanical Toner** *($14.50 for 6.5 ounces)* is a good, irritant-free toner that contains some good anti-irritants and water-binding agents. This does contain coloring agents.

☹ **Oil Balancing Toner** *($16 for 6.5 ounces)* lists alcohol as the second ingredient, which makes this too drying and irritating for all skin types.

☺ $$$ **Best Defense Daily Facial Moisturizer Oil-Free with SPF 15** *($26 for 2 ounces)* is a good, in-part avobenzone-based sunscreen for normal to oily skin. It does contain some good antioxidants and water-binding agents. The tiny bit of lanolin is not enough to be a problem for someone with normal to oily skin, but calling this oil free when it contains an emollient waxy ingredient like lanolin is misleading.

☺ $$$ **Best Defense Fragile Eye Moisturizer** *($22.50 for 0.5 ounce)* is a good emollient moisturizer that contains a good assortment of water-binding agents, but only minimal amounts of antioxidants. It is still an option for normal to dry skin anywhere on your face.

☺ $$$ **Best Defense Line Smoothing Complex** *($32 for 0.5 ounce)* is a decent lightweight moisturizer for normal to slightly dry or oily skin that has a good mix of water-binding agents, but it lacks any significant antioxidants.

✔☺ **Best Defense Moisture Balance Restorative Overnight Liposome Complex** *($29.75 for 2 ounces)* would be a good emollient moisturizer for someone with dry skin. It contains mostly water, slip agent, plant oils, water-binding agents, film-forming agent, antioxidants, emollients, preservatives, and fragrance.

✔☺ **Hydronamins Moisturizing Vitamin Therapy Day Creme SPF 15** *($29.75 for 1.9 ounces)* is a good, in-part avobenzone-based sunscreen for normal to dry skin. It also contains a good assortment of water-binding agents and antioxidants.

✔☺ **Hydronamins Moisturizing Vitamin Therapy Night Creme** *($36.75 for 2 ounces)* is similar to the Vitamin Therapy Day Creme above only without sunscreen. It has a very good mix of water-binding agents, antioxidants, and plant oils. It would be a great option for normal to dry skin.

☹ **Best Defense Tri-Activating Skin Clarifier** *($34.75 for 1 ounce)* contains plant extracts that sound as if they are related to AHAs, but they have no exfoliating properties. This product has no other redeeming features, and it won't clarify even one skin cell.

☺ **$$$ Oil Balancing Serum** *($19.75 for 0.45 ounce)* is just absorbent with film-forming agent and some very good water-binding agents. That won't balance skin but it is a good option for someone with normal to slightly oily skin.

☹ **Best Defense Sportscreen SPF 15** *($19.50 for two 3-ounce tubes)* doesn't contain the UVA-protecting ingredients of avobenzone, titanium dioxide, or zinc oxide, and is not recommended.

☹ **Best Defense Sportscreen SPF 30** *($15 for two 3-ounce tubes)* doesn't contain the UVA-protecting ingredients of avobenzone, titanium dioxide, or zinc oxide, and is not recommended.

☹ **Best Defense Five-Minute Revitalizing Masque** *($7.50 for 2.65 ounces)* is a standard clay mask that includes eucalyptus, balm mint, pine needle, sage, and thyme, all potential skin irritants. The mask also contains some water-binding agents and a detergent cleansing agent. The water-binding agents are nice, but the detergent cleansing agent is sodium lauryl sulfate, which can be a skin irritant.

☹ **Best Defense Tender Lip Care SPF 15** *($14.50 for two 0.5-ounce tubes)* doesn't contain the UVA-protecting ingredients of avobenzone, titanium dioxide, or zinc oxide, and is not recommended.

☺ **Self-Adjusting Tinted Moisturizers SPF 15** *($22.50)* is another moisturizer that claims to intuitively know where skin is dry and where it's oily, and to perform as needed to benefit whatever skin type it's used on. It makes great ad copy, but the truth is there is no way for one emulsified moisturizer to address the night-and-day differences between oily and dry skin. This is merely a lightweight, silicone-based moisturizer that also contains aluminum starch and talc for a somewhat dry finish. No significant UVA protection is provided, so if you opt to use one of the three peachy (but sheer) colors you will need to use a separate sunscreen—so much for an all-in-one product.

☺ **Under Eye Concealer** *($14)* comes in a tube and is "designed" to work with their "patented Hydron moisturizing system." This creamy concealer will work with (or without) anyone's moisturizer, although it will crease slightly no matter what you use (or don't use) underneath. A high concentration of titanium dioxide lends each of the three shades a chalky appearance that can be difficult to blend away, especially on medium to dark skin tones.

IGIA

There probably isn't a woman in the United States right now who hasn't seen the ads for this line. Whether it is for the IGIA Hair Removal System, the IGIA Sun System Facial Tanner, the IGIA Clear Blemish Remover, or the IGIA Epil-Stop, these IGIA promotions seem to have perfected the art of convincingly selling miraculous-sounding, but useless, beauty products. All the products are widely advertised in fashion magazines, on television, and in mail-order catalogs throughout the United States and Canada. For more information about IGIA, call (800) 716-8667 or visit www.igia.com.

Let's start with the IGIA Sun System because this product speaks to the ethics of the company more than any other item they sell. The other products, while useless, at least aren't harmful.

☹ **Sun System Facial Tanner** *($149)* claims to let you "[do] in minutes what usually takes hours to acquire. Compact, easy to use, and safe. Comes with a convenient 30-minute timer so there's no need to worry about burning. You control the amount of color you receive, while its four UV lamps help you get that even tan. Stop wasting money on unhealthy tanning salons and get better results in the privacy of your own home with the IGIA Sun System." Using the same type of UV lights for the face that tanning beds use is dangerous and unhealthy for skin! According to the FDA (www.fda.gov), the FCC (Federal Communications Commission), the American Academy of Dermatology (www.aad.org), and the Skin Cancer Foundation (www.skincancer.org), tanning beds are nothing more than skin cancer machines and should be made illegal. Tanning beds are set up to radiate the most damaging effects of the sun only inches away from your body, and, worse, they are available day after day, month after month. In addition, they allow body parts that are usually covered to be exposed. They pose the same or increased risk of skin cancer that unprotected exposure to the sun allows (Sources: *Journal of the American Academy of Dermatology,* May 2002, pages 706–709, and May 2001, pages 775–780; *Journal of the National Cancer Institute,* February 2002, pages 224–226; and *Pediatrics,* June 2002, pages 1009–1014). It is senseless to make this machine readily available to an unsuspecting public that believes something is safe when the contrary is true. There is no such thing as a safe tan generated by any kind of UV exposure, whether from a light bulb indoors or from the sun outside. This machine alone casts a great shadow over IGIA. In fact, trust is the one thing this kind of company is *not* radiating.

☹ **Epil-Stop and Foam** *($19.95 for 4 ounces)*, and **Epil-Stop and Silk** *($19.95 for 4 ounces)*. The FDA issued a recall on September 13, 1997, for this product, which is manufactured by International Chemical Corporation, Amherst, New York. Previously, on September 4, 1997, the California Poison Control Office had issued a press release warning that Epil-Stop "is adulterated in that it has high pH levels which may cause skin irritation and burning." Check out the FDA home page at www.fda.gov for more information.

IGIA Epil-Stop products were advertised on television, in magazines, and over the Internet, with claims about removing hair and stopping hair growth naturally and painlessly. If all that were true, my midweek leg stubble would be a thing of the past. It isn't. Epil-Stop is a horrendous example of marketing-claim abuse, which isn't surprising, at least not to this cosmetics watchdog. It turns out that Epil-Stop works like any other drugstore depilatory: by dissolving hair with a high-pH ingredient base. Unlike other drugstore products, however, Epil-Stop took the pH to a much higher level, eating away not only the hair but the skin as well. The company has since reformulated them and the products should perform less caustically, but there is still no reason to use these over Neet or Nair, which are available at the drugstore.

☹ **IGIA's Hair Removal System** *($119)* is supposed to be a "painless home electrolysis system that helps keep hair from growing back! Unlike common [tweezing] depilatory devices that can cause skin irritation, this system uses mild radio frequency pulses that [are] absolutely safe and delivered through the tweezers to remove hair without touching the skin." Well, that much is true. This overpriced machine delivers low-wattage radio waves through the hair shaft. Does that kill off a hair follicle? There is no research indicating that these machines do anything but tweeze the hair. The low voltage may make these machines ineffective, but they are also extremely low risk in comparison with the other IGIA products; this one is the safest in the bunch. Keep in mind that these kinds of self-electrolysis machines have been advertised for years and years. I remember them from when I was a kid. The chances of operating them successfully yourself are at best slim. You probably would end up just tweezing instead of zapping the hair, because getting the device to work right is extremely tricky and incredibly time-consuming. Yet, given the time it takes for a hair to grow back, it could take months before you knew if it was really working. What a waste.

☹ **BioTonic Blemish Remover** *($99)*, while more benign than the Sun System above, is a shocking waste of money. Here's the marketing language used in the brochure: "The IGIA Clear Blemish Remover uses a non-invasive process [a dull, metal-tipped, plastic wand] that produces negative ions to destroy bacteria and remove unattractive blemishes within seconds. Once the bacteria [are] destroyed the natural healing process can occur through the pores. The IGIA Clear Blemish Remover works best on small raised spots and typical skin problems such as pimples, blemishes, blackheads, ingrown hairs, and mild acne." The brochure carries on further, saying "this is the safe, painless way to remove unsightly skin spots and let your natural beauty shine through. Includes one bottle of cleanser and one moisturizer lotion, and comes in an attractive, slim, white plastic case." The idea that ions (which are nothing more than a group of atoms with a positive, negative, or neutral electric charge) can penetrate a pore and kill blemish-causing bacteria is preposterous. Even if ions could do that, bacteria are only part of the reason a blemish occurs. This expensive little implement doesn't address hormonal issues, the pore lining, oil production, or the use of skin-care products that can clog pores and cause breakouts. All it will remove is money from your wallet.

☺ **Epil Stop & Blond** *($24.95 for 4 ounces)* is a decent hair bleach that will lighten hair, though it tends to turn it a bit more yellow as opposed to white blond, which is preferred for lightened hair on the face or body.

☹ **Veinaway** *($8.99 for 2 ounces)* is supposed to be the miracle answer for getting rid of surfaced veins and capillaries. According to IGIA, it was previously only available in doctor's offices. That isn't true, and there isn't one shred of evidence that this product has even a modicum of benefit for the problem of surfaced capillaries and varicose veins. This is merely a standard emollient moisturizer that contains minimal antioxidants, which have no impact on surfaced veins and capillaries anyway. Veinaway also contains vitamin K, a supplement necessary for blood clotting, but there is no research showing that to be effective for stopping varicose veins or surfaced capillaries (Source: *Archives of Dermatology*, December 1998, pages 1512–1514). The horse chestnut in this product has some limited ability to help venous insufficiency when taken orally, but there is no research showing it can have any effect in that regard when applied topically.

☹ **Facial Gym** *($19.95)* is supposed to be "Your Secret Weapon Against Aging Facial Muscles!" And how does this tiny plastic contraption do that? Here's the mythology. According to IGIA, "Unfortunately as we age, face and neck muscles begin to droop and sag. Many experts agree that proper exercise is one way to stretch, tone and tighten all areas of the face and neck. The patented Facial Gym uses special isometric exercises for the lips and mouth to help prevent sagging, double chins, lines and creases." Now for the reality: For the most part, facial exercises of any kind are more likely a problem for skin than a help. The reason facial exercises can have little to no benefit is because loss of muscle tone is not a major cause of wrinkles or sagging skin. In fact, muscle tone is barely involved in these at all. The skin's sagging and drooping—and almost every facial wrinkle— are caused by four major factors: (1) deteriorated collagen and elastin (due primarily to sun damage); (2) depletion of the skin's fat layer (a factor of genetic aging and gravity); (3) repetitive facial movement (particularly true for the forehead frown lines and for smile lines from the nose to the mouth); and (4) muscle sagging due to the loosening of facial ligaments that hold the muscles in place.

It turns out that facial exercise is not helpful for worn-out collagen, elastin, or the skin's fat layer because none of that is about the muscles; it's strictly about layers of skin and fat tissue. It is especially not helpful for the lines caused by facial movement! Rather, facial exercises would only make those areas appear more lined. The reason Botox injections into the muscles of the forehead, laugh lines, and lines by the temple and eye do work at smoothing out lines in those places is because Botox *prevents* the muscles from moving! (It actually stops muscle movement of any kind, including movements like squinting and raising the eyebrows that create wrinkles in those areas.) Nor will facial exercises reattach facial ligaments; that is only possible via surgery. One step involved in a surgical face-lift is to actually re-drape the muscle of the cheek and the jaw, drawing it upward and then literally stitching it back in place where it used to be. If facial exercise could positively impact the muscle tone of the cheek and jaw it would cause a bulge in the wrong place. That's because exercise doesn't move and reattach the ligaments. If it worked, it would just tone the sagged muscle, making it appear fuller lower down, and that would only make skin look more droopy in that area.

☹ **Facial-Glo Micro-Dermabrasion Plus** *($39.95)*. I wonder if the marketing folks at IGIA sat around one day and decided to take an ordinary, battery-operated facial brush and cleansing scrub, give them a name that sounded like a pricey salon or medical procedure, and then smiled knowing that they could sucker the consumer into buying this completely ordinary product. This is nothing more than a topical scrub and rotary brush. It has no association with or resemblance to microdermabrasion whatsoever.

ILLUMINARE (MAKEUP ONLY)

Illuminare is a fledgling cosmetics company impassioned about sun protection. Ruthie Molloy, a former physical therapist and part-time makeup artist, was inspired to create what could be called a "liquid mineral makeup." What Molloy created is a smart, simple, and reasonably easy-to-use makeup line where high levels of sun protection are the rule rather than the exception. The ongoing emphasis is on developing products with as few ingredients as possible to minimize or eliminate irritating or sensitizing reactions. Has she succeeded? Although Illuminare products are not without their drawbacks, the line's steadfast commitment to sun protection as well as its fine-tuned selection of foundation, blush, and eyeshadow tones is admirable. Every product carries an SPF, and all of them use only titanium dioxide and zinc oxide as the active ingredients. Illuminare also wisely avoids using common irritants, fragrances of any kind, and (this point is shocking for a cosmetics company) shuns the term "hypoallergenic" because it is not an FDA-regulated term. Now that's refreshing!

So what's not to like about this niche line? Ironically, the one major drawback of titanium dioxide and zinc oxide (namely their heavy, occlusive, and dry nature) is the very thing that creates difficulty when it comes to blending these products. Even though Illuminare uses microfine versions of these mineral sunscreens (as do many other companies), that does not eliminate the somewhat dry finish and semi-opaque look these have on the skin. Although Illuminare's technology can be wonderful, no matter how you slice it, any product with 7% zinc oxide along with titanium dioxide is going to have some tactile issues that may not be to everyone's preference. Yet the trade-off is worth it, espe-

The Reviews I

cially if you have rosacea or sensitive skin and need your foundation to be as mild and gentle as possible while still providing significant coverage. In fact, the entire makeup collection is a boon for anyone with sensitive skin. For more information about Illuminare, call (866) 999-2033 or visit www.illuminarecosmetics.com.

☺ <u>FOUNDATION:</u> This is Illuminare's main focus, and each foundation contains zinc oxide and titanium dioxide as the UVA-protecting sunscreens. Although they claim the shades are the same for each foundation, I found enough differences among them to warrant avoiding a shade in one formula but not another. Each foundation is packaged in a squeeze tube. ✔☺ **Ultimate All Day Foundation/Concealer Matte Finish Makeup SPF 21** *($20, $2.50 trial size)* starts out disarmingly thick and a bit dry, but blends surprisingly well and has an incredibly smooth, ultra-matte finish that does not budge once it has dried. Without a doubt oily to very oily skin types will love this foundation's inordinately long-wearing formula, and the coverage, though medium to opaque, is relatively natural-looking (this is still makeup, after all). Removing it takes some effort, and is easiest with a silicone-based or mineral oil–based cleanser and a washcloth. The five shades are all excellent and best for fair to medium skin. This is far too matte for those with normal to dry skin to contemplate. For that skin type, ☺ **Fantastic Finish Moisturizing Sunscreen Makeup SPF 21** *($20, $2.50 trial size)* will work much better. This moist, creamy makeup also begins thick and can be a bit tricky to blend over the skin, but with patience (and some moisturizer underneath), it works well, providing light to medium coverage and a satin finish. Of the five shades, Sienna Sun and Florentine Fair are a touch too peach for most light skin tones. ☺ **Extra Coverage Foundation/Concealer Semi-Matte Finish Sunscreen Makeup SPF 21** *($20, $2.50 trial size)* is identical in texture, finish, and application to the Fantastic Finish above, but, true to its name, this offers full coverage and tends to work best as a spot concealer rather than as a full-face foundation. Still, if you have normal to dry skin and need the coverage, this is a good choice, and of the five colors, only Florentine Fair is too peach to work for most light skin tones.

☺ $$$ <u>BLUSH:</u> **Perfect Color Blush SPF 21** *($20)* is identical in texture, application, and finish to the Fantastic Finish foundation, except that these are natural (and beautiful) blush tones that add a healthy glow to the cheeks. The sunscreen is titanium dioxide and zinc oxide, and the formula is concentrated, so only a tiny dab is needed for soft, sheer color. This leaves a moist finish that is ideal for normal to dry skin. Oily skin will likely not enjoy this blush's finish and feel on the skin. **Perfect Color Blush Ultimate SPF 21** *($20)* has an identical texture, application, sunscreen, and finish as the Ultimate All Day Foundation above. This makes it an excellent counterpart to any matte or ultra-matte foundation for those who prefer a nontraditional blush option. The colors are all top-notch, and these wear extremely well without fading or slipping.

<u>EYESHADOW:</u> ✔☺ $$$ **All Day Eye Colors SPF 15** *($15)* are creamy, thick-textured eyeshadows that come in a squeeze tube and can be applied with fingertips, a sponge, or a synthetic brush. You only need a little of this potent formula to get a soft wash of color

that blends decently and that, once it sets, lasts all day without fading or creasing. These really do wear amazingly well, and the colors are exceptionally neutral. Perla Bianca and Perla Rossa have a soft shimmer, but this is clearly indicated and easy to sidestep if you're so inclined. Although I am not a proponent of this type of eyeshadow, this is one of the best formulas I have come across, and the matte finish is sorely missing among others of its kind.

IMAN

Only a handful of women are known by their first name alone—Madonna, Cher, Ann-Margret, and, of course, the exquisite, regal Iman. As her story goes, she was singled out as a teen from the streets of Nairobi, Kenya, to become a model. From that point on Iman broke the fashion color line, along with model Beverly Johnson, gracing the covers of fashion magazines and runways that had previously deemed black women unacceptable as cover models.

Venturing into the world of makeup seemed a natural for this elegant, savvy aristocrat. Originally, Iman achieved breakthroughs for women of color that other cosmetics lines could learn from, and over the years, a few did. Today, although there are still some beautiful options to consider, Iman's makeup line needs to be updated. The colors themselves aren't the weak spots. Rather, the products' textures and application are simply less elegant than what many other companies are sporting, including Iman's own Sephora-exclusive line, I-Iman, reviewed in this chapter.

Where Iman's line loses considerable ground is in its skin-care products, called Liquid Assets. Regrettably, whoever put these products together doesn't seem to have had a plan, or to have realized that there are different skin types. The cleansers are disappointing, the toners are mediocre, the AHA products are limited, and the oil-free products are too emollient and may cause breakouts. Additionally, not one of the daytime moisturizers contains sunscreen, even though women of color are also subject to sun damage. In fact, sun damage can make darker skin tones become ashen, and lighter-skinned women of color also run a risk of skin cancer. Like most of the skin-care lines glutting the cosmetics market today, these products have the requisite plant extracts. But don't get too excited if you're a consumer who thinks plant extracts are what good skin-care is all about; most of the green stuff is listed after the preservatives, which means there isn't much of it there. For more information about Iman, visit www.i-iman.com. **Note:** All Iman skin-care products contain fragrance.

IMAN SKIN CARE

☹ **Cleansing Bar with Grapefruit Normal/Oily Skin Formula** (*$8.50 for 3.5 ounces*) is a standard, detergent-based cleansing bar with some plants and grapefruit. This is a fairly drying bar cleanser, and that doesn't help any skin type.

☹ **Cleansing Bar with Rose Petal** (*$8.50 for 3.5 ounces*) is almost identical to the Cleansing Bar with Grapefruit (including the grapefruit) above, only the fragrance is different. The same basic comments apply.

☺ **Liquid Assets Gentle Cleansing Lotion** *($14.50 for 4 ounces)* is a standard, detergent-based, water-soluble cleanser that would work well for most skin types. It does contain a small quantity of plant extracts that can be skin irritants, but probably not enough of them to be of concern for most skin types.

☹ **Liquid Assets Skin Refresher Lotion** *($14.50 for 6 ounces).* The orange oil and menthol in this lotion are skin irritants and not refreshing for skin in the least.

☹ **Perfect Response Oil-Free Cleanser, for Acne Prone, Very Oily Skin** *($15 for 4 ounces)* includes sodium C14-16 olefin sulfate as the primary detergent cleansing agent, plus peppermint extract and lemon extract, and all of these are exceedingly irritating. This product is not recommended for any skin type.

☹ **Perfect Response Gentle Toner for Acne Prone, Very Oily Skin** *($15 for 6 ounces)* contains witch hazel, which is mostly alcohol, and that's not gentle, plus several of the plant extracts can be skin irritants. The amount of tea tree oil it contains is not enough to make it effective as a disinfectant.

☹ **Perfect Response Oil-Free Hydrating Gel for Acne Prone, Very Oily Skin** *($18 for 2 ounces)* is a lightweight gel that contains some very good water-binding agents and antioxidants. Unfortunately, it also contains some significant irritants, including sulfur and arnica, which makes it a problem for all skin types.

☹ **Perfect Response Blemish Gel for Acne Prone, Very Oily Skin** *($12 for 0.5 ounce)* would be a great 5% benzoyl peroxide gel to disinfect blemishes, except that it also contains peppermint and lemon, which are unnecessary irritants that can make acne-prone skin redder and more inflamed, and that can also hurt the skin's healing process.

☹ **Perfect Response Clay Masque for Acne Prone, Very Oily Skin** *($12 for 4 ounces)* is an OK clay mask with 2% salicylic acid and a small amount of charcoal. It doesn't have a low enough pH for the BHA to be effective as an exfoliant, but the clay mask can absorb oil. It also contains a small amount of peppermint and lemon, which are unnecessary skin irritants.

☺ **Perfect Response Even-Tone Fade Gel with AHA** *($20 for 1.7 ounces).* The plant extracts in this gel are meant to sound as if they are AHAs, but they have no exfoliating properties for skin. The hydroquinone it contains can have melanin-inhibiting properties and that's worth checking out.

☹ **All Day Moisture Complex SPF 15** *($17.50 for 3 ounces)* doesn't contain the UVA-protecting ingredients of avobenzone, titanium dioxide, or zinc oxide, and is not recommended.

☺ **Time Control Renewal Complex** *($29.50 for 1 ounce)* contains only about 3% to 4% AHA in a base with a pH that's too high to make this an effective exfoliant. However, it is a good lightweight moisturizer for normal to dry skin with some good antioxidants and water-binding agents.

☺ **Time Control Firm Defense Eye Cream** *($22 for 0.5 ounce)* contains nothing that will control one second of time on your face or firm one skin cell. This is merely a gel-style lotion that contains a teeny amount of water-binding agents. The bearberry extract may have some melanin-inhibiting properties, but other than that, there's not much this product has to offer for skin.

☹ **Oil-Free Advanced Moisture Complex SPF 15 Normal to Oily Skin** *($17.50 for 3 ounces)* doesn't contain the UVA-protecting ingredients of avobenzone, titanium dioxide, or zinc oxide, and is not recommended.

☺ **Perfection Even-Tone Fade Cream** *($20 for 2 ounces)* is a standard 2% hydroquinone product (which does inhibit melanin production when used with an effective sunscreen) in a good emollient base for normal to dry skin. It also contains a tiny amount of lemon and grapefruit, but probably not at a high enough concentration to be a problem for most skin types. The sunscreen ingredient is ineffective for UVA protection and isn't enough for reliable UVB protection either.

☹ **Under Cover Agent Oil-Control Lotion** *($16 for 1 ounce)* is a liquid version of Phillips' Milk of Magnesia that uses magnesium aluminum silicate instead of magnesium carbonate to absorb oil. It would do the trick, but it also contains balm mint and camphor, which are skin irritants.

☹ **Sun Defense Lip & Eye Stick SPF 15** *($15 for 0.14 ounce)* doesn't contain the UVA-protecting ingredients of avobenzone, titanium dioxide, or zinc oxide, and is not recommended.

☹ **Sun Defense Lotion SPF 25** *($20 for 4 ounces)* doesn't contain the UVA-protecting ingredients of avobenzone, titanium dioxide, or zinc oxide, and is not recommended.

IMAN MAKEUP

In Iman's makeup line you will find a decent number of attractive matte eyeshadows, all appropriate for a wide range of skin colors, from Asian to Latin and all shades of African-American skin. Then there are the powder blushes, which all have subtle to in-your-face shine. In other areas, however, the line is more short-sighted, including limited concealer colors, lack of a good foundation for drier skin, and disappointing mascara. Iman's makeup tester unit is nicely organized, but you need a salesperson's assistance to try anything. On balance, between the mostly stellar foundation shades, a reasonable price point, and richly pigmented eyeshadows, Iman remains a contender for women of color and is in many ways a distinct improvement over Fashion Fair and Flori Roberts.

FOUNDATION: ☺ **Second to None Cream to Powder Foundation** *($18.50)* has a beautiful texture, a smooth application, and a slightly powdery finish. This type of foundation would work well for normal to slightly dry or slightly oily skin types. The coverage is light to medium, and out of 15 shades, there are only a few—Sand 5 (too peach), Earth 3 (slightly red), and Clay 4 (red)—that should be avoided; all of the other colors are exquisite.

☺ **Second to None Oil-Free Makeup SPF 8** *($16.50)* has an embarrassingly low SPF that lacks UVA protection, but this product is a decent foundation for oily skin. Far from being the ideal, this water, clay, and talc-based makeup's texture can't compare to the silky-smoothness of dry-finish silicones, which are the basis for most modern foundations. This offers light to medium coverage and a soft, long-lasting matte finish. One caution: The formula dries quickly, so deft blending is essential. The only colors to consider avoiding are Clay 2, Sand 2, Sand 4, and Earth 3. The other shades are recommended for medium to dark skin.

☹ <u>CONCEALER:</u> **Corrective Concealer** *($12)* is a lightweight, noticeably greasy formula that tends to stay "wet" and will assuredly crease into any lines around the eyes. That's a shame, because the three colors available (no shades for dark skin tones) are superb.

<u>POWDER:</u> $$$ Both the ✔☺ **Luxury Loose Powder** *($17.50)* and the ✔☺ **Luxury Pressed Powder** *($18)* are standard, talc-based powders with a wonderfully soft, silky texture, flawless application, and a good selection of sheer matte shades that are appropriate for medium to very dark skin tones. The only color to avoid is Clay Medium, which is very orange.

☹ **Oil-Blotting Pressed Powder** *($19.50)* is talc-based, and oily skin will be appreciative of its dry but smooth texture. How sad that the five attractive shades go on so unevenly and tend to streak. **Sheer Finish Bronzing Powder** *($16)* comes in two gorgeous bronze tones, but both are iridescent. These may work for a nighttime walk on the beach, but in daylight it will look like you ran into some glitter.

☺ <u>BLUSH:</u> **Luxury Blushing Powder** *($15)* isn't as stunning as it once was, and its texture pales in comparison to the superior blush options from NARS, Bobbi Brown, and Cargo. However, the color range is impressive. All of the shades have some amount of shine, but the majority show just a hint of it. Amazon Lily and Tigress have glaring shine, while Freesia is too dark brown to work as blush, though it's fine as contour color for almost-ebony skin. **Cream Highlighter** *($15)* is very slick and gleams with iridescence, but it does blend well. Don't expect this to stay put for long, as it tends to slide all over, taking the shine with it.

☺ <u>EYESHADOW:</u> **Luxury Eyeshadow** *($10)* has the same slightly dry texture as the blush. The eyeshadows apply and cling well, but just aren't as stunning as the suede-like options from Estee Lauder and Lancome, to name two. Yet there are enough rich, matte shades here to justify a visit to the Iman counter. The matte shades to try include Almond, Onyx, Plum, Vanilla, Cedar Chip, and Mahogany. The remaining shades are pretty, but each has some amount of shine.

<u>EYE AND BROW SHAPER:</u> ☺ **Perfect Eye Pencil** *($8.50)* is indeed perfect if you prefer a creamy pencil with a slight powder finish that could easily smudge. **Luxury Brow Gel** *($14.50)* is a non-sticky, lightweight brow gel with a mediocre brush and two sheer, shiny colors, including metallic bronze, which is just odd.

☺ **Perfect Eyebrow Pencil** *($12.50)* is standard, but nice. It goes on well, isn't greasy, and should stay around for a while. There is a brush at the end of the pencil for softening the color. The single color is fine for brunettes.

☹ **Luxury Liquid Eyeliner** *($12)* has a nice, fine-tipped brush and applies evenly, but it's extremely prone to smudging and chipping.

LIPSTICK AND LIP PENCIL: ☺ **Luxury Moisturizing Lipstick** *($12)* is a creamy lipstick that has a light, slick feel and soft, glossy finish. The color range is stunning, and includes a number of dark purple, chocolate brown, red, and mahogany tones that nicely complement dark skin and have a good stain. **Luxury Lip Gloss** *($10)* is indeed quite luxurious. The texture is smooth and non-sticky, and so for gloss aficionados this is a find! The only drawback is the small selection of colors.

☺ **Perfect Lip Pencil** *($11)* is similar to the Eye Pencil above and the same comments apply. These are too creamy to prevent lipstick from feathering, though the colors are bold, which is great for naturally dark lips. **Dual-Tone Lipstick** *($11.50)* is a standard creamy lipstick that has a light and a dark half in colors such as silver and black. These really have no purpose, although the claim is that this helps "adjust the intensity of your lipstick." Save your money and blot with a tissue instead, or just choose a different color. **Lip Even** *($12)* is supposed to serve as a base coat for unevenly pigmented lips, but is too sheer and slippery to work well, especially when compared to what a not-too-creamy lip pencil can do.

☹ **Luxury Lip Shimmer** *($15)* is a standard, iridescent wand-applicator gloss that isn't sticky, but the large glitter particles make this feel grainy on the lips.

☹ **MASCARA: Perfect Mascara** *($12)* isn't perfect in the least, unless your definition of mascara perfection is one that builds barely discernible length and absolutely no thickness.

☹ **SPECIALTY: Luxury Face Palette** *($22.50)* is a collection of eight shades for cheeks, lips, and eyes, all housed in one large compact. Not only are the colors contrasting and not complementary, the cream-to-powder formula has a rough, grainy texture that is only enhanced by the heavy-handed shine present in each shade.

I-IMAN (MAKEUP ONLY)

I-Iman Makeup is essentially a spin-off of Iman's original namesake makeup line. It is available primarily at select Sephora stores and on their Web site, and is described as "flashy, trashy, glamorous, and great. [With] bold, uninterrupted color." Such disparate adjectives are not typically attached to makeup, but Iman clearly has a wild side, and it is on full display here, most notably in the blush, eyeshadow, and lipstick shades the line features. Although there are some conventional colors, the majority of hues scream color. Yet that can be a good thing for darker skin tones, as they require deep, often bold hues if the product is to show up and last on the skin. I-Iman wins high marks for making sure darker skin tones have an ample color selection. That benefit is somewhat diminished, though, as most of the colors are also the embodiment of sparkling iridescence.

The true star attractions in I-Iman cosmetics are the foundations, concealers, and pressed powders. Once again, Iman has presented a beautiful range of skin tone–correct shades that go from light to dark with nary a misstep along the way. The rest of the line, however, is hit-or-miss. If you're a woman of color, there is no doubt you should take a close look at many of the options here. However, it's up to you to decide if the rich but natural colors that complement your skin tone are right for you, or if the ones that seem to be more for shock value than anything else are the way to go. I'm all for the occasional accent of color in makeup, but not if the color upstages the woman, because that can work to her disadvantage. You may want to view I-Iman as an extension of the wonderful foundation options that began with the original Iman line. Even if there are only a few of the classic color choices that made it such a boon (and not only for women of color) are left, it's still a good option for all skin tones looking for richly pigmented makeup. For more information about I-Iman, call (877) 850-8887 or visit www.i-iman.com.

FOUNDATION: ☺ $$$ **Stick Foundation** *($30)* is silicone-based stick makeup that has a thick, slightly dry texture and powder finish. This is not nearly as slippery or creamy as many other stick foundations, so application can be trickier. The overall texture and finish make this one to consider for women with normal to oily skin who prefer medium to full coverage. This would also make an excellent concealer for dark circles, with minimal risk of creasing. There are 18 shades, and only a few are less than stellar; #4, #6, #10, and #14 are a bit too peach or red for most skin tones. **Liquid Foundation** *($27)* has a fluid, moist texture and a natural matte finish that provides medium coverage. This formula for normal to slightly dry skin comes in a pump bottle and features 16 mostly beautiful shades. Only #3, #4, #5, and #12 are too orange or peach for most skin tones. The deepest shades do not have a hint of ashiness, which is a huge plus for the darkest skin tones.

☺ $$$ **Matte Spray** *($27)* is a unique product that comes in a spray bottle and is basically a clear, alcohol-free gel that uses magnesium aluminum silicate as the absorbent. Although it feels slightly sticky at first, it has a nice dry finish. It also can be used over or under foundation, and should do a reasonably good job of keeping excess shine at bay. By the way, if you're wondering what the ingredient Hyasol-BT is, it's just another name for the water-binding agent hyaluronic acid.

☹ $$$ **I-Luminous** *($27)* is a sheer liquid foundation infused with pink or bronze iridescence. The shine you get from this is more intense than many others, and there's no reason to consider this over the countless less expensive options available everywhere.

☺ $$$ **CONCEALER:** I-Iman's **Concealer** *($18)* is a silicone-based liquid concealer that comes with a wand applicator and has a creamy, easy-to-blend texture. Coverage is smooth and even, though it does have a slight tendency to crease into lines under the eye. Of the six shades, five are superior for medium to dark skin tones; only #3 is the exception, and it is too peach for most skin tones.

POWDER: ☺ $$$ **Pressed Powder** *($25)* is talc-based, with a slightly thick, yet very silky, texture that enables you to achieve a smooth matte finish and light coverage. The range of ten shades is superior for light to dark skin tones—only shade #7 is too orange to pass muster. **Bronzer** *($27)* has a texture similar to the Pressed Powder, and offers an easy application with a smooth matte finish.

☺ $$$ **Loose Powder** *($25)* is a talc-based powder that has an excellent, finely milled texture, but unfortunately it comes in five unconventional colors, all replete with shine. These may work for some as a shiny blush, but anyone hoping to find a flesh-toned color should look elsewhere. **I-Shimmer** *($25)* has a texture and base identical to the Loose Powder above, but this is even shinier, with large glitter particles mixed in with the talc. Shades 05 and 06 are worth considering if you want to add a layer of sheer glitter to your face or body.

☺ $$$ <u>**BLUSH:**</u> **Stick Blush** *($20)* is a wax-based, traditional creamy blush that features mostly vivid and some "I can't believe this is supposed to be blush" hues. The rich colors to consider for those with dark skin who prefer a sheer cream blush are #3, #5, and #6. Shade #4 is pure neon orange, and is a difficult color to work with to say the least!

☹ <u>**EYESHADOW:**</u> **Dual Eyeshadow** *($25)* are more or less only for those who believe shadowing and shading the eye means lots of glittery shine and stark, contrasting colors. These duos offer powder or powder-with-cream eyeshadow options, and none of the pairings are what I would call workable. Plus, the texture and application fall far short of Iman's original Luxury Eyeshadow. **Eye Kit** *($30)* comes with nine cream eyeshadows in a compact, and not only are the very shiny colors awful, but the formula creases easily, too.

<u>**EYE AND BROW SHAPER:**</u> ☺ **Eye Pencil** *($14.50)* is a standard pencil with a soft, creamy texture that glides well over the skin. All of the colors have a subtle iridescence, and it's enough to emphasis a less-than-taut lashline. **Eyebrow Stencil and Color Kit** *($25)* features two matte shades of brow powder in a compact, along with two very tiny and uncomfortably stiff brushes and three reusable eyebrow stencils, labeled as Full, Natural, and Fine. The stencils are more silly than practical, but I suppose they can be somewhat helpful if you really want to duplicate these particular brow shapes. I would suggest forgoing the gimmick and instead investing in a single effective matte brow powder.

<u>**LIPSTICK AND LIP PENCIL:**</u> ☺ **Lipstick** *($16)* is a full-coverage lipstick that has a thick, greasy texture and some incredibly rich (and very dark) colors, most of which are frosted. Although this is not a poor lipstick, there are certainly more elegant textures out there to consider. **Lip Kit** *($25)* includes nine frosted lip colors in one compact. The colors are a mix of the familiar and the exotic, and they have the same formula as the regular Lipstick. If you can see yourself using most of these colors, this is an option—but there is only a minuscule amount of each color.

☺ **Lip Shine** *($15)* is an emollient, non-sticky lip gloss that offers opaque and semi-opaque colors, most of which are quite nice. **Lip Pencil** *($14.50)* is just a standard lip pencil that is about as ordinary as they come.

☹ <u>**MASCARA:**</u> **I-Iman Lash** *($18)* builds substandard length and thickness while smearing along the way.

☺ $$$ <u>**SPECIALTY:**</u> **I-Makeup Kit** *($27)* takes some of the creamy eyeshadows from the Eye Kit along with some shades from the Lip Kit and packages them in one compact. The color combinations are strange, and due to the poor eyeshadow formula, this is only half good, and all too easy to pass up.

JAFRA

When it comes to in-home lines of makeup and skin-care products, it barely matters which one you choose to try out, because the demonstration for all of them begins the same way. An array of products is set in front of you, and a presentation placard of information is placed next to the salesperson or, to use the preferred term, "beauty consultant." You are then taken through a rather fun, hands-on demonstration of products and uses after your skin type has been assessed. Of course, skin typing is almost always hit-or-miss, but I'll get to that in a minute. The skin-care routine generally involves a minimum of six products and, more often than not, "if you really want great skin," an average of seven products, although that rarely includes an adequate sunscreen. Once your face is clean and loaded up with several moisturizers, including an exfoliator, "firming" gel, protective cream, and eye lotion, the makeup application begins.

Jafra's routine is no exception, and this just as accurately describes the techniques of Mary Kay, Shaklee, Amway, and all the others. Like its peers, Jafra offers some products that are great, some that are good, some that are bad, and some that are really bad. Jafra's real insult to skin is that the majority of their sunscreens lack UVA-protecting ingredients or even adequate SPF ratings. Jafra claims that they have "quality product formulations incorporating the latest technologies and ingredients available in the beauty industry. Our expert, scientific team is tightly networked with other worldwide leading beauty developers to produce outstanding product choices for total beauty care." I don't know who they've been talking to, but most of their sunscreens fall far short of responding to the information from any current research, and that means all the studies that have taken place over the past ten years. Other shortcomings are their AHA products, which have pH levels that make them ineffective for exfoliation, and their blemish-fighting products, which are laden with skin irritants. I won't even get started on their royal jelly products!

What you will find to your skin's advantage are a few well-formulated moisturizers that are filled with state-of-the-art water-binding agents, antioxidants, and anti-irritants. However, it would not be skin-wise to rely on Jafra for one-stop shopping to cover all your skin-care needs. For more information about Jafra, call (800) 551-2345 or visit www.jafra.com.

JAFRA SKIN CARE

☺ **Balancing Foam Cleanser** *($14 for 4.2 ounces)* uses TEA-lauryl sulfate as the main detergent cleansing agent, which is potentially too drying and irritating for all skin types. The small amount of salicylic acid is not effective as an exfoliant due to the high pH of the cleanser.

☺ **Cleansing Gel for Oily Skin** *($14 for 4.2 ounces)* is a good, though very standard, water-soluble, detergent-based cleanser for someone with normal to oily skin. It is fragrance-free.

☺ **Cleansing Lotion for Dry to Normal Skin** *($12.50 for 8.4 ounces)* is a plant oil–based cleanser that can be an option for someone with normal to dry skin. It is more of a basic cold cream than anything else.

☺ **Cleansing Lotion for Normal to Oily Skin** *($4 for 8.4 ounces)* is meant to be wiped off with a washcloth, and that's essential, because it won't come off with simple splashing. This cleanser is an option for someone with normal to dry skin, not normal to oily skin.

☺ **Cleansing Cream for Dry Skin** *($14 for 4.2 ounces)* is a thicker version of the Cleansing Lotion for Dry to Normal Skin above only in cream form. The same basic comments apply.

☹ **Original Formula Cleansing Cream** *($14 for 3 ounces)* is cold cream, and it is thick, heavy, and greasy. It contains mostly mineral oil, wax, lanolin, plant oil, and preservative. It can leave a greasy film on the skin and is only an option for very dry skin.

☹ **Purifying Gel Cleanser** *($14 for 4.4 ounces)* is a standard, detergent-based, water-soluble cleanser that also contains a small amount of salicylic acid, though the pH of the base is too high for it to be an effective exfoliant. It does contain eucalyptus and juniper, which can be skin irritants, though the amounts are so small, they probably won't negatively affect skin.

☹ **Replenishing Cream Cleanser** *($14 for 4.4 ounces)* is a wipe-off cleanser that is an option for someone with normal to dry skin. It does contain lemon extract but in too small an amount to have an impact on skin.

☹ **Soothing Results Cleansing Lotion** *($14 for 8.4 ounces)* is a wipe-off makeup remover that contains lemon peel, which can be an irritant, and is not soothing for the skin.

☺ **$$$ Dual-Action Eye Makeup Remover** *($9 for 2 ounces)* is a silicone-based eye-makeup remover that also contains plant oils. It can leave a slightly greasy film on the skin but it will remove eye makeup.

☹ **$$$ Gentle Exfoliating Scrub for All Skin Types** *($14 for 2.5 ounces)* isn't all that gentle and it can be slightly greasy. It contains standard synthetic scrub particles (ground-up plastic), plus several plant oils and other emollient thickeners that make it very hard to rinse off. It also contains several plant extracts that can be skin irritants, including balm mint, sage, nettle, coltsfoot, and rosemary.

☹ **Original Formula Skin Freshener** *($15 for 8.4 ounces)* contains mostly water and alcohol, as well as menthol, which makes it too irritating for all skin types.

☹ **Skin Freshener for Dry to Normal Skin** *($15 for 8.4 ounces)* is similar to the Original Formula above and the same comments apply.

☹ **Skin Freshener for Dry Skin** *($15 for 8.4 ounces)* could have been a very good toner for someone with normal to dry skin, but the ivy, ammonium, alum, and rose oil are all potential skin irritants.

☹ **Skin Freshener for Normal to Oily Skin** *($15 for 8.4 ounces)* contains mostly alcohol, which can dry and irritate the skin, and is not recommended.

☹ **Skin Freshener for Oily Skin** *($15 for 8.4 ounces)* is similar to the Skin Freshener for Normal to Oily Skin above and the same comments apply; plus this contains lemon extract and menthol, which only add fuel to the fire.

☺ **Stimulating Tonic Spritzer** *($15 for 6.7 ounces)* is just glycerin and water with some fragrant plant extracts. The teeny amounts of water-binding agents are barely worth mentioning.

☺ **Soothing Results Calming Toner for Sensitive Skin** *($15 for 8.4 ounces)* is a good toner for most skin types.

☹ **Soothing Results Day Cream SPF 6 for Sensitive Skin** *($16 for 1.7 ounces)*. Although this does contain titanium dioxide as the active ingredient, the SPF 6 falls painfully short (meaning sun damage–causing short) of the SPF 15 minimum set by the American Academy of Dermatology and the Skin Cancer Foundation, and it is not recommended.

☺ **Soothing Results Night Cream, for Sensitive Skin** *($17.50 for 1.7 ounces)* is a simple, but decent, moisturizer for normal to dry skin with a tiny amount of water-binding agents and a teeny amount of an antioxidant.

☹ **Rediscover Alpha Hydroxy Complex** *($35 for 1 ounce)* contains several fruit extracts, but sugarcane extract and apple extract are not related to AHAs. This moisturizer cannot exfoliate skin, and that is the only real purpose of a well-formulated AHA product. It also lacks any significant water-binding agents or antioxidants.

☹ **Day Cream Moisturizer SPF 6 for Dry to Normal Skin** *($16 for 1.7 ounces)* has an SPF 6, and that's inadequate for daily protection from sun damage, and it doesn't contain the UVA-protecting ingredients of titanium dioxide, zinc oxide, or avobenzone. This is absolutely not recommended.

☹ **Day Cream Moisturizer SPF 6 for Dry Skin** *($16 for 1.7 ounces)* is similar to the SPF 6 for Dry to Normal Skin version above and the same comments apply.

☹ **Day Lotion SPF 6 for Normal to Oily Skin** *($16 for 4.2 ounces)* is similar to the SPF 6 for Dry to Normal Skin version above and the same comments apply.

☹ **Day Lotion SPF 6 for Oily Skin** *($16 for 4.2 ounces)* is similar to the SPF 6 for Dry to Normal Skin version above and the same comments apply.

☺ **Lipid Intense Hydrator SPF 12** *($23 for 1.7 ounces)* is a good, in-part zinc oxide–based sunscreen, but an SPF 15 would be far better for skin. This isn't an intense hydrator, but it is a good moisturizer for normal to dry skin that contains some very good water-binding agents. It does contain fragrance.

☺ **Moisture Manager Hydrator SPF 12** *($16 for 1.7 ounces)* is a good, in-part zinc oxide–based sunscreen, but an SPF 15 would be far better for skin. The rather boring moisturizing base is mostly water and thickeners, making this a less than stellar product all around.

☺ **Moisture Response Hydrator SPF 12** *($19 for 1.7 ounces)* falls short of the essential need for an SPF 15 or greater, plus it does not contain the UVA-protecting ingredients of titanium dioxide, zinc oxide, or avobenzone; it is, therefore, not recommended.

☹ **Oil Control Hydrator SPF 12** *($16 for 1.7 ounces)* is similar to the Moisture Response version above and the same comments apply.

✓☺ $$$ **Time Protector Daily Defense Cream SPF 15** *($38 for 1.7 ounces)* is a very good, in-part zinc oxide–based sunscreen with some good water-binding agents and antioxidants. It would be a very good (though pricey) option for someone with normal to dry skin. It does contain fragrance.

✓☺ $$$ **Time Corrector Firming Moisture Cream** *($38 for 1.7 ounces)* won't correct one minute on your face, or firm anything, but it is a very good moisturizer for dry skin.

☺ **Time Protector Eye Cream** *($21 for 0.5 ounce)* is a good moisturizer for normal to dry skin with small amounts of water-binding agents, antioxidants, and anti-irritants. It does contain fragrance.

☺ $$$ **Time Protector Skin Firming Complex** *($35 for 1 ounce)* is a good, light-weight moisturizer for normal to slightly dry skin that contains an impressive mix of water-binding agents, but it lacks any significant antioxidants or anti-irritants.

☺ **Night Cream for Dry Skin** *($17.50 for 1.7 ounces)* is an OK moisturizer for normal to dry skin that contains tiny amounts of some very good water-binding agents and antioxidants.

☺ **Night Cream Moisturizer for Dry to Normal Skin** *($17.50 for 1.7 ounces)* is similar to the Night Cream for Dry Skin above, but this version contains a better mix and concentration of water-binding agents and antioxidants.

☺ **Night Cream for Normal to Oily Skin** *($17.50 for 1.7 ounces)* is an OK moisturizer for normal to slightly dry skin with a small amount of some good water-binding agents and an even smaller amount of an antioxidant.

☺ **Night Lotion for Oily Skin** *($17.50 for 4.2 ounces)* is an OK moisturizer for someone with normal to dry skin (not normal to oily) that contains some very good water-binding agents.

✓☺ $$$ **Elasticity Recovery Hydrogel** *($35 for 1 ounce)* is a very good moisturizer for normal to dry skin that contains a good combination of water-binding agents and antioxidants.

☺ **Extra Care Cream** *($9.50 for 0.5 ounce)* is just Vaseline, mineral oil, lanolin, wax, soybean oil, and preservatives. This would be an option for someone with very dry skin, but it lacks any state-of-the-art water-binding agents or antioxidants, which would have really made it "extra care."

☺ **Intensive Retinol Treatment** *($40 for 30 capsules)*. Each capsule contains mostly silicones, retinol, fragrance, tiny amounts of vitamins E and C, and film-forming agent. If you are looking for a retinol product this is an option, but it holds no advantage over the versions from L'Oreal or Cetaphil available at the drugstore for far less money.

✓☺ $$$ **Optimeyes Eye Treatment** *($21 for 0.5 ounce)* is a very good moisturizer for normal to slightly dry skin that contains a good mix of antioxidants and water-binding agents. It does contain fragrance.

☺ **Overnight Moisture Recovery Cream** *($25 for 1.7 ounces)* is a very basic, ordinary moisturizer for normal to dry skin. It does contain fragrance.

☹ $$$ **Royal Jelly Milk Balm Moisture Lotion, Original Formula** *($65 for 1 ounce).* You may be wondering why this standard moisturizer sells for $65 an ounce. The answer is royal jelly, which is supposed to be a miracle ingredient. The salesperson told me it could heal burns, eliminate scars, and erase wrinkles. It sure sounds like a miracle. Is it? Well, bee larvae who get fed *fresh* royal jelly turn into queen bees. But if you try to sneak *stored* royal jelly into them, they don't turn into queens. As natural and interesting as all that bee-feeding sounds, there is still no research showing that royal jelly has any miracle benefit for the skin. Several other moisturizers in the Jafra lineup are far more interesting than this one.

☹ $$$ **Royal Jelly Milk Balm Moisture Lotion, Original Unscented** *($65 for 1 ounce)* is similar to the Royal Jelly Original Formula above and the same comments apply.

☹ $$$ **Royal Jelly Milk Balm Moisture Lotion Dry and Normal to Dry** *($65 for 1 ounce)* is an OK moisturizer for normal to dry skin with a small amount of water-binding agents and antioxidants. The price tag is all about the royal jelly, but that gimmick doesn't translate to good skin care.

☹ **Clear Blemish Treatment** *($11 for 0.5 ounce)* contains 2% salicylic acid and has a pH of 3, which is great for effective exfoliation. However, it also contains alcohol, which makes this too irritating and drying for all skin types, and it can hurt the skin's healing process.

☹ **Clear Pore Clarifier** *($16.50 for 1.7 ounces)* has a pH close to 5, which means it isn't low enough for the BHA (salicylic acid) to be an effective exfoliant. This product also contains eucalyptus and clove oils, which are skin irritants.

☺ **Deep Cleansing Mask for Normal to Oily Skin** *($14 for 2.5 ounces)* would be an OK clay mask for someone with normal to oily skin. The teeny amount of tea tree oil isn't enough to make it effective as a topical disinfectant. It does contain fragrance.

☺ **Refreshing Moisture Mask for Dry and Dry to Normal Skin** *($14 for 2.5 ounces)* contains small amounts of clay and talc along with several emollients and small amounts of water-binding agents. It is an option as a mask for normal to dry skin. It does contain fragrance.

☺ $$$ **Soothing Results Cooling Yogurt and Honey Mask, for Sensitive Skin** *($12.50 for 2.6 ounces)* is a clay mask with several plant oils, thickeners, water-binding agents, and anti-irritants. Clay isn't the best thing for sensitive skin, but this could be a good mask for someone with normal to dry skin.

☺ **Cooling Hydration Mask** *($15.50 for 4.4 ounces)* contains mostly film-forming agents, which allow it to be peeled off the face when it dries. Other than that, it lacks any significant amounts of ingredients beneficial for skin.

☺ **Ecko the Gecko Kids Sunblock SPF 35** *($10 for 3.5 ounces)* is a good, in-part avobenzone-based sunscreen in a standard moisturizing base. There is absolutely nothing in this sunscreen that makes it more appropriate for children than for adults.

☹ **Protector Stick SPF 15** *($7 for 0.14 ounce)* does not contain the UVA-protecting ingredients of avobenzone, titanium dioxide, or zinc oxide, and is not recommended.

☹ **Sunscreen Cream SPF 8** *($12.50 for 4.2 ounces)*. While this does contain avobenzone for UVA protection, the SPF 8 falls far below the SPF 15 recommended by the American Academy of Dermatology and the Skin Cancer Foundation. It is not recommended.

☺ **Sunblock Cream SPF 15** *($12.50 for 4.2 ounces)* is a very good, in-part avobenzone-based sunscreen that would be appropriate for normal to slightly dry skin.

☺ **Sunblock Cream SPF 30** *($12 for 4.2 ounces)* is similar to the Sunblock Cream SPF 15 above, only with longer sun protection, and the same basic comments apply.

☺ **Sunless Tanner for Body** *($11.50 for 4.2 ounces)* and **Sunless Tanner for Face** *($10.50 for 1.7 ounces)* both contain dihydroxyacetone, the same ingredient as all self-tanners, to affect the color of skin. These would work as well as any.

JAFRA MAKEUP

Jafra's color collection has a few fairly interesting selections, and the packaging has been given a fairly impressive face-lift. It is still a rather straightforward line, with all the basics and some good options for a wide range of skin tones. The color line is divided into Warm, Cool, and Neutral, which is helpful, except that some of the Neutrals tend to be warm rather than truly neutral. The real challenge with this makeup is finding a Jafra salesperson with enough experience to guide you toward the best colors. The salespeople only receive training on how to sell the products, and the ones I dealt with were clearly uncomfortable recommending shades, not to mention the hit-or-miss prospect of available testers for every color.

<u>FOUNDATION:</u> ☹ **Moisturizing Makeup SPF 6** *($13)* does not offer UVA protection, and even if it did, the SPF 6 is embarrassingly low. This does have a very smooth texture that provides medium coverage, but on the whole the range of 12 shades is too peach, pink, or rose for most skin tones. The only shade to consider is Cashmere, which may work for someone with darker skin. **Oil-Controlling Makeup SPF 6** *($13)* has four fewer shades than the one above, and the same problems with overly peach, pink, or rose colors. The texture is great, but that's no consolation for a lack of neutral, flesh-toned shades and a dismal SPF with inadequate UVA protection.

☺ **Always Color Stay On Makeup SPF 10** *($16)* now lists titanium dioxide as the active sunscreen, but SPF 15 is still the minimum recommended. This lightweight, ultra-matte finish foundation dries quickly and provides semi-opaque coverage. The 20 shades are largely disappointing; the only colors to consider are for darker skin tones, and they include Golden Tan, Warm Ginger, Espresso, Rich Mahogany, and Chestnut.

☺ **Stick Makeup SPF 15** *($15)*. Jafra finally gets the sunscreen right with this in-part zinc oxide foundation. This creamy stick makeup has a minimal powder finish and offers light to medium coverage while blending superbly over the skin. What a shame this only comes in four shades, though three of them are quite good, if a tad peach. Spice is the one shade to avoid.

CONCEALER: ☹ **Cream Concealer** *($10)* comes in stick form and offers six mediocre colors. The dark shades are decidedly more neutral than the lighter tones, which are too peachy pink to look natural. On top of that, the texture makes creasing all too easy. **Total Concealer SPF 12** *($10)* comes in a tube with a wand, and the two shades aren't much better than those for the Cream Concealer above and, therefore, are not the best option for most skin tones. The SPF number is meaningless, as this product does not list any active sunscreen ingredients.

☺ **White Souffle Highlighter** *($9.50)* is a liquid concealer that is indeed white, but it goes on very subtly, requiring just a tiny bit to lighten a shadow under the eye or along the corners of the mouth or nose. It can be used under or over foundation for highlighting without iridescence.

☺ POWDER: **Translucent Face Powder** *($14)* is talc-based and has an incredibly soft and smooth feel. The super-light finish is not as dry as most powders, making it a good choice for normal to dry skin. The seven colors are good, although the lighter shades are slightly peach, so be careful, although the sheer finish can negate that concern. The darkest colors are wonderful. **Pressed Powder** *($14)* is identical to the Translucent Face Powder above in terms of texture, finish, and smooth application. This one features five shades, each with a subtle peach tint that shouldn't be cause for concern.

☺ BLUSH: **Powder Blush** *($12)* has a great soft texture that blends on smoothly and evenly without grabbing or streaking. All of the colors are great, too, but be aware that Bronze and Soft Peach are shiny. There are some good options for darker skin, such as Terra Cotta, Desert, Brownstone, and Copper.

☺ EYESHADOW: Jafra offers **Eyeshadow Duos** *($13)* and **Trios** *($14)* with a texture that is best described as thick and slightly "wet"; almost every shade is shiny, or else the color combinations are too bright or contrasting. There are a handful of surprisingly neutral, workable groups, but most of these have a shine that is too strong for daytime makeup. The only matte combinations to consider are Caravan and Neutral Ground. Color-wise, the best Duos are Cappuccino, Moonshadow, and Portofino, but each features at least one extremely shiny shade, which I'll leave to your taste.

☺ EYE AND BROW SHAPER: **Eye and Brow Pencils** *($8)* are both standard pencils with a creamy application and dry finish. The colors are fine, but for the Eye Pencils, avoid the silver, green, and blue shades. **Liquid Eyeliner** *($10)* has a very thin, soft brush that tends to make the application spotty and more difficult than usual. **Inkwell Eyeliner** *($10)* is a better choice than the Liquid Eyeliner above for liquid liner, and has a brush that is soft but firm enough to get the job done without incident. The only drawback is that it takes some time to dry, so you risk smearing. **Automatic Eyeliner** *($8.50)* is a standard, twist-up, retractable pencil that applies smoothly but stays slightly creamy, so smudging may be an issue. Platinum is deceptively shiny.

☺ <u>LIPSTICK AND LIP PENCIL:</u> **Treatment Lipsticks SPF 15** *($9)* are basic creamy lipsticks with a slightly glossy finish. The color selection is wonderful, but the sunscreen lacks UVA protection. **Always Color Stay-On Lipstick** *($10)* is Jafra's version of Revlon's ColorStay lipstick. This one works quite well, with a soft and opaque ultra-matte finish. The best part is that these tend not to flake or peel off like a lot of ultra-matte lipsticks do. **Lip Lacquer** *($8.50)* is a smooth, slightly sticky lip gloss with some strong, opaque colors. It will last longer than traditional gloss because it has more pigmentation. **Lip Pencil** *($8)* is reasonably priced for a very standard, slightly creamy pencil, and the color selection is plentiful. **Automatic Lip Pencil** *($8.50)* is a creamy, soft, twist-up pencil that glides on, but it won't help keep lipstick in place for long if you're prone to colors bleeding. The six colors are very good.

<u>MASCARA:</u> ☹ **Conditioning Mascara** *($8.50)* and **Volume Building Mascara** *($8.50)* are, at best, mediocre mascaras that never really take lashes beyond average length. Neither provides any thickness, though they do not clump.

☹ **Waterproof Mascara** *($8.50)* builds good length and noticeable thickness though it can feel sticky and heavy when applied. Plus, if this gets even slightly wet, you'll see what a joke the waterproof claim is.

☹ <u>BRUSHES:</u> Jafra's brush sets tend to come and go, but they regularly feature the **Retractable Blush Brush** *($7)*, which would be OK in a pinch, but it's too small and loose to achieve professional results.

JAN MARINI SKIN RESEARCH

Jan Marini Skin Research, Inc., was founded, of course, by Jan Marini, who originally started out marketing products for M.D. Formulations. Thus, it isn't surprising to find that her own line is also aimed at dermatologists and plastic surgeons, much the way M.D. Formulations is. In direct contrast to many of the other skin-care lines reviewed in this book, Marini's line stands out with its selection of far more realistic and varied skin-care products. First, there are no spiraling-out-of-control ingredient listings where everything is thrown in except the kitchen sink. More important, there are some well-formulated products that include sunscreens, an acne formulation, skin-lightening options, and good glycolic acid–based alpha hydroxy acid (AHA) products and beta hydroxy acid (BHA) products. Two additional strong points are that many of the products are fragrance free, while all are free from coloring agents!

For good or bad, there are also some of the current trendy ingredient offerings, ranging from retinol to vitamin C and growth factors, along with a smattering of exotic plant extracts. It is interesting to observe that Marini attributes the research for her "topical form of lipid (fat) soluble Vitamin C that is stable and able to be absorbed" to the form "developed in conjunction with physician researcher Nicholas Perricone, M.D." Now that Perricone has his own version of vitamin C products (quite similar to Marini's, by the way, using ascorbyl palmitate and magnesium ascorbyl palmitate), and given that he claims his are the best ever with the highest concentration of the stuff, I wonder if she would now agree with his findings? Does that mean we should all buy Perricone's products? Or do they both get rid of wrinkles and Perricone is wrong about the superiority of his products? Stay tuned as the saga of the cosmetics and vitamin C wars continues.

As I discussed earlier in this book, there is no conclusive research about vitamin C eliminating even one wrinkle on the skin, something Perricone concludes in his own writings. I've also discussed at length the limited research (and thus my resulting skepticism) about the value of vitamin A (retinol) cosmetics products on the skin. If you still want in on either vitamin C or vitamin A, this line definitely has some pricey versions to consider. Ironically, the claims made by the world of cosmetics for vitamin C and vitamin A are almost identical. So once again you have to wonder, if vitamin C gets rid of wrinkles, why would you need vitamin A? It never fails to amaze me that women still have wrinkles with all these antiaging products!

Marini uses "growth factor" in a group of products called "Transformation." The actual ingredient is transforming growth factor (TGF beta-1), which is a complex protein known to bring about changes in connective tissue. TGF is a human growth factor responsible primarily for wound healing. It stimulates collagen production, or, a far better description, according to Dr. Bruce A. Mast, M.D., Division of Plastic and Reconstructive Surgery, Department of Surgery, University of Florida, Gainesville, would be that TGF beta-1 "is a proscarring component of healing." Mast explained that in order for a wound to heal, the body has to be able to create scar material, or collagen, for skin. But that kind of collagen production is not related to the skin's intrinsic support structure. Mast's concern in regard to TGF beta-1 in skin-care products is that if it really worked, it could encourage scar formation on the surface of the skin, and that doesn't improve the appearance of wrinkles.

For the most part, Marini's professional information packet is exceptional, offering a wealth of accurately stated facts about skin care and the effect products have on the skin. The information about vitamin A, vitamin C, and the growth factors is overblown, but it is nevertheless in essence accurate. For example, one of the information sheets for the Marini line explains that "approximately 90% to 95% of what we think is inevitable aging is the result of cumulative sun damage. Most of this damage is programmed into the skin in childhood, but it takes many years to manifest itself." No one argues with this fact. It then goes on to say that most of that damage is reversible by using these products. Wouldn't that be nice! But then it would also be true for other products on the market that contain similar, if not identical, formulations, in all price ranges.

For more information about the availability of Jan Marini Skin Research products, call (408) 362-0130 or (800) 347-2223, or visit www.jmskinresearch.com.

JAN MARINI AGE INTERVENTION

It is somehow ironic that the two Age Intervention products would boast that none of them contain "AHA. Not Vitamin C. Not Vitamin A. [And these are] a dramatic new concept in antiaging technology created especially for a woman's facial skin." Ironic be-

The Reviews J

cause several of Marini's other products do contain AHA and vitamins C and A, which makes it hard to see why the line continues to sell them if those aren't the answer for a woman's skin. What these two products contain that is different from the other products in Marini's line is pregnenolone acetate, progesterone, and estradiol. This is the first cosmetic product I've seen that contains estradiol. However, the other two ingredients are not unique to Marini's line. Actually, Revlon sold products for years that contained pregnenolone acetate, and there are many products that contain progesterone.

Pregnenolone acetate is a precursor (trigger to create) to other hormones; it can affect levels of progesterone and estrogen in the body when taken orally. When applied to skin, it may work as a water-binding agent, but there is no information on whether it can be absorbed through skin, and there is no research showing it can change skin.

Concerning progesterone, a study published in the *American Journal of Obstetrics and Gynecology* (June 1999, pages 1504–1511) states that "In order to obtain the proper (effective) serum levels with use of a progesterone cream, the cream needs to have an adequate amount of progesterone in it [at least 30 milligrams per gram]. Many over the counter creams have little [for example, 5 milligrams per ounce] or none at all." Marini does not provide information about how much progesterone her products contain.

Estradiol is definitely unique to Marini products. The body produces three main forms of estrogen—estrone, estradiol, and estriol—and estradiol is the most physiologically active form. Decreased production of estrogen by the ovaries can lead to symptoms such as hot flashes, night sweats, vaginal dryness, urinary tract infections, depression, and irritability. Estrogen replacement can help relieve these symptoms. Although estrogen offers many benefits, it is not indicated for everyone and women should evaluate their individual risks versus benefits with their physician or health-care provider. Whether or not natural estrogens are safe has not been well-researched and the FDA considers the claims and safety of cosmetics containing them to not be proven.

Marini's information about her Age Intervention products states that they contain interferon, although that ingredient does not show up on the list of ingredients. Interferon is an immune modulator used to treat varying diseases, ranging from warts to cancer. The product information for the Age Intervention products states that "Some researchers believe topically applied interferon may significantly reduce the appearance of fine lines and wrinkles associated with cumulative sun damage. It is speculated that interferon appears to have a substantial repair mechanism on compromised cells, enabling them to perform in a younger and healthier manner." If any of that is true, Marini doesn't support those contentions with documented studies or published research of any kind, and there is none to be found elsewhere.

Applying hormones topically to skin is something I strongly suggest should not be taken lightly. These are not benign cosmetic ingredients, and there is limited research establishing either benefits or risks. The same can be said for interferon. To sum up, aside from the serious nature of these other ingredients, $$$ **Age Intervention Face Cream**

($75 for 1 ounce) and $$$ **Age Intervention Face Serum** *($75 for 1 ounce)* are good emollient moisturizers for dry skin that contain a good mix of water-binding agents and antioxidants. It's the hormones and interferon that I'm concerned about, and they are of concern because the risks for long-term use are not known.

JAN MARINI ANTIOXIDANT GROUP

☺ $$$ **Antioxidant Group Skin Silk Protecting Hydrator** *($40 for 1 ounce)* is an interesting name for a product that doesn't contain any significant amounts of antioxidants. This is an emollient moisturizer for normal to dry skin that contains some good emollients and water-binding agents, but the antioxidants are all but absent. It does contain a small amount of arnica, but probably not enough to be a problem for skin.

☺ $$$ **Antioxidant Group Recover-E** *($40 for 1 ounce)* is a lightweight gel that contains a good mix of antioxidants and water-binding agents. For the money, though, this isn't quite the impressive formulation of antioxidants you may be counting on.

☹ **Antioxidant Group Body Block SPF 30** *($25 for 4 ounces)* doesn't contain the UVA-protecting ingredients of titanium dioxide, zinc oxide, or avobenzone, and is not recommended.

☹ **Antioxidant Group Daily Face Protectant SPF 30** *($45 for 2 ounces)* doesn't contain the UVA-protecting ingredients of titanium dioxide, zinc oxide, or avobenzone, and is not recommended.

JAN MARINI BENZOYL PEROXIDE GROUP

☹ **Benzoyl Peroxide Wash 2.5%** *($25 for 8 ounces)* is a cleanser, and because a cleanser is washed away, the benzoyl peroxide (the effective ingredient), which should stay on the skin to work, would be rinsed down the drain. For most skin types, any of the following three benzoyl peroxide products would be a far better consideration.

✓☺ **Benzoyl Peroxide 2.5%** *($25 for 4 ounces)* is a reliable topical disinfectant to use for fighting breakouts, but there are similar, if not identical, versions available for far less.

✓☺ **Benzoyl Peroxide 5%** *($25 for 4 ounces)* is similar to the 2.5% version above, just a more potent concentration.

✓☺ **Benzoyl Peroxide 10%** *($25 for 4 ounces)* is similar to the 5% version above, only in a more potent concentration.

JAN MARINI BIOGLYCOLIC GROUP

☺ **Bioglycolic BioClean Cleanser** *($25 for 8 ounces)* is a standard, detergent-based, water-soluble cleanser that would work well for most skin types.

☺ **Bioglycolic Facial Cleanser** *($25 for 8 ounces)* is a standard, detergent-based, water-soluble cleanser that includes AHA. While AHAs are great for exfoliating, their effectiveness as an exfoliant in this product would be rinsed down the drain, and it would be problematic if it got into the eyes on the way. Thankfully, the pH of this product is too high for it to be effective as an exfoliant, and so it doesn't pose much risk.

The Reviews J

☺ **Bioglycolic Oily Skin Cleansing Gel** *($25 for 8 ounces)* is similar to the Facial Cleanser above except that it contains a higher concentration of detergent cleansing agents. The same basic comments apply.

☺ $$$ **Bioglycolic Cream** *($60 for 2 ounces)*. This is a well-formulated AHA moisturizer that would be good for normal to dry skin. It does contain sodium hyaluronate, but that is just one of many good water-binding agents for skin and doesn't make this a superlative formulation. Among AHA products, there are many far less expensive options to consider, particularly from Alpha Hydrox, at the drugstore.

✓☺ $$$ **Bioglycolic Facial Lotion** *($45 for 2 ounces)* is similar to the Cream above only in lotion form. The same basic comments apply.

☺ $$$ **Bioglycolic Facial Lotion SPF 15** *($45 for 2 ounces)* is a good, titanium dioxide–based sunscreen for someone with normal to slightly dry skin. It has about an 8% to 10% AHA content (glycolic acid); however, the pH of 4 to 5 makes it minimally effective for exfoliation. Using an expensive sunscreen can also be problematic because, as is true for all sunscreens, a liberal application is essential to receive the SPF number on the label, and expensive ones tend to make users reluctant when it comes to applying sunscreen generously. There is nothing about this formulation worth the price tag.

☺ $$$ **Bioglycolic Eye Cream** *($33 for 0.5 ounce)*. The pH of 4.5 to 5 is too high for this AHA product to be effective as an exfoliant. The moisturizing base is lackluster, with only minimal water-binding agents and no antioxidants.

☺ **Bioglycolic Lightening Gel** *($35 for 2 ounces)* includes AHA, although the pH is too high for that ingredient to be effective as an exfoliant. This product also contains kojic acid, which has some effect in reducing melanin production, but it is considered unstable and a potentially irritating ingredient.

☺ $$$ **Bioglycolic BioClear** *($50 for 1 ounce)* contains about 8% to 10% AHA and about 1% BHA in a fairly basic, lightweight moisturizing formula. It would work well for exfoliation for someone with normal to dry skin. Generally, though, the combination of AHA and BHA isn't the best option. BHA can exfoliate both in the pore and on the surface of skin, so it isn't necessary to have the AHA, which only affects the surface. Given that BHA can cover both territories, using it alone is the best way to reduce the risk of irritation. This also contains azelaic acid (a component of grains such as wheat, rye, and barley), which has been shown to be effective for a number of skin conditions when applied topically in a cream formulation at a 20% concentration (Source: *International Journal of Dermatology*, December 1991, pages 893–895). However, other research suggests that azelaic acid is more irritating than hydroquinone mixed with glycolic acid or kojic acid (Source: *eMedicine Journal*, www.emedicine.com, November 5, 2001, volume 2, number 11). Regardless, this product contains far less than 20% azelaic acid, so it is hard to say what, if any, effect it would have on skin.

☹ **Bioglycolic Acne Gel I** *($35 for 2 ounces)* contains a mixture of AHA and BHA, but alcohol is the first ingredient in this product, and that can cause dryness and irritation, making breakouts worse.

☹ **Bioglycolic Acne Gel II** *($35 for 2 ounces)* is almost identical to the Acne Gel I above and the same comments apply.

☺ **Bioglycolic Sunless Self Tanner** *($25 for 4 ounces)* is a standard, dihydroxyacetone-based self-tanner, and although this product contains AHA, it has a high pH that makes it ineffective as an exfoliant. Actually that is preferred, because otherwise you would simply be exfoliating away the tan you just applied.

JAN MARINI C-ESTA GROUP

☺ $$$ **C-Esta Cleansing Gel** *($25 for 6 ounces)* is a standard, detergent-based, water-soluble cleanser. For the money, if you want vitamin C on your skin it would be better to get it in a form that stays on the skin rather than in a cleanser that you rinse down the drain, though this product doesn't contain much vitamin C anyway.

✓☺ $$$ **C-Esta Cream** *($75 for 1 ounce)* contains a good amount of vitamin C in the form of ascorbyl palmitate in a rather standard emollient moisturizer for normal to dry skin. It also contains some good water-binding agents and a small amount of other antioxidants. If you are looking for vitamin C this is fine, though overpriced for what you get, especially considering that vitamin C in any form is not a panacea for skin care. Obviously that's something Marini agrees with as well, because not all of her products contain vitamin C.

✓☺ $$$ **C-Esta Eye Contour Cream** *($40 for 0.5 ounce)* is similar to the C-Esta Cream above, though it doesn't contain as much vitamin C. The same basic comments apply.

✓☺ $$$ **C-Esta Eye Repair Concentrate** *($55 for 0.5 ounce)* is similar to the C-Esta products above, only in a gel-like lotion, and it's better for normal to slightly dry skin. The same basic comments apply.

✓☺ $$$ **C-Esta Serum** *($75 for 1 ounce)* is a lightweight lotion that contains a good amount of water-binding agents as well as vitamin C, but other than its texture it does not differ significantly from the other C-Esta products. It is an option for normal to slightly dry skin.

☺ $$$ **C-Esta Facial Mask** *($50 for 2 ounces)* contains an impressive mix of water-binding agents, anti-irritants, and a small amount of antioxidants. It will feel good as a mask but offers no benefit over and above the other C-Esta products.

☺ $$$ **C-Esta Lips** *($40 for 0.5 ounce)* assumes that none of the other C-Esta products can be used around the mouth, so now you have one just for the lips. But it's similar to the C-Esta products above for skin, and the same comments apply. This version does contain fragrance.

JAN MARINI FACTOR-A GROUP

☺ $$$ **Factor-A Cream** *($45 for 1 ounce)* is a good consideration for a product containing retinol, though there are far less expensive options available. This version does contain a good mix of water-binding agents and a small amount of additional antioxi-

The Reviews J

dants. A few of the plant extracts are skin irritants, but they are present in such small amounts that they are not of much concern for skin.

☺ $$$ Factor-A Plus Cream *($45 for 1 ounce)* would have been a good option if you were looking for a combination of vitamin A and AHA, but the pH is too high to make this an effective exfoliant.

☹ Factor-A Plus Lotion *($40 for 1 ounce)* contains alcohol as the second ingredient, which can be a problem for skin.

☺ $$$ Factor-A Lotion *($40 for 1 ounce)* is a lightweight lotion that contains some good water-binding agents and, of course, retinol. This is an option for normal to slightly dry skin.

JAN MARINI TRANSFORMATION

☺ $$$ Transformation Cream *($60 for 1 ounce)*. The big-deal ingredient in this product is transforming growth factor (TGF beta-1). As described above, the claims for what this ingredient can do are at best exaggerated, and its effectiveness is not established in skin-care products. This also contains some good water-binding agents and a small amount of antioxidants. It does contain fragrance.

☺ $$$ Transformation Eye Cream *($40 for 0.5 ounce)*. Like the Cream above, this version also contains TGF beta-1, and the same comments apply. This one also contains sugarcane extract, but that is not an AHA, nor is the pH appropriate for exfoliation. This version does contain a more impressive mix of water-binding agents and antioxidants. It would receive a happy face except for the unknown risk of the TGF ingredient, which makes it too uncertain to recommend.

☺ $$$ Transformation Serum *($50 for 1 ounce)* is similar to the Eye Cream above, only this version is lighter in weight and contains some potentially irritating plant extracts.

JAN MARINI PROTEOLYTIC ENZYMES

☺ $$$ Clean Zyme Papaya Cleanser *($20 for 4 ounces)*. Despite all the fancy words about how papaya (a source of the enzyme papain) works, there is no research showing it to have exfoliating properties on skin, and definitely none showing it to be preferred over AHAs or BHA.

☺ $$$ Day Zyme *($40 for 1 ounce)* is similar to the Papaya Cleanser version above, only in a slightly thicker form for someone with normal to slightly dry skin.

☺ $$$ Night Zyme *($40 for 1 ounce)* is similar to the Day Zyme above, only with slightly more emollient. It would be an option for someone with normal to dry skin.

☺ Skin Zyme *($35 for 2 ounces)* is almost identical to the Night Zyme above, and the same comments apply.

JANE (MAKEUP ONLY)

Jane, under the ownership of parent company Estee Lauder (it was purchased by Lauder in 1997), is still going strong as a drugstore cosmetics line aimed at young girls.

The Reviews J

What does it mean to be a teen? In Jane's lexicon, being a teen is all about experimenting with makeup while discovering the "real you." According to their Web site, "…whether your eyes are blue or brown or your hair is blonde or bright green, whether you've got a bazillion freckles or what seems like a gigunda nose, there's something interesting (pretty) about you. That's why we say THERE'S NO SUCH THING AS A PLAIN JANE." Naturally, for all of the impressionable young girls out there, Jane has a bevy of products that promise to help them stand out from the crowd. Jane maintains that "feeling good about yourself is way sexy," but the underlying implication is clearly that feeling good about yourself requires makeup. The feeling sexy part is somewhat disturbing, especially since pre-teens are regularly seen clustered around Jane's cosmetics, and these very same young girls are at an age where their self-esteem is extremely fragile and vulnerable. In today's social climate, teens are maturing faster than ever, and I can't help but wonder how much cosmetics companies like Jane have encouraged this through their ad copy and fun-loving, empowerment-masked-as-cosmetic-adornment philosophy.

The last couple of years have seen the launch of several new Jane makeup products and the disappearance of just as many, such as all of the concealers, the original mascaras, and some of the inexpensive gems that gave similar department-store products a run for their money. Perhaps most obvious is that Jane's makeup products are individually packaged and their in-store display units have been simplified. The makeup selection is now heavily centered on all manner of lipsticks and glosses, with the choices rivaling gloss-centric lines like Bonne Bell.

Although Jane's teen appeal is obvious, the simple packaging, neutral colors, and vivid, creamy lipstick colors are more in alignment with what adults would be interested in. However, the prices are more than reasonable and many of the colors are appropriate for a wide range of skin tones. What is certainly aimed at pre-teens and teenagers are Jane's flavored lip products that taste like vanilla, butterscotch, pineapple, peach, cinnamon, and several others. It's almost an unwritten rite of passage that a girl's first experiences with lipsticks or glosses involves choosing what taste she wants as she licks her lips, as opposed to what color or finish is most flattering. It amounts to choosing makeup based on novelty instead of practical allure, and that's not necessarily the best way to discover yourself. For more information about Jane, visit www.janecosmetics.com.

☺ **FOUNDATION:** Jane's foundation formulas do not have any colors suitable for darker skin tones, so this is clearly a line aimed at fairer-skinned youth and definitely not African-Americans. **Oil Free Foundation** *($3.47)* features six mostly neutral shades and a soft matte finish. The formula has apparently been tweaked for the better, as my past complaints about this blending on in a choppy fashion no longer apply. The only shade to watch out for is Soft Beige, which is too rose for most light skin tones. **Stay Calm Face Makeup SPF 8** *($4.99).* Whether or not your face is or isn't calm, which this makeup won't change one iota, this foundation has a fluid, silky texture that melts into skin for a beautiful, long-wearing, soft matte finish. The sunscreen is without adequate UVA protection and the SPF 8 is simply infuriating, as it gives the teenagers this line is aimed at an introduction to skin health that could be detrimental to them in the long run. However, that doesn't mean this isn't a foundation to consider for anyone of any age if you have a fair to light complexion and normal to oily skin and you're willing to wear a separate sunscreen underneath! There are six shades altogether, but the following three are embarrassingly peach and inappropriate for all skin tones: Dream Cream, Open Sesame, and Sunny Honey.

☺ **POWDER:** **Oil-Free Finishing Powder** *($3.47)* is a talc-based pressed powder with a soft, silky-dry texture that applies sheer and even, and three colors that are decidedly peach-toned. Lighter skin tones may want to try Colorless or Fair, but should still be cautious. **Staying Powder Loose Powder** *($3.47)* is a very good, dry-finish, exceedingly standard talc-based powder, that would be best for someone with oily skin. The colors (three in all) are a bit too orange or peach to satisfy anyone hoping for truly neutral colors. **True to You Sheer Finish Powder** *($3.47)* is identical to the Staying Powder in all regards except that this one offers a tiny bit less coverage. **Radiation All-Over Glimmer** *($2.84)* is simply loose, iridescent powder in both flesh-toned and vivid shades. If you want to perpetuate the shine trend, this is a cheap way to go about it.

☺ **BLUSH:** **Blushing Cheeks** *($3.22)* all have a soft, smooth texture and go on quite sheer. The color range is impressive, and although a few of the colors have noticeable shine, the majority are matte. These would be excellent for very light to medium skin tones.

EYESHADOW: ☺ **Eye Zing Shadow** *($2.99)* is a collection of powder eyeshadows that have a soft, easy-to-blend texture. Many of the shades are shiny, so choose carefully (if you have lines, these will make them more apparent), and you're bound to be pleased with both performance and price! **Fabulizer for Eyes** *($3.99)* is a cream-to-powder eyeshadow in a pen dispenser that feeds the product onto an angled sponge tip. The packaging is very cool, but the sheer pastel, shimmery colors are unflattering.

☹ **Iced Shadow** *($2.84)* is a water-based, loose-powder eyeshadow that does feel wet and cooling as it is applied, but the color tends to grab on the skin, does not blend easily or evenly, and tends to flake off. Adding another element to this messy contrivance are the colors, which are all glaringly shiny. **Glimmeratzi Sheer Color Eye Gloss** *($3.49)* are slick, glitter-infused eyeshadows that leave a slightly sticky finish. When is this glossy eye look going to be over? Are women just looking for a makeup challenge? Apparently so, since products like this keep popping up.

☺ **EYE AND BROW SHAPER:** The fairly standard **Gliding Eye Pencil** and **One Liners Eye Pencil** (automatic pencils) *($2.99 each)* go on well without being greasy, dragging, or looking choppy. They would be an option for anyone, regardless of age. If you prefer using pencils to matte powder eyeshadows, these are as good as any you'll find. **Going Steady Eye Definer Pencil** *($2.84)* is just a standard pencil with a cream-to-powder texture and a sheer, iridescent finish. It works as well as much more costly versions, and is worth considering if shiny pencils are what you're after. **Fan Club Lash & Brow**

Mascara *($3.22)* is a lightweight, clear brow gel that also works to add very subtle definition to the lashes. It does not contain film-forming agents, so it's non-sticky, but it is not the best choice if you have unruly brows that need to be held in place.

LIPSTICK AND LIP PENCIL: Jane must know that teenagers can't help but buy lipsticks and glosses, because there are an astounding number of options for lips from this otherwise small line of products. ☺ **Lip Huggers Satin Lipstick** *($2.84)* may be too creamy and opaque for teens and too glossy and slippery for adults. The colors are fine, but this is one slippery, glossy lipstick. **Barely Lips Sheer Lipstick** *($2.84)* is right up a teen's alley and may work for adults looking for an emollient, glossy lipstick with only a hint of color. **Hip Lips Lipstick** *($2.84)* has a creamy, smooth texture and a fair amount of stain. There are only a few shades, but these are worth a look, and the Pez-style dispenser is truly unique and fun. **Quik Stix** *($2.84)* are the traditional chubby lip pencils that seem like a good idea at first, but end up being just a slightly greasy lipstick you have to sharpen. At this low price, however, that may not be such a bad trade-off! **One Liners Lip Liners** *($2.84)* are automatic, retractable lip pencils that have a smooth texture and a great color selection. **Double Talk Smoochable Lip Color** *($4.99)* is Jane's take on Max Factor's Lipfinity. This two-part product contains a base lip color that goes on easily and with less intense color saturation than you might expect. You're supposed to give the base color two minutes to dry, then you can apply a glossifying top coat—which you will need, as the base color gets very dry and tight on its own. Unlike Lipfinity, the color is not transfer resistant—you'll still see lip prints on coffee cups or anyone you smooch and it is easy to remove.

☺ **MegaBites Flavorful Lip Color** *($2.84)* are standard creamy lipsticks that are either fruit-, drink-, or dessert-flavored, and the taste may seem inviting or repulsive, depending on your mood. ☺ **MegaBites Mega Lip Shimmer** *($3.49)* is another assortment of flavored lipsticks (Jalapeno Grape, anyone?) that have a slick, light application and glossy, soft iridescent finish. This easily creeps beyond the lip line even if you don't have lines around your mouth, but I don't think the target audience for this lipstick is too concerned with longwearing, stay-in-place colors. **LipKick Energizing Liquid Lipstick** *($2.84)* is an intensely flavored sheer lipstick that you apply with a wand. These are more akin to lip gloss than lipstick. **Lickety Stix Lip Gloss** *($2.84)* are two flavored, Chap Stick–style lip balms with a slight tint. If you like the idea of tasty lipsticks, that's one issue; the other is that ingesting any large amount of lipstick is not a good idea, and these kinds of products encourage young girls to do just that. **Shine Language Lip Gloss** *($2.84)* is a semi-sheer emollient pot gloss that keeps lips moist and wet-looking while providing a hit of teen-appeal flavor. **Megabites Glossy Gloss** *($2.84)* and **Megaswirls Lip Gloss** *($2.84)* offer even more flavored gloss options, with slightly thick textures and the requisite shiny, wet finish. **Fabulizer for Lips** *($2.99)* are only fabulous if you define that word as glittery, sheer lip color that comes in an assortment of food flavors. I think "frivolous" is a more fitting term!

☹ **WeatherWear Lipstick SPF 15** *($3.49)* is a small collection of standard creamy lipsticks that have more of a waxy feel than many others. Sadly, the sunscreen does not provide adequate UVA protection, and the small amount of peppermint extract can be a problem for the lips and offers no significant benefit. Revlon, Cover Girl, and Almay all have better lipstick with sunscreen options.

MASCARA: ✓☺ **Fan Club Curling Mascara** *($3.22)* applies smoothly and easily builds noticeable length and lift, with minimal thickness. It is a pleasure to use, does not clump or flake, and lasts all day—a winner for lengthening and defining! ✓☺ **Fan Club Waterproof Mascara** *($3.22)* shares all of the same traits as the Fan Club Curling Mascara above and holds up very well in the waterproofing department. And at this price, this should definitely be considered before most other waterproof choices, as the performance matches the best of them.

☺ **BRUSHES:** Jane's brushes aren't awful, they are just the wrong shape and tend to have a poor consistency. The eyeshadow brushes are too small and thin, while the powder and blush brushes are soft enough but aren't the best sizes and don't have the best density of bristles for proper application. The prices are rock bottom, but the performance is not impressive.

☺ **SPECIALTY:** **Glimmeratzi Glitter Gel** *($2.84)* is a sheer, water-based gel infused with lots of sparkles. These brightly packaged tubes are bound to catch a teen's eye (and many young women's, too), and they are a great, inexpensive way to add glaring glitz to your skin.

JANE IREDALE (MAKEUP ONLY)

Jane Iredale's color line is advertised as "The Skin Care Makeup," but it isn't skin-care-like in the least. Ingredients like bismuth oxychloride, mica, and iron oxides have no benefit for skin, and they are the primary ingredients of Iredale's powders. A few of the products do include excellent sunscreens along with a smattering of antioxidants, and the ingredient lists are relatively short (which is beneficial for those with sensitivities), but that's about as skin-caring as this line gets. Marketing sound bites aside, there are some very good products to consider, especially if you prefer the look of a powder foundation over traditional liquids, creams, or cream-to-powders. When it comes to foundation colors, this line has some truly exceptional choices for all skin tones.

Regrettably, many of the claims surrounding the products walk the line between fact and fiction, with a clear preference for the mild scare tactics used by other lines with a "natural" angle. For example, Iredale's Web site states, "Many lip products, especially glosses and balms, contain petroleum products. Petroleum draws oil out of the lips and, therefore, causes them to dry and chap." That is entirely untrue. Not only is petroleum as such not in any lip products (only its purified hydrocarbon derivative, petrolatum [Vaseline] is), but also lips do not have oil glands (a fact also mentioned on Iredale's site)—so how can any topical ingredient draw oil *out* of the lips? It can't.

Here's another debatable claim: "Because our bases are concentrated pigment, the coverage we can achieve is far superior to normal makeup with a minimum amount of product. This is why mineral makeup should always look sheer and natural." These powders can be applied sheer, but the very nature of their ingredients results in a heavy-textured product that, like it or not, does look powdery and "made-up" on the skin. This is especially true if you have any dry patches on the skin, because these mineral powders, which also claim to "trap moisture," will exacerbate any dryness and can look caked and change color over very oily areas. Actually, they do trap moisture, but they trap it away from the skin. That's the nature of any powdered mineral, they are extremely absorbent and drying. Iredale denigrates talc, dismissing it as cheap filler material, but talc serves as the essential backbone for a number of the most luxurious-feeling powders you will find, some of which have a softness and virtually seamless finish on the skin that other lines (including Iredale's) should envy.

Still, if the concept of a type of powdered makeup that is different from the traditional talc-based powders you've seen at the cosmetics counters or drugstores appeals to you, then this line presents some fine choices. I recommend using caution when you read (or are told) about the inflated benefits of some rather ordinary, but nevertheless effective, ingredients, but there is certainly nothing in these straightforward formulations that's harmful or irritating, and that's always beneficial. For more information about Jane Iredale, call (800) 817-5665 or visit www.janeiredale.com.

☺ $$$ <u>FOUNDATION:</u> **Amazing Base Loose Mineral Powder Base SPF 20** *($42)* lists titanium dioxide and zinc oxide as its active sunscreen ingredients and these same ingredients also contribute to the powder's opacity, cling, and long-wearing capabilities. This loose powder foundation is talc-free and has a very smooth texture and a dry finish that tends to get drier in feel and appearance the longer it is worn. Use it dry, or mix it with a moisturizer to approximate a liquid foundation or to allow for easier application over drier skin (keep in mind that this will diminish the powder's sunscreen properties). Either method can be messy, which is true for any loose powder application, and that's a definite drawback. Amazing Base provides medium to full coverage and is not as natural-looking as the brochure claims. The smooth, dry texture and comparatively lighter finish (though this still looks like powder makeup) with a faint bit of shine is preferable to the loose mineral foundations from Youngblood, philosophy, and bare escentuals. Iredale's ten shades are mostly neutral but some go on a bit darker than they appear. The only shade to be careful of, due to its slight peach-rose tone, is Honey Bronze. There are no colors in this version for darker skin tones. **PurePressed Base SPF 17** *($48)* is a pressed-powder version of the Amazing Base and this one is more matte and not as thick, so oilier skin will be less likely to experience a heavy, caked look once the skin's oil and the powders mix. The sunscreen is pure titanium dioxide and zinc oxide. The same basic comments made for the Amazing Base apply here as well; however, this offers a considerably more tidy application and a much broader range of shades, including some exemplary options

The Reviews J

586 Don't Go to the Cosmetics Counter Without Me

for darker skin tones called **Global Shades.** These are richly pigmented and as a result do not look as ash or gray on deeper skin tones as many other powders can. Of the 18 shades, the only ones to consider avoiding are Natural, Honey Bronze, and Teakwood. The vast majority of skin-true shades here are gorgeous.

<u>CONCEALER:</u> ☹ **Circle/Delete** *($29)* comes in a pot with two colors; one is lighter and the other is a medium tone. The texture is quite thick and creamy, and you will get opaque coverage. This will definitely crease, and applying one of the mineral powders over it tends to look heavy and obvious. Over and above that, the three duos have colors that are mostly a far cry from real skin tones.

☺ $$$ **CoverCare** *($20)* is a full-coverage, matte-finish concealer with a dry texture that can make it difficult to blend on evenly. The consistency is actually semi-solid, and when it's squeezed out of the tube (which takes some effort), it tends to come out (and fall off) in chunks. If you have the patience to use this and can apply it quickly, it can be an option. It is unlikely it will crease, although the dry, somewhat powdery finish will accentuate any prominent lines around the eyes. All three available colors are neutral, and would work quite well over blemishes or red discolorations.

☺ $$$ <u>POWDER:</u> **Pure Matte Finish** *($33)* feels matte and has a light, dry texture oily skin will love, but it contains more shine than both of the Base powders above. There is one shade, and it's suitably neutral, though limited to light skin. The rice starch is not an ideal ingredient to use over blemishes. **24-Karat Gold Dust** *($34)* is simply mica, iron oxides, and real gold flakes. Combined, they make this simply a shiny loose powder whose glistening effect works nicely for evening glamour. The price is steep considering the wealth of shiny powders available at the drugstore.

☺ $$$ <u>BLUSH:</u> **PurePressed Blush** *($26)* has a silky texture that goes on exceedingly smoothly. The color range is impressive for a niche line, with equally good options for light and dark skin tones.

☺ $$$ <u>EYESHADOW:</u> **PurePressed Eyeshadows** *($17.50)* are sold as singles and have a silky texture that is slightly drier than the PurePressed Blush. There are some worthwhile matte shades that go on sheer, blend well, and stay put; the shiny shades are clearly marked as shimmer or pearlescent, so you can pick and choose accordingly. **Duo Eye Shadows** *($27)* offer some attractive pairings, including three matte duos that should appeal to anyone seeking an understated yet defined look. Avoid Dusky Blue/Charcoal.

<u>EYE AND BROW SHAPER:</u> ☺ **Eye Pencils** *($9)* are creamy, run-of-the-mill pencils that apply well, but smudge easily.

✓☺ $$$ **PureBrow Colour** *($20)* is a tinted brow mascara that is a breeze to apply and that ably enhances the brows with five superior shades. It does not get sticky or make brows look greasy or too thick, and though the price is high, this is an easy recommendation. ✓☺ $$$ **PureBrow Fix** *($20)* is a standard, PVP-based clear brow gel that will work as well as the one from Cover Girl, which sells for under $5. The only advantage this has are the two brushes that come with it, though most will find one end preferable.

LIPSTICK AND LIP PENCIL: ☺ **$$$** PureMoist LipColours *($17)* are standard, but very good, creamy lipsticks that have a slightly glossy finish and medium coverage. **PureMoist LipSheres** *($17)* are sheer lipsticks that have less pigment than the LipColours above, so count on minimal staying power, as with most sheer lipsticks. **PureGloss for Lips** *($14.50)* is a lightweight, emollient gloss that's non-sticky and comes in a nice range of shades. This does contain a tiny amount of tangerine peel oil and ginger, and both can be lip (and skin) irritants.

☹ **Lip Pencils** *($9)* have a creamy texture and great colors, but are otherwise quite boring, and they need regular sharpening.

☹ **$$$ MASCARA:** PureLash Lengthening Mascara *($16)* builds moderate length with a very clean, clump-free application. Thickness is scarce, and this isn't what I would call dramatic mascara, but it does the job and stays on all day. **PureLash Mascara** *($16)* offers decent, but unimpressive, length with a soft curl. This doesn't thicken lashes in the least, but wears well and removes easily.

☺ **BRUSHES:** The brushes available are mostly excellent, and the ones to consider for their workable shapes and soft, but firm, feel are the **Chisel Powder** *($24.50)*, **Eye Shader** *($9)*, and **Eye Contour** *($9.50)*; **Dual Eye Liner/Brow** *($12)* and **Camouflage** *($15)* are options as well, and both are synthetic. The **Handi Brush** *($39)*, which is recommended for applying Jane Iredale's powder bases, is cut straight across and applies the powder much like a sponge would, and may be worth a test to see how you like the results. The **Sable Lip Brush** *($15)* is OK but does not include a cap, while the **White Fan Blush** *($12)* has little practical purpose and is easily replaced by other brushes.

JASON NATURAL (SKIN CARE ONLY)

As the name implies, Jason Natural is about—surprise!—"natural" ingredients. According to their brochure, "We believe consumers must have a reliable natural alternative to chemically synthesized, technical grade products, and to that end we are devoted to developing and manufacturing a wide range of personal care and beauty care products that are truly botanical in origin." While there are natural ingredients in these products, there are also lots of synthetic ones, including laureth sulfosuccinate, lauramide DEA, cocamidopropyl betaine, triethanolamine, formaldehyde releasing preservatives, and artificial coloring agents.

This line also wants you to know that its information dates back to the ancient Egyptians and that much of their "knowledge of the healing power of herbs and their special effects on the skin was gathered into books during medieval times." Is there really anything from ancient Egypt or medieval Europe that would be of interest to us today? After all, they didn't have sunscreens, they didn't have antibiotics, and they had no knowledge of antioxidants. While the notion of ancient folklore is romantic, it is nonsense when it comes to the health of your skin.

Still, there are some good, and even great, products in this line, particularly moisturizers containing all the antioxidants you could ever want. For a line with great prices, that's really impressive. Given the price point, I would consider a closer look. But ignore the claims—even Jason Natural cosmetics can't keep its own ingredients and claims straight. For more information about Jason Natural, call 1-800-JASON-05 or visit www.jason-natural.com. **Note:** All Jason Natural products contain fragrance.

☹ **Clean Start Refreshing Cleanser for Normal Skin** *($9.50 for 8 ounces)* is a standard, detergent-based, water-soluble cleanser that also contains mixed citrus oils and several fragrant plant extracts high up on the ingredient list, which means that this can be irritating to the eyes and skin.

☹ **D-Clog Naturally Balancing Cleanser** *($9.69 for 8 ounces)* contains several ingredients that can be problematic for all skin types, including cornstarch, flour, and camphor.

☺ **Fresh Face Rehydrating Cleanser** *($9 for 8 ounces)* is a standard, plant oil–based, wipe-off cleanser. It can leave a greasy film behind on the skin, but it is an option for dry skin.

☹ **Satin Soap Natural Tea Tree Oil, Anti-Bacterial Liquid Soap** *($5.50 for 16 ounces)* contains tea tree oil, which can be useful as an antibacterial agent, but there is not enough of it in this cleanser for it to be effective. It also contains triclosan, an effective topical disinfectant, but there is no research showing that it can be effective for blemishes. And it also contains eucalyptus, which is too irritating for all skin types.

☺ **Satin Soap Natural Aloe Vera Liquid Soap** *($5.50 for 16 ounces)* is a highly fragrant, detergent-based cleanser, though it can still be an option for normal to oily skin.

☺ **Satin Soap Natural Apricot Liquid Soap** *($5.50 for 16 ounces)* is similar to the Natural Aloe version above except that this one contains plant oils, which makes it better for normal to dry skin.

☺ **Satin Soap Natural Chamomile Liquid Soap** *($5.50 for 16 ounces)* is similar to the Natural Aloe version above and the same comments apply.

☺ **Satin Soap, Natural Glycerin and Rosewater Liquid Soap** *($5.50 for 16 ounces)* is similar to the Natural Aloe version above and the same comments apply.

☺ **Satin Soap, Natural Herbal Extracts Liquid Soap** *($5.50 for 16 ounces)* is similar to the Natural Aloe version above and the same comments apply.

☺ **Satin Soap, Natural Lavender Liquid Soap** *($5.50 for 16 ounces)* is similar to the Natural Aloe version above and the same comments apply.

☺ **Quick Clean Eye Makeup Remover for All Skin Types, Oil Free** *($7.49 for 75 pads)* is a standard, detergent-based eye-makeup remover that will work as well as any, and they left most of the fragrant ingredients out of this one.

☺ **Citrus 6-in-1 Facial Wash & Scrub with Ester-C** *($6 for 4.5 ounces)* is supposed to contain AHAs and BHA, but it doesn't, which is good, because it would all just be rinsed away in a cleanser product, along with the vitamin C. Aside from that, it is a mild, detergent-based cleanser with soft scrub particles that can be good for exfoliation.

☺ **Original Apricot Scrub Facial Wash and Scrub** *($4.50 for 4.5 ounces)* is a detergent-based cleanser that uses ground-up nuts and shells as the exfoliant. It is an option as a topical scrub.

☺ **Beta-Gold Rehydrating Freshener** *($9 for 8 ounces)* is a basic, OK toner of water and glycerin with a teeny amount of water-binding agents and antioxidants. This supposedly contains AHAs, but they are not listed on the ingredient label, though even if they were present the pH isn't low enough for them to be effective as an exfoliant. It also contains citrus oils, added mostly for fragrance, but the amount is tiny.

☹ **Fruit Cooler Refreshing Toner for Normal Skin** *($8.49 for 8 ounces)* lists witch hazel (which contains alcohol) as the second ingredient, and that means that it can be too irritating for most skin types.

☹ **Vegee Tonic Balancing Astringent** *($9.50 for 8 ounces)* contains alcohol and is not recommended.

☺ **70% Aloe Vera All Purpose Moisturizing Creme** *($5.50 for 4 ounces)* is an emollient moisturizer for normal to dry skin. The amount of aloe sounds impressive, at least to those who think aloe is a miraculous ingredient, but the aloe gel is more water than aloe.

☺ **84% Aloe Vera All Purpose Moisturizing Creme** *($7 for 4 ounces)* is similar to the 70% Aloe Vera above and the same comments apply.

☺ **98% Aloe Vera Super Gel** *($7 for 8 ounces)* is indeed mostly aloe, with some thickening agents and preservatives. The price isn't bad, but for those looking for aloe, pure aloe from the health food store may be of more interest, and that wouldn't contain preservatives or thickening agents.

☺ **Aqua Moist Balancing Moisture Lotion SPF 12** *($9.50 for 4 ounces)* would be far better with an SPF 15, but it is an in-part titanium dioxide–based sunscreen that would be good for someone with normal to slightly dry skin.

☺ **Hemp Plus Oil Enriched with Natural EFA's Moisturizing Creme** *($9 for 1 ounce)* has a good blend of plant oils and antioxidants. It would be a good moisturizer for normal to dry skin, although the hemp oil is not any better for skin than any other emollient plant oil.

☺ **Hemp Plus Oil Enriched with EFA's** *($9.50 for 4 ounces)* is a good blend of plant oils and antioxidants and would be a very good moisturizer for dry skin.

☺ **Natural Cocoa Butter All Purpose Moisturizing Creme** *($5.50 for 4 ounces)* is a basic moisturizer for dry skin.

☺ **Natural NaPCA Moisturizing Creme** *($7 for 4 ounces)* contains mostly water, aloe, plant extracts, thickeners, water-binding agents, vitamins, and preservatives. This would be a very good, lightweight moisturizer for normal to slightly oily skin.

☺ **Nature's Exotic Moisturizer with Mango Butter** *($6.50 for 2 ounces)* is a basic emollient moisturizer for dry skin, though it is neither exotic nor unusual.

☺ **Nature's Exotic Moisturizer with Shea Butter** *($6.50 for 2 ounces)* is similar to the Mango Butter version above and the same comments apply.

The Reviews J

☺ Nature's Rich Moisturizing Blend, A-Pex3, with Avocado, Almond, and Apricot *($6.50 for 2 ounces)* is an emollient moisturizer for dry skin.

☺ Perfect Solutions Ester-C Moisture Creme, Daily Age Defense *($16.50 for 2 ounces)* is a good moisturizer for dry skin, though there's nothing in it that can defy age. The vitamin C, vitamin A, and other antioxidants are good for skin, but they won't change or stop wrinkling.

☺ Perfect Solutions Ester-C Moisture Lotion, Daily Age Defense *($16.50 for 4 ounces)* is an emollient moisturizer for normal to dry skin that contains some good plant oils, but only teeny amounts of antioxidants.

☺ Moisture Plus SPF 15 *($9 for 4 ounces)* is a good in-part titanium dioxide–based sunscreen in a standard, matte-finish lotion base. It would be an option for normal to oily skin.

☹ Quick Recovery Rehydrating SPF 12 Lotion *($9 for 4 ounces)* is a good, in-part titanium dioxide–based sunscreen, but the too-low SPF 12 makes it not worth the trouble, especially considering that this line has so many good sunscreens with SPF 15 or greater; so there is no reason to even consider this one.

☺ Suma Moist Active Creme Concentrate with Live Yeast Cell Extracts *($9 for 2 ounces)*. Yeast can be good as an antioxidant, but there is little to no research about its effect (alive or dead) on skin. Suma is a plant extract with a sparse amount of research showing it to have anti-inflammatory properties. Other than that, this is a good moisturizer for dry skin.

☺ Super E Creme, Super Moisture Creme, 25,000 I.U. *($11 for 4 ounces)* isn't all that super—the 25,000 IU of vitamin E in it comes to only 0.67 ounce. This is just a good emollient moisturizer with plant oils and some good antioxidants, just not very much of them. See the comments for the Pure Vitamin E Oil 14,000 I.U. below.

☺ Vitamin E All Purpose Moisturizing Creme, 5,000 I.U. *($6 for 4 ounces)* is similar to the Super E Creme above and the same comments apply, only this contains 0.1 ounce of vitamin E.

☺ Pure Vitamin E Oil 14,000 I.U. *($6 for 1 ounce)* is just vitamin E and some plant oils. That makes it a good, though greasy, moisturizer for dry skin. While 14,000 IU sounds like a lot, it ends up being less than 0.33 ounce. How much of any antioxidant skin needs is unknown, but this makes it sound like you're getting a whole lot when you're not. Research has shown that vitamin E is not helpful for healing scars.

☺ Vitamin E Oil 5,000 I.U. *($6 for 4 ounces)* is similar to the Pure Vitamin E Oil above, and the same comments apply, only this one contains 0.1 ounce of vitamin E.

☺ Vitamin E Oil Blend 45,000 I.U. *($10.50 for 2 ounces)* definitely contains more vitamin E (about 1 ounce) than the two products above, and if that's what you're interested in, then this is the preferred option.

☺ Vitamin K Creme with Bioflavonoids and Calendula *($20 for 2 ounces)* would be a very good moisturizer for normal to dry skin, but the claims it makes about vitamin

K improving circulation and eliminating surfaced capillaries are unsubstantiated. It does contain methylsulfonylmethane (MSM); please refer to Chapter Seven, *Cosmetics Dictionary*, for more information about MSM.

☺ **Super Anti-Oxidant Youth Enhancing Tea Time Antiaging Moisturizing Creme** (*$4.99 for 4 ounces*) claims that this can eliminate free-radical damage, but that would mean you would never again get another wrinkle or skin discoloration in your life. If that were the case, Jason Natural should stop selling all their other products because this one would be the fountain of youth. All for only $4.99! While this is a good moisturizer for dry skin, with plant oils and some antioxidants, exactly how much antioxidant it takes to even reduce free-radical damage is unknown, and this product doesn't contain all that much of it anyway.

☹ **Woman Wise 1,000 mg Progesterone Max Comfort and Balancing Creme** (*$18.99 for 2 ounces*). Please refer to Chapter Seven, *Cosmetics Dictionary*, for information regarding products making claims about their progesterone and wild yam content.

☹ **Woman Wise 10% Wild Yam Balancing and Moisturizing Creme** (*$9.99 for 4 ounces*) Please refer to Chapter Seven, *Cosmetics Dictionary*, for information regarding products making claims about their progesterone and wild yam content.

☺ **SPF 16 Sun Block** (*$8 for 4 ounces*) is a great, part titanium dioxide and zinc oxide sunscreen for normal to dry skin.

☺ **SPF 26 Sun Block Sport Stick** (*$9 for 4 ounces*) is similar to the SPF 16 Sun Block above, and the same comments apply.

☺ **SPF 26 Total Sun Block** (*$8 for 4 ounces*) is similar to the SPF 26 Sun Block Sport Stick above, and the same comments apply.

☺ **SPF 36 Family Sun Block** (*$10.50 for 4 ounces*) is similar to the SPF 26 Total Sun Block above, and the same comments apply.

☺ **SPF 40 Active Sun Block** (*$10.75 for 4 ounces*) is similar to the SPF 36 Family Sun Block above, and the same comments apply.

☺ **SPF 46 Kids Sun Block** (*$11 for 4 ounces*) is similar to the SPF 40 Active Sun Block above, and the same comments apply.

☺ **SPF 20 Natural Lip Protection on a String** (*$5 for 0.16 ounce*) is a great, in-part titanium dioxide and zinc oxide sunscreen (there are also other sunscreen agents in this formula) for normal to dry skin.

☹ **Sunless Maxi Tan SPF 16** (*$9 for 4 ounces*) contains dihydroxyacetone, the same ingredient all self-tanners use to affect the color of skin. While this would work well for that, the active ingredients for the sunscreen aren't listed and, therefore, this cannot be relied on for sun protection.

☹ **Fresh Papaya-Pineapple Facial Peel & Mask** (*$8 for 4.5 ounces*) contains several plant extracts that can be skin irritants. In addition, it contains papain and bromelain, but neither of these ingredients have research showing them to be effective as exfoliants for skin.

☹ **Meditation Masque, Anti-Stress Aromatherapy, Soothing, and Refreshing Masque** *($9.50 for 4 ounces)* is a standard clay mask that contains menthol, which isn't refreshing, it's just irritating for skin.

☹ **T-Zone Ultimate Balancing Clay Oil-Control Aromatherapy Masque** *($9.50 for 4 ounces)* is similar to the Meditation Masque above, only this one includes camphor, and that can be too irritating for all skin types.

JASON NATURAL TOPICAL VITAMIN C PRODUCTS

☺ **Super-C Cleanser Gentle Face Wash** *($10 for 6 ounces)* is a standard, detergent-based, water-soluble cleanser that can be a good option for someone with normal to oily skin. It contains a host of antioxidants, but in a cleanser their benefit is just rinsed down the drain.

☺ **C-Light Skin Tone Balancer** *($19.99 for 1 ounce)* contains a good amount of vitamin C in a standard moisturizing base that would be good for someone with normal to dry skin. The pH of this product is too high for the BHA (salicylic acid) to be an effective exfoliant. Also, this product contains kojic dipalmitate, a melanin inhibitor, and that may have benefit as a skin lightener. However, all skin-lightening products are useless without the consistent daily use of a good sunscreen. This also contains tiny amounts of water-binding agents and other antioxidants.

✓☺ **$$$ Hyper-C Serum Antiaging Therapy** *($50 for 1 ounce)* contains nearly every form of vitamin C imaginable in a lotion of plant oil and water-binding agents along with other antioxidants. One concern is that this product also contains cornstarch, which can be a problem on skin. If you're looking for vitamin C, though, this is an option to consider.

✓☺ **$$$ Ultra-C Eye Lift Treatment** *($20 for 0.5 ounce)* contains mostly water, glycerin, plant extracts, thickeners, water-binding agents, silicone, preservatives, and fragrance. There are several forms of vitamin C in this product, so if you are looking to cover your vitamin C bases, you might as well consider this one.

☹ **Deep-C Orange Peel, Peel Off Masque** *($17.50 for 2 ounces)* contains alcohol and witch hazel, which can be too irritating for all skin types.

☺ **Vita-C Max One Minute Facial** *($30 for 4 ounces)* is a very good emollient mask that contains several antioxidants, water-binding agents, and emollients. This is a fine option for dry skin.

☹ **"C" My Lips Protector SPF 15** *($8 for 0.47 ounce)* doesn't contain the UVA-protecting ingredients of titanium dioxide, zinc oxide, or avobenzone, and is not recommended.

JASON NATURAL NEW CELL THERAPY

☹ **New Cell Therapy 7 1/2 Plus Balancing Cleansing Pads with Alpha/Beta Hydroxy Acids** *($10 for 50 pads)* contains about 4% AHAs (as glycolic acid), but the other plant ingredients, sugarcane and sugar maple extract, are not AHAs. It also contains

BHA, but the pH of this product is not low enough for any of these to be effective as exfoliants. Plus, it contains several irritating ingredients, including witch hazel, lemon extract, and alcohol, and that makes it a problem for all skin types.

☺ **New Cell Therapy 6 Plus Daytime Moisturizing Emulsion with Alpha Hydroxy Acids** *($10 for 2 ounces)* contains about 2% to 3% AHA, which isn't enough for this to work as an exfoliant, and the plant extracts it contains are not effective as exfoliants.

☺ **New Cell Therapy 12-1/2 Plus Moisturizing Oil-Free Gel with Alpha Hydroxy Acids** *($20 for 1.1 ounces)* contains about 4% AHA, but the product's pH isn't low enough for it to be an effective exfoliant and the "fruit acids" are not effective as exfoliants at any pH.

☺ **New Cell Therapy 12-1/2 Plus Protective Moisturizer SPF 12 with Alpha Hydroxy Acids** *($20 for 1.6 ounces)* does contain titanium dioxide as one of the active sunscreen ingredients, but the SPF 12 falls short of the SPF 15 standard. Given that this line has so many excellent sunscreens with SPF 15 or greater, why waste your time with something below standard?

☺ **New Cell Therapy 10 Plus Nighttime Creme with Alpha Hydroxy Acids** *($15 for 1 ounce)* contains about 2% to 3% AHA, which isn't enough for it to be an exfoliant. Aside from that, this is just an ordinary emollient moisturizer for dry skin.

☺ **New Cell Therapy 3-1/2 Plus Gentle Eye Gel with Alpha Hydroxy Acids** *($12.99 for 1 ounce)* contains "mixed fruit acids," but these are not effective for exfoliation. And with a less than 2% concentration of lactic acid, there isn't enough to make this effective as an exfoliant. It is a good lightweight moisturizer for slightly dry skin, though.

☹ **New Cell Therapy 5-1/2 Plus Fast Acne and Blemish Relief with Alpha Hydroxy Acids** *($9 for 1 ounce)* contains both lemon and orange extract high on the ingredient list, making it too irritating for most skin types. And it does not contain any AHAs (the plant extracts listed are not the same thing as glycolic or lactic acids) and that is not helpful for fighting blemishes. The tiny amount of tea tree oil is not enough to be effective as a disinfectant.

JASON NATURAL SKIN-AMINS ORGANIC TOPICAL VITAMIN THERAPY

☺ **Skin-amins Topical Vitamin Therapy Hi-Vitamin A Complex with MSM, 10,000 I.U.** *($10 for 2 ounces)*. While this product can be a very good moisturizer for someone with dry skin (it contains several good water-binding agents, antioxidants, and anti-irritants), the claims about improving acne and age spots are bogus. There are no such things as age spots—they are sun-damage spots, resulting in hypermelanin production—so the term is very misleading. The ingredients are great for dry skin, but they can be a problem for breakouts, and there are no melanin-inhibiting ingredients in this product. The 10,000 IU of vitamin A listed sounds impressive, but that adds up to only 0.000106 of an ounce, barely a dusting.

☺ **Skin-amins Topical Vitamin Therapy Hi-Vitamin B Complex with MSM, 3,000 milligrams** *($10 for 2 ounces)* is similar to the Skin-amins Topical Vitamin Therapy Hi-

Vitamin A Complex above except that this one contains vitamin Bs, and the same basic comments apply.

☺ Skin-amins Topical Vitamin Therapy Hi-Vitamin C Complex with MSM, 3,000 milligrams *($10 for 2 ounces)* is similar to the Skin-amins Topical Vitamin Therapy Hi-Vitamin A Complex above except that this one contains several forms of vitamin C as the showcase ingredients, and the same basic comments apply. The 3,000 milligrams equate to 0.1 ounce of vitamin C, as in barely a drop of orange juice.

☺ Skin-amins Topical Vitamin Therapy Hi-Vitamin D Complex with MSM, 12,000 I.U. *($7.99 for 2 ounces)* is similar to the Skin-amins Topical Vitamin Therapy Hi-Vitamin A Complex above and the same basic comments apply, although the benefits of vitamin D applied topically on skin are unknown. If you're choosing, there is abundant research extolling the benefits of vitamins E, C, and B for skin. Actually, sticking all of them in one product would have saved buying different products.

☺ Skin-amins Topical Vitamin Therapy Hi-Vitamin E Complex with MSM, 10,000 I.U. *($7.99 for 2 ounces)* is similar to the Skin-amins Topical Vitamin Therapy Hi-Vitamin A Complex above except that this one contains vitamin E, and the same basic comments apply.

☺ Skin-amins Topical Vitamin Therapy Hi-Vitamin H, F, K, Complex with MSM, 6,000 mg *($11.99 for 2 ounces)* is similar to the Skin-amins Topical Vitamin Therapy Hi-Vitamin A Complex above and the same basic comments apply. Vitamin F refers to the essential fatty acids of linoleic acid and linolenic acid, which have emollient and antioxidant properties for skin. Vitamin H is biotin, part of the vitamin B family, and it has no reported benefit for skin when applied topically. The only research on vitamin K's effectiveness on skin or surfaced spider veins comes from the companies that sell the vitamin.

JEANNETTE GRAF, M.D.
(SEE DR. JEANNETTE GRAF, M.D.)

JOEY NEW YORK

So who's Joey? Her name is Joey Roer, and that's all the Web site for this line wants you to know about the founder. Joey's main claim to fame seems to be a very hip New York location that is described as being "…among America's premiere destinations for world-class therapeutic skin care treatments and beauty enhancement products. All of Joey New York products contain only all-natural quality ingredients." This may indeed be a premier destination—it's located at 24 West 57th Street, Suite 503, New York City—and the products do get some attention in fashion magazines, but none of that explains the primarily problematic formulations this line struggles with.

First, these aren't natural in the least. A mere cursory look at the ingredient lists easily proves that, with ingredients like imidazolidinyl urea, PEG-100 stearate, carbomer, tetrasodium EDTA, and triethanolamine. Plus, the plant extracts that are present occur in such minute amounts that they are barely worth mentioning. Even more significant is that while some of the plants used do have anti-irritant properties (licorice and chamomile), many others have an irritating effect on skin (including camphor, peppermint, yarrow, coltsfoot, pine, lemon, and grapefruit). What a waste. The Pure Pore products have a good amount of salicylic acid (BHA), but not one has an appropriate pH to make it an effective exfoliant, and including peppermint, camphor, sulfur, and alcohol in several of these can cause unnecessary inflammation and irritation, which only makes matters worse for skin. Many of the claims for the Joey New York products are over the top, even for the cosmetics industry.

There are a few positives in this line to note, however. The sunscreens are well formulated and there are a couple of well-formulated moisturizers, but that's about it. For the most part, Joey New York has a far better location than it has formulations. For more information about Joey New York, call (800) 563-9691 or visit www.joeynewyork.com.

JOEY NEW YORK SKIN CARE

☺ **Extra Gentle Eye Makeup Remover** *($17 for 6 ounces)* is just a very standard, detergent-based cleanser that would do fine for removing makeup. This does not contain fragrance and that's a plus.

☺ **Gentle Makeup Remover Pads** *($12 for 50 pads)* is identical to the Extra Gentle Eye Makeup Remover above except that the cloths for wiping off your makeup are provided.

☹ **Firm and Tone Eye Cream** *($20 for 0.5 ounce)* contains several problematic ingredients, including arnica and ivy. It is also a mediocre formulation that won't firm anything.

☺ $$$ **Lift Up Eye Gel** *($20 for 0.5 ounce)* is a very good lightweight moisturizer that contains some impressive water-binding agents and antioxidants.

☹ **Line Up** *($40 for 1 ounce)* is supposed to be the safe alternative to Botox. First, Botox isn't unsafe; and second, not only can't this perform even a fraction like Botox, the comparison is actually inane and misleading. In fact, the second ingredient listed is sodium silicate, a highly alkaline earth mineral that has absorbing properties, but that is also a strong skin irritant. The fourth ingredient is magnesium aluminum silicate, which also has absorbing properties. None of that is helpful for skin, particularly when it comes to wrinkles. The irritation, along with the spackle effect of this formulation, is not the answer to anyone's skin-care needs. The teeny amount of collagen has no effect on the collagen in your skin, and the plant extracts are a mix of anti-irritants and irritants.

☺ $$$ **Double Stuff Day and Night Moisturizer** *($40 for 1 ounce of Green Tea with Multivitamins SPF 30 and 1 ounce of Red Marine Algae Vitamin Enriched Moisturizer).* The Green Tea with Multivitamins SPF 30 is a good, in-part zinc oxide–based sunscreen in a standard moisturizing cream for normal to dry skin that contains a small amount of antioxidants and water-binding agents. The Red Marine Algae Vitamin Enriched Moisturizer is a good emollient moisturizer for normal to dry skin that contains a nice mix of water-binding agents and antioxidants.

☺ **$$$ Double Stuff Eye Masque and Face Masque** *($32 for 0.5 ounce of Eye Masque and 1.7 ounces of Face Masque).* The fourth ingredient listed in the Eye Masque is alcohol, and that's not great for skin anywhere on the face, much less the eye area. The Face Masque part of this two-part system is mostly just water, glycerin, film-forming agent, and some anti-irritants. That's OK, but not really worth the time and trouble to apply it.

☺ **$$$ Microdermabrasion Facial Peel** *($40 for 1.7 ounces of Facial Peel and 1 ounce of Sealant).* The Facial Peel contains synthetic wax (paraffin) and ground-up plastic (polyethylene) along with preservatives. The Sealant that you put on after the scrub is just a good emollient moisturizer for dry skin. There is nothing about this product that mimics any aspect of true microdermabrasion. It is little more than an exceedingly standard scrub you rub over skin that will remove some excess skin, and then a follow-up moisturizer.

☺ **Outdoor Activities SPF 20** *($22 for 4 ounces)* is a very good, in-part avobenzone-based sunscreen in an exceptionally standard lotion base. This offers no advantage to Ombrelle products that are available at the drugstore for half the price.

JOEY NEW YORK PURE PORES

☺ **Pure Pores Cleansing Gel with Vitamin C** *($22 for 8 ounces)* is a standard, detergent-based cleanser that also contains plant oils and about 1% salicylic acid (BHA), although the pH of the product isn't low enough for the BHA to be effective as an exfoliant or pore cleanser. The jojoba oil can be a problem for oily skin types, and the grapefruit and orange oils can be skin irritants. The amount of vitamin C is a mere dusting and not worth mentioning, much less naming the product after it.

☺ **Pure Pores One Step Toner and Moisturizer** *($22 for 8 ounces)* contains about 3% glycolic acid (an AHA), but the pH of the product is too high for it to be effective as an exfoliant. Other than that, this contains a teeny amount of water-binding agents and minimal antioxidant, while two of the plant extracts can be skin irritants.

☺ **Pure Pores Vitamin Toner with Ginseng** *($18 for 8 ounces)* is just water, slip agent, plant extracts, and small amounts of antioxidants. That's good, but not great, and it won't change the status of anyone's pores.

☺ **$$$ Pure Pores Crushed Almond and Honey Scrub** *($28 for 4 ounces)* is just what the name implies, a honey and almond meal scrub that also contains clay, making it slightly difficult to rinse off. It's an option, but it doesn't really get much more standard than this when it comes to a scrub, and you could do just as well by adding ground-up almonds to any cleanser you are already using.

☺ **Pure Pores Oil-Free Moisturizer with Ginseng** *($24 for 2 ounces)* contains several thickening agents high up on the ingredient list that would be problematic for someone with breakouts. Other than that, it is an OK moisturizer for someone with normal to slightly dry skin.

☹ **Pure Pores Pore Tightener and Filler Serum** *($30 for 1 ounce)* contains mostly deodorant (aluminum chlorohydrate) and alcohol. A formula like this would be better under your arms than on your face, but it would probably be too irritating even for that area!

☹ **Pure Pores Blackhead Remover and Pore Minimizer Gel** *($20 for 2 ounces)* contains about 1% BHA, but the pH of this product isn't low enough for it to be effective as an exfoliant. It also contains something called "fruit acids," but these aren't the same as AHAs or BHA, they are merely sound-alikes that lead you to believe this product contains something it does not. There are also a handful of potentially irritating plant extracts, including balm mint and fennel, so this just adds up to a product with more potential problems than benefits.

☹ **Pure Pores Masque and Blemish Treatment** *($22 for 2 ounces)* contains too much alcohol, as well as sulfur and camphor, making this seriously irritating for all skin types. Sulfur can be a mild disinfectant, but the irritation it can cause makes it more of a problem for skin than a help.

☹ **Pure Pores Roll on Blemish Fix** *($18 for 3.3 ounces)* contains too much alcohol, as well as camphor, making this too irritating for all skin types.

☹ **Pure Pores Hide and Heal** *($16 for 0.5 ounce)*. The salicylic acid in this product can't exfoliate because of the product's high pH, and it is no more effective as a concealer than any other. This version also contains menthol, camphor, eucalyptus, and peppermint, which, because of the irritation and inflammation they cause, can actually damage the skin's healing process.

☹ **Chin Breakout Relief** *($25 for 2 ounces)* is supposed to be all-natural, but this contains nylon-12, a synthetic polymer. That's not bad, but making the claim of "all-natural" is just so irritating. In addition, this contains alcohol and peppermint, which does make this product irritating for skin.

JOEY NEW YORK CALM AND CORRECT

☺ **Calm & Correct Gentle Soothing Cleanser** *($24 for 8 ounces)* is a good, gentle, detergent-based cleanser that would work well for most skin types. It would have been far more soothing, however, without the fragrant oil and artificial coloring agents.

☺ **Calm & Correct Gentle Soothing Toner** *($24 for 8 ounces)* is an OK, though highly fragrant, toner.

☺ **$$$ Calm and Correct Moisturizer** *($40 for 1 ounce)* is supposed to "diminish the appearance of dark circles under the eyes, spider veins on the face and legs, and the redness that results from laser treatments and chemical peels." As if any of those things are related! Not surprisingly, the fish cartilage and seaweed in this product can't do any of that. Aside from the hyped claims, this is a good moisturizer for normal to dry skin with a nice assortment of water-binding agents and antioxidants.

☺ **$$$ Calm and Correct Serum** *($38 for 1 ounce)*. The only reason to consider this product would be if you agreed with the notion that fish cartilage (the second ingredient listed) is a great ingredient for skin, because that is really the only unique aspect of the formulation. Aside from that, this is just an OK lightweight moisturizer for normal to dry skin. The fish cartilage may be a good water-binding agent for skin.

JOEY NEW YORK MAKEUP

When it comes to Joey New York's makeup, perhaps the best advice would be to run, don't walk, past the beckoning tester unit. Their concept is to make "truly different, innovative, and needed products," but what they've come up with is a mishmash of staggeringly poor and stunningly basic products, all bearing premium price tags. Perhaps Joey didn't survey the vast cosmetic landscape to see what the competition was doing, because nothing here bests what you will find from other lines. In fact, almost every single product seems like a misguided spin-off. You may find that the far-reaching claims for some of these products pique your interest, but then be disheartened upon using them. There are a couple of gems, but they're not worth investigating if you think you can't restrain yourself enough to avoid the pitfalls that abound with the other products of this line.

☹ **FOUNDATION: Pure Pores Pore Minimizer Foundation** *($35)* is a silicone-based makeup with a super-slick texture that dries instantly. You're left staring back at a solid, very dry matte finish that provides medium coverage and can, for a brief period of time, make pores *appear* smaller. This can quickly break down once your skin's oil mixes with it, however, just as the foundation separates readily in the bottle. A select few with oily skin may find this useful, but there are far more elegant matte-finish foundations available, and almost all of them give you at least some amount of time to blend them on before they set. **Pure Pores Tinted Moisturizer SPF 15** *($34)* has three very sheer colors that barely tint the skin, and the sunscreen does not have adequate UVA protection. If the base formula were interesting, this would merit a better rating. As it stands, there is no reason to choose this over tinted moisturizers (with effective sunscreens) from Bobbi Brown, Aveda, or Neutrogena.

☺ $$$ **CONCEALER: Pure Pores Hide and Heal** *($16)* is an opaque, matte-finish concealer that has a thick-as-toothpaste texture and comes in three good colors. This contains 0.5% salicylic acid, a concentration too low to affect blemishes (but the pH of the product is too high for it to be effective anyway). Hide and Heal functions as a concealer, but blending is difficult and it is too dry and heavy to use under the eyes.

☺ $$$ **POWDER: Finishing Powder** *($26)* is an inordinately smooth, talc- and mica-based pressed powder that comes in seven beautiful colors. The mica adds noticeable shine, so this isn't advised for anyone looking to blot oil or shine. Those with normal to dry skin may appreciate the satin finish, but check this in the daylight to be sure you don't mind the sparkles.

☹ **BLUSH: Chiseled Cheeks** *($35)* is a three-part, modular blush that gives you a cream-to-powder highlighting shade along with powder blush and contour shades. The idea is to use the three shades in tandem to create the look of high, sculpted cheekbones, yet this is too contrived to look convincing, especially given the artificial shimmer and the fact that the contour color is pigment-rich while the blush is sheer. I understand the concept, but the application looks more paint-by-the-numbers than artistic.

☹ <u>EYESHADOW:</u> **Opti-Brite Eye Color** *($40)* is packaged just like the Chiseled Cheeks set above, except that with this one you get three eyeshadow colors: Eye Base, Eye Contour, and Eye Lift (a dark shade). Although these have a smooth texture, they tend to drag over the skin and don't blend as well as they should. I also take issue with the fact that the contour color is only a notch darker than the pale base colors. This seems extraneous, given that you could lightly apply the darkest shade as a soft crease color and use the same shade for eyelining. And at this price you don't want anything to be extraneous!

☺ $$$ <u>EYE AND BROW SHAPER:</u> **State of the Arch Kit** *($28)* features a shiny brow powder that goes on reasonably well, if a bit too powdery, and a dual-sided brush to define and fill in the brows. This kit can work if you don't mind the shine, but please be advised that there are better and less costly brow powders and brushes available.

<u>LIPSTICK AND LIP PENCIL:</u> ☺ $$$ **Opti-Brite Lipstick Swirl** *($17)* gets its alleged brightening effect from a blend of "blue botanicals" (borage, cornflower, and safflower) that "give teeth a whiter look." Now I've heard everything. Of these three botanicals, only cornflower is actually blue, and none of them can overpower the synthetic dyes used to create each lipstick's color. This is strictly an ordinary cream lipstick with a glossy finish and a nicely varied shade selection. **Opti-Brite Lip Shine** *($18)* pleases with its smooth, lightweight, and completely non-sticky texture, but the displeasing price should inspire you to look elsewhere for what amounts to plain lip gloss. Contrary to its claim, this will not make teeth look whiter. **Opti-Brite Lip Pencil** *($16)* works very well as a standard lip pencil, but so do others that sell for less. The one unique aspect is the unconventional, but workable, range of colors.

☹ **Super Duper Lip Kit** *($25)* is sold to women with the claim that it can dramatically enhance lips, "making them fuller, smoother, softer" and, of course, plump. This is serious snake oil salesmanship, since all that the Super Duper Lip Kit contains is sugar, glycerin, honey, and a tiny amount of AHA. As you can imagine, it is a thick, sticky gel that's a mess to use and absolutely does not make lips fuller or plump. It will make lips softer, but what a sticky way to go about getting soft lips! The Kit throws in a standard nude pink lip pencil, but that's little consolation for the uninformed consumers who buy (literally and figuratively) into this utter work of fiction. **Delipcious Lip Balms SPF 15** *($12)* lack UVA protection and impart the most pungent flavors and tastes (bordering on distasteful tastes) from such sweet-sounding temptations as Banana Cream Pie and Pina Colada. You've been warned!

JURLIQUE INTERNATIONAL (SKIN CARE ONLY)

Jurlique is supposed to be the "purest skin care on earth, suitable for all skin types, and completely nonacnegenic. No chemicals, artificial preservatives, colors, or fragrance added." The products, however, don't seem as important as the faith and virtue and environmental sensibility projected in the claims. Though all of the plants in Jurlique products sound really nice and most have strong evidence of their potent antioxidant or anti-irritant properties (such as turmeric, grape, green tea, evening primrose oil, and rose hips oil), many also have a large amount of research showing that they are either skin irritants or are seriously problematic for skin (such as rosemary, sage, gromwell, peppercorn, quince, rose, and arnica).

Despite Jurlique's claims of being nonacnegenic, many of the ingredients (including waxy thickening agents and some plant oils) in these products can indeed clog pores and cause breakouts. Furthermore, these products absolutely do contain fragrance. What do the owners of Jurlique think lavender oil and geranium oil are for? You can attribute any miracle to these ingredients you like, but they are potentially skin irritants and there is no research showing them to have any balancing benefit for skin.

When you get through all of Jurlique's hype, which borders on the cultish, what is most disappointingly fascinating is that these products do not use a reliable preservative system. Luckily, the products do come in tiny containers, so you may very well use them up in one or two weeks, before they have a chance to become contaminated. Of course, that makes your yearly expenditure on skin care rather steep.

Furthermore, the formulas are astonishingly similar. Product after product contains the same oils and plant combinations. There is only one sunscreen in the line (and it contains synthetic sunscreen agents, too, which is surprising for this line), and that is a serious shortcoming, and none of the day creams in this line have sun protection. Additionally, I am really concerned about the lack of preservatives. Setting all that aside, if you are looking for natural, and you have a sizable budget to boot, Jurlique offers enough natural products to satisfy the most devout natural activist. For more information about Jurlique International, call (800) 854-1110 or visit www.jurlique.com. **Note:** All Jurlique products are highly fragranced.

☹ **$$$ Cleansing Lotion Makeup Remover** *($29 for 3.4 ounces)* is mostly thickeners, plant oil, and fragrant plant extracts. Several of the plant extracts can be skin irritants, and overall there is little benefit to using this cold cream–style cleanser versus plain safflower oil (the third ingredient) to remove your makeup.

☹ **$$$ Face Wash Cream Deep Cleansing Treatment** *($23 for 1.4 ounces)* uses crushed almonds and oat bran as the abrasive, along with plant oils and thickening agents. It is an option as a scrub for normal to dry skin. The plant extracts are mostly anti-irritants and antioxidants, but their benefit would be rinsed down the drain. Mixing some crushed almonds into whatever cleanser you're presently using would net similar benefits to this one.

☺ **$$$ Tea Tree and Lavender Foaming Facial Cleanser** *($33 for 6.8 ounces)* is a standard, detergent-based cleanser. It contains a minuscule amount of tea tree oil, but not enough for it to be effective as a topical disinfectant.

☹ **$$$ Aromamists** *($24 for 1.7 ounces)* are available in seven different versions, each with a different fragrance blend: Pampering, Romance, Tranquility, Energizer, Travel, Party, and Clarity. The fragrance is added to a base of water and glycerin. The teeny amount of lactic acid in these products is not there in sufficient concentration to have exfoliating properties. This is not very different from applying eau de cologne to your skin.

☺ **$$$ Floral Waters** *($19 to $32 for 1 ounce to 3.4 ounces)* is available in ten different fragrant combinations: Rosewater, Chamomile, Jasmine, Lavender, Lemon, Neroli, Orange, Geranium, Sandalwood, and Ylang-Ylang. They are all in the same water and glycerin base, making these identical to the Aromamists above, and the same comments apply.

☹ **Day Care Conditioner Herbal Water** *($32 for 3.4 ounces)* lists the second ingredient as grape alcohol, and alcohol in any form is drying and irritating for skin.

☺ **$$$ Herbal Extract Recovery Mist for Ageless Normal Skin** *($43 for 1 ounce)* is a rather simple mix of water, plant extracts, glycerin, slip agents, fragrant oil, and vitamin C.

☺ **$$$ Herbal Extract Recovery Mist for Delicate Sensitive Skin** *($43 for 1 ounce)*. For the most part this is an OK toner for normal to dry skin, but the quince, rose, and grapefruit make it inappropriate for sensitive skin.

☺ **$$$ Herbal Extract Recovery Mist for Moisture Depleted Skin** *($43 for 1 ounce)* is almost identical to the Herbal Extract for Delicate Sensitive Skin above, and the same comments apply.

☺ **$$$ Herbal Extract Recovery Mist for Oily Problem Skin** *($43 for 1 ounce)* is almost identical to the Herbal Extract for Delicate Sensitive Skin above, and the same comments apply. How it's possible that almost the exact same ingredients said to be good for sensitive and moisture-depleted skin can be appropriate for oily skin is anyone's guess.

☹ **Pure Rosewater Freshener Spray** *($28 for 3.4 ounces)* contains quince, rose oil, and grape alcohol, and that makes this too drying and irritating for all skin types.

☹ **Chamomile Rose Aromatic Hydrating Concentrate, Dry Sensitive and Mature Skin** *($42 for 1.7 ounces)* is mostly rosewater and grape alcohol, which makes it too drying and irritating for all skin types.

☹ **Lavender Lavandin Aromatic Hydrating Concentrate, Normal to Dry Skin** *($42 for 1.7 ounces)* is similar to the Chamomile Rose version above and the same comments apply.

☺ **$$$ Calendula C-Cream** *($28 for 1.4 ounces)* is an emollient moisturizer for normal to dry skin that contains some good plant oils and anti-irritants, although it lacks any significant amount of water-binding agents or antioxidants.

☺ **$$$ Day Care Face Cream** *($30.50 for 1.4 ounces)* doesn't contain sunscreen and should not be used during the day unless an additional effective sunscreen is worn. It is a very good emollient moisturizer with several antioxidants and a tiny amount of water-binding agents. Some of the plant extracts can be skin irritants.

☺ **$$$ Day Care Face Lotion** *($33 for 1 ounce)* is similar to the Day Care Face Cream above only in lotion form, and the same basic comments apply.

☺ **$$$ Day Care Face Oil** *($35 for 1 ounce)* is supposed to be "Perfect for use on oily skin, and has a soothing calming effect on overactive skin." This contains safflower, avocado, macadamia, and jojoba oils along with shea butter and triglyceride, all emollients that are problematic for oily skin.

☺ $$$ **Eye Gel** *($65 for 0.53 ounce)* is a lightweight gel moisturizer for normal to slightly dry or oily skin. It contains some very good antioxidants and anti-irritants. The tiny amounts of arnica and rose are probably too minimal to be a problem for skin.

☺ $$$ **Herbal Extract Recovery Gel** *($61 for 1 ounce)* is similar to the Eye Gel above and the same basic comments apply.

☹ **Lemon Lime Aromatic Hydrating Concentrate, Normal to Oily Skin** *($42 for 1.7 ounces)* contains grape alcohol, lemon oil, and lime oil, and that makes this too irritating and drying for all skin types.

☹ **Pine Needles Aromatic Hydrating Concentrate, Suits All Skin Conditions** *($42 for 1.7 ounces)* contains mostly water, slip agent, pine oil, and plant extracts. You're supposed to dilute this before using it, and that would be wise given that it would otherwise be similar to using furniture polish. Pine oil can have disinfecting properties, but it is also a significant skin irritant.

☹ **Rosemary Sage Aromatic Hydrating Concentrate, Oily, Non-Sensitive Skin** *($42 for 1.7 ounces).* The rosemary and sage oil plus the grape alcohol in this can all be skin irritants, and are not appropriate for any skin type.

☺ $$$ **Wrinkle Softener Beauty Cream** *($24 for 0.3 ounce)* is a very good emollient moisturizer with a good amount of antioxidants and anti-irritants.

☺ $$$ **Skin Bronzer** *($34 for 1 ounce)* is a lightly tinted moisturizer similar to the Wrinkle Softener above.

☺ $$$ **Sun Cream SPF 30+** *($36 for 3.5 ounces)* is a very good, in-part avobenzone- and titanium dioxide–based sunscreen.

☹ **Blemish Cream** *($24 for 0.3 ounce)* contains several thickeners that can be a problem for blemishes. Tea tree oil has not been shown to be effective as a topical disinfectant for acne, and especially not in such a tiny amount. The colloidal silver can have disinfecting properties, but it can be irritating to skin, cause silver toxicity, and prolonged contact can turn skin grayish blue.

☹ **Facial Steam Concentrate** *($28 for 3.4 ounces).* Steaming the skin causes capillaries to surface or makes existing ones more pronounced. Heat is damaging to skin and, with or without a product like this, it should never be considered a skin-care treatment.

☺ $$$ **Deep Penetrating Cream Mask** *($36 for 1.7 ounces)* is a standard clay mask that contains plant oils and plant extracts and a small amount of vitamins that can be potent antioxidants. This is an option for someone with normal to slightly oily or combination skin.

☺ $$$ **Moor Purifying Mask** *($35 for 1.7 ounces)* is similar to the Deep Penetrating Cream Mask above and the same basic comments apply. It contains Moor extract, a trade name for silt extract, which is another way of saying clay, and it has no special properties for skin.

☺ **$$$ OPC Beauty Face Mask** *($68 for 4.2 ounces)* is a standard clay mask with several emollient plant oils, water-binding agents, and antioxidants. It is a good option for normal to slightly dry or slightly oily skin.

☹ **$$$ Lip Care Balm** *($20 for 0.3 ounce)* is a very good basic lip balm that contains a small amount of pepper oil, which can be a significant skin irritant.

JURLIQUE ULTRA-SENSITIVE SKIN CARE

All of Jurlique's Ultra-Sensitive products contain Szechuan peppercorn extract and gromwell extract (Latin name *Lithospermum officinale*). Szechuan peppercorn is a significant skin irritant and gromwell extract can cause cell damage (Source: American Herbal Products Association (AHPA), http://www.ahpa.org). None of the following products are recommended for any skin type, much less for sensitive skin:

☹ **Ultra-Sensitive Face Wash** *($38 for 6.8 ounces).* See comments above.

☹ **Ultra-Sensitive Makeup Remover** *($42 for 3.4 ounces).* See comments above.

☹ **Ultra-Sensitive Hydrator/Toner Gel** *($28 for 3.4 ounces).* See comments above.

☹ **Ultra-Sensitive Day Moisturizing Lotion** *($68 for 3.4 ounces).* See comments above.

☹ **Ultra-Sensitive Aromatic Hydrating Concentrate** *($42 for 1.7 ounces).* See comments above.

☹ **Ultra-Sensitive Night Treatment Gel** *($70 for 3.4 ounces).* See comments above.

☹ **Ultra-Sensitive Nurturing Mask** *($60 for 5.5 ounces).* See comments above.

KARIN HERZOG SKIN CARE

It is strange to review a cosmetics line whose primary formulations are based on a major premise most researchers and I personally disagree with, but Karin Herzog's line of skin-care products is just that. Most of the skin-care products are based on the notion that oxygen in creams, lotions, and masks can help skin in regard to improving circulation. The theory is that the oxygen in these formulations can penetrate from the surface into the circulatory system and thereby get rid of wrinkles, cure acne, and heal rosacea and an assortment of other skin ills. Based on this assumption, almost all of the Herzog products contain hydrogen peroxide as the source of oxygen. The notion of oxygen in skin care is a spurious concept, and the reasons for that, not the least of which is its function as a major cause of free-radical damage and the resulting breakdown of collagen, but it is also detrimental to skin-cell growth (Sources: *Journal of Investigative Dermatology,* August 2002, pages 489–498; *Free Radical Research,* May 2002, pages 555–566; *Human and Experimental Toxicology,* February 2002, pages 61–62; and *Journal of Trauma,* November 2001, pages 927–931).

The confusion about the skin and oxygen is complicated by what the skin does need when healing chronic wounds. The demands of regenerating the tissue can require increased topical oxygen, as in a hyperbaric chamber. However, this method of wound care lacks research showing it to be effective or the best option for skin (Source: *Annals of the*

New York Academy of Sciences, May 2002, pages 239–249). Further, skin problems are unrelated to ulcerated wounds that don't heal.

It is important to point out that Herzog's use of hydrogen peroxide does have some support in the area of alternative medicine. Still, there are no long-term studies in regard to its effect on skin, and the risk of free-radical damage is never explained.

Apart from the oxygen issue, another Herzog claim I find disturbing is that her "products are so pure, and the quality standards so rigorous, that many of the Karin Herzog products require no preservatives." A head of lettuce can be entirely pure and natural, too, yet give it a week or two in your refrigerator and it will begin to break down as mold and bacteria grow. Not a pretty picture, and extremely bad for skin and eyes. Bacteria, mold, and fungus can begin to contaminate a cosmetic from the second it is formulated; however, and fortunately, only a handful of Herzog's products don't list preservatives, the others do contain preservatives.

I know it may get boring to hear me carry on about sunscreen, but here is yet another "scientifically designed" line talking about its vast research and product superiority, yet all the while ignoring the skin's need for sun protection. Further, a quick and cursory look at the ingredient labels lets you catch on to the repetitive nature of the formulations; one after the other has almost the same combination of ingredients—water, mineral oil, Vaseline, hydrogen peroxide, thickeners, vitamins, and fragrance. So if you thought one of these moisturizers was good, there would be absolutely no reason to buy the others because they are all so similar. By the way, the Vaseline and mineral oil make these products suitable only for those with dry skin. Herzog's reasoning for the Vaseline is that it keeps the hydrogen peroxide stable and helps force it into the skin, but there is no research or information to confirm that claim.

For more information about Karin Herzog Skin Care, call (800) 261-7261 or visit www.karinherzog.ch.

☺ $$$ **Cleansing Milk** *($30 for 7.05 ounces)* is just thickeners and a small amount of detergent cleansing agent. It can be a decent option for someone with normal to dry skin, though it's incredibly overpriced for such an ordinary formulation.

☺ $$$ **Cleansing Cream** *($32 for 1.76 ounces)* is one of the more overpriced cold creams I've seen. It can leave a greasy film on the skin. The brochure brags that this product doesn't contain preservatives, and it doesn't, but then neither does Vaseline, which is what you are mostly buying when you buy this cleanser.

☹ $$$ **Mild Scrub** *($34 for 1.76 ounces)* contains mostly marble powder and mineral oil. This can be pretty scratchy stuff and doesn't rinse very well. There is little about using this that baking soda and a gentle cleanser wouldn't easily replace.

☹**Additional Day Cream** *($30 for 1.76 ounces)* doesn't have an SPF and lists only octyl methoxycinnamate (a UVB-protecting ingredient) in the regular list of ingredients, so this product should absolutely not be relied on for sun protection. It's exceedingly ordinary and shockingly overpriced for what you get.

☺ **$$$ Additional Night Cream** *($32 for 1.76 ounces)* is similar to the Day Cream above except that it contains a good water-binding agent and a small amount of retinol. As a retinol product, it is a fine option.

☹ **Eye Cream 0.5% Oxygen** *($46 for 0.6 ounce)*. It's interesting to consider buying an eye cream that contains the warning "rinse immediately if in contact with eyes." Other than that, this merely contains water, mineral oil, glycerin, thickeners, plant oil, vitamin E, hydrogen peroxide, retinol, fragrance, and plant extracts. Given that retinol is unstable in the presence of oxygen, this product only gets more confusing. And the purpose of vitamin E is as an *anti*oxidant to undo the effect of the hydrogen peroxide. Very strange and very expensive.

☹ **Oxygen Face Cream** *($34 for 1.76 ounces)* contains—yes—more hydrogen peroxide, in water, with mineral oil and thickeners. For some reason this one is recommended for teenagers to control acne—but mineral oil for blemishes? They've got to be kidding. Hydrogen peroxide does have antibacterial properties, but there would be no reason to use this when a bottle of hydrogen peroxide is available at the drugstore for less than a dollar. However, because of free-radical damage, I do not recommend using hydrogen peroxide, either in these products or in the little brown bottle you buy at the drugstore.

☹ **Vita-A-Kombi 1, Vita-A-Kombi 2,** or **Vita-A-Kombi 3** *(#1, $50 for 1.94 ounces; #2 $53 for 1.94 ounces; #3 $56 for 1.94 ounces)*. The varying numbers for these products indicate the concentrations of hydrogen peroxide—1%; 2%, and 3%. These standard, mundane moisturizers are hardly worth the money. On the other hand, if you want to believe the hype about hydrogen peroxide, you could just go to the drugstore and buy 3% hydrogen peroxide for 89 cents and some Vaseline and have the same thing. These do contain retinol and vitamin E, the same as the Eye Cream above, and the same comments apply.

☹ **Vita-A-Kombi Fruit Acids 1% Oxygen** *($50 for 1.94 ounces)* is similar to the Vita-A-Kombi above only with the addition of AHAs. However, the concentration of AHAs (less than 2%) and the high pH of the base means these will not be effective for exfoliation.

☺ **$$$ Vitamin H Cream** *($48 for 1.94 ounces)*. Vitamin H refers to biotin, of which this product contains only a minuscule amount. That isn't really a problem, because there is no research showing it to have benefit when applied topically to skin. However, the other vitamin B ingredient in this product, riboflavin, may be a problem for skin when exposed to sunlight (see vitamin B2 in Chapter Seven, *Cosmetics Dictionary*).

☹ **Oxygen Sun & Solarium Cream** *($30 for 5.17 ounces)*. While many products sold by cosmetics companies are disappointing or ineffective, few are downright offensive. This one, however, falls in the offensive category. It is "Specially designed for solarium tanning [tanning beds, and], this product acts as a tanning accelerator during the solarium session while simultaneously hydrating the skin." Encouraging in any way the use of tanning beds is unconscionable for a skin-care company, especially one that uses a great deal of rhetoric about their research and information about wrinkles and the health of skin. According to the FDA (www.fda.gov), the FCC (Federal Communications Commission), the American Academy of Dermatology (www.aad.org), and the Skin Cancer Foundation (www.skincancer.org), tanning beds are nothing more than skin-cancer machines and should be made illegal. Tanning beds radiate the most damaging effects of the sun only inches away from your body, and, worse, they are available day after day, month after month. In addition, they allow parts of the body that are usually covered to be exposed to damaging radiation. They pose the same or increased risk of skin cancer that unprotected exposure to the sun does (Sources: *Journal of the American Academy of Dermatology*, May 2002, pages 706–709, and May 2001, pages 775–780; *Journal of the National Cancer Institute*, February 2002, pages 224–226; and *Pediatrics*, June 2002, pages 1009–1014).

☺ $$$ **Facial Oil** *($21 for 0.49 ounce)* is mostly emollients and a small amount of retinol and vitamin E. The clear packaging, which allows light to penetrate, offers no protection to help keep the retinol stable.

☹ **Essential Mask** *($38 for 1.76 ounces)* is virtually identical to many of the moisturizers in this line, containing mostly water, mineral oil, thickeners, hydrogen peroxide, retinol, and fragrance.

KIEHL'S (SKIN CARE ONLY)

Kiehl's independent, small-town image went by the wayside in April 2000 when it was purchased by L'Oreal. How did this very expensive, obscure skin-care line become so well known? Especially when you consider that the company doesn't advertise (although it does have a PR firm that handles its press relations, which has garnered it a lot of attention in fashion magazines). Kiehl's has definitely gotten value out of its attention-getting media mentions.

The line has been around for quite some time; it has its origins in a family-owned pharmacy. Still, the products hardly warrant excitement or even mild enthusiasm, and most are surprisingly ordinary, with a dusting of natural ingredients almost always at the very end of the ingredient list, well past the preservatives. That amounts to little more than a token attempt to make the products appear more natural to the consumers who want to believe a plant or vitamin must somehow be better for the skin than something that sounds more chemical. Nevertheless, that token amount is enough to allow Kiehl's to brag about how its products nourish the skin or are more environmentally friendly.

Aside from the allure of the natural, this line consists of totally ordinary and often completely unnatural ingredients. More disheartening for skin is that many of the ingredients are questionable for sensitive-skin types or for oily skin, and in some instances would be irritating for any skin type; and most of the sunscreen products are a serious problem for reliable sun protection. For more information about Kiehl's, call (800) KIEHLS-1 or visit www.kiehls.com.

☹ **Foaming Non-Detergent Washable Cleanser** (*$14.50 for 8 ounces*) is not in the least a non-detergent cleanser because the second ingredient listed is sodium C14-16 olefin sulfate, a detergent cleansing agent (technically called a surfactant) that is an ingredient in shampoos that is known for stripping hair color. By any dictionary definition, this is a standard detergent cleanser and it can be drying and irritating for skin.

☺ **Gentle Foaming Facial Cleanser for Dry to Normal Skin Types** (*$14.50 for 8 ounces*) is a fairly gentle, though standard, detergent-based, water-soluble cleanser that also contains a tiny amount of plant oils. It is a good option for normal to slightly dry or slightly oily skin.

☺ **Oil-Based Cleanser and Makeup Remover** (*$11.50 for 4 ounces*) actually isn't oil-based because what it mostly contains are some very emollient thickening agents. There are small amounts of plant oil and lanolin oil. This product is little more than cold cream, and is an option for very dry skin.

☺ **Rare-Earth Oatmeal Milk Facial Cleanser #1 (Mild)** (*$18.50 for 8 ounces*) doesn't contain any earth that is remotely rare, just standard kaolin and bentonite, better known as clay. But I guess if you want to charge this kind of money for clay and standard detergent cleansing agents, you have to call it rare. Clay can be slightly tricky to rinse off skin but it does leave skin soft and is an option for someone with oily skin.

☺ **Rare-Earth Oatmeal Milk Facial Cleanser #2 (Medium Strength)** (*$18.50 for 8 ounces*) is very similar to Facial Cleanser #1 (Mild) above and the same comments apply.

☺ **Ultra Moisturizing Cleansing Cream** (*$17.50 for 8 ounces*) is a very ordinary, lotion-type cleanser with oils that is an option for normal to dry skin.

☺ **Washable Cleansing Milk a Moisturizing Cleanser for Dry or Sensitive Skin** (*$14.50 for 8 ounces*) is a lotion cleanser that can be an option for normal to dry skin, though it isn't all that washable without the help of a washcloth. The trace amounts of milk and vitamins in this product are barely detectable.

☹ **Milk, Honey, and Almond Scrub** (*$19.50 for 6 ounces*) is a scrub that uses ground almonds as the abrasive. It also contains a large amount of flour and starch, which can be a problem for blemish-prone or oily skin.

☺ **Ultra Moisturizing Buffing Cream with Scrub Particles** (*$11.50 for 4 ounces*) is a scrub that uses a synthetic scrub ingredient (ground-up plastic). It also contains thickening agents and oils, and would be suitable for someone with very dry skin.

☹ **Pineapple and Papaya Facial Scrub Made with Real Fruit** (*$28 for 4 ounces*) is a standard detergent cleanser with cornmeal as the abrasive. The teeny amounts of pineapple and papaya have no exfoliating properties for skin.

☹ **Blue Astringent Herbal Lotion** (*$13.50 for 8 ounces*). Not only is the alcohol in this product drying and irritating, but the aluminum chlorohydrate (yes, the same stuff used in antiperspirants) in it can add to that irritation.

☹ **$$$ Calendula Herbal Extract Toner Alcohol-Free** (*$34 for 8 ounces*) is a standard toner of water, slip agent, plant extracts, and preservatives. The plant extracts are mostly anti-irritants, which is nice, but this lacks any antioxidants or water-binding agents and if you're going to spend this kind of money on a toner it should contain all the elements skin needs.

☹ **Cucumber Herbal Alcohol-Free Toner for Dry or Sensitive Skin** *($14.50 for 8 ounces)* is alcohol-free, but not irritant-free. It contains balm mint, pine needle, arnica, and camphor, all of which can be serious irritants. There is nothing about this product appropriate for sensitive skin, or any skin type for that matter.

☹ **Herbal Toner with Mixed Berries and Extracts** *($19.95 for 8 ounces)* does have berries in it, but it also has peppermint and lemongrass, which can be irritating for skin.

☹ **Rosewater Toner #1** *($13.50 for 8 ounces)* is mostly alcohol with rose fragrance. It can be irritating and drying and is completely useless for skin.

☹ **Rosewater Facial Freshener-Toner** *($13.50 for 8 ounces)* is almost identical to the Rosewater Toner #1 above and the same comments apply.

☹ **Tea Tree Oil Toner** *($24 for 8 ounces)* lists eucalyptus second and grapefruit third on the ingredient list, making this a skin irritation waiting to happen. The teeny amount of tea tree oil in this product isn't enough for it to be an effective disinfectant for blemishes.

☺ **$$$ Anti-Oxidant Skin Preserver** *($57.50 for 1.5 ounces)* contains mostly thickeners, plant oils, and small amounts of vitamins E, A, and C. This is a very emollient, though ordinary, moisturizer for normal to dry skin. The vitamins are decent antioxidants, though they're hardly unique to this product—and for this price there isn't very much of them in here.

☺ **$$$ Creamy Eye Treatment with Avocado** *($22.50 for 0.5 ounce)* is an OK, basic moisturizer for normal to dry skin. Nothing in here makes this preferred for the eye area.

☺ **Creme d'Elegance Repairateur Superb Tissue Repairateur Creme** *($26.50 for 2 ounces)*. Regardless of what language you say it in, this cream will not repair skin. It is just a very simple moisturizer of thickeners and plant oil that is an option for dry skin. The teeny amounts of water-binding agents and antioxidants are barely detectable.

☺ **Panthenol Protein Moisturizing Face Cream** *($23.50 for 4 ounces)* is a good moisturizer for dry skin that contains water-binding agents and antioxidants.

☺ **Sodium PCA Oil-Free Moisturizer** *($22.50 for 4 ounces)* is an OK, though basic, moisturizer for normal to dry skin. The tiny amounts of water-binding agents and antioxidants are insignificant.

☺ **Lycopene Facial Moisturizing Lotion** *($35 for 1.7 ounces)* doesn't contain lycopene, but it does contain tomato extract, which has lycopene as a component. The tomato plant extract itself actually has weak antioxidant properties (Source: *Free Radical Research,* February 2002, pages 217–233), but lycopene is better all by itself as an antioxidant (Source: *American Journal of Clinical Nutrition,* 1997, volume 66, number 1, pages 116–122). This is just an OK moisturizer for normal to dry skin with small amounts of water-binding agents and minuscule amounts of antioxidants.

☺ **$$$ Lycopene Facial Moisturizing Cream** *($60 for 1.4 ounces)* is almost identical to the Lycopene Facial Moisturizing Lotion above and the same comments apply.

☺ **$$$ Light Nourishing Eye Cream** *($17 for 0.5 ounce)* is an exceptionally standard, boring moisturizer for normal to dry skin. It does contain vitamins, but the amounts are insignificant.

☹ **$$$ Moisturizing Eye Balm with Pure Vitamins A & E** *($16.50 for 0.5 ounce)* is a decent, extremely emollient, and somewhat heavy moisturizer for dry skin. It does contain some vitamin A and E, but lacks any water-binding agents (if it had them it would have netted a much happier face).

☹ **Ultra Facial Moisturizer** *($12 for 2 ounces)* is not ultra in the least. This is just a very standard moisturizer for normal to dry skin. It contains minuscule amounts of vitamins A and E.

☹ **Ultra Facial Moisturizer SPF 15** *($27 for 4 ounces)* doesn't contain the UVA-protecting ingredients of titanium dioxide, zinc oxide, or avobenzone, and is absolutely not recommended.

☹ **Ultra Protection Moisturizing Face Gel SPF 15** *($29 for 0.5 ounce)* doesn't contain the UVA-protecting ingredients of titanium dioxide, zinc oxide, or avobenzone, and is absolutely not recommended.

☹ **Dermal Protection Face Cream with SPF 8** *($42 for 4 ounces)* has an SPF that is far below the standard minimum of SPF 15 set by the American Academy of Dermatology and the Skin Cancer Foundation, and it doesn't contain the UVA-protecting ingredients of titanium dioxide, zinc oxide, or avobenzone. It is absolutely not recommended.

☺ **$$$ Algae Masque** *($24 for 2 ounces)* is a good mask for someone with dry skin, but the algae has no magical benefit. It is an antioxidant, but no better than lots and lots of antioxidants that show up in skin-care products, and this one doesn't contain very much of it anyway.

☹ **Imperiale Repairateur All-Day Treatment Masque (Oily/Acne)** *($14.50 for 1 ounce)* contains several plant oils, and that makes it completely inappropriate for someone with oily skin, plus there is nothing in it of benefit to someone with breakouts or acne, such as a disinfectant or exfoliant.

☹ **Imperiale Repairateur All-Day Treatment Masque (Normal to Oily)** *($22.50 for 2 ounces)* is similar to the Oily/Acne version above and the same comments apply.

☺ **$$$ Moisturizing Masque** *($37 for 2 ounces)* is indeed moisturizing and good for someone with dry skin.

☹ **Rare-Earth Facial Cleansing Masque** *($17.50 for 5 ounces).* There is nothing rare about the clay in here—it is just standard bentonite and kaolin. This also contains cornstarch, which can be a problem for skin, and several plant oils that can be problematic for oily skin.

☹ **Rare-Earth Face Masque (Gently Astringent for Oily-Acne Skin)** *($14.50 for 4* *ounces)* is a sulfur-based clay mask. There is nothing gentle about sulfur, and although it is a disinfectant, it happens to be a very irritating one.

☺ **Soothing Gel Masque** *($14.95 for 8 ounces)* is just a layer of film-forming agent, which you apply over the skin, and some plant extracts. That can feel OK, and peeling off the layer of plastic will make skin feel temporarily smoother, but for the most part this is really just a waste of time.

☹ **Drawing Paste with Azulene** *($13.50 for 0.5 ounce)* is supposed to "…draw oils and impurities to the surface to help prevent blemishes. [And offer] control of surface oiliness and the maintenance of skin integrity." This product contains several plant oils and lanolin oil, which makes it completely inappropriate for oily skin. There are absorbents in this product, but their action is hindered by the very oils this product contains. This also includes sulfur, which is a significant skin irritant.

☹ **Treatment and Concealing Stick for Blemishes** *($24 for 0.18 ounce)* contains more ingredients that are problematic for breakouts than you can imagine, including zinc oxide, lanolin oil (can you believe lanolin oil in a product for acne?), isopropyl palmitate, and carnauba wax (that's car wax).

☺ **Lip Balm #1** *($4.95 for 0.7 ounce)* is a very emollient lip gloss that contains mostly Vaseline, plant oils, lanolin, and preservatives.

☺ **All-Sport "Non-Freeze" Face Protector SPF 30** *($15 for 1.4 ounces)* is a good, in-part avobenzone-based sunscreen in an ordinary emollient, wax-based balm. This would only be an option for very dry skin.

☹ **Ultra Protection Water Based Sunscreen Lotion SPF 25** *($26 for 4 ounces)* doesn't contain the UVA-protecting ingredients of titanium dioxide, zinc oxide, or avobenzone, and is absolutely not recommended.

☹ **Sunscreen Creme SPF 15** *($23 for 8 ounces)* doesn't contain the UVA-protecting ingredients of titanium dioxide, zinc oxide, or avobenzone, and is absolutely not recommended.

☺ **Klaus Heidegger's All-Sport Water-Resistant Skin Protector with SPF 25** *($19 for 4 ounces)* is a good, in-part titanium dioxide–based sunscreen that would be good for normal to slightly dry skin.

KINERASE

☺ $$$ **Kinerase Lotion** *($99 for 3.73 ounces)* and **Kinerase Cream** *($99 for 2.82)* were developed by Senetek PLC (www.senetekplc.com) and are distributed by ICN Pharmaceuticals, Inc. Kinerase contains a plant growth hormone called N6-furfuryladenine, also called kinetin. Kinerase is not the only product that contains kinetin; it is also used in Almay's Kinetin Skin Care products and The Body Shop's Skin Re-Leaf products, both available at a fraction of the price of Kinerase. For more information about kinetin see Chapter Seven, *Cosmetics Dictionary*. For more information about Kinerase, call (877) 546-3727 or visit www.kinerase.com.

KISS ME MASCARA

☺ $$$ **Kiss Me Mascara** *($24)* begs you to "stop painting your lashes—tube them!" and what they mean by that is the single unique selling point for this otherwise lackluster mascara. Instead of using a traditional mascara base of water, oils, waxes, and film-forming agents, Kiss Me uses a water base with a standard, water-soluble film-forming agent (a hairstyling ingredient). When the mascara is brushed on lashes, it forms tiny "tubes" around each lash, and these can only be removed with water and friction. According to Blinc, the makers of Kiss Me, this mascara is water-resistant, yet comes off easily with water. How can this be? How can mascara claim to be water-resistant and be removable *with* water? It turns out that water alone is not enough to remove the mascara. You need some form of friction (such as your fingers) to get this mascara off, and as it breaks down it can become stringy and streaky—almost like having spider webs on your lashes as the tubes dissolve. You can get some lengthening, but no thickness to speak of. It does stay on well, and does not clump or flake. This ends up being a fairly expensive mascara whose payoff is minor. And the rationale for its use is a bit strained—after all, other than leaving out waxes and oils (which are not harmful to lashes) this is a very basic mascara formula whose only major plus is easy removal. For more information about Kiss Me Mascara, call (877) 454-7763 or visit www.kissmemascara.com.

KISS MY FACE (SKIN CARE ONLY)

I love the name of this skin-care line. It evokes a sense of tenderness and affection that is sweet and caring. You may have run into these products in health food stores and the occasional drugstore. It is particularly hard for teens to ignore. And perhaps even more beguiling than the name are the incredibly low prices. I only wish the thoughtful name translated into thoughtful products, but I'm not sure what this company was thinking. Despite the claims about the line not using any unnecessary chemicals, there are plenty of them in these products. Actually, their brochure states that the products contain "no synthetics or chemicals, artificial preservatives or fragrances of any kind.… All the ingredients coming from renewable resources are environmentally sound. Many of the herbs are grown or harvested by indigenous people, helping preserve their way of life." Triethanolamine, propylparaben, propylene glycol, or sodium lauryl sulfate are about as natural as plastic. And no fragrance? These products are highly fragranced!

Further, this line seems to have a penchant for lime, lemon, camphor, eucalyptus, grapefruit, and peppermint, which serve no purpose for skin other than to cause unnecessary irritation, which impedes the skin's healing process.

While the prices are more than reasonable, there are other aspects of this line that leave much to be desired, such as cleansers with sodium lauryl sulfate as the main cleansing ingredient, AHA products with either minimal concentrations of AHA or a pH that's too high for them to work, blemish products with extremely irritating ingredients, lots of fragrant, sensitizing plant oils, and several poorly formulated sunscreens. For more information about Kiss My Face, call (800) 262-KISS or visit www.kissmyface.com.

☹ **Original Moisture Soap** *($4 for 9 ounces);* **Almond Creme Moisture Soap** *($4 for 9 ounces);* **Fragrance Free Antibacterial Moisture Soap** *($4 for 9 ounces);* **Orange Blossom Moisture Soap** *($4 for 9 ounces);* **Peaches & Creme Moisture Soap** *($4 for 9 ounces);* **Pear Antibacterial Moisture Soap** *($4 for 9 ounces);* **Peaceful Patchouli Moisture Soap** *($4 for 9 ounces);* **Summer Melon Moisture Soap** *($3.99 for 12 ounces);* and **Tea Tree Moisture Soap** *($4 for 9 ounces)* all list sodium lauryl sulfate as the second ingredient, which means they pose a high risk of irritation for all skin types. **Chamomile Olive Soap Bar** *($2.99 for 8 ounces);* **Pure Olive Oil Soap Bar** *($2.99 for 8 ounces);* **Olive & Aloe Soap Bar** *($2.99 for 8 ounces);* **Olive & Herbal Soap Bar** *($2.99 for 8 ounces);* and **Olive & Honey Soap Bar with Calendula** *($2.99 for 8 ounces)* all have a standard soap base that can be drying for most skin types.

☹ **Citrus Cleanser** *($7 for 3.75 ounces)* is a standard wipe-off, cold cream–type cleanser with additions of lime oil, lemon oil, and other plant extracts that are completely unnecessary skin irritants.

☹ **Foaming Facial Cleanser** *($10 for 4 ounces)* contains lime oil, lemon oil, and other plant extracts that are completely unnecessary skin irritants.

☹ **Exfoliating Face Wash** *($10 for 4 ounces)* contains oils of lemon, grapefruit, tangerine, lemongrass, orange, and lime. All are irritating, and useless for the skin.

☺ **Gentle Face Cleanser for Normal to Dry** *($10 for 4 ounces)* is a relatively rinseable cleanser with plant oils and detergent cleansing agent. The orange oil isn't the best, but it's probably not enough to be a problem for the skin. This could be an option for someone with dry skin.

☺ **Shea Butter Eye Makeup Remover** *($8 for 1.5 ounces)* is a plant oil–based makeup remover that also contains witch hazel in an alcohol-base, not the best for the eye area.

☺ **Daily Scrub/ Weekly Masque** *($7 for 4.5 ounces)* is just oatmeal, almond meal, cornmeal, and some slip agents and thickeners. It would work for normal to oily skin.

☹ **Organic Jojoba & Mint Facial Scrub** *($10 for 2 ounces).* Between the mint, peppermint, eucalyptus, camphor, and bergamot oils, this is an irritation waiting to happen.

☹ **Aloe & Chamomile Toner for Normal/Dry Skin** *($9 for 4 ounces)* does contain aloe and chamomile, but it also contains witch hazel and tea tree oil, which are both out of place in a product for dry skin. Tea tree oil can be a good topical disinfectant, but not when it's present in such a small amount, and the witch hazel is in an alcohol-base and can be drying and irritating for most skin types, especially for dry skin.

☹ **Aloe & Tea Tree Astringent for Normal/Oily Skin** *($9 for 4 ounces)* is similar to the Aloe & Chamomile Toner above only with the addition of camphor, which adds to the irritation.

☹ **Citrus Essence Astringent for Oily and Combination Skin Types** *($5 for 8 ounces)* contains witch hazel and lemon juice, along with extracts of more citrus fruits. This is a problem waiting to happen.

☺ **Flower Essence Toner** *($5 for 6 ounces)*. Several of the fragrant plant extracts in this product can be skin irritants, but aside from that it is a basic toner.

☺ **Alpha + Aloe Oil Free Moisturizer 5% Alpha Hydroxy Acid Fragrance Free** *($9.95 for 16 ounces)* is indeed oil free, but it does contain other ingredients such as isopropyl palmitate and emulsifying wax that can be a problem for oily skin. While this product contains a concoction of AHAs, it would be far better if it only contained lactic acid and/or glycolic acid (they perform the best for skin). Regardless, the pH of this product isn't low enough to make it an effective exfoliant, though this would be a good moisturizer for dry skin. And this product is highly fragranced!

☺ **Alpha + Aloe Oil Free Moisturizer Vanilla Scent 5% Alpha Hydroxy Acid** *($9.95 for 16 ounces)* is similar to the Alpha + Aloe Oil Free version above and the same comments apply.

☹ **Aromatherapeutic Alpha Hydroxy Creme** *($15 for 1 ounce)* contains about 1% of something called natural mixed fruit acids, which aren't at all the same as an alpha hydroxy acid, and even if you could rely on this amorphous mixture, there isn't enough of it to be effective as an exfoliant. This also contains several irritating plant oils, including lemon, lime, tangerine, orange, and grapefruit, which makes it too potentially irritating for all skin types.

☺ **Peaches & Creme Moisturizer 8% Alpha Hydroxy for Face and Neck** *($8.95 for 4 ounces)*. The forms of AHAs used in this product are nicely identified mixed fruit acids, including citric acid, malic acid, and tartaric acid. However, glycolic acid and lactic acid are considered the better forms of AHAs for exfoliation of skin. But the point is moot because the pH of this product is too high for it to be an effective exfoliant anyway. There are fewer irritating plant extracts in this product than in most of the Kiss My Face products, which makes this an OK emollient moisturizer for dry skin.

☺ **Peaches & Creme Moisturizer 4% Alpha Hydroxy Moisturizer** *($8.95 for 4 ounces)* is almost identical to the Peaches & Creme Moisturizer 8% version above, and the same comments apply.

☺ **All Day Moisture Creme** *($10 for 3.75 ounces)* has no sunscreen, so you wouldn't want to use this during the day. It is simply a standard, exceedingly ordinary moisturizer for dry skin with teeny amounts of vitamins A and E.

☺ **All Night Olive & Aloe Moisture Creme** *($10 for 3.75 ounces)* is a very good emollient moisturizer for dry skin that contains several plant oils, antioxidants, and a small amount of water-binding agent.

☺ **Chinese Botanical Moisturizer** *($4 for 4 ounces)* is similar to the All Night Olive & Aloe Moisture Creme above and the same basic comments apply. The plant extracts it contains all have Chinese names, but they all correlate to the better-known plant extracts that have some antibacterial, anti-inflammatory, and also potentially irritating effects.

☺ **Fragrance Free Oil Free Moisturizer with NaPCA** *($9 for 16 ounces)* is basically just water, wax, fragrance, preservatives, and a tiny amount of something called NaPCA, which is short for sodium pyrrolidone carboxylic acid. It is a good water-binding agent, but nothing to get excited about, and there's not enough of it in here to make this otherwise ordinary, waxy moisturizer worth considering. This product absolutely contains fragrance!

☺ **Fragrance Free Olive & Aloe Moisturizer for Extra Sensitive Skin** *($9 for 16 ounces)* contains extracts of sage, orange blossom, lavender, and fennel, and so I would hardly consider this fragrance-free, and those are all potential skin irritants. Extra-sensitive skin will be in for a shock with this emollient, though ordinary, moisturizer.

☹ **Olive & Aloe Moisturizer for Sensitive Skin** *($9 for 12 ounces)* is almost identical to the Fragrance Free Olive & Aloe version above and the same comments apply.

☹ **Honey & Calendula Moisturizer for Extra Dry Skin** *($9 for 16 ounces)* is almost identical to the Fragrance Free Olive & Aloe version above and the same comments apply.

☹ **Ultra Light Facial Creme for Normal to Oily Skin** *($10 for 4 ounces)* is a basic moisturizer for dry skin that contains a tiny amount of tea tree oil, but not enough to be effective as a disinfectant.

☹ **Vitamin A & E Moisturizer** *($9 for 12 ounces)* is a basic emollient moisturizer with a tiny amount of retinol, sold in packaging that won't keep it stable. The product claims to contain 25,000 IU of vitamin A and 5,000 IU of vitamin E, but that only adds up to about 0.1 ounce of vitamin E and far less of vitamin A.

☺ **Vitamin C & A Ultra Rich Moisturizer** *($15 for 1 ounce)* is a good emollient moisturizer for dry skin.

☺ **A, C, & E Eye Opener** *($15 for 0.5 ounce)* is a good emollient moisturizer for normal to dry skin.

☹ **Anti-Ox Facial Serum** *($15 for 1 ounce)* contains lime, lemon, and grapefruit oils, and is not recommended.

☹ **Everyday SPF 15 Moisturizer** *($12 for 11 ounces)* doesn't contain the UVA-protecting ingredients of titanium dioxide, zinc oxide, or avobenzone, and is not recommended.

☹ **Spray On Sun Block SPF 30** *($9 for 4 ounces)* doesn't contain the UVA-protecting ingredients of titanium dioxide, zinc oxide, or avobenzone, and is not recommended.

☹ **Sunswat SPF 15** *($9 for 4 ounces)* doesn't contain the UVA-protecting ingredients of titanium dioxide, zinc oxide, or avobenzone, and is not recommended.

☺ **Certified Organic Lip Balm SPF 15** *($3.50 for 0.15 ounce)* is a good, in-part titanium dioxide–based sunscreen in a very good emollient base.

☺ **Hot Spots Certified Organic Formula Sunscreen SPF 30** *($9 for 0.5 ounce)* is a good, in-part avobenzone-based sunscreen in a very good emollient base.

☺ **Instant Sunless Tanner** *($10 for 4 ounces)* contains dihydroxyacetone, the same active ingredient used in all self-tanners. It would work as well as any.

☺ **Oat Protein Sunblock SPF 18** *($9 for 4 ounces)* is a very good, titanium dioxide–based sunscreen in an emollient base for dry skin, though it does go on rather white and heavy.

☺ **Oat Protein Sunblock SPF 30** *($10 for 4 ounces)* is a good, in-part titanium dioxide–based sunscreen in a very good emollient base for normal to dry skin.

☹ **Deep Pore Cleansing Masque Normal/Oily Skin** *($10 for 2 ounces)* contains peppermint, grapefruit, clove, lemongrass, and witch hazel. Ouch!

☹ **Ester-C Serum** *($15 for 1 ounce)* does contain vitamin C, but it also contains several irritating plant extracts.

☺ **Lemongrass Souffle Masque** *($10 for 2 ounces)* is a standard clay mask with almond oil, which makes it OK for normal to slightly dry or combination skin.

☺ **Organic Botanical Lifting Serum** *($12 for 1 ounce).* The ingredients in this serum won't lift the skin anywhere, though it is a good emollient moisturizer for dry skin.

☹ **After Sun Aloe Smoother with Jewelweed and Yucca** *($6 for 4 ounces)* is 95% pure aloe, which is nice and can be soothing; however, it also includes mint oil, which can turn the soothing effect into irritation. You would be far better off with no additives and pure aloe, which is available at most health food stores. Jewelweed is often recommended for reducing complications from poison ivy; however, research has proven that jewelweed is no better than a placebo for dermatitis or topical itching.

☹ **Botanical Acne Gel** *($16 for 1.7 ounces)* contains witch hazel, peppermint oil, and camphor oil, which will only make acne worse by making skin redder and more irritated.

L'OCCITANE

With a very lush French accent and an inviting boutique that evokes an atmosphere reminiscent of southern France, L'Occitane also emanates wafting fragrances from the moment you pass through its doorway. L'Occitane started out as a fragrance company that moved on to aromatherapy and then ventured into skin care. The staples of the line are shea butter and essential oils. Shea butter is indeed a good emollient for dry skin, but it is not a cornerstone or must-have by any means, and it is a must-not for oily or combination skin types. Essential oils are lovely to inhale, but they are problematic for skin when it comes to their high risk of irritation or causing an allergic reaction. Several of the moisturizers, though basic, are OK for dry skin, but some of the sunscreens are poorly formulated and are accompanied by dangerous information such as "helps to fight harmful rays while allowing a natural suntan to develop." If you are tanning, the harmful rays of the sun are causing serious and most likely irreversible damage. There are some decent options in this line, but L'Occitane is mainly just another highly fragranced line of skin-care products, extolling their "natural" contents when they are anything but all-natural. All in all, this line seems to have very little available for what it really takes to create healthy skin for a wide range of skin types. For more information about L'Occitane, call (888) 623-2880 or visit www.loccitane.com. **Note:** All L'Occitane products are highly fragranced.

The Reviews L

☺ **Dermatological Soap** (*$10 for 3.5 ounces*) is supposed to be a gentle bar soap. It isn't alkaline, and that's good, but the cornstarch in it can be a problem for skin. There is little reason to consider this over the Dove bar cleanser available at the drugstore.

☹ **Cold Cream Soap** (*$7 for 5.3 ounces*) is a standard bar soap loaded with fragrance, and it contains mint, too, which adds to the irritation of the cleansing agents.

☺ **Refreshing and Cleansing Cloths** (*$10 for 20 cloths*) is mostly fragrance with detergent cleansing agents and some emollients. That will remove makeup, but it isn't particularly refreshing or helpful for skin.

☺ **Extra Gentle Cleansing Milk** (*$18 for 8.4 ounces*) is a plant oil–based cleanser that is more cold cream, only in lotion form. It can be an option for normal to dry skin.

☺ **Extra Gentle Cleansing Water** (*$16 for 8.4 ounces*) contains mostly fragrance, water, slip agent, detergent cleansing agents, emollient, preservatives, and more fragrance. The tiny amount of antioxidant has little benefit for skin. This will clean the skin and can be an option for someone with normal to oily skin.

☺ **Foaming Milk** (*$22 for 6.7 ounces*) is an extremely standard, detergent-based cleanser that would be an option for normal to oily skin, although the cornstarch can be a problem for the skin.

☹ **Purifying Foaming Gel** (*$21 for 8.4 ounces*) is a standard, detergent-based, water-soluble cleanser that would work well for normal to oily skin. However, the problematic plant extracts of lemon, cypress, peppermint, niaouli, and ylang-ylang give it more risks than positives.

☺ **Very Mild Cleansing Lotion** (*$20 for 8.4 ounces*) is supposed to be for sensitive skin, but this highly fragranced, wipe-off, cold cream–style cleanser is especially inappropriate for sensitive skin.

☹ **Clarifying Toner** (*$26 for 2.6 ounces*) is just water, plant extracts, fragrance, and preservatives. The plant extracts can be skin irritants, and this ends up being just too ordinary for words.

☺ **Essential Water for the Face** (*$20 for 6.7 ounces*) contains mostly water, slip agent, plant extracts, glycerin, preservatives, and fragrance. The small amount of plant extracts present can have antioxidant properties.

☹ **Lavender Vinegar** (*$15 for 5.1 ounces*) contains alcohol and camphor—ouch! The vinegar, which can also be an irritant, is incidental to the other ingredients.

☺ **100% Pure Shea Butter** (*$32.50 for 4.9 ounces*) is, as the name says, pure shea butter. That is a good emollient for dry skin, but it lacks any water-binding agents and antioxidants that would have made it add up to a much better product for dry skin.

☺ **$$$ Elixer** (*$38 for 1 ounce*) could have been a great emollient moisturizer for dry skin, but the grapefruit oil is listed high up on the ingredient list, which gives this product a potential for irritation that your skin just doesn't need.

☺ **$$$ Precious Cream** (*$35 for 1.7 ounces*) is a rather ordinary, though emollient, moisturizer for dry skin. It does contain grape seed oil, which can be a good antioxidant, but that isn't all skin needs to be healthy. State-of-the-art water-binding agents would have made this a great moisturizer.

☺ $$$ **Essential Lotion** *($32 for 1 ounce)* is similar to the Precious Cream above and the same comments apply.

☺ $$$ **Protective Lotion SPF 15** *($34 for 1 ounce)* is a very good, in-part avobenzone-based sunscreen in a lightweight lotion base that would be an option for normal to slightly dry skin. The teeny amounts of antioxidants in this product are barely worth mentioning.

☺ $$$ **Eye Balm** *($24 for 0.5 ounce)* is an OK, film-forming-agent–based lotion that contains small amounts of antioxidants and water-binding agents. The cornstarch can be a problem for skin.

☹ **Rebalancing Cream-Gel** *($21 for 1.4 ounces)* contains peppermint, lemon, and cypress, which makes it too potentially irritating for all skin types. It also contains a large amount of sunscreen (the UVB-type), but this gel doesn't have an SPF rating.

☹ **Ultra Moisturizing Daycare SPF 15** *($25 for 2.6 ounces)* doesn't contain the UVA-protecting ingredients of titanium dioxide, zinc oxide, or avobenzone, and is not recommended.

☺ $$$ **Ultra Moisturizing Night Care for Dry Skin** *($28 for 2.6 ounces)* is an OK, though exceedingly standard, emollient moisturizer for normal to dry skin.

☹ **Dry Oil Sun Care Spray SPF 8** *($25 for 8.4 ounces)* has a dismally low SPF, although it does contain avobenzone (for UVA protection), but a sunscreen needs to have both the appropriate UVA ingredients and an SPF of 15 or greater to be beneficial for skin.

☺ $$$ **Sun Block Cream SPF 30** *($21 for 2.6 ounces)* is a very good, in-part titanium dioxide–based sunscreen in an emollient moisturizing base that would be good for normal to dry skin.

☺ **High Protection Sun Lotion SPF 20** *($27 for 8.4 ounces)* is similar to the Sun Block Cream SPF 30 above only in lotion form. The same basic comments apply.

☹ **Reparative After Sun Balm** *($23 for 8.4 ounces)* is a very ordinary, though emollient, moisturizer for dry skin. The peppermint oil is irritating to skin and that is a problem for all skin types. There is nothing in this product that can repair even a minute of sun damage.

☹ **Self Tanning Cream SPF 8** *($25 for 5.2 ounces)* has a dismally low SPF, although it does contain avobenzone (for UVA protection). (A sunscreen needs to meet both UVA and UVB standards to be beneficial for sun protection.) It does contain dihydroxyacetone, the same ingredient all self-tanners use to affect the color of skin.

☹ **Clarifying and Exfoliating Face Mask** *($28 for 2.6 ounces).* The peppermint and lemon it contains make this very ordinary mask of detergent cleansing agent and a small amount of water-binding agents too irritating for all skin types.

☺ $$$ **Moisturizing Mask** *($25 for 2.6 ounces)* is a good emollient mask for dry skin that contains emollients, water-binding agents, and small amounts of antioxidants.

☺ **$$$ Soothing Exfoliating Face Mask** (*$26 for 2.6 ounces*) is a standard clay mask with plant oil, soothing agent, thickeners, and way too much fragrance. This can be an option for normal to slightly dry skin.

L'OREAL

Does anyone else think that L'Oreal's "Because I'm worth it" tag line is ingenious? Perusing the packages for all of their products, this mantra pops up everywhere, and almost subliminally reinforces not only that L'Oreal products are elite, but also that you *deserve* to use them. You owe it to yourself, you are making the right choice, and you *will* become beautiful as a result. What powerful feelings and images those four words stir! It's too bad that the slogan doesn't carry over to the majority of L'Oreal's skin-care products.

As they stand, there is little about these products that's "worth" your attention. Particularly inexcusable are several sunscreens without UVA-protecting ingredients. (L'Oreal has known for years about the issue of UVA protection. Not only do their products sold outside the United States usually contain UVA-protecting ingredients—titanium dioxide, zinc oxide, and avobenzone—but they also own a patent on Mexoryl SX, a UVA-protecting sunscreen ingredient used only outside the United States.) Their toners are almost all alcohol-based, and the moisturizers are long on fantastical claims and short on fulfillment or state-of-the-art formulations. There are a few shining stars, but you have to search for them amidst a parade of underachievers. Still, the best of L'Oreal's skin care is amazingly similar to what you will find at the Lancome counter. (L'Oreal is Lancome's parent company.) I find it amusing that, more often than not, when I compare Lancome and L'Oreal products by price it is apples to oranges. But when you examine the formulas, you'll see a rose by any other name is still a rose, even though it is being sold at the drugstore. For more information about L'Oreal, call (800) 322-2036 or visit www.lorealparisusa.com. **Note:** All L'Oreal products are highly fragranced unless noted otherwise.

L'OREAL SKIN CARE

☺ **HydraFresh Deep Cleanser Foaming Gel for Normal to Oily Skin** (*$4.99 for 6.5 ounces*) is a very good, very basic, detergent-based, water-soluble cleanser that would work well for someone with normal to oily or slightly dry skin.

☺ **HydraFresh Cleanser Foaming Cream for Normal to Dry Skin** (*$4.99 for 6.5 ounces*) is a standard, detergent-based cleanser that can be too drying for someone with normal to dry skin, but is still an option for someone with normal to oily skin.

☺ **Shine Control Foaming Face Wash with Pro-Vitamin B5** (*$5 for 6 ounces*) is virtually identical to the Hydra Fresh Cleanser Foaming Cream above, minus the plant oil. That is helpful for oily skin, but other than that, this is just a cleanser and it doesn't control shine in the least. The tiny amount of vitamin B5 in this cleanser is barely detectable.

☺ **RevitaClean Cold Cream for Dry or Maturing Skin** *($5.29 for 5 ounces)* is a mineral oil– and Vaseline–based cleanser that can be an option for dry skin, but it can leave a greasy feel on the skin. The teensy amount of retinyl palmitate (a form of vitamin A) has no effect on skin.

☺ **RevitaClean Gentle Foaming Cleanser** *($5 for 6 ounces)* is a very good, very basic, detergent-based, water-soluble cleanser that would work well for someone with normal to oily or slightly dry skin. The teeny amounts of vitamin A and sunflower oil can have little to no impact on skin.

☹ **Refreshing Eye Makeup Remover** *($4.99 for 4.2 ounces)* contains mostly water, slip agent, detergent cleansers, preservatives, and fragrance. This is a standard eye-makeup remover, though it can be more drying than most.

☺ **Turning Point Instant Facial Scrub** *($8.99 for 1.7 ounces)* is a basic scrub that uses a synthetic abrasive in a fairly emollient gel base that includes thickeners, silicone, and mineral oil. This does contain salicylic acid, but the pH is too high to let it be effective for exfoliation. This would work just fine for someone with normal to dry skin.

☹ **HydraFresh Toner** *($4.99 for 8.5 ounces)* is an alcohol-based toner with a small amount of salicylic acid (BHA). There is never a reason to use alcohol on the skin, and the pH of this toner is too high for the salicylic acid to be effective for exfoliation.

☹ **Shine Control Double-Action Toner Oil Free** *($4.99 for 8.5 ounces)* is an alcohol-based toner, and that can be drying and irritating for all skin types.

☹ **Shine Control Oil-Free Toner** *($5.99 for 4 ounces)* is similar to the Double-Action Toner above and the same comments apply.

☹ **Active Daily Moisture Lotion SPF 15, with UVA/UVB Sunscreen, for All Skin Types** *($7.39 for 4 ounces)* doesn't contain the UVA-protecting ingredients of titanium dioxide, zinc oxide, or avobenzone, and is absolutely not recommended.

☺ **Active Daily Moisture Lotion for Normal to Dry Skin** *($5.99 for 4 ounces)* is an exceptionally mediocre emollient moisturizer for dry skin.

☹ **Age Perfect Day Anti-Sagging & Rehydrating Cream SPF 15** *($15.99 for 2.5 ounces)* doesn't contain the UVA-protecting ingredients of titanium dioxide, zinc oxide, or avobenzone, and is absolutely not recommended.

☺ **Age Perfect Night Cream Anti-Sagging & Rehydrating Cream** *($15.99 for 2.5 ounces)*. While this is an OK moisturizer for dry skin there is nothing in it that can keep the skin from sagging. The skin's sagging is a function of the fat content of skin (and this isn't going to add fat to the skin), the fact that skin keeps growing (is any cream going to claim it will stop skin from growing?), and that the face muscles shift position downward (no cream can affect the position of muscles). This does contain BHA, but the pH of this product makes it ineffective for exfoliation. This also contains niacinamide, the same B-vitamin ingredient that shows up in Olay's Total Effects moisturizer and that can be a good ingredient for skin (refer to Chapter Seven, *Cosmetics Dictionary,* for details). Given how much more of the showcased niacinamide that is present in Olay's version, you would be better off with it than with this L'Oreal version.

☺ **Age Perfect Skin Illuminator & Age Spot Diffuser** *($15.99 for 2 ounces)* has a pH of 5, and that means that the exfoliating properties of the salicylic acid in this product will be ineffective. Other than that, it is just a standard moisturizer with some mica that gives it a subtle iridescent finish, but it does nothing to change the brown discolorations you may see on the back of the hand. The same comments made about niacinamide for the Anti-Sagging version above also apply here.

✔☺ **Age Perfect Anti-Sagging and Ultra-Hydrating Cream Eye** *($13.99 for 0.5 ounces)* is an emollient moisturizer for dry skin that has some interesting water-binding agents and antioxidants. It also contains wild yam extract, but that does not have any hormonal benefit for skin.

☹ **Excell A³ Alpha Hydroxy Cream SPF 8 with Triple Fruit Acid** *($11.99 for 1.7 ounces)* has an SPF that is far below the standard SPF of 15 set by the American Academy of Dermatology and the Skin Cancer Foundation. It also doesn't contain the UVA-protecting ingredients of titanium dioxide, zinc oxide, or avobenzone, and is absolutely not recommended.

☺ **Eye Defense with Liposomes** *($9.99 for 0.5 ounce)*. Liposomes are a delivery system (not an ingredient) and are capable of holding other ingredients and releasing them once the liposome is absorbed into the skin (Source: *Journal of Pharmaceutical Sciences,* March 2002, pages 615–622). However, it is helpful for there to be worthwhile ingredients like antioxidants and water-binding agents for the liposomes to deliver into the skin, elements this moisturizer doesn't contain much of.

☺ **Future E Moisture + A Daily Dose of Pure Vitamin E Normal to Dry Skin** *($8.99 for 4 ounces)* is just an OK moisturizer with small amounts of vitamin E and water-binding agent. The pH of this product is too high for the salicylic acid to be effective for exfoliation.

☺ **Future E Moisture + A Daily Dose of Pure Vitamin E Oil Free** *($9.99 for 4 ounces)* is similar to the Vitamin E Normal to Dry version above and the same basic comments apply.

☹ **Future E Moisture + A Daily Dose of Pure Vitamin E for Your Skin SPF 15 Normal to Dry Skin** *($9.99 for 4 ounces)* doesn't contain the UVA-protecting ingredients of avobenzone, titanium dioxide, or zinc oxide, and is not recommended.

☹ **Future E Moisture + A Daily Dose of Pure Vitamin E Oil Free SPF 15** *($9.99 for 4 ounces)* doesn't contain the UVA-protecting ingredients of avobenzone, titanium dioxide, or zinc oxide, and is not recommended.

☹ **HydraFresh Moisturizer for Normal to Oily Skin SPF 15** *($8.99 for 2.5 ounces)* doesn't contain the UVA-protecting ingredients of avobenzone, titanium dioxide, or zinc oxide, and is not recommended.

☹ **Hydra Fresh Mineral Charged Moisturizer for Normal to Dry Skin SPF 15** *($9.99 for 2.5 ounces)* doesn't contain the UVA-protecting ingredients of avobenzone, titanium dioxide, or zinc oxide, and is not recommended.

☺ **Hydra Fresh Circle Eraser** *($9.99 for 0.5 ounce)* is supposed to eliminate puffy circles under the eyes, but there is nothing in here (or anywhere) that can do that. The tiny amount of caffeine can't reduce swelling from overnight fluid retention or fat deposits. This is a standard emollient moisturizer with tiny amounts of water-binding agents and antioxidants.

☹ **Hydra Renewal Daily Dry Skin Cream with Pro-Vitamin B5** *($5.99 for 1.7 ounces)* is an extremely standard, emollient moisturizer for dry skin. It contains tiny amounts of vitamin E and vitamin B5, but too little to have much effect. The urea can have exfoliating and water-binding properties similar to those of an AHA product. It contains the preservative Kathon CG, which is not recommended for use in leave-on products.

☺ **Line Eraser Pure Retinol Concentrate** *($14.99 for 1 ounce)* is another product joining others on the retinol bandwagon. This one from L'Oreal is in a rather simple, but good, moisturizing base and contains about 0.25% retinol, which is the same amount as most retinol products being sold. It is good for someone with normal to dry skin. The packaging is the kind that ensures the retinol will be stable.

☹ **Line Eraser Pure Retinol Concentrate SPF 15** *($16.99 for 1.2 ounces)* doesn't contain the UVA-protecting ingredients of avobenzone, titanium dioxide, or zinc oxide, and is not recommended.

☺ **Overnight Defense** *($11.99 for 1.7 ounces)* is an OK emollient, but standard, moisturizer for dry skin.

☺ **Wrinkle Defense** *($11.99 for 1.4 ounces)* contains nothing that has any chance of defending against wrinkles. It is a simple moisturizer for dry skin, with minimal amounts of water-binding agents and antioxidants. It also contains UVB sunscreen ingredients, but is not rated with an SPF.

☺ **Revitalift Anti-Wrinkle Firming Cream with Pro-Retinol A & Par-Elastyl, for Face and Neck** *($9.99 for 1.7 ounces)*. This product does not contain retinol; rather, it contains retinyl palmitate, which is a form of vitamin A that can be an effective antioxidant, only there isn't very much of it in here. There is no such chemical or compound as par-elastyl, that is merely a marketing term L'Oreal created to make a rather basic moisturizing formula sound more exotic. It does contain sunscreen ingredients (UVB only), but is not rated with an SPF.

☺ **Revitalift Eye Anti-Wrinkle and Firming Cream** *($9.99 for 0.5 ounce)* is similar to the Face and Neck version above, and the same comments apply.

☺ **Revitalift Oil-Free Anti-Wrinkle + Firming Lotion** *($10.69 for 1.7 ounces)* is just an OK moisturizer with a rather ordinary formulation for normal to slightly dry skin.

☹ **Revitalift Complete Multi-Action Treatment SPF 18** *($11.99 for 1.7 ounces)* doesn't contain the UVA-protecting ingredients of avobenzone, titanium dioxide, or zinc oxide, and is not recommended.

☺ **Revitalift Slim Face Contouring and Toning Solution** *($10.49 for 1.7 ounces)* has a name that should at least raise your eyebrows (if not your skin), with a formulation that has mostly water and alcohol plus some silicone, glycerin, slip agents, caffeine, water-binding agent, and film-forming agent. This is one to leave on the shelf, though I suspect it will be hard to pass up given the claims that Revitalift Slim is supposed to "combat the numerous factors that affect the look and feel of aging skin. For many women over 40, that means sagging, slackening, or puffiness around the jawline and neck." The truth is that caffeine can't undo that and neither can L'Oreal's other showcased ingredient, par-elastyl. It is interesting to note that there is nothing in this product called "par-elastyl," though I suspect it refers to the soybean protein, because the L'Oreal Web site defines "par-elastyl" as being derived from vegetable protein. Any form of protein makes for a good water-binding agent, but it doesn't have special properties that make it capable of altering the shape of skin.

☺ **Visible Results Skin Renewing Moisture Treatment SPF 15 Fragrance Free** *($18.96 for 1.6 ounces)*. Finally L'Oreal has a sunscreen with UVA protection! This is a good, in-part titanium dioxide–based sunscreen in a standard emollient base that would be an option for normal to dry skin. However, this is absolutely not fragrance free; it contains lavender oil, and without question that ingredient adds fragrance.

☹ **Plenitude Turning Point Instant Facial Cream** *($11.99 for 1.7 ounces)* is similar to many moisturizers in the L'Oreal product group, yet is even more mediocre. The pH of this product isn't low enough to allow the salicylic acid to act as an effective exfoliant.

☹ **Plenitude Visible Results Skin Renewing Treatment Eye** *($16.96 for 0.42 ounces)* is a silicone-based, very mundane moisturizer that contains a bit of shimmer and little else. It contains a tiny amount of Vitamin C but nothing else of particular interest for the eye area or anywhere else on the face.

L'OREAL PURE ZONE

☹ **Pure Zone Anti-Breakout Cleanser Cream** *($7.99 for 5 ounces)* is a 2% salicylic acid cleanser in a lotion form that isn't the best for normal to oily skin, but that may possibly work for dry skin. However, the pH (over 5) is too high for the BHA to be effective as an exfoliant. It also contains menthol, and though it's probably not enough to be a problem for skin, it is a waste to have it in here at all. It does contain fragrance.

☹ **Pure Zone Anti-Breakout Cleanser Foaming** *($7.99 for 5 ounces)* is a standard, detergent-based cleanser that contains 2% salicylic acid, though the pH (over 5) isn't low enough for it to be effective as an exfoliant. It does contain small amounts of menthol and fragrance.

☹ **Pure Zone Anti-Breakout Cleanser Scrub** *($7.99 for 6.7 ounces)*, with alcohol and menthol in the mix, adds up to being more irritating than your skin bargained for. The pH of this product makes the salicylic acid ineffective. It does contain fragrance.

☹ **Pure Zone Skin Relief Oil Free Moisturizer** *($7.99 for 2.5 ounces)* is an interesting option for a "moisturizer." This silicone-based, 0.6% salicylic acid lotion is mostly water, silicone, glycerin, clay, thickeners, preservatives, and fragrance. It will leave a matte feel on skin and the 0.6% solution would be suitable for someone with normal to dry skin and minimal problems with breakouts. However, the pH of 5 makes the salicylic acid ineffective for exfoliation.

☹ **Pure Zone Pore Tightening Astringent** *($7.99 for 6.7 ounces)* lists alcohol as the second ingredient, which makes it too irritating and drying for all skin types. That is unfortunate as this is the only salicylic acid product in the Pure Zone group (all of these contain it) that has a pH of 3.5 and is, therefore, an effective exfoliant.

☹ **Pure Zone Spot Check** *($7.99 for 0.5 ounce)* is similar to the Tightening Astringent above and the same comments apply.

L'OREAL MAKEUP

L'Oreal's extensive makeup collection has evolved into something spectacular. The foundations have not only shown improved textures and smoother than ever applications, but the color range is also (slowly) improving. There are still a fair number of peach and pink shades to watch out for (Lancome's foundations still offer superior colors), but the effort is being made. The rest of the makeup offers a series of pleasant surprises, from superior concealers to silky powder blushes, superior eyelining options, and some of the best-performing mascaras available at the drugstore or anywhere else for that matter. You will also find L'Oreal's lipsticks are competing every step of the way with Lancome's lip formulas, for only one-third the price. Turning this line around was no short order, but category for category L'Oreal's makeup has now become the most reliable line at the drugstore. If their foundations followed Revlon's lead and featured effective sunscreens, and the eyeshadows were improved, it would be almost impossible to resist.

FOUNDATION: ☺ **Ideal Balance Balancing Foundation for Combination Skin** *($11.99)* is another foundation claiming to moisturize dry areas while keeping shine in check over oily ones. Considering the number of women who readily identify with the combination skin profile, it's not surprising that products with promises to reconcile the demands of that two-part condition keep appearing. Despite the name, this makeup is not capable of balancing anything, though the slightly thick, noticeably silky texture glides on and feels smooth. This has a soft matte finish that won't hold back excess oil for long—you can almost sense the moisture in the formula at war with an army of dry-finish ingredients. Overall, this formula is best for someone with normal to slightly oily skin, because it's matte enough to look unflattering over any dry or flaky patches. If you decide to try this, the best almost-neutral shades from the assortment of 12 colors are Soft Beige, Beige, Buff, Tan, Caramel, and Cappuccino (the last two are excellent for dark skin tones). The remaining colors are unabashedly pink or peach. **AirWear Breathable Long-Wearing Foundation SPF 14** *($11.99)* has a wonderfully light, ultra-silky texture and a soft powdery finish that would make it a good choice for someone with normal to oily skin seeking light to medium coverage. Regrettably, the sunscreen does not contain any UVA-protecting agents, but if you're willing to wear a sunscreen underneath this, it is worth considering. The range of nine shades is mostly impressive, with choices for light

The Reviews L

to dark (but not very dark) skin tones. The only shades to consider avoiding are Cream (pink) and Caramel (may be too golden orange for some skin tones). By the way, there is absolutely nothing in this formula that provides oxygen to the skin, which is actually good news, because oxygen triggers free-radical damage and that's why "antioxidants" (think anti-oxygen) are good for skin. **AirWear Breathable Long-Wearing Powder Foundation SPF 17** *($11.69)* is a soft, smooth-textured, talc-based powder foundation that applies and blends nicely, affording sheer to light coverage. Typically of L'Oreal, this pressed-powder foundation doesn't contain the UVA-protecting ingredients of titanium dioxide, zinc oxide, or avobenzone. But, sun-protection gripes aside, the six available colors are all very good, especially Tan and Caramel, which are good shades for darker skin tones. **Quick Stick Long Wearing Foundation SPF 14** *($10.99)* is a reasonably smooth stick foundation that includes a titanium dioxide sunscreen, and an SPF that's almost to the benchmark of SPF 15. The smooth application dries to a solid, unmovable, difficult-to-remove matte base. If matte, full coverage is what you're after, this one would be an option. One caution: This has a strong silicone base that absolutely does not blend over a silicone-based moisturizer or especially over a silicone serum. The formula works best for normal to oily skin. There are 12 shades to consider, but 5 are a problem for most skin tones: Soft Ivory, Nude Beige, Buff, Golden Beige, and Cocoa are all too pink or peach. There are, however, some good choices for dark skin tones. **Visible Lift Line Minimizing Makeup SPF 12** *($10.29)* has made a dismaying switch to octyl methoxycinnamate as its only active sun-protecting ingredient—so this is no longer a sufficient option as a foundation with sunscreen. However, it does have a silky texture that melds with the skin and dries to a soft matte finish. Coverage runs from light to medium and despite the fact that the target market for this is women with dry skin, the non-emollient formula is best for normal to oily skin. The antiwrinkle claims surrounding this one are dubious. It can help to smooth out skin to some degree, but that is the nature of most foundation applications. There are 15 shades to consider, including options for very light skin tones. The following shades should be avoided by most skin tones: Pale, Buff, Creamy Natural, Golden Beige, Sand Beige, Sun Beige (just slightly peach), Cocoa, and Cappuccino. The other shades are worth testing, but what a shame the sunscreen has been downgraded. **Feel Naturale Compact Light Softening One-Step Makeup SPF 15** *($11.29)* is a very good cream-to-powder makeup that has a wonderfully smooth, creamy application and a soft, slightly matte finish along with phony claims that it can manipulate light to create flawless skin. The duality of this type of makeup is that it's creamy enough to slip into any lines on the face and at the same time powdery enough to exaggerate any dry, flaky skin. Normal to slightly dry skin would fare best with this. Although the label makes the ubiquitous "oil-free" claim, this does have waxes that will likely aggravate the situation for those prone to breakouts. If you thought the sunscreen had adequate UVA protection, you don't know L'Oreal. Strangely, a few of the darkest shades do not list *any* SPF or active ingredients.

The 12 shades feature some remarkably neutral choices; the ones to avoid are Sand Beige, Golden Beige, Buff (can be too peach), Soft Ivory (slightly pink), Sun Beige (too peach), and Cocoa (ashy red).

☺ **Translucide Naturally Luminous Makeup SPF 18** *($11.99)* has a fantastic texture that's easy to blend to a soft matte finish with light to medium coverage, and contains the smallest amount of vitamin C imaginable. The nine shades available (with nothing for very light or dark skin tones) weigh in a bit too heavily on the peach or pink side, although they may still work for some skin tones. The following shades should be considered with caution: Soft Ivory, Nude Beige, Natural Beige, Caramel Beige, and Cappuccino. As expected, the sunscreen is incomplete when it comes to UVA protection. **Visible Lift Extra Coverage Line Minimizing Makeup SPF 12** *($10.29)* does not contain adequate UVA protection, though you may notice that titanium dioxide is listed as the third ingredient on the regular ingredient listing. However, if it is not listed as "active ingredient," that doesn't count for UVA protection. Despite the sun-protection problems, this silky, creamy formula lives up to its extra-coverage claim. The finish is natural matte, making this a good choice for someone with normal to slightly dry skin who is willing to wear a separate sunscreen underneath. There are nine shades available, but almost all of them are too peach or pink and they look incredibly artificial given the opaque nature of this foundation. The only contenders are Nude Beige, Natural Beige, and Golden Beige. **Feel Naturale Makeup SPF 15** *($10.99)* has no reliable UVA protection and the application might make you want to sing Paul Simon's "Slip Slidin' Away," but the sheer-coverage, light-matte finish, and improved selection of colors make this a possibility for normal skin willing to pair this with an effective sunscreen. Oily skin won't enjoy the slickness of this product. Of the 12 shades, the ones to leave on the shelf include Pale, Nude Beige, Sand Beige, Buff, and Cappuccino.

☹ **Mattique Oil-Free Matte Makeup** *($8.79)* is L'Oreal's oldest foundation, and compared to their latest creations this is subpar. The fairly matte texture is accompanied by a slightly sticky feel, which someone with oily skin might not like. As for the nine colors, with the possible exception of Nude Beige, all are too peach or pink to recommend.

CONCEALER: ☺ ✓**AirWear Long-Wearing Concealer** *($9.89)* is a smooth, silicone-based concealer that glides on and covers well without looking heavy or thick. It has a crease-free matte finish that is a pleasure to blend, and it layers beautifully for areas that need more intense camouflage. Of the six colors, avoid Corrector (too yellow), Brightener (too pink), and Deep (may turn ash on some darker skin tones). ✓☺ **Visible Lift Line Minimizing Concealer** *($9.99)* has an elegant, creamy application that dries to a soft matte finish and it doesn't crease into the lines around the eyes. It is very similar to Lancome's ever-popular Effacernes Concealer ($21), check it out for yourself. The four skin-tone shades are beautiful, though Medium-Deep won't work very well for darker skin tones. Avoid the overly yellow Neutralizer and white Lightener shades. If you want to test the line-minimizing claim, use this concealer around one eye and leave the other

The Reviews L

bare. Now tell me which side has fewer apparent lines, the one with the concealer has more lines, right?

☺ **Feel Naturale Concealer** *($7.69)* has a lot of initial slip, so keeping the coverage where you want it can be a challenge. This dries to a soft matte finish and provides decent sheer-to-medium coverage without creasing. The three shades are workable, but Deep may be too peach for some skin tones. **Cover Expert Exact Match Concealer** *($8.99)* features two cream-to-powder concealers in one pot. You can use the light or dark shade as needed, or blend them to create the closest match. The color combinations are very good, but there are only two duos available, with nothing for light or dark skin tones. Those who fall in the happy medium will be pleased with the colors and will find that this one has a smooth, silky texture reminiscent of Lancome's Photogenic Concealer. The formula is easy to apply, blends very well, and provides excellent coverage for dark circles or other imperfections.

POWDER: ☺ **Visible Lift Line Minimizing Powder** *($11.99)* is a translucent, talc-based powder with a silky, very sheer finish that has a hint of sparkling shine. It won't diminish one line on your face, but it nicely sets makeup and could work for all skin types. All but one of the shades is excellent, just avoid Colour Lift, a pink tone that no one should be dusting all over their face. **Feel Naturale Ultrafine Light Softening Powder SPF 15** *($11.59)* has been reformulated numerous times, and this latest version provides an undeniably silky texture and superior application. Sunscreen-wise, this misses the mark for UVA protection, but is still a great pressed-powder option. Of the three shades, Deep is the only dud. **On the Loose Shimmering Powder** *($5.99)* comes in small pots and creates an intense, though smooth, application of shiny powder. This wins major points for its superior ability to cling to the skin. For evening, it's an option, and will give you the appropriate glittering shine everyone else seems to be wearing. I would suggest avoiding the orange Five Alarm and blue Diva Down unless your music video is in heavy rotation on MTV. ✔☺ **Translucide Naturally Luminous Powder** *($9.89)* is a talc-free loose powder that has a marvelous, powdered-sugar texture and a smooth, even finish. It feels like silk on the skin and comes in four shades, of which only Deep is a bit too coppery for most darker skin tones. This fragranced powder is perfect for those who hate to look powdered but want to look polished.

BLUSH: ✔☺ **Feel Naturale Light Softening Blush** *($10.99)* is a great collection of blushes with beautiful colors, textures, and an application that is strikingly similar to Lancome's Blush Subtil ($25.50). It should suit all skin types very well. The following shades are quite shiny, and best for evening, if at all: Charmed Peach, Mauvelous, Mocha Rose, and Plume. ☺ **Translucide Luminous Gel Blush** *($9.49)* is an interesting option for a sheer, tinted-gel blush. The six shades range from barely to moderately shiny finishes, but each blends out exceptionally sheer to almost no color at all. The application is wet-feeling and then dries to a matte (in feel) finish. It would be hard to make a mistake with this one, since the color is so soft, yet it takes patience to blend it on and wait for it to dry; and if you want noticeable color, it can take a lot of trouble to build up much intensity. Still, this minimalist blush does have its purposes.

☺ **Cheek to Cheek Sculpting Blush Duet** *($9.89)* is a dual-sided powder blush that offers a light and medium blush tone for highlighting and "sculpting" the face. This has a smooth, but slightly too-thick, texture. Application can be spotty or it can go on too sheer, requiring repeated applications to build anything close to sculpture! Besides, the best way to sculpt (read: contour) the face is with a matte, tan-brown or golden brown color. The Blissful Bronzes shade comes close, but is too soft to adequately contour. **Blush Delice Sheer Powder Blush** *($7.99)* may be sheer when it comes to color impact, but not when it comes to shine. This is one of the shiniest blushes at the drugstore! Wearing any one of the five shades is more about adding iridescence over color, but if that's your goal or you have a disco night planned, this smooth blush won't disappoint. **Touch-On Colour Lips, Eyes, Cheeks** *($9.89)* shares the same general comments as the Blush Delice above, only this has a slightly grainy cream-to-powder texture and softer (but still quite shiny) colors. This does not feel great over the lips, and the colors are a bit too harsh for the eye.

☺ **EYESHADOW: Wear Infinite Long-Wearing Silky Powder Eyeshadow** *($3.79 singles, $4.69 duos, $6.59 quads)* are a reformulation of L'Oreal's former Soft Effects eyeshadows. The colors are still divided into perle (noticeably shiny) and matte (true matte to subtle shine) finishes, but the color selection has improved. For example, there are a number of viable options among the quads, though (with the exception of Wood Rose) each one has at least one shiny shade. The formula is very silky, but also very sheer and almost waxy-feeling. Don't count on anything close to infinite wear from these, but for very soft color and easy application, they'll do. The best matte Singles to consider are Sable, Bark, Chocolat, Raven, and Sand. From the Duos, only Classic Khakis is matte. **Colour Fresco Refreshing Creme Eyeshadow** *($6.59)* is a twist-up, cream-to-powder eyeshadow that has a cool, wet feel and glides on almost too well. It dries to a powder finish and tends not to smudge, which is nice. Application can be tricky because these colors are all shiny and tend to go on strong, which can make blending an even trickier proposition. They will need to be softened quickly unless a bold stripe of shimmery color is your goal.

EYE AND BROW SHAPER: ✓☺ **Line Intensifique Extreme Wear Liquid Liner** *($7.89)* is an outstanding liquid liner that is relatively easy to apply (for liquid liner) and it holds up well—no smearing, chipping, or flaking all day long. The brush is almost too flexible, but it does work well. Give this a try if you're a fan of Lancome's Artliner ($25).

☺ **Super Liner Perfect Tip Eyelining Pen** *($7.19)* must have been tweaked, because now it is almost as good as the newer Line Intensifique. This has an identical brush and equally good application, but doesn't quite have the latter's extra long wear. **Wear Infinite Silky Powder Eye Liner** *($6.89)* is a standard pencil that has a swift, smooth application and a reliable powder finish. If you prefer pencils, this is one to consider, as it is less likely to smudge or fade than many others. However, the color selection is mostly shiny, and there are several hues that are inappropriate for lining the eyes, unless you're going for all-out techno-glamour or are auditioning for the role of Cleopatra. **Le Grande Kohl Line and Define Pencil** *($6.79)* is an extra-long standard pencil very reminiscent of Lancôme's Le Crayon Kohl ($18). This applies smoothly without being greasy and blends well without streaking. Many of the colors have shine, but Black Sable and Onyx are safe bets. **Brow Stylist Sculpting Brow Mascara** *($7.49)* is a very good, sheer brow tint that features a dual-sided brush with long and short bristles, a feature that makes this type of product useful in grooming and defining both full (think Brooke Shields) and sparse or thin (Bette Davis) brows. There are two colors plus a Clear version, and all are options for subtle brow enhancement.

☺ **Pencil Perfect Automatic Eye Liner** *($6.79)* isn't what I would call perfect; if anything, it tends to go on creamier than most, and that means a greater risk of smearing. As a plus, it doesn't need sharpening. **Eye Smoker Line and Shadow Crayon** *($8.39)* is a chubby pencil that goes on creamy, and also features shiny colors. It has the odd quality of smudging in place rather than smearing, but I suppose that's the intended effect. **Brow Colourist Colour and Highlighting Pencil** *($8.39)* is a standard, slightly creamy brow pencil that is not preferred to the Brow Powderist described below. There is a shiny highlighting powder eyeshadow at the other end of the pencil that isn't really necessary, but I suppose it adds some appeal to this otherwise ho-hum pencil. **Brow Powderist Redefining Powder** *($7.29)* is a sheer, dry-textured brow powder that includes two coordinating colors in one compact. The colors are suitable and allow for a custom match, though each has an understated shine. The powder has a tendency to flake unless you are diligent about knocking all of the excess off the brush before applying. That means the final result will take longer, but the flaking should be minimal. The brush that comes with this is terrible and should be discarded immediately.

☹ **Lineur Intense Defining Liquid Liner** *($7.19)* is a traditional liquid liner that goes on like the name says—intense—but compared to the Line Intensifique above, this takes too long to dry and smudges before the day is done.

<u>**LIPSTICK AND LIP PENCIL:**</u> ☺ **Endless Comfortable 8-Hour LipColour** *($7.89)* is remarkably similar to Lancôme's Rouge Attraction Lipcolour ($20). Both share the same lightweight, creamy-smooth texture and selection of opaque, mostly iridescent colors. Perhaps most telling is that both use the same technology. L'Oreal refers to theirs as "Soft-Seal," while Lancôme calls it "StayPut." Either way, if you're curious to test the long-wear claims, your financial bottom line will be better if you start with L'Oreal's version, and don't count on either the long-wear or "stay put" claim working out. It's just a lightweight, softly creamy lipstick with more marketing finesse than technological flair. **Endless Comfortable 8-Hour Liquid LipColour** *($7.89)* is a semi-opaque liquid lip gloss that feels extra light and has a glossy, smooth finish. This silicone-based product has a good stain, but will last eight hours only if you refrain from eating, drinking, or speaking

too much! Otherwise, expect to touch this up about as often as a creamy lipstick. **Shine Delice Sheer Shimmering LipColour** *($6.99)* is a slick, glossy lipstick that comes in a marvelous selection of colors that aren't all that sheer. This is perfect for subdued lipstick, but the fragrance is intense. **Colour Endure Stay On LipColour** *($9.39)* is similar to Revlon's ColorStay, except L'Oreal's tends to wear better without chipping. Both go on matte, and stay in place. However, regardless of the claims about not feeling dry there is no emollient feel to this at all. The color selection has been reduced somewhat, but the choices are still numerous for fans of ultra-matte lipsticks. **HydraSoft Deeply Softening LipColour SPF 12** *($10.39)* doesn't contain UVA protection, but it is a very good, standard, glossy lipstick in a slim container. This one has no distinct advantage over dozens of other creamy, sheer lipsticks. If anything, Revlon and Almay have the edge when it comes to lipsticks with effective sunscreens.

✓☺ **Colour Riche Rich Creamy LipColour** *($7.19)* is rich in every way except price, which is a boon for you! This decadently creamy lipstick offers intense colors that have admirable staying power, though it is creamy enough to slip into lines around the mouth. You will find this to be almost identical to Lancome's Rouge Sensation LipColour ($19.50), right down to the fragrance. ✓☺ **Colour Riche Crystal Shine LipColour** *($7.19)* is identical to the Colour Riche lipstick above, only these shades are infused with loads of iridescence for ultra-sparkly lips. ✓☺ **Rouge Pulp Anti-Feathering Lip Liner** *($8.49)* is an automatic, nonretractable pencil that comes in six very good shades and really is impressive at keeping lipstick in place. This is a keeper! ✓☺ **Glass Shine High Shine Lip Gloss** *($7.99)* is a standard, non-sticky lip gloss that comes in an aluminum tube reminiscent of Stila's popular Lip Gloss ($17). Most of the gorgeous shades offer semi-opaque color and a slight stain, but it's still gloss, so be prepared for frequent touch-ups.

☺ **Rouge Pulp Liquid Lipcolour** *($8.39)* is the precursor to Glass Shine, and remains a fine, non-sticky, wand-type lip gloss that includes some vivid, splashy colors. This is not as glossy as the High Shine Lip Gloss above. **Colour Riche Rich Creamy Lipliner** *($7.19)* is a standard, twist-up, retractable pencil that has a built-in sharpener. The sharpener part isn't necessary given the finer point that most twist-up pencils like this one already have, plus after one use the shavings clog in the sharpener and that's that. The application is smooth and creamy, and the available colors are versatile. **Crayon Petite Automatic Lip Liner** *($6.89)* is a standard twist-up lip pencil that is definitely creamier than most and offers some good colors, including a Clear version. **Lip Duet Lip Liner and Colour Crayon** *($8.89)* gives you a standard lipliner and lip color in one thick, dual-sided pencil. This has the edge over other crayon-type lipsticks due to its smooth application, well-coordinated colors, and non-greasy finish. If this concept appeals to you, this version won't disappoint.

<u>MASCARA:</u> ✓☺ **Lash Intensifique Lash by Lash Body Building Mascara** *($6.69)* is indeed intense, and is dramatically similar to Lancome's Amplicils ($20). Both go on quite heavily, and build admirable length and copious thickness. Clumping can be a

The Reviews L

problem if this is applied too eagerly, and the large brush may be a problem for getting to those hard-to-reach lashes—yet for lash impact, this should be on your short list of contenders! ✔☺ **Lash Intensifique Curved Brush Mascara** *($6.69)* is identical to the Lash by Lash Body Building Mascara above, only the curved brush allows you to create maximum impact a bit faster. ✔☺ **Lash Intensifique Waterproof Mascara** *($6.69)* is way above average for waterproof mascara. This builds remarkable length, lift, and curl while keeping your lashes at their best through tears or a swim. ✔☺ **Lash Architect 3-D Dramatic Mascara** *($7.49, straight or curved brush)* is amazing mascara! Talk about long, thick lashes. With just a few strokes you can actually look like you're wearing false eyelashes. As enthusiastic as I am about this one, there is one downside: It can be clumpy and uneven, and has a tendency to flake (though not smear) during the day, especially if you over-apply, which is easy to do because it builds length so fast. If your goal is ample length with thickness, then the Lash Intensifique above is the way to go. ✔☺ **Le Grand Curl** *($7.39)* is still one of the best mascaras that goes on well without clumping, holds up through the entire day, remains smear-free, and, oh yes, lengthens and thickens with ease. It will lift and curl as you apply it, but that is the nature of any good mascara, and this is no exception. ✔☺ **Le Grand Curl Waterproof Mascara** *($5.99)* builds fantastic length, lift, and curl. You lose some thickness, but that's the sacrifice with most waterproof mascaras, and this one does not give in when lashes get wet.

☺ **Superior Longitude Extreme Lengthening Mascara** *($9.29)* isn't what I would consider extreme, especially after trying the cream of L'Oreal's mascara crop above. However, this does lengthen without much effort and builds subtle thickness. It lasts all day without flaking, but can smear slightly during application. **Lash Out Curved Brush** *($5.99)* has a better brush than the original Lash Out mascara below, and that enables you to build a touch more length with a softer, cleaner separation. Thickness is not in this mascara's bag of tricks, but if that's not what you need or prefer, this is fine. **Voluminous Volume Building Mascara** *($6.69, straight or curved brush)* remains a superior lengthening mascara, but it doesn't build the same thickness or create the same all-out drama that it did before. It doesn't clump or smear, however, and it does hold up beautifully throughout the day. **Voluminous Mascara Curved Brush** *($5.99)* is nearly identical to the Volume Building version above, only this goes to great lengths faster, thanks to a longer-bristled brush.

☺ **Lash Out Lengthening and Separating Mascara** *($5.99)*. Given the enticing name, this isn't too impressive. It's OK, but not on a par with L'Oreal's best. Lash Out does lengthen well, but as it separates the lashes it also tends to stick them together, which can create long lashes with sparse body. **Longitude Lash Out Extra Lengthening Waterproof Mascara** *($5.99)* is just a very mediocre mascara that can take up to 15 coats before you see much length or thickness, and even then the results are mediocre. It does hold up underwater, but unless you're willing to settle for less, skip this one in favor of Le Grand Curl Waterproof above for best results. **FeatherLash Softly Sweeping Mascara** *($6.19)* ends up being a patchy application of mascara that builds uneven length and minimal thickness. It won't smear and doesn't clump, which is great, but the payoff is not what I have come to expect from a L'Oreal mascara. Still, for minimal lash enhancement, it works. **FeatherLash Mascara Curved Brush** *($6.19)* has the same traits as the original FeatherLash, but the brush makes it easier to apply an even, sheer layer for barely defined lashes. **FeatherLash Water Resistant Mascara** *($6.19)* is marginally adept at lengthening, but gets a thumbs-down for thickness. It goes on easily, with no globs or clumps, but be prepared to work for anything more than a subtle effect. What's best about this mascara is that lashes stay soft to the touch and the formula nicely resists water, yet is easily removed with a water-soluble cleanser. **Voluminous Waterproof Mascara** *($5.99)* is rather lackluster when compared to the waterproof Le Grand Curl and (especially) Lash Intensifique mascaras, but it does the job with noticeable length and definition, plus it holds up underwater.

LA MER

What can $530 buy you? It can buy you a night out on the town, including limo, dinner for two, and a nice dress. Or you can decide to spend it on three pairs of really nice designer shoes. Another option is a rather elegant designer necklace, earring, and bracelet set. Or if you were someone who is seduced by distorted cosmetics advertising, you could waste your money on four or five skin-care products from the La Mer line.

The original Creme de la Mer was launched by Estee Lauder as a miracle product for wrinkles based on research from Max Huber, a NASA scientist. How does space technology relate to wrinkles? Well, it doesn't. Huber at one time suffered severe burns in an accident and then, according to the Max Huber Laboratories, it took 12 years and 6,000 experiments to come up with the cream, "which he made through an arcane and lengthy process." That was over 30 years ago. Of course, given that none of this self-experimentation was ever documented, there is no way to know what Huber was using before or what else could have produced whatever results he was so happy about.

It turns out that Creme de la Mer was, and still is, almost exclusively water, thickening agents, and some algae. But this miracle product wasn't enough, at least not for the Lauder company, which was selling a lot of products and clearly understood that, in the world of skin care, if one product sounds good women will buy other unrelated products that carry the same name. With the expanded range of La Mer products, Estee Lauder has added a slew of hocus-pocus ingredients to the continuing list of concoctions that were never in Huber's original formula; so much for that mythic story having any real credibility. These supplementary products contain powdered silver, diamond dust, something called declustered water, and a semiprecious stone, tourmaline, that is supposed to have magnetic properties. Wow! It's almost too outlandish to even begin explaining, but I'll do my best. And do keep in mind that if these products were the be-all and end-all for the Estee Lauder company, why is it selling all those other products it makes for the dozen or so other lines it owns just around the counter or next door?

The Reviews L

Supposedly, the La Mer products are worth the money because some of them contain magnetized tourmaline, colloidal silver, and declustered water. Declustered water is water manufactured to have smaller ions, which supposedly makes the water penetrate the skin better. There is no proof that this synthetic water does what the company claims, but even if the water could penetrate better, is that better for skin? There is definitely research indicating that too much water in the skin can make it plump, but that could also prevent cell turnover and renewal, and inhibit the skin's immune response. Either way, the skin likes taking on water—it plumps to a thousand times its normal size just from taking a bath—and it doesn't need help to do any more, nor would that be good for skin in the long run.

Tourmaline does have unique electrical properties and is used in some machinery to control the direction of light. While that might sound like it can throw light away from the face, it doesn't change the appearance of wrinkles. After all, it would take a great deal of lighting (take it from someone who has been involved with fashion photography makeup) to hide wrinkles, and then you would still need to digitally improve the picture and erase the wrinkles. Even if this ingredient could have that effect, in a cleanser the tourmaline would just be wiped or rinsed away. The other claim is that this magnetized crystal somehow attracts the iron in blood and helps pull the blood to the surface. I won't get into the argument about the issue of magnets for sports injuries (which, from the research I've seen, is bogus), but for the face, if the tourmaline could have that effect, that could cause too much blood flow to tiny capillaries and the risk of them appearing on the surface of the skin.

As for the colloidal silver, that simply refers to ground-up silver being suspended in solution. Silver can have disinfecting properties, but prolonged contact with it can be irritating to skin and even turn skin grayish blue. That can't help erase wrinkles, heal skin, or provide any benefit. Silver is better worn as jewelry, though if you are allergic to silver you will be allergic to the silver in this product as well.

The other gimmicky ingredients include fish cartilage, algae (explained in the Creme de la Mer review below), minerals (copper, sodium, calcium, quartz), and other forms of algae. While all of these may have some water-binding properties (all except the minerals, which have little benefit for skin care and are barely present in these formulations), the fiction that any of them could have an impact on wrinkles is not substantiated in any published scientific study.

For more information about La Mer, call (212) 572-4200 or visit www.neiman marcus.com or www.elcompanies.com. **Note:** All La Mer products contain fragrance.

LA MER SKIN CARE

☺ $$$ **The Cleansing Lotion** (*$65 for 6.7 ounces*). Supposedly, this milky emulsion derives its remarkable cleansing powers from magnetized tourmaline, colloidal silver, and declustered water, but see the comments in the introductory paragraphs above for an explanation about this bravado. What you can most certainly expect is a standard, wipe-off cleanser for dry skin that is not all that different from Neutrogena's Extra Gentle Cleanser (for a fraction of the price).

☺ $$$ **The Cleansing Gel** *($65 for 6.7 ounces)* is an exceptionally standard, detergent-based cleanser that would be an option for normal to oily skin. But at this price, can anyone's skin feel better? The tiny amount of silver in here can be a skin irritant.

☹ **The Mist** *($75 for 6.7 ounces)* contains a eucalyptus extract, which is a skin irritant. It would have been a good toner without that irritant, but the price is a joke given the basic ingredients and the small amounts of antioxidants.

☹ **The Oil Absorbing Tonic** *($60 for 6.7 ounces)* is a toner that contains mostly alcohol, and, at any price, much less for this amount of money, that's an irritation for skin.

☺ $$$ **The Tonic** *($60 for 6.7 ounces)* would be a good, though average, toner for most skin types—that is, if the price doesn't get you first. It also has declustered water, colloidal gold, and sea plant extracts. While that keeps with the ocean theme and may have some antioxidant properties for skin, it still doesn't warrant the price tag. After all, we're talking about algae and seaweed. The gold can be a contact allergen, but probably not when present in such a small amount, which is not enough to create a ring for an ant.

☹ **Creme de la Mer** *($165 for 2 ounces; $1,000 for 16 ounces)* is the original product created by Max Huber, as described above in the introduction for La Mer. As enticing as this dramatic story sounds, the reality is that this very basic cream doesn't contain anything particularly extraordinary or unique, unless you want to believe that seaweed extract (sort of like seaweed tea) can in some way heal burns and scars. Even if it could, burns and scars don't have much to do with wrinkling, and this product is now being sold as a wrinkle cream. According to Susan Brawley, professor of plant biology at the University of Maine, "Seaweed extract isn't a rare, exotic, or expensive ingredient. Seaweed extract is readily available and [is] used in everything from cosmetics to food products and medical applications." Creme de la Mer contains mostly seaweed extract, mineral oil, Vaseline, glycerin, waxlike thickening agents, plant oils, plant seeds, minerals, vitamins, more thickeners, and preservatives. This rather standard moisturizer contains some good antioxidants (but for the money, a surprisingly small amount), but these ingredients are also found in many other moisturizers that cost a *lot* less. This also contains a eucalyptus extract that can be a skin irritant, as well as Kathon CG, a preservative that is recommended for use only in rinse-off products.

☺ $$$ **Serum de la Mer** *($175 for 1 ounce).* You would think that for $165 the original Creme de la Mer above would be enough, but no, it now takes more, because this product is supposed to prepare your face for the Creme. This is a very good lightweight moisturizer for normal to dry skin with some good water-binding agents and antioxidant, but the price, even if fish cartilage was something special, is just unwarranted.

☺ $$$ **Eye Balm** *($95 for 0.5 ounce).* The miraculous claims about this moisturizer go on and on. It is a good moisturizer for normal to dry skin, but the benefits of fish cartilage and malachite are up to you to decide, because there is no research showing them to be worth this kind of investment for skin. What should give you something to think about is the inclusion of a eucalyptus extract and mint, which are unnecessary and potentially irritating. This is otherwise an emollient moisturizer with some good antioxidants and water-binding agents.

☺ $$$ **The SPF 18 Fluid** *($50 for 1 ounce)* is a good, in-part avobenzone-based sunscreen in a rather standard emollient base that would be an option for normal to dry skin. Remember, you have to use sunscreen liberally to gain the SPF benefit. How liberally are you going to apply this product when it would take a couple of jars a month or more if used properly?

☹ $$$ **Moisturizing Lotion** *($140 for 1.7 ounces)* would make a good moisturizer for dry skin, though the price is just bizarre. However, what makes this product not good for skin is the inclusion of lime and eucalyptus extract, which are potentially irritating and sensitizing for all skin types.

☹ $$$ **Oil Absorbing Lotion** *($140 for 6.7 ounces)* uses a film-forming agent, like most lotions with oil-absorbing claims do. Oh, it still has the algae and water-binding agents, but like the Moisturing Lotion above, it also includes irritating ingredients that are not helpful for skin.

☺ $$$ **Refining Facial** *($75 for 3.4 ounces)* is a relatively standard clay mask. The sea stuff is in here, as are tourmaline and diamond powder. If you feel that scrubbing with microscopic amounts of gemstones (and then rinsing them down the drain) is the way to go, then nothing I can say about this marketing gimmick is going to deter you.

☹ $$$ **The Lip Balm** *($40 for 0.32 ounce)* could have been a very good, albeit expensive, Vaseline-based lip balm with some very good water-binding agents and antioxidants, but it contains a eucalyptus extract that can be a skin irritant.

LA MER MAKEUP

It should come as no surprise that La Mer's makeup collection, called SkinColor, features products that carry the same "do you believe in miracles?" claims that the rest of the ever-expanding line espouses. Isn't it funny that not long ago all you needed (according to the company) was the original Creme de la Mer to achieve skin-care nirvana—and today there is a whole collection of products that supposedly enhance and "work intuitively with" the Creme de la Mer? For a small fortune, you can now leave the La Mer counter with not only skin-care products, but also foundation, concealer, and powder. The prices are outlandish, the claims are extraordinary, and although the makeup products are indeed impressive, they are not the revolutionary breakthrough they're made out to be.

The concept behind La Mer SkinColor revolves around using bioluminescent sea proteins and gemstones to "create and capture light energy … that provides protective green light antioxidant benefits" to the skin. Taking the concept of color and light to a new plateau seems to be the goal of La Mer, as they maintain that "the full spectrum of colored light from gemstones in tandem with colored light from transparent micronized pigments [creates] a whole new translucent color palette—visibly correcting imperfections while adding dimension and life to the skin." Estee Lauder (owner of the La Mer line) uses similar claims for their own LightSource moisturizers and Lauder-owned Aveda is big on gemstones, too, or at least tourmaline. Although there is not a shred of published research pointing to sea proteins and gemstones capturing and harnessing light energy for skin, if you buy into these assertions, you can consider the considerably less expensive options from Lauder and Aveda before taking out a second mortgage in order to outfit your vanity or makeup case with all things La Mer.

☺ $$$ **The Foundation SPF 15** *($65)* has a light, undeniably silky-smooth texture and provides even, light to medium coverage with a soft matte finish, making this a contender for those with normal to slightly oily or slightly dry skin. It is almost identical to Estee Lauder's Equalizer Makeup SPF 10, though Lauder's sunscreen includes titanium dioxide. This La Mer foundation banks on the supposition that its buzz ingredients will offset the fact that it does not contain adequate UVA protection. Sixty-five dollars and you'll still need a separate sunscreen! There are eight shades available, with no options for very dark skin. The majority of shades are beautiful—only Sunswept Beige (too pink) and Drift Bisque (peach) should be considered with caution.

☺ $$$ **The Concealer** *($50)* comes in a squeeze tube and has a creamy-smooth texture that spreads easily over skin and offers medium to full coverage with a soft matte finish. This poses minimal risk of creasing, and the eight shades nicely complement the foundation colors. Sunswept Beige is slightly peach and Sunset Bronze is too gold for most medium skin tones, but if cost is not a deciding factor, the remaining shades are worth considering.

☺ $$$ **The Powder** *($60)* has an incredibly light, talc-based texture and offers imperceptibly sheer coverage in four excellent shades. This applies flawlessly and were it not for the price, I would recommend it without reservation. For comparable loose powders, take a look at the options from Laura Mercier, L'Oreal, and Sonia Kashuk before investing in this one. This type of loose powder is best for normal to dry skin because of its soft, "moist" feel and finish.

☺ $$$ **The Pressed Powder** *($55)* claims it has a "buttery smooth texture," and this you can bank on! This talc-based powder blends seamlessly over the skin and does not look dry or chalky. The five neutral shades are uniformly workable, with Sand Bronze being a great (albeit expensive) bronzing powder color.

LA PRAIRIE

La Prairie has been at the forefront of expensive antiaging products for more than three decades. Many of the products in this originally Swiss skin-care line are called "cellular treatment." After a while, it all starts sounding silly. Even the mascara is named "Cellular Treatment Intensified Mascara." Aligning these products with the concept of being able to affect the cellular level of skin or eyelashes is overdone and over the top. If your skin could improve with these products, the prices alone might cause premature aging. So what do the women who can safely afford these products get for their money? The prestige of knowing they can afford them, period. High-priced skin-care lines attract women who think that the dollars they spend will buy them something special that most other women can't afford. To some extent, they're right: other women can't afford these. Yet anyone who reads and understands the ingredient lists would find the prices as ludicrous for the contents as they actually are.

In years past La Prairie claimed spleen and placenta extract got rid of wrinkles. Now those ingredients are history, replaced by new ingredients that carry the same promise of wrinkle-free skin. In retrospect, perhaps La Prairie finally realized those ingredients were jokes and couldn't change any aspect of skin. What an expensive waste of time for a lot of women.

If you can choke past the prices there are some excellent moisturizers in this line brimming with noteworthy antioxidants, water-binding agents, and anti-irritants, and there are some well-formulated sunscreens with UVA-protecting ingredients, although selling sunscreens at $125 an ounce should be illegal. Given that a generous application is the cornerstone for getting correct sunscreen coverage, this price almost guarantees that you will not be using enough to get the essential protection from sun damage that the skin really needs and that the label indicates. There are also some exceedingly average products to wade through, but that isn't hard to do. For more information about La Prairie, call (800) 821-5718 or visit www.laprairie.com. **Note:** All La Prairie products contain fragrance.

La Prairie Skin Care

La Prairie Cellular

☹ **Purifying Systeme Cleansing Gelle** *($60 for 5 ounces)* contains TEA-lauryl sulfate as the main detergent cleansing agent, which makes it potentially too irritating for all skin types.

☺ **$$$ Foam Cleanser** *($60 for 4 ounces)* is a standard, detergent-based, water-soluble cleanser that is about as ordinary as they come. It does contain some Vaseline and silicone to blunt the drying effect of the rather strong cleansing agents, as well as some anti-irritants, but those are nothing special either, and it would just be better if this product didn't contain such drying detergent cleansing agents.

☺ **$$$ Purifying Creme Cleanser** *($60 for 6.8 ounces)* is meant to be rinsed off, but it actually requires a washcloth. It is merely a very expensive cold cream in lotion form. It is a decent cleanser for normal to dry skin, but there is little advantage in using this cleanser over Neutrogena's Extra Gentle Cleanser for one-sixth the price.

☺ **$$$ Cellular Eye Make-Up Remover** *($45 for 4.2 ounces)* is a standard, silicone-based, wipe-off cleanser that contains some plant extracts (some that can be irritants and others that can be anti-irritants). That's nice, but I wonder if the executives in these companies laugh about the women who believe they're getting something special when they spend this kind of money for such an ordinary product.

☺ $$$ **Essential Exfoliator** *($60 for 7 ounces)* is an extremely basic scrub that contains thickeners, plant oils, and detergent cleansing agents. The abrasive is ground-up apricot seeds. This is a good scrub for dry skin, but is overpriced for what you get.

☹ **Cellular Purifying Systeme Dual Phase Toner** *($65 for 8.4 ounces)* is a standard, alcohol-based toner that makes it too drying and irritating for all skin types.

✓☺ $$$ **Cellular Refining Lotion** *($65 for 8.2 ounces)* would be a good toner for most skin types, with a decent amount of antioxidants and water-binding agents, though for the money it should be overflowing with those types of ingredients. The plant extracts are a mixture of anti-irritants and irritants, but they are present in such tiny amounts that they probably have no effect on skin. The tiny amount of urea works as a water-binding agent, not as an exfoliant.

✓☺ $$$ **Cellular Brightening System Day Emulsion with SPF 15** *($125 for 1 ounce)* is a good sunscreen with titanium dioxide for an absurd amount of money. And for skin lightening, it is essential to correctly and religiously wear a sunscreen. This product does contain magnesium ascorbyl phosphate, a form of vitamin C that can have some skin-lightening effect, but the research shows that for it to work it takes at least a 3% concentration and this product contains less than 1%. It's a good moisturizing base, but there are far better ways to deal with skin discolorations than this one.

☺ $$$ **Cellular Retinol Complex PM** *($150 for 1 ounce)* is an emollient moisturizer with a small amount of water-binding agents and antioxidants, and, of course, retinol (the same amount that almost every other company uses). There's no advantage to be gained in spending this kind of money on a retinol product when lines from L'Oreal to Lancome and Lauder have their versions for far less (even Lauder's, which is better formulated than this one, costs about a third less).

✓☺ $$$ **Cellular Hydrating Serum** *($150 for 1 ounce)* is a very good emollient moisturizer for normal to dry skin loaded with antioxidants, water-binding agents, and anti-irritants.

✓☺ $$$ **Cellular Moisturizer SPF 15 The Smart Cream** *($140 for 1 ounce)* is a very good, in-part avobenzone-based sunscreen in an emollient base that contains an impressive mix of antioxidants, water-binding agents, and anti-irritants. The tiny amount of balm mint should not be a problem for skin. However, what isn't smart about this product is the price. Sunscreen must be applied liberally to obtain the benefit of the SPF on the label. How likely are you to apply this liberally when it would be gone in about a month, which would add up to about $1,600 a year to protect your face from the sun? There is no question this is overpriced for what you get.

✓☺ $$$ **Cellular Eye Moisturizer SPF 15 The Smart Eye Cream** *($125 for 0.5 ounce)* is almost identical to the Cellular Moisturizer SPF 15 version above and the same comments apply. There is nothing in this that makes it more appropriate for the eye area.

☺ $$$ **Cellular Purifying Systeme Hydrating Fluid SPF 15** *($100 for 1.7 ounces)* is an avobenzone-based SPF 15 sunscreen for $100! I'm just speechless. I know there are women who are going to buy this, and probably under-use it (Sunscreen requires liberal application and is anyone going to apply this overpriced sunscreen liberally?) and then not even get the full SPF protection on the label. While some of the plant extracts may add some soothing benefits and the neem extract some antimicrobial activity, there are others that are irritants. The water-binding agents are nice, but again, the amounts are very small, at least for the amount of money you're spending.

☹ **C Energy Cellular Serum** *($150 for 1 ounce)* lists alcohol as its second ingredient, and that makes it too drying and irritating for all skin types. The third ingredient is ascorbic acid, an effective form of vitamin C for its antioxidant properties, but it can also be a skin irritant. If you are going for vitamin C, there are better products than this one.

☺ $$$ **Cellular Day Creme** *($110 for 1 ounce)* is a lot of money for a product that is mostly thickeners and Vaseline, but I think La Prairie was hoping you wouldn't notice. Plus, without a sunscreen it is a definite no-no for daytime. It would be good for dry skin, but doesn't compare to some of the other more interesting products in this line, because it lacks any of the antioxidants, water-binding agents, and anti-irritants the others contain.

☺ $$$ **Cellular Eye Contour Creme** *($95 for 0.5 ounce)* weighs in at $3,040 per pound, yet it is nothing more than a Vaseline-based moisturizer with small amounts of water-binding agents. Most of the interesting ingredients are listed well after the preservatives. It is a decent emollient moisturizer for someone with dry skin, but is basically ordinary.

☺ $$$ **Cellular Lipo-Sculpting Systeme Eye Gel** *($125 for 0.5 ounce)* lists alcohol as the fourth ingredient, which may make this potentially drying and irritating. The handful of plant extracts are a strange mix of anti-irritants and potentially very irritating ones. There is also a cornucopia of water-binding agents and antioxidants, but for those you'll find better options in this line than this one.

✓☺ $$$ **Cellular Lipo-Sculpting Systeme Face Serum** *($125 for 1 ounce)* is a light-weight lotion that won't sculpt or change puffiness. However, this is still a very good moisturizer for normal to slightly dry skin that is loaded with antioxidants and water-binding agents. The caffeine has weak antioxidant properties, but the tannin can be a skin irritant.

☺ $$$ **Cellular Night Cream** *($110 for 1 ounce)* is a rather emollient, though extremely standard, moisturizer for dry skin. This boring, Vaseline-based moisturizer would be OK for someone with dry skin, but the cost is just a burn for what isn't as well formulated as many products available for a fraction of this price.

☺ $$$ **Cellular Wrinkle Cream** *($110 for 1 ounce)*. If this is a wrinkle cream, what are all the other products for? It is similar to the Night Cream above and the same basic comments apply.

☺ $$$ **Cellular Skin Conditioner** *($70 for 4 ounces)* is similar to the Night Cream above, minus the Vaseline, but the same basic comments apply.

☺ $$$ **Cellular Neck Cream** *($110 for 1 ounce)*. There is nothing in this product that is special for the neck. In fact, it is quite similar to the Night Cream above, and the same comments apply.

☺ $$$ **Cellular Purifying Systeme Hydro Repair** *($125 for 1 ounce)* is a good 8% AHA and about 0.5% BHA exfoliant in a good, lightweight moisturizing base for someone with normal to dry skin. It contains some good antioxidants and water-binding agents, but not enough of them for what you are paying.

☹ **Cellular Purifying Systeme Normalizing Serum** *($150 for 1 ounce)* lists alcohol as its fourth ingredient, and that won't normalize anything, at least not at this price, which is truly abnormal for what you get.

☺ $$$ **Cellular Time Release Moisturizer-Intensive** *($125 for 1 ounce)* is a good moisturizer for normal to dry skin, but this is a lot of money for a castor oil–based moisturizer! The water-binding agents are good, but are not unique to this formulation, and overall this isn't as impressive as many of the other La Prairie moisturizers.

✓☺ $$$ **Cellular Time Release Moisture Lotion SPF 15** *($125 for 1.7 ounces)* is a good, in-part avobenzone-based sunscreen that contains almost everything but the kitchen sink when it comes to noteworthy antioxidants and water-binding agents. It does add up to a good lightweight moisturizer for normal to dry skin. Remember you have to apply sunscreen liberally to obtain the full SPF benefit, and you need to consider how likely that is when you're paying this much for sunscreen.

✓☺ $$$ **Cellular Desensitizing Serum** *($150 for 1 ounce)* is an impressive, lightweight lotion with an excellent mix of antioxidants, water-binding agents, and anti-irritants. It is a very good option for normal to slightly dry or slightly oily skin.

☺ $$$ **Normalizing Serum** *($150 for 1 ounce)* lists alcohol as the fourth ingredient, which makes this lotion too potentially irritating for all skin types, and that isn't normalizing in the least. The teeny amount of salicylic acid and the high pH make this ineffective for exfoliation.

☺ $$$ **Cellular Balancing Mask** *($110 for six 0.12-ounce ampoules)* is a two-part mask that you mix together. Minuscule amounts of aloe vera and baking soda along with talc, clay, rice starch, and film-forming agent are not going to balance anyone's skin.

☺ $$$ **Cellular Cycle Ampoules for the Face** *($275 for seven 0.1-ounce treatments)* is a two-part, self-mixed treatment that contains the most ordinary assembly of ingredients you could imagine, and it prices out to about $5,700 a pound! They can't be serious. This isn't even as interesting as a lot of other La Prairie products.

☺ $$$ **Cellular Moisture Mask** *($65 for 1 ounce)* is an OK, emollient mask for someone with dry skin, but it lacks any significant amounts of antioxidants or water-binding agents.

☺ $$$ **Cellular Purifying Systeme Regulating Mask** *($100 for 2.6 ounces)* is a standard clay mask with a huge ingredient list. The tiny quantity of AHAs in it are insufficient to act as exfoliants, the plant extracts are a mixture of irritants and anti-irritants, and the water-binding agents are nice, but useless in a clay (absorbing) mask. It's a good basic mask, but for the money, a true "Why bother?" product.

☹ **Cellular Purifying Systeme Blemish Control** *($65 for 0.5 ounce)* does contain salicylic acid, but the first ingredient is alcohol, which not only is too irritating and drying for all skin types but also can impede the skin's healing process.

LA PRAIRIE AGE MANAGEMENT

☺ $$$ **Age Management Balancer** *($70 for 8.4 ounces)* is a good, irritant-free toner, but hardly worth the price tag. There is nothing in it that will manage age, and though it contains some good water-binding agents and antioxidants, the amounts are less than what you would expect given the cost. The lactic acid (AHA) is present in too minute a concentration to be effective for exfoliation.

☹ **Age Management Intensified Emulsion with SPF 8** *($100 for 1.7 ounces)* is an embarrassing product and offensive in defining itself as a skin protector, especially given the other far better (though exceedingly overpriced) SPF 15 sunscreens La Prairie has that do contain avobenzone.

✓☺ $$$ **Age Management Eye Repair** *($100 for 0.5 ounce)* has a huge ingredient list that is like throwing in the kitchen sink plus everything in the refrigerator. What you end up with is a very good moisturizer with impressive water-binding agents, antioxidants, and anti-irritants. It would work great for normal to dry skin. The 3% concentration of AHAs is not enough to have exfoliating properties, plus the pH is too high for the AHAs to work even if the concentration were high enough.

☺ $$$ **Age Management Night Cream** *($125 for 1 ounce)*. The pH of this moisturizer is too high for the AHA it contains to be effective as an exfoliant. It would be good for someone with dry skin. While there are a lot of interesting ingredients listed, there's mostly just a dusting of each.

☹ **Age Management Retexturizing Booster** *($150 for 1 ounce)* contains mostly alcohol, which is too drying and irritating for any skin type, and it is not recommended.

☺ $$$ **Age Management Stimulus Complex for the Eyes** *($125 for 0.5 ounce)* is an emollient moisturizer that contains a small amount of antioxidants and water-binding agents. The showcased ingredients are vitamin K and retinol. The retinol can be a good antioxidant and helpful for skin, but there is no research showing vitamin K to be of benefit for skin (at least other then the company selling vitamin K). For a retinol product this is just fine, but it would be an understatement to say that there are less expensive and better-formulated versions than this one.

✓☺ $$$ **Age Management Stimulus Complex SPF 25** *($150 for 1 ounce)* is a very good, in-part avobenzone-based sunscreen in an emollient base with some good water-binding agents and antioxidants. The fancy-sounding ingredients are so far toward the end of the ingredient list you aren't even getting a few cents worth of the stuff. This does contain retinol, and if that sounds like it's worth the money to you, go for it.

LA PRAIRIE SKIN CAVIAR

☺ $$$ **Essence of Skin Caviar Cellular Eye Complex** *($95 for 0.5 ounce)* is an OK, rather standard, lightweight moisturizer for someone with dry skin. It does contain 0.04% caviar, which amounts to about half of one fish egg—now, isn't that exciting? The notion that this is an instant face-lift in one minute doesn't hold water, and this isn't anywhere near as impressively formulated as several of the La Prairie Cellular moisturizers above.

☺ $$$ **Extrait of Skin Caviar Firming Complex** *($100 for 1 ounce)* contains mostly water, silicones, glycerin, thickeners, caviar extract, water-binding agents, antioxidants, preservatives, fragrance, and coloring agents. Several of the plant extracts can be skin irritants, but they are present in such small amounts that they probably won't have an impact on skin. This is a good moisturizer for normal to dry skin but it won't firm your skin in any way, shape, or form.

☹ **Skin Caviar** *($125 for 2 ounces)* is mostly silicone, some water, alcohol, a tiny amount of antioxidant, and even less water-binding agent. There is little reason to consider this for any aspect of skin care.

☺ $$$ **Skin Caviar Luxe Cream** *($300 for 1.7 ounces).* If you were going to spend an unseemly amount of money to get a great skin-care product, choosing this incredibly mundane formulation would not be the way to do it. The plant extracts are a waste, with some being incredibly irritating (such as horsetail, arnica, and sage), and there's not enough of the mulberry root to have any skin-lightening effect. The water-binding agents are nice, but are so far toward the end of the ingredient list that there's only a trace of them. The vitamins are good antioxidants, but not unique, as they show up in an endless array of other products, and there is only a very small amount of them, too. And, for the minuscule amount of caviar, you're better off picking up some at the grocery store and having it on toast rather than on your skin.

☹ **Skin Caviar Firming Mask** *($125 for two-piece set, including 0.35 ounce of Penetrating Serum and 1 ounce of Skin Caviar Firming Complex).* The Penetrating Serum is a blend of standard plant oils (like those from your kitchen cupboard) and fragrant oils. The Firming Complex part is mostly alcohol, and that adds up to irritation and dryness regardless of the sprinkling of other ingredients.

LA PRAIRIE SUISSE

☺ $$$ **Suisse De-Sensitizing Systeme Cleansing Emulsion** *($60 for 5 ounces)* is a ridiculously expensive lotion cleanser that can be an option for dry skin. The plant extracts can be anti-irritants, but they are present in incredibly small, barely detectable amounts.

☺ $$$ **Suisse De-Sensitizing Systeme Soothing Mist** *($65 for 4 ounces)* could have been a very good, silicone-based toner for dry skin, but the balm mint, horsetail, and rose extracts are potential skin irritants, while the other plant extracts are anti-irritants. I suspect that there isn't enough of any of these to make a difference, but at this price and given the claims, it's disappointing.

☹ **Suisse De-Sensitizing Systeme Nurturing Cream** *($125 for 1.7 ounces)* contains several potentially irritating plant extracts high up on the ingredient list, which isn't de-sensitizing at all, and it contains a poor showing of antioxidants and water-binding agents. There is little else of interest in this un-nurturing moisturizer.

☺ **$$$ Suisse De-Sensitizing Systeme Barrier Shield SPF 15** *($100 for 1 ounce)* is a very good sunscreen that contains only titanium dioxide and zinc oxide as active ingredients, which indeed makes it fine for sensitive skin, but the price is shocking for this unbelievably basic group of ingredients. Not to mention that some the plant extracts can be skin irritants!

☹ **Suisse De-Sensitizing Systeme Exfoliating Enzyme Mask** *($100 for 1.7 ounces)*. The purported enzymes in this product are papaya extract and pineapple extract, but these aren't enzymes, they're just irritating plant extracts. Enzymes like papain or bromelain can exfoliate skin, but they're not the same as these extracts. And several of the other plant extracts present can also be skin irritants.

LA PRAIRIE SOLEIL SUISSE

☺ **$$$ Soleil Suisse Cellular Anti-Wrinkle Sun Cream SPF 30** *($100 for 1.7 ounces)* is a titanium dioxide–based sunscreen that would be good for someone with dry skin. It is a basic moisturizer with a sprinkling of plant extracts (some that can be irritants), water-binding agents, and antioxidants. That's good, but if you aren't using this product liberally (and all sunscreens must be applied liberally), all of those ingredients are pointless because you won't be getting adequate sun protection.

☺ **$$$ Soleil Suisse Cellular Anti Wrinkle Sun Block SPF 50** *($125 for 1.7 ounces)* is similar to the Sun Cream SPF 30 above. This product will be going by the wayside when the FDA's new ruling on SPF limits takes place. While an SPF 50 sounds like you are getting more complete protection, all you are really getting is more *hours* of protection, and there just isn't that much sunlight in a day. Not to mention you still have to reapply it if you are perspiring or swimming. An SPF 50 does protect from 98% of the sun's rays, but that's identical to what an SPF 30 does.

☹ **Soleil Suisse Cellular Self Tan for the Body Spray Auto-Bronzant SPF 15** *($75 for 5 ounces)* contains, as all self-tanners do, the active ingredient dihydroxyacetone. It will turn skin brown exactly the same way a $10 self-tanner will. However, the sunscreen in this product doesn't include the UVA-protecting ingredients of titanium dioxide, zinc oxide, or avobenzone, and this is not recommended.

☹ **Soleil Suisse Self Tanner for Face SPF 15** *($75 for 1.7 ounces)* is similar to the Body Spray above and the same comments apply.

LA PRAIRIE MAKEUP

Colorwise, La Prairie makeup leaves much to be desired, especially given the high to ludicrous prices for what amount to ordinary cosmetics. A few of the products exhibit supple, silky textures, but the expense is hard to justify when similar items are available for substantially less from so many other lines. Perhaps most troubling, and a sure sign that this company pays more attention to extolling fad ingredients than to technical skincare research, is the lack of effective sunscreens in almost all of their foundations. Carrying on about the so-called antiaging benefits of their makeup without getting this fundamental concern right is kind of like saying that smoking cigarettes is harmless as long as you don't inhale.

FOUNDATION: La Prairie does not offer shades for darker skin, but their foundations are relatively easy to test without asking a salesperson for assistance. ☺ $$$ Skin Caviar Concealer/Foundation SPF 15 ($150) is the most expensive foundation in this book, and it pains me to give this a smiling face rating. It claims to have a "new technology" that "forms a continuous matrix of treatment and colour that lasts all day." When it comes to makeup, technology does not have to be so pricey, and this straightforward, minimal-frills, silicone-based foundation is no exception. The sunscreen lacks UVA protection, though the foundation part has a liquid silk texture that blends well and offers medium coverage and a matte finish. The concealer is housed in a compact that is built into the foundation's cap, and has a creamy texture that melts into skin, but can crease. If you decide to open your pocketbook for this one (though I implore you to think twice before you do), avoid Peche, Soleil Peche, and Honey Beige. Cellular Treatment Foundation Satin SPF 15 ($60) has a good, partially titanium dioxide–based sunscreen and a lightweight, but slick, texture that can provide sheer to light coverage with a satin finish. This is best for normal to dry skin. Of the nine shades (with nothing for darker skin tones), five are best avoided: 1.0, 3.2, 3.5, 4.0, and 4.5. Cellular Treatment Powder Finish SPF 10 ($60) is a wet/dry powder foundation that has a wonderfully smooth texture and a gorgeous silky finish. It would work best for normal to slightly dry or slightly oily skin types. What a shame the price is so ridiculous, and that no active ingredients are listed for the sunscreen (though titanium dioxide is the second ingredient). Four of the six shades are great, but avoid Rose Beige (too rose) and Soleil Beige (too peach).

☹ $$$ Cellular Treatment Foundation Flawless SPF 8 ($75) is outrageously priced, especially with no effective UVA-protecting ingredients and an embarrassingly low SPF, despite its claims of retexturizing skin to near perfection. If you're somehow still intrigued, this has a rich, creamy texture and provides medium to full coverage with a satin matte finish. It can easily look heavy on the skin, but normal to dry skin will appreciate the feel. Of the eight shades, the following are too pink, peach, or rose for most skin tones: #100, #400 (slight rose), #500, and #600.

☹ Cellular Treatment Foundation Naturel SPF 8 ($60) has a dismally low SPF that does not list the active sunscreen ingredients. Even though this creamy-textured, satin-finish foundation is ideal for dry skin, all eight of the sheer to light coverage shades are too peach, pink, or rose to recommend. Perfecting Primer ($55) is a barely shiny, semi-opaque white liquid that leaves an obvious whitish cast on the skin. If you think giving your face an opalescent white cast will "perfect" your look, this is for you, but hopefully most will recognize what a waste this is. **Cellular Energizing Colour Finish SPF 15** *($65)* is a very sheer tinted moisturizer that is positioned to appeal to the affluent, outdoorsy type, which makes it inexcusable that it doesn't contain UVA-protecting ingredients. The colors are borderline rose, peach, and orange, though this is too sheer for that to matter. This is not recommended over the superlative versions, which do have adequate sun protection, from Clinique, Aveda, Bobbi Brown, and Lancome.

☹ <u>CONCEALER:</u> **Professional Cover Cream SPF 15** *($40)* has a reliable, titanium dioxide–based sunscreen with an SPF 15, which is great, but it also has a creamy (bordering on greasy) texture, with an opaque, thick finish that can easily crease into lines. Two of the four colors are good, but not *that* good, given the price tag. **Cellular Treatment Concealer** *($30)* has a decent creamy formula that offers a natural finish and medium coverage, but the three colors are woefully poor.

<u>POWDER:</u> ☹ **Cellular Treatment Loose Powder** *($40)* is a sheer, talc-based powder that claims it leaves a "fresh, natural matte finish," but La Prairie should revisit that claim given that this one has a noticeably shiny finish and ends up being anything but matte.

☺ $$$ **Cellular Treatment Pressed Powder** *($36)* is just a regular talc-based pressed powder with a nice silky feel. It has a soft finish that normal to dry skin will appreciate. The three shades are slightly peachy pink, but are sheer enough to work for most light skin tones. **Les Bronzes Bronzing Powder** *($50)* is a pressed-powder bronzer with two flattering shades in one compact, but both are too shiny, especially if you have noticeable wrinkles.

☺ $$$ <u>BLUSH:</u> **Cellular Treatment Blush** *($37.50)* has a slightly grainy, but overall smooth, texture that applies and builds well. The colors look vivid, but go on sheer, and all of them have shine, though for most it's subtle. Avoid the Persimmon and Vin shades.

☺ $$$ <u>EYESHADOW:</u> **Cellular Treatment Eye Color** *($32)* is only good at treating the eyes to a halo or shadow of iridescence. These single eyeshadows feel soft and apply well, but unless your eyelid and brow bone are perfectly taut, you're not likely to love the line-emphasizing final result. The same comments hold true for the **Ensemble de Couleur** *($50)*, a kit of two eyeshadow colors and a powder eyeliner. The eyeshadows are identical to the one above, and since the eyeliner part is very dry it tends to work best with a wet (damp) brush.

<u>EYE AND BROW SHAPER:</u> ☺ $$$ **Long Lasting Creamy Eye Definer** *($25)* and **Versatile Brow Definer and Styling Brush** *($25)* are standard pencils that are dressed up in elaborate packaging. Please don't be fooled: The packaging doesn't affect performance, and why waste your money for something so ordinary?

☺ $$$ **Cellular Treatment Wet/Dry Eyeliner** *($32)* presents classic black and brown shades in a very good, deeply pigmented formula that works best when used wet. The finish is mostly matte, but you will notice a bit of shine, which La Prairie can't seem to help itself from using.

<u>LIPSTICK AND LIP PENCIL:</u> ☺ $$$ **Cellular Treatment Lip Colour** comes in two formulas. The **Sheers** represent over half of the color range and they're glossy and

iridescent. The **Creams** have a greasy, wet finish and will bleed into lines almost faster than you can apply them, though the colors are opaque.

The ☺ **$$$ Lip Pencils** *($25)* are in the same boat as the eye and brow pencils, and it's best to let them just sail on by.

☹ **Cellular Treatment Lip Enhancer** *($40)*. This slightly dry, waxy lipstick claims to ambush every lipstick pitfall at the pass, but it's just a barely passable concealer that can lightly smooth the lip's surface. Don't bother with this unless you get a thrill out of wasting money.

☺ **$$$ MASCARA: Cellular Treatment Intensified Mascara** *($25)*. The knock-your-socks-off price of this mascara doesn't even compare to the completely lackluster performance, though the lashes do stay soft and pliable.

☺ **$$$ BRUSHES:** La Prairie has added a few token Brushes *($28–$65, $125–$250 for collections)*. What's frustrating is that only four of the nine brushes are sold separately. If you want more than that, you have to buy one of the kits. In or out of the kits, these brushes are nicely shaped and look elegant, but you will find similarly priced and far more appealing brushes from Trish McEvoy and Stila. The best single brush to consider from La Prairie is the **Professional Concealer Brush** *($30)*, which can double as an eyeshadow brush.

LA ROCHE-POSAY (SKIN CARE ONLY)

La Roche-Posay has been owned by L'Oreal since 1989, and its products have been available primarily in Europe and Canada, selling both in drugstores and department stores. Recently a merger took place between La Roche-Posay and BioMedic (also reviewed in this book); together, the lines will become known as La Roche-Posay BioMedic. Exactly which products stay and which ones go as these two lines commingle their identities is yet to be seen. As things change and improve (or worsen, you never know), I will report on them in my online newsletter *Cosmetics Counter Update*. From La Roche-Posay's viewpoint, merging with BioMedic will create "...the ultimate skincare specialists."

For now, the existing La Roche-Posay products (sold in Canadian drugstores, and available in dermatologist and plastic surgeon offices in the United States) are extremely simple and completely uninspiring. For the most part they lack any significant water-binding agents, antioxidants, or anti-irritants. Plus there are no sunscreens of any kind, and not even products for blemish-prone skin. Despite the company's claim that they are "dedicated to serving all skincare physicians," no self-respecting dermatologist would recommend these products. At least not one who had any insight into current research regarding skin-care product formulations. The quality of La Roche-Posay's current products is far below any state-of-the-art products being sold by lines from Clinique to Neutrogena, or even BioMedic (maybe that's why they're merging). For more information about La Roche-Posay and BioMedic, call (800) 736-5155 or visit www.laroche-posay.com or www.biomedic.com.

The Reviews L

☺ **Effaclar Purifying Foaming Gel** *($14.95 for 5 ounces)* is a standard, but good, detergent-based cleanser that would work well for most skin types except dry skin. It contains fragrance.

☺ **Surgras Cleansing Bar** *($6.95 for 4 ounces)* is a standard, detergent-based cleansing bar that can be fairly drying for most skin types. It contains fragrance.

☺ **Toleriane Dermo-Cleanser** *($12.95 for 6.76 ounces)* is a simple lotion cleanser that is suitable for normal to dry skin. It does not contain fragrance.

☺ **Toleriane Foaming Cleanser** *($12.95 for 3.38 ounces)* is a fairly drying, detergent-based cleanser that may be an option for oily skin.

☺ **Toleriane Eye Make-Up Remover** *($15.95 for 30 capsules)* is a standard, detergent-based makeup remover that also contains a good water-binding agent, which would make it easier for the skin around the eyes.

☹ **Thermal Spring Water** *($4.95 for 1.76 ounces)* is just water and nitrogen. The thermal spring water is supposed to be "rich in selenium, a powerful antioxidant." Whether or not that is true (pure selenium as a supplement would be better, though) is irrelevant, because the nitrogen that is used as a propellant to create a mist of water can generate free-radical damage and cause cell death (Sources: *Mechanisms of Ageing and Development,* April 2002, pages 1007–1019 and *Toxicology and Applied Pharmacology,* July 2002, pages 84–90).

☺ **Active C Day/Night Emulsion** *($27.75 for 1 ounce)* contains mostly water, silicones, ascorbic acid, thickener, slip agent, plant oil, preservatives, and fragrance. Vitamin C is a good antioxidant, but it is not the one be-all and end-all ingredient. This one-note product is OK, but needs more to warrant a stronger recommendation.

☺ **$$$ Active C Eyes** *($27.95 for 0.5 ounce)* is almost identical to the Active C Day/Night Emulsion above and the same comments apply.

☺ **$$$ Active C Facial Skincare** *($34.95 for 1 ounce)* is similar to the Active C Day/Night Emulsion above except that this one has 5% L-ascorbic acid, which is considered a more bioavailable form of vitamin C. For a vitamin C product both this concentration and price are impressive, but a more complex formulation that included water-binding agents and anti-irritants would be far better for skin. It is an option for normal to slightly oily or slightly dry skin.

☺ **$$$ Active C Light Facial Skincare** *($34.95 for 1 ounce)* is similar to the Active C Facial Skincare above and the same basic comments apply. It is an option for normal to slightly oily or slightly dry skin.

☹ **Hydranorme Facial Skincare** *($14.95 for 1.37 ounces)* is a dated formulation that is embarrassingly mundane and ordinary.

☹ **Hydraphase Facial Moisturizer** *($17.95 for 1.7 ounces)* is a silicone- and film forming agent–based moisturizer with alcohol and thickeners and a teeny amount of an antioxidant. It is a poor formulation and is not recommended.

☹ **Toleriane Facial Skincare** *($17 for 1.35 ounces)* is an exceptionally dull moisturizer that lacks even a dusting of antioxidants, water-binding agents, or anti-irritants. This product is not recommended.

☹ **Toleriane Soothing Protective Facial Cream** *($15.95 for 1.35 ounces)* is similar to the Toleriane Facial Skincare above and the same comments apply.

☹ **Toleriane Soothing Protective Light Facial Fluid** *($16.95 for 1.35 ounces)* is similar to the Toleriane Facial Skincare above only in lotion form, and the same basic comments apply.

☺ **Ceralip** *($8.95 for 0.5 ounce)* is a standard emollient lip balm similar to Chap Stick.

☹ **Effaclar K Acne Treatment Fluid** *($22.95 for 1 ounce)* is a mediocre, matte-finish moisturizer with 1.5% salicylic acid, though the pH isn't low enough for it to be effective for exfoliation.

LAC-HYDRIN (SKIN CARE ONLY)

Lac-Hydrin products were the original AHA products sold anywhere! They have been in drugstores for years, and much of what we know about how AHAs act is a result of these formulations. Lac-Hydrin Five (stands for 5% lactic acid) and Lac-Hydrin 12 (this one is prescription-only and contains 12% lactic acid) offer AHAs in bases that have the correct pH for them to be effective exfoliants. These aren't elegant formulations, but they are some of the best AHA exfoliants available. For more information about Lac-Hydrin, call Bristol-Meyers Squibb Company at (800) 332-2056 or visit www.drugstore.com.

☺ **Lac-Hydrin Five Lotion** *($10.99 for 8 ounces)* and **Lac-Hydrin 12 Lotion** *($34.98 for 7.6 ounces)* are both good AHA products containing lactic acid in a standard, Vaseline-based moisturizer. Both versions are appropriate for someone with dry skin and both are fragrance-free.

LANCASTER

You may not be familiar with the Lancaster name, but chances are you have heard of one or more of the lines that their parent company, Coty, owns, including Germaine Monteil, Isabella Rossellini's Manifesto, Rimmel, Davidoff, and Joop. Considered Coty's prestige brand, Lancaster markets only fragrances in the United States; they sell their skin-care and makeup products in Canada and Europe, primarily at department stores. While there are some decent options to consider in the makeup products, overall the skin-care products are lackluster, with some extremely dated formulations. Some of the moisturizers are little more than water, silicone, and wax. Others have a long list of water-binding agents and antioxidants, but they are listed well after the preservatives and are present in quantities hardly worth mentioning. While the line is swimming in a sea of moisturizers there isn't a sunscreen to be found, and the selection of products for normal to oily or blemish-prone skin will only make matters worse for those skin types. For more information about Lancaster, call (800) 961-3872 or visit www.mjmfragrances.com.

The Reviews L

Note: All of the prices are in US dollars. All Lancaster products contain fragrance unless otherwise noted.

LANCASTER SKIN CARE

LANCASTER AQUAMILK (ALL SKIN TYPES)

☺ $$$ **Eye & Face Cleansing Water** *($26 for 6.7 ounces)* is a standard, detergent-based cleanser that uses sodium lauryl sulfate, a strong skin irritant, as one of the cleansing agents. There probably isn't much of it in here, but for this price, there shouldn't be any.

☺ **Fresh Foaming Cleanser** *($26 for 13.5 ounces)* is a standard, detergent-based cleanser that would work well for normal to dry skin. The tiny amount of water-binding agents and plant oils won't have much effect on skin.

☺ **Soft Milk Cleanser** *($26 for 13.5 ounces)* is a standard, mineral oil–based cleanser that is more of a cold cream than anything else. It is an option for someone with normal to dry skin, but this is pricey for such a basic formulation.

☹ **Fresh Toner (with Alcohol)** *($26 for 13.5 ounces)* is an alcohol-based toner, and that makes it too irritating and drying for all skin types.

☺ **Soft Toner (Alcohol Free)** *($26 for 13.5 ounces)* is a very standard, mediocre toner of water, glycerin, slip agent, and anti-irritant, though several plant extracts in this product are irritants, making the anti-irritant completely useless.

☺ **Soft Touch Exfoliant** *($28 for 3.4 ounces)* is a standard emollient scrub that uses synthetic scrub particles as the abrasive. It would be an option for normal to dry skin.

☺ $$$ **Absolute Eye Cream** *($28 for 0.5 ounce)* is an absolutely ordinary, silicone-based moisturizer that would be OK for normal to dry skin. It contains the most minuscule amount of antioxidants and water-binding agents imaginable.

☺ **Absolute Moisture Cream** *($32 for 1.7 ounces)* is similar to the Eye Cream above and the same comments apply.

☺ **Absolute Moisture Light Cream** *($32 for 1.7 ounces)* is similar to the Eye Cream above and the same comments apply.

☺ **Absolute Moisture Rich Cream** *($32 for 1.7 ounces)* is similar to the Eye Cream above and the same comments apply. The teeny amount of coffee oil adds no special benefit to this mediocre moisturizer.

☺ **Absolute Moisture Mask** *($26 for 2.5 ounces)* is an emollient clay mask that would be an option for someone with normal to dry skin.

☺ $$$ **Clear-It-All Mask** *($26 for 2.5 ounces)* is a standard clay mask containing nothing that can get rid of blemishes or blackheads, though it can temporarily make oily skin feel soft.

☹ **Instant Reviving Mask** *($26 for 2.5 ounces)* lists alcohol as the second ingredient, and it also contains menthol. That adds up to a mask that is too drying and irritating for all skin types.

LANCASTER SKIN MAXIMIZER (ALL SKIN TYPES)

☺ **Energizing Cleansing Foam** *($22 for 6.7 ounces)* is a standard, detergent-based cleanser that can be an option for someone with normal to oily skin.

☹ **$$$ Energizing Toning Water-Gel** *($22 for 6 ounces)*. There is nothing energizing about this very ordinary toner. The menthol will make skin tingle, but that is irritation, and it can hurt the skin's healing process.

☹ **$$$ Long Lasting Radiance Fluid** *($40 for 1.7 ounces)* is a very ordinary moisturizing lotion that contains mostly silicone and waxes. The minuscule amounts of water-binding agents and antioxidants are barely detectable. It also contains a teeny amount of glycolic acid, which is not enough for it to be effective as an exfoliant.

☹ **$$$ Long Lasting Eye Cream** *($40 for 0.5 ounce)* is similar to the Radiance Fluid above, except that the second ingredient on the list is aluminum starch octenylsuccinate, an absorbent that is the last thing you want to do for the skin around the eyes. This does have a long list of water-binding agents and antioxidants, but in total the amount is so small as to be merely a dusting.

☺ **$$$ Long Lasting Night Care** *($50 for 1.7 ounces)* is similar to the Long Lasting Radiance Fluid above and the same comments apply.

☺ **$$$ Long Lasting Radiance Moisturizer** *($40 for 1.7 ounces)* is similar to the Long Lasting Radiance Fluid above and the same comments apply.

☹ **$$$ Long Lasting Radiance Rich** *($40 for 1.7 ounces)* is similar to the Long Lasting Radiance Fluid above and the same comments apply.

LANCASTER SKIN PURE (OILY SKIN)

☹ **Face and Eye Cleansing Gel Cream** *($20 for 13.5 ounces)* lists alcohol as the second ingredient, which makes this too drying and irritating for all skin types.

☹ **Matifying/Purifying Bi-Phase Toner** *($20 for 13.5 ounces)* lists alcohol as the second ingredient, which makes this too drying and irritating for all skin types.

☺ **Moisture Fluid Oil Free** *($22 for 1.7 ounces)* is a lightweight, matte-finish lotion that contains clay, which can be a good absorbent, but so can a pressed powder. This adds no real benefit to the skin because it lacks antioxidants and water-binding agents.

☺ **Matifying Cream Oil Free** *($22 for 1.7 ounces)* is similar to the Moisture Fluid Oil Free version above and the same comments apply.

☺ **$$$ Clarifying Mask** *($20 for 1.7 ounces)* is an extremely standard clay mask that can be an option for normal to oily skin.

☹ **Matte T-Zone Stick** *($15)* contains several ingredients that are problematic for oily skin, including several waxes, plant oils, and castor oil.

LANCASTER SURACTIF (NORMAL TO DRY SKIN)

☺ **Cleansing Treatment** *($35 for 13.5 ounces)* contains mostly water, mineral oil, thickeners, water-binding agent, preservatives, and anti-irritants. There's little reason to use this instead of just plain mineral oil. It is an option for normal to dry skin, but it's simply not worth the money.

☺ **Preparation Lotion** *($35 for 13.5 ounces)* is as ordinary as toners get, and that won't prepare your skin for anything but disappointment.

☹ $$$ **Eye Treatment Plus** *($50 for 0.5 ounce)* is a standard, silicone-based moisturizer that contains fractional amounts of water-binding agents and antioxidants.

☹ $$$ **Facial Treatment Plus** *($60 for 1.7 ounces)* is similar to the Eye Treatment Plus above and the same comments apply. The teeny amount of glycolic acid in this product is not enough to make it effective as an exfoliant.

☹ $$$ **Firming Serum** *($55 for 1 ounce)* is an emollient moisturizer for normal to dry skin that contains a small amount of antioxidants, plant oils, and water-binding agents.

☹ $$$ **Lightweight Cream** *($60 for 1.7 ounces)* is similar to the Eye Treatment Plus above and the same comments apply.

☹ $$$ **Neck and Decollete Treatment** *($55 for 1.7 ounces)* is similar to the Eye Treatment Plus above and the same comments apply.

☹ $$$ **Excellence Lifting Revitalizer Cream** *($135 for 1.7 ounces)*. With 78 different ingredients, this moisturizer definitely excels when it comes to numbers. What is anything but excellent are the sunscreen ingredients. They include avobenzone, but the product does not have an SPF rating so you can't rely on it for sun protection. This also suffers from minimal amounts of the good stuff, as do most Lancaster products. The truffle and champagne extract in here is almost silly, but the quantities are so insignificant it isn't worth discussing why they have no benefit for skin. There are a few problematic fungus extracts and a teeny amount of plant extracts that might be skin irritants, but again they don't add up to much so there isn't much to worry about, except for the money you would be wasting on this product.

☹ $$$ **Night Firming Treatment Plus** *($65 for 1.7 ounces)* is a basic emollient moisturizer for normal to dry skin with minute amounts of interesting water-binding agents and antioxidants.

☹ $$$ **Retinol Plus Retexturizer** *($55 for 1.7 ounces)* actually doesn't contain any retinol, though it does contain a trace amount of retinyl palmitate. This is a very basic, mediocre moisturizer for dry skin.

☹ $$$ **Rich Facial Treatment Plus** *($60 for 1.7 ounces)* is an emollient, but very boring, moisturizer for normal to dry skin.

☹ $$$ **Relaxing Masque** *($35 for 1.7 ounces)* is an ordinary emollient mask with teeny amounts of anti-irritants and antioxidants.

☹ $$$ **Lip Conditioning Cream** *($25 for 0.5 ounce)* is a simple, but emollient, lip moisturizer. The clay adds a matte finish, but it also absorbs moisture, which is just not the best thing for lips.

LANCASTER RE-OXYGEN

Most skin-care products these days, just like those from Lancaster, contain antioxidants, which are ingredients that reduce the negative effect of oxygen or oxidative substances on skin. At the same time, companies sell products that contain oxygen-releasing ingredients, which supposedly deliver oxygen molecules when they come into contact with skin. But that generates free-radical damage (Source: *Human and Experimental Toxicology*, February 2002, pages 61–62). Oxidative stress is an unavoidable consequence of life in our everyday, oxygen-rich atmosphere. The "oxygen paradox" is that oxygen is dangerous to the very life forms for which it has become an essential component of energy production. Cells, tissues, organs, and organisms have multiple layers of antioxidant defenses, as well as damage removal and replacement or repair systems to cope with the stress and damage that oxygen causes (Source: *Journal of the International Union of Biochemistry and Molecular Biology*, October-November 2000, pages 279–289). Oxygen is a problem for skin and these products can only make matters worse.

☹ **Care for Eyes** *($32 for 0.5 ounce)*, **Relax, Refresh 02 Emulsion** *($70 for 1.7 ounces)*, and **02 Cooling Mask** *($32 for 1.7 ounces)* are not recommended due to their oxygen content.

LANCASTER MAKEUP

You will find several Lancaster makeup items have, for the most part, competitive textures, finishes, and colors that you would be remiss not to consider, especially if this line is sold in your city. However, I wouldn't get swept away by what the rest of the color line has to offer, which is mostly sheer to all-out glittery shine. There is not a single matte blush or eyeshadow to be found, the eye and brow pencils are hopelessly ordinary, and the mascaras are wholly unimpressive. If anything, a cursory view of the user-friendly tester unit quickly demonstrates that this line's major strong point is neutral foundations, with the weak point being the overflow of teen-appeal, glitter-infused novelty products. Still, if you avoid those and focus on what's best, there's no reason you cannot leave the Lancaster counter as a satisfied customer.

FOUNDATION: None of the Lancaster foundations offer options for dark to very dark skin tones. Each formula blends extremely well, making these a pleasure to work with. ☺ $$$ **Light Enhancing Cream Compact Foundation** *($30)* has a smooth, but thick, slightly powdery texture and offers medium coverage and a semi-matte finish. If you have normal to slightly dry skin, the five shades are worth a look, though M03 is too rosy for most skin tones. **Light Enhancing Adaptive Foundation SPF 6** *($30)* does not contain any active ingredients, so the SPF claim is without merit (not to mention that it's so low it's dangerous for the health of your skin). Despite this failing, the foundation does have a beautifully soft, creamy feel. Coverage is in the light to medium range, and this has a natural matte finish that feels a bit moist, so those with oily areas shouldn't expect much shine control. If you have normal to dry skin, the seven mostly neutral shades are splendid—only L03 may be too pink for some skin tones. ✓☺ **Light Enhancing Matte Finish Foundation** *($28)* is a wonderful matte-finish foundation that has a delicate, light texture and sheer to light coverage. The eight shades are exceptional, though M07 is slightly peach. This is highly recommended for those with normal to oily skin.

☺ $$$ **Skin Feel Revealing Powder-Veil Foundation** *($30)* has a concentrated, silicone-based formula that comes out thick but feels surprisingly light on the skin, blending down to a soft matte finish with medium coverage. The only drawback is that the formula tends to separate in the tube, and no amount of shaking helps. Of the six shades, avoid D10, which is too orange for most skin tones. **Oxygen Foundation** *($30)* claims to provide a rush of oxygen to the skin, but that's not a good thing, since oxygen generates free-radical damage. Still, any oxygen this foundation provides is gone as soon as you press the pump dispenser. This is merely a very good foundation for those with dry skin. It has a silky, moist texture that blends to a natural satin finish and provides sheer, skin-enhancing coverage. The six shades have a couple of peachy rose options (03 and 05), but this is really too sheer to make them worth avoiding. **Skin Pure Mattifying Compact Treatment** *($20)* is a matte-finish, cream-to-powder makeup that goes on sheer and does a reasonably good job of keeping excess shine at bay. However, the thickeners in this formula can be problematic for those who are battling blemishes. If you have oily, blemish-free skin (which is rare), the three slightly peach, but sheer, shades are all options.

CONCEALER: ☺ $$$ **Light Enhancing Cream Concealer** *($14.50)* is a great creamy concealer that has a semi-liquid texture that can make blending a bit difficult, but it does have an attractive finish and only a slight tendency to crease into lines around the eyes. Of the three shades, D08 is too peach to look convincing on dark skin.

☹ **Skin Pure Blemish Treatment Tinted Pencil** *($12)* is an automatic, retractable pencil that is just what the doctor did *not* order, especially for blemishes. Who thought putting a peach-tinted layer of castor oil and waxes over already clogged pores would be a good idea? Nothing in this pencil will treat blemishes, but it may very well make matters worse.

POWDER: ☺ $$$ **Light Enhancing Loose Powder** *($26)* is talc-based and has a soft, slightly dry application and sheer matte finish. Each of the three shades is fine, though the darkest color won't work for dark skin. **Light Enhancing Pressed Powder** *($24)* is a very standard, but effective, talc-based powder that has a soft, dry texture and very sheer coverage. The three shades deposit minimal color on the skin, but will keep shine at bay.

☺ $$$ **Light Enhancing Bronzing Powder** *($24)* is a pressed bronzer with a dry texture and a sheer, smooth application. The two shades have a soft shine and are more peachy than bronze. **Luminizer Magic Powder** *($24)* is a loose, golden bronze glitter powder housed in a saltshaker container. It's overindulgent shine at a premium price, and tends to go everywhere but where you want it.

BLUSH: ☺ $$$ **Light Enhancing Powder Blush** *($20)* has a sheer, dry texture that applies smoothly. Each shade is laced with iridescence and the colors tend to go on brighter than they appear—even the neutral tones take on a brighter edge once blended on the skin, so choose carefully—or simply look to other product lines for more reliable color-true matte blush.

☹ **Luminizer Stick** *($21)* is a water-to-powder glitter stick that imparts a sheer layer of gaudy glitter that tends to stick to the skin. A product like this lowers my estimation of this makeup line.

EYESHADOW: The ☹ **Light Enhancing Eye Shadows** *($15.50)* are sold as singles, and each has a dry, slightly grainy texture and semi-smooth application. The colors are mostly bright and shiny, which is distracting and unattractive. This is not the line to shop for neutral eyeshadows, but if shiny is your thing, other lines' eyeshadows easily outperform this formula. **Automatic Cream to Powder Eye Shadow** *($13)* is exactly what it says, and these come packaged in the click-pen applicators seen in many other lines. The brush on this one is short and blunt, and the product's slick texture and intensely shiny colors are not at all appealing.

☺ **Cream Eye Shadow Crayon** *($13)* are jumbo standard pencils that are an interesting option for eyeshadow. The soft, creamy texture is easy to apply, blends well, and has a slight powder finish. All of the nude to pastel shades have a subtle shine, and these can crease, but if the novelty appeals to you, they may have potential.

EYE AND BROW SHAPER: ☺ **Eye Enhancing Pencil** *($13)* and **Brow Enhancing Pencil** *($13)* are both standard pencils that are nothing special, unless creamy pencils that smudge are what you're after.

☹ **Eye Enhancing Liquid Liner** *($14.50)* has everything going for it and performs beautifully until the formula sets—then the smearing begins and there's no looking back.

LIPSTICK AND LIP PENCIL: ☺ **Moisture Enhancing Lipstick** *($14.50)* is a creamy bordering-on-greasy lipstick that won't last too long but that does provide a smooth feel and comes in a generous assortment of colors. ✓☺ **Velvet Matte Comfort Lipstick** *($14.50)* is a superior semi-matte lipstick that has a wonderfully smooth application, opaque, long-lasting colors, and does not feel dry on the lips. This is one to check out!

☺ **Sheer Lipstick** *($14.50)* works well as a sheer, glossy lipstick that's assuredly fleeting, but it does provide a soft, casual look. **Shine Enhancing Lipcolor** *($13)* is a lipstick/lip gloss hybrid that is essentially a lip gloss with a decent amount of pigment. This is slightly sticky and quite glossy. **Luminizer Magic Lip Gloss** *($13)* is just a sheer, non-sticky, glitter-packed gloss that has a good brush applicator.

☺ **Lip & Cheek Crayon** *($13)* is your average chubby lip pencil popularized by the Lauder-owned lines. Just like almost all the others, this one's soft tip and greasy texture make sharpening a daily occurrence, and this simply can't compare with a good lipstick.

MASCARA: ☺ **Lash Volumizing Mascara** *($15)* is hardly volumizing. It builds some length and a touch of thickness without clumping, but it's unusually boring and not worth auditioning.

☹ **Lash Enhancing Mascara** *($15)* is terrible, unless you are wearing mascara for no added emphasis or definition, preferring instead to downplay the lashes. What a do-nothing disappointment!

☺ **$$$ BRUSHES:** Lancaster does offer a **Brush Set** *($40)* that features workable, soft Powder, Blush, and Eyeshadow brushes. A relatively useless Fan Brush and scratchy Brow/Lash Brush are included, but are best tossed aside to make room for more practical brushes. These aren't top-of-the-line brushes, but the price is more than reasonable.

LANCOME

This very French line maintains a more casual ambience when compared to the other French lines sold at department stores such as Yves St. Laurent, Orlane, Givenchy, Guerlain, and Chanel, whose elitist airs are so thick you can cut them with a knife. Over the years, Lancome has done a noteworthy job of making sure its image and products radiate a contemporary elegance. Owned by L'Oreal, one of the top cosmetics companies in the world, Lancome has the advertising dollars to keep its "high-end" image in consumer's minds as one of the standards for beauty products. In tandem with the air of European style that Lancome exudes, its products have always been aimed at baby boomers and anyone else concerned with the "ravages of time."

Lancome's skin-care line includes a vast group of products, yet in the area of interesting water-binding agents, antioxidants, and anti-irritants they fall astoundingly short. Cosmetics companies such as Estee Lauder are so far ahead of Lancome it is almost shocking. Another fact that is likely to be of some interest to the consumer is that Lancome is owned by L'Oreal, and you can often find L'Oreal products that are virtually identical to the Lancome products—the products are first launched at the L'Oreal shelves and then turn up at the Lancome counters a month or two later. In terms of quality, both L'Oreal and Lancome lag behind, though if you think Lancome has the answers for you, try L'Oreal first. Just be warned: Their products are highly fragranced, a very French thing to do. For more information about Lancome, call (800)-LANCOME or visit www.lancome.com. **Note:** All Lancome products contain fragrance.

LANCOME SKIN CARE

☺ **Ablutia Fraicheur Purifying Foam Cleanser** *($21.50 for 6.4 ounces)* is a very standard, detergent-based, water-soluble cleanser that can be drying for some skin types, but it's appropriate for someone with normal to oily skin.

☺ **Clarifiance Oil-Free Gel Cleanser** *($21.50 for 6.8 ounces)* is a standard, detergent-based, water-soluble cleanser that would work well for most skin types except for dry skin.

☹ **Vinefit Cleansing Bar** *($13 for 4 ounces)* is an extremely standard bar cleanser that contains the tiniest amount of grape extract and oil. It can be drying for most skin types.

☺ **Clarifiance Oil-Free Gel Cleanser** *($21.50 for 6.8 ounces)* is a very basic, though good, detergent-based cleanser that would work well for most skin types except for dry skin.

☺ **$$$ Gel Controle** *($19.50 for 4.2 ounces)* is a standard, detergent-based cleanser that would work well for normal to oily skin. It contains a tiny amount of salicylic acid, but the high pH of this cleanser makes it ineffective for exfoliation.

☺ $$$ **Mousse Controle** *($19.50 for 4.2 ounces)* is a detergent-based cleanser that dispenses like a mousse hair-styling product. The clay in it has some oil-absorbing properties. Of interest is the arginine, an amino acid, listed as the third ingredient. Arginine can be effective in wound healing, but in a cleanser it would just be rinsed away before it had much of a chance to be of help. This product also contains salicylic acid, but the pH of the mousse isn't low enough for it to be effective as an exfoliant.

☺ **Galatee Comfort Milky Creme Cleanser** *($37.50 for 13.5 ounces)* is supposed to be a splash-off or tissue-off cleanser for all skin types, but it ends up being a standard, mineral oil–based, wipe-off cleanser that can leave a greasy film on the skin. It may be good for extremely dry skin, although it needs to be wiped off to remove both the makeup and the cleanser.

☺ $$$ **Gel Clarte** *($19.50 for 4.2 ounces)* is a standard, detergent-based cleanser that can be an option for normal to oily skin. The papaya and pineapple extracts have no exfoliating properties.

☺ **Mousse Clarte** *($25 for 6.8 ounces)* is similar to the Gel Clarte above, only in a mousse dispenser, and the same basic comments apply.

☺ $$$ **Mousse Confort** *($19.50 for 4.2 ounces)* is a standard, detergent-based cleanser that can be an option for normal to oily skin. It would be too drying for dry skin.

☺ $$$ **Bi-Facil Double-Action Eye Makeup Remover** *($20 for 4 ounces)* is a very standard, silicone-based, wipe-off cleanser, nothing more. It would work as well as any.

☺ $$$ **Effacile Gentle Eye Makeup Remover** *($17.50 for 4 ounces)* is a detergent-based eye-makeup remover that isn't all that gentle, but it will take off eye makeup.

☹ **Eau de Bienfait Cleanser Water with Vitamins for Face and Eyes** *($23.50 for 6.8 ounces)* is a standard, detergent-based makeup remover that would be gentler than the Effacile above, except that the pineapple and papaya extracts are inappropriate for the eye area.

☺ $$$ **Exfoliance Delicate Exfoliating Gel** *($21 for 3.5 ounces)* is a standard, detergent-based scrub that uses ground-up plastic (polyethylene) as the abrasive, which is fairly gentle for normal to oily skin. This does contain a tiny amount of salicylic acid (BHA), but the pH is too high for it to have any benefit for exfoliation.

☺ $$$ **Exfoliance Confort** *($21 for 3.4 ounces)* is similar to the Exfoliance Delicate Exfoliating Gel above only in a far more emollient base and without the BHA, which means this is far better for normal to dry skin.

☺ $$$ **Exfoliance Clarte Clarifying Exfoliating Gel** *($21 for 3.4 ounces)* is similar to the Exfoliance Delicate Exfoliating Gel above only with more detergent cleansing agents, which does make it better for normal to oily skin. The same comments apply about the BHA.

☹ **Tonique Controle Toner for Oily and Normal to Oily Skin** *($19.50 for 6.8 ounces)* is basically just alcohol, and that is too irritating and drying for all skin types.

☹ **Tonique Clarte** *($19.50 for 6.8 ounces)* is similar to the Tonique Controle above and the same comments apply.

The Reviews L

☺ **Tonique Douceur Non-Alcoholic Freshener for Dry/Sensitive Skin** *($27.50 for 13.5 ounces)* is indeed alcohol-free, but it's also little more than applying fragrant water to your skin. This is a very average, do-nothing toner with almost nonexistent antioxidants and water-binding agents, and way too pricey for such a mundane formulation.

☹ **Vitabolic Clarifier Radiance Boosting Tonic** *($27.50 for 3.4 ounces)* is basically just alcohol, along with some potentially irritating plant extracts that just boost the risk of skin irritation and dryness. The pH is too high for the BHA it contains to be effective for exfoliation.

☺ **Tonique Confort** *($19.50 for 6.8 ounces)* is an OK toner with a small, but OK, amount of water-binding agents and an antioxidant. It is an option for normal to dry skin.

☺ $$$ **Absolue Absolute Replenishing Cream SPF 15** *($90 for 1.7 ounces)*. Considering that this is one of Lancome's most expensive skin-care products they had to put some effort into explaining why paying $90 for a 1.7-ounce product made it better for skin than the other products they sell to produce the same benefit—namely, getting rid of wrinkles. It does contain an in-part avobenzone sunscreen, but this is merely a good, largely silicone-based moisturizer that contains a small amount of antioxidants and even less water-binding agent. It will work well for normal to dry skin. This cream claims it "replenishes skin's appearance that has changed as a result of chronological aging, sun exposure, and hormonal fluctuations" by addressing three primary concerns: dryness, diminished radiance, and loss of elasticity. However, claiming that these concerns can be remedied by the teeny amount of wild yam, soy extract, and sea algae this contains is sheer fantasy. Wild yam does not behave like progesterone in the skin. (It also doesn't appear to do so when eaten or taken in supplements either. As Dr. Andrew Weil states on his Web site, www.drweil.com, "All sorts of claims have been made about wild yam because it contains a precursor of steroid hormones called diosgenin, which was used as the starting material for the first birth-control pill. But diosgenin itself has no hormonal activity. Nor can the human body convert it into something that does.") Soy does have antioxidant properties, but its documented effects on estrogen, when taken orally, do not give the same results as when it is applied topically to skin, or at least there is no research establishing that to be the case.

What about the sea algae? Is this Lancome's attempt to compete with Lauder's Creme de La Mer skin care? Sea algae (seaweed) can function as an antioxidant and water-binding agent, and it costs only pennies to include it in a cosmetic product. For the money, a product brimming with antioxidants and water-binding agents would have been far more impressive.

Finally, remember that sunscreens must be applied liberally if you are to obtain the SPF benefit on the label. At this price you may be reluctant to do that.

☺ $$$ **Absolue Absolute Replenishing Lotion SPF 15** *($90 for 1.7 ounces)* is virtually identical to the Cream version above, only in lotion form, and the same basic comments apply.

☺ $$$ **Absolue Eye** *($60 for 0.5 ounce)* is just an OK, emollient, silicone-based moisturizer that would work well for normal to dry skin. It contains mostly water, glycerin, silicones, plant oil, emollient, thickeners, mica (shine particles), algae, preservative, wild yam, more preservatives, and soybean extract. See the comments for the Absolue Replenishing Cream SPF 15 above concerning those ingredients.

☺ $$$ **Bienfait Total Fluide SPF 15** *($55 for 3.4 ounces)* is a very good, in-part avobenzone-based sunscreen. So why the neutral face rating? Now that so many products contain UVA-protecting ingredients, you can be more picky about what you choose, and this formulation lists alcohol as the third ingredient. That can be drying and irritating for most skin types—not to mention that the price is completely unwarranted.

☺ $$$ **Bienfait Total UV Eye SPF 15** *($28.50 for 0.5 ounce)* is a good, in-part titanium dioxide–based sunscreen that contains a small amount of antioxidants, but lacks water-binding agents. For the price you would expect full benefits. However, the sun protection is very good.

☹ **Bienfait Total Day Creme SPF 15** *($36 for 1.7 ounces)* does not contain the UVA-protecting ingredients of titanium dioxide, zinc oxide, or avobenzone, and is not recommended.

☺ $$$ **Impactive Multi Performance Silkening Moisturizer** *($38 for 1.7 ounces)* is a silicone-based moisturizer that does leave a silky feel on the skin and that contains some good antioxidants and water-binding agents. It is a good option for someone with normal to dry skin.

☹ **Hydra Controle Oil-Free Hydrating Gel** *($35 for 1.7 ounces)* lists alcohol as the fourth ingredient, which can be a problem for skin. It contains only negligible amounts of water-binding agents, antioxidants, and anti-irritants. The triclosan in this product is a topical disinfectant, but there is no research showing it to be effective for controlling blemishes.

☺ $$$ **HydraZen for Normal/Combination Skin** *($44 for 1.7 ounces)* is supposed to be relaxation in a jar, or at least that's what the name and ad copy suggest. It's "stress relief for your skin" and contains something called "Acticalm." Even if you could apply something to the face to make it calmer, according to HydraZen that would only take a moisturizer, because that's all this product is. The only unique thing about HydraZen is the name. If mind over matter works, then you will feel calmer, but it probably isn't from applying this good, but rather ordinary, ho-hum, silicone-based, lightweight moisturizer that contains minimal water-binding agents and antioxidants. Some of the plant extracts can be irritants.

☺ $$$ **Hydra Zen Cream for Normal to Dry Skin** *($44 for 1.7 ounces)* is similar to the HydraZen for Normal/Combination Skin above except that this one contains several plant oils, which does make it better for dry skin. Still, it lacks the amounts of antioxidants and water-binding agents that would have warranted a better rating.

☺ $$$ **Hydra Zen Cream for Very Dry Skin** *($44 for 1.7 ounces)* is similar to the Hydra Zen Cream above and the same basic comments apply.

The Reviews L

☺ **$$$ Hydra Zen Skin De-Stressing Anti-Puffiness Eye Treatment** *($36 for 0.5 ounce)* is an OK, emollient, silicone-based moisturizer that contains a decent amount of antioxidants and water-binding agent, though it's not exactly brimming over with them. The caffeine it contains can't depuff the eye and the plant extracts are a mix of irritants and anti-irritants.

☺ **$$$ Niosome + Perfected Age Treatment** *($68 for 2.5 ounces)* is a good basic moisturizer for dry skin. There are some antioxidants, but such negligible amounts that they don't count for much.

☺ **$$$ Nutribel Nourishing Hydrating Emulsion** *($40 for 2.5 ounces)* is a very emollient moisturizer for dry skin that contains mostly water, plant oils, glycerin, mineral oil, thickeners, urea, water-binding agents, and preservatives. This isn't exciting, but it is good.

☺ **Nutrix Soothing Treatment Creme** *($32 for 1.9 ounces)* costs a lot of money for what you get, which is primarily mineral oil, Vaseline, lanolin, waxes, and tiny amounts of water-binding agents. It is an option for very dry skin. However, lines from Lubriderm to Eucerin offer similar formulas for far less money.

☺ **Trans-Hydrix Multi-Action Hydrating Creme** *($36.50 for 1.9 ounces)* is a very basic, ordinary, emollient moisturizer for dry skin.

☹ **Progres Counter des Yeux Eye Creme** *($37.50 for 1.5 ounces)* is a thick, heavy eye cream of mostly thickeners, Vaseline, and emollient. It also contains preservatives that are recommended for use in rinse-off products only, and, as such, is not recommended.

☺ **$$$ Primordiale Intense Creme** *($74 for 1.7 ounces)*. There is simply nothing intense about this silicone-based moisturizer for dry skin except the price. The plant extracts it contains are meant to sound like they can perform like AHAs, but they have no exfoliating properties. The teeny amount of vitamin E is barely detectable, and there are no water-binding agents of any consequence.

☺ **$$$ Primordiale Intense Eye** *($46 for 0.5 ounce)* contains mostly water, silicones, glycerin, film-forming agent, plant oils, slip agent, vitamin E, preservatives, caffeine, wound-healing agent, algae, fragrance, and water-binding agent. The teeny amounts of vitamin E and plant extracts can't provide much benefit and caffeine can be a skin irritant, though when present in such a small amount that's unlikely. This would have been better if it had much larger amounts of antioxidants and water-binding agents.

☺ **$$$ Primordiale Lip** *($29 for 0.5 ounce)* is an emollient, clear, somewhat glossy lipstick—period. It isn't concentrated in the least.

☺ **$$$ Primordiale Intense Night Renewing Age Defense Treatment** *($63 for 1.7 ounces)* is virtually identical to Lancome's former Primordiale Nuit; the only noticeable difference on the ingredient list is a different form of silicone. Despite the fantastic claims, this remains a rather ordinary moisturizer for dry to very dry skin.

☹ **Renergie Lift Contour Skin Firming and Conditioning Complex** *($54 for 1 ounce)* is, with only minor differences (and I mean really minor differences), virtually identical to L'Oreal's Revitalift Slim Face Contouring and Toning Solution. The major difference? L'Oreal's is $10.49 for 1.7 ounces, which means a possible savings to you of more than $60 if you give the L'Oreal version a try instead of this one from Lancome. That is, if you really want to buy into the claim that these two primarily alcohol-based products can reduce facial puffiness and firm and lift skin. Not only is that unlikely, but the alcohol when present in this amount can be drying, and the *Terminalia sericea* plant extract can be a skin irritant. This one is up to you, but there are better products than this from both Lancome and L'Oreal to consider.

☺ $$$ **Renergie Double Performance Treatment Anti-Wrinkle and Firmness** *($80 for 2.5 ounces)* contains nothing that can firm or have any impact on stopping wrinkles. This very basic moisturizer includes mostly water, thickeners, silicone, Vaseline, water-binding agents, sunscreen ingredient, fragrance, vitamin E, caffeine, preservatives, and coloring agents. This is mediocre and repetitive, just like many of the Lancome moisturizers.

☺ $$$ **Renergie Emulsion Oil-Free Lotion, Double Performance, Anti-Wrinkle, Firming** *($65 for 1.7 ounces)* is even more empty of beneficial skin-care ingredients than the Renergie Double Performance above. This version takes out the Vaseline, which makes it better for oily skin, and adds a tiny amount of cornstarch, but even the trace amount of vitamin E is gone, replaced with a minuscule amount of vitamin A. Otherwise, the same basic comments apply, but for the money this is truly a serious disappointment for any skin type.

☺ $$$ **Renergie Eye** *($46 for 0.5 ounce)* is similar to the Renergie Double Performance Treatment above and the same basic comments apply.

☺ $$$ **ReSurface** *($52.50 for 1 ounce)* is Lancome's contribution to the retinol bandwagon, only L'Oreal beat Lancome to the punch a few months earlier with its Line Eraser Pure Retinol ($12.89 for 1 ounce). These products are virtually the same, with the same retinol, the same small amount, the same lightweight lotion formulation, and the same airtight packaging (which is necessary to keep the retinol stable). If you're thinking of retinol, despite the meager evidence that there is any reason to use it, why would you choose the Lancome version over the L'Oreal version? Keep in mind that the only benefit to using this product *is* retinol, because it comes up short for any other worthwhile skin-care ingredients.

☺ $$$ **ReSurface Eye** *($44 for 0.5 ounce).* If you thought Lancome's Re-Surface retinol moisturizer was a necessity, then of course the eye version would be part of the package. At least that's what Lancome is hoping you believe about this moisturizer with retinol. However, if retinol is the ingredient you're after, the original ReSurface above, at $52.50 for 1 ounce, could absolutely be used around the eyes and be a significant savings. However, you do remember that L'Oreal's version, Line Eraser Pure Retinol ($12.89 for 1 ounce), is an equally good option for a retinol product?

☺ $$$ **Vinefit Complete Energizing Lotion SPF 15** *($37.50 for 1 ounce).* The best part of this overpriced sunscreen is the sunscreen, which is an appropriate SPF 15 with an in-part titanium dioxide–based sunscreen. Other than the touted grape seed oil and grape

The Reviews L

extract, which are good antioxidants, this product does contain niacinamide. There is research showing that niacinamide is effective in the production of ceramides (a vital component of skin) and in reducing the negative effects of sun exposure (which suppresses the skin's immune response). Whether or not niacinamide can do that when applied topically is unknown, but it is still an intriguing ingredient to consider using on skin. However, Olay has far better products that include this ingredient than Lancome. Overall, the moisturizing base, for normal to dry skin, is exceptionally ordinary.

☺ $$$ **Vinefit Cream SPF 15** *($37.50 for 1.7 ounces)* is a cream version of the Vinefit Complete version above and the same basic comments apply.

☺ **Vinefit Cool Gel** *($26 for 1.7 ounces)* has grape extract and a tiny amount of vitamin E and niacinamide, but it also lists alcohol as the fourth ingredient, and that's not cooling, that's irritating for skin.

☹ **Vinefit Lip SPF 8** *($14.50 for 0.5 ounce)* is a poorly formulated sunscreen with no UVA-protecting ingredients and an abysmally low SPF 8, far below the standard of SPF 15 set by the Skin Cancer Foundation and the American Academy of Dermatology. This is just embarrassing.

☹ $$$ **Vitabolic Dark Eye Circle Treatment** *($46 for 0.5 ounce)* is yet another addition to the world of vitamin C skin-care products. Vitabolic uses ascorbic acid. Refer to Chapter Seven, *Cosmetics Dictionary,* for more details about ascorbic acid and vitamin C. Basically, with only ascorbic acid, and no other antioxidants or water-binding agents, this is a one-note product. All in all, Avon's vitamin C product is far more interesting (it even has the same form of vitamin C) for less money.

☹ $$$ **Vitabolic Deep Radiance Booster** *($45 for 1 ounce)* is almost identical to the Vitabolic Dark Eye Circle version above and the same basic comments apply.

☹ $$$ **Vitabolic Oil Free** *($49 for 1 ounce)* is almost identical to the Vitabolic Dark Circle Eye version above, except that they took out the plant oil, though the same basic comments still apply.

☹ $$$ **Complexion Expert** *($46 for 1 ounce)* is supposed to lighten skin discoloration. This very standard, extremely ordinary emollient moisturizer may just do that because it does contain kojic acid, along with the exceptionally standard emollients and plant oil and teeny amounts of vitamins E and C. There is definitely convincing research, both in vitro and in vivo, and in animal studies, showing that kojic acid is effective for inhibiting melanin production (Sources: *Biological and Pharmaceutical Bulletin,* August 2002, pages 1045–1048; *Analytical Biochemistry,* June 2002, pages 260–268; *Cellular Signaling,* September 2002, pages 779–785; *American Journal of Clinical Dermatology,* September-October 2000, pages 261–268; and *Archives of Pharmacal Research,* August 2001, pages 307–311). So why doesn't this ingredient show up in more skin-lightening products (most use hydroquinone, or plant extracts that have arbutin as one of their components)? It's because kojic acid is an extremely unstable ingredient in cosmetic formulations. Upon exposure to air or sunlight it turns a strange shade of brown and loses its efficacy, and it is also considered extremely irritating as well (Source: www.emedicine.com, "Skin Lightening/Depigmenting Agents," November 5, 2001).

☹ **Pure Empriente Masque Purifying Mineral Mask with White Clay** *($24 for 3.4 ounces)* is a standard clay mask that contains camphor, making it too irritating for all skin types.

☹ **Hydra Intense Masque** *($24 for 3.4 ounces)* lists alcohol as the second ingredient, and that makes it completely hydra un-intense and not recommended.

☹ **Pore Controle Masque** *($24 for 3.4 ounces)* is a standard clay mask with some salicylic acid, but the pH of the base is too high for it to be an effective exfoliant. It also contains menthol, which won't help skin in the least; it is just irritating and a problem for all skin types.

☺ **$$$ T. Controle Oil-Free Powder Gel Instant T-Zone Matifier** *($22.50 for 1 ounce)* is an interesting product made of silicone and film-forming agent, period—there is no powder in here. It will put a silky film over the skin, but don't count on this helping your oily skin because there is nothing in this product that can hold back oil. It is a decent lightweight silicone moisturizer, but that's about it. Definitely test it before you even consider purchasing this misleading product. If anything, it will make someone with oily skin feel somewhat oilier!

LANCOME OLIGO MINERAL

Lancome has been quietly selling this small collection of products exclusively at Neiman Marcus, and no wonder! Neiman's is known for carrying upscale (read: very expensive) cosmetics, and pride themselves on their select menagerie of skin-care and makeup lines. I suspect that one of the reasons the Oligo Mineral line is not available in "mainstream" department stores is because the products are almost identical to Lancome's other products; the major difference is that these carry lofty, needlessly marked-up price tags. Naturally, the hook that supposedly justifies the hefty price is the inclusion of several minerals, from copper to zinc. Yet even if such an assortment of minerals had some extraordinary benefit for topical use on the skin, Lancome adds them in such small amounts that their impact (if any) would be nominal. Leaving aside the illusion of affluence that purchasing these products may convey, there is no reason to stop by the Neiman Marcus Lancome counter to check these out. If Lancome is where you want to spend your cosmetics dollars, your skin won't notice the difference if you ignore this sub-line and focus on their Nordstrom or Macy's department-store offerings. The only difference you will notice is in your budget.

☺ **$$$ Oligo Mineral Cleanser** *($48.50 for 4 ounces)* is an extremely standard foaming cleanser that can be quite drying for most skin types, though it certainly does clean well. The fragrance comes way before the fountain-of-youth minerals, which means their presence is more for show than effect.

☹ **Oligo Mineral Toner** *($40 for 6.8 ounces)* is an embarrassing formulation that lists alcohol as the second ingredient. That makes it too drying and irritating for all skin types, and Lancome knows better (at least they do in their less expensive toners). What a shame, because sans alcohol, this would have been a very good moisturizing toner for dry skin.

☺ $$$ **Oligo Mineral Fortifying Cream** *($125 for 2.6 ounces)* is a silky, emollient moisturizer that would be a fine option for normal to dry skin, but there is nothing especially unique in this that makes it worth the investment. It does contain some good antioxidants, but the amounts are minuscule, and for this price, it should be overflowing with them.

☹ $$$ **Oligo Mineral Eye Cream** *($75 for 0.5 ounce)* is almost identical to, but less elegant than, the Fortifying Cream above, and the same basic comments apply. This does have a tiny amount of caffeine, but it's not enough to be a significant problem for irritation, and it won't wake up the eye area either.

☺ $$$ **Oligo Mineral Lotion** *($95 for 1.7 ounces)* is a very good lightweight lotion for normal to slightly dry skin, featuring an effective blend of water, silicones, slip agent, mineral oil, anti-irritant, vitamins E, C, and A (antioxidants), minerals, preservatives, and fragrance. But save your money. Lancome's Vinefit Complete Energizing Lotion SPF 15 ($37.50 for 1.7 ounces) offers an even silkier formula with equally good antioxidants and effective sun protection to boot, yet costs almost two-thirds less.

LANCOME SUN PRODUCTS

☺ **SPF 15 Face and Body Lotion with Pure Vitamin E** *($25 for 5 ounces)* is a very good, avobenzone-based sunscreen in a lightweight lotion base for someone with normal to dry or slightly oily skin. It is a very basic moisturizer with a minuscule amount of vitamin E.

☺ $$$ **UV Expert SPF 15 Water Light Fluid** *($31 for 1 ounce)* is similar to the SPF 15 Face and Body Lotion above only in a matte finish, lotion base, and the same basic comments apply.

☺ **SPF 25 Face and Body Lotion with Pure Vitamin E** *($25 for 5 ounces)* is similar to the SPF 15 Face and Body Lotion above and the same review applies.

☺ **Water-Light Spray SPF 15 with Pure Vitamin E** *($25 for 5 ounces)* is a very good avobenzone-based sunscreen that is mostly slip agents, film-forming agent, and plant oil. It should work well for someone with normal to dry skin.

☺ $$$ **High Protection SPF 30 Face Creme with Pure Vitamin E** *($24 for 1.7 ounces)* is similar to the lotions above, but there is nothing unique or special about this one that warrants the far smaller amount of sunscreen product for the same price.

☺ $$$ **Soleil Expert Sun Care SPF 30 High Protection Sun Stick** *($19.50 for 0.26 ounce)* is an avobenzone-based sunscreen, and the amount you get for the price is ludicrous given that this is simply a good sunscreen in an ordinary emollient lipstick-type base.

☺ $$$ **Soleil Ultra Eye Protection SPF 40** *($25 for 0.5 ounce)* is a good, but extremely overpriced, sunscreen that includes titanium dioxide and zinc oxide as two of the active sunscreen ingredients. This combination is not unique to Lancome and the use of an SPF 40 sounds like you are getting "more" protection, but all you would be getting is longer protection, and there just isn't that much sunlight in a day. (SPF ratings over 30 are not going to be around after the FDA's new sunscreen regulations take effect.) Nothing about this sunscreen makes it preferred for the eye area; if anything, the talc and other active ingredients (octyl methoxycinnamate and oxybenzone) can be irritating if they get in the eye. This is an ordinary moisturizer for normal to dry skin.

☺ $$$ **Soleil Ultra Face and Body Lotion SPF 40** *($25 for 0.5 ounce)* is similar to the Soleil Ultra Eye Protection above minus the talc, and the same comments apply. Actually, these two products are so similar there is no reason to spend more money on the version above.

☺ $$$ **Soleil Cool Comfort After Sun Rehydrating Face and Body Lotion** *($25 for 5 ounces)* is a very basic, ordinary moisturizer for normal to dry skin with tiny amounts of antioxidants and fractional amounts of anti-irritants. Mica adds a small touch of shine to the skin.

☺ $$$ **Flash Bronzer Self Tanning Face Gel with Pure Vitamin E,** available in **Medium, Deep,** and **Extra Deep** *($24 for 1.7 ounces)*; **Flash Bronzer Oil Free Tinted Self Tanning Face Lotion for the Face with Vitamin E** available in **Medium** or **Dark** *($24 for 1.7 ounces)*; and **Flash Bronzer Tinted Self Tanning Mousse** *($27 for 5 ounces)* all contain dihydroxyacetone, the same ingredient all self-tanners use to affect the color of skin. These would work as well as any, but there is nothing in these formulations that makes them preferred over far less expensive versions available in drugstores.

☹ **Flash Bronzer Instant Self Tanning Body Spray with SPF 15 and Pure Vitamin E** *($27 for 4.2 ounces)* doesn't contain the UVA-protecting ingredients of titanium dioxide, zinc oxide, or avobenzone, and is not recommended.

LANCOME MAKEUP

In contrast to their rather lackluster skin-care products, Lancome's French-bred, American-made makeup is a stellar collection that, in some categories, continues to set precedents as new technology evolves. Their selection of everything from foundations to lipsticks is enormous—and there are prime picks in every category. I don't know how the counter personnel keep track of everything, but for the most part Lancome's sales force is adept at navigating through the products. In contrast to the staff at Estee Lauder, Lancome's representatives maintain a more passive-aggressive, casual approach, which can still be unnerving but is definitely less intense. Although the makeup tester units still do not divide colors into logical groups (such as pinks and plums), the specific products are distinguished and grouped together, so you're not left to guess which lipstick formula you're sampling or which concealer you're blending.

If you're looking for a force to reckon with for foundations, Lancome is a must-see. They continue to offer some of the most elegant, silky formulas anywhere and in a color range that is overwhelmingly neutral, whether your skin is porcelain or ebony. The only troubling aspect is that most of Lancome's foundations with sunscreen do not contain adequate UVA protection. Considering that Lancome obviously knows about the risks with this issue, I recommend these foundations with mixed emotions. The fact that they continually launch new foundations with incomplete sun protection is tantamount to a company like Ford knowingly selling new cars without air bags. Beyond this major gripe, you will discover that Lancome has a well-deserved reputation for their fantastic mascaras, and their latest powder-based products apply with a silkiness that makes them gratifying to work with. The rest of the makeup comprises some completely valid options, but before you commit to Lancome, consider the similar options available for less from sister companies L'Oreal and Maybelline. Striking a balance between the best of each of these lines will give you first-class makeup that beautifies without breaking the bank.

FOUNDATION: ✔☺ **$$$ Dual Finish Versatile Powder Makeup** *($31)* is a talc-based wet/dry powder foundation that offers a soft matte finish and a beautiful selection of colors. The application, especially when used dry, is smooth and even, although this type of foundation is best for normal skin; dry skin may find this too dry and oily skin may find it too cakey after it is applied. I would avoid wet application since this type of product tends to go on choppy and streak. The only disappointing color among the 16 is Matte Miel Fonce IV, which may turn orange on some skin tones. Matte Porcelaine Delicate and Matte Rose Clair are slightly pink, but not enough to show on lighter skin. ✔☺ **Maquicontrole Oil-Free Liquid Makeup** *($32.50)* is Lancome's original ultra-matte foundation (launched over 17 years ago, well ahead of its time) and it has remained an exceptional oil-free foundation that offers medium to full coverage and a true matte finish. It has incredible staying power and is ideal for oily to very oily skin. Of the ten shades, avoid Beige Natural III and Beige Bisque III. ✔☺ **Teint Idole Enduringly Divine Makeup** *($32.50)* is one of the best (and last) ultra-matte makeups. It has a decent slip, but blending must still be precise because it dries quickly and doesn't budge. The smooth texture offers medium to full coverage, and this wears beautifully. Of the 15 shades, only Bisque 0, Suede 0, and Suede 2 are problematic. Suede 10 is perfect for dark skin, while Ivoire 0 would work for the fairest complexion. ✔☺ **Bienfait Total UV Tinted SPF 15** *($36)* is an excellent option for a lightweight, sheer, tinted moisturizer for normal to oily skin types. The texture has a soft, creamy slip that blends beautifully on the skin and it sets to a soft matte finish. Of course, any shine-prone areas will show through relatively quickly, but for those who prefer a light wash of color with an in-part titanium dioxide sunscreen, this is brilliant. The four shades are mostly winners—only Tawny may be too peach for some skin tones, but just barely.

☺ **$$$ Photogenic Skin-Illuminating Makeup SPF 15** *($32.50)* is divine, with a light, fluid texture that blends to a soft, natural finish with light to medium coverage. The 19 shades are mostly wonderful, and this blends with ease. If Lancome would just add some UVA protection, Photogenic would be a great recommendation for normal to slightly dry or slightly oily skin types. If you're willing to wear sun protection underneath this, there are some superior colors to consider for both light and dark skin tones (but not for very dark skin). The following shades are too pink, peach, or copper for most skin tones: Bisque 2 (slightly pink), Bisque 4, Bisque 8, Suede 4 (slight copper), and Suede 6. **Photogenic Ultra-Comfort Skin Illuminating Makeup SPF 15** *($32.50)* is a marvelous-feeling foundation that is piggybacking off the success of Lancome's original Photogenic makeup. This version is designed for normal to dry skin and it shows. The silicone-based formula feels silky and airy on the skin while imparting light coverage and a soft, natural finish that blends easily. Of the ten shades available, only Ultra Bisque 2 and Ultra Bisque 4 (both slightly peach) should be considered with caution. The other eight colors are true to Lancome's usually excellent neutral foundation palette. The only drawback that keeps this from being a Paula's Pick is the sunscreen, which does not contain UVA-protecting ingredients. If you're willing to wear an effective sunscreen underneath this, it is whole-heartedly recommended! **Maqui-Libre Skin-Liberating Makeup SPF 15** *($32.50)* offers sheer coverage and a natural finish with its lightweight, fluid texture that blends easily. If only the sunscreen contained effective UVA protection, this would be a slam-dunk for casual weekend makeup for those with normal to dry skin. If you're willing to pair this with a reliable sunscreen, you will find most of the seven shades are superior. Rose Clair II and Beige Bisque III are too pink and rose, respectively. **Teint Optim' age Minimizing Makeup SPF 15** *($32.50)* claims it is "makeup for a new age," yet it contains no UVA-protecting ingredients, which borders on archaic. If sun protection isn't your goal, this enviably smooth makeup blends on superbly, offering sheer to light coverage with a soft matte finish. It is best for normal to dry skin. The claims about "age minimizing" are bogus—there is nothing in here to support that and it won't make one wrinkle on your face look less noticeable—but it is still an excellent foundation. Be careful with the following shades: Beige Bisque III (may turn slightly pink) and Beige Dore III (just slightly peach). **Maquivelours Hydrating Foundation** *($32.50)* is an emollient, demi-matte-finish formula that is best for normal to dry or very dry skin seeking medium coverage. Of the nine shades, the ones to avoid are Rose Clair II, Beige Rose III (both too pink), and Beige Bisque III (peachy).

☹ $$$ **Imanance Tinted Day Creme SPF 15** *($36)* is an in-part titanium dioxide–based SPF 15 tinted moisturizer. The coverage is sheer and the emolliency makes it suitable for normal to dry skin only. The only useful skin-tone color is Bisque; the three remaining shades are all orange or red, though Tawny may work for some medium skin tones.

<u>CONCEALER:</u> ✓☺ $$$ **Effacernes Waterproof Protective Undereye Concealer** *($21)* has a lush, creamy texture that provides superior coverage and allows smooth blending. The squeeze tube takes some getting used to (it's easy to squeeze out too much product), but once you acclimate, this concealer is an ace in the hole, and it doesn't crease! The four shades are quite nice, though Porcelaine I is slightly pink. Contrary to the name, this concealer is not waterproof. ✓☺ $$$ **Photogenic Skin-Illuminating Concealer SPF 15** *($21)* is one of the best concealers available. First, it has an all titanium dioxide–based sunscreen, which makes this a wonderful counterpart to your regular sun

protection, whether from a moisturizer or your foundation. Second, it has an incredibly soft, ultra-light texture that blends beautifully—almost melting into the skin—yet covers quite well. The finish is soft matte, and it has only a slight tendency to crease into lines. The six colors are mostly superb. Only Correcteur (slightly yellow) and Camee (too peach) should be avoided, and bronze may be too copper for very dark skin tones.

☺ $$$ **Maquicomplet Complete Coverage Concealer** *($21)* has taken a turn for the worse. This smooth, liquidy concealer with excellent, crease-free coverage now features seven shine-laden shades. How maddening! With all of the other shiny products in the Lancome lineup, why adulterate a perfectly good concealer? This is still worth considering, but please realize that the shiny finish does nothing to minimize wrinkles, nor does it look good over blemishes. **Palette Mix Complexion Kit** *($30)* is a compact with three different flesh-toned shades that you use in combination to get just the right color for your skin. Although this cream-to-powder formula has a superbly smooth finish, most women will have difficulty combining colors like this on their face. It isn't a bad idea, just more time-consuming than a makeup application should be.

<u>POWDER:</u> ✓☺ $$$ **Photogenic Sheer Loose Powder** *($30)* and ✓☺ $$$ **Photogenic Sheer Pressed Powder** *($25)*. These talc-based powders have replaced Lancome's Poudre Majeur, and claim to contain the "Photo-Flex Complex of 2-D reflecting powders and 3-D diffusing powders." I guess when you're charging upwards of $25 for something as basic as powder you need a good hook. Admittedly, both of these powders have a soft, finely milled, sumptuous texture and a smooth, dry finish (the Pressed Powder version is slightly drier), but the special effects are nothing more than subtle iridescence, plain and simple. Although the shine is barely discernible, those hoping to reduce shine may want to look elsewhere. Both powders offer seven shades, and almost all of them are beautifully soft and neutral, including options for darker (but not very dark) skin tones. Only Soft Bronze stands out as too orange for dark skin, and Deep Bronze would make a great bronzing powder. Note: A major plus for the Loose Powder version is its packaging, which adds a powder screen to prevent flyaway loose powder from getting all over everything. ✓☺ **Matte Finish Shine Control Sheer Pressed Powder** *($22)* has a stunningly smooth texture and an even application that does not look powdery or thick on the skin. This talc-based powder comes in six gorgeous colors (though Suede may be too copper for dark skin) and is best for normal to oily skin looking to tame shine without a powdered appearance.

☺ $$$ **Poudre Blanc Neige Light-Reflecting Compact Powder** *($30)* is a standard pressed powder with a smooth, silky finish and a truly soft shine. For a subtle amount of shine, which is a welcome change of pace from the glitter in most products, this is an option. The one shade is a sheer, very pale yellow.

☺ $$$ **Poudre Soleil Sun-Kissed Bronzing Powder** *($30)* is a pressed-powder bronzer with an OK, sheer application and three overly shiny, unnaturally copper colors. This is far from a natural-looking bronzer, and at this price, you can confidently ignore it. **Star**

Bronzer Bronzing Powder for Face & Body SPF 8 *($35)* is similar to the Bronzing Powder above, except this comes in an oversized compact and features a paltry sunscreen that lacks UVA protection. Both shades are shiny, and a bit too peach (Dore) or copper (Intense) to be considered a top choice.

BLUSH: ✓☺ $$$ **Blush Subtil Delicate Oil-Free Powder Blush** *($25.50)* is a talc-free powder blush that has an enviably soft texture and even application. The color selection is beautiful, but each one has at least some shine. The prime offenders in regard to shine are the ultra-sparkly Miel Glace, Bronze Glow, Pink Parfait, Pink Pool, and Soiree. Rouge Glow is a great shade for darker skin, while Bronze Brule is excellent for contouring. ☺ **Couleur Flash Blush Stick** *($28.50)* is a twist-up, cream-to-powder blush with a creamy slip-on application that quickly dries to a soft, sheer powder finish. This has been pared down to a single shade, a pale plum that would work for light skin tones.

☹ **Blush Focus Exceptional Wear Sheer Cheek Color** *($19.50)* is meant to combine the one-touch application of a cream blush with the long wear and soft finish of a powder blush, but it fails to perform well in either category. The texture is hard to explain, but I'll do my best. It's semi-creamy with the dryness of a powder, yet tends to flake and chip right out of the container. What's more confounding is that while it is difficult to pick up color with a brush, using your finger picks up too much color and makes it hard to apply with a light touch. It also applies unevenly, looking sheer in spots and intense in others. Perhaps what's most distressing about this blush is that it took the place of Lancome's far superior cream-to-powder blush Pommette. Lancome, what were you thinking?

EYESHADOW: ☺ $$$ **Colour Focus Exceptional Wear EyeColour** *($16.50)* at last allows Lancome to offer single powder eyeshadows instead of just duos. In comparison to their MaquiRiche eyeshadows, this formula is undeniably silkier and not nearly as powdery. It applies evenly and easily, with just enough color saturation so that successive applications are not necessary before you can build any intensity. What is frustrating is that almost all of the 35+ shades have either a soft shimmer or a traffic-stopping shine! Couldn't just a few matte shades exist for those who aren't interested in the trend? Consider the following colors almost matte due to their extremely soft shine: Daylight, Positive, Peep, Scene, and Horizon. By the way, the flying saucer–style compact houses a tiny curved eyeshadow applicator that is truly bizarre and unusable, though it does look cool!

☺ $$$ **MaquiRiche CremePowder EyeColour Duo** *($26 for duo with compact)* are Lancome's powder eyeshadow selections, and you get to create your own compact by selecting two eyeshadow colors of your choice. It's a great concept, but it would be better if there were some basic matte choices. As is, every color is noticeably shiny. This formula has a creamier, more powdery feel than the Colour Focus above, and has a greater tendency to flake during application. **Ombre Couture Multi-Effect EyeColour Trio** *($31.50)* provides two eyeshadows and a powder eyeliner in one sleek compact. The trios are well-coordinated and blend beautifully, though the texture is a bit slippery and several strokes are required for color intensity. Two of the three shades in every set are exceedingly shiny, so these are best ignored if you have any lines or sagging around the eye area. **Aquatique Waterproof EyeColour Base** *($19)* is billed as "foundation for eyes." You're supposed to believe you need a separate product (beyond foundation or concealer) to even out the skin tone on the eyelid and to prevent eyeshadows from creasing. This offers an opaque, thick formula that most certainly can crease, and what's worse is that the single color is strongly peach, not exactly what all women need or want. **Ombre Perfecteur Perfecting EyeShadow Base** *($20)* is a waterproof concealer for the eyelid area that is also supposed to extend the wear of eyeshadows. The nude, matte color is applied from a pen outfitted with an angled sponge tip. It tends to go on thick, but does blend evenly. It's OK, but not really necessary if you already use a matte-finish concealer. **L'Ombre Style Duo EyePowder Pen** *($25 for applicator pen with two colors)* is a unique concept: This is a dual-ended pen with each end holding a sponge-tip applicator that is "fed" with powder color from the base. However, several shades labeled as matte have obvious shine. Only Matte Fumee (charcoal gray) and Matte Brun (chocolate brown) are truly matte. For a simple eye design, this could work—but the delivery system is not for everyone.

<u>EYE AND BROW SHAPER:</u> ☺ $$$ **Le Crayon Kohl** *($18)* is a standard eye pencil in a nice range of colors. This one is longer than most, so it may seem clumsy at first. These are no better than many others that go for far less money (particularly those from L'Oreal). **Brow Artiste** *($28)* offers two matte-finish, powder-type brow colors in a compact. While most women need only one brow color and mixing takes time, these are still a viable option and have a nice dry texture and matte finish.

✔☺ $$$ **Artliner Precision Point EyeLiner** *($25)* is excellent for a liquid eyeliner that maintains an easy-to-apply, quick-drying, long-lasting formula and has a good brush. For considerably less money, you can get the same results (sans some of the funkier colors) from L'Oreal's Line Intensifique. ✔☺ **Le Crayon Poudre for the Brows** *($19.50)* is one of the best needs-sharpening brow pencils. It goes on easily, if a bit creamy, and the colors are matte and soft. There's even a good brush at one end for softening and blending the color.

☹ $$$ **Le Stylo Waterproof Long Lasting EyeLiner** *($19.50)* is a smooth-textured, twist-up eye pencil with mostly shiny colors that all tend to smudge, though no more so than most creamy pencils. This is fine for a smoky look, and it is reasonably waterproof. **Modele Sourcils Brow Groomer** *($17.50)* is a rather sticky brow gel available in clear or tinted versions. This has a thick, bushy brush that can coat the brows with too much product, which only increases the unpleasant stickiness. This remains an option for full, unruly brows.

☹ **Maquiglace Lumineuse Automatic Eyeliner** *($20)* is no match for the Artliner Precision Point Eyeliner above. The salesperson steered me away from this, commenting that it is very difficult to apply evenly. She was right, plus the two shades are intensely shiny.

<u>LIPSTICK AND LIP PENCIL:</u> ☺ $$$ **Rouge Attraction Lasting Impact LipColour** *($20)* boasts about the StayPut technology it uses to keep the color on the lips as long as possible, but I'll wager you will find this doesn't make it until lunchtime before needing

a touch-up. Although it does have a beautifully smooth, silky texture and the shades are richly pigmented, the finish is too slippery and creamy to make most women's expectations of long wear a reality. The colors offer some striking choices—including glitter, metallic, and hologram finishes, in case you're feeling impetuous the next time you're visiting a Lancome counter. **Rouge Sensation Multi-Sensation LipColour** *($19.50)* has a supremely creamy texture and soft glossy finish. This isn't as greasy as it used to be, though it will still travel into lines around the mouth. The opaque colors are simply stunning. **Rouge Absolu Creme Absolute Comfort Moisturizing LipColour** *($19.50)* is about as creamy as Rouge Sensation above, but with a noticeably slicker feel that easily slips off the lips and into lines around the mouth. If feathering is not an issue for you, this is as comfortable as a cream lipstick gets. **Sheer Magnetic Extra Shine Weightless LipColour** *($19.50)* is a relatively standard, semi-sheer lipstick that has a lot of slip and maintains a glossy finish while imparting subtle (often iridescent) color. **Lip Dimension Lasting Liquid Lip-Shaping Colour** *($20)*. If it weren't for the high price, I would wholeheartedly recommend this lipstick/lip gloss hybrid. It has a silky-smooth, lightweight texture, easy application, and a brilliant selection of sophisticated, opaque colors. For those of you looking for a less expensive alternative, check out L'Oreal's Glass Shine High Shine Lip Gloss ($7.99). **Lip Brio Lastingly Brilliant Lip Lacquer** *($20)* is assuredly overpriced, but this smooth gloss has been around for years, so someone must be buying it! For light-coverage colors and a lower-wattage glossy finish, this wand-applicator gloss wins high marks to match its high price. **Le Crayon Lip Contour** *($18.50)* is a standard automatic, retractable lip pencil with good colors and a smooth application. You will notice little difference between this and L'Oreal's Colour Riche Rich Creamy Lipliner ($7.19). **Le Lipstique LipColouring Stick with Brush** *($19.50)* is a standard pencil with a blending brush at the other end. That's convenient, but not worth the price. This does have some staying power, leaving a slight stain on the lips. The texture is drier than the Le Crayon version above, and that can reasonably help prevent feathering.

☺ **Juicy Tubes Ultra Shiny Lip Gloss** *($14.50)* has a thick, viscous application and a sticky, high-gloss finish. It comes in a squeeze tube and offers a range of sheer, trendy colors, but putting up with stickiness and intense fragrance may not be your cup of tea.

MASCARA: Lancome calls itself "the world's mascara leader," and if you take into account their superior options along with those from sister companies L'Oreal, Maybelline, and Helena Rubinstein, it's hard to dispute this claim!

✓☺ $$$ **Definicils High Definition Mascara** *($20)* is Lancome's perennial top seller, and it is easy to see why. This is an excellent lengthening mascara that builds some thickness with minimal to no chance of clumping. ✓☺ $$$ **Intencils Full Intensity Mascara** *($20)* builds extremely thick, full lashes, but also has a slight tendency to clump. If you have a lash comb handy, this mascara is great for all-out drama. ✓☺ $$$ **Magnificils Full Lash Precision Mascara** *($20)* builds magnificent length and definition without a clump or smear. I once recommended passing on this mascara, but not anymore. This wears all day and keeps lashes incredibly soft, too! Lancome insists this is the original formula, but I'm skeptical.

☺ $$$ **Flextencils Full Extension Curving Mascara** *($20)* claims that its "ultra-curving PowerSHAPE formula with patented brush gives lashes up to 30% more visible length with an eye-opening 30° curve." They then go on to say the claim is based on an in vitro (test tube) study, which is curious since one wonders whose eyelashes were used in this manner! Flextencils ends up being less impressive than most of Lancome's mascaras. It lengthens moderately and does add a soft curl, but it doesn't have the same "wow factor" as the ones above. **Amplicils Panoramic Volume Mascara** *($20)* has a name that probably sounds more intriguing to an audiophile than to a cosmetics customer, but the communication is clearly about making lashes more than they are. This is a respectable mascara, but it's not Lancome's best (for that, Definicils and Intencils are still preferred). Amplicils doesn't achieve quite the length the others do and it can clump if you're not careful. Yet if you use restraint and carefully wipe down the wand a bit, you'll find you can create relatively long lashes with thickness to spare. For a more refined, Paula's Pick version of this mascara, L'Oreal's Lash Intensifique Mascara ($6.69) is a must-try.

☺ $$$ **Eternicils Enduring Mascara Waterproof** *($20)* works very well (almost *too* well!) as a waterproof mascara, and it provides decent length and thickness. However, this is unusually difficult to remove, and is best reserved for occasional use. **Aquacils Waterproof Mascara with Keratine** *($20)* is currently not sold at Lancome counters, but it can be special ordered and is available on their Web site. This remains a fine waterproof mascara that lasts whether you're caught in a drizzle or a downpour.

☺ $$$ **Forticils Fortifying Lash Conditioner** *($16.50)* is a lash primer that is supposed to be applied before mascara. This will not condition the lashes at all, but it will add an extra layer, which may help; but if you need this product, it just means you bought an inferior mascara to start with.

☺ $$$ <u>**BRUSHES:**</u> Lancome offers a decent assortment of **Brushes** *($13–$52.50)* with a gorgeous feel and softness, though they are truly overpriced for what you get. Although the bristles may feel great, the shapes and sizes of many of the brushes are not the best for most face shapes and they can be awkward to work with. When you're considering spending $25 and up on an eyeshadow brush, it should be perfect. For the money, you would be far better off shopping at Bobbi Brown, Trish McEvoy, Laura Mercier, or Stila for brushes. If you wish to remain Lancome-loyal, the best brushes to consider are the **Le Bronzer Bronzing Powder Brush** *($35),* **Le Lip, Lip Brush** *($20),* and **La Brosse Precise Eye Makeup Brush** *($16.50).* Avoid the **Pinceau Lustrage Face Fiber Optic Brush** *($25),* which looks cool but serves little purpose and, according to the Lancome consultants I spoke to, doesn't last long. **Star Bronzer Magic Bronzing Brush** *($29.50)* is a soft, tapered powder brush whose handle is a reservoir for a sheer, shiny golden bronze powder. A push button at the base of the handle shoots powder into the brush, and from there it can be dusted over the face or body. A clever execution to be sure, but this pricey product has little impact other than the sparkling shine it leaves.

LAURA MERCIER

Laura Mercier has become a familiar name not only to beauty aficionados but also to cosmetics consumers at large. If you've flipped through almost any fashion magazine recently, it is hard to overlook her handiwork, either on the cover or mentioned in editorials. She is a formidable, in-demand makeup artist who has successfully shown us her capabilities.

Whereas Mercier's makeup collection is a strong point, her skin-care products leave much to be desired. Most of the formulations are good, but hardly groundbreaking when it comes to satisfying a range of skin types. One positive is that the two face sunscreens are nicely formulated with avobenzone and the products are fragrance-free. Overall, the only unique aspect of this group worth mentioning is that most of the products include emu oil. There is research showing it to be a good emollient that may be able to heal skin, but there is no research showing it to have antiaging or antiwrinkling effects. However, not everyone agrees that emu oil has no effect. A study published in *Plastic and Reconstructive Surgery* (December 1998, pages 2404–2407) concluded that applying emu oil on a fresh wound actually delayed wound healing. Emu oil's reputation is driven mostly by cosmetics company claims and not by any real proof that emu oil is an essential requirement for skin. For more information about Laura Mercier, call (888)-MERCIER or visit www.lauramercier.com.

LAURA MERCIER SKIN CARE

☺ $$$ **One Step Cleanser** *($35 for 8 ounces)* is an extremely standard, detergent-based, water-soluble cleanser that would work as well as any for most skin types, except for extremely dry skin. It does contain coloring agents.

☺ $$$ **Eye Make Up Remover** *($18 for 4 ounces)* is a standard, detergent-based eye-makeup remover that would work as well as any. This version does have some good anti-irritants, which is helpful.

☺ $$$ **Face Polish** *($24 for 3.7 ounces)* is a standard, detergent-based scrub with some plant oil that uses ground-up plastic (polyethylene) as the abrasive. This does contain some irritating plant ingredients, but in such small amounts they won't be a problem for skin. This is an option for normal to dry skin.

✓☺ $$$ **Eyedration Firming Eye Cream** *($35 for 0.5 ounce)* is a very good moisturizer with several antioxidants, anti-irritants, and water-binding agents that would work well for normal to dry skin, although there is nothing firming about it or special for the eye area.

☺ $$$ **Mega Moisturizer Cream with SPF 15** *($38 for 2 ounces)* is a good, avobenzone-based sunscreen for normal to dry skin in an emollient moisturizing base with a teeny amount of water-binding agent. The price is out of line for what you get.

☺ $$$ **Moisturizer Cream with SPF 15** *($38 for 2 ounces)* is almost identical to the Mega Moisturizer Cream version above and the same comments apply.

The Reviews L

☹ **Lip Balm SPF 15** *($20 for 0.12 ounce)* does not contain the UVA-protecting ingredients of titanium dioxide, zinc oxide, or avobenzone, and is not recommended.

☺ **$$$ Lip Silk** *($17 for 0.4 ounce)* is supposed to retexture lips, but this very standard, Vaseline-based moisturizer can't do that. The teeny amounts of AHAs and BHA and the product's pH of 6 mean that this can have no exfoliating properties.

LAURA MERCIER MAKEUP

What sets Mercier's well-organized makeup line apart from the rest is her trademark "flawless face." Mercier believes that perfecting the complexion is the most important step to makeup application, and her line presents some incredible options for doing just that. Much like her competitors, Mercier has continued to expand her cosmetics offerings, segueing from a soft, neutral palette to a blitz of shine and shimmer. As a trendsetter, Mercier is in a position of influence, yet she has clearly pandered to what consumers want. Isn't it ironic that almost all of her magazine covers feature celebrities (such as Julia Roberts and Meg Ryan) wearing barely a hint of shine? Rather, their features are beautifully enhanced with artistic shading, subtle highlighting, and mostly soft, understated shadows that are immaculately blended. The only real shine comes from the lips, and that is attractive and a look many women love. Clearly, Mercier plays down shine in her own work, despite the dominance it has among the powder blushes and eyeshadows at her cosmetics counters.

You will discover that Mercier's makeup products, particularly her foundations, are in many ways a step above the rest. The tester unit is very user-friendly and the counter staff I've come across really have their act together, merging makeup skill with an obvious affection for the line's namesake. Mercier herself regularly makes special appearances at her counters, and my guess is that sitting in her chair would be an experience you wouldn't soon forget.

FOUNDATION: ✔☺ **$$$ Oil-Free Foundation** *($38)* is a superlative foundation for normal to slightly oily skin. The texture is very smooth and it blends out to a seamless, soft matte finish with medium coverage. This simply looks great on the skin. There are 12 shades, with options for very light but not for very dark skin tones. The only one to consider avoiding is Shell Beige (slightly pink). ✔☺ **$$$ Moisturizing Foundation** *($38)* would be suitable for normal to dry skin seeking medium coverage. The texture is elegantly light and creamy, leaving a beautiful, natural finish. All six colors are excellent, although shades for darker skin tones are absent. ✔☺ **$$$ Foundation Stick to Go** *($35)* presents yet another twist-up stick option. Thankfully, Mercier's formula is sheer and light, with a cream-to-powder texture that meshes well with the skin instead of sitting on top of it. All five shades are superb, but there are no options for very light or dark skin tones. This type of foundation works best on normal to slightly oily skin that is not prone to breakouts. Other skin types can consider using one of the shades as a light-coverage concealer. ✔☺ **Foundation Powder** *($38)* is a superlative powder foundation that comes in seven gorgeous shades, including options for light and dark (but not very dark) skin tones. This talc-based powder offers a suede-smooth texture, even application, and light to medium coverage when used dry. If you use it wet it provides fuller coverage, but you also run the risk of streaking if you're not careful. If the price isn't too off-putting and you have normal to oily skin, this is a must-try the next time you're near a Mercier counter.

☺ $$$ **Tinted Moisturizer SPF 20** *($38)* has no reliable UVA protection, but is still a decently creamy, very sheer moisturizer that blends on effortlessly. Of the four shades, be careful with Almond and Tan—both can be too coppery for most skin tones, though the sheerness doesn't really emphasize this. **Foundation Primer** *($28)* is a very thin, lightweight, clear gel of silicone and film-forming agent. It's supposed to contain light-reflecting ingredients that protect the skin, but it doesn't (unless you consider the emollient shine from the finish protecting). It can be a good, simple, matte-finish moisturizer for someone with slightly oily skin but that's about it. **Secret Finish** *($25)*. The real secret is that this ordinary, overpriced, lightweight moisturizer will not make a discernible difference in how your makeup wears. It is merely water, slip agent, thickener, rice starch (for a soft matte finish), plant extracts (including witch hazel, an irritant), vitamins, preservatives, more silicone, fragrance, and coloring agents. If anything, this formula isn't nearly as modern or effective as the less pricey handful of silicone-based mattifiers sold by M.A.C., Neutrogena, and Prescriptives.

☺ $$$ <u>CONCEALER:</u> **Secret Camouflage** *($27)* is a two-sided compact concealer with a thick, dry texture and truly opaque camouflage coverage. All of the duos have yellow to beige or peach to copper colors that can work if they are mixed in the right proportions, but why would you want to do that (and use two separate brushes for the task, as is recommended at the Mercier counter) when there are so many excellent one-step concealers available? Secret Camouflage was designed as a cover-up for facial blemishes or birthmarks, and if all else has failed, it can be an option. SC4, 5, and 6 are too peach or copper to recommend. For the eye area, there is **Secret Concealer** *($20)*, which is far more user-friendly than the Secret Camouflage. It comes in a small pot and offers three decent shades, each with a very creamy-smooth texture. It covers well but it does tend to crease on and off during the day. Give this a test run before you decide to purchase.

<u>POWDER:</u> ✓☺ $$$ **Loose Powder** *($30)* has an out-of-this-world silky texture that blends beautifully over the skin and leaves a satiny-smooth, dry finish. All of the shades are workable and have a subtle yellow undertone. Only Star Dust and Sun Dust are too shiny to recommend, although both would work for a glistening evening look. Caution: The cornstarch in this product could cause irritation or breakouts for those who are sensitive to it. ✓☺ **Pressed Powder** *($28)* has many of the same qualities as the Loose Powder above, minus the cornstarch. The texture is smooth and dry and all of the colors are outstanding.

☺ $$$ **Shimmer Pressed Powder** *($32)* is simply Mercier's wonderful Pressed Powder with added shine. If you're not using powder to tone down shine, you'll love this, despite the price.

✔☺ $$$ **Bronzing Stick** *($30)* has a soft, emollient texture that blends superbly over skin and leaves a moist, sheer bronze finish. There is only one shade, but it's top-notch.

☺ $$$ **Bronzing Powder** *($30)* produces a great soft tan color, but the amount of shine is too distracting to look natural. **Loose Pearls** *($20)* are small containers of loose, iridescent powders that change color depending on what direction the light hits them. They're messy, but they do cling well and produce intense shine, which some women undoubtedly want.

<u>BLUSH:</u> ☺ $$$ **Cheek Colour** *($20)* has a great texture, a soft, even application, and features a small selection of beautiful colors—but all of them have shine. It's not overpowering, but this is one area where you may want to sneak over to peek at Bobbi Brown and Stila's matte blush options.

✔☺ $$$ **Cheek Colour Stick to Go** *($26)* is a swivel-up blush stick with a creamy-soft texture and three great, sheer colors. It actually blends quite well and is an excellent (though pricey) option for those who prefer this type of product.

☺ $$$ **Face Tint** *($20)* is Mercier's Loose Powder formula, with blush colors. This is not as easy to use as a pressed-powder blush, but the few colors are matte and add a sheer, healthy flush to the cheeks.

<u>EYESHADOW:</u> ☺ $$$ **Eye Colour** *($18)* has an adequate assortment of both matte and subtle to glaring shiny shades. The texture is slightly dry and the colors tend to go on softer than you might expect, but you can build intensity if needed. **Eye Paints** *($50)* is a sleek compact containing ten of Mercier's eyeshadows. The colors are attractive, with half being shiny. This is not a refillable compact, so it's only a worthwhile investment if you will use all (or almost all) of the eyeshadows. **Eye Basics** *($22)* are liquid eyeshadows that come in a tube with a sponge-tip applicator. These have been reformulated and no longer have the unpleasant thick, sticky formula they once did. They now have a lightly creamy, sheer texture that blends easily and dries to a natural matte finish. The three shades are neutral and this works almost as well as a matte-finish concealer over the eyelids.

☹ $$$ **Creme Eye Colour to Go** *($19)* applies with a wand applicator and has a very slick texture that can make blending a challenge. All four shades are extremely shiny and have a creamy, slippery finish.

<u>EYE AND BROW SHAPER:</u> ☺ $$$ **Eye Pencil** *($16)* and **Brow Pencil** *($16)* are both utterly standard, with traditional colors, and are not worth more than a fraction of this price. Mercier apparently developed "an exact texture" for these, but there isn't a difference between these and most other pencils sold. **Brow Powder Duos** *($23)* features two dry-textured brow powders in one compact. The color combinations are quite good, and there are suitable options for redheads and blondes, along with traditional options for brunettes—but all of the colors are sparkly. Why the eyebrows need to shine is beyond me, but if this appeals to you, these brow powders do apply and blend well. **Eye Liner** *($20)* is a standard powder-cake liner that must be used wet with an eyeliner brush. The texture is the same as most cake liners, except that these all have a bit of sparkle to

them and the shiny particles can flake off and get into the eye, which is annoying to say the least.

☺ $$$ **Eye Brow Gel** *($18)* is basic clear brow gel. It's a great way to keep unruly brows in place, but there is no reason to spend this much when there are equally good options available from Cover Girl, Maybelline, and Sonia Kashuk.

LIPSTICK AND LIP PENCIL: ☺ $$$ **Lip Colour** *($18)* is divided into Cremes and Shimmers, which are iridescent. Supposedly, these can "fill in ridges and lines," but that's something these fairly greasy lipsticks simply cannot do. Both are just standard lipsticks with an excellent range of colors and a slight stain. **Lip Sheer** *($18)* is exactly that, a sheer lip color with a glossy finish and marvelous colors that all have a slight stain. **Matte Lipstick** *($18)* is not matte in the true sense of the word, but compared to Mercier's other lipsticks, this is definitely less glossy and greasy. The small color range is gorgeous— it has some of the best warm-toned reds anywhere. This goes on easily and feels wonderfully creamy on the lips, providing rich, opaque coverage. **Lip Paints** *($50)* provides you with ten lip colors, all housed in a slim silver compact that includes a great lip brush. There are various palettes available, from Laura's favorites to a combination of Lip Sheers and Cremes. If you like Mercier's lipstick textures and colors, this is a must-see. **Lip Pencil** *($16)* has a standard creamy texture and dry finish. The color range has expanded and now offers better options to coordinate with the lipsticks. Less expensive pencils abound, but these work well. **Lip Glamour** *($18)* is liquid lipstick/gloss hybrid that is more emollient than sticky and provides intense color with high-wattage shine. As usual, Mercier's colors are bound to please.

☹ $$$ **Lip Gloss** *($18)* is outrageously expensive for what amounts to a standard, very sticky gloss.

MASCARA: ☹ $$$ **Mascara** *($18)* sweeps on much lighter than it used to, creating subdued definition and average length. Thickness is a foreign concept to this mascara, and overall the payoff isn't worth the price.

✓☺ $$$ **Thickening and Building Mascara** *($19)* is a notable improvement over Mercier's original mascara. This formula is a pleasure to apply, and it builds impressively long, lifted lashes with a fair amount of thickness. Lashes look full, soft, and fringed—all without clumping or smearing.

☺ $$$ BRUSHES: Mercier has done her homework when it comes to **Brushes** *($20–$52; $100–$250 for Travel, Mini, or Master Sets with portfolio)*. Most of these are masterfully shaped and are dense enough to hold and deposit color evenly on the skin. Almost every brush is available with a long or short handle, which is an attractive option. The best ones among this collection of either natural or synthetic hairs are the **Powder Brush** *($52)*, **Camouflage Powder Brush** *($28)*, which is more appropriate for eyeshadows, and the **Cheek Colour Brush** *($42)*. Almost all of the **Eyeshadow Brushes** *($25–$29)* are worth a closer look; only the **Crew Cut Brush** *($29)* is superfluous. The rest are worth testing, but you may find them too small, scratchy, or stiff for comfort.

☺ **$$$ SPECIALTY:** Mercier also sells a handsome assortment of **Brush Cases** *($40–$50)* and a practical **Travel Tote** *($65)*. Although I am not a fan of curling the eyelashes, this line has a **Precision Lash Curler** *($32)* that expertly curls the lashes at the outer corner of the eye, where conventional lash curlers cannot easily reach. If you must curl your lashes, this is a gentler way to go about it.

LINDA SY

Linda Sy Fang is a California-based dermatologist whose namesake skin-care line has been quietly establishing a following since 1981. Sy was one of the first dermatologists to put her name on a product line, long before any other dermatologist would even have considered it. According to the company, the goal of Linda Sy Skin Care is to keep the formulations simple, functional, and elegant. The products are indeed simple, with most containing less than ten ingredients, and all are admirably fragrance and colorant-free. However, what passed for elegant 20 years ago seems antiquated and inelegant by today's standards. Most of Linda Sy's products contain no antioxidants and anti-irritants and the most inconsequential amounts of water-binding agents. There's nothing in this line that can't easily be replaced by products available at the drugstore that are both more elegant and more reasonably priced.

Knowing this line is from a dermatologist, it is surprising to find that only two of the four available sunscreens contain adequate UVA protection, and that the acne products are just irritations waiting to happen. The moisturizers are OK options for those with dry skin, and Sy does have an all-zinc-oxide sunscreen that goes on quite sheer and light, which is great for sensitive skin (including those with rosacea), but that's about it. Overall, there is nothing exceptional and nothing worth considering over the countless other options available at drugstores and department stores. For more information about Linda Sy Skin Care, call (877) 546-3279 or visit www.lindasy.com.

LINDA SY SKIN CARE

☹ **Unscented Superfatted Soap for Dry, Sensitive Skin** *($7 for 3.5 ounces)* is a standard bar soap (tallow based) that contains plant oil—but not enough to cut the drying effects that soap can have, especially on dry, sensitive skin.

☹ **Unscented Soap for Normal or Oily Skin** *($7 for 3.5 ounces)* is almost identical to the Unscented Superfatted Soap above, and nothing about this, including the olive oil it contains, is appropriate for someone with oily skin.

☺ **Oil-Free Cleansing Lotion** *($11 for 8 ounces)* is basically formulated like Cetaphil Lotion, but even simpler. It would work well as a gentle, water-soluble cleanser for normal to dry or sensitive skin, but like the original Cetaphil, it will not be very effective in removing makeup.

☹ **Astringent** *($11 for 8 ounces)* is an alcohol-based toner with no other redeeming feature whatsoever, which makes it too irritating and drying for all skin types, and it is not recommended.

☹ **Facial Lotion with 10% Lactic Acid** *($19 for 2 ounces)* does contain 10% AHA (lactic acid), but the base has a pH of 5, which makes it ineffective for exfoliation. This is a basic liquid formula that also contains a small amount of clay, which can be drying for skin.

☺ **Moisture Lotion for Dry Skin** *($16 for 4 ounces)* is about as basic and boring as a moisturizer gets. There is little reason to consider this over almost anything you would find at a drugstore, ranging from Eucerin to Vaseline Intensive Care. It would be an OK option for someone with dry to very dry skin. It contains mostly water, mineral oil, lanolin, thickeners, plant oil, a water-binding agent, and preservatives. Contrary to the claim, this will leave a greasy residue on the skin, because that's what the main ingredients in this product do.

☺ **Moisture Lotion for Normal/Combination Skin** *($16 for 4 ounces)* is almost identical to the Moisture Lotion for Dry Skin above, just a little lighter in texture. It can feel slightly sticky on the skin and, contrary to the claim, that is a problem for acne-prone skin. Why would anyone with combination skin or acne want to put greasy-feeling Vaseline or lanolin derivatives on their face?

☺ **Moisturizing Oil for Face & Body** *($18 for 8 ounces)* is a basic combination of plant oils, Vaseline, silicone, and preservatives. It would definitely be an option for dry, chapped, or irritated skin, but no better than using plain almond, olive, or safflower oil from your kitchen cabinet.

☺ **Vita-Oil for Delicate Skin** *($19 for 1 ounce)* is recommended for the eye area and face, but except for teeny additions of vitamins C, A, and D (antioxidants) this is really just plain old jojoba oil and lecithin. Keep in mind that plain jojoba oil or lecithin from the health food store can do the same thing this product does, and for a lot less money.

☺ **Protective Cream** *($23 for 3 ounces)* is an exceedingly tedious formulation containing water, glycerin, thickeners, silicones, tiny amounts of water-binding agents, and preservatives.

☺ **$$$ Superior Cream** *($25 for 2 ounces)* is an ironic name for what is a completely mediocre moisturizing cream for normal to dry skin. It contains mostly water, thickener, Vaseline, more thickeners, and preservatives. There is nothing about this formula that Eucerin or Aquaphor at the drugstore can't replace for far less money.

☹ **Optimal Moisturizing Sunscreen SPF 15** *($23 for 8 ounces)* does not contain the UVA-protecting ingredients of avobenzone, titanium dioxide, or zinc oxide, and is not recommended.

☹ **Optimal Light-Textured Sunscreen Lotion SPF 15** *($18 for 4 ounces)* does not contain the UVA-protecting ingredients of avobenzone, titanium dioxide, or zinc oxide, and is not recommended.

☺ **Recreational Sunscreen SPF 30** *($22 for 4 ounces)* does contain avobenzone, though the amount is lower than average for all-day UVA protection. Still, this would be an option for normal to dry skin as a daytime moisturizer.

✔☺ **ZincO Cream SPF 20 Regular or Tinted** *($28 for 3 ounces)* is one of the few sunscreens available that uses only zinc oxide as the active ingredient. This formula uses 14.5% zinc oxide, a higher than average amount that will assuredly provide excellent UVA and UVB protection. What's surprising is that with this much zinc oxide the product applies easily and leaves only a minimal white cast on the skin. This is one to consider, especially if you have dry, sensitive skin. The tinted version looks a bit odd (it's kind of grayish pink), but it blends easily into the skin and imparts a touch of bronze color.

☹ **Acne Oil Control Gel** *($22 for 2 ounces)* does contain 2% salicylic acid, but the pH of 6 is too high for it to be effective as an exfoliant. Equally problematic is the alcohol base, which makes this too irritating and drying for all skin types.

☹ **Acne Cover Lotion** *($14 for 2 ounces)* claims it "helps teenagers gain confidence while waiting for their acne treatments to work," yet this confusing cocktail of alcohol, clay, titanium dioxide, zinc oxide, and sulfur will only keep them irritated while they're waiting (and why should you wait anyway?). The pink tint of this product is not the color you want to use over a red, inflamed blemish.

LINDA SY MAKEUP

While Linda Sy's skin care has its share of effective options, the makeup selection comes off as a slipshod afterthought. It is clear that Sy knows about sunscreen formulary standards for UVA protection, yet none of her foundations offer an effective combination of active ingredients. The powders are also subpar, and for both foundation and powder the majority of the colors are far-from-neutral castaways.

☹ **FOUNDATION: Liquid Makeup Sunscreen SPF 15** *($25)* is a watery foundation that blends decently and dries to a semi-opaque, soft matte finish. It does not contain adequate UVA-protecting sunscreen ingredients of avobenzone, zinc oxide, or titanium dioxide. (Titanium dioxide is listed as one of the regular ingredients, but unless it is on the active ingredient list its presence is meaningless.) There are five colors, but all of them except Golden Light are too peach or pink. **Essential Cream SPF 15** *($25)* is a very thick, emollient cream foundation that only comes in one shade (Medium), which is a sheer pink tone. The same sunscreen comments for the Makeup Sunscreen above apply to this one as well. For those with dry skin looking for a rich foundation, Origins' Dew Gooder Makeup is a much more elegant option.

POWDER: ☹ **Concealing Loose Powder** *($32)* is a talc-free powder that goes on dry, tends to grab onto the skin, and provides opaque coverage with a shiny finish. There is only one color available, and it is way too peach for most skin tones. And why powder with anything that adds shine to your skin? **Bronzing Loose Powder** *($32)* is identical to the Concealing Loose Powder above, except for the color. It's a shame this powder applies so thickly and unevenly, as the bronze tone would work well on light to medium skin.

☺ **$$$ Translucent Loose Powder** *($18)* is much lighter in texture and application than the powders above, and leaves a soft matte finish on the skin. There are two colors available, and both would be good choices for fair to light skin tones.

LIP INK (MAKEUP ONLY)

Lip Ink guarantees indelible lip color, or as close to it as you can get anywhere in the cosmetics world. Well, hold on to your lips, because this product delivers, maybe not as well as the claims profess, but nevertheless it is impressive. Despite the name, it's not ink—just a very strong, semipermanent lip stain that doesn't easily rub or wear off. Mine lasted a full day and a half—through meals, a shower, bedtime, and past the next morning—but you may find it doesn't wear quite that long, at least not without needing some maintenance. Lip Ink is a quick-drying liquid lip color that feels very wet when applied, and after it dries—and you must let it dry—it feels like nothing on the lips. What you then see are fully colored, dyed lips! Unfortunately, Lip Ink doesn't add a drop of moisture, so if you have dry, cracked lips, using Lip Ink will give you fully colored, dyed, dry, cracked lips, too. Putting the Lip Ink Shine over it helps a lot, but the initial appearance and wear isn't the best if you have any dry skin on your lips. For more information about Lip Ink, call (800) 496-9616 or visit www.lipink.com.

☺ $$$ **Lip Ink Starter Kit** *($45)* includes **Lip Ink Shine**, which is an emollient lip gloss, to keep the lips from drying out. Just like Max Factor's Lipfinity Moisturizing Top Coat, this gloss doesn't compromise the staying power of the lip color, but it will rub off on anyone you are snuggling with! It is available in colorless or tinted versions. By the way, Lip Ink claims that Lip Ink Shine contains light reflectors to erase signs of sun damage. Any gloss can provide a dewy, moist surface that looks smoother, but that claim makes their silicone-based gloss sound uniquely beneficial, and it isn't.

I know this all sounds great, but I have a few warnings about this product. Primarily, it isn't that easy to use. Here are some excerpts from the instructions that come with the kit: "Always start with clean, dry lips. Then, before applying Lip Ink Color, massage a small amount of Lip Ink Shine into the lips until the shine disappears. [This isn't necessary if your lips aren't dry, and it can make the color bleed.] Shake the vial against the palm of your hand before using. Wipe all excess from applicator wand. Apply with gentle pressure using long, smooth strokes. Move in one direction only. Allow color to dry (10-20 seconds) with lips in a slightly parted, relaxed position. Repeat for a total of three layers of color. Finish with a final coat of shine moisturizer." For a product sold with claims of being a time-saver, this product definitely takes work! And you have to be careful about applying it perfectly or your mistakes will be semipermanent, too!

I was also disturbed by a few of Lip Ink's claims, such as its being the only healthy alternative to lipstick. Lip Ink believes, because their products do not contain waxes or animal fats (which are ingested in small amounts when one wears traditional lipstick), that they are healthier. Yet these products have a preponderance of synthetic ingredients, including everything from synthetic dyes to propylene glycol, phenoxyethanol, and on and on. The herbs and botanicals are simply window dressing to give consumers what they want, which is plants aplenty. In addition, ingredients like rosemary oil, peppermint, and sage oil are potent irritants. Yes, we do ingest a fair amount of lipstick, but the ingredients in most lipstick colors are quite harmless and are readily destroyed by stomach acids before they have a chance to do any harm.

You may be wondering how Lip Ink products compare to Max Factor's Lipfinity and Cover Girl's Outlast lip colors. All three share the same principles of all-day wear complete with a gloss-like product to enhance comfort. However, I give the edge to Lipfinity and Outlast for three reasons: (1) the colors are easier to apply and offer almost full coverage instantly, (2) the formulas do not contain any irritants, and (3) they cost less. Lip Ink's only advantage is that you can create a sheer stain or full-coverage color. That may be enough of a plus to make the choice easier, but when an irritant-free alternative exists at your local drugstore, you'd be foolish not to check it out. Variations on the original Lip Ink (using the same formula) include ☺ **Lip Ink Aliens Color** *($15)*, which is a collection of mostly odd colors like gray, green, and blue. They're a kicky alternative to the straightforward Lip Ink colors. **Lip Ink Ultra** *($15)* is a small collection of understated colors, each with more pigment, which further enhances the original Lip Ink's inordinately long wear. Finally, the Lip Ink formula is available as a **Liquid Lip Liner** *($15)* that you apply with a thin brush. The same pros and cons that apply to the full-fledged Lip Ink colors apply here as well.

☺ **Eye Liner** *($15)*, **Miracle Brow Liner** *($15)*, and **Miracle Brow Tint** (with mascara brush) *($15)* are all liquid-based and very waterproof. They stay and stay and stay and stay. Because your eyes are less inclined to come in contact with liquids and food than your mouth, the liner and brow color could probably stay on for days! However, there are problems with the application that make these products tricky to use. The first ingredient is alcohol, and among the extracts are rosemary oil, peppermint, and arnica, which explains why it burns and why Lip Ink includes a warning about not using it over broken skin. The other issue is the liquid, runny consistency of the product itself. You will want to practice on your hand before you consider using this on your eyes. It can be hard to get the watery finish to go on dark enough or thin enough, so it tends to spread and is hard to control. You need to wait a minute or so for it to dry, and don't blink or you can end up with liner or brow color where you don't want it. The color selection for both products is quite good. **Brow and Lash Conditioner** *($15)* is just silicone-based clear mascara that will groom the brows and barely enhance the lashes without feeling stiff or sticky. However, the silicones do not dry down, so this can feel a bit slick and can make thin or sparse brows look greasy. **Magic Powder** *($15)* is described in groundbreaking terms, but is simply an iridescent loose powder that, like many others, changes color depending on what light (or angle) you're viewing it in.

☺ **$$$ Tinted Waxless Lip Balm** *($40 for kit with three colors)* is a collection of three tinted, silicone-based glosses. Although these do not contain wax, few glosses do (wax is primarily used in lipsticks to create their texture and shape), and anyway there is nothing wrong with using wax in lip products. These are fine for slick, non-sticky pot glosses, though the price is steep.

☺ **Tinted Shine Moisturizer** *($15)* is a silicone-based wand-type lip gloss that comes in an enticing, largely iridescent range of colors. This is fine as far as gloss goes, and it can be used over any Lip Ink color without disrupting the design.

☹ **Lash Tint** *($15)* contains the same basic ingredients found in Lip Ink, and this is just too much alcohol (among other irritants) to put anywhere near the eyes. This very thin mascara tints the lashes and stops there. Lip Ink recommends following this with your regular mascara, but I recommend skipping this product altogether.

LIP LAST (SEE ENGLISH IDEAS)

LIZ EARLE NATURALLY ACTIVE SKIN CARE

The name Liz Earle may not sound familiar, but her appearances on QVC are creating quite a stir, at least for those women who are writing me to ask, "Do those products work?" Every time a new infomercial airs, I get hundreds of immediate requests to review those products and to determine whether or not the products are "really worth it." You all know that it is astounding to me that women wonder who is really telling the truth about any product being advertised by the cosmetics industry, but even more so in the world of infomercials. Given the large number of celebrities or made-for-infomercial-celebrities endorsing cosmetics, that alone should give one pause. What about all the other TV lines? Is Jennifer Flavin-Stallone (Serious Skin Care) telling the truth? What about Joan Rivers (Results)? Linda Evans (Rejuvenique)? Kathie Lee Gifford (Natural Advantage Antiaging System and the since defunct Mon Amie, and from 1993 the Timeless Essence Night Recovery Cream—Gifford has been very free with her endorsements)? Or Marilyn Miglin (her own line), Adrien Arpel (Signature Club A), Diane Young, and Victoria Principal (Principal Secret)—need I go on? The never-ending question—"Are any of these really worth the money?"—is easily answered by saying "no," at least not the way the products are represented in the ads and commercials. So what about Earle's products already?

Liz Earle is a former beauty editor. Using this experience and working with a skin-care product manufacturer, she has arrived at these products bearing her name. There isn't much else to discuss except the products, which are fairly basic and offer no sunscreens (though her line does have sunscreens available in England). If you're in the mood to consider a new group of skin-care products, this isn't the one to contemplate, so you may as well switch channels now. For more information about Liz Earle, visit www.lizearle.com or www.iqvc.com.

☹ **Cleanse & Polish** *($14.50 for 3.4 ounces)* has a wafting smell of eucalyptus that penetrated through the box I received. That can irritate the eyes and skin. Other than that, this is more of a cold cream and can leave a slightly greasy film on the skin.

☺ **Instant Boost Skin Tonic** *($12.69 for 6.8 ounces)* is an OK toner for normal to dry skin, if you can get past the fragrance. The plant extracts it contains can be good anti-irritants, but it contains only a teeny amount of vitamin E and water-binding agents.

The Reviews L

☺ **$$$ Daily Eye Repair** *($21.68 for 0.5 ounce)* does contain a teeny amount of AHA, but it's not enough for exfoliating purposes. If you are looking for a vitamin E cream, this is one to consider; just remember that although it is a good antioxidant the vitamin does not repair skin. It would be a good moisturizer for normal to dry skin, though there is nothing in this product that makes it better for the eye area.

☺ **Skin Repair for Dry/Sensitive Skin** *($14.96 for 1.7 ounces)* is an OK moisturizer for normal to dry skin, although the fragrance makes it inappropriate for sensitive skin types. It contains some good plant oils, but only teeny amounts of water-binding agents and antioxidants.

☺ **Skin Repair for Normal/Combination Skin** *($14.96 for 1.7 ounces)* is similar to the Skin Repair for Dry/Sensitive Skin above only with fewer plant oils. This moisturizer is still too emollient for combination skin types.

☹ **Smoothing Line Serum** *($21.30 for 0.5 ounce)* contains menthol, and that can be a potential skin irritant.

☹ **Brightening Treatment** *($13.54 for 1.7 ounces)* contains camphor; that won't brighten skin, but it can cause redness and irritation.

☹ **Intensive Nourishing Treatment** *($12.11 for 1.7 ounces)*. Talc is listed as the second ingredient, which makes this anything but nourishing. The plant extract (comfrey) can be, at the very least, irritating to skin, and it contains no significant water-binding agents or antioxidants. This product has more negatives than positives and is not recommended.

☺ **$$$ Superbalm Concentrate** *($23.51 for 0.34 ounce)* contains mostly emollient plant oils and fragrance. It is an option for dry skin, but there is nothing in it that makes it worth the price tag. You could easily replace this with hazelnut oil from the health food store and avoid the fragrance.

☺ **Superbalm** *($17.81 for 1 ounce)* is similar to the Concentrate version above except that this one contains thickeners that give it a solid form.

☹ **Spot–On** *($9.26 for 0.2 ounce)* contains balm mint and lavender oil, which means this is more like wearing fragrance than using skin care. This can be irritating for all skin types. It does contain tea tree oil, but the other ingredients get in the way of that being helpful for blemishes.

LORAC

Makeup artist Carol Shaw is the creator of the Lorac line (it's her first name spelled backwards). Independently owned, Lorac has always been primarily about color, and against formidable competition, it is "the little line that could." The line's major claim to fame is Carol Shaw's celebrity clients. Shaw's celebrity portfolio has done almost as much to make Lorac a beauty magazine staple as the products themselves. In contrast to the many makeup artistry lines that have been snatched up by the cosmetics giants and that have subsequently watched their inventory and exposure increase exponentially, Lorac has stayed the course and launched new products slowly, each with a bit of innovation on an otherwise standard theme. Product-wise, Lorac has its share of highs and lows. The handful of skin-care products are not worth mentioning. Just ignore those and move on to the makeup, something Shaw clearly knows something about.

There are certainly some good Lorac products, though the skin-care products are dismal, with only six options, which means women with oily skin and women with very dry skin would be using the same products. However, the lack of varied color options when compared to Lorac's competitors, from M.A.C. to Bobbi Brown, Stila, Trish McEvoy, NARS, Vincent Longo, and on and on, makes this a line you could easily overlook and not feel as though you've missed out on looking like an'"A-list star"! For more information about Lorac, call (800) 845-0705 or visit www.loraccosmetics.com.

LORAC SKIN CARE

☺ **Oil-Free Face Wash** *($17 for 8 ounces)* is a very basic, detergent-based, water-soluble cleanser that can work for most skin types, except for dry skin.

☺ **Oil-Free Makeup Remover** *($17 for 6.5 ounces)* is a fairly standard eye-makeup remover that will indeed take off eye makeup.

☻ **Makeup Remover** *($17 for 6.5 ounces)* is just a standard, detergent-based makeup remover similar to the Oil-Free Makeup Remover above. It will work as well as any.

☹ **Alcohol-Free Toner** *($18 for 4 ounces)* contains menthol, which makes it too irritating for all skin types.

☻ **Moisturizer** *($37.50 for 2 ounces)*. This remarkably ordinary moisturizer would be OK for someone with normal to dry skin, and for this amount of money it should contain unique or state-of-the-art ingredients. Unfortunately, it only contains trace amounts of water-binding agents and vitamin E, and some of the plant extracts it contains can be skin irritants.

☺ **Vitamin E Stick** *($16 for 0.12 ounce)* contains almost no vitamin E to speak of. It's just a basic, greasy, clear lipstick that contains mostly castor oil, waxes, and Vaseline. It's good for dry lips, but there is nothing even vaguely unique in here.

LORAC MAKEUP

Compared to Bobbi Brown or Stila, Lorac doesn't offer the same caliber of foundation colors or the array of products. However, Lorac holds their own when it comes to blush, eyeshadow, lipstick, and makeup brush options. Shaw has named quite a few of her lipsticks after the celebrity who inspired that color. Women are undeniably drawn to this, and admittedly it is kind of fun to see how Susan Sarandon or Nicole Kidman's "color" will look on you. Novelty aside, Lorac has a fair share of worthwhile choices, but it's certainly not the only game in town.

FOUNDATION: ☺ $$$ **Oil-Free Makeup** *($30)* is a darling of *In Style* magazine's beauty editors, and this foundation does have its strong points. The fluid, lightweight texture blends very well, merging into skin to create a natural finish with sheer coverage.

The Reviews L

I wish the colors were better, but you'll be able to tell which are the best ones by noting which tester bottles are empty or nearly so! Each shade tends to go on lighter than it looks and the ones to avoid due to peach or strong yellow tones are S5, S6, and S8. Shades S4 and S7 are borderline, but may work for some skin tones. **Translucent Cream Makeup** *($35)* is a creamy compact makeup that stays moist on the skin and offers sheer to almost no coverage. For normal to dry skin, this is an option, and the five shades are fairly good, though CM3 and CM5 are too peach for most skin tones.

✔☺ **$$$ Satin Makeup** *($35)* has a sheer, elegantly moist texture that is a treat for normal to dry skin. This one offers better coverage than the Oil-Free Makeup, but still blends well. Again, the colors tend to go on lighter than they appear. To avoid an overly jaundiced or peachy look, avoid M6, M7, and M8. ✔☺ **$$$ Oil-Free Wet/Dry Makeup** *($35)* is fantastic. This ultra-smooth, almost creamy, pressed-powder foundation is a joy to apply. It blends imperceptibly over the skin and creates a sheer, polished finish. All five shades are superior. This isn't much for oil control, but it makes no claims in that regard, either!

<u>CONCEALER:</u> ☹ **Coverup** *($16)* comes in a pot and offers great emollient coverage, but it also tends to crease almost immediately and keeps on creasing. If creasing isn't a concern for you, there are a few good shades to consider, but there are also some to avoid, such as C4 and C7.

☹ **Oil-Free Neutralizer** *($28)* is supposed to even out any blue or red discolorations. The color is greenish yellow, and the coverage is too sheer to make a difference one way or the other.

☺ **$$$ Quick Fix** *($25)* borrows from the tag line of Bounty paper towels, calling itself the "quicker-fixer-upper." This kit features four colors in one split-pan compact. You get a yellow-toned concealer, an iridescent pink highlighter, an emollient lip balm, and a lip/cheek tint. This isn't that bad if you have use for the colors, but it's not what I would call universally appealing.

<u>POWDER:</u> The ☺ **$$$ Face Powder** *($28)* is a talc-based loose powder that has a very dry texture, smooth finish, and some workable colors. Although it looks fairly heavy on the skin, it does provide decent coverage. This is not recommended for normal to dry skin. Of the five shades, avoid P3 and P5, which are too golden orange.

☺ **$$$ Perfect Powder** *($32)* is a pressed powder with minimal coverage. It makes a big deal about being talc-free, which is strange, since other Lorac powders do contain talc. What this does contain, however, is mica, a shiny mineral pigment that negates the purpose of powder, which is to reduce shine. It's an OK option, but offers minimal payoff compared to almost every other pressed powder out there, though the colors are quite neutral. **Bronzer** *($28)* is a pressed-powder bronzer with a silky feel and sheer finish, but like so many others of its ilk, it is very shiny—which doesn't add up to a natural-looking tan.

✔☺ **$$$ Translucent Touch Up Powder** *($32)* is a talc-based powder that has a smooth-as-silk texture and three very good colors. It provides a bit more coverage than traditional pressed powder, and blends on easily. If the price weren't so prohibitive, it would be an excellent option. As is, this is preferred to the Perfect Powder above.

BLUSH: Shaw's powder ✔☺ $$$ **Blush** *($16)* offers a small, but very good, palette of colors. Plum, Rose, Tan, Peach, and Earth are particularly great. Avoid Desire, unless the goal is extreme shimmer on your cheeks. The texture and application are beautiful. Pink and Red are brighter colors that work well on darker skin. ☺ $$$ **Sheer Wash** *($24)* is another liquid lip and cheek stain to consider. Lorac has the edge with their application and color selection—where most lines offer one shade, they have four. The liquid is dispensed through a deodorant-sized roller-ball applicator that nicely covers the cheek area, but it can release too much and in the wrong place if you aren't careful. Applying it with precision to the lips is almost impossible (whose lips are the size of this roller-ball applicator?). As is true for all liquid stains, this dries almost immediately and tends to work best on smooth, flawless skin. If you can master the application quirks inherent to this product, the colors are beautiful, and this lasts all day without fading.

The ☹ **Lip/Cheek Tint** *($15)* is a pot of color that goes on somewhat greasy and then dries to a smooth, slightly dry-looking finish. There are three shades and all are better suited for lips due to their high concentration of pigment and the difficulty in blending this type of product over skin. This contains isopropyl myristate as the second ingredient, and, therefore, is not recommended for anyone who is battling breakouts.

☺ $$$ **EYESHADOW:** For this entire mostly shiny collection of **Eye Shadows** *($16)*, the best part is their superb blendability. These go on incredibly smooth and a bit on the sheer side, but building intensity is easy enough. If only there weren't such an overwhelming assortment of intensely shiny shades, this would be a slam-dunk recommendation. The best options (still with slight shine) include Beige, Black, Cappuccino, Dark Brown, Light Brown, Nude, Sentimental, Smokin', and Suede.

☺ **Jewel Eye Shadow Box** *($37.50)* is a collection of four shimmery pastel eyeshadows Lorac recommends for highlighting. These apply easily but the shine is obvious. Still, it's an option for teens and twenty-somethings with perfectly taut brow lines.

EYE AND BROW SHAPER: The ☹ **Eye Pencils** *($12)* are standard fare and more or less available to appease pencil lovers. You can find comparable pencils that don't need routine sharpening at the drugstore.

☹ $$$ **Brow Wax** *($16)* is basically a soft brow pencil color in a pot. In contrast to pencils, this starts moist and dries to a soft powder finish, but can still go on heavier than a matte brow powder. The three available colors are excellent, particularly the Blonde/Tan and Auburn/Brown—but this type of product won't be to everyone's taste and really isn't worth the expenditure over just a plain appropriate shade of matte powder eyeshadow.

☹ **Cream Eyeliner Collection** *($28)* is a palette of eight traditional cream eyeliners, and by traditional, I mean smudge-prone and thick. All but two of the shades are strongly iridescent and one of the two "matte" shades is blue, which leaves you with black unless you want shiny, smeary eyeliner.

LIPSTICK AND LIP PENCIL: The ✓☺ $$$ **Cream Lipstick** *($17.50)* selections are no longer being described as matte, which is great because they never were. This is a light, decadently creamy lipstick with a slightly greasy finish that goes on smoothly and imparts rich color. The large selection of celebrity-inspired shades is stunning. ✓☺ $$$ **Matte Lips** *($17.50)* are not matte, but these do have a less creamy texture that the Cream Lipstick above, and offer more intense colors that last without feeling dry or cakey on the lips. Although the color selection is limited, Explore and Inspire are two of the best red hues you'll find.

☺ $$$ **Sheer Lipstick** *($17.50)* is the exact same formula as the Cream Lipstick, but with less pigment, so these tend to fade quickly. The colors are fine, but not exceptional. **Lip Palette** *($25)* offers four of the Sheer Lipsticks and four Lip/Cheek Tints in one thin palette. A synthetic, nicely shaped lip brush is included, and this is an all-out bargain if you happen to like all of these Lorac colors. **Lip Gloss** *($15)* is a standard slick pot gloss that is highly fragrant. It would work as well as any other gloss, and this is less sticky than most, though it is very slippery. The same lip gloss formula is also available as **Refresh** or **Reflect Lip Gloss Quads** *($28.50)*, which come in a larger pot divided into sections. **Lip Polish** *($17.50)* is, by any other name, just lip gloss. The twist with this one is its fluid texture and that it comes in a tiny nail-polish bottle. You apply the color with the built-in brush and you're left with smooth, sheer color and a slightly sticky finish. **Lip Pencil** *($12)* is just a standard pencil with a great color selection that coordinates nicely with the majority of Lorac's lipsticks.

☹ $$$ **Tinted Vitamin E Stick** *($16)* isn't really tinted, it's just an emollient lipstick that's loaded with white iridescence. Used alone, this can make lips look ghostly. **Lip & Eye Duo** *($24)* is a gimmicky product that features an overly iridescent lip gloss on one end and a cream-to-powder iridescent eyeshadow on the other. Neither part of this duo product has much going for it, but for maximum shine with minimal effort, and for decent staying power, this will do the job.

☺ $$$ **MASCARA:** **Lorac Lashes** *($17.50)* goes on well and lengthens beautifully, with minimal to no clumping. It offers very little in terms of thickness, but for a natural lash look, it is an option. The Aubergine color is an attractive deep plum shade for those who want a more experimental color.

☺ **BRUSHES:** Another strong point of the Lorac line is the excellent assortment of **Brushes** *($9–$35)*. The eyeshadow brushes are very workable and nicely shaped, and the **Brush 103 Coverup** *($24)* works well for more detailed concealer or blending jobs if this kind of brush is of interest to you. Avoid the **Brush 110 Powder** *($35)* and **Brush 109 Eye Contour** *($25)* brushes, both of which are floppy and hard to control. **Brush 111** *($9)* is just a mascara wand you can create for free once your mascara is used up, just use that brush, which is the exact same thing.

☺ $$$ **SPECIALTY:** Shaw has launched a few of her key colors as **Greatest Hits CDs** *($48)*. These cleverly named color collections feature four eyeshadows, one blush, one lip/cheek tint, and a lip gloss. Not bad, considering that purchasing these items as singles (instead of as an "album") would cost over twice as much.

LUBRIDERM (SKIN CARE ONLY)

For more information about Lubriderm, call (800) 223-0182 or visit www.skin help.com.

☹ **Moisturizing Body Bar** *($2.49 for 4 ounces)* is a standard, detergent-based cleansing bar that contains tallow. The bar also contains some Vaseline and mineral oil to soften the dryness, but they aren't much help in the long run.

☺ **Moisturizing Lotion, Advanced Therapy for Extra-Dry Skin** *($7.59 for 16 ounces)* is an exceptionally standard moisturizer that contains mostly water, thickeners, glycerin, mineral oil, silicone, water-binding agent, preservatives, teeny amounts of antioxidants, and fragrance. There is little reason to consider this an option for good skin care, given the lack of water-binding agents, antioxidants, and anti-irritants.

☺ **Moisturizing Lotion, Fresh Scent** *($5.29 for 10 ounces)* is a mundane moisturizer for dry skin that contains mostly water, mineral oil, Vaseline, thickeners, lanolin, silicone, thickeners, and fragrance.

☺ **Moisturizing Lotion, Seriously Sensitive** *($5.99 for 10 ounces)* is similar to the Moisturizing Lotion, Fresh Scent above, only minus the scent, and the same basic comments apply.

☺ **Skin Therapy Moisturizing Lotion, Fragrance-Free** *($5.29 for 10 ounces)* is similar to the Moisturizing Lotion, Fresh Scent above, only minus the scent, and the same basic comments apply.

☹ **Daily UV Moisturizer Lotion with Sunscreen SPF 15** *($5.29 for 10 ounces)* doesn't contain the UVA-protecting ingredients of titanium dioxide, zinc oxide, or avobenzone, and is not recommended.

☺ **Skin Firming Body Lotion** *($7.99 for 10 ounces)* has a pH of 4.5, and that precludes the tiny amount of AHA in here from having any exfoliating properties. This not only won't firm skin, it lacks any beneficial ingredients for skin whatsoever.

LUBRIDERM SKIN RENEWAL

The big-deal ingredient in all of the Skin Renewal products is a polyhydroxy acid (PHA) known as gluconolactone. This is supposedly a nonirritating alternative to AHAs, and is described as working well for all skin conditions, from dry and sensitive skin to those with rosacea and atopic dermatitis (eczema). Gluconolactone is a water-binding agent composed of a carbohydrate (glucuronic acid) and lactic acid. Its ability to exfoliate is about the same as that of other AHAs, such as glycolic acid. But the fact remains that skin cannot tell the difference between AHAs and PHA, it only responds by being exfoliated, assuming that the pH of the product is low enough for that to occur. In the case of Lubriderm's Skin Renewal products, the pH of all of them ranges from 4.5 to

6—too high to allow exfoliation. A recent study published in *Cosmetic Dermatology* (September 2001, pages 24–38) states that gluconolactone is effective at a pH of 3.5, and when it comes to performance there is a huge difference between effectiveness at a pH of 4.5 and a pH of 3.5. In addition, that study states that another PHA, lactobionic acid, was shown to be even more effective than gluconolactone when used at the correct pH. While PHA is an option for skin, this one from Lubriderm doesn't quite fit the bill.

☺ **Skin Renewal Anti-Wrinkle Day/Night Cream** *($11.79 for 1.7 ounces)* contains about 6% gluconolactone in a very ordinary, mediocre emollient base. This would be an OK moisturizer for dry skin, but with a pH of 4.5, don't expect much in terms of exfoliation or skin-renewing.

☺ **Skin Renewal Anti-Wrinkle Eye Cream** *($11.79 for 0.5 ounce)* contains about 4% gluconolactone in a standard moisturizing base. The pH of 4.5 makes this ineffective for exfoliation.

☹ **Skin Renewal Anti-Wrinkle Facial Lotion SPF 15 Fragrance Free** *($11.79 for 3.38 ounces)* doesn't contain the UVA-protecting ingredients of titanium dioxide, zinc oxide, or avobenzone, and is not recommended. (Even if the PHA in here did work, whatever effect it had would be completely nullified without an appropriate UVA-protecting sunscreen.)

☹ **Skin Renewal Anti-Wrinkle Facial Lotion SPF 15 Scented** *($11.79 for 3.38 ounces)* doesn't contain the UVA-protecting ingredients of titanium dioxide, zinc oxide, or avobenzone, and is not recommended.

☹ **Skin Renewal Age Defying Hand Cream SPF 15** *($8.75 for 3.38 ounces)* doesn't contain the UVA-protecting ingredients of titanium dioxide, zinc oxide, or avobenzone, and is not recommended.

☺ **Skin Renewal Firming Body Lotion** *($8.75 for 6.77 ounces)* contains about 8% gluconolactone in a lightweight moisturizing base with a pH of 5, which doesn't make it effective for exfoliation.

LUSH (SKIN CARE ONLY)

Originating in Canada, and with a handful of boutiques in other parts of the world, Lush is a concept store trying to go one better than The Body Shop. "Natural" is a major theme here, and I mean major. Essential oils and perfumes are infused into everything; walking into one of these stores will knock you over if you have allergies or a sensitive nose. The unique angle you'll find is that Lush sells skin-care products the way grocery or health food stores let you shop for bulk food items. You can scoop the stuff up yourself from bins and tubs or buy prepackaged items. Even more eye-catching are the shapes, sizes, and decorations for the numerous Lush bar cleansers. These are nothing short of artwork and are either beautiful or fetchingly cute. As clever as all that is, none of it is helpful for skin in the least.

There is no benefit to be gained from scooping cosmetics out of a bin, and besides, I would be very concerned about bacterial contamination. As for natural—OK, you already know this one—with ingredients like sodium lauryl sulfate, TEA-lauryl sulfate, propylene glycol, triethanolamine, tetrasodium EDTA, and preservatives, these products are loaded with very unnatural stuff. Actually, what is a bit startling is that this company includes ingredients that many cosmetics companies have abandoned (or are trying to—especially sodium lauryl sulfate, which shows up in most of the cleansers).

I feel badly that the claims this company makes are so disingenuous and artificial because the names of the products are just adorable: Baby Face, Demon in the Dark, Angels on Bare Skin, and Draught of Immortality are my absolute favorites. But cute names and concepts are not the best way to make a decision about your skin care, and Lush products end up having more problems than serious answers for skin. For more information about Lush, call (888) 733-LUSH or visit www.lushcanada.com. **Note:** All prices are in Canadian dollars.

☹ **Pineapple Grunt** *($5.95 for 100 grams)*; **Bohemian** *($6.95 for 100 grams)*; **Figs and Leaves** *($6.95 for 100 grams)*; **Banana Moon** *($6.25 for 100 grams)*; **Honey Waffle** *($5.80 for 100 grams)*; **Alkmaar** *($5.95 for 100 grams)*; **Sea Vegetable** *($6.25 for 100 grams)*; **Red Rooster** *($6.95 for 100 grams)*; **The Buddah Bar** *($7.95 for 100 grams)*; **Sunny Citrus** *($6.65 for 100 grams)*; **Plantational** *($6.95 for 100 grams)*; **Coal Face** *($9.95 for 100 grams)*; and **Demon in the Dark** *($6.25 for 100 grams)* are standard detergent-based bar cleansers that all contain sodium lauryl sulfate as the main cleansing agent, which is a potent skin irritant and is not recommended for any skin type. They also all have wafting fragrance and a cornucopia of potentially irritating plant extracts, which can create additional problems for most skin types.

☺ **Baby Face** *($7.95 for 35 grams)* is a bar cleanser that contains several emollients that can help cushion the drying effect of the cleansing agents it contains. It is an option for normal to dry skin, but not a very good option.

☹ **Sweet Japanese Girl** *($9.95 for 35 grams)* is a bar cleanser that contains emollients, including cocoa butter, shea butter, and plant oil, which help cushion the drying effect of the cleansing agents it contains. It also contains scrub particles from almond and beans as well as a teeny amount of tea tree oil, but not enough for it to be effective as a disinfectant. Recommending this for oily skin is a joke because the emollient in it can clog pores.

☹ **Queen of Hearts Complexion Soap** *($6.80 for 100 grams)* is a fragrant bar cleanser that contains a good deal of fragrant oils and drying detergent cleansing agents.

☹ **Fresh Farmacy** *($6.95 for 100 grams)* is a bar cleanser with calamine powder, sodium lauryl sulfate, and fragrant oils. It can be extremely drying, and calamine is a skin irritant not meant for frequent use.

☹ **Seaweed Sushi** *($7.95 for 100 grams)* is a bar cleanser that contains ground-up rice and claims that it is helpful as a scrub, but the fragrant plant oils (sage, lime, and pine) can be skin irritants and the detergent cleansing agents are also drying for skin.

☹ **Ultra Bland** *($10.95 for 60 ml)* contains mostly peanut oil, fragrance, thickener, borax, and preservatives. Borax has fungicide, preservative, insecticide, herbicide, and disinfectant properties. It also can act as a bleach by converting some of its water molecules to hydrogen peroxide (H_2O_2), but that generates free-radical damage, which isn't good for skin. The pH of borax is about 9.5, making it a skin irritant. None of this product is particularly bland.

☺ **Spring Cleanser for All Skin Types** *($11.95 for 240 grams)* is mostly almond oil and thickener with a great deal of fragrance. It is more of a cold cream and your skin would be far better off with just plain almond oil.

☺ **Angels on Bare Skin** *($7.95 for 100 grams)* is a scrub that contains ground-up almonds and clay, and a great deal of fragrance. It's not bad, but your skin would be far better off with just plain ground-up almonds you buy from the grocery store without the wafting fragrance.

☺ **Draught of Immortality** *($16.95 for 250 grams)* is supposed to be a moisturizer and cleanser in one. It ends up being just a basic wipe-off cleanser of plant oil and cocoa butter, and that can leave a greasy film on the skin.

☺ **Ocean Salt** *($14.95 for 120 grams)*, just as the name indicates, contains mostly salt. It also contains thickening agents to suspend the salt, as well as irritating plant extracts. If you're looking for a scrub, plain salt is an option, though an irritating one (ever hear the saying "as painful as rubbing salt in a wound"?). Plain baking soda would work far better and be better for skin.

☹ **Enzymion** *($29.95 for 45 grams)*. The tiny amount of papaya in this product is not effective for exfoliation, and the lemon and lime can be skin irritants.

☹ **Eau-Roma Water** *($12.95 for 250 grams)* is a toner that contains fragrant water and preservatives. This serves no purpose for skin other than as a potential irritant.

☺ **Breeze on a Sea Air** *($13.95 for 250 grams)* contains mostly water, aloe vera, fragrance, and preservatives. It lacks any antioxidants or water-binding agents and applying this to your skin ends up being almost like applying cologne to your skin. If you are looking for aloe vera, your skin would be much better off with plain aloe vera from the health food store.

☹ **Tea Tree Water** *($12.95 for 250 ml)* contains mostly tea tree water and grapefruit. Tea tree oil can be a disinfectant, but tea tree water is too diluted to be effective, and grapefruit is just a skin irritant and has no helpful skin properties.

☹ **Angelicum for Oily Skin** *($19.50 for 50 grams)* contains a lot, and I mean a lot, of plant oils, lavender water, preservatives, fragrance, and pine oil. This is so inappropriate for oily skin! And what's the purpose of the pine oil—is someone polishing furniture with this stuff?

☺ **Celestial for Sensitive Skin** *($15.95 for 50 grams)*. Finally a product in the Lush lineup with minimal fragrance! Though it still contains vanilla water and orchid extract, I imagine that it contains the least amount of fragrance of all the products they sell. But while this may be the least for Lush, it isn't little enough to make this a good moisturizer because it doesn't contain one water-binding agent, antioxidant, or anti-irritant.

☹ **Imperialis for All Skin Types** *($14.95 for 50 grams)*. The amount of emollients in this product makes it unsuitable for all skin types, except dry skin, but the amount of fragrance is a problem waiting to happen.

☺ **Skin Drink for Dry Skin** *($11.95 for 55 grams)*. The emollients are great, but this product misses the boat by leaving out any antioxidants, water-binding agents, or anti-irritants.

☹ **Mask of Magnanimity** *($16.95 for 325 grams)*. The peppermint oil in this product makes it a problem for all skin types.

☺ **Skin's Shangri La** *($39.95 for 45 grams)* is an extremely emollient moisturizer for dry skin that contains some good plant oils and a tiny amount of antioxidants. The fragrance is a bit much, but not terrible.

☺ **After Life** *($39.95 for 45 grams)* is similar to the Skin's Shangri La above and the same comments apply.

☺ **Enchanted Eye Cream** *($18.95 for 45 grams)* is simply fragrance, thickeners, plant oil, and preservatives, making it an ordinary emollient moisturizer for dry skin with too much fragrance, especially for the eye area.

☺ **Mirror Mirror Neck Cream** *($18.95 for 50 grams)* contains far more fragrance than beneficial ingredients for skin. It's emollient, but ordinary, and not worth the trouble of applying it.

☺ **Lip Service** *($7.95 for 20 grams)* is an OK emollient balm for dry lips. It does contain borax, which can be a skin irritant.

☺ **Lite Lip Balm** *($7.95 for 12 grams)* is a very good emollient balm for dry lips with some great plant oils and lanolin.

☺ **Love Lettuce Facial Exfoliator and Mask** *($7.95 for 180 grams)* is mostly clay and some ground-up almond shells. It is an option for normal to oily skin.

☹ **Cosmetic Warrior Mask** *($7.45 for 180 grams)* contains mostly clay, grapes, eggs, honey, corn flour, garlic, tea tree oil, and fragrance. This sounds more like lunch then a skin-care product. Food on skin can encourage bacteria growth, which is a problem for blemish-prone skin, the very skin type that this mask is aimed at. There is not enough tea tree oil for it to be effective as a disinfectant.

☺ **Wow Wow Face Mask** *($7.25 for 180 grams)* is supposed to be for dry, mature skin with broken veins. There is nothing in this product that can affect surfaced capillaries. It is just a fragrant clay mask and while that may be an option for oily skin, it is a problem for dry skin.

☹ **Coolie-O Face Mask** *($6.95 for 180 grams)* contains mint, spearmint, and peppermint, and while those may be great in chewing gum, they are potent skin irritants.

☺ **Aromabread Mask** *($6.95 for 100 grams)* is just a clay mask with some flour, yogurt, avocado, bread crumbs, and fragrance. Food is a problem for encouraging bacteria growth and the avocado can be a skin irritant.

The Reviews L

☺ **Ayesha** *($7.95 for 180 grams)* is a clay mask that also contains some honey, plant extracts, asparagus, kiwi, and fragrance. Other than the clay absorbing oil, the other ingredients are not helpful for skin and the kiwi may be a skin irritant.

M.A.C.

Once the new kid on the block as a start-up cosmetics company with edge and attitude, M.A.C. (Makeup Art Cosmetics) is now a serious contender in the prestigious world of department-store cosmetics. In fact, M.A.C.'s rampant success clearly paved the way for every other artistry line that took the "imitation is the sincerest form of flattery" concept to dizzying new heights. But this Toronto-based company, now under the ownership of Estee Lauder, is well funded and is launching new products that keep it nicely up to date with its more elegant neighbors at the high-end cosmetics counters. Especially when it comes to packaging and marketing pieces, the line is now much more attractive. And, in many respects, M.A.C. continues to set precedents that leave other lines scrambling to catch up.

One clear sign that Estee Lauder is now at the helm of M.A.C. is how the selection of skin-care products has improved over the past few years. Though there are no surprises at M.A.C. (at least not based on the other lines Lauder owns), the skin-care products have some great antioxidants and water-binding agents and, of particular interest, finally, there is a well-formulated sunscreen. Despite these improvements, this is still not a comprehensive line to consider for skin care. A limited selection of sunscreens, no products for blemish-prone skin, and a lack of toners make the selection pale in comparison to many other lines, including those owned by Lauder. By and large the main reason (but it's a very important reason) to shop M.A.C. is for their makeup, which remains a strong specialty. For more information about M.A.C., call (800) 387-6707 or visit www.maccosmetics.com. **Note:** All M.A.C. skin-care products contain fragrance.

M.A.C. Skin Care

☺ **Cold Cream Cleanser** *($15 for 4 ounces)* is an accurate name for this standard, cold-cream cleanser (a jar that you dip your hand into, not the most sanitary option) that is quite similar to Pond's Cold Cream, which costs far less. It can be an option for dry skin.

☺ **Everyday Lotion Cleanser** *($15 for 5 ounces)* is virtually identical to Neutrogena's Extra Gentle Cleanser ($6.06 for 6.7 ounces). Both are indeed gentle, neither removes makeup very well, and both can leave a slightly greasy film on the skin. Still, this can be an option for someone with dry skin.

☹ **Green Gel Cleanser** *($15 for 5 ounces)* is a standard, detergent-based, water-soluble cleanser that can be an option for someone with normal to oily skin, though the third ingredient is TEA-lauryl sulfate, which can be an irritant for some skin types.

☺ **Super Cleansing Oil** *($15 for 5.1 ounces)* actually contains only a teeny amount of sesame oil. This is mainly just waxy emollients that need to be wiped off. It is an option for normal to dry skin.

☺ **Wipes** *($12.50 for 45 sheets)* are basically silicone with some thickening agents soaked onto disposable sheets. These will wipe off makeup, but for the money, this isn't all that much better or more effective than baby wipes, which you can get fragrance-free, unlike this version that contains fragrance.

☺ **Pro Eye Makeup Remover** *($15 for 5 ounces)* is a standard, detergent-based makeup remover similar to almost every one of its kind in this book. It would work as well as any.

☺ **$$$ Scrub Mask** *($16.50 for 3.6 ounces)*. This very standard clay mask is an option for exfoliating, but the menthol is an unnecessary, risky skin irritant.

✓☺ **Day SPF 15 Light Moisture** *($22 for 1.7 ounces)* is a very good, in-part titanium dioxide–based sunscreen that contains some impressive water-binding agents and antioxidants.

☹ **$$$ EZR (Eye Zone Remoisturizer) Day/Night Emulsion** *($28 for 1 ounce)*. The interesting ingredients are listed so far at the end of the list they're barely detectable. There is more sunscreen in this product than there are water-binding agents or antioxidants; and what is a sunscreen agent doing in a product meant to be worn at night? This isn't a bad moisturizer, just not as impressive as many, many others.

☺ **$$$ Moisture Feed Eye** *($25 for 0.5 ounce)* is an emollient moisturizer with some very good water-binding agents and anti-irritants, but only small amounts of antioxidants, which precludes a Paula's Pick checkmark, but this one was close. There is also caffeine, and the tannin in the caffeine constricts skin, which can make skin look temporarily smoother, although it can also cause irritation; it will not in any way make eyes look more awake, but the amount of caffeine is so small that it will have little to no effect on skin.

✓☺ **$$$ Fast Response Eye Cream** *($25 for 0.5 ounce)* is a very good, silicone-based moisturizer for dry skin that also contains caffeine, just like the Moisture Feed above, and those comments apply as well. This also contains an array of antioxidants and water-binding agents.

☺ **Oil Control Lotion** *($22 for 1.7 ounces)*. The salicylic acid in this product cannot control oil, nor can any other ingredient it contains. This is just a good BHA product in a lotion with a pH that lets the BHA exfoliate skin and make it feel smoother. It also contains some great water-binding agents and a tiny amount of antioxidants.

☺ **Studio Moisture Fix** *($22 for 1.7 ounces)* is a very good moisturizer for dry skin with some excellent water-binding agents, but minuscule amounts of antioxidants.

✓☺ **Strobe Cream** *($25 for 1.7 ounces)* is a very good moisturizer for dry skin that contains some very good antioxidants and water-binding agents. The AHA amounts to less than 2%, which means it's ineffective for exfoliation.

☹ **Fix +** *($11.50 for 5 ounces)* is supposed to set makeup, but this ends up being an unnecessary extra step. It is just a toner, nice, but not great.

☺ **Lip Conditioner** *($8 for 0.5 ounce)* is a very good, emollient, Vaseline-based balm that even has a small amount of antioxidants and vanilla flavoring. Not bad, and a great price!

The Reviews M

☹ **Radically Clear Acne Treatment** *($11.50 for 0.05 ounce)* is supposed to "treat and conceal," but it does neither very well. This product doesn't contain one effective ingredient to "treat" blemishes. There is neither a disinfectant that can kill the bacterium that causes acne nor an exfoliant that can unclog pores. The green color of this can't hide the red of irritated skin nearly as well as a flesh-tone concealer or foundation. It also contains menthol, which can make skin redder. Altogether, it's a completely ill-conceived product.

M.A.C. MAKEUP

M.A.C. claims that many professional makeup artists use its products, and in my experience that is true. Lots of professional makeup artists prefer neutral-toned foundations and matte eyeshadows and blushes (despite the ongoing iridescent craze), and this line has a generous offering in each category. In fact, the color selection for everything from lipsticks to pencils is exceptional. Also, most of the makeup brushes are beautiful, full, and soft, as well as properly sized to fit the contours of the face and eyes. For the most part, you will find it a pleasure to shop this line, and M.A.C.'s salespeople are sometimes trained as makeup artists, too, though they have lots of corporate pressure now to meet sales quotas. M.A.C. is now firmly entrenched in the Lauder "Power of Three" scripted method of selling. For example, if you visit the M.A.C. counter looking for mascara, the counterperson is required to show and recommend at least two other products, such as an eye cream or a liquid liner. This follows suit with any other product that may catch your eye, so be prepared to deflect or ignore what you know isn't necessary—too many "yes" responses can add up fast. The user-friendly tester units are divided by product type, but not consistently by texture or finish. It's easy to get overwhelmed by the wide range of choices, but once you get acclimated, making sense of it all is not too difficult.

FOUNDATION: ☺ $$$ **Studio Tech Foundation** *($26)* is a new breed of cream-to-powder foundation that offers a lighter, almost weightless texture, smooth application, and a soft, satin finish that tends not to grab onto dry areas. It combines the super-light feel of a water-to-powder makeup with the slip and smoothness of silicone-based cream-to-powder makeups. Studio Tech applies easily and provides light to medium coverage. There are 18 shades available, with suitable options for very light (NC15, NW15) and darker (NW50, NW60) skin tones. Although the majority of the 18 shades lean toward neutral, four of them are bound to be too orange or rose for their intended skin tones: NC45, NW25, NW30, and NW45. This formula is best for normal to slightly dry and dry skin—the non-matte, nonpowdery finish won't do much to temper shine, and even though this is not traditional cream-to-powder makeup, there are enough waxes and thickeners present to make it problematic for those battling blemishes. If your skin fills the bill for this makeup, it's certainly worth a test run.

☺ **Studio Finish Satin Foundation SPF 8** *($19.50)* does not provide UVA protection and the sunscreen level would be too low even if it did. This is still an excellent fluid foundation for normal to dry skin. It leaves a moist, satin finish and provides sheer to light coverage. The 17 shades nicely represent most skin tones, although very dark skin tones may still have some challenges. The following shades are too pink, rose, or peach for most skin tones: NC45, NW20 (slight pink), NW25, NW35, and NW40. **Studio Finish Matte Foundation SPF 8** *($19.50)* does not provide UVA protection and the sunscreen level would be too low even if it did. It comes in a long tube that makes it a bit tricky to control the amount you use. This has a blendable, smooth texture with lots of slip, and it dries to a minimal matte finish that is similar to the Finish Satin foundation above. The 19 shades are quite wonderful, providing light to medium coverage, but test the following colors with caution: NW25 (just slightly pink), NW30, NW40, NW45, and NC50. **Matte Creme Matifiance** *($16.50)* has its strong points. It's a thick, silicone-based liquid that has a matte-cream texture reminiscent of a soft spackle. It can definitely give the appearance of smoother skin, but the effect is temporary, lasting only a few hours depending on what you wear over it and how much you move your face. Still, it's worth a test run to see if it works for you.

✓☺ **StudioFix Powder Plus Foundation** *($22.50)* is easily one of the top pressed-powder foundations available. It has an exceptionally silky texture that applies and blends like a dream. As usual, wet or dry application is possible, though using this wet poses the risk of streaking. Dry application provides light to medium-full coverage. If you prefer this type of foundation and have normal to slightly dry or slightly oily skin, consider this a must-try. Almost all of the 36 colors are impressive (albeit repetitive) for a broad range of skin tones, but the following shades are best avoided: NW20, NW25, NW30, NW37, NC40 (slight peach), NC42, W15, W25, W40 (remember, all W shades are available in M.A.C. stores only). The M.A.C. stores also sell a range of color-correcting StudioFix shades, and the only one that really works is Fragile Peach.

☺ **Hyper Real Foundation** *($24)* has a gorgeously smooth application and feels more elegant than either of the Studio Finish Foundations above. Yet in an effort to "mimic skin's natural dimensions," M.A.C. has spiked this with bluish pink iridescence. This may look appropriate in photographs, but tends to look sparkly and artificial in daylight. The six shades are beautiful and offer light coverage. There are also additional shades of pale, shiny Violet, Green, and Bronze that are adept at creating a soft shimmer effect wherever you put them.

☹ **Gloss** *($16.50)* is supposed to add a polished glow to the skin, but this effect can be achieved with any of M.A.C.'s shiny powders and you won't have to cope with this thick, sticky texture that undermines any other makeup it's combined with.

<u>CONCEALER:</u> ☺ **Concealer SPF 15** *($12.50)* has been reformulated and is not quite as thick as it used to be, but is still a substantially creamy concealer. Even coverage remains the strong point for this formula, though it can crease into lines under the eye unless it's set with powder. The sunscreen is now in-part (as opposed to all) titanium dioxide, and the additional synthetic sunscreen may cause problems if it gets too close to the eye. This is still a viable option, and of the 15 shades, only 4 are below par; avoid

The Reviews M

NW20, NW25, NW30, and NW45. Shade W55 is an excellent option for very dark skin. ✓☺ **Select Cover-Up** *($12.50)* is a brilliant alternative to M.A.C.'s mainstay Concealer SPF 15 above, as this version is significantly lighter in texture and much easier to work with. Lightly creamy with a natural matte finish, Select Cover-Up provides good camouflage with minimal risk of creasing. Eleven mostly neutral shades are available, plus five color correctors, which I recommend avoiding because almost all of them are too obviously pink, green, orange, or yellow to look convincing, although peach is an OK option for the color correctors. Of the regular shades, the ones to be cautious with are NC42, NC45, NW35, and NW45.

POWDER: ☺ $$$ **Studio Finish Face Powder** *($18.50)* is a very soft, talc-based powder that comes in a tub and has an excellent texture and natural matte finish. The shade selection has been edited down to 11 suitable colors, with equally good options for fair and dark skin tones. **Studio Finish Pressed Powder** *($18.50)* is also talc-based, with a silky-smooth texture and sheer finish. There are 18 shades to consider, and only NC45, NW35, NW45, and W60 are too rose, peach, or ash for most skin tones. **Blot Powder** *($15)* is talc-based and comes in only three colors, all fine. It has a drier texture than the Studio Finish Pressed Powder above, and gives a translucent matte finish. This pressed powder is best for normal to oily skin types looking more for shine control than coverage.

☺ $$$ **Iridescent Powder** *($18.50)* comes in a tub and is appropriately named. The small collection of sheer colors does well in terms of providing high shine. **Sheer Shimmer Powder** *($16)* is nothing more than a talc-based iridescent pressed powder. The shine is fairly intense, so this is best for evening special effects. **Bronzing Powder** *($16)* is a pressed-powder bronzer that comes in four utterly believable tan shades, three of which have an iridescent finish. Matte Bronze is truly matte, though for the money I wouldn't choose this over Wet 'n' Wild's Bronzer ($2.99).

BLUSH: ☺ $$$ **Blush** *($16)* is your everyday pressed-powder blush with a smooth, dry texture that can feel a bit grainy. The colors are divided into Mattes, Satins (minimal shine), and Frosts (high shine), but do not apply as true as they once did. If anything, the colors tend to go on soft, but you can build on the intensity. **Cheekhue** *($17.50)* comes in small tubes of cream-to-powder blush that are mostly bright hues of pink, red, plum, and violet. The colors go on quite strong, but do blend out to a soft, sheer powder finish with a subtle shine. If you can master the application and don't mind mildly sparkling cheeks, these are a good cream blush option. And who can resist a blush shade named Velvet Elvis? **Sheertone Blush** *($16)* is a pressed powder blush that is very similar to M.A.C.'s longstanding powder blush, only these are more refined. They feel silkier, go on easier, and blend better—but you sacrifice color, since these are remarkably soft. Many women will appreciate this sheerness, and M.A.C.'s enticing initial lineup of colors are almost all matte.

☺ **Cream Colour Base** *($14)* comes in compacts of slick, creamy color that can be used on the lips, eyes, or cheeks, but there are clearly colors that will only work on the eyes and nowhere else, and the same for the lips and cheeks, unless your blush color of choice is iridescent silver. Fresco and Quartz are affable cheek colors, but the rest of the lot are quite shiny and they're immensely crease-prone if used as eyeshadow.

EYESHADOWS: The ☺ Eye Shadows ($12.50 small, $14 large) maintain the same almost-smooth, dry texture they've had for the past several years. The only real difference this time around is that many of the colors go on softer and more sheer. You'll notice less of this with the medium to dark shades, which tend to go on grainier and deeper than they look, and just don't blend out like the best eyeshadows do, though there is minimal flaking. These are not the smoothest shadows in town, but they do the job. Although the shades are labeled as Satin, Frost, Matte, and Velvet (which are extremely shiny), they are arranged haphazardly on the tester unit. However, it is quite easy to determine which shades have shine, though many of the Matte shades sneak in a bit of low-key sparkle, too. M.A.C. stores carry an extended selection of shocking shades such as opaque orange, taxicab yellow, and vivid green, but avoid these unless you're the newest theatrical makeup artist for *Into the Woods*. **Paints** *($15)* make many M.A.C. makeup artists giddy as they go on and on about how much they *love* these tiny metal roll-up tubes that dispense a thick, but light-textured, cream. Most of the nearly opaque colors supply intense shine, though there are a few sleeper shades that can work for a mildly shiny look. Paints can be used alone or mixed with other products, and they sheer out well if you prefer a subtle wash of color. What really makes the M.A.C. staff (and customers) happy is that these tend not to crease. **Colour Theory No. 9** *($15)*. These are powder eyeshadows whose odd, largely unappealing colors just happen to have the best texture and smoothest application of all M.A.C.'s eyeshadows. They blend magnificently, though the iridescent colors go on very sheer. **Sheer Colour Extract** *($12.50)* has a liquid-cream texture that's light as silk and, as the name states, provides sheer color. This formula dries almost instantly, and has a slight shimmering finish that does not budge all day. These are an option if you need long-wearing eye makeup, but blending them on right will take practice and patience!

☹ **Eyeglass** *($21)* is a thick, sticky, colored gloss for the eyelids that understandably looks cool in photos, but is terribly uncomfortable and impractical for regular use. The bold primary colors are a kick, but no one at the M.A.C. stores recommended this for anything more than a lark.

EYE AND BROW SHAPER: The ☺ Eye Pencils *($11.50)* are utterly standard (right down to the commonplace colors) and comparable to most other pencils out there. For lining the eyes, M.A.C.'s matte eyeshadows are a better alternative. **Eye Kohls** *($12.50)* are an unnecessary addition to the Eye Pencils, but here's one more twist on the creamy, standard pencil formula. The chance of smearing is slightly less than for the Eye Pencils above, but don't bet on them not smearing.

✔☺ **Eye Brow Pencils** *($12.50)* have been improved. These automatic, ultra-sleek pencils apply easily and impart soft color without being greasy or smudging. The colors are brow-perfect, but don't ask me to explain the sexually-charged names such as Stud, Lingering, and Fling!

☺ **Creme Liner** *($11.50)* is an ultra-dramatic liner that comes in a pot. Use this with a damp brush for best results. Once it sets, it stays on quite well. M.A.C. stores carry an extended array of metallic colors for those so inclined. **Liquid Liner** *($15)* is fairly straight-forward, applying nicely with a decent brush and drying quickly without flaking or smearing. **Brow Set** *($12)* is just a basic brow gel that can double as clear mascara. It's not too sticky and works well for both purposes, and the brush is great. **Colored Brow Set** *($12)* is identical to the regular Brow Set, only this features three tints that work well for blondes and brunettes.

LIPSTICK AND LIP PENCIL: M.A.C.'s ☺ **Lipsticks** *($14)* are one of the major attractions of this line. The majority of the formulas have lush textures and feel comfort-able, and the color range is nearly unparalleled. Here is how they break down. ✓☺ Satins are softly creamy with a rich, opaque texture and moist finish. This is the best compromise of long wear and desirable creaminess. ☺ **Creams** are similar to the Satins, but offer less color and a glossier finish. ☺ **Frosts** are simply Creams with iridescence, and are available in over 50 colors. ✓☺ **Mattes** are not true mattes, but come pretty close with their deeply pigmented, full-coverage colors and non-glossy finish. ✓☺ **Retro Mattes** are the real deal and come in a limited selection of colors for true matte lipstick fans. **Lustres** are creamy lipsticks that feel slick and leave a glossy finish. The colors offer semi-opaque coverage, and these can easily slip into lines around the mouth. **Sheers, Tones,** and **Glazes** all offer minimal color payoff and varying degrees of gloss and shimmer. These will eventually be phased out in favor of the Lustres.

☺ $$$ **Lacquer** *($16)* is a thick-textured liquid lipstick that has a sticky, high-gloss finish and a tantalizing range of medium-coverage colors. The wand applicator has a brush instead of an angled sponge tip, and the brush holds up well without splaying.

☺ **LipGlass** and **LipGlass Tinted** *($10)* are very thick, tenacious glosses whose heavy, syrupy texture is not for everyone. The tinted version comes in a tube with a wand appli-cator. **Lip Pencils** *($11.50)* have a superior color selection; but that's the only thing that separates these standard pencils from the pencils found in almost every other line. **Clear Lipstick** *($14)* and **Lip Treatment** *($14)* are both colorless, emollient lip balms that are great for dry lips and add a soft, glossy finish.

MASCARA: ☹ **Mascara S** *($12)*. The "S" stands for sheer, and this boring mascara assuredly is. Unless you want the smallest bit of lash enhancement, stay away from this.

☺ **Mascara N** *($12)* is slightly better than the one above. It builds decent length and a touch of thickness without clumping, but tends to break down and smear before the end of the day. **Mascara X** *($12)* is billed as M.A.C.'s most dramatic mascara, and it certainly provides more oomph than the two above, yet it takes considerable effort to build lots of length and decent thickness. L'Oreal makes several mascaras that run circles around this. **Pro Longlash Mascara** *($9.50)* is touted as extreme lengthening mascara, and it does lengthen—just not that well or that fast. It provides no thickness, and finishes lashes with a soft curl, but for all the promises, it just doesn't have that "wow" factor that the Pro Lash Mascara below does.

✔☺ **Pro Lash Mascara** *($9.50)* is in a league all its own! This home-run mascara builds dramatic thickness and length while being only slightly difficult to control. It's almost too easy to over-apply this mascara, so be sure to exercise some restraint to avoid a heavy, clumped appearance. Otherwise, you will be impressed at how quickly this revs up your lashes!

☺ **Pro Lash Colour** *($9.50)* is mascara for lashes and brows that comes in bright, bold colors like green, red, and platinum. The formula is identical to the tamer Pro Lash Mascara above, so it performs well, but none of the colors are suitable for eyebrows, at least not if your goal is natural-looking color. For a colorful twist or for Halloween, this is an option.

☺ $$$ <u>BRUSHES:</u> As stated in previous editions of this book, M.A.C. has one of the best selections of brushes you'll find anywhere *(over 30 different brushes, ranging from $8.50 to $62.50)*. The big brushes are a little pricey, but they last forever if you take care of them. Though there are indeed good, inexpensive brushes to be found, if you're going to splurge, this is one area where the extra expense won't be wasted. Be sure to check out M.A.C.'s variety of eyeshadow brushes, particularly the ✔☺ **#275 Medium Angled Shading Brush** *($23)*, an excellent, versatile eyeshadow brush. Also, test the ✔☺ **#216 Blending Brush** *($18)*. The only brushes to really avoid are the **#201 Sponge Tip Applicator** *($8.50)*, which comes free in most eyeshadow kits, the **#204 Lash Brush** *($8.50)*, which is easily duplicated by washing off an old mascara wand, and the **#207 Duster** *($18)*, which is a fantail brush that I'm sure has some function but is truly not imperative for daily makeup application. The freestanding M.A.C. stores sell pricier brushes known as M.A.C. Pro brushes, and these are definitely worth a look, especially if you're a working makeup artist with a generous budget.

M.A.C. PROFESSIONAL STUDIO MAKEUP

In addition to the familiar line of M.A.C. makeup products available at department stores across the country, M.A.C. also has several freestanding boutique cosmetics stores in a handful of cities in Canada and the United States. These stores carry all of the products found at the department-store M.A.C. counters and a few extras and main-line product extensions that are interesting to check out. For a full exposure to everything M.A.C. has to offer, these stores are definitely worth a visit.

☺ $$$ **Face and Body Foundation** *($28.50)* comes in a 4-ounce bottle and is very liquidy and sheer. It takes some patience to blend on, as it tends to slide around a lot before drying. This can be layered for more coverage (as can most foundations) and is reasonably waterproof. For body makeup it can be a problem, however, as it can come off on clothes, and it's not a great choice for major flaws you want to fully conceal. There are 18 shades, and most are neutral and workable. The deeper shades can be sketchy because most of them have a slight peach to red cast that won't work for many skin tones.

☺ **Sheer Coverage Foundation SPF 15** *($22)* has an updated formula that is jojoba oil– and shea butter–based, so this compact foundation is more emollient than ever be-

The Reviews M

fore. It does not dry to a powder finish, but stays moist (almost greasy) on the skin and is best for dry to very dry skin seeking sheer to light coverage. The SPF is now in-part titanium dioxide, and the range of 26 shades is one of the largest selections of foundations you will find. The following colors are too pink, peach, orange, red, or ash for most skin tones: C40, NC50, NC55, NC65, NW25, NW30, NW40, W40, and W45.

☺ **Full Coverage Foundation SPF 15** *($24)* has been reformulated, but is still a wax-based emollient foundation that offers substantial coverage and lends a rather heavy appearance to the skin. You can manipulate the application to look somewhat natural, but it will still feel thick and creamy. For a concealer, it works quite well, and the range of 35 shades is extensive to say the least. The sunscreen is in-part titanium dioxide. There are colors for very light to very dark skin tones, but the following shades are too pink, peach, orange, red, copper, green, or ash for most skin tones: NC45, NW20, NW25, NW30, NW35 (slightly peach), NW45, NW50, C50, W20, W25, W30, W40, and W55 (slightly red, but may work for some very dark skin tones).

☺ **Tint** *($10)* is a collection of liquid color correctors and highlighters (gold, white, bronze) that can be used alone for a soft shine or mixed into a foundation or with any other color product. The only thing the color-correcting tints do is place a noticeable layer on the skin that looks strange, and the highlighters are merely another way to incorporate shine into your makeup routine. **Glitter** *($10)* comes in small jars of loose glitter particles that represent an extremely messy method of shining yourself up. **LipGlass Stain** *($13)* comes in a squeeze tube and offers intense, glossy color that shares the same basic texture as the LipGlass above.

Lipmix *($10 per tube, $9 for Lipmix tray)* is a collection of mostly iridescent, intensely pigmented colors that can be used alone or mixed with an existing lipstick to create a custom shade. It's an intriguing option, and I wish there were more practical shades to experiment with, but as it stands now many of the colors are odd and are easily passed up in favor of M.A.C.'s brilliant assortment of lipsticks. Caution: These products can stain, and it takes some effort to remove them from skin and lips; on the plus side, that can be construed as a benefit for the lips! For makeup artists who are passionate about experimenting with lip color, it doesn't get much better than this.

☺ **$$$ Pigment** *($18)* comes in small jars of shiny loose powder, available in almost every color imaginable and with a shininess scale that goes from sheer to POW! However, there is little benefit to using this product over similar versions from L'Oreal, for one-third the price, and they are inherently messy to use.

MAKE UP FOR EVER (MAKEUP ONLY)

This Paris-based makeup collection traces its roots to theatrical and fashion makeup, with the concept being that a professional makeup artist not only desires, but also needs, every conceivable color and texture to create the broadest range of looks. Since 1984, Make Up For Ever creators Dany Sanz and Jacques Waneph have been doing their best to meet these criteria. Through the years this line has gone from offering a tremendous array of colors in their own boutiques to a more streamlined, "everyday" collection of products in selected department stores and at Sephora. Make Up For Ever has an intriguing blend of classic, workable shades positioned next to some truly unique hues and finishes that only those involved with theatre or the most flamboyant "anything goes" makeup artist (or diva) would covet. A major plus for this line is that the majority of colors are densely pigmented and work beautifully on medium to deep skin tones. The drawback is that fair and lighter skin tones may be left feeling that most of the color choices are too intense for them, especially if their goal is a soft, natural makeup application. Still, for those who literally want it all when it comes to possible shades, this line more than delivers what it takes to please.

The foundation colors are a classic case of not judging a book by its cover. Upon first glance, many of the liquid foundation shades appear too peach, orange, or pink. Yet application on the skin proves that these morph into neutral, flesh-tone shades that offer substantial, yet natural-looking, coverage. The concealers are a bit on the weak side, as the two main options leave you deciding between a greasy, full-coverage option and a dry-textured pencil that works but is not worth choosing over more user-friendly liquid or cream-to-powder concealers. The rest of the line offers some viable options for pencils, liquid liners, lipsticks, glosses, decent mascaras, and exquisite makeup brushes. There are more than a handful of intensely shiny or glittery products, but if that's what you're into, Make Up For Ever will not disappoint. In addition to the vast color palette, the overall mix of product formulas offers a bit of the tried-and-true with some rather innovative alternatives. The tricky part is getting used to applying and blending deeply pigmented colors and wading through some of the weaker choices to find what really works for you. This line is worth seeking out if you want exposure to the types of richly pigmented colors that M.A.C. used to offer but has slowly phased out since Estee Lauder has been at the helm. And if you're a theatrical or fashion makeup artist, this line is a must-see. For more information on Make Up For Ever, call (877) 757-5175 or visit www.makeupforever.fr (this Web site has an English translation).

FOUNDATION: ✓☺ **$$$ Face and Body Liquid Makeup** *($37)* is a liquidy, water-based foundation that also contains a blend of silicone and mineral oil, so this has a good amount of slip on the skin yet blends readily to a natural matte finish. Coverage can go from sheer to medium, and allows you to build coverage without looking thick. The collection of 12 shades is deceiving, as many of them look too peach or pink in the container, but all of them end up being soft and neutral on the skin—plus there are equally good options for light and dark skin tones. This can be used on the body if desired, but it isn't as tenacious or clingy as products like DermaBlend, so the results can be mixed. This lightweight formula works best for normal to slightly dry or slightly oily skin. ☺ **$$$ Powder Foundation** *($40)* is talc-based with a hint of mica, so it does have a slightly shiny finish. It also has the requisite smooth, dry texture and offers sheer to light coverage. The six shades are all slightly yellow, but should work for most skin tones. **Mat Velvet Oil-Free Foundation SPF 20** *($36)* contains effective sunscreen agents, but they're not listed as active so they cannot be relied on for daily protection. That's a shame, because this offers a great smooth texture, soft matte finish, and light to medium coverage that would appeal to those with oily skin. The seven colors are very good—only Matte Beige 5 is too peach to look convincing on the skin. Note: This starts out thick, but quickly sheers out as it is blended.

☺ **$$$ Metalizer** *($19)* is sheer liquid shimmer that's available in an array of metallic colors. The shine is low-key, especially if this is mixed with a foundation, but this is still a look best reserved for evening or special effects.

☹ **$$$ Corrective Makeup Base SPF 18** *($20)* is essentially a lightweight, slightly moist liquid foundation that comes in color-correcting shades of green, purple, white, blue, yellow, and orange. The sunscreen is in-part titanium dioxide, which is great, but I am just not a fan of color correctors, so this is hard to recommend. However, because these colors are very sheer, mesh quite well with the skin, and leave a soft matte finish, the corrective effect is all but gone once foundation, concealer, and powder are applied on top. If you're curious to see how a product like this would work for you, definitely test it before purchasing. The Yellow and White shades could work as stand-alone foundations for very light skin. **Pan Stik** *($30)* is reminiscent of the type of full-coverage, slightly greasy foundations often used for theatrical makeup. This traditional, oil-and-wax–based stick foundation has a soft, creamy finish and OK colors, but the final result on skin is not what I would call subtle or natural.

CONCEALER: ☹ **Pencil Concealer** *($17)* is a dual-sided pencil that comes in two different skin tones, one for lighter skin and one for darker skin. Neither offers great shades and this style of concealer is no match for a good liquid or cream concealer.

☺ **$$$ Lift Concealer** *($18)* comes in a squeeze tube and is basically a sheer-coverage concealer with a matte finish and pale or mid-pink colors that are not too useful for most skin tones. However, this could work as a highlighter if you can adapt to the pinkish tones. **5-Camouflage Cream Palette** *($30)* claims it is a custom concealer for blemishes and scars, and there is no doubt you can achieve full coverage with this thick-textured creamy concealer, though putting this talc-and-wax–based product over a blemish is likely to prolong its unwelcome stay! The palette includes four flesh-toned colors that veer slightly to the peachy side, along with a green color corrector. You can blend the shades together to create a custom match, but unless you need significant coverage and are willing to put up with this difficult texture, this is easy to pass up. Again, theatrical makeup artists will likely find more uses for this than the average cosmetics consumer.

POWDER: ☺ **$$$ Compact Powder** *($28)* is talc-based and has a silky, dry texture and sheer finish that doesn't look chalky or too powdery on skin. The four shades are all decent options. **Sun Tan Bronzing Powder SPF 8** *($30)* is a very good bronzing powder that comes in believable tan shades and has only a hint of shine. No active ingredients are listed to back up the SPF claim, but it takes more than a dusting of bronzing powder for substantial sun protection anyway. **Shine-On Powder** *($25)* has an honest name, as most powders with shine also claim to keep skin matte while concurrently adding sparkles to the skin. This loose powder has a pleasant texture and softly shiny shades that can work well for an evening look. ✔☺ **Super Matte Loose Powder** *($28)* has an incredibly light, silky texture that affords a seamless matte finish. The available shades are excellent, and although this is pricey, it's a great option for oily skin.

☹ **Star Powder** *($17)* is simply very shiny loose powder that comes in a wide variety of shades, from gold and silver to lots of pastel hues. For versatile iridescent shimmer, look no further. If you want to go even shinier, consider **Glitter** *($19),* but be prepared for a messy proposition.

☺ **$$$ BLUSH: Powder Blush** *($15)* comes in a bountiful array of shades, from the pinkest pinks to the most understated neutrals. These are strongly pigmented shades, and without careful, sheer application they tend to grab on the skin, which is a side effect of this blush's drier texture. Use restraint, and you're likely to be pleased with the results and the long wear. **Blush Cream** *($18)* is an emollient creamy blush that is a good option for those with dry skin who have been unhappy with the results they get with a powder blush. The eight shades are fine (though shades 1 to 3 are shimmery), and they go on less intensely than the Powder Blush above. ✔☺ **Blush Pencil Mat** *($14)* is a standard chunky pencil that is an overall gimmicky way to use blush, but this works surprisingly well, blending on thick at first but spreading out easily over the skin for a sheer, flushed effect and a soft matte finish.

EYESHADOW: ☺ **$$$ Eyeshadow** *($15)* has a texture, application, and intensity that are identical to the Powder Blush above. The range of shades is staggering, with some of the most imaginative (and largely unnecessary) shades right next to the earth and neutral tones that are universally flattering. These do provide opaque coverage and can drag a bit over the skin if you don't use a good eyeshadow brush, but they last without creasing or fading.

☺ **$$$ Pearly Waterproof Eyeshadow Pencil** *($17)* is a standard chubby pencil with a creamy texture that slides onto the skin and imparts sheer, shimmering color. This pencil is not preferred to the Eyeshadow above, but some will undoubtedly find it intriguing, and the formula is waterproof.

EYE AND BROW SHAPER: ☹ **$$$ Eye Pencil** *($16)* is a standard pencil that has a very creamy texture and more than its fair share of opaque blue and green hues that can be striking but do little to complement or shape the eye.

☺ **$$$ Color Liner** *($19)* is a good liquid eyeliner that features a soft but firm-textured brush and a formula that applies easily and dries quickly. There are lots of iridescent shades to wade through, but the classic colors are just fine, though they call for more than one swipe along the lashline for maximum effect. This eyeliner does last well without chipping or smearing. **Pearly Waterproof Eyeliner Pencil** *($16)* is a standard, creamy eye pencil that's easy to apply, and also extremely waterproof. Removing this long-wearing eye pencil will require a silicone- or oil-based cleanser.

LIPSTICK AND LIP PENCIL: All of Make Up For Ever's lipsticks in standard twist-up packaging have identical ingredient lists and, therefore, all five formulas have a similar texture; the differences are in the opacity of the colors and the addition of iridescence. ☺ $$$ **Matte Lipstick** *($16)* is in no way a true matte lipstick. It's merely a good creamy lipstick with full-coverage colors. **Pearly Lipstick** *($16)* is identical to the Matte Lipstick except these come in frosted, mostly pastel colors. **Sheer Lipstick** *($16)* is not that sheer. It's more of a semi-opaque lipstick with rich colors and a glossy finish. **Lacquered Lipstick** *($16)* has the richest, most opulent colors of the bunch, and a standard creamy feel and finish. ✔☺ **Super Lip Gloss** *($16)* is one of the smoothst, least sticky glosses you're likely to find. It comes in a tube and is silicone-based, so it can feel slippery (and can encourage lipstick feathering if you're prone to that), but women who have a problem with bleeding lipstick should stay away from glosses in the first place. The available shades are beautiful. ✔☺ **Rouge Pinceau Mat Lipstick and Brush** *($19)* is an excellent matte lip product that comes in a compact that includes a cleverly concealed, built-in lip brush. This has a featherlight, silky-feeling texture and lovely semi-opaque colors. This is a rather unique product, and fans of matte lipstick should check it out. ✔☺ **Liquid Lip Color** *($18)* is awesome, especially if you like intense, opaque color and a completely non-sticky, high-gloss finish. This lipstick/gloss hybrid comes in a tube with a brush applicator, and the opening of the tube is large enough to prevent the brush from splaying—a major plus. The colors are riveting and have great staying power, though these don't last quite as long as the Rouge Pinceau above.

☺ **5-Color Lipstick Palette** *($35)* includes five lip colors (identical in formula to the regular lipsticks) in a sleek, mirrored compact. The combination of shades is actually quite good, and if you can see yourself using the preselected shades, this type of product can be considered a safe bet.

☺ $$$ **Lip Pencil** *($16)* is a standard pencil that has the same texture as the Eye Pencil above, and the wide selection of shades is commendable.

MASCARA: ☹ $$$ **Mascara Volume** *($16)* offers a clean application but it takes awhile to produce acceptable length and an OK amount of thickness. It does not clump, smear, or flake—a significant plus—but there are better mascaras out there if you want thick, dramatic lashes.

The regular ☺ $$$ **Mascara** *($16)* is a fine lengthening mascara, but isn't as impressive as it could be. It applies evenly without a trace of clumpiness, and stays on well throughout the day. Shade #8 is a standard clear gel formula that can be used on lashes or for brow grooming.

☹ **Waterproof Mascara** *($16)* is indeed waterproof and builds decent length and some thickness. Unfortunately, it tends to flake and smear throughout the day because of its creamy formula. This is a great example of how "waterproof" does not necessarily mean "smearproof."

BRUSHES: You will find Make Up For Ever's ✔☺ Brushes *($13–$54)* have something to offer everyone, whether you're a makeup brush neophyte or connoisseur. The brushes include both natural and synthetic hair options, and the majority are expertly shaped and appropriately sized for their intended purpose. There are some superfluous ones to consider carefully, but that chiefly depends on what your needs are. All in all, the choices are plentiful and the prices are comparatively reasonable.

☺ $$$ SPECIALTY: Aquarelle *($18)* is an intensely shiny liquid that is a mixture of water, clay, alcohol, slip agent, film-forming agent, and iridescent pigments. For a nighttime look or for special effects with opaque iridescence, these are one of the easier-to-control options; for daytime, the shine is too distracting. The formula tends to hold well on the skin without flaking or smearing, and the color range is typical Make Up For Ever (read: extensive).

MARCELLE (CANADA ONLY)

Nestled among the flashier lines filling the shelves and display cases of Canadian drugstores is the unassuming, attractively priced Marcelle line. The packaging is simple and some of the products are fragrance-free, which is a definite strong point. However, while many of the products don't include fragrance, lots do. Ingredients like lavender are more recognizable as fragrant additives, but there are others you won't recognize, such as floralozone and hedione. The claim that these products are hypoallergenic isn't accurate in the least. There is no way any company can know what your skin may be allergic to, and fragrance is not the only culprit that can cause allergic reactions. Many of these products contain ingredients that have a high potential for irritation or a sensitizing reaction, or can cause breakouts, such as witch hazel, several of the sunscreen ingredients, plant extracts, plus menthol, alcohol, a form of tallow, sodium lauryl sulfate, and isopropyl myristate. For more information about Marcelle, call (800) 387-7710 or visit www.marcelle.com. **Note:** All prices listed for Marcelle products are in Canadian dollars.

MARCELLE SKIN CARE

☺ **2 in 1 Face and Eye Cleanser** *($11.25 for 170 ml)* is a simple lotion cleanser that is meant to be wiped off. It works OK for removing makeup, as would any lightweight, lotion-style, cold-cream cleanser, but it isn't the best way to "clean" skin. It is an option for dry skin. The algae in this product may have some antioxidant properties, but in a cleanser it's just wiped off before it can have any effect.

☺ **Aquarelle Oil-Free Purifying Cleansing Gel for Oily Skin** *($11.95 for 170 ml)* is a good, standard detergent cleanser for most skin types. It won't purify anything, but it can clean the skin without irritation or dryness, and it won't irritate the eyes.

☹ **Cleansing Cream** *($14.50 for 240 ml)* is a mineral oil–based detergent cleanser that can leave a greasy film on the skin. Calling this product hypoallergenic is stretching the truth to the point of breaking because it contains sodium lauryl sulfate, an ingredient well known for being a serious skin irritant (it is the sensitizer that is used as the standard in dermatologic skin irritation tests).

☺ **Cleansing Milk Combination Skin** *($11.25 for 240 ml)* is a standard, detergent-based, water-soluble cleanser that would work well for normal to dry skin, but not for combination skin. It contains a tiny amount of lactic acid that probably isn't enough to be a problem for the skin or eyes, but there are several waxes that might present a problem for those with blemish-prone or oily skin (and also problematic for combination skin).

☺ **Cleansing Milk Oily Skin** *($11.25 for 240 ml)* is almost identical to the Combination Skin version above and the same comments apply.

☺ **Cleansing Milk for Dry to Normal Skin** *($11.25 for 240 ml)* is a mineral oil–based cleansing lotion that needs to be wiped off. It is an option for normal to dry skin.

☺ **Gentle Foaming Wash All Skin Types** *($10.95 for 170 ml)* isn't all that gentle, but it is a good, standard, detergent-based, water-soluble cleanser that can be an option for normal to oily skin. It does contain a small amount of sodium lauryl sulfate, but not enough to be a problem for most skin types.

☺ **Hydractive Water Rinseable Cleansing Lotion for Dehydrated/Normal to Dry Skin** *($11.95 for 180 ml)* is an emollient cleanser with a tiny amount of detergent-cleansing agent. It is a very good option for dry skin.

☺ **Eye Make-Up Remover Pads** *($8.50 for 60 pads)* are mineral oil–soaked pads. This is one way to get waterproof makeup off, but it is only minimally different from buying a bottle of mineral oil and using some cotton pads.

☺ **Creamy Eye Make-Up Remover** *($6.99 for 50 ml)* is basically just mineral oil, some thickeners, slip agents, and Vaseline, and it will wipe off makeup.

☺ **Eye Make-Up Remover Lotion Oil-Free** *($8.50 for 120 ml)* is a standard, detergent-based makeup remover that works as well as any reviewed in this book.

☺ **Gentle Eye Make-up Remover—Sensitive Eyes** *($9.98 for 120 ml)* is a very good, standard, silicone- and mineral oil–based makeup remover.

☹ **Scrub Wash for All Skin Types** *($10.95 for 100 ml)* is a clay-type cleanser that also contains witch hazel (which itself contains mostly alcohol), more alcohol, and menthol, and that makes it too potentially irritating for all skin types.

☹ **Aquarelle Oil Normalizing Toner Alcohol-Free for Oily Skin** *($11.95 for 240 ml)*. There is nothing in this product that can control oil in the least, plus the witch hazel in it contains a good amount of alcohol and that is drying and irritating for skin.

☺ **Hydra-C ComplexE Tonifying Lotion** *($11.50 for 200 ml)* is an exceptionally basic toner of water, slip agent, glycerin, preservatives, and the smallest amount of vitamin E imaginable.

☺ **Hydractive Reviving Toner, Dehydrated and Normal to Dry Skin** *($11.25 for 180 ml)* is a good toner for most skin types with a small amount of water-binding agents. It is an option for normal to dry skin.

☹ **Skin Freshener Combination Skin** *($11.25 for 240 ml)* is mostly just alcohol and glycerin along with a small amount of menthol, and that makes it potentially too irritating and drying for any skin type.

☹ **Skin Freshener Normal to Dry Skin** *($11.25 for 240 ml)* is similar to the Skin Freshener Combination Skin above, and the same basic comments apply. This product also contains aluminum chlorohydrate, a key ingredient in underarm deodorant, which can cause breakouts and allergic reactions.

☺ **Alpha-Radiance Cream Normal to Dry and Sensitive Skin** *($15.95 for 60 ml)* contains less than 3% AHAs, and that quantity isn't enough to make it effective as an exfoliant. Other than that, it is just a mediocre moisturizer for normal to dry skin. The fragrances are definitely not appropriate for sensitive skin.

☺ **Alpha-Radiance Lotion, Combination to Oily and Sensitive Skin** *($15.95 for 120 ml)* is almost identical to the Normal to Dry version above and the same comments apply.

☹ **Hydra-C Complex E** *($16.95 for 50 ml)* is a poor formulation with negligible amounts of vitamins C and E, and a fractional amount of water-binding agent. On top of that, it also contains menthol, which is irritating to skin.

☺ **Aquarelle Aqua-Matte Hydrating Fluid** *($14.95 for 120 ml)* is a matte-finish moisturizer that contains only minuscule amounts of water-binding agents and antioxidants, beneficial additions that all skin types need. However, the second ingredient is farnesol, primarily a fragrance component in cosmetics. A small number of in vitro research and animal studies show that farnesol does have antibacterial and antioxidant properties, but there is no research showing that it has those effects on skin.

☺ **Hydractive Eye Contour Gel** *($11.95 for 15 ml)* is a simple lightweight moisturizer for normal to slightly dry skin that contains mostly water, glycerin, water-binding agent, film-forming agent, and preservatives. There is nothing in this product that makes it unique for the eye area.

☺ **Hydractive Hydra-Repair Night Treatment for All Skin Types** *($17.95 for 60 ml)* is a good emollient moisturizer for someone with dry skin. It contains some good water-binding agents, but only a minuscule amount of antioxidants.

☺ **Hydractive Hydra-Replenishing Cream** *($15.95 for 40 ml)* is a very ordinary, boring moisturizer for dry skin with negligible amounts of water-binding agents and antioxidants. The Hydra-Repair Night Treatment above is a far better and more interesting formulation for dry skin.

☺ **Moisture Cream** *($14.50 for 60 ml)* is an exceptionally mundane moisturizer for dry skin. It contains mostly waxes and mineral oil, and a tiny amount of lactic acid (AHA), but not enough to have exfoliating properties.

☺ **Moisture Lotion** *($14.75 for 120 ml)* is similar to the Moisture Cream above, only in lotion form, and the same basic comments apply.

☺ **Night Cream** *($10.75 for 40 ml)* is almost identical to the Moisture Cream above, and the same basic comments apply.

The Reviews M

☺ **Eye Care Cream, Ultra-Light** *($8.95 for 15 ml)* is an OK moisturizer for normal to dry skin. It contains a small amount of water-binding agents and an antioxidant.

☺ **Eye Cream Ultra Rich** *($8.75 for 15 ml)* is nothing more than mineral oil, Vaseline, and wax. It's emollient, but it's also an exceptionally dated, obsolete formulation.

☺ **Dry Skin Lubricating Cream** *($10.50 for 120 ml)* is almost identical to the Eye Cream Ultra Rich above, and the same comments apply.

☺ **Anti-Wrinkle Cream with Collagen & Elastin** *($15.75 for 40 ml)* is a good, but simple, emollient moisturizer for normal to dry skin. The collagen and elastin are good moisturizing ingredients, but they have absolutely no effect on the collagen and elastin in your skin. This also contains an antioxidant.

☺ **Moisture Cream Eye with Gingko Biloba SPF 15** *($12.50 for 15 ml)* contains titanium dioxide and zinc oxide as the sunscreen ingredients, which makes this a great sunscreen. Other than that, the base is incredibly ordinary and nothing in it, including the gingko, makes this preferred for the eye area.

☹ **Multi-Defense Cream Daily Moisturizer SPF 15** *($15.75 for 60 ml)* doesn't contain the UVA-protecting ingredients of avobenzone, zinc oxide, or titanium dioxide among the active ingredients, and it is not recommended.

☹ **Oil-Free Multi-Defense Lotion Daily Moisturizer SPF 15** *($15.75 for 120 ml)* doesn't contain the UVA-protecting ingredients of avobenzone, zinc oxide, or titanium dioxide among the active ingredients, and it is not recommended.

☺ **Protective Block No Chemical Sunscreen Cream SPF 25** *($12.95 for 50 ml)* is an excellent sunscreen that contains both titanium dioxide and zinc oxide as the active ingredients in a very standard moisturizing base that would be OK for someone with normal to slightly dry skin.

☺ **Protective Block No Chemical Sunscreen Lotion SPF 25** *($12.95 for 120 ml)* is almost identical to the Cream SPF 25 above, only in lotion form, and the same basic comments apply.

☺ **Protective Block No Chemical Sunscreen Spray SPF 15** *($12.95 for 120 ml)* is similar to the Lotion SPF 25 version above, but with only titanium dioxide as the active ingredient, and the same basic comments apply.

☹ **Sun Block Cream SPF 15** *($8.95 for 90 ml)*, **Sun Block Cream SPF 20** *($8.95 for 90 ml)*, **Sun Block Lotion SPF 15** *($8.95 for 120 ml)*, and **Sunblock Lotion SPF 20** *($8.95 for 120 ml)* do not contain the UVA-protecting ingredients of avobenzone, zinc oxide, or titanium dioxide among the active ingredients, and they are not recommended.

☺ **Self-Tanning Lotion with Alpha-Hydroxy Acid Moisturizing Formula for Face** *($11.25 for 50 ml)* is a standard, dihydroxyacetone-based self-tanner that would work as well as any. It contains about 2% to 3% AHA, which isn't enough for it to be effective as an exfoliant, and besides the pH is too high for it to achieve that purpose.

☺ **Self-Tanning Spray with Erythrulose** *($13.95 for 120 ml)* does use erythrulose, which is chemically similar to the self-tanning agent dihydroxyacetone that is used in most self-tanners. Depending on your skin color, there can be a difference in the color erythrulose produces. However, dihydroxyacetone completely changes the color of skin within two to six hours, while erythrulose needs about two to three days for the skin to show a color change.

☺ **Clay Mask with Kaolin** *($10.95 for 100 ml)* is a standard clay mask, but the witch hazel in it can be a skin irritant.

☺ **Gentle Purifying Mask** *($10.95 for 50 ml)* is a standard clay mask that also contains some plant oil and water-binding agents to help reduce the drying effect of the clay. This can be good for someone with normal to dry skin.

☹ **Time Release Hydrating Mask** *($10.95 for 50 ml)* is a clay mask with several water-binding agents, thickeners, and preservatives. This includes a tiny amount of fruit extracts, and although they sound like they are AHAs, they are not. This product also contains menthol, which can be a skin irritant, and that's too bad, because the moisturizing ingredients here are good ones.

MARCELLE MAKEUP

When it comes to makeup, Marcelle's options include a disproportionate number of boring to just plain awful products. The high points among the many lows include a couple of excellent foundations that now come in an improved shade range, along with eye and brow pencils that outperform many others in any price range. The blush, eyeshadow, and lipstick are nice but about as exciting as Meatloaf Mondays, and this company tops my list for putting out some of the worst mascaras ever. I know this sounds a bit grim, but the good news is that Marcelle's best products are really wonderful and something any self-respecting Canadian cosmetics consumer need not hesitate to investigate.

<u>FOUNDATION:</u> ☺ **Moisture Rich Makeup** *($10.25)* has a great moist texture and creamy application that those with dry skin will flip over, but of the seven shades, the only passable choice is Naturel, which would work for light skin only. **Oil-Free Matte Finish Makeup** *($10.25)* is a good matte-finish makeup that blends well but feels a bit sticky once it dries. This provides light to medium coverage, and the color range has been improved—now instead of avoiding all seven shades, you can consider the neutral Almond and Naturel if you have light skin. **Sheer Tint Fluid Moisturizer SPF 15** *($11.95)* comes without reliable UVA protection and is otherwise just a basic tinted moisturizer that has sheer, almost translucent coverage from four shades. Avoid Bronze, as it is still too peach. **Le Stick Perfect Radiance Foundation** *($14.95)* is a silicone-based stick makeup that dries to a slightly thick powder finish as soon as it's blended. Don't expect any playtime with this one! It's not as elegant as many other stick foundations, and the six shades are barely to noticeably peach. Linen, Soft Beige, and Barely There are the best of the lot, but I would encourage you to explore the options from L'Oreal or Clinique before this one.

☺ **True Radiance SPF 15 Oil-Free Liquid Makeup** *($10.25)* lacks UVA protection, but it does have an even, light texture that blends well and provides light to medium coverage. The six shades have been tweaked, and are now an impressive selection of neutral tones for light to medium skin. **Dual Cream Powder Makeup** *($12.25)* is briefly creamy, but dries very quickly to a sheer matte finish. Significant shine control is iffy, but it will go further than most cream-to-powders do for oily skin. This is really best for normal skin, and the six shades are now excellent.

☹ <u>**CONCEALER:**</u> **Cover Up Stick** *($7.75)* is a standard, lipstick-style concealer that's greasy and comes in four terrible colors that would be a challenge for any skin tone. **Concealer Crayon** *($7.95)* is a creamy, chubby pencil concealer that applies smoothly and blends well, but it tends to migrate into lines and the coverage can fade shortly after it's applied.

<u>**POWDER:**</u> ☺ **Face Powder Loose** *($10.50)* has a soft, slightly dry, talc-based texture and a sheer finish. It's available in six mostly attractive colors; only Rosy Peach should be left on the shelf.

☹ **Pressed Powder** *($10.50)* and **Silky Finish Powder** *($8.75)* are also talc-based, and almost all the shades are too pink or peach to recommend. The only passable shade of each is Translucent.

☺ **Pressed Bronzing Powder** *($10.50)* comes in only one shade, and it's a great tan color that loses points for the subtle shine it imparts, which is not the goal if you're trying to fake a tan.

☺ <u>**BLUSH:**</u> **Velvety Powder Blush** *($7.75)* has an incredibly sheer, even application as well as an agreeable soft texture. Of the six shades, all are shiny except Blushing Bronze. **Cream Blusher** *($9.50)* is a traditional cream blush, meaning it has a slightly greasy feel and stays moist on the skin. The shade selection is pleasant, but they are all infused with shine, and that can be too distracting. **Light Effects Cheeks, Lips, Eyes** *($9.50)* are pairs of cream-to-powder blushes and highlighters in one compact. Each duo deposits more shine on the skin than actual color, which is disappointing unless all you're after is the sparkles. **Le Stick Perfect Radiance Blush** *($14.95)* is an emollient, twist-up stick blush that has a barely detectable powder finish and comes in a series of iridescent colors.

<u>**EYESHADOW:**</u> ☺ **Eyeshadow Singles** *($6.25)* apply softly and evenly, and neutral colors outweigh the vivid hues. Many of the shades appear to be matte, but all of them have at least a bit of shine.

☹ **Duet Eyeshadow Pencil Crayon** *($9.95)* is a too-creamy, dual-sided standard pencil whose colors are mismatched and intensely shiny.

<u>**EYE AND BROW SHAPER:**</u> ✔☺ **Kohl Eye Liner** *($7.50)* is similar to many other pencils on the market, though this edges out your everyday pencil with its slightly drier texture and color intensity that makes one-stroke application a reality. It also wears well without smearing, which is unusual for a pencil. ✔☺ **Accent Eyebrow Crayon** *($7.50)* is a standard brow pencil that is a breeze to apply, is not greasy, and comes in great colors. There is a brush on one end to soften the color, and if you prefer brow pencil to powder, this is one to try.

☺ **Waterproof Eyeliner** *($7.50)* is a standard eye pencil that goes on creamy and soft; it does stay on well when wet, but so do most eye pencils.

☹ **Powder Eye Liner** *($7.50)* is just terrible. This standard pencil will need constant sharpening because the tip breaks off every time it's used. *Every time!* This is one to avoid.

LIPSTICK AND LIP PENCIL: ☺ **Rouge Vitality Lipcolour** *($8.50)* is a basic, creamy lipstick with a middle-of-the-road texture and medium coverage. The color range is divided into four groups—Brown, Neutral, Red, and Mauve—which is helpful, though the Neutral group merely features lighter versions of colors from the Mauve and Brown categories. **Lip Definition Contour Crayon** *($9.25)* is a standard pencil with a nice range of colors, and it applies quite smoothly.

☺ **Liquid Lipgloss** *($8.75)* is a rudimentary wand-type gloss with sheer, iridescent colors and a moderately sticky finish. **Duet Lip Pencil Crayon** *($9.95)* has a better application than the Duet Eyeshadow Pencil above, but only because the emollient texture is better suited to lips. Still, this is just another dual-ended lip crayon that needs sharpening.

MASCARA: ☹ **Superlash Mascara** *($9.25)* won't take your lashes up, up, and away and, in fact, it takes a long time to build even slight length. **Ultimate Lash Mascara** *($9.25)* is ultimately disappointing if you expect anything more than minimal length and no thickness. **WaveLength Waterproof Mascara** *($9.49)* goes on thick and wet, tends to stick lashes together and to the skin (which isn't pretty), and also tends to run if it gets wet. On top of this, it is a chore to remove! **Lash Extreme Lengthening Mascara** *($9.25)* is one of the most do-nothing mascaras I have ever tried. What little definition this does build is hindered by the formula's tendency to smear.

☺ **Healthy Lash Mascara** *($9.25)* is a distinct improvement over the above fiascoes, but remains an average lengthening mascara that doesn't show a trace of thickening ability.

MARILYN MIGLIN (SKIN CARE ONLY)

Marilyn Miglin found her niche in the world of television home shopping with skin-care products and promises of younger-looking skin. Her products have evolved over the years from oxygen-laced products to vitamin C–based products and now to soy-based skin-care products that promise to add estrogen topically to skin. Aside from the fact that adding oxygen to skin would generate free-radical damage and would negate the beneficial effects of any antioxidants in the products, Miglin doesn't seem so enamored with antioxidants these days anyway, now that soy is the latest miracle ingredient for skin.

What is most stunning, after all her effusiveness about getting rid of wrinkles and restoring youthful skin, is that there is no sunscreen anywhere to be found in this line, a completely unacceptable omission. Making claims about products imbued with the latest technology and research and omitting sunscreens is a farce. Sunscreen *is* the latest technology and the apex of research when it comes to preventing wrinkles and retaining skin's youthfulness. Miglin's products aren't bad, they're just incapable of living up to even a fraction of the claims being professed for them. For more information about Marilyn Miglin, call (800) 322-1133 or visit www.marilynmiglin.com or www.hsn.com. **Note:** All Marilyn Miglin products are fragranced unless otherwise noted.

☺ $$$ **Cleantone** *($25 for 4 ounces)* is a standard, wipe-off makeup remover that contains a long list of vitamins and water-binding agents. You are still just wiping off makeup, though, and that can be an option for someone with dry skin.

☺ **Skin Vitality Cleanser** *($24 for 7 ounces)* is a standard, detergent-based, water-soluble cleanser that would be an option for normal to oily skin. The minute amount of minerals in this product would be rinsed away before they had a chance to have any benefit for skin.

☺ $$$ **Moisture Cleanser** *($20 for 4 ounces)* is just a mineral oil– and Vaseline-based, cold cream–style, wipe-off cleanser. It can be an option for very dry skin, though Pond's cold cream would work as well. It is fragrance-free.

☺ $$$ **Water Activated Cleanser** *($20 for 4 ounces)* is a lanolin oil–based cleanser with a tiny amount of detergent cleansing agent. It is an option for very dry skin.

☺ **Delicate Eye Make Up Remover** *($18 for 6 ounces)* is a standard, detergent-based eye-makeup remover, identical to most of its kind reviewed in this book. It would work as well as any.

☹ **Laser Lotion I** *($25 for 6 ounces)* is a detergent-based toner that contains less than 2% lactic acid in a pH that is not low enough for it to be effective as an exfoliant. It also contains a small amount of very irritating plant extracts.

☹ **Laser Lotion II** *($25 for 6 ounces)* is similar to the Laser Lotion I above and the same comments apply.

☹ **Priming Lotion I** *($22.50 for 8 ounces)* is an OK toner that contains some very good water-binding agents, but the witch hazel contains a good deal of alcohol and that can be drying and irritating for all skin types.

☹ **Priming Lotion II** *($22.50 for 8 ounces)* is similar to the Priming Lotion I above only with the addition of a detergent cleansing agent, and it contains fewer water-binding agents.

☺ **Daily Moisture Lotion** *($25 for 1.7 ounces)* is a mediocre, very emollient, mineral oil– and lanolin oil–based moisturizer that contains nothing of value to skin. It is about as dated a formulation as you can imagine.

☺ $$$ **Tissue Cream** *($25 for 0.5 ounce)* is similar to the Daily Moisture Lotion above and the same basic comments apply.

☺ $$$ **Hylagen Nutrients** *($55 for 1 ounce)* is a lightweight gel, film-forming-agent–based moisturizer that contains some very good water-binding agents, but lacks any antioxidants.

☺ $$$ **Hylagen Night Treatment** *($42 for 1 ounce)* is almost identical to the Hylagen Nutrients above except in cream form, and the same basic comments apply.

☺ $$$ **Eye 31** *($27.50 for 0.5 ounce)* is supposed to contain "31 proven ingredients to minimize fine lines and combat dryness, pollution and stress." There aren't even 31 interesting ingredients in this moisturizer and none that are proven to combat pollution or stress. However, this very basic moisturizer of plant oil, mineral oil, and lanolin, along with insignificant amounts of antioxidants, will be helpful for dry skin. All in all, however, this is a boring formulation.

☺ **Restore** *($25 for 4 ounces)* is a very good moisturizer for normal to dry skin, although some of the plant extracts, which are rather high on the ingredient list, can be skin irritants.

☺ **Skin Lift** *($25 for 1 ounce)* won't lift skin anywhere, but the large amount of film-forming agents can make skin look temporarily smoother. This could have been a very good moisturizer for someone with normal to dry skin, but the oxygenated water negates any of the benefit the antioxidants would have provided.

☺ **Perfect Balance Oxygen 600** *($37.50 for 4 ounces)* contains a small amount of oxygenated water (though *all* water is oxygenated and what little can be added under pressure would be released when you opened the jar). It does contain minuscule amounts of very good water-binding agents and antioxidants. This product claims to be super-oxygenating for the skin, amplifying the skin's oxygen intake. Even if it were possible to improve the skin's appearance by delivering oxygen to it, there isn't enough oxygen in this product to duplicate the amount of oxygen from a single breath or to impact one skin cell. In the long run, "extra" oxygen just triggers extra free-radical damage.

☹ **Liquid Veil** *($25 for 4 ounces)* is an alcohol-based facial mask with a film-forming agent (polyvinyl alcohol) that dries into a plastic-like layer over the skin that you then peel off. Alcohol can dry and irritate the skin and the polyvinyl alcohol when peeled off can make skin feel temporarily smoother, but that's about it. The brochure says, "The tingling tells you it is working." What all the tingling really communicates is irritation and dryness.

☺ $$$ **Natural Mineral Mask** *($27 for 4 ounces)* is a standard clay mask and little else. It is an option for normal to oily skin.

☺ $$$ **Natural Soothing Mask** *($25 for 4 ounces)* is a sticky gel-type moisturizer with some good water-binding agents. It is an option for normal to dry skin.

MARILYN MIGLIN ESTROSOY

As the name indicates, Estrosoy products contain soy extracts. While eating soy-based food products can provide phytoestrogenic properties for the body, there is no research showing that to be the case when they are applied topically. These products also contain red clover, an herb that is sold as a supplement for relief of menopausal symptoms such as hot flashes and vaginal dryness. Red clover does contain high concentrations of four major isoflavones (similar to soy) that have been shown to have estrogenic properties. However, the research on red clover also found that it was no better than a placebo for alleviating menopausal symptoms (Sources: *Harvard Women's Health Watch*, Decem-

The Reviews M

ber 2001, http://www.health.harvard.edu/medline/Women/W1201e.html and *Natural Medicines Comprehensive Database,* http://www.naturaldatabase.com). There is also no research showing red clover to have benefit when applied topically on skin, though, as with soy, it may have anti-inflammatory and antioxidant properties.

☺ **Estrosoy Foaming Facial Cleanser with Collagen** *($20 for 6.75 ounces)* is a standard, detergent-based, water-soluble cleanser that would be an option for normal to oily skin. The negligible amount of soybean oil present is not enough to have benefit for skin as an emollient and there is no research showing that it has estrogenic properties when applied topically.

☺ **Estrosoy Replenish Lift** *($35 for 2 ounces)* is an emollient moisturizer for dry skin that contains soybean oil and soybean protein. Those ingredients have no estrogenic properties when applied topically to skin, though they do have water-binding benefits. This product does contain a tiny amount of antioxidants, so it does add up to being an OK moisturizer—but it won't lift skin anywhere. All in all, you would be far better off eating soy products than putting this on your skin.

☺ **Estrosoy Neckline Firmer** *($20 for 1 ounce)* is similar to the Estrosoy Replenish Lift above and the same comments apply. There is nothing in this product that makes it specially suited for the neck.

☺ $$$ **Estrosoy Eye Creme** *($20 for 0.5 ounce).* If soy is the goal then the Replenish Lift above has more to offer than this film-forming-agent– and Vaseline-based moisturizer does. It is just an OK moisturizer for normal to dry skin.

☺ $$$ **Estrosoy Concentrate with Collagen** *($35 for 0.5 ounce)* is a good, emollient moisturizer for normal to dry skin that contains some good plant oils, water-binding agents, and a small amount of antioxidants, although none of these ingredients will impart estrogenic benefit for skin.

MARILYN MIGLIN PERFECT C

☹ **Perfect C Cleanser** *($20 for 4 ounces)* is a wipe-off makeup remover that contains lemongrass, lime, spearmint, bergamot, and tangerine. All of these are potent skin irritants.

☹ **Perfect C Cleansing Bar** *($20 for three 4.2-ounce bars)* is a standard bar cleanser that can be fairly drying for most skin types. The amount of vitamin C is barely worth mentioning.

☺ **Perfect C Skin Toner** *($20 for 6 ounces)* is a good, relatively irritant-free toner. However, the way this is packaged ensures that the vitamin C will not remain stable even before you open it up.

☹ **Perfect C Firming Creme, Daily Anti-Oxidant Skin Protection** *($20 for 2 ounces)* contains several plant oils that are fairly potent skin irritants, including orange, lime, lemon, bergamot, and spearmint. In addition, the type of packaging means that the tiny amount of antioxidants that are present will be unstable and useless. This product offers zero protection for skin.

☺ $$$ **Perfect C Firming Eye Creme** *($20 for 0.5 ounce)* is an OK moisturizer for dry skin that contains minuscule amounts of vitamin C and water-binding agents.

☺ **Perfect C Radiance Skinglo** *($25 for 1 ounce)* contains sparkles, and they're the only thing in this product that makes the skin glow. This is mostly just a mediocre moisturizer for normal to dry skin with tiny amounts of antioxidants.

☻ **Perfect C Serum, Nightly Free-Radical Neutralizer** *($35 for 0.85 ounce)* contains a good amount of vitamin C and a water-binding agent, but the irritating plant oils, including bergamot, lemon grass, lime, and spearmint, make this problematic for skin in the long run.

MARIO BADESCU

Fashion magazines have been mentioning Mario Badescu products for some time, and in New York the Badescu salon has been around for more than three decades. These products sing an old familiar song, with lyrics telling you they are supposed to be all-natural skin-care treatments, and actors and supermodels touting their benefits. I can't confirm whether or not celebrities really use these products, but even if there are some who do, there are lots of other celebrities using lots of different products, so that's no way to make a trustworthy skin-care decision.

It probably goes without saying, or at least you won't be surprised when I mention it, that none of these products are natural in the least. They contain all the same old standard ingredients that show up in almost every product line I've ever reviewed.

One major attraction for Badescu is that the prices are more than reasonable, especially in comparison to other spa or boutique skin-care lines. The downside is that the products themselves have some of the most lackluster formulations I've seen. The sparse amounts of water-binding agents, antioxidants, and anti-irritants used in the preponderance of products here is shocking. The cleansers are unimpressive, the acne products are an irritation waiting to happen, and the AHA moisturizers either don't contain AHAs or they don't have enough of the ingredient or a low-enough pH to be effective as exfoliants. Most appalling are the sunscreens, which have no UVA-protecting ingredients.

Several of the Badescu products contain an ingredient called "seamollient." As exotic as the name sounds, it's just a fancy term for water and algae. Given that the Creme de la Mer products also brag about algae (and charge an astronomical sum for it), if you want algae on your skin, you may as well put it there via the Badescu products for far less. (Why algae has a cult following of any kind for skin care is a mystery, as there is no research substantiating the fascinating claims made for it.)

An interesting note for those consumers who are becoming more aware of and paying more attention to ingredient lists: I'm concerned about a new bit of deception taking place on ingredient labels, which the Badescu line demonstrates quite nicely. For example, rather than listing mineral oil or Vaseline in their products, manufacturers may use names such as Sonojell or Protol, which are nothing more than trade names for

The Reviews M

Vaseline and mineral oil, respectively. Further, and most distressing, is that Badescu's products don't meet FDA labeling criteria. This trend of cloaking ingredients in trade names and ignoring FDA labeling guidelines doesn't help the consumer, though it does help the cosmetics companies make their ordinary products sound more mysterious and natural. For more information about Mario Badescu, call (800) BADESCU or visit www.mariobadescu.com.

☹ **Cucumber Cream Soap** *($10 for 6 ounces)* isn't soap in the least. It's just a standard, detergent-based, water-soluble cleanser, though the second ingredient is alcohol, and that makes it too drying and irritating for all skin types.

☺ **Seaweed Cleansing Soap** *($12 for 8 ounces)* isn't soap, but rather an exceptionally standard detergent cleanser with small amounts of seaweed. It can be good for someone with normal to oily skin.

☺ **Orange Cleansing Soap** *($12 for 8 ounces)* is a simple, standard detergent cleanser that can be an option for normal to oily skin.

☺ **Keratoplast Cream Soap** *($10 for 8 ounces)* is a standard, detergent-based, water-soluble cleanser. It is an option for normal to oily skin. Keratoplast is the trade name for isodecyl salicylate, but the pH of this cleanser is too high, which negates any potential exfoliating properties.

☺ **Enzyme Cleansing Gel** *($12 for 8 ounces)* is a standard, detergent-based, water-soluble cleanser that also contains grapefruit and papaya extracts. Neither of these extracts have any exfoliating properties, though they can be potential skin irritants.

☺ **Cleansing Milk with Carnation & Rice Oil** *($10 for 4 ounces)*. You would be far better off using canola oil than this greasy and waxy cold cream–type concoction.

☺ **Botanical Face Gel** *($12 for 8 ounces)* doesn't clean very well, as it is just a very simple mix of gel thickening agents that can feel light on oily skin. Why it doesn't contain any cleansing agents to get through makeup and oil is a good question.

☺ **Glycolic Foaming Cleanser** *($15 for 6 ounces)* is a standard, detergent-based cleanser, and while it does contain glycolic acid, the amount is so minuscule and the pH of this product is so high that it won't deliver any exfoliating benefits.

☺ **Carnation Eye Makeup Remover Oil** *($6 for 2 ounces)* is, as the name says, carnation oil. But there is little reason to use this to wipe off makeup instead of the sunflower, canola, or olive oil you have in your kitchen cabinet.

☺ **Cucumber Makeup Remover Cream** *($10 for 4 ounces)* is a standard cold cream that contains mostly mineral oil and Vaseline. It can be an option for dry skin.

☺ **Eye Make Up Remover Gel (Non Oily)** *($6 for 2 ounces)* contains mostly water, Vaseline, glycerin, carnation oil, and preservatives. Calling this non-oily is just bizarre, because it's just a standard, greasy, wipe-off eye-makeup remover.

☹ **Special Cleansing Lotion "C"** *($15 for 8 ounces)* contains mostly alcohol and sodium sulfate, a highly alkaline salt. The only thing special about this is how drying and irritating it can be for skin.

☹ **Cucumber Cleansing Lotion** *($15 for 8 ounces)* is a mix of drying and irritating extracts and alcohol. This is a toner to avoid.

☺ **Seaweed Cleansing Lotion** *($15 for 8 ounces)* is an ordinary toner of aloe and seaweed extracts. The witch hazel in it contains a good deal of alcohol and that can be problematic for all skin types.

☹ **Keratoplast Cleansing Lotion** *($17 for 8 ounces)*. The lemon and pollen in this product are an irritation or allergic reaction waiting to happen. Keratoplast is the trade name for isodecyl salicylate, but the pH of this cleanser means it won't have any exfoliating properties.

☹ **Aloe Lotion** *($15 for 8 ounces)* contains alcohol, making it too drying and irritating for all skin types.

☺ **Almond & Honey Non-Abrasive Face Scrub** *($15 for 4 ounces)* uses cornmeal as the abrasive. It also contains talc and clay, which are good absorbents, but in addition it contains zinc oxide, which isn't the best for blemish-prone skin. This has ingredients with conflicting properties that make it a problem for normal to dry skin and normal to oily skin.

☺ **Strawberry Face Scrub** *($15 for 4 ounces)* isn't much of an exfoliant, but it is a standard, detergent-based cleanser that smells of strawberries.

☺ **Glycolic Acid Toner** *($18 for 8 ounces)* contains less than 1% glycolic acid, which isn't anywhere near enough to provide exfoliating properties.

☺ **Aloe Vera Toner** *($15 for 8 ounces)* is just water, aloe, and preservatives. Watered-down, preserved aloe is not an improvement over the pure aloe vera you can find at any health food store.

☹ **Oil Free Moisturizer SPF 17** *($20 for 2 ounces)* doesn't contain the UVA-protecting ingredients of titanium dioxide, zinc oxide, or avobenzone, and is not recommended.

☹ **Aloe Moisturizer SPF 15** *($20 for 2 ounces)* doesn't contain the UVA-protecting ingredients of titanium dioxide, zinc oxide, or avobenzone, and is not recommended.

☺ **Seaweed Night Cream** *($20 for 1 ounce)* is a simple emollient moisturizer with a tiny amount of water-binding agents.

☺ **Vitamin A E D Neck Cream** *($18 for 1 ounce)* is a very ordinary, emollient moisturizer for dry skin with the tiniest amounts of vitamins A, E, and D imaginable.

☹ **AHA & Ceramide Moisturizer** *($20 for 2 ounces)* doesn't contain any AHAs. The lemon extract it contains isn't an AHA, though it can be a skin irritant. It doesn't even contain ceramide! This is just thickeners and slip agents. What a waste of time and money.

☺ **Cellufirm Drops** *($25 for 1 ounce)* contains some very good water-binding agents and antioxidants in a lightweight lotion form. It is an option for skin that is slightly dry or normal to oily.

☺ **Herbal Hydrating Serum** *($30 for 1 ounce)* is a fairly ordinary lotion of glycerin, teeny amounts of water-binding agents, and minuscule amounts of plant extracts.

☺ **Buttermilk Moisturizer** *($18 for 2 ounces)* includes a teeny amount of lactic acid, but not enough to have exfoliating properties, and other than that this is just water, plant oil, thickeners, and preservatives.

☺ **Honey Moisturizer** *($25 for 2 ounces)* is a simple moisturizer of thickeners, plant oil, and a teeny amount of honey.

☹ **The Moisture Magnet (Pentavitin) SPF 15** *($22 for 2 ounces)* doesn't contain the UVA-protecting ingredients of titanium dioxide, zinc oxide, or avobenzone, and is not recommended. Pentavitin is the trade name for a type of saccharide, and it is a decent water-binding agent, but no better than dozens of other types of saccharides that are also excellent water-binding agents.

☺ **Kera Moisturizer** *($20 for 2 ounces)* contains a form of salicylic acid (trade name Keratoplast), but the pH of this moisturizer is too high for it to have exfoliating properties. Other than that, there is nothing of interest for skin in this mediocre moisturizer.

☺ **$$$ Glycolic Eye Cream** *($20 for 0.5 ounce)* is an ordinary, though emollient, moisturizer that contains mostly plant oils, Vaseline, thickeners, vitamin E, and a tiny amount of glycolic acid. The amount of AHA is insignificant, so this won't have any exfoliating properties.

☺ **$$$ Ceramide Eye Gel** *($18 for 0.5 ounce)* is an OK, lightweight gel moisturizer that contains some good water-binding agents but lacks any antioxidants. It does contain ceramide (a very good water-binding agent), but little else.

☺ **$$$ Ceramide Complex with NMF and AHA** *($35 for 1 ounce)*. This is a good moisturizer for normal to dry skin with a decent mix of water-binding agents and antioxidants, although it does not contain ceramides or AHAs, despite its name.

☺ **$$$ Ceramide Herbal Eye Cream** *($18 for 0.5 ounce)* is an emollient moisturizer that contains a small amount of a water-binding agent.

☺ **$$$ Dermonectin Eye Cream** *($18 for 0.5 ounce)*. Dermonectic is a trade name for hydrolyzed fibronectin, a type of protein similar to the collagen and elastin found in the skin's intercellular matrix. Sun damage and other factors cause the fibronectin in your skin to deteriorate, which plays a role in skin aging and wrinkling. As is true for all proteins, regardless of their origin, it is probably a good water-binding agent for skin, but applying fibronectin topically on skin doesn't help reinforce or rebuild the fibronectin in your skin. This is a good, though not exciting, moisturizer for dry skin, with some antioxidants, plant oils, and fibronectin as the water-binding agent.

☺ **Orange Protective Cream** *($18 for 1 ounce)* is a mundane emollient moisturizer that contains mostly water, plant oil, algae, thickeners, silicone, fragrant extract, and preservatives.

☺ **Vitacel Moist Cream** *($18 for 1 ounce)* contains salicylic acid, but the pH of the cream isn't low enough for the AHA to be effective as an exfoliant. It does contain some good water-binding agents and antioxidants, and would be an option for normal to dry skin. The RNA in here cannot affect the genetic coding of skin, which is a good thing.

☺ **Bee Pollen Night Cream** *($18 for 1 ounce)* is an emollient, plant oil– and mineral oil–based moisturizer that lacks any water-binding agents and antioxidants. The insignificant amount of bee pollen present has no benefit for skin.

☺ **Ginseng Moisturizing Cream** *($18 for 2 ounces)* is just a barely passable moisturizer for normal to dry skin.

☺ **Hydrating Moisturizer with Biocare and Hyaluronic Acid** *($20 for 2 ounces)* is an emollient moisturizer that contains small amounts of water-binding agents and vitamin A.

☹ **$$$ Hyaluronic Eye Cream** *($18 for 0.5 ounce)* is an emollient moisturizer for normal to dry skin with a negligible amount of hyaluronic acid and nothing else of much value for skin.

☺ **Hyaluronic Day Cream** *($18 for 1 ounce)* is similar to the Eye Cream version above and the same comments apply.

☹ **Hyaluronic Moisturizer SPF 15** *($22 for 2 ounces)* doesn't contain the UVA-protecting ingredients of titanium dioxide, zinc oxide, or avobenzone, and is not recommended.

☺ **Caviar Night Cream** *($20 for 1 ounce)* contains some good water-binding agents and a fractional amount of caviar, but lacks any antioxidants. It is an option for normal to dry skin.

☺ **$$$ Revitalizing Night Cream** *($40 for 1 ounce)* is a plant oil– and Vaseline-based moisturizer for normal to dry skin that also contains some good antioxidants and a small amount of water-binding agents.

☹ **Buffering Lotion** *($17 for 1 ounce)* contains mostly water, alcohol, and sodium sulfate. The alcohol and the alkalinity of the sodium sulfate make this a serious problem for skin.

☹ **Drying Lotion** *($17 for 1 ounce)* is an incredibly accurate name for this product that contains mostly alcohol, calamine, camphor, and sulfur, all exceedingly drying and irritating ingredients. You can't heal skin by drying and irritating it; that only hinders the skin's healing process. Skin must be intact to heal. Plus these ingredients will only make skin red and risk causing capillaries to surface. Calamine, by the way, contains about 5% zinc oxide (which can clog pores) and a good deal of phenol, which is extremely toxic to skin. In 1992, the FDA actually tried to ban calamine altogether, but that didn't happen. Absorbing oil and reducing the swelling of blemishes is impossible with these ingredients.

☹ **Drying Cream** *($8 for 0.5 ounce)* can definitely dry the skin because it contains sulfur, which is a strong irritant and disinfectant. Meanwhile, the zinc oxide, beeswax, octyl palmitate, and mineral oil can clog pores and make skin feel oily! Why would anyone make a drying product (assuming that drying will stop breakouts, which it won't) in the form of a cream that is similar to diaper rash ointment? This is a very confused product that will confuse all skin types.

☹ **Healing Cream** *($20 for 1 ounce)* lists the first ingredient as balsam of Peru, a fatty resin that, when applied topically, can cause allergic skin reactions and contact dermatitis. It also has the potential to cause photodermatitis and phototoxicity. In addition, balsam of Peru, due to its high incidence of causing skin reactions, is used as a standard substance that is used in patch tests for skin sensitivity (Sources: *Natural Medicines Comprehensive Database*, http://www.naturaldatabase.com and *Journal of the American Academy of Dermatology*, December 2001, pages 836–839). This product won't help heal skin.

☹ **Control Moisturizer for Oily Skin** *($18 for 2 ounces)* lists balsam of Peru as the second ingredient. Refer to the Healing Cream review above for information about that ingredient.

☹ **Control Cream** *($17 for 1 ounce)* is similar to the Control Moisturizer above only with plant oil and film-forming agent, but the same basic comments apply.

☹ **Eye and Lip Sunscreen SPF 15** *($17 for 0.5 ounce)* doesn't list active ingredients on the label and so can't be relied on for effective sun protection.

☹ **All Purpose Sun Tan Milk SPF 12** *($18 for 8 ounces)* has a substandard SPF 12, lists no active ingredients on the label, and so can't be relied on for effective sun protection.

☹ **Self Tanning Lotion SPF 15** *($12 for 4 ounces)* doesn't contain the UVA-protecting ingredients of titanium dioxide, zinc oxide, or avobenzone, and is not recommended. It uses dihydroxyacetone, the same ingredient all self-tanners use to affect the color of skin.

☹ **Body Sun Block SPF 30** *($10 for 6 ounces)* doesn't list any active ingredients on the label and so can't be relied on for effective sun protection.

☹ **Suncare SPF 30** *($22 for 4 ounces)* doesn't list any active ingredients on the label and so can't be relied on for effective sun protection.

☹ **Azulene Calming Mask** *($18 for 2 ounces)* is a mask that forms a plastic-like layer over the face. It also contains some castor oil and clay. That wouldn't be a problem for the skin, although it's not very helpful, but this product also includes wheat starch, which can clog pores, and balsam of Peru, which can be a skin irritant. This won't calm anything, especially not your skin!

☺ $$$ **Strawberry Tonic Mask** *($18 for 2 ounces)* is a standard clay mask. The fractional amount of strawberry extract serves no purpose for skin. The wheat starch in it can be a problem for irritation and potentially can clog pores.

☺ $$$ **Gingko Mask** *($22 for 2.5 ounces)* is an emollient mask that can be an option for normal to dry skin.

☺ $$$ **Normalizing Mask with Cotton Milk** *($25 for 2.5 ounces)* is a slightly sticky emollient mask that would be an option for normal to dry skin. This doesn't contain cotton milk, but it does contain cottonseed oil.

☺ $$$ **Rolling Cream Peel with AHA** *($18 for 2.5 ounces)*. The teeny amount of lactic acid in here can have no exfoliating properties. This is just a thick, waxy cream you massage over skin that removes some skin with it as you rub it off. It would be better for the knees, lips, elbows, and feet than for the face.

☺ $$$ **Cucumber Tonic Mask** *($18 for 2 ounces)* is a clay mask with film-forming agent, wheat starch, thickeners, and a teeny amount of cucumber extract. The wheat starch is a problem for breakouts and skin sensitivity.

☺ $$$ **Enzyme Revitalizing Mask** *($20 for 2 ounces)* is a plasticizing mask with some papaya extract. There is no research showing papaya extract to have exfoliating properties for skin. If anything, it can be a skin irritant.

☹ **Drying Mask** *($18 for 2 ounces)* contains mostly film-forming agent, calamine lotion, and sulfur. Both the calamine and sulfur can be skin irritants. Calamine lotion has no efficacy against blemishes and sulfur is more irritating than it is disinfecting against the bacterium that causes breakouts.

☹ **Flower and Tonic Mask** *($18 for 2 ounces)* lists balsam of Peru as the second ingredient, a significant skin irritant. See the review of the Healing Cream above for comments about balsam of Peru.

☹ **Special Mask for Oily Skin** *($18 for 2 ounces)* is a standard plasticizing peel-off mask that also contains some clay and calamine. Calamine is a skin irritant. This mask has little benefit of any kind for skin.

MARY KAY

In the winter of 2001, at the age of 83, Mary Kay Ash passed away, leaving behind a cosmetics empire bearing her name. Hers was one of the original home-sales cosmetics companies. It began in 1963, when Mary Kay Ash (with her son's help) created a company that evolved to include more than 300,000 salespeople. Ash's trademark style, as has also happened with the other grande dames of cosmetics (Helena Rubinstein, Marcella Borghese, and Elizabeth Arden), has become infused with her memory and is now part of her company.

With all due respect to Ash's fortitude and rallying presence, and as impressive as her business acumen proved to be, the average Mary Kay salesperson's income is only about $5,000 to $10,000 a year. Obviously, the ability to sell does not come naturally to every member of the sales force.

In regard to the products, much of the Mary Kay lineup is a mixed bag of strong and weak points and the weak points are really weak. Skin Revival has been discontinued, though it was heralded by the company initially as a skin-care miracle; but miracles in the cosmetics industry do tend to come and go. TimeWise is now supposed to be the answer to speedy skin care, with only two steps that clean, tone, and fight aging. But TimeWise doesn't include a sunscreen, which makes this pair of products time-foolish. The basic Mary Kay skin-care routine is a dated mix of greasy cleansers, irritating toners, and daytime moisturizers with poorly formulated SPFs. Wading through this mix of products is cumbersome, but there are a few new state-of-the-art formulations worth checking out. For the most part, though, this is a line in need of fresh air and a fresh face. For more information about Mary Kay, call (800) 627-9529 or visit www.marykay.com.

The Reviews M

MARY KAY SKIN CARE

☺ **Gentle Cleansing Cream Formula 1** *($10 for 4 ounces)* is a traditional, greasy, mineral oil– and Vaseline-based cold cream. It might be gentle, but it is also quite heavy, and can leave a greasy film on the skin. It is an option for very dry skin.

☺ **Creamy Cleanser Formula 2** *($10 for 6.5 ounces)* is a mineral oil–based, wipe-off cleanser that can leave a greasy film on the skin. It is less heavy than the Gentle version above and is an option for someone with dry skin.

☺ **Deep Cleanser Formula 3** *($10 for 6.5 ounces)* is an extremely standard, but good, detergent-based, water-soluble cleanser that is an option for most skin types except dry skin.

☹ **Velocity Facial Cleanser** *($10 for 5 ounces)* lists TEA-lauryl sulfate as the second ingredient, which makes this potentially too irritating and drying for all skin types.

☹ **Purifying Bar** *($12 for 4.2 ounces, $10 for refill)* is a standard bar cleanser that won't purify anything, at least not any better than Dove bar cleanser. Mary Kay's version contains eucalyptus, which is a skin irritant.

☺ **Oil-Free Eye Makeup Remover** *($14 for 3.75 ounces)* is a standard, silicone-based eye-makeup remover that will work as well as any reviewed in this book.

☹ **Hydrating Freshener Formula 1** *($11 for 6.5 ounces)* contains a small amount of menthol, arnica, and peppermint, which can all seriously irritate the skin.

☹ **Purifying Freshener Formula 2** *($11 for 6.5 ounces)* contains mostly water and alcohol, which can irritate and dry skin.

☹ **Blemish Control Toner Formula 3** *($11 for 6.5 ounces)* lists alcohol as the second ingredient, and it also contains eucalyptus, making this too irritating for words regardless of your skin type.

☺ **Moisture Rich Mask Formula 1** *($12 for 4 ounces)* is a very emollient, very ordinary cream for dry skin. It contains an insignificant amount of antioxidants, but it also contains a small amount of menthol, which can be a skin irritant.

☺ **Revitalizing Mask Formula 2** *($12 for 4 ounces)* is a standard clay mask that also contains ground-up walnut shells. It can be a good exfoliant, but the waxes in this product (carnauba wax, in particular) can be a problem for blemish-prone skin. It is also hard to rinse off.

☺ **Clarifying Mask Formula 3** *($12 for 4 ounces)* is a standard clay mask that can be an option to absorb oil for normal to oily skin.

☺ **Indulging Soothing Eye Mask** *($15 for 4 ounces)* is a decent mask with some good anti-irritants and a tiny amount of a water-binding agent.

☺ **Enriched Moisturizer Formula 1** *($16 for 4 ounces)* isn't all that enriched or all that different from the Balancing and Oil-Control versions below. This is an extremely standard, mundane moisturizer for normal to dry skin.

☺ **Balancing Moisturizer Formula 2** *($16 for 4 ounces)* is a very boring, basic, mineral oil–based moisturizer. This is OK for normal to dry skin, but there are far better options for skin than this humdrum choice.

☺ **Oil-Control Lotion Formula 3** *($16 for 4 ounces)* is a lightweight, silicone-based moisturizer. Nothing in this product can control, change, or affect the amount of oil your skin produces. It is just an OK moisturizer for slightly dry skin with a matte finish and that's about it.

☺ **Oil Mattifier** *($15 for 1 ounce)* is similar to the Oil-Control Lotion above and the same comments apply.

✓☺ **Acne Treatment Gel** *($7 for 1.25 ounces)* contains 5% benzoyl peroxide in a non-irritating gel formulation. This would work fine as a disinfectant for acne-prone skin.

☹ **Velocity Lightweight Moisturizer** *($12 for 4 ounces)*. With alcohol listed as the third ingredient and some plant extracts that can be irritating for skin, this moisturizer can be a heavyweight problem for skin.

☹ **Daily Protection Moisturizer with Sunscreen SPF 15** *($16 for 4 ounces)* doesn't contain the UVA-protecting ingredients of avobenzone, zinc oxide, or titanium dioxide, and is not recommended.

☺ $$$ **Day Solutions SPF 15** *($30 for 1 ounce)* is a good, in-part avobenzone-based sunscreen in an emollient base that includes a long list of antioxidants and water-binding agents, and it would work well for normal to dry skin. However, the antioxidants and water-binding agents are listed so far after the preservatives that they barely amount to more than a dusting. This also contains some plant extracts that are potentially irritating, but thankfully, there are not much of those in here either.

☹ **Night Solution** *($30 for 1 ounce)* lists alcohol as the second ingredient and also contains several plant extracts that are potential skin irritants, and though this gel-based moisturizer with AHA and BHA has a good concentration of each and a relatively low pH of 3.5 to 4, the alcohol is no solution for any skin type.

☺ **Nighttime Recovery System** *($25 for 2.8 ounces)* is a rather unimpressive light-weight moisturizer for normal to slightly dry skin.

☺ **Advanced Moisture Renewal Treatment Cream** *($19 for 2.5 ounces)* is an emol-lient, mineral oil– and Vaseline-based moisturizer that contains tiny amounts of antioxidants and water-binding agents. It is an OK option for dry skin.

☺ **Calming Influence** *($20 for 1 ounce)* contains the most minute amounts of anti-irritants and even less than that of water-binding agents. This also contains some plant extracts that can be skin irritants, making this a poor influence for everyone.

☺ **Extra Emollient Night Cream** *($11 for 2.5 ounces)* is a very standard, very emol-lient moisturizer that contains mostly Vaseline, mineral oil, waxes, fragrance, and preservatives. It does contain menthol, which can be a skin irritant, though the amount is so small it probably doesn't affect skin in the least.

☺ **Instant Action Eye Cream** *($15 for 0.65 ounce)* is an emollient moisturizer for dry skin that contains a good mix of antioxidants, water-binding agents, and anti-irri-tants, but there is nothing about it that is special for the eye area or that will do anything but moisturize skin.

☺ $$$ **Lumineyes Dark Circle Diminisher** *($28 for 0.5 ounce)* is an emollient moisturizer that contains vitamin K and retinol. There is no research showing that retinol can affect dark circles. The only information showing that vitamin K may affect dark circles is from the company selling the ingredient. This is as good a moisturizer as any if you are interested in a retinol product, and there's even some vitamin E and C in here as well, so this may be considered a grand slam.

☺ $$$ **Spot Solution Skin Lightening Cream** *($28 for 0.5 ounce)* is a hydroquinone-based skin lightener, but there is no information as to how much of it this product contains. Hydroquinone is effective for skin lightening and a 2% concentration is best, but there is no way to tell if that's what you are getting. This may be a good option and the formulation is a good one (including retinol), but there is no way to know for sure, hence the neutral face.

☺ **Triple-Action Eye Enhancer** *($15 for 0.65 ounce)* claims to have more benefits in one little product than almost any other I've ever seen. According to the company's magazine, it has much more than just triple action; I lost count after six benefits. It has free-radical scavengers, AHAs, and light-diffusing ingredients; it can be used as an eyeshadow base or as an under-eye concealer; it reduces puffiness and increases skin firmness; and, finally, it reduces the appearance of wrinkles. What's in this little miracle? Mostly silicone, film-forming agent, clay, several thickeners, and preservatives. There are tiny amounts of vitamins E and A, but they appear at the end of the ingredient list and so are completely insignificant. Then what about those benefits? Well, there aren't enough AHAs in this product to exfoliate skin (less than 2% lactic acid). It doesn't have light-diffusing properties, unless you consider a little shimmer a camouflage. The film-forming agents can form a tight layer over the skin, giving the illusion of smoother skin. This product is a poor under-eye concealer. And as an eyeshadow base it's too emollient, which would just help makeup settle into creases.

☺ **Triple Action Lip Enhancer** *($15 for 0.5 ounce)* is a very good emollient moisturizer for the lips, but the amount of AHA in it is minimal, and the triple benefit it should have contained, but doesn't, is sunscreen.

☹ **Satin Lips** *($18 for 0.15 ounce of Lip Mask and 0.15 ounce of Lip Balm)*. This could have been a great topical exfoliant and emollient balm for lips, but both the Lip Mask and Lip Balm contain menthol and that can make chapped lips worse, not better.

☹ **Sun Essentials Ultimate Protection Sunblock SPF 30** *($9.50 for 4.5 ounces)* doesn't contain the UVA-protecting ingredients of avobenzone, zinc oxide, or titanium dioxide, and is not recommended.

☹ **Sun Essentials Sensible Protection Sunblock SPF 15** *($9.50 for 4.5 ounces)* doesn't contain the UVA-protecting ingredients of avobenzone, zinc oxide, or titanium dioxide, and is not recommended.

☹ **Sun Essentials Lip Protector Sunblock SPF 15** *($6.50 for 0.16 ounce)* doesn't contain the UVA-protecting ingredients of avobenzone, zinc oxide, or titanium dioxide, and is not recommended.

☺ **Sunless Tanning Lotion** *($10 for 4.5 ounces)* uses dihydroxyacetone, the same ingredient in all self-tanners, which affects the color of skin. This would work as well as any.

MARY KAY TIMEWISE

☹ **$$$ TimeWise 3-in-1 Cleanser** *($18 for 4.5 ounces)* is a standard, mineral oil–based cleanser with a small amount of detergent cleansing agents. It is an option for dry skin. The plant extracts are a mix of anti-irritants and irritants.

☺ **TimeWise Age Fighting Moisturizer** *($20 for 3.3 ounces)*. While there are some good water-binding agents in here, they are present in the smallest amounts imaginable. This is a good basic moisturizer for someone with normal to dry skin, but that's about it.

MARY KAY MAKEUP

Mary Kay's makeup products have been renamed MK Signature, and along with the name change, there have been several improvements in a few categories. Accompanying the positives, however, are many familiar negatives, including foundations that still have embarrassingly low levels of sun protection, not to mention more than a handful of unacceptable colors. The concealers have markedly improved, and the blushes and eyeshadows offer more elegant textures and fashion-forward colors than before (though you still need to watch out for way too much shine and some truly dated shade couplings). The remaining color products reflect Mary Kay's history of providing OK to very good makeup that rarely completes that last lap to superiority—a feat that a select few companies routinely accomplish. Mary Kay claims "We're a company that knows what women want…" and they are clearly doing something right, especially when you consider the entire line generated sales of $1.4 billion in 2001 (Source: *The Rose Sheet*, August 26, 2002). However, impressive sales figures do not necessarily equate to the best products or mean that this is *the* cosmetics line for you. MK Signature shows promise, but still has a way to go before it is a line that makes it worth calling a Mary Kay representative.

FOUNDATION: ☹ **Day Radiance Cream Foundation with Sunscreen SPF 8 Dry Skin** *($14)* is only for those with dry skin who prefer a thick, creamy, full-coverage foundation. This blends decently, but lacks the smoothness of foundations from Estee Lauder, Origins, Bobbi Brown, and Lancome, to name a few. The SPF 8 is too low (SPF 15 is the minimum recommended by the American Academy of Dermatology and the Skin Cancer Foundation), but it is a titanium dioxide–based sunscreen. The following colors are too peach, pink, ash, yellow, or copper for most skin tones: Blush Ivory, Delicate Beige, Mocha Bronze, Bittersweet Bronze, Rich Bronze, Toasted Beige, and Cocoa Beige.

☺ **Day Radiance Liquid Foundation with Sunscreen SPF 8 Normal/Combination Skin** *($14)* feels light and moist and blends easily to a light-coverage, natural finish. The SPF is identical to that of the foundation above, and the same comments apply. The following colors are too peach, pink, ash, yellow, or copper for most skin tones: Soft Ivory, Blush Ivory, Delicate Beige, Toasted Beige, Mocha Bronze, Rich Bronze, Walnut

The Reviews M

Bronze, Bittersweet Bronze, and Mahogany Bronze. **Day Radiance Oil-Free Foundation** (*$14*) is a very good, matte-finish foundation that has adequate slip for easy blending. This is ideal for those with oily skin who are looking for sheer to light coverage, though the finish is a bit sticky. The following colors are too peach, pink, ash, yellow, or copper for most skin tones: Delicate Beige, Toasted Beige, Blush Ivory, Mocha Bronze, Bittersweet Bronze, Walnut Bronze, and Rich Bronze. **Creme-to-Powder Foundation** (*$14 for foundation, $9 for refillable compact*) has a great, smooth, soft finish without feeling greasy or too thick, and provides medium coverage with an effect that's not too powdery or too creamy. There are 11 shades, and among them Ivory 2, Beige 2, Bronze 1, Bronze 1.5, and Bronze 2 are best avoided.

☺ $$$ **TimeWise Dual Coverage Powder Foundation** (*$14 for foundation, $9 for refillable compact, $4 for powder brush*) has the requisite smooth, dry texture that characterizes most pressed-powder foundations, but this goes on sheer and blends exceptionally well, leaving a satin finish. The nine shades aren't the most neutral around, but the majority pass muster and they're really too sheer to be problematic. The only significant drawback is the shiny particles added to this powder. They are clearly visible on the skin, especially in daylight, which may not be the result you want.

<u>CONCEALER:</u> ✔☺ **MK Signature Concealer** (*$9.50*) comes in a squeeze tube and is very concentrated. This has an improved, silicone-enhanced texture that blends without slip-sliding all over your face, which is a huge plus. It provides almost full coverage without looking thick or creasing, so it's a top choice if you have very dark circles. The six colors are fairly good, with the best ones being Light Ivory, Ivory, and Beige. Avoid Yellow—the name says it all.

<u>POWDER:</u> ☺ **MK Signature Loose Powder** (*$12.50*) is a talc-based powder with a soft, dry consistency. This goes on sheer, and four of the five colors are quite good—only Bronze can be too peach for most skin tones.

☹ $$$ **Highlighters Bronzing Beads** (*$18, $10 for Retractable Powder Brush*) are iridescent powder beads that provide a soft wash of shiny bronze color. For the money, this doesn't hold any advantage over The Body Shop's Brush-On Bronze ($16.50).

☺ <u>BLUSH:</u> **MK Signature Cheek Color** (*$9 for blush tablet, $8 for refillable compact*) has a smooth, dry texture and an application that begins sheer, but builds nicely for color that is more vibrant. However, many of the shades are quite sparkly, and that's too distracting for daytime wear. The matte options include Nutmeg, Desert Bloom, Maple Walnut, Just Peachy, and Cranberry Bold.

<u>EYESHADOW:</u> ☺ **MK Signature Eye Color** (*$6.50 for each eyeshadow, $8–$38 for the various compacts*) are utterly silky, and these apply beautifully without flaking or streaking. They are pigment-rich, too, so it only takes a tiny amount to shape and shade the eye. How disappointing that almost all of the single shades are inordinately shiny. The **Eye Color Duets** (*$6.50*) are all shiny and feature a few of the most unattractive, dated color selections ever. The sole matte options are White Sand and Hazelnut.

☺ **MK Signature Eyesicles Eye Color** *($10)* are slick, cream-to-powder eyeshadows that leave more of a sheen than a shine. They are quite easy to blend, though a bit hard to control when it comes to placement. Still, they're one of the better options for fans of this type of eye makeup.

EYE AND BROW SHAPER: ☺ **MK Signature Eyeliner** *($9.50)* is a standard, twist-up, nonretractable pencil that has a smooth finish and a reasonable price. This product makes waterproof and smudgeproof claims and although it does hold up underwater, it will eventually smudge. Avoid Indigo and Violet unless you want people to notice your eyeliner more than your eyes. **MK Signature Brow Liner** *($9.50)* is a very good automatic, nonretractable brow pencil that comes in four great colors and is relatively easy to apply, though it's still not preferred to a brow powder or brow mascara.

☺ **Brow Definer Pencil** *($7.50)* is a standard pencil that must be a holdover, as this rather slick pencil only comes in one color, best for blonde brows.

☹ **MK Signature Liquid Eyeliner** *($10.50)* isn't something I'd want to put *my* signature on. This takes longer than usual to dry, tends to smear, and can ball up and roll off as it's worn. On top of all that, the brush is difficult to control.

LIPSTICK AND LIP PENCIL: ☺ **MK Signature Creme Lipstick** *($12)* leans heavily toward the greasy side of creamy, and has a semi-opaque, soft gloss finish. The range of over 35 shades has been modernized and is now handily divided into Berries, Reds, Neutrals (which are not neutral at all—they are popular cool tones), Metals (which are largely unattractive), Pinks, and Chocolates. **MK Signature Lip Liner** *($9.50)* is a good, automatic, nonretractable lip pencil that does not distinguish itself from most other pencils, except for a preponderance of drab or deep brown tones.

✔☺ **MK Signature Lip Gloss** *($12)* is a semi-fluid, syrupy lip gloss that is barely sticky and leaves an ultra-wet glossy finish. The striking shades aren't for the sheer-and-soft crowd, but those who appreciate a kick of color won't be disappointed. A colorless version is also available.

MASCARA: ☺ **Flawless Mascara** *($8.50)* is only flawless if you have minimal expectations from mascara. This goes on sheer and thin, so building any thickness is impossible, but you will get meager length with no clumps or smearing. **Waterproof Mascara** *($8.50)* takes several sweeps before you get anything close to a noticeable difference, and that's a generous comment. At least this is waterproof and tends not to clump.

☺ **Endless Performance Mascara** *($8.50)* has been improved and is now recommended as an acceptable lengthening mascara that defines lashes quickly without clumps or flaking. It's not on a par with the best lengthening mascaras at the drugstore or department store, but it's still worth considering if your lashes do best with modest enhancement.

MAX FACTOR (MAKEUP ONLY)

Max Factor earned his place in cosmetics history as *the* makeup artist for movie stars and the rich and famous of the 1920s and beyond. Among his many credits, Max Factor

The Reviews M

developed innovative makeup colors and textures that were unheard of (and sorely needed) at the dawn of cinema's Technicolor era. Movie studios and Hollywood's elite relied on his expertise to create all manner of makeup, from the line's still-available Pan Cake Makeup and Erace Secret Cover Up to the very first lip gloss, circa 1930. (I don't recommend Pan Cake foundation for anyone, but it's nice to recognize the roots of the makeup we are all wearing.) Another little-known, but monumentally important, contribution made by Factor was his Theory of Color Harmony. This theory referred to the art of selecting and blending colors based on a woman's skin tone, eye color, and hair color, and today you would be hard-pressed to find a cosmetics company that doesn't use some incarnation of this idea to coordinate makeup palettes.

Although this line's namesake is highly regarded, most of today's Max Factor products are either decades out of date or modern-day blunders. This line was close to drowning until parent company Procter & Gamble resuscitated it with the launch of the remarkable Lipfinity. For the first time in a long time, lipstick lovers everywhere found themselves clamoring for this innovation, or at least were curious about its claim of "lasts all day" color. As you will see in the review below, this momentous product really does live up to the hype, although not without a few caveats. Other than Lipfinity, however, and a few nice mascaras, I cannot come up with a convincing reason to shop this line. The prices are reasonable, but Factor's competition at the drugstore is eons ahead of this once-groundbreaking line. For more information about Max Factor, call (800) 526-8787 or visit www.maxfactor.com.

MAKEUP REMOVER: ☺ **Remover for Long Lasting Makeup** (*$3.99 for 2 ounces*) is a very standard, mineral oil–based lotion that will definitely remove just about any makeup, but plain, fragrance-free mineral oil will, too, and for mere pennies.

FOUNDATION: ☺ **Facefinity Long Lasting Makeup with PermaWear SPF 15** (*$8.99*) is an intriguing option for an ultra-matte foundation, and one that leaves me ambivalent. On the one hand, it does have a smooth texture that spreads evenly and allows enough time for careful blending, which is essential (but not always a reality) for an ultra-matte makeup. Facefinity provides medium to full coverage and offers a solid, slightly powdery matte finish, and the sunscreen is pure titanium dioxide, which is great. What's not appealing is how obvious this looks on the skin—no matter how little you use, this tends to create a "made-up" look that is not flattering, and it often looks pasty or chalky on the skin. And there are just too many superior foundations available that match Facefinity's best qualities without announcing their presence on the skin. If you decide to audition this one, be aware that it is strictly for normal to oily skin—the slightest hint of dry skin will be magnified by this makeup. This does indeed hold up well throughout the day, while still being easy to remove with a water-soluble cleanser. As far as the nine colors go, they are mostly quite good, which is almost surprising from Max Factor, whose foundations typically tend to lean toward the peach and pink side. What's odd is that the three lightest colors are all extremely light—almost white, and appropriate only for very fair skin. The remaining six colors are best for fair to medium skin tones; only Cool Bronze and Cream Beige are too pink or peach for most skin tones. Rose Beige is slightly pink, but may work for some light skin tones.

☹ **Pan-Cake Makeup** *($6.99)* and **Pan-Stik Makeup** *($6.99)* are both packaged in sealed plastic wrap that prevents you from viewing the colors (and testers are routinely absent). For that reason alone, these are difficult for me to recommend, but in addition, the textures of both foundations are too heavy, thick, or greasy, and almost all of the colors are strongly peach or pink. **Whipped Creme Makeup** *($6.79)* is hands down the worst foundation at the drugstore. No other makeup comes close to offering such shockingly awful colors, and with a rather inelegant texture to boot. **Lasting Performance Stay Put Makeup** *($7.99)* served as the precursor to Facefinity, and although it does stay put, the unpleasantly dry texture and stiff, chalky finish make this a weak entry in the ultra-matte foundation category. If you decide to try it anyway, avoid Cream Beige and Natural Honey. **Powdered Foundation** *($7.44)* works better as a talc-based pressed powder than as a foundation. Although the colors are reasonably good, this tends to be too powdery and cakey on the skin. **Silk Perfection Liquid to Powder Makeup** *($6.99)* desperately needs the axe or a reformulation. This old-fashioned cream-to-powder makeup is too waxy, looks artificial on the skin, and comes in only one salvageable color, Light Champagne.

☹ <u>CONCEALER:</u> **Erace Secret Cover Up** *($4.49)* was the staple of my first makeup experiences. The coverage with this one was and still is good, with a creamy consistency that doesn't get greasy, but the strong fragrance and turn-for-the-worse color selection is not what I would choose today.

☹ <u>POWDER:</u> **Lasting Performance Pressed Powder** *($6.99).* The texture of this is silky, yet it's a strangely waxy powder that takes forever to show anything on the skin, and the four talc-based colors are strongly peach or pink.

☺ <u>BLUSH:</u> **Natural Brush-On Satin Blush** *($6.49)* is a soft, exceedingly smooth blush in a subtle range of pastel and earth tones, each with its share of obvious shine. This is an option, though far from the best.

☺ <u>EYESHADOW:</u> **Lasting Color Eyeshadows** *($3.79)* are single pressed-powder eyeshadows that have a great texture and blend well, but watch out for flaking. The color mix is primarily pale pastels alongside bright shades, and all of them have shine.

<u>EYE AND BROW SHAPER:</u> ☺ **PenSilks Glide On Eye Pencil** *($5.49)* is an automatic, nonretractable eye pencil and one end is a sponge tip to soften the line after you apply it. While this does glide on easily it stays relatively creamy, which means it will also smear easily. There is a sponge tip at one end to smudge the line before that happens naturally. **Eyebrow** and **Eyeliner** *($5.39)* are just standard pencils that are a tad too greasy to choose over those from Revlon, L'Oreal, or Cover Girl.

☹ **Linemaker Eyeliner** *($5.39)* is a liquid eyeliner that is applied with a felt-tip pen applicator, which works well, but it takes a bit too long to dry and is prone to some initial chipping.

LIPSTICK AND LIP PENCIL: ✓☺ **Lipfinity** *($8.99)* may be the biggest lipstick launch ever. It is one of two lipstick products (the other is Cover Girl's Outlast) that uses PermaTone technology. What's PermaTone? According to Max Factor's Web site, it is a "revolutionary new color bond complex which provides semi-permanent color by gently attaching color pigments to lips in a 'flexible mesh' effect." The formula, researched and developed by Procter & Gamble, consists of complex pigments and silicone-based polymers that resist normal wear and tear and will not come off while you are eating, drinking, or even kissing. In fact, according to Max Factor, Lipfinity gives you "perfect, non-budge color for an amazing eight hours!" Sounds too good to be true doesn't it? Well, for the most part, Max Factor, in this case, is not stretching the truth. This really is a breakthrough lipstick in terms of long and comfortable wear, though you need to remember a few important tips, because this isn't traditional lipstick you just put on and go. Lipfinity consists of a lip gloss–like product that puts a layer of opaque color over the lips accompanied by a top coat that's similar to Chap Stick (but more emollient feeling). The colored portion of the product is applied separately to the lips with a sponge-tip applicator and then the color needs about a minute or two to dry completely. Once dry, you can slick on the top coat, and voilà—you get the long wear and coverage of an ultra-matte lipstick and the familiar feel of a traditional creamy lipstick.

However (you knew that was coming, didn't you?), along with the pros, there are some considerable cons to keep in mind before trying Lipfinity. First, application of the "paint" layer can be tricky. The color goes on thick and opaque and must be smoothed out immediately or you will be left with an uneven layer. Application needs to be almost perfect, as any irregularity can quickly turn into a permanent mistake, though mistakes and the entire lip color can be removed with pure mineral oil or plain Vaseline. Finally, your lips must be absolutely clean, smooth (any flaking, no matter how minor, will be greatly exaggerated), and dry before you use this. The moisturizing top coat does indeed make this feel great, and for the most part the color stays on and stays true, even through meals (as long as they aren't greasy or oily meals). You may notice some color fading toward the inner part of the lips, but you weren't expecting perfection were you? A few more minor drawbacks include the lack of testers, coupled with the fact that the color swatch on the box (and the product itself) does not provide an accurate indication of what the actual color will look like once applied. Although you should not need to touch up the color for most of the day (really!), the top coat does need to be reapplied at regular intervals to avoid dry lips. If you can find a color you like and you're not prone to dry, chapped lips, this is definitely worth a try! The **Lipfinity Moisturizing Top Coat** *($5.99)* is now sold separately, which is convenient, as you will likely go through this long before the partnered lip color is gone. For a touch of pizzazz, you may want to consider the glistening **Lipfinity Top Coat Shimmer Finish** *($6.39)*.

☺ **Lasting Color Lipstick** *($6.49)* has a lush, creamy finish, but it's doubtful you'll find it lasting longer than any other creamy lipstick, and the strong fragrance can be off-putting.

MASCARA: ✔☺ **2000 Calorie Mascara** *($3.97)* is a masterful, all-purpose mascara that provides equal amounts of length and thickness, with only a minor tendency to clump if you overdo it.

☺ **S-T-R-E-T-C-H Mascara** *($3.97)* is the diet version of 2000 Calorie Mascara. You can add clump-free length with this one, but it's lean on thickness and drama. **Lash Enhancer No. 1 Mascara** *($3.97)* is a no-frills mascara that works well for a natural look, and it lasts all day without incident. **2000 Calorie Aqualash Mascara** *($3.97)* builds enough length and thickness to be satisfactory for those occasions that call for reliable waterproof mascara. ✔☺ **Lashfinity Mascara** *($5.99)* is above-average waterproof mascara that applies cleanly and evenly, building nice length and a touch of thickness. It stays on beautifully throughout the day, looking perfect from morning until nighttime removal, which is quite easy using a water-soluble cleanser. Keep in mind that waterproof mascaras are not the best choice for everyday mascara. Max Factor does not claim that this is waterproof, but it definitely is, and the ingredient list is nearly identical to that of most other mascaras that are labeled as waterproof.

☺ **No Color Mascara** *($3.99)* is identical to Cover Girl's CG Smoothers Natural Brow & Lash Mascara ($5.49), and the same review applies—but notice the lower cost for this one.

☹ **BRUSHES:** There is only one option here, and it's the paltry, might-work-in-a-pinch **Blush Brush** *($4.49)*, if you don't mind a brush that splays and isn't all that soft.

MAYBELLINE (MAKEUP ONLY)

Maybelline is one of the best-known and most recognized mass-market makeup lines in the world—it's available in 90 countries. Throughout its long history, which began in 1915 when T. L. Wilson founded the company and named it after his sister, Mabel, the company has prided itself on bringing innovative products to cosmetics consumers. Today, Maybelline is still going strong and has shown a marked improvement in its products since it was bought by L'Oreal in early 1996. With improved product selection and modern textures, it is getting harder to tell the difference between L'Oreal and Maybelline products, though Maybelline has a lower price point and offers more glittery, teen-appeal products. Both specialize in offering a large selection of lipsticks, nail polishes, and mascaras, and their foundations share the same strengths and weaknesses (smooth textures and finishes, but often-poor colors, plus the inclusion of sunscreens that are often without much-needed UVA-protecting ingredients). The pressed powders, mascaras, pencils, and matte-finish concealers are impressive and inexpensive. With a little caution, there's no reason you can't come away from Maybelline with some great bargains and a beautiful look. For more information about Maybelline, call (800) 944-0730 or visit their interactive Web site at www.maybelline.com.

MAKEUP REMOVER: ☹ **Expert Eyes 100% Oil-Free Eye Makeup Remover** *($3.99 for 2.3 ounces)* is a very standard, liquid eye-makeup remover that contains boric acid as one of the main ingredients, which is a problematic antiseptic that should be kept away from the eyes.

☺ **Expert Touch Moisturizing Mascara Remover** *($3.69 for 2.3 ounces)* is an incredibly simple concoction of mineral oil, emollient thickener, lanolin oil, and preservative. This greasy liquid will indeed remove mascara and most other makeup as well—but the greasy film it leaves behind is not something most women would want to put up with.

FOUNDATION: Typically, no testers are available for any of Maybelline's foundations, making it difficult to recommend even the ones I liked a lot, which have good textures and color choices. Without being able to test the color first, you can easily end up with the wrong color and with makeup that looks unnatural and mask-like. Your best bet when shopping for foundation at a drugstore or mass-market store is to make sure you can return the makeup if it is not exactly right. Otherwise, it can become a costly venture.

☺ **EverFresh Makeup SPF 14** *($7.49)* is a replacement for Maybelline's Non-Stop All Day Makeup. In contrast to that formula, this foundation has more of a liquid texture, but feels slightly heavier on the skin. It blends quite well for an ultra-matte foundation, and provides natural-looking medium coverage. Unfortunately, the sunscreen lacks adequate UVA protection, so this would need to be used with a separate sunscreen, which is not the best option for those with oily skin. There are 12 shades, including some excellent options for dark skin tones. The fair to light shades have a faint to objectionable peach cast, and the ones to pass on include Natural Beige, Soft Cameo, Fawn, and Sand. **True Illusion Makeup SPF 10** *($8.49)* is attractively packaged, and closely resembles a Lancome foundation bottle. Although this has a smooth, sheer application, it lacks reliable UVA-protecting ingredients and the SPF 10 is meager for a full day of protection. If you're willing to wear an SPF 15 lotion with UVA-protecting ingredients underneath, this may be an option, because several of the colors are great, the texture is impressive for someone with normal to dry skin, and the price is almost a steal. Of the ten mostly neutral shades, the following are too orange or peach for most skin tones: True Buff, True Beige, True Golden, and True Sand. **PureStay Powder Plus Foundation SPF 15** *($7.19)* is a standard pressed powder with slightly heavier coverage so it can double as a foundation. It has a superior, smooth texture, an even application, and a soft matte finish that can go from sheer to medium coverage. The expanded range of 12 shades is a mixed bag, with seven of them (Buff, Cream, Soft Cameo, Natural Beige, Fawn, Sand, and Caramel) being a bit too peach or pink on the skin. If the sunscreen provided adequate UVA protection, this would be an across-the-board winner for normal to oily skin. If you're willing to wear a separate sunscreen or foundation with sunscreen underneath (which is a problem for those with oily skin), this is worth looking into, but watch out for those peachy pink shades. **3 in 1 Express Makeup SPF 15** *($8.39)* is the one to choose if you want a stick foundation that goes on creamy and dries to a soft powder finish with a reliable, all titanium dioxide–based SPF 15. This would work well for normal to slightly oily or slightly dry skin that needs sheer to medium coverage. As with most stick foundations, the waxes that keep this in stick form are not great for oily skin that is prone to breakouts. There are 12 shades, but the best ones are strictly for light to medium skin tones—all of the darker shades, from Tan on down, are just too peach or copper for most women of color. **Express Makeup Shine Control SPF 15** *($8.39)* is another stick foundation with a creamy application that blends out to a powder finish. It's quite similar to the 3 in 1 Express Makeup above. This spin-off foundation has an equally smooth application and provides the same light to medium coverage, but it has a more solid matte finish that can feel somewhat drying on all but oily skin. The sunscreen is pure titanium dioxide, which is great, though it is not the best for breakout-prone skin. Still, this is worth a test run, and the nine colors present options for all but very light and deep skin tones. The only colors to consider avoiding due to peach or pink overtones are Buff, Soft Cameo, and Natural Beige. **Shine Free Oil Control Makeup** *($6.49)* has a very smooth, liquidy, silicone-based texture that blends easily and dries to a solid matte finish. For normal to slightly oily skin types, this could work well, although the all-day shine control claim won't hold for those with very oily skin. The ten shades present some viable options for light to medium skin tones that prefer light to medium coverage. Avoid Light Ivory/ Buff—it is too peach for most skin tones. The other fair to light shades have a soft peach cast, but not enough to make you pass this up if your skin type and preferences match this foundation's capabilities.

☺ **Smooth Result Age Minimizing Makeup SPF 18** *($6.99)* is yet another foundation that does not contain adequate UVA protection. Smooth Result is indeed smooth, and provides light to medium coverage. What's not so smooth is that among the 12 shades, the lighter colors have a slight peach or pink tint that shows up on the skin. Nude is an excellent neutral color, and the darker shades are striking—but Soft Cameo, Fawn, and Sand are not the shades you want to take home. This foundation is best for normal to dry skin, but must be worn with an effective sunscreen for daytime protection.

<u>CONCEALER:</u> ✔☺ **Great Wear Concealer** *($5.19)* is an excellent, non-creasing concealer that goes on matte, but smoothly, without looking dry or heavy. It comes in four superb shades and is best for someone with normal to oily skin.

☹ **True Illusion Undetectable Concealer SPF 10** *($5.19)* has no UVA-protecting ingredients and the SPF 10 is too low for all-day protection, so it is unreliable for sunscreen; but it is a very good concealer with a smooth texture and a semi-opaque, natural matte finish. It blends easily and does not crease; however, the bad news is that only two of the six shades look like skin. Those are Ivory/True Ivory and Light Beige, both of which are great options for light skin tones. **Coverstick** *($4.19)* is an OK, lipstick-style concealer that is now packaged so that you can see the colors. Although most of the shades are workable, this dated formula is too greasy to stay put for long, and it creases easily. This is only recommended for those who prefer this type of concealer to all others and are willing to put up with the drawbacks inherent to the formula.

☹ **Shine Free Blemish Control Concealer** *($5.19)* lists salicylic acid as its active ingredient, and while that certainly has its place in the battle against blemishes, it takes more than a 0.65% concentration to have an effect, plus the pH is too high to allow exfoliation. Besides, all four shades of this tube concealer are glaringly peachy pink, and would only draw attention to what you're trying to hide. **Smooth Result Age Minimizing Concealer SPF 18** *($5.99)* is an undeniably smooth, cream-to-powder textured concealer packaged in a lipstick-style tube. Despite the texture, this has a slightly dry, pasty finish and offers no effective UVA protection. All of the four shades have a pink to peach tinge, with Light Beige and Medium Beige being the most obvious. **Corrector Concealer Cover Stick** *($5.29)* is a creamy, opaque stick concealer in yellow or green. As a whole, color-correcting products such as this just add another step to makeup application and rarely look convincing or natural.

POWDER: ☺ **True Illusion Pressed Powder SPF 10** *($6.99)* has a disappointing SPF number, but it does have a great titanium dioxide–based sunscreen. It can make a nice addition to an effective sunscreen or foundation with sunscreen, but should not be used alone during the day. This talc-free powder has a soft, silky feel and some lovely colors for very light to medium/dark skin tones; avoid True Beige, which is too pink for most complexions. **Shine Free Translucent Pressed Powder** *($5.19)* can't control shine anymore than most powders can, but it is a wonderfully soft, dry powder that applies smooth and sheer and is indeed oil-free. It's talc-and-kaolin (clay) based, and comes in five colors. Deep Beige/Caramel and Natural Beige are too orange, especially for those battling excess oil, but the other three shades are fine. **Finish Matte Pressed Powder** *($5.89)* is an exceptional talc-based powder with three beautiful colors and a silky, even texture. It does contain a tiny bit of mineral oil, but not enough for your skin to notice one way or another. This is best for normal to slightly dry skin that is fair to light.

☺ **Shine Free Oil Control Loose Powder** *($5.89)* comes in two shades, but it is impossible to see them through the unopened package, and that makes this talc-based, dry-finish powder hard to recommend. **Smooth Result Age-Minimizing Pressed Powder** *($6.99)* claims to "smooth away the appearance of first lines" while "providing natural coverage that creates younger looking skin." I suppose if this ordinary talc-based powder can make such enticing claims, then all other pressed powders should be in everyone's antiaging arsenal! This does have a fairly soft, almost creamy feel, but can go on a bit too powdery and tends to settle into, rather than "float" over, lines and wrinkles. The six shades present some attractive options, though Beige and Medium Beige are too peach. Smooth Result is best for normal to slightly oily skin, but is in no way a superior powder to consider for camouflaging wrinkles, be they your first or fiftieth line.

☹ **Corrector Powder** *($6.29)* is a dry-textured pressed powder in pale pink or yellow, and neither shade will serve to correct anything—though they will lend a chalky, pastel look to the skin.

BLUSH: ☺ **Brush/Blush** *($5.19)* is a standard powder blush that comes in an enticing array of colors and has a silky-soft texture that provides a sheer color application with a bit of sheen. The sparkly shades to watch out for are Mocha Velvet, Pink Tangerine, Mambo Mauve, Plushed Plum, and Beach Club. **Express Blush** *($7.29)* is a nice partner to Maybelline's 3 in 1 Express Makeup. This is a cream-to-powder stick blush that goes on sheer and soft, creating a gentle wash of blendable color. There are eight beautiful shades, of which three have a slight amount of shine. The colors are nicely grouped into warms and cools. This would work for those with normal to slightly dry skin who have the patience to blend this on evenly.

☺ **Cool Effect Blush** *($5.99)* is a shimmery liquid blush that comes in a nail polish–style bottle replete with a brush applicator. It applies easily enough without the brush, which is the preferred method of application, rather than the strange blush-that-looks-like-it's-a-nail-polish gimmick. When used with a sponge or fingertips, this imparts sheer color that's heavy on the sparkling shine but dries to a matte (in feel) finish. This would do the trick for an evening that calls for sparkling cheeks.

EYESHADOW: ☹ **Expert Eyes Eyeshadow Singles** *($3.39)*, **Duos** *($4.09)*, **Trios** *($4.89)*, **Quads** *($5.59)*, and **8-Pans** *($7.29)* are mostly shiny shades or dreadful color combinations, with a texture that clings unreliably and is just all-around messy. To top that off, these have almost no staying power to speak of. There are a few attractive color combinations, but the flaky eyeshadow formula leaves much to be desired.

☺ **Cool Effect Cooling Cream Eyecolor** *($5.59)* has no cooling effect whatsoever, but what it does have is opaque, intense shine that can go on as thick as gold lamé or just sheer, but intensely shiny. For an evening look, it has possibilities, but the mood has to be right. **Cool Effect Cooling Eyeshadow/Liner** *($5.59)* is a chubby eyeshadow pencil that goes on somewhat wet, which means it glides easily, and then dries to a matte finish that doesn't smear or move all day. I only wish the mostly pastel colors were more varied and that you could actually see the color before purchasing it; you have to judge this one by a color swatch on the end of the needs-sharpening pencil. **Crystal Glitters Shadow Pencil** *($5.99)* is another standard, chubby pencil that has a creamy texture that borders on greasy. These have a shiny finish, but none of the colors are glittery, just a soft shimmer that should be set with powder if you want them to last. **Roller Color Loose Powder Eye Shadow** *($5.49)* comes in a small vial and has a roller-ball applicator, so despite the name, this is not a messy way to apply eyeshadow. However, it is an extremely shiny way, and as you roll the color on it does not blend at all, so you're stuck with a sheer stripe of glitter.

EYE AND BROW SHAPER: ✓☺ **Expert Eyes Defining Liner** *($5.09)* is a great automatic, retractable eye pencil that comes in appropriate black and brown shades. The dry finish isn't as smudge-prone as most eye pencils, though it's not quite as worry-free as lining with a matte powder eyeshadow. Definitely worth a look for pencil lovers! ☺ **Expert Eyes Brow and Liner Pencil** *($5.09)* is an automatic pencil that can be sharpened (the sharpener is built into the pencil) to a finer tip than most. Other than that, it's just a standard pencil with a dry texture, which means less smudging. **Smoked Kohl Liner** *($5.59)* is a standard pencil that has a smudge tip at one end, and is as reliable as anything you'll find at the department store, right down to the plethora of colors. **Ultra-Brow Brush-On Brow Color** *($5.59)* is a standard, matte brow powder that comes packaged with the standard hard brush that you should toss away and replace with a good soft professional brush. There are two shades, which is limited to say the least, but what's available works if it matches your brow color. **Brow Styling Gel** *($5.59)* is a standard brow gel that is very easy to apply and feels light and non-sticky. There are two sheer colors, which would work for dark blondes and brunettes, as well as a clear shade for just holding unruly brows in place. It's a good inexpensive option if you're looking to tame your brows or add a soft sheen. **Expert Eye Twin Brow and Eye Pencil** *($3.09)* is much less greasy than the last time I reviewed it, and although Maybelline claims it has not changed the formula, I suspect something was tweaked along the way. This is still a standard small pencil whose dry, stiff texture is best for brows—this would hurt if you used it for eyelining. There are ample colors for all brow colors, from blonde to black, and the dry finish really stays put.

☺ **Lineworks Washable Liquid Liner** *($6.19)* is a basic liquid liner that dries to a smooth, flat finish. Unfortunately, it applies a bit unevenly and mistakes are hard to correct. For those who can ace the application, it does wear well during the day. **Lineworks Felt-Tip Eyeliner** *($6.19)* is just like a felt-tip pen, and it delivers a liquid liner that dries to a smooth, matte finish that doesn't budge once it's in place—so applying this is serious and it can be unforgiving. However, the end result is a dramatic line that doesn't chip or flake during the day. **Expert Eyes Softlining Pencil** *($4.09)* is a standard "sharpen me again" pencil that goes on creamy and stays that way. It smudges and smears easily. **Great Wear Water Proof Eyeliner** *($6.29)* is a standard, twist-up pencil that glides easily over the skin and draws a thick line. The texture is creamy, but the tacky finish it has doesn't feel great. This does hold up really well, and resists smudging, but it is no more waterproof than most pencils. **Eye Duets Liner/Shadow** *($6.29)* is an exceptionally standard dual-sided pencil. I would love to say these are in some way an improvement over the numerous other dual-sided pencils out there, but they are just mediocre. The eyeliner end is creamy and prone to smudging, and the eyeshadow end, while sheer and powdery, is extremely shiny and tends to flake.

☹ **Eye Express Easy Eyelining Pen** *($6.19)* does go on easily, and it takes a while to dry. Actually, it never quite set itself the way I was expecting, and it stayed tacky to the touch for quite a while. If you accidentally touch it later in the day, it can come off in pieces—so it may be best to pass up this Express. **Lineworks Ultra-Liner Waterproof Liquid Liner** *($6.19)* is just a standard liquid liner that has good staying power underwater, but it tends to peel or smudge if accidentally rubbed. **Line Works Waterproof Liquid Eye Liner** *($6.29)* claims to offer all-day smudgeproof wear, and fails on both counts. This standard liquid liner has a large brush tip, so creating a fine line is difficult. If you prefer thicker lines, it does the job, but the slightest hint of water or moisture around the eye will lead to an early, unbecoming demise of your design. L'Oreal's Line Intensifique Extreme Wear Liquid Liner is a much better option in the same price range as this one.

LIPSTICK AND LIP PENCIL: ☺ **Moisture Whip Lipstick** *($6.39)* has been around for decades and remains a rich, creamy, slightly glossy lipstick that's not for those prone to lip color feathering or bleeding. **Wet Shine Wet Look Lipcolor** *($5.19)* is extremely similar to L'Oreal's So Delice lipstick, as both share the same slick, light texture, soft colors, and high-gloss finish. This version is slightly more sheer than L'Oreal's, but, unlike So Delice, it is fragrance-free! **Wet Shine Diamonds** *($5.19)* is identical to the original Wet Shine Lipstick, only this is infused with loads of sparkles, which can lend a slight grainy feel to the lips. **Wear 'n Go Long Wearing Lipcolor** *($6.99)* offers a beautiful palette of 36 shades that claim to "go on with lip liner precision," yet it takes only one application to see they go on like almost every other lipstick, and the precision part has to come from your application technique! With that said, this is a basic, creamy lipstick with a slick finish that can be fleeting. Most of the colors go on opaque, and a few have a slight frost, which, for some women, can be an attractive finishing touch. **Gloss Twist Lip Shine** *($5.99)* is another gloss pen that requires you to click up the color into the brush tip. This formula feels great on the lips and imparts sheer, glossy color that's slightly sticky. I doubt you will be able to tell the difference between this one and those from the Stila line, which sell for three times the price.

☹ **Moisture Whip Lip Liner** *($5.19)* is a standard lip pencil that has a thick, creamy texture and strong colors. This applies easily, but the pencil's soft consistency makes it difficult to draw a thin line. **Lip Express Lipstick 'n Liner in One** *($5.49)* is an oversize (width-wise) lip pencil that is supposed to do double duty as lipstick and lipliner. To some extent, that's exactly what it does, just not very well. Like all chubby pencils, this is difficult to sharpen, and the creamy color part is so soft it's impossible to keep a decent tip on the end without perpetual sharpening, which causes you to go through the product much faster than you would with an ordinary lipstick. **Lip Polish Hi-Shine Color** *($5.49)* provides a somewhat creamy, but also powdery, texture that spreads sheer, colored glitter over the lips. It isn't as greasy or messy as some glosses, but it also isn't as smooth—it just has lots of sparkle. **Wear 'n Go Long Wearing Lip Liner** *($5.49)* is an automatic lip pencil that has a soft texture and provides sheer, short-lived color. Funny that the Wear 'n Go Lipstick has a lipliner partner, as that lipstick is supposed to apply with "lip liner precision." Wouldn't that mean no lipliner is necessary?

MASCARA: ☺ **Lash Expansion Mascara** *($5.59)* has a "lash-wrapping" brush that supposedly covers every lash for thicker, longer lashes—but so does any good mascara, and this is no exception. Lash Expansion lengthens and provides moderate thickness without clumping or smearing. It's an in-between option if Maybelline's Illegal Lengths makes your lashes too long (is that possible?) or Volum' Express makes them too thick. **Illegal Lengths Mascara** *($5.09)* has been reformulated and still comes in as one of the better lengthening mascaras around. What you'll notice with this latest version is a bit more thickness and a slightly greater tendency to smear while applying, as this formula is quite "wet." Overall, this remains an excellent lengthening mascara. **Illegal Lengths Waterproof Mascara** *($5.09)* is still a good choice for nicely waterproof mascara that lengthens lashes with ease and that wears well through several laps around the pool. ✓☺ **Full 'n Soft Mascara** *($6.39 regular or curved brush)* is a very good mascara. It doesn't build much thickness, but it does quickly build long lashes without clumping or smearing. ✓☺ **Lash Discovery Mascara** *($5.99 regular or curved brush)*. They say that good things come in small packages, and although this mascara's very small brush made me skeptical initially, I was surprised at how adept it let me be at not only getting to each and every lash but also expertly lengthening, separating, and providing appreciable thickness without clumping or smearing. For those of you still hooked on Maybelline's substandard Great Lash mascara, try this one instead. ✓☺ **Volum' Express Mascara** *($4.69; regular or curved brush)* is the Maybelline mascara to choose if thick, dramatic lashes are your goal. The full brush builds thickness and some length quickly, and without clumping. It lasts throughout the day and removes easily, but overzealous application can cause some smearing. ✓☺ **Wonder Curl Waterproof Mascara** *($5.09 regular or curved brush)* provides excellent length and a soft, fringed curl, all while being remarkably waterproof. This will require a silicone- or oil-based product for removal, but for those times when a long-wearing, waterproof mascara is called for, this shines! ✓☺ **Volum' Express Waterproof Mascara** *($4.69)* builds quickly and thickens well for a waterproof mascara without clumping. It stays on underwater, too!

☺ **Wonder Curl Mascara** *($5.09, regular or curved brush)* doesn't perform any better than others in the arena of making lashes curl more. This is an OK, almost boring mascara in terms of length and overall performance, and isn't as impressive as the L'Oreal or Lancome versions. **Full 'n Soft Waterproof Mascara** *($6.39)* builds excellent length and noticeable thickness, but be prepared to work at it. This is a rather wet formula, and will smear during application if you're not very careful. It is waterproof and a bit more stubborn to remove than most. **Lash Discovery Mascara Waterproof** *($5.99, regular or curved brush)* isn't as exciting as its non-waterproof counterpart, but it's still worthwhile if you're looking for a good lengthening mascara that lasts all day and holds up nicely if your lashes get wet. As is true for most waterproof mascaras, thickness is minimal at best.

☹ **Great Lash Mascara** *($3.59; regular or curved brush)* builds some length, though it takes a good deal of effort to get anywhere. The big drawbacks are that it does not build any thickness and it has a tendency to smear. Its continual mention in beauty magazines' "best-of" lists astonishes me, as it does every makeup artist I've ever interviewed. It may (shockingly) be the #1–selling mascara, but that doesn't mean it's the best. **Great Lash Waterproof Mascara** *($3.59)* is an utterly boring mascara that takes lots of effort for an "is that all there is?" result. It stays on in the rain or pool, but so do Maybelline's other waterproof mascaras—all of which are preferred to this one.

☺ **BRUSHES:** Maybelline's name may not be synonymous with brushes, but if you're on a budget and are ready to toss out your miniature sponge applicators and other inferior tools, you'll find the **Eyeshadow Brush** *($4.39)*, **Blush Brush** *($4.89)*, and **Face Brush** *($7.99)* are extremely soft, but firm, and work surprisingly well. The **Eye Contour Brush** *($4.99)* is an option for brows or eyelining, but it's too small for eyeshadow, and the **Retractable Lip Brush** *($4.99)* is a standard lip brush that travels well. Last, the **Brush 'n Comb** *($3.89)* is a standard, feasible brow and lash comb that's affordably priced.

M.D. FORMULATIONS (SKIN CARE ONLY)

Cosmetics companies buy and sell other cosmetics companies all the time. and that often ends up creating what could only be called strange bedfellows. In the fall of 2001, M.D. Formulations and bare escentuals merged to become one company—M.D. Formulations—thus marrying a line with a clearly medical orientation to an all-natural, new age–aimed company. If you happen into a bare escentuals boutique, you will find spa-styled products radiating aromatherapy and bouquets of plant extracts side-by-side with the ultra-serious, nonfragranced line of skin-care products called M.D. Formulations. Adding to the confusion is the fact that the M.D. Forte line of products, which was once part and parcel of M.D. Formulations, was sold to Allergan (www.allergan.com) and is now retailed as an entirely separate entity with the original packaging still in place. (The M.D. Forte product reviews follow directly after this one.)

What has remained the same, aside from M.D. Formulations' business acquisition of bare escentuals, is that M.D. Formulations far surpasses its competition in the area of serious AHA products, offering the widest range of glycolic acid–based AHA products on the market. Not only are most of the products formulated with a range of 8% to 20% AHAs (5% to 10% is the standard percentage in most other well-made AHA products), but the pH of the products is generally also appropriate for effective exfoliation. There is a great deal of research showing that AHAs in effective formulations can improve photodamaged skin, and they also have been reported to normalize hyperkeratinization (that is, to reduce overthickened outer skin) and to improve the function of the intercellular matrix in deeper skin layers (Sources: *Cutis,* August 2001, pages 135–142; *Journal of the European Academy of Dermatology and Venereology,* July 2000, pages 280–284; *American Journal of Clinical Dermatology,* March-April 2000, pages 81–88; *Skin Pharmacology and Applied Skin Physiology,* May-June 1999, pages 111–119; *Dermatologic Surgery,* August 1997, pages 689–694; *Journal of Cell Physiology,* October 1999, pages 14–23; and *British Journal of Dermatology,* December 1996, pages 867–875).

I encourage you to look into M.D. Formulations, though with a few caveats. This is because I do not encourage or recommend the use of AHA products with over a 10% concentration on a daily or even semi-regular basis (nor does the FDA, at www.FDA.gov, or the European Union Commission's Scientific Committee on Cosmetic Products, in a report dated August 8, 2000). Further, AHAs are not the only ingredients that are of value to skin—lots of others play a vital role. Most important, you don't need for every skin-care product you use—cleanser, toner, scrub, moisturizer, or treatment product—to contain AHA. Just one per face or body, used once or twice a day, is plenty. After all, you only have so much skin to remove before you start taking off too much and causing problems. Another issue to be extra cautious about is the use of a well-formulated sunscreen. This is because when AHAs exfoliate they return the skin to some amount of its pre-sun-damaged level and it is vital to protect the skin from exposure to more damage.

M.D. Formulations also makes several products that are problematic for skin because they contain unnecessarily irritating ingredients, and some of the AHA moisturizers are fairly ordinary and absurdly overpriced for what you get. Despite those reservations, and the fact that these products are incredibly overpriced, if you pick and choose carefully you stand to find some very good AHA products. For more information about M.D. Formulations, call (800) MD-FORMULA or visit www.mdformulations.com.

☺ $$$ **Facial Cleanser Sensitive Skin Cleanser** *($32 for 8 ounces)*. A skin cleanser for sensitive skin that contains AHAs is an oxymoron. And to recommend more than one product with AHAs, as this line does (a cleanser, toner, *and* moisturizer for one face) is a problem for irritation and too much exfoliation. There are only so many skin cells that need to come off the face! However, this cleanser has a pH of about 4.5, and that makes it less than effective for exfoliating and gives it a much lower risk of causing irritation. Other than that, this is just a standard, detergent-based, water-soluble cleanser with thickening agents and preservatives. To suggest that there are cheaper, more gentle ways to clean the skin is an understatement.

☺ **Facial Cleanser Basic** *($18 for 8 ounces)* is a gentle, water-soluble cleanser for most skin types. But wait before you buy, because this product is pretty much a knock-off of Cetaphil Gentle Skin Cleanser, which is less than half the price of this one for twice the amount of product.

☹ $$$ **Facial Cleanser Oily and Problem-Prone Skin** *($32 for 8 ounces)* is a standard, detergent-based cleanser that contains 12% glycolic acid in an effective pH. This much AHA in a cleanser that might get into the eye area is a bad idea and since no one needs to use lots of products that exfoliate skin, it'd be a better idea to use an AHA product where there is less chance that you'll get it in your eye.

☹ $$$ **Facial Cleanser** *($32 for 8 ounces)* is similar to the Facial Cleanser for Oily and Problem-Prone Skin above, and the same comments apply.

☹ $$$ **Facial Cleanser Sensitive Skin Formula** *($32 for 8 ounces)* is similar to the Facial Cleanser for Oily and Problem-Prone Skin above, only this version has a pH of about 4.5, which makes it less effective for exfoliation. That is relatively good news, but the risk to the eyes when splashing this water-soluble, detergent-based cleanser off the skin is a problem, and it's not a good idea for sensitive skin either.

☹ $$$ **Face and Body Scrub** *($35 for 8.3 ounces)* is a detergent-based scrub that uses ground-up plastic (polyethylene) as the abrasive. It also contains 15% glycolic acid with an effective pH. Talk about AHA overkill!

☹ **Glycare Lotion** *($43.75 for 4 ounces)* contains mostly alcohol as well as eucalyptus, making this a careless toner and potential irritant for any skin type.

✓☺ $$$ **Moisture Defense Antioxidant Spray** *($28 for 6 ounces)* is a glycerin- and detergent-based toner that also contains a good assortment of water-binding agents, antioxidants, and anti-irritants.

✓☺ $$$ **Moisture Defense Antioxidant Creme** *($55 for 1 ounce)* is filled with very good antioxidants, water-binding agents, and anti-irritants. It also contains a good amount of urea (it's the fourth ingredient), which is a component of urine, though synthetic versions are used in cosmetics. In small amounts urea has good water-binding and exfoliating properties for skin (Sources: *Skin Pharmacology and Applied Skin Physiology*, January-February 2002, pages 44–54 and *American Journal of Clinical Dermatology*, 2002, volume 3, number 3, pages 217–222). If you are using this moisturizer with other AHA products, keep in mind that you only have so much skin and that too much exfoliation can be a problem.

✓☺ $$$ **Moisture Defense Antioxidant Hydrating Serum** *($42 for 1 ounce)* is similar to the Antioxidant Creme above, only in a lotion form, and the same basic comments apply. This one does add lactic acid to the mix with an effective pH for exfoliation.

☺ $$$ **Moisture Defense Antioxidant Treatment Masque** *($26 for 2.5 ounces)* has the same impressive mix of antioxidants and water-binding agents as the other Moisture Defense products. This once-a-week step will do little for your face, as it is the benefit you receive from daily use of these ingredients that may be significant for skin.

☺ $$$ **Advanced Hydrating Complex Cream Formula** *($44 for 1 ounce)* is an OK, though very basic, moisturizer with minimal water-binding agents and minuscule amounts of antioxidants. It is ok for normal to dry skin.

☺ $$$ **Advanced Hydrating Complex Gel Formula** *($44 for 1 ounce)* is more of a toner for normal to slightly dry or slightly oily skin than anything else. It contains a good amount of water-binding agents, but minimal to no antioxidants.

☺ $$$ **Facial Lotion with 12% Glycolic Compound** *($53 for 2 ounces)* is just AHAs with a thickener and preservatives. This is a very good, well-formulated (and potent) AHA lotion. However, this product contains no emollients, water-binding agents, antioxidants, or anti-irritants. Using this concentration of AHA daily is potentially an unknown, long-term problem for skin (Source: www.fda.gov).

☺ $$$ **Facial Cream with 14% Glycolic Compound** *($53 for 2 ounces)* is similar to the 12% Glycolic Compound above, only with a slightly higher AHA content and a thicker base, but it offers minimal moisturizing benefit for dry skin. The effect of using this amount of AHA daily is unknown, but it is potentially a long-term problem for skin (Source: http://www.fda.gov).

☺ **Facial Lotion Sensitive Skin Formula** *($36 for 2 ounces)* has a pH of about 4.5 and a 12% concentration of glycolic acid, but because the pH is so high (over 4), it is not as effective for exfoliating, and that's good news for someone with sensitive skin. But then what does your $36 get you? This is an amazingly boring moisturizer for normal to slightly dry skin that can still have a sting.

☺ $$$ **Facial Cream Sensitive Skin Formula** (*$36 for 1 ounce*) is similar to the Lotion Sensitive Skin Formula above and the same basic comments apply.

☺ $$$ **Smoothing Complex with 10% Glycolic Compound** (*$35 for 0.5 ounce*) includes 10% AHAs in a pH effective for exfoliation. For an AHA product it's great, and the 10% concentration of AHA is far less risky for skin, though the moisturizing formula is standard and ordinary.

☹ **Vit-A-Plus Clearing Complex** (*$39 for 1 ounce*) is a gel lotion that contains mostly alcohol—a lot of it—which makes this too irritating and drying for all skin types.

☺ $$$ **Vit-A-Plus Illuminating Serum** (*$65 for 1 ounce*) contains 15% glycolic acid with a pH that makes it effective for exfoliation. It also contains retinol, other antioxidants, anti-irritants, small amounts of water-binding agents, and plant extracts that may have melanin-inhibiting properties. There is no research showing that retinol is stable at this pH or in combination with an AHA. For an AHA product it is an option, but the efficacy of the other ingredients is unknown.

☺ $$$ **Vit-A-Plus Night Recovery Complex** (*$50 for 1 ounce*) is a mixture of 8% AHA, 2% BHA, and a small amount of vitamin A (retinyl palmitate); it has a pH of 4, which is just borderline for an effective exfoliant. For an exfoliating moisturizer with small amounts of water-binding agents and antioxidants, this is an option.

☺ $$$ **Vit-A-Plus Revitalizing Eye Cream** (*$53 for 0.5 ounce*) contains 8% AHA, but the pH of 4.4 means it definitely has a reduced ability, if any, to exfoliate. As a simple moisturizer, it's fine, but this is a poor choice for the eye area.

☺ $$$ **Vit-A-Plus Antiaging Lotion** (*$50 for 1 ounce*) contains 10% AHA with some good antioxidants, though the pH of 4.5 makes this not very effective for exfoliation. The antioxidants, water-binding agents, and the AHA with an effective pH in the M.D. Formulations Moisture Defense group of products make them far better choices for skin than this.

☺ $$$ **Vit-A-Plus Intensive Antiaging Lotion** (*$55 for 1 ounce*) is similar to the Vit-A-Plus Antiaging Lotion above and the same basic comments apply. This version has 20% AHA, though the pH of the base is still too high for it to be all that effective for exfoliation.

☺ $$$ **Vit-A-Plus Hydra-Firming Masque** (*$36 for 4 ounces*) is a standard clay mask with AHA and BHA, but the pH of 4.5 makes these mostly ineffective for exfoliation. For a basic clay mask it's an option, but it is really more of a "Why bother?" than anything else.

☹ **Sun Protector SPF 20** (*$24 for 4 ounces*) doesn't contain the UVA-protecting ingredients of avobenzone, titanium dioxide, or zinc oxide, and is not recommended.

☺ $$$ **Total Daily Protector SPF 15** (*$20 for 2.5 ounces*) is a good, in-part zinc oxide–based sunscreen in a rather mundane moisturizing base of just thickeners and silicone.

☺ **$$$ Total Protector 30** *($22 for 2.5 ounces)* is similar to the Total Daily Protector SPF 15 above, and the same basic comments apply.

☺ **$$$ Total Protector Color Tint SPF 30**, comes in **Light**, **Medium**, and **Dark** *($22 for 2.5 ounces)*; the colors aren't the best and the emollient base is extremely standard, but the sun protection is stellar, with in-part zinc oxide protection.

✓☺ **Benzoyl Peroxide 5%** *($20 for 4 ounces)* is a good benzoyl peroxide topical disinfectant in an extremely lightweight base for someone with problem skin.

✓☺ **Benzoyl Peroxide 10%** *($20 for 4 ounces)* is a good benzoyl peroxide topical disinfectant in a higher concentration than the 5% version above in an extremely lightweight base for someone with problem skin.

☹ **Glycare Acne Gel Acne Medication** *($30 for 2 ounces)* contains alcohol as the second ingredient, and it is not recommended.

☹ **Skin Bleaching Gel** *($40 for 1.5 ounces)* is a standard 2% hydroquinone product with a 10% AHA content, although the pH of 4.5 makes the AHA fairly ineffective for exfoliation. It also contains vitamin C, which can help inhibit melanin production. This might still be an option, but the high alcohol content makes it unnecessarily drying and irritating.

M.D. FORTE (SKIN CARE ONLY)

Once a part of M.D. Formulations (preceding review), M.D. Forte is now owned by Allergan, the pharmaceutical company that distributes Botox. Due to Allergan's established emphasis on selling to physicians, M.D. Forte will most likely retain its role as a skin-care line sold through doctors' offices. Is there a difference between M.D. Formulations and M.D. Forte? In essence, their products are almost impossible to tell apart, with virtually identical formulations. The only difference is that M.D. Forte has even stronger concentrations of AHA in their products. Please refer to the introductory material for M.D. Formulations above for the general information about AHA formulations and the role of AHAs in skin care. For more information about M.D. Forte, call (714) 246-4500 or visit www.skinstore.com or www.allergan.com.

☺ **Facial Cleanser I, 12% Glycolic Compound** *($21 for 8 ounces)* is a standard, detergent-based cleanser that contains 12% AHA in an effective pH. This much AHA in a cleanser that might get into the eye is a bad idea, and since no one needs lots of products that exfoliate skin, it'd be better to use another AHA product where it is less likely to get into the eye.

☺ **Facial Cleanser II with 15% Glycolic Compound** *($21 for 8 ounces)* is similar to the Facial Cleanser I above, and the same basic comments apply.

☺ **Glycare for Oily Skin Cleansing Gel** *($24 for 8 ounces)* is similar to the Facial Cleanser I above, and the same basic comments apply.

☹ **Glycare I for Oily Skin** *($17 for 2 ounces)* contains 15% AHA, but it also contains a great deal of alcohol as well as some eucalyptus, making this a careless toner and potentially irritating for all skin types.

The Reviews M

☹ **Glycare II for Oily Skin** *($17 for 2 ounces)* is almost identical to the Glycare I above, and the same comments apply.

☹ **Glycare Perfection** *($16 for 1.7 ounces)* contains 35% alcohol, and that is perfectly irritating and drying for all skin types.

☺ **Facial Lotion I, 15% Glycolic Compound** *($36 for 2 ounces)* is just AHAs with a thickener and preservatives. This is a basic AHA toner for most skin types, if you can handle this much AHA on your skin. Keep in mind that the effects of using this amount of AHA daily is unknown, and potentially a long-term problem for skin.

☺ $$$ **Facial Lotion II, 20% Glycolic Compound** *($47 for 2 ounces)* is similar to the Facial Lotion I above, and the same comments apply.

☺ **Facial Cream I, 15% Glycolic Compound** *($25 for 1 ounce)* is just AHAs with a thickener and preservatives. This is a basic AHA product for most skin types (although the long-term effects of using this amount of AHA on skin are unknown), but don't count on it for any other benefit as it contains no emollients, water-binding agents, or antioxidants.

☺ $$$ **Facial Cream II, 20% Glycolic Compound** *($35 for 1 ounce)* is similar to the Facial Cream I above, only with a higher concentration of AHAs, and the same comments apply. This product is pretty intense and definitely not for everyone. The long-term effects of using this much AHA on skin are unknown.

☹ $$$ **Facial Cream III, 30% Glycolic Compound** *($45 for 1 ounce)* is similar to the Facial Cream I above only with a higher concentration of AHAs, and the same comments apply. This product is not recommended. The long-term effects of using this much AHA are unknown and this much irritation on a daily basis is a definite risk to skin.

☺ **Advanced Hydrating Complex Cream** *($33 for 1.7 ounces)* is an OK, though very basic, moisturizer for normal to dry skin with minimal water-binding agents and a minuscule quantity of antioxidants.

☹ **Advanced Hydrating Complex Gel Formula** *($37 for 1.7 ounces)* is a very overpriced, ordinary gel with too much alcohol, and that isn't hydrating, just very drying.

✓☺ $$$ **Replenish Hydrating Cream** *($39 for 2 ounces)* is a silicone-based moisturizer with some very good water-binding agents, antioxidants, and anti-irritants. It is an excellent option for someone with normal to dry skin.

☺ $$$ **Rejuvenating Eye Cream** *($46 for 0.5 ounce)* is an 8% AHA moisturizer. Thankfully, the pH of 4.4 makes it minimally effective for exfoliation, and that's good news for the delicate eye area. The emollient base does contain some good antioxidants and retinol.

✓☺ $$$ **Skin Rejuvenation Lotion I, 5% Glycolic Compound** *($34 for 1 ounce)* is an excellent, effective AHA lotion for sensitive skin. It does contain small amounts of good water-binding agents and antioxidants.

☺ $$$ **Skin Rejuvenation Lotion II, 20% Glycolic Compound** *($49 for 1 ounce)* is almost identical to the Rejuvenation Lotion I above except that it contains a much higher concentration of AHA. The 20% concentration is a concern because the long-term effects of using this high a concentration of AHA are unknown.

☺ $$$ **Skin Rejuvenation Lotion III, 30% Glycolic Compound** *($49 for 1 ounce)* is almost identical to the Rejuvenation Lotion II above except that it has a still higher concentration of AHA. The 30% concentration is a concern because the long-term effects of using this high a concentration of AHA are unknown.

☹ $$$ **Skin Bleaching Gel** *($28 for 1.5 ounces)* is a standard 2% hydroquinone product with a 10% AHA content, although its pH of 4.5 makes the AHA fairly ineffective for exfoliation. It also contains vitamin C, which can also help inhibit melanin production. This would be an option nevertheless, but the high alcohol content makes it unnecessarily drying and irritating.

☹ $$$ **Skin Rejuvenation Hydra-Masque** *($24.50 for 4 ounces)* is a standard clay mask with AHA and BHA, although the pH of 4.5 makes them ineffective for exfoliation. For a basic clay mask it's an option, but it is really more of a "Why bother?" than anything else.

☹ **Sun Protector SPF 20** *($17 for 4 ounces)* doesn't contain the UVA-protecting ingredients of avobenzone, titanium dioxide, or zinc oxide, and is not recommended.

☺ **Total Daily Protector SPF 15** *($13 for 2.5 ounces)* is a good, in-part zinc oxide–based sunscreen in a rather mundane moisturizing base of just thickeners and silicone.

☺ **Environmental Protector SPF 30** *($18 for 2.5 ounces)* is similar to the SPF 15 version above and the same basic comments apply.

MEDERMA

Selling products that promise to get rid of scars is getting to be big business. With that kind of popularity, and given how hard it is to get rid of scars (just like it is so difficult to get rid of wrinkles, cellulite, and breakouts), it isn't surprising that a product called ☹ **Mederma** *($24.95 for 1.76 ounces)* is available, touting its ability to get rid of scars, diminish redness, and make skin look smooth and flawless.

How does Mederma do this? Mederma uses onion extract as the scar-changing ingredient. It contains water, thickeners, onion extract, fragrance, and preservative, and it seems that only Mederma believes their claim. An article in the *Archives of Dermatology* (December 1998, pages 1512–1514, "Snake Oil for the 21st Century") from the Department of Dermatology, Harvard Medical School, stated that "With the current promulgation of skin 'products' and their promotion and even sale by dermatologists, and the use of treatments of no proven efficacy, this association between dermatology and quackery is set to continue well into the 21st century. The list of offending treatments includes silicone gel sheets and onion extract cream (Mederma) for keloids...."

Another study in *Cosmetic Dermatology* (March 1999, pages 19–26) compared the results of Mederma to those of a placebo. The results were as follows: "Treated [Mederma] and placebo [untreated] subjects were compared on all covariants: age, gender, ethnicity, scar age, and use. No significant difference exists between treated and placebo groups for any of these variables.... More placebo patients than treated patients reported improvement with a less noticeable scar [after] 1 week and a less red scar after 1 month." Interestingly, "More treated patients reported improvement with a softer scar after 2 months. There were no differences in improvement for either of the physician-related measures between the two groups."

Recently, a study in *Plastic and Reconstructive Surgery* (July 2002, pages 177–183) stated that "Computer analysis of the scar photographs demonstrated no significant reduction in scar erythema [redness] with Mederma treatment." The study did note a minimal increase in collagen production, but then, collagen is what scars are made of. And that's not exactly the cure for scars Mederma presents. For more information about Mederma, call (888) 925-8989 or visit www.merzusa.com.

MERLE NORMAN

Merle Norman began with a background in cosmetics chemistry, and began making her first products in her kitchen before opening her Studio in 1931. Her famous "Try Before You Buy" philosophy was an industry first, and is still a mainstay feature of the Merle Norman stores—they have samples aplenty. History aside, many of Merle Norman's boutiques are still in dire need of some serious cosmetic surgery, not just a face-lift year after year (all of the stores I visited have a slightly worn, fairly antiquated feel), and most of the skin-care products seem to be stuck in a time warp. The display units (and not all stores have them) are still poorly organized and not very user-friendly; in fact, they appear almost haphazard.

I admit this all sounds pretty dismal, but with some tweaking this line could really be a contender. Merle Norman needs to take a look at itself through more contemporary, fashionable glasses if it has any hope of joining the rest of the cosmetics world in this new millennium. For more information about Merle Norman, call (800) 40-MERLE or visit www.merlenorman.com. **Note:** Since the Merle Norman boutiques are privately owned and operated, each one can set prices as they see fit, so the prices listed below may vary from store to store. Also, all Merle Norman products contain fragrance unless otherwise noted.

MERLE NORMAN SKIN CARE

☺ **Cleansing Lotion** *($16.50 for 14 ounces)* is just a mineral oil–based, wipe-off cleanser with a small amount of detergent cleansing agent. It also contains Vaseline and lanolin, and adds up to be little more than cold cream.

☺ **Cleansing Cream** *($12.50 for 7.5 ounces)* is a thick, greasy, mineral oil–based cleanser, very reminiscent of similar versions sold in the '50s, but for a cold cream for dry skin it will work.

☹ **Special Cleansing Bar** *($8.50 for 4 ounces)* contains sodium lauryl sulfate as one of the main cleansing agents, making it too potentially irritating and drying for all skin types.

☺ Instant Eye Makeup Remover *($8.50 for 3 ounces)* is a standard, detergent-based eye-makeup remover that would work as well as any reviewed in this book.

☺ Very Gentle Eye Makeup Remover *($8.50 for 2 ounces)* is nothing more than mineral oil and thickening agents, so it is gentle, but greasy, way to take off makeup.

☹ Fresh 'n Fair Skin Freshener *($10.50 for 5.5 ounces)*. Alcohol is the second ingredient listed, which makes this product too drying and irritating for all skin types.

☺ Refining Lotion *($10.50 for 5.5 ounces)* is an exceedingly ordinary toner that can be an option, albeit a poor one, for most skin types.

☺ Aqua Lube *($10.50 for 2 ounces)* is mostly mineral oil, Vaseline, and lanolin, making it a greasy, boring option for dry skin.

☺ Super Lube *($14.50 for 2 ounces)* is a greasy, boring option for dry skin.

☺ Intensive Moisturizer *($13.50 for 1.25 ounces)*. The only thing intense about this moisturizer is its dated formulation of mineral oil, thickeners, plant oil, lanolin oil, and preservatives.

☺ Moisture Emulsion *($14.50 for 3 ounces)* is an exceedingly ordinary moisturizer of mineral oil, slip agent, and thickeners.

☺ Moisture Lotion *($13 for 3 ounces)* is similar to the Moisture Emulsion above and the same comments apply.

☹ Protective Veil *($12 for 3 ounces)* is just water, thickeners, preservatives, and fragrance, and is not protective or helpful in any way for skin.

☹ Sun Defense Sunscreen for Face and Body, SPF 25 *($11.50 for 4 ounces)* doesn't contain the UVA-protecting ingredients of avobenzone, titanium dioxide, or zinc oxide, and is not recommended.

☺ Sun Free Self Tanning Creme Light *($12.50 for 4 ounces)*, like all self tanners, contains dihydroxyacetone, the ingredient that turns skin brown. It works as well as any.

MERLE NORMAN LUXIVA

☺ Luxiva Collagen Cleanser *($18.50 for 6 ounces)* is just a mineral oil–based, wipe-off cleanser with a small amount of detergent cleansing agent. It also contains Vaseline and lanolin, and adds up to be little more than cold cream. The teeny amount of collagen has no effect on the collagen in your skin.

☺ $$$ Luxiva Foaming Cleanser for Dry Skin *($18 for 4 ounces)* is a detergent-based cleanser that is far better for normal to oily skin than for dry skin. The plant extracts can be anti-irritants. This does contain coloring agents.

☹ Luxiva Foaming Cleanser for Oily Skin *($18 for 4 ounces)* is almost identical to the Dry Skin version above, only this one contains eucalyptus and lemon, which are drying and irritating problems for all skin types.

☺ Luxiva Dual Action Eye Makeup Remover *($14.50 for 4 ounces)* is a very standard, but good, silicone-based eye-makeup remover that also contains a small amount of detergent cleansing agents.

☹ **Luxiva Skin Refining Cleanser** (*$19.50 for 4 ounces*) won't refine anyone's skin. It has some synthetic scrubbing beads (polyethylene), which are OK for mechanical exfoliation, but it also contains a fair amount of potassium hydroxide, making it extremely alkaline, which can be a skin irritant. This product has more problems than benefits.

☺ **Luxiva Polished Perfection Facial Scrub** (*$19.50 for 4 ounces*) is a standard, detergent-based cleanser that uses crushed apricot seeds as the abrasive. It is an option for normal to dry skin.

☹ **Luxiva AHA Toner Normal to Oily Skin** (*$14 for 6 ounces*) is mostly alcohol, and it also contains a small amount of menthol, which makes it mostly irritating for all skin types.

☹ **Luxiva AHA Toner for Dry Skin** (*$14.50 for 6 ounces*) doesn't contain AHA. Although the plant extracts are meant to sound like they may have exfoliating properties, they don't. It also contains menthol, and that can be a skin irritant.

☹ **Luxiva Collagen Clarifier** (*$15 for 6 ounces*). This definitely contains collagen, and while collagen is a good water-binding agent, it offers no other benefit for skin. This also contains menthol, which makes it potentially irritating for all skin types.

☹ **Luxiva AHA Intensive Complex** (*$32 for 1 ounce*) contains about 7% lactic acid, which would be great except that the pH of 5 is too high for it to be effective as an exfoliant, and it contains no discernable amounts of antioxidants or water-binding agents.

☺ $$$ **Luxiva Changing Skin Treatment SPF 15** (*$42 for 1 ounce*) is a very good, though overpriced, in-part zinc oxide–based sunscreen that is good for someone with normal to dry skin. It does have an abundance of interesting water-binding agents, but the gimmick here is that it also contains soybean and wild yam extract. See Chapter Seven, *Cosmetics Dictionary* for more information about the claims attached to these ingredients. This does contain menthol, but probably in such a tiny amount it won't affect skin.

☺ **Luxiva Preventage Firming Defense Creme for Oily and Normal/Combination Skin Types SPF 15** (*$38 for 2 ounces*) is a very good, in-part titanium dioxide–based sunscreen in a good moisturizing base that includes water-binding agents, anti-irritants, and antioxidants. It is good for normal to slightly dry or combination skin, but there is nothing about this product that is appropriate for oily skin types. This does contain witch hazel distillate, which is mostly alcohol, but the amount probably isn't enough to be a problem for skin.

✔☺ **Luxiva Preventage Firming Defense Creme for Dry Skin SPF 15** (*$38 for 2 ounces*) is similar to the Oily and Normal/Combination Skin Types version above, and the same comments apply, only this version is better for normal to dry skin.

✔☺ $$$ **Luxiva Preventage Firming Eye Creme SPF 15** (*$21.50 for 0.5 ounce*) is similar to the Preventage Firming Defense Creme for Dry Skin above, and the same basic comments apply.

☺ **Luxiva Collagen Support** (*$20 for 2 ounces*) is an OK lightweight moisturizer for normal to dry skin. It does contain collagen and elastin, which are good water-binding agents, but they have no effect on the collagen and elastin in your skin. Though this contains several good water-binding agents, it lacks any antioxidants.

☹ **Luxiva Day Creme with HC-12** *($23 for 2 ounces)* is a rather ordinary moisturizer for normal to dry skin. It does contain some good plant oils, but only a teeny quantity of water-binding agents and even fewer antioxidants. The plant extracts are a mix of anti-irritants and irritants. Without sunscreen, this is inappropriate for daytime.

☺ **Luxiva Delicate Balance Moisturizer, for Sensitive Skin** *($38 for 1.7 ounces)* is a very good moisturizer with several excellent water-binding agents. The lack of fragrance does make it better for sensitive skin, but that also makes it better for normal to dry skin, too.

☺ $$$ **Luxiva Energizing Concentrate** *($37.50 for 1 ounce)* is a good, though simple, lotion that contains some very good water-binding agents. It is an option for normal to slightly dry skin.

✓☺ $$$ **Luxiva Fine Line Minimizer** *($44.50 for 1 ounce)* is a good lightweight moisturizer that contains some very good antioxidants and a water-binding agent for someone with normal to slightly dry skin.

☺ **Luxiva Firming Neck and Chest Creme** *($34.50 for 2 ounces)* contains a tiny amount of salicylic acid, but the pH is too high for it to be effective as an exfoliant. Overall, this is a good moisturizer for normal to dry skin, with an impressive list of water-binding agents and antioxidants. A few of the plant extracts may be irritants, but the amounts are probably too insignificant to make them a problem for skin. There is nothing in this product that makes it preferred for the neck or chest.

☺ **Luxiva Moisture Rich Facial Treatment** *($20 for 3 ounces)* is similar to the Luxiva Firming Neck and Chest Creme above, and the same comments apply.

☹ $$$ **Luxiva Hydrosome Complex** *($34.50 for 1 ounce)* is a good, emollient moisturizer for dry skin that contains a small amount of antioxidants and water-binding agents.

✓☺ **Luxiva Nighttime Recovery Creme** *($38 for 2 ounces)* is a very good moisturizer for normal to dry skin with many state-of-the-art ingredients.

☹ **Luxiva Protein Creme** *($39.50 for 4 ounces)* is a very ordinary, Vaseline-based moisturizer for dry skin. It does contain teeny amounts of collagen and water-binding agent, but not enough to make this of interest for skin.

☹ **Luxiva Shine Control Hydrator** *($34.50 for 2 ounces)* contains grapefruit, eucalyptus, witch hazel distillate, and lemon peel. All together, that adds up to irritation and dryness, and you will still have oily skin!

☹ **Luxiva Shine Control Lotion** *($17 for 1 ounce)* is similar to the Shine Control Hydrator above, and the same comments apply.

☺ $$$ **Luxiva Triple Action Eye Gel** *($18.50 for 0.5 ounce)* is a very good lightweight gel moisturizer that would work for normal to slightly dry or slightly oily skin; it has a good mix of water-binding agents and antioxidants. Some of the plant extracts may be skin irritants, but the amounts are probably not enough to make them a problem for skin.

The Reviews M

☺ **Luxiva Lip Revive** *($15 for 0.5 ounce)* is just a good moisturizer for dry skin. It is supposed to help prevent lipstick from feathering, but it does a poor job of that. It does contain salicylic acid, but the pH is too high for it to be effective as an exfoliant, which is something lips don't need anyway.

MERLE NORMAN MIRACOL

☹ **Miracol Booster Revitalizing Lotion Concentrate** *($10.50 for 1.25 ounces)* is mostly water, alcohol, a form of milk, and preservatives. If this didn't have a price tag on it I would have thought it was a joke. Not only is this drying and irritating for skin, but it is also one of the more useless skin-care products in this entire book.

☹ **Miracol Revitalizing Cream (Mask)** *($14 for 6 ounces)* is mostly water, egg white, fragrance, and preservatives. The question is, "Why bother?"

☹ **Miracol Revitalizing Lotion (Mask)** *($13 for 5.5 ounces)* is similar to the Cream version above, only in lotion form, and a complete waste.

MERLE NORMAN MAKEUP

There is little to love or even like within Merle Norman's decades-old makeup line. I am almost amazed at how so many unreliable, dated products have stayed on the market for so long, but I think I have the answer. More so than many other lines, the experience of Merle Norman is a family affair. Chances are good that if you use Merle Norman today, it's not because you saw a seductive ad or heard your friend raving about her "perfect" foundation. Rather, Merle Norman fans are introduced to the line by their mothers, sisters, or grandmothers—because these are the products they have used unfailingly since they were young. It's a slice of something akin to an American cosmetic rite of passage.

In the previous edition of this book, I commented that this line needed a makeover, and it still does, desperately so. Although some improvements have been made, for the most part the makeup leaves much to be desired. If you want to see what I mean when I recommend avoiding peach, pink, rose, and orange foundations (plus concealers and powders) look no further—Merle Norman foundations are saturated with those exact shades. If you visit one of Merle Norman's many Cosmetic Studios, you're bound to feel like you've stepped back in time, and not in that quaint, apple-pie-cooling-on-the-windowsill way. From displays to packaging and just about everything in between, this is a line that seems blissfully unaware that Jimmy Carter is no longer president. What's ironic is that beneath this dated veneer there are some products that could really shine (no pun intended) if they were modernized just a bit. In the meantime, this line's unintentional retro products are best left back in the era whence they came.

FOUNDATION: ☹ **Liquid Makeup SPF 16** *($16.50)* is an extremely light, but emollient, foundation; however, the sunscreen contains no UVA-protecting ingredients and the somewhat opaque finish along with 25 shades that are almost all too peach, pink, orange, or ash make this impossible to even suggest as a possibility. **Luxiva Ultra Powder Foundation** *($23.50)* is a standard, talc-based powder foundation that goes on slightly grainy, but still has a sheer finish. The texture could easily look cakey if you overdo it. The 17 shades are OK—they are sheer enough so that the really bad colors aren't so obvious—but in this price range, you will be far more pleased with the elegantly modern powder foundations from Chanel, M.A.C., Lancome, or Estee Lauder. **Luxiva Lasting Foundation SPF 12** *($28)* has a slick, almost greasy, texture that has enough slip so you can blend this evenly before it dries to a light-coverage, ultra-matte finish. The sunscreen is all titanium dioxide, which is commendable, but the majority of the 21 shades are overwhelmingly pink, peach, rose, or orange. The only colors that look like skin are Palest Ivory, Ivory, and Ecru. Cafe Beige is OK, but may be too red for some skin tones. **Luxiva Face the Day Creme-to-Powder Makeup SPF 25** *($26)* has a slightly grainy, but still smooth, texture and a solid-powder finish. Titanium dioxide is the only active sunscreen agent, but once again the ten shades are shockingly poor. **Total Finish Compact Makeup** *($20)* is as close to greasepaint as you're likely to find, but even greasepaint isn't *this* greasy. The salesperson confided that everyone calls this the "Tammy Faye Bakker" foundation, and all of the 24 shades are as far from natural skin tones as you can get. **Powder Base Foundation** *($14.75)* is creamier, actually greasier, than it is powdery, and has an almost sticky feel and 26 mostly embarrassing shades. It finally blends out smooth and sheer, but with almost no powder feel, so the name is misleading. Plus, it is so thick that it tends to stain the skin. **Luxiva Ultra Foundation with HC-12** *($23.50)* claims it contains a "special treatment complex" of HC-12, which stands for Hydrating Complex, and it seems to be a combination of plant oils, water-binding agent, plant extracts, and vitamins. If you have very dry skin, this will help to moisturize, but that's about it. This has a creamy texture and sheer finish, so the mostly poor colors aren't as apparent as they are in the other formulas. If you're set on trying a Merle Norman foundation and have dry skin, you may be able to find a worthwhile color among the 21 shades, but this is really stretching it.

☺ **Aqua Base Foundation** *($14.50)* is an extremely creamy, rather thick foundation that is supposed to provide matte coverage. It is somewhat matte, but it can feel more thick and heavy than matte, especially if you don't blend it out carefully. If you want medium coverage with a silky feel and have normal to dry skin, this is the only real foundation option in the Merle Norman lineup, with some of the better skin tones to consider among the 24 shades. The following colors are inordinately peach, pink, rose, or yellow: Translucent, Palest Porcelain, Cream Beige, Bamboo Beige, Fawn Beige, Delicate Beige, Champagne Beige, Porcelain, Taffy Cream, Golden Birch, Bronze Glow, and Gentle Tan.

☹ **CONCEALER: Cover Up** *($11)* can be a decent option for an opaque, soft matte–finish concealer, if you can find a reliable skin tone shade among the 14 choices. The majority of them are too pink, peach, or rose, and there are a handful of color correctors (yellow, green, lavender) that add a strange cast to the skin. The best options for this one are Warm Light, Olive, and Warm Medium, but make sure you sample before buying to make sure the color looks even remotely natural. **Retouch Cover Creme** *($11)* has atrocious pink and peach shades, and can crease into the lines around the eyes.

Oil-Free Concealing Creme *($11)* is oil-free, but still has a fairly emollient texture. It does go on drier than the Retouch Cover Creme above, but the colors are just really bad. **Luxiva Smooth Touch Concealer** *($14.50)* is a twist-up stick concealer with titanium dioxide as its main ingredient. Titanium dioxide is a wonderful sunscreen agent, but its prominence in this product lends a thick, difficult-to-blend texture and chalky, opaque coverage that is much less than what most other concealers achieve. What a shame, as two of the five colors actually resemble skin.

POWDER: ☹ **Remarkable Finish Pressed Powder** *($14.50)* and **Remarkable Finish Loose Powder** *($15)* are both talc-based powders that go on soft and smooth, but the seven colors are mostly too peach or pink to recommend. **Remarkable Finish Pressed Powder Gold Compact** *($26)* is identical to the Finish Pressed Powder above, save for an elegant compact and the fact that there is only one shade available. It is sheer, but still has a noticeably pink tone. **Sheer Face Powder** *($20)* is another talc-based loose powder and, like the Gold Compact version above, has only one available shade. Despite the sheerness, it can still add a peach tone to skin.

☺ **Duskglo Highlighting Powder** *($14)* comes in a small pot and is just a very shiny loose powder that can be messy to use, but it will indeed add lots of sparkles.

☺ BLUSH: **Luxiva Creme Blush** *($14.50)* has a soft, smooth texture and a sheer finish. The color range is very good, and if you prefer a traditional cream blush (meaning one that stays creamy), this is a surprisingly good option, though don't expect it to not move as the day wears on. **Luxiva Lasting Cheekcolor** *($14.50)* has an attractive smooth-textured powder that evenly applies soft but visible color. There are quite a few matte shades available for both fair and darker skin.

EYESHADOW: Merle Norman has their share of shiny eyeshadows, but the shine tends to separate from the color, which is something those who crave glimmering eyes may not have bargained for. ☺ **Luxiva Lasting Eyecolor** *($12.50)* has a silky texture that goes on sheer—so building any intensity or drama from these shadows takes work. But there are some workable matte options to investigate, such as Linen, Almond, Cashew, Mink, Cappuccino, Blackberry, Bark, and Smoke. The rest of the shades are too shiny or pastel to seriously consider. **Luxiva Lasting Eyecolor Duet** *($15)* are just pairs of the same eyeshadow formula above. Although most of the color pairings make sense, all except Linen/Mink are noticeably shiny. **Luxiva Lasting Eyecolor Trios** *($15.50)* vary from season to season, and share the same formula as the other eyeshadows. Each trio tends to have one odd shade that you're not likely to get much use from. **Crease Resistant Shadow Base** *($10.95)* is a cream-to-powder concealer for the eyelids. It may work for some, but won't hold up nearly as well as a matte finish concealer.

☹ **Automatic Shadow Base** *($10.95)* comes in a compact and is too creamy to even stand a chance at preventing your shadows from fading or creasing. **Shimmerstick Creme Eyeshadow** *($12.95)* is a cream eyeshadow in pencil form that is intensely shiny, blends out to nothing, and is hard to sharpen. **Luxiva Creme Eyelites** *($12.50)* are tubes of very sparkly cream-to-powder eyeshadows. The sparkles tend to separate from the color and get everywhere.

EYE AND BROW SHAPER: ☺ **Automatic Definitive Eye Pencil** *($12)* is a standard, twist-up, nonretractable pencil that has a soft, creamy texture and does dry to a transfer-resistant finish with impressive staying power. **Tinted Brow Sealer** *($12.95)* is a lightweight mascara for the brows that comes in six excellent sheer colors. This works well to softly define and groom the eyebrows, and is not sticky. A clear version is also available. **Only Natural Brow Powder** *($12)* is a group of matte brow powders that come with a stiff brush. Forget the brush, but the powders work well to create a defined brow that doesn't appear artificial or drawn on.

☺ **Automatic Eyeliner** *($12)* and **Waterproof Eyeliner** *($12)* are standard liquid eyeliners with stiff applicators. They work for a dramatic look, but the shade selection is limited, and the stiff brush can make application trickier than it needs to be. The waterproof version is quite tenacious, so count on it lasting under most conditions. **Definitive Eye Pencil** *($12)* is a standard pencil that needs sharpening and has a soft texture that smooths on without being greasy. Basic, but unexciting. **Definitive Brow Pencil** *($12)* is a basic brow pencil with the usual dry finish. It will work as well as any. **Automatic Fine Brow Pencil** *($12)* doesn't need sharpening, but the fragile tip breaks off easily, and it's not retractable. It is otherwise an unremarkable way to draw on or fill in brows. **Luxiva Eye Ink** *($12.50)* is a distinct improvement over Merle Norman's other liquid eyeliners. This has a flexible precision brush that is easy to work with and the formula dries fast. Unfortunately, it has a slight tendency to smear.

LIPSTICK AND LIP PENCIL: ☺ **Lipstick** *($12)* is a traditional, creamy, semiopaque lipstick that has a slight stain to keep the color around longer. The color selection consists primarily of pinks and fuchsias. **Luxiva Ultra Lipcolor SPF 15** *($13)* does not contain UVA-protecting ingredients. It offers slightly more coverage than the Lipstick above, while feeling lightweight on the lips. **Moist Lip Color** *($10.95)* is a lip gloss with slightly more color than is typical, and it works well for a reasonably non-sticky, glossy finish. **Lip Pencil Plus** *($12.95)* is a fat, two-sided pencil: one end has a matte finish and functions as a lipliner, the other end is creamy with a "lipstick" finish. I find these types of products more gimmicky than useful, and keeping the pencil sharpened can be a pain, but it's a fun product to check out. ✓☺ **Definitive Lip Liner** *($12)* has a soft, slightly creamy application that dries to a transfer-resistant finish. It comes in a twist-up, nonretractable container and really does have impressive staying power.

☹ **Luxiva Lasting Lipcolor** *($15)* is an ultra-matte lipstick that applies beautifully and sets to a solid, weightless matte finish. Regrettably, it fades quickly after it sets, and what's left of the color tends to ball up and feel uncomfortable. Revlon's ColorStay Lipcolor is still the way to go for ultra-matte lipstick.

MASCARA: ☺ **Creamy Flo-Matic Mascara** *($13)* is Merle Norman's oldest mascara. It doesn't clump, but it's also not the one to choose if you prefer any sort of thickness.

For length and lash definition, it should please, but mascaras that cost less can do even more. **Luxiva Ultra Mascara** *($14)* manages to make lashes feel incredibly dry, although it builds ample length and a decent amount of thickness without clumps. If the dryness weren't so noticeable, this would earn higher marks. **Ultra Thick Mascara** *($14.50)* is not a bad choice for a thickening mascara, and does not instantly clump as it has in the past. Still, it makes lashes feel very dry, too, and is no match for Maybelline's Volum' Express Mascara ($5.39).

☹ **Supreme Lash Mascara** *($14.50)* is not supreme in the least. This subpar mascara does little to impress, but it does clump a bit. As one of Merle Norman's newer mascaras, this is a real disappointment.

☺ **Waterproof Mascara** *($13.50)* builds average length and enough thickness to qualify for those occasions where waterproof mascara is a must, and this is extremely waterproof! The only downside is trying to remove it, which will take more than one attempt, regardless of which type of remover you use.

BRUSHES: Merle Norman's brush selection has some great shapes and sizes, but the ☹ **Powder** *($20)* and **Blush Brush** *($15)* bristles are too sparse and stiff to be of much use, and they don't feel very nice against the skin. ☺ **Makeup Artistry Brush Set** *($50)* seems like a bargain, as you get all 13 Merle Norman brushes, yet the ones to avoid are the highest priced, so you can just pick and choose from the good ones and still come out ahead in terms of price.

The best brushes to consider in this group are the three ☺ **Eyeshadow Brushes** *($5.50–$6.50)* and the **Concealing Brush** *($6.50),* which is the only synthetic brush but can be an option for either concealer or eyeshadow.

METROGEL, METROLOTION, AND METROCREAM

These three prescription-only drugs are applied topically to treat rosacea. They contain the active ingredient metronidazole, an antimicrobial thought to combat the cause of rosacea. For many people, this is in fact an optimal way to treat rosacea, and it is considered the place to start when putting together an effective skin-care program for that skin disorder (Sources: *Journal of Cutaneous Medicine and Surgery,* May 13, 2002; www.pubmed.com; *Skin Therapy Letter,* January 2002, pages 1–3; *Advances in Therapy,* November-December 2001, pages 237–243; and *American Journal of Clinical Dermatology,* May-June 2000, pages 191–199). MetroCream contains the active ingredient (metronidazole) in a simple emollient base that is best for someone with dry skin; MetroGel contains it in a simple, water-based gel formula that is excellent for someone with oily skin; and MetroLotion is great for someone with normal to dry skin. As another option, metronidazole is also found in the prescription-only topical drug Noritate. For more information about these products, call (800) 582-8225 or visit www.metrocream.com.

MOISTUREL (SKIN CARE ONLY)

For more information about Moisturel, call (800) 494-7258 or visit www.bms.com.

☺ **Sensitive Skin Cleanser** (*$8.49 for 8.75 ounces*) is a good, though extremely basic, detergent-based, water-soluble cleanser for normal to dry skin.

☺ **Therapeutic Cream** (*$15.49 for 16 ounces*) is a Vaseline-based moisturizer that also contains silicone, glycerin, and thickeners. This is an extremely standard, mediocre moisturizer for dry skin.

☺ **Therapeutic Lotion** (*$11.99 for 14 ounces*) is similar to the Cream above, only in lotion form and with less Vaseline, and the same basic comments apply.

MORGEN SCHICK

Morgen Schick, as effervescent as any TV talk-show host, is a former model for the prestigious Ford agency. Her image has graced the cover of more than 50 magazines; she has made appearances as "The Makeover Queen" on *The Montel Williams Show, Entertainment Tonight,* and *Good Morning America,* and she appears regularly on E! Entertainment's *Fashion Emergency.* She has also written a book, *Your Makeover: Simple Ways for Any Woman to Look Her Best.* Her namesake cosmetics line is sold on the Home Shopping Network and online at www.hsn.com.

Of course, given Schick's modeling background, the first assumption many consumers might make is that she knows all about makeup application and artistry, and skin care, too, after all, she does look beautiful. It's possible that Schick does know about makeup application and artistry, but more often than not for most models quite the opposite is true, they are no better or worse at applying makeup than the average person, and they are always beholden to their natural beauty and to their makeup artists, stylists, hairstylists, lighting specialists, and photographers. While Schick may very well be talented at applying her own or others' makeup, I just don't think a consumer is thinking it through if they accept the "well, she was a model, so she must know all about makeup and skin care" approach to shopping for cosmetics. Besides, even with her credentials, what matters most is the quality of the products that bear her name. The skin-care products are an embarrassment, with very little to offer and no sunscreens anywhere to be found. And overall, the makeup disappoints, although there are a few highlights such as the brushes, liquid blushes, and lip colors. As entertaining as infomercials can be, this line isn't a reason to stay tuned. For more information about Morgen Schick, visit www.hsn.com.

Note: Almost all of the following products are sold separately or as part of a kit. As is typical for "as seen on TV" lines, the kits sell for significantly less than the individual products. In addition, not all of the products reviewed below may be consistently available, as the products' rotation seems to change frequently. All Morgen Schick products contain fragrance.

MORGEN SCHICK SKIN CARE

☺ **Marine Wash** *($19.95 for 4 ounces)* is a standard, detergent-based cleanser that contains some good anti-irritants, though their effectiveness in a wash-off cleanser is limited.

☺ **Perfectly Gentle Eye Makeup Remover** *($10 for 2 ounces)* is a standard, detergent-based eye-makeup remover similar to almost every other one reviewed in this book.

☺ **Skin Prep Pre-Makeup Primer** *($18 for 2 ounces)* is just thickening agents with some film-forming agent and lots of fragrance (the teeny amounts of vitamins in here are insignificant for skin). This is an unnecessary extra step that doesn't help prime skin for makeup. What would have made this a great primer is an effective sunscreen, something this line doesn't offer.

☺ **Hydrating Lotion** *($22 for 2 ounces)* is a mineral oil–based moisturizer that contains a decent mix of plant extracts, which, for the most part, can be anti-irritants, even though it lacks any water-binding agents or antioxidants.

☹ **Supple Balm Lip Balm** *($12 for 1 ounce)* contains camphor, a skin irritant that is not helpful for lips or for skin anywhere on your body.

☺ **Halo Anti-Wrinkle Firming Brightening Kit** *($42 for* **Halo Retouch Serum** *1 ounce;* **Halo Triple Performance Facial Cream** *1.7 ounces;* and **Halo Triple Performance Eye Treatment** *0.5 ounce).* All of Schick's Halo products list boron nitride as the second ingredient. Boron nitride is a synthetic powder that is supposed to hide wrinkles by causing some kind of an optical illusion. According to the ingredient's manufacturer, "Wrinkles and fine lines in human skin are visible primarily because light is not reflected out of them. [Boron nitride has] the ability … to hide fine wrinkles using optical effects." It only takes one side-by-side application with almost any other moisturizer to notice that these products won't hide anything on your face, "fine wrinkles" or otherwise. If anything, because boron nitride is an absorbent, similar to talc, it soaks up moisture—the opposite of what dry skin really needs. There is absolutely no reason to buy the kit, because the serum, facial cream, and eye treatment are virtually identical, with only small differences between their thickening agents. These all have a similar matte finish due to the large amount of boron nitride, though they do contain some very good water-binding agents and a small amount of antioxidants. They are an option for normal to slightly dry skin, but if you're interested, you only need to try one of these products. The Serum and Eye Treatment are also sold individually.

MORGEN SCHICK MAKEUP

☹ **FOUNDATION: Hide or Highlight Makeup & Concealer** *($25, or $39.95 as part of the Perfect Face Kit)* consists of two thick, dry-textured concealers that can also be used as foundation, and a creamier, peach-toned concealer for use under the eyes. Each kit has three different shades that you can use alone or customize to match your skin tone, or whatever it is you're trying to hide (or highlight). Schick is not an advocate of a full-face foundation application, believing instead that spot coverage is all that's needed for many women, especially those who don't like feeling too made-up. Yet the colors in each of the three kits (Light, Medium, and Dark) are just too peach, orange, or yellow to possibly look natural over bare skin, regardless of your skin color or how well you blend the colors together. Plus, spot application of makeup, almost without exception, even on flawless skin, tends to look—well, spotty.

The concept of having all you need for facial makeup in one compact is enticing, but this product is more trouble than it's worth. The only useful part is the under-eye concealer, but only if you don't mind the faint peach cast and its tendency to crease into any lines under the eye!

<u>POWDER:</u> ☺ $$$ **Whisper Set Powder** *($20, or $39.95 as part of the Perfect Face Kit)* is a very soft, talc-based loose powder that has a smooth, shiny finish. If you don't mind the shine and have very light skin, this may be an option. It almost goes without saying that there are better, much less expensive powder options.

☹ **Sculpting Powder** *($19.50 when sold alone—it is also part of the Sculpting Kit)* is meant to be used on the flat parts of the face to shadow and sculpt the features, but you can do that with any soft tan or golden brown blush or powder; it doesn't take a specially designated product. Plus, this talc-based pressed powder has a poor, unappealing dry/waxy texture that makes it difficult to pick up much powder on your brush. This product is not recommended.

<u>BLUSH:</u> ☺ $$$ **Light Ups** *($18, or $21.50 as part of the Light Ups Twin Pack)* are wax-based, cream-to-powder shimmer products that apply easily and blend well, leaving a very soft, subtle shine on the skin. For an evening look, these would be a worth a try, but you may find Revlon's SkinLights line more enticing in terms of price, local availability, and color selection. **Cream Cheek Color** *($16.50)* is an OK option for a soft, creamy blush. However, since the moist formula provides a glow on its own, the iridescence seems like overkill.

☺ **Schick Stick** *($15)* is a liquid lip and cheek stain housed in a pen-style applicator that features a soft, appropriately sized felt-tip sponge. This applies easily enough and does create an attractive, reddish brown stain. However, like similar liquid blushes, it must be used with a deft hand because it dries quickly and then cannot be easily blended away. **High Roller** *($15)* is a bronze-toned liquid stain designed to be used on the lips, eyes, and cheeks. If you can master the application, this will work well. If not, you'll be reaching for your cleanser, as this can go on streaky and uneven if you aren't careful.

☺ $$$ <u>EYESHADOW:</u> **6-Piece Eye Color Kit** *($27.50)* comes with two brushes and a four-color powder eyeshadow set. The shadows are also available separately as an **Eye Color Compact** *($24.50)*. While the eyeshadows do have a soft, smooth texture, they apply quite sheer, so building any coverage takes some effort. Of the four colors, two are matte and two are shiny, and the color combinations are not what I would call workable. The **Crease Brush** and **Flat Liner Brush** are both excellent, although the Crease Brush can be too large for some eye shapes. For more workable quad eyeshadows, check out the options available from Physician's Formula or Estee Lauder.

<u>LIPSTICK:</u> ☺ **Lip Color** *($13.50, or $26.50 as part of the Lip Kit)* is a standard, but very good, creamy lipstick that comes in a limited selection of colors and has a soft, slightly glossy finish.

☺ **Lip Shine** *($14.50, or $26.50 as part of the Lip Kit)* is a standard lip gloss that has a light, minimally sticky feel and a reasonable selection of colors. They offer decent color saturation for a gloss, but beware: the formula contains peppermint extract, which can be quite irritating to the lips.

☺ <u>MASCARA:</u> **Perfect Lash Mascara** *($15)* is hardly perfect. It's reasonably decent at providing length, but the formula goes on quite wet, and it takes several attempts to make lashes look, well, close to perfect.

<u>BRUSHES:</u> The ☺ **$$$ Sculpting Brush** *($42.50)*, ☺ **Powder Set Brush** *($13)*, **Hide or Highlight Brush** *($13)*, **Flat Liner Brush**, and **Crease Brush** *($27.50 as part of the Midnight Eye Color Kit)* are wonderfully shaped brushes that offer a dense, soft feel and elegant look. The Sculpting and Eyeshadow Brushes are natural hair, the others are made of Taklon, a synthetic material that is quite workable and a good choice for using with creamy or emollient products.

MURAD (SKIN CARE ONLY)

Like M.D. Formulations, Neostrata, SkinCeuticals, Cellex-C, BioMedic, Dr. Mary Lupo, N.V. Perricone, M.D., and other lines of skin-care products created by or aimed at physicians, the Murad line, from Dr. Howard Murad, wants you to believe that his products are completely about science and sound medical advice. They aren't. Although there are some good products, they are just cosmetics, and there is nothing medicinal about them in any way, shape, or form.

Murad was one of the first doctors to appear on an infomercial selling his own line of skin-care products, and quite successfully so. At the beginning, Murad's products were all about AHAs and his products were indeed well-formulated in this regard. But Murad also had poorly formulated products (now there are even more) that contained alcohol and other irritating ingredients, ranging from arnica to citrus oils. Some of the sunscreens offered now have SPFs of less than 15, and some still have no UVA-protecting ingredients. What is most objectionable is the endless parade of products claiming they can stop, get rid of, or reduce wrinkles and aging.

Regardless of whether dermatologists know best about lotions and potions, no conscientious doctor would or should be selling products using the ludicrous claims that are made for Murad's products. Almost every product has the same hype, the same unsubstantiated claims, the same exaggeration about the beneficial effects of ingredients that are often present only in the tiniest amounts, without even a mention of the standard or potentially irritating ingredients that are also present. There are some good products in this line, but there are also some utter disappointments as well. In this case, as is true with many physician-oriented lines, the doctor doesn't always know best. For more information about Murad, call (888) 99-MURAD or visit www.murad.com. **Note:** All Murad products contain fragrance unless otherwise noted.

☺ **$$$ AHA/BHA Exfoliating Cleanser, Deep Cleansing for All Skin Types** *($25 for 6 ounces)* is a standard, detergent-based, water-soluble cleanser that contains plant oil, synthetic scrub particles, and about 2% AHA and 0.5% salicylic acid (BHA). AHAs and BHA are a problem in cleansers because you don't want to get them in your eye, and because their effectiveness is washed down the drain, although the pH of this product is too high for them to be effective as exfoliants anyway.

☹ **Clarifying Skin Cleanser** *($20 for 6 ounces)* is a standard, detergent-based, water-soluble cleanser that would have been a decent option for most skin types except that it also contains menthol, bitter orange, citronella, lemon, and lime oils, which make it potentially too irritating for all skin types.

☺ **Moisture Rich Skin Cleanser** *($22 for 6 ounces)* is a standard, detergent-based, water-soluble cleanser with thickening agents and a small quantity of water-binding agents. It isn't what anyone would call "moisture rich," though it is a good cleanser for someone with normal to oily skin.

☺ **Refreshing Skin Cleanser** *($22 for 6 ounces)* is an extremely standard, detergent-based, water-soluble cleanser for someone with normal to oily or combination skin. It does contain a tiny amount of glycolic acid (AHA), but both the too-small amount of AHA and the too-high pH make it ineffective for exfoliation.

☺ **$$$ Environmental Shield Vitamin C Daily Cleanser** *($30 for 6 ounces)* is a standard, detergent-based, water-soluble cleanser with too much fragrance. The water-binding agents and antioxidants are good, but they would be rinsed down the drain before they had a chance to be of any benefit for skin.

☺ **Energizing Pomegranate Cleanser** *($20 for 5.1 ounces)* is a standard, detergent-based cleanser that contains a tiny amount of pomegranate, a good antioxidant, but whose benefit would be rinsed down the drain before it could work. The witch hazel distillate, which contains a large amount of alcohol, may be drying and irritating for skin.

☺ **Gentle Make-Up Remover** *($16.50 for 4.2 ounces)* is a standard, detergent-based, wipe-off makeup remover with tiny amounts of antioxidants and anti-irritants. It also contains a small amount of glycolic acid, but thankfully the pH isn't low enough to make it active on the skin; that would be a huge mistake in something that might get in the eye!

☹ **Clarifying Toner** *($14.50 for 6 ounces)* contains mostly witch hazel distillate, whose main component is alcohol, as well as some menthol and lemon; all are completely unnecessary skin irritants.

☹ **Hydrating Toner** *($16 for 6 ounces)* contains mostly witch hazel distillate, whose main component is alcohol. It also contains a tiny amount of AHA, less than 2%, which means this is not effective as an exfoliant.

☹ **Environmental Shield Activating Toner** *($28 for 6 ounces)* contains mostly witch hazel distillate, whose main component is alcohol, along with menthol, balm mint, and citrus oils. That won't shield anything, but it can cause irritation and inflammation. What a shame, because there are some very good water-binding agents in this formula.

☹ **Combination Skin Formula** *($48 for 3.3 ounces)* is a lightweight lotion that contains about 7% AHAs and about 1% BHA. It also contains a good deal of alcohol, which makes it a problem for all skin types.

☺ **Acne Management Gel Moisturizer** *($32 for 2.5 ounces)* is a silicone-based, lightweight lotion moisturizer that contains 0.5% BHA, although the pH is too high for it to be effective as an exfoliant. As a lightweight moisturizer with some good antioxidants and water-binding agents it is an option, but there is nothing in it that will prevent breakouts.

☹ **Advanced Oily Prone Skin Formula** *($48 for 3.3 ounces)* does contain BHA, but it also contains a lot of alcohol, which only exacerbates the potential for breakouts from irritation.

✓☺ **$$$ Advanced Sensitive Skin Smoothing Cream** *($48 for 3.3 ounces)* is about a 6% glycolic acid–based moisturizer that also contains small amounts of antioxidants, water-binding agents, and anti-irritants. As an exfoliant for normal to dry skin it would be a very good option.

☹ **Age Spot and Pigment Lightening Gel** *($48 for 1.4 ounces)* would be a decent skin-lightening product with its 2% hydroquinone and 8% AHA content, but it also contains a lot of alcohol, and that can cause unnecessary skin dryness and irritation and won't help skin or sun-damage spots (there are no such things as age spots).

☺ **$$$ Cellular Serum** *($42 for 1.4 ounces)* is a very good, lightweight lotion that contains an impressive mix of water-binding agents and antioxidants. It also contains some plant extracts that can be skin irritants.

☹ **Clarifying Gel** *($48 for 1.4 ounces)* contains mostly alcohol, which makes it too drying and irritating for all skin types.

☺ **Energizing Pomegranate Moisturizer SPF 15** *($25 for 2 ounces)* is a very good, in-part avobenzone-based moisturizer in an emollient base that contains some good antioxidants and anti-irritants, just not very much of them. Pomegranate does have some antioxidant properties when ingested, but there is no research showing that it has those properties when applied to skin.

☺ **Energizing Pomegranate Treatment** *($30 for 0.5 ounce)* is a silicone-based moisturizer, although the fourth ingredient is boron nitride, an earth mineral that is an absorbent with some antibacterial properties. There are some good antioxidants and a tiny amount of water-binding agents, but for the most part it is very hard to decide what sort of treatment this would offer, though it may be an option for normal to oily skin.

☹ **Environmental Shield Age Proof Eye Cream SPF 15** *($50 for 0.5 ounce)* doesn't contain the UVA-protecting ingredients of avobenzone, zinc oxide, or titanium dioxide, and is not recommended.

☺ **$$$ Environmental Shield Essential Day Moisture SPF 15** *($44 for 1.4 ounces)* is a good, titanium dioxide–based sunscreen, though the second ingredient is alcohol, which can be a problem for skin.

✓☺ **$$$ Environmental Shield Essential Night Moisture** *($48 for 1.4 ounces)* is a very good moisturizer for normal to dry skin, with a good mix of antioxidants and water-binding agents.

☺ **$$$ Environmental Shield Daily Renewal Complex** *($80 for 1.4 ounces)* is a silicone-based moisturizer with an impressive mix of antioxidants and plant oil, though several of the plant oils are also fragrances and can be skin irritants.

☺ **$$$ Eye Complex SPF 8** *($50 for 0.5 ounce)* has a dismal SPF rating and cannot be relied on for adequate daily protection even though it contains titanium dioxide as one of the sunscreen ingredients. With so many good SPF 15 products around, why bother with this one when it comes to protecting your skin from sun damage? And particularly when sunscreen is the most vital part of any skin-care routine, and most likely the only one that really makes a significant difference in the health of skin?

☺ **$$$ Night Reform** *($52.50 for 1.4 ounces)* is a good 8% AHA in a lightweight, slightly moisturizing base. It does contain a small amount of antioxidants and water-binding agents.

☹ **Perfecting Day Cream SPF 15** *($32 for 2.25 ounces)* doesn't contain the UVA-protecting ingredients of avobenzone, zinc oxide, or titanium dioxide, and is not recommended. So much for the concept of perfecting skin!

✓☺ **Perfecting Night Cream** *($34 for 2.25 ounces)* would be a very good moisturizer for normal to dry skin. It contains several state-of-the-art antioxidants and water-binding agents.

✓☺ **$$$ Perfecting Serum** *($52 for 1 ounce)* is a lightweight lotion of water-binding agents, antioxidants, and plant oils. It is a very good moisturizer for someone with normal to slightly dry skin.

☺ **Skin Perfecting Lotion** *($27 for 2 ounces)* is a matte-finish moisturizer that contains retinol along with other very good antioxidants and water-binding agents. However, there is nothing in it that will perfect skin. It does contain arnica, a possible skin irritant.

☹ **Skin Smoothing Cream SPF 8** *($48 for 1.7 ounces)* has a too-low SPF rating and no UVA-protecting ingredients. It is inconceivable that any line endorsed by a physician would sell a product with an SPF of less than 15 and that did not include UVA-protecting ingredients.

☺ **Skin Soothing Formula** *($10.50 for 0.5 ounce)* is merely Vaseline, lanolin, vitamin E, waxes, and a tiny amount of BHA. It doesn't have the right pH for the salicylic acid to be effective as an exfoliant.

The Reviews M

✔☺ **Environmental Shield Oil Free Sunblock SPF 15** *($20 for 2 ounces)* is a very good, titanium dioxide–based sunscreen that also contains some very good antioxidants and a water-binding agent. This is an excellent option for normal to dry skin.

✔☺ **Environmental Shield Hydrating Sunscreen SPF 15** *($23 for 4.2 ounces)* is a very good, in-part avobenzone-based sunscreen that contains an impressive mix of antioxidants and water-binding agents. It is a very good option for normal to dry skin.

✔☺ **Environmental Shield Waterproof Sunblock SPF 30** *($25 for 4.2 ounces)* is similar to the Hydrating Sunscreen SPF 15 above and the same basic comments apply, though this does contain a film-forming agent that creates a water-resistant application.

☺ **Environmental Shield Age Proof Self Tanner SPF 15** *($25 for 4.2 ounces)* is a good, in-part avobenzone-based sunscreen that also contains dihydroxyacetone, the same ingredient used in all self-tanners to affect skin color.

☹ **Acne Management Formula** *($13 for 0.5 ounce)* contains AHA and BHA, though the pH is too high for them to be effective as exfoliants, and so this won't manage breakouts.

☹ **Acne Prone Skin Formula** *($48 for 3.3 ounces)* lists alcohol as the second ingredient, and that makes it too drying and irritating for all skin types.

☹ **Hydrating Gel Masque** *($25 for 2.25 ounces)*. This peel-off mask wouldn't be a problem, but several of the plant extracts, including arnica, ivy, and pellitory, can be irritating for most skin types.

☺ **Purifying Clay Masque** *($22.50 for 2.25 ounces)* is a standard clay mask with some very good water-binding agents and antioxidants.

NAD'S GEL HAIR REMOVAL

Nad's Gel Hair Removal *($29.95 for one kit)* is a hair remover that uses a method known as sugaring. Sugaring involves the use of sugars with a caramel-like consistency instead of wax to remove hair. That is, it works identically to regular waxing, only instead of spreading a wax substance over the skin, you're spreading caramel.

I have to say this is one of the first products I've ever run into where the claim of being 100% natural and organic is 100% true. Nad's ingredients are honey, molasses, fructose, vinegar, lemon juice, water, alcohol, and food dye. Nothing synthetic there! But does that make it better than waxing, as the company claims? First, waxing isn't unnatural because wax is a natural substance. And as far as hair removal is concerned, the effect is identical. You spread the Nad's caramel gel over the hair you want removed (there needs to be some hair length or there won't be anything for it to grab on to). Then you rip it off and out comes the hair, same as waxing.

The two main positives to sugaring over waxing are, first, sugaring's mess washes away, while wax has to be peeled or scratched off (and that isn't easy). Plus caramel doesn't have to be heated, while wax does! Easy cleanup and a relatively easier application are the incredible benefits of sugaring.

But before you jump on the bandwagon of Nad's or other sugaring hair-removal systems, there are several concerns about the veracity of the claims that accompany the sugaring method for getting rid of unwanted hair. Nad's states "when you use Nad's, the hair is extracted, including the roots so re-growth is softer, finer and slower." That isn't true. Hormones and genetics determine hair growth and hair thickness, not hair removal. What does happen when you "tweeze" or otherwise pull out hair is that because it has been removed closer to the root the next hair takes longer to get back to the top. This is unlike shaving, which removes hair only from the surface, so the hair pops back out faster. Also, because each hair follicle has a different rate of growth, the hair can seem softer because there will be less of it as it grows back than what was present when you first waxed or sugared.

There are also claims about sugaring preventing ingrown hairs. Ingrown hairs are unrelated to the way hair is removed. Ingrown hairs occur because after a hair has been removed below the skin's surface, the new hair sometimes has trouble finding its way back to the surface. That applies to hair removal in general, regardless of whether you shave, tweeze, sugar, wax, or use depilatories.

Another claim: "Because of the natural substances in Nad's, there is little chance of irritations. Redness for a short time is normal, depending on how sensitive your skin is." Natural or not, ripping out hair hurts, and for some skin types that can be a problem. Sugaring does not require heating, so it's less irritating than hot waxing—but that isn't about natural. For more information about Nad's, call (800) 653-9797 or visit www.nads.com.

NARS

Francois Nars, a French-born makeup artist and accomplished photographer, started his cosmetics line later in the game compared to his contemporaries (everyone from M.A.C. to Stila) at a time when anyone hoping to join the established makeup artistry lines needed a good hook. NARS met that challenge by offering richer, bolder colors that were unabashedly shiny and often glittery. Mass quantities of party-time shine and fashion magazine "must-have" color mandates were bound to get attention, and soon every Park Avenue diva worth her weight in Manolo Blahniks shoes or Prada handbags was clamoring for blushes with names like Orgasm and Mata Hari, and sinfully deep red lipsticks dubbed Fire Down Below and Scarlet Empress. It also helped that NARS products were sold in trendy stores like Barneys New York, and that Francois Nars regularly made appearances at his counters. The attention and press eventually caught the eye of Shiseido, which purchased the NARS line in 2000. With considerable financial backing, NARS was able to extend their color line as well as launch a skin-care collection, not to mention increase the NARS presence in dozens more department stores. Francois also published a cleverly designed, mostly practical book, *Makeup Your Mind,* which competes nicely with similar tomes from Bobbi Brown and the late Kevyn Aucoin.

Much can be said about the makeup side of this cosmetics line, but there is little to be said about the skin-care products other than "Why bother?" or better yet, "What were they thinking?" The cleansers are drying, the toners are dated formulations of alcohol and other irritants, and the moisturizers are mundane, poorly conceived and dated formulations. A little grape juice won't save a mix of alcohol, film-forming agent, and waxes, especially not at these inflated prices. And sunscreen? Forget about it! For more information about NARS, call (212) 941-0890 or (888) 903-NARS, or visit www.narscosmetics.com.

NARS Skin Care

☹ **Purifying Soap** *($19 for 6.7 ounces)* is a standard, detergent- and tallow-based, highly alkaline soap that can be drying and irritating for most skin types.

☺ **$$$ Balancing Foam Cleanser** *($30 for 4.2 ounces)* is a standard, detergent-based cleanser that can be more drying than most.

☺ **$$$ Gentle Cream Cleanser** *($32 for 4.2 ounces)* is almost identical to the Balancing Foam Cleanser above, and the same comments apply.

☹ **Hydrating Freshening Lotion** *($35 for 6.7 ounces)*. Both the second and fifth ingredients are alcohol, and that is neither hydrating nor refreshing. What an extremely dated and poorly conceived formulation this is, for any skin type.

☹ **Balancing Toning Lotion** *($32 for 6.7 ounces)* is similar to the Hydrating Freshening Lotion above, and the same comments apply. This one adds camphor and eucalyptus to the mix, which is like adding fuel to a burning fire.

☹ **Essential Vitamin Serum** *($70 for 2.5 ounces)* lists alcohol and film-forming agent as its primary ingredients, and then there are some thickeners, a tiny bit of vitamin A, more alcohol, potassium hydroxide (that's lye), fragrance, and a minuscule amount of vitamin E. The only thing essential about this product is the need not to use it.

☺ **$$$ Hydrating Moisture Cream** *($65 for 3.4 ounces)* contains mostly water, plant oil, thickeners, slip agents, silicones, Vaseline, vitamin A, fragrance, film-forming agent, potassium hydroxide, grape oil, a minute amount of vitamin C, and preservatives. This boring moisturizer is not worth your time or money.

☹ **Balancing Moisture Lotion** *($50 for 2.5 ounces)* contains more alcohol and potassium hydroxide than it does any beneficial ingredients. The teeny amounts of antioxidants are meaningless for skin.

☺ **$$$ Aqua Gel Hydrator** *($70 for 3.4 ounces)* is a silicone-based moisturizer with many of the same problems the other moisturizers in this line have. The only difference is that this one contains a teeny bit more antioxidants, but not enough to warrant using it. The claim that it contains 87% water is basically letting you know that there isn't much of anything else in here. Plus your skin doesn't need water (healthy skin is only 10% water, and too much water destroys the skin's structure). Rather, the skin needs ingredients that support its structure, antioxidants to reduce free-radical damage, and sunscreen to prevent sun damage—something this line almost completely ignores.

☺ **$$$ Lip Conditioner** *($21 for 0.12 ounce)* is a standard emollient lip balm that contains a small amount of antioxidants.

NARS MAKEUP

Although Francois Nars's use of color is unconventional and does more to shock than to enhance, his general application tips are beneficial and his book *Makeup Your Mind* clearly puts his products to good use on a wide variety of skin tones, from ghostly pale to deep ebony. He has beautifully demonstrated what he is capable of, and has some admirable products to back his skills. Personal talent aside, when you get right down to it, the NARS makeup has as many strengths as weaknesses. It reaches its zenith with blushes, foundation shades, brushes, and lipsticks, but fails to rise above the horizon when it comes to eyeshadows, concealers, pencils, and mascaras. This isn't a line to shop if your makeup tastes are conservative or if you prefer a wide selection of matte shades, but everyone else will be in their glory, especially if the price tags don't stop them.

One bonus of shopping most makeup artist–styled lines is that you are more likely to find an educated sales staff with some makeup application and artistry skills, and NARS is such a line. If you ask, you may receive a makeup lesson with one of the line's onsite artists. As long as you're comfortable with this, and keep the emphasis on technique as opposed to multiple sales, it can be an invaluable experience.

FOUNDATION: There are two types of liquid foundation available, each housed in a pump bottle that can take some getting used to when it comes to controlling how much you use. ☺ $$$ **Balanced Foundation** *($38)* is a very standard, oil-based foundation that has a rich, creamy feel and finish. This is appropriate only for normal to very dry skin that prefers medium coverage. The color range is superior, but avoid Sahara (slightly pink) and Sedona and Santa Fe (both slightly peach). There are some good options for darker skin tones. **Gel Fraicheur** *($30)* is really more of a lightweight tinted moisturizer than a foundation. The texture is slightly creamy, blending on very sheer and drying to a soft powder finish. This would be suitable for all but very oily skin, and of the four shades, only Antilles is too orange to recommend. This lists SPF 10 on the product, but no active ingredients are present, so do not rely on this for any sun protection.

☺ $$$ **Oil Free Foundation** *($38)* claims its finish is semi-matte, but it is actually true matte. This may be an option for normal to oily skin, but the texture is rather heavy, lending itself to medium coverage, and the short-lived matte finish is slightly sticky. The best attribute of this makeup is the impressive selection of colors—just avoid Sahara and Santa Fe, which are too pink and peach for most skin tones. **Makeup Primer** *($28)* is just an ultra-light moisturizer that supposedly "primes" the skin for foundation. There is no reason to layer this many products on your face (moisturizer, often specialty treatments, then makeup primer, and then foundation); it doesn't help the makeup perform or hold up any better on the skin. As a moisturizer, it lacks any state-of-the-art water-binding agents or antioxidants.

☺ $$$ **CONCEALER:** The lipstick-style **Concealer** *($16.50)* provides creamy, opaque coverage. NARS claims this is "creamy yet crease-resistant," but it can indeed slip into the lines around the eyes. If you prefer creamy, lipstick-style concealers, there are some colors to consider, but avoid Honey, Praline (both too pink), Custard (too peach), and Toffee (too orange).

<u>POWDER:</u> ☹ $$$ **Pressed Powder** *($24)* is a talc-free formula with a soft texture that crumbles easily, but does afford a silky-smooth finish with a touch of shine. It looks much better on the skin if applied with a brush (which is true of most powders).

☺ $$$ **Loose Powder** *($30)* is messier than usual, but that is a packaging issue that will hopefully be addressed soon. This is otherwise a gorgeous powder that looks beautifully natural on the skin, with only a trace of shine. The five shades are exemplary—Snow is ideal for very fair skin, but watch out for Mountain, which can be too ash on dark skin tones. The **Bronzing Powder** *($24)* makes me think I may eventually have to concede that all bronzing powders should have shine, since countless cosmetics lines offer just that, and NARS is no exception. If you want a soft shine from your bronzer, this is an attractive, sheer-finish option that applies softly.

<u>BLUSH:</u> NARS has an impressive, attractive selection of ✔☺ $$$ **Blush** *($20)*. They have a splendid texture and there are some viable options for a matte or shiny finish. Caution: Most of the colors are very strongly pigmented, so use the least amount possible and build from there. Many of these colors would be gorgeous on darker skin tones. Desire and Mata Hari are two of the best true pink blushes out there. The distractingly shiny shades include Orgasm, Silvana, and Sin. ✔☺ **Color Wash** *($24)* is NARS's version of BeneFit's BeneTint liquid blush, but the NARS product bests BeneFit by offering more color choices, and each one is suitable for a natural, flushed appearance or subtle lip stain.

☹ $$$ **The Multiple** *($33)* is a chunky, wind-up stick that has a creamy, somewhat greasy texture and soft, sheer colors that would work for cheeks, eyes, and, in some cases, lips. Although all of the colors have varying degrees of shine, these are an option for a fun evening look, though the price is extraordinary for what amounts to sheer, shiny color. Shop around before making a final decision on this one.

☹ <u>EYESHADOW:</u> Both the **Single Eye Shadow** *($17)* and the **Eye Shadow Duos** *($27)* have an OK, slightly dry texture and are very pigmented, which causes them to blend on unevenly, not to mention that the shine flies everywhere. With colors this strong, you need a smooth, silky texture to artfully apply and blend them. There are a few almost matte duos to consider, but I wouldn't label any of these a must-have—the majority of shades are too Technicolor-bright or too intensely shiny for daytime wear. **Cream Eye Shadow** *($17)* eyeshadows are exceedingly shiny and have a smooth texture that stays moist, so they won't stay in place and will fade. If creamy eyeshadows are what you're after, look to BeneFit or M.A.C. first.

<u>EYE AND BROW SHAPER:</u> The four ☹ $$$ **Eye Liner Pencils** *($16.50)* and four waxy ☹ **Eyebrow Pencils** *($16.50)* are as standard as they come (the Eye Liner Pencils are slightly more creamy than the drier-finish Eyebrow Pencils), and absolutely not worth the price. **Glitter Pencil** *($24)* is a fairly creamy, thick pencil infused with flecks of glitter. The glitter tends to chip off onto the face and the price tag on this is just absurd. **Liquid**

Liner *($27)* is insanely priced given the number of superior liquid liners available for less than $10. NARS's version comes in a nail-polish bottle and features an OK brush and mostly wild colors that go on sheer. Repeated applications are necessary to build intensity, and that increases the odds against precise, even application. Why anyone would bother with this is beyond me—if you want to spend this kind of money on liquid liner, I suggest Lancome's fantastic Artliner ($25).

LIPSTICK AND LIP PENCIL: The NARS lipstick collection is supremely good, and if you're willing to tolerate the costs you won't be disappointed by the opulent colors and reasonable wear time. Although there are three kinds of lipsticks, the NARS counter display doesn't separate them, which is frustrating. However, if you shop this line at Sephora, you'll find that the various formulas are grouped together and a pleasure to navigate. The ☺ $$$ **Satins** *($21)* are creamy, bordering on greasy, and are fairly opaque. The **Sheers** *($21)* are quite glossy and offer coverage that is light rather than sheer. The colors are great. The ✓☺ **Semi-Mattes** *($21)* are the real standouts here; they have an opaque, slightly creamy finish and a good stain. Creamy lipsticks don't get much better than this, and this formula comprises the bulk of the NARS lipstick colors.

☺ $$$ **Lip Gloss** *($20)* features some bold colors in a sticky, thick formula whose price is unwarranted for what you get, which is just a gloss, and a rather tacky-feeling one at that. **Lip Therapy** *($21)* is just a glossy, emollient lipstick available in a colorless or barely-there pink shade. This lists an SPF 20, but no active ingredients accompany the sunscreen claim, so that means it's null and void.

☺ $$$ **Lip Lacquer** *($20)* is an improvement over the Lip Gloss above, with a much smoother, less sticky texture. If you must spend this kind of money for standard lip gloss, choose this one and delight in the gorgeous colors that go from mild to wild. **Lip Liner Pencil** *($16.50)* claims it won't bleed or feather, and although that won't hold true for everyone, this one does have a drier finish that should keep those problems in check for a few hours, at least. The color selection is small but good.

☹ **MASCARA:** NARS's **Mascara** *($19)* should, at this price, be the gold standard. Instead, it's merely substandard, taking too much effort to build much length or thickness. It stays wet on the lashes for far too long, and some smearing is inevitable. **Waterproof Mascara** *($19)* shares similar traits, only this one tends to stick the lashes together and creates a spiky look. This is hardly waterproof either, which is a real letdown given the price.

☺ $$$ **BRUSHES:** The **Brushes** *($18–$50)* almost all have a lovely, soft feel and are appropriately shaped for a variety of application techniques. The only ones to steer clear of are the **Brow Brush** *($20)*, which is too scratchy, along with the **Lip Brush** *($18)* and **Retractable Lip Brush** *($18)*, which are really too small for most women's lips. The **Push Eyeliner** *($24)* is identical to those found in many other lines, except that NARS charges more. The best brushes are the ✓☺ **Point Concealer** *($22)*, ✓☺ **Flat Concealer** *($25)*, ✓☺ **Angular Eye Shader** *($24)*, the pricey, but luxurious ✓☺ **Eye Shader** *($55)*, and the ✓☺ **Liquid Eyeliner** *($20)*.

☺ **$$$** <u>SPECIALTY</u>: **Body Glow** *($55)* comes in a heavy glass bottle and is just coconut oil with golden bronze shimmer and potent fragrance. This would be an expensive way to complete your St. Tropez tanned look, which I hope was also from a bottle and not from the sun! **Face Glow** *($30)* is less shiny and fragrant than the Body Glow, but is rather expensive for a shimmery face lotion; not to mention that it lists an SPF of 10 without any active sunscreen ingredients (a disturbing trend in this line). Revlon SkinLights Face Illuminator SPF 10 ($13.99) works just as well, and comes in several shimmery shades. **Nail Polish** *($15)* truly offers something for everyone, with a color range that goes from classic red to icy silver. Finding a nail color to coordinate with your lipstick is almost always chic, and you won't be disappointed here. **Artist's Palette** *($53–$67)* is the NARS take on Trish McEvoy's makeup planners, only with hers you get to choose the colors. These are overpriced, preselected colors that have limited appeal unless you prefer almost all of your makeup colors to be shiny; however, for the twenty-something Disco Queen on the run, these may be just the ticket. If you're curious to try these, the smartest, most workable colors are in the Lust for Life and Erotica palettes.

NATURA BISSE (SKIN CARE ONLY)

If you've heard of or sampled Natura Bisse, I suspect that must mean you've been hanging out at the Neiman Marcus makeup counters where this overpriced, pointless line is sold. It is hyped (and I mean overhyped) as an AHA product line that is supposed to provide the highest concentration of AHAs you can buy. That does seem to be the case, but as you will see from the reviews, it is likely that they do not have the concentration stated on the label or they could pose a serious risk to skin.

There are a host of other gimmicks lurking in this line, ranging from thymus extract to amniotic fluid, horse protein serum, and a handful of plant extracts, none of which can benefit skin in any substantial way. There are also products claiming to add oxygen to the skin, but none of them contain enough to give air to one skin cell. For all the hoopla this line makes about advanced skin-care formulations, the SPFs are dismal, and for the most part the sunscreens don't contain UVA-protecting ingredients. So much for up-to-date research on the part of this line! Natura Bisse may have an elite air about it, but many of the products are poorly formulated. If you're going to overspend on skin care, this is not the place to waste your money. For more information about Natura Bisse, call (800) 7-NATURA or visit www.naturabisse.com. **Note:** All Natura Bisse products contain fragrance unless otherwise noted.

☺ **$$$ China Clay Cleanser Purifying and Cleansing Paste** *($37 for 4.2 ounces)* is a standard, detergent-based, water-soluble cleanser that contains some clay (China clay is merely a trade name for standard clay, nothing as interesting as the name implies), fragrance, and preservatives, and that's it. It's an exceptionally overpriced cleanser that is still an option for normal to oily skin.

☺ $$$ **Oily Skin Milk Cleanser** *($28 for 6.5 ounces)* is simply cleanser with several ingredients that are extremely problematic for oily skin, including Vaseline and potentially irritating plant extracts. This can be an option for normal to dry skin, but mostly it is just ill-advised.

☺ $$$ **Dry Skin Milk Cleanser** *($24 for 6.5 ounces)* is an extremely basic, mineral oil– and Vaseline-based wipe-off cleanser that is an overpriced option for dry skin.

☺ $$$ **Facial Cleansing Gel Foaming Cleanser** *($28 for 7 ounces)* is a standard, detergent-based, water-soluble cleanser that is an option for normal to oily skin.

☺ $$$ **Facial Cleansing Gel + A.H.A. for Normal to Oily Skin** *($36 for 6.5 ounces)* is a standard, detergent-based cleanser that contains about 4% AHA. However, the pH of the product is 5, which makes it ineffective for exfoliation. This also contains a small amount of sodium lauryl sulfate as one of the cleansing agents and that may be potentially too irritating for all skin types, and at this price there shouldn't be any mistakes for your skin to worry about.

☺ $$$ **Facial Cleansing Cream + A.H.A. for Dry Skin** *($36 for 6.5 ounces)* is a standard, detergent-based cleanser that contains about 4% AHA; however, the pH of 5 makes it ineffective for exfoliation.

☺ $$$ **Eye Make-Up Remover Hypo-Allergenic Lotion** *($25 for 3.3 ounces)* is just water, a detergent cleansing agent, plant extracts, alcohol, and fragrance. Between the alcohol and fragrance, this is anything but hypoallergenic, and although it will take off eye makeup, using this around the eyes is not the best idea.

☹ $$$ **Dry Skin Toner Moisturizing Toner** *($27 for 6.5 ounces)* is an OK, ordinary toner that is primarily water, slip agent, amniotic fluid, castor oil, and preservatives. I won't even get into the nonsense about the amniotic fluid, but this contains Kathon CG, a preservative that is not recommended for use in leave-on products such as this one. For more specific information about Kathon CG refer to Chapter Seven, *Cosmetics Dictionary*.

☹ **Oily Skin Toner, Astringent** *($27 for 6.5 ounces)* is mostly alcohol and is not recommended for any skin type.

☹ **Action Complex Facial Fluid with Vitamin A+C+E** *($102 for 1 ounce)* lists alcohol as the second ingredient, which makes this potentially irritating and drying for all skin types. This also contains Kathon CG, a preservative that is not recommended for use in leave-on products such as this one.

☹ **Double Action Hydroprotective Day Cream for Dry Skin SPF 10** *($63 for 2.5 ounces)* has an unacceptably low SPF of 10, and that's bad enough, but this product also doesn't contain the UVA-protecting ingredients of avobenzone, titanium dioxide, or zinc oxide, and is not recommended.

☺ $$$ **Elastin Refirming Night Cream for Deeply Dry Skin** *($56 for 2.5 ounces)* is a mediocre moisturizer for normal to dry skin. The elastin is a good water-binding agent, but it can have no effect on the elastin in the skin.

The Reviews N

☺ $$$ **Essential Shock Night Cream for Dry Skin** *($95 for 2.5 ounces)* is almost identical to the Elastin Refirming Night Cream above, and the same basic comments apply.

☹ $$$ **Essential Shock Concentrate** *($160 for 2 sets of 12 0.1-ounce vials)* is a two-part product, with the ampoules containing amniotic fluid and alcohol, and the bottle containing water-binding agents. The only shocking thing about this is that there are women buying this stuff who think it will be helpful for skin.

☹ **Essential Shock Eye and Lip Treatment SPF 15** *($52 for 0.5 ounce)* doesn't contain the UVA-protecting ingredients of avobenzone, titanium dioxide, or zinc oxide, and is not recommended.

☹ **Eye Contour Cream SPF 10** *($65 for 0.8 ounce)* has an inadequate SPF number and it doesn't contain the UVA-protecting ingredients of avobenzone, titanium dioxide, or zinc oxide, and is not recommended. It isn't even a very interesting moisturizer on top of the disappointing SPF.

☹ **Stimul-Eye Complex** *($62 for 1 ounce of Active Gel, 0.8 ounce of Active Lotion, and 24 eye pads).* The Active Gel is applied to the eye area and then you soak the little pads (they're cut in the shape of the eye area) with Active Lotion and place that over the eye. Don't worry, you don't have to go out like this, it is meant as a treatment you leave on for 15 minutes. You then remove the pads and massage the rest into the skin. The Active Gel contains mostly water, seaweed, slip agent, water-binding agent, and preservative, which makes it a rather boring moisturizer for normal to oily skin. The Active Lotion is mostly water, glycerin, fragrant plant extracts, slip agents, castor oil, a teeny amount of water-binding agent, and preservatives, which makes it a substandard toner. All together, that adds up to an overpriced, rather useless product. It also contains Kathon CG, a preservative that is not recommended for use in leave-on products such as this one.

☹ **Hydra Complex SPF 10** *($118 for 1.7 ounces)* has an inadequate SPF number and it doesn't contain the UVA-protecting ingredients of avobenzone, titanium dioxide, or zinc oxide, and is not recommended.

☺ $$$ **Hydroprotective Concentrate for Dry Skin** *($78 for 1.2 ounces)* is just thickeners with lanolin and a tiny amount of water-binding agents and antioxidants, when for the money you would expect much more. Instead, you end up getting way too little of the stuff that skin really needs.

☺ $$$ **Rose Mosqueta Oil for Dry Aged Skin** *($45 for 1 ounce).* Rose mosqueta oil is another name for rose hip oil, but this doesn't contain all that much of it, as there are also thickening agents in here. Rose hip oil is a good antioxidant, but there are lots of good antioxidants, like vitamin E oil capsules, which are available for a lot less money and without the added fragrance and thickening agents.

☹ **Special Lift Immediate Firming Concentrate** *($45 for 0.6 ounce).* What can I say about a product that contains mostly amniotic fluid, serum protein, and alcohol? Other than "what a waste of money," I can tell you that amniotic fluid and serum protein are good water-binding agents, but the alcohol undoes any benefit you might get from them.

☹ **Stabilizing Concentrate** *($92 for 12 0.1-ounce ampoules)* won't stabilize anything, and with alcohol as the third ingredient this is primarily drying and irritating for all skin types. It does contain some good water-binding agents, but their effectiveness is negated by the alcohol.

☹ **Stabilizing Gel Cream for Oily Skin** *($46 for 2.5 ounces)* contains mostly alcohol, which won't stabilize anyone's skin, though it can be extremely irritating and drying. Aside from that, it is a very mundane, lightweight moisturizer with a small quantity of water-binding agents and fractional amounts of antioxidants.

☹ **Titian Neck and Chest Firming Serum** *($80 for 1.7 ounces)* is similar to the Stabilizing Concentrate above, and the same review applies.

☺ **$$$ Green Tea Extract Facial Phyto-Firming Serum** *($46 for 1 ounce)* is just water, slip agent, green tea, alcohol, thickener, and preservatives. I'm sure there is some reason for this ordinary gel lotion, but I can't think of one. It would be far healthier for you to just drink a cup of green tea than to bother with this.

☹ **Vital Gel Cream for Mature Skin SPF 10** *($80 for 2.5 ounces)* has a too-low SPF of 10, which is bad enough, but it also doesn't contain avobenzone, titanium dioxide, or zinc oxide for UVA protection, and is not recommended. How un-vital can you get?

☺ **$$$ Ananas Finishing Mask, for Mature Skin** *($40 for 4.2 ounces)* includes anana, a fancy name for pineapple extract, which can be a skin irritant, though there's not much of it in here so it probably isn't a problem. Other than that, it's just a bunch of thickening agents and not one other beneficial ingredient for skin, which makes it a do-nothing kind of mask.

☺ **$$$ Stimul-Eye Mask** *($38 for 1 ounce)* is an emollient moisturizer with a film-forming agent to give it that "mask" feel on skin. It does contain small amounts of water-binding agents and anti-irritants, but overall it is just OK and not worth taking the time to sit through the application process.

☺ **$$$ Thermal Mud Finishing Mask for Oily Skin** *($38 for 4.2 ounces)* doesn't contain any mud whatsoever. This is just a bunch of thickening agents with some magnesium aluminum silicate. Almost all of the thickening agents are problematic for oily skin, and while the magnesium aluminum silicate can absorb oil from skin, the thickening agents can be a problem; using generic milk of magnesia from the drugstore will provide far better results.

NATURA BISSE SENSITIVE LINE

The Sensitive Line products all contain white willow (another name for willow bark) and green tea, both of which are good anti-irritants (willow bark is the source of salicylates, which are related to aspirin). However, almost all the items in this Sensitive Line group of products also either contain significant skin irritants or simply lack much else of particular interest for skin. It is also important to mention that those two ingredients, as well as other effective anti-irritants, are found in lots and lots of products that are far less pricey than these.

☺ $$$ **Sensitive Cleansing Cream for All Skin Types** *($34 for 6.5 ounces)* is an incredibly standard, overpriced, detergent-based, water-soluble cleanser that would be good for most skin types. It contains a small amount of papaya extract, which can be a skin irritant, but there probably isn't enough of it to affect skin negatively.

☹ $$$ **Sensitive Toner for All Skin Types** *($22.50 for 6.5 ounces)* is a good, though exceedingly boring, toner for most skin types. This does contain Kathon CG, a preservative that should not be used in products meant to be left on the skin, and that is definitely not appropriate for sensitive skin.

☹ $$$ **Sensitive Concentrate Calming Concentrate for All Sensitive Skin Types** *($120 for 1.7 ounces)* is a rather standard lotion moisturizer that contains Kathon CG, a preservative that should not be used in products meant to be left on the skin.

☹ $$$ **Sensitive Soothing Gel Cream for All Skin Types** *($60 for 2.5 ounces)* is an exceptionally ordinary moisturizer for normal to dry skin with a mere dusting of antioxidants and water-binding agents. This also contains Kathon CG, a preservative that should not be used in products meant to be left on the skin.

☹ $$$ **Sensitive Soothing Night Cream for All Skin Types** *($70 for 2.5 ounces)* is similar to the Sensitive Gel Cream above, and just as boring, with minimal interesting ingredients and the same Kathon CG preservative issue.

☹ $$$ **Sensitive Eye Gel Calming Gel for the Eyes** *($52 for 0.8 ounce)* is similar to the Sensitive Soothing Gel Cream above, and poses the same concerns.

☺ $$$ **Sensitive Soothing Mask for All Skin Types** *($32 for 2.5 ounces)* is basically just thickening agents and film-forming agent, with some plant extracts. It does contain a tiny bit of papaya extract, which can be a skin irritant for most skin types, but probably not enough to affect the skin. There are also small amounts of plant extracts that can be anti-irritants, but they are barely present in this formulation and can have little to no impact on skin.

NATURA BISSE OXYGEN LINE

☹ **Oxygen Cream for All Skin Types** *($65 for 2.5 ounces)*. You have to sit down for this one. This contains a very standard group of thickening agents with some egg yolk, lanolin, and hydrogen peroxide (that's right, the stuff you buy at the drugstore for 89 cents for 8 ounces). Most important, hydrogen peroxide does have an unstable oxygen molecule that can impact skin, but that generates free-radical damage, greatly reducing the production of healthy new skin cells. The cumulative problems that can stem from impacting the skin with a substance that is known to generate free-radical damage and impair the skin's healing process, cause cellular destruction, and reduce optimal cell functioning, means this is an ingredient it is best to avoid using (Sources: *Carcinogenesis,* March 2002, pages 469–475; *Anticancer Research,* July-August 2001, pages 2719–2724; and *Plastic and Reconstructive Surgery,* September 2001, pages 675–687). Please refer to information about free-radical damage in Chapter Seven, *Cosmetics Dictionary,* for more specifics.

☹ **Oxygen Concentrate for All Skin Types** *($120 for 12 ampoules totaling 1.2 ounces)* is similar to the Oxygen Cream above, except that the second ingredient listed in this one is alcohol, so this is irritating, drying, potentially damaging to skin, and a waste of money. This product is a contender for the most useless and potentially most skin-damaging product in this entire book.

☹ **Oxygen Finishing Mask, for All Skin Types** *($32 for 4.2 ounces)* is a standard clay mask with alcohol as the second ingredient, plus hydrogen peroxide for the oxygen.

NATURA BISSE GLYCO LINE

These glycolic acid–based products are a mixed bag; some have pH levels that are effective for exfoliation and some do not. Other than the AHA these products contain, they are not specially formulated in any way, and are not preferred over Alpha Hydrox products, which are available at the drugstore. What is of most concern are the two AHA treatment products that not only claim to have a glycolic acid content of 25% and 50%, but also claim that they do not cause photosensitivity. According to the FDA's *Backgrounder* report (July 7, 1997, www.fda.gov), "[AHAs are] safe for use in cosmetic products at concentrations less than or equal to 10 percent, at final formulation pHs greater than or equal to 3.5, when formulated to avoid increasing the skin's sensitivity to the sun, or when directions for use include the daily use of sun protection. [For salon use, AHA products are] safe for use at concentrations less than or equal to 30 percent, at final formulation pHs greater than or equal to 3.0, in products designed for brief, discontinuous use followed by thorough rinsing from the skin, when applied by trained professionals, and when application is accompanied by directions for the daily use of sun protection." For more details, see my comments in the introduction to the Natura Bisse line.

☹ **Glyco-Balance** *($75 for 3.3 ounces)* is just water, alcohol, AHA, pH balancer, thickeners, and preservatives. This basic AHA product contains too much alcohol, making it too irritating and drying for all skin types at any price. The pH of 4 does mean that this AHA product will be effective for some amount of exfoliation, but there are AHA products that have far more elegant and non-irritating formulations than this one, and for far less.

☺ $$$ **Glyco-Eye Exfoliating Eye Contour Cream** *($67 for 0.8 ounce)* has a pH of 5, which means that the 12% concentration of AHAs will not be effective for exfoliation, but that's probably good news for the eye area. Other than the AHAs, this has only a negligible amount of antioxidants and a water-binding agent. The minuscule amount of thymus extract in this product has no impact on skin. Overpriced and completely not worth the money sums this one up quite nicely.

☺ $$$ **Glyco-Face Exfoliating Cream with Glycolic Acid for Normal to Dry Skin** *($75 for 2.5 ounces)* is virtually identical to the Glyco-Eye version above, and the same comments apply.

☺ $$$ **Glyco-Peeling 25%** *($122 for 12 0.1-ounce ampoules)* contains mostly alcohol, which can be drying and irritating for skin. However, as an AHA product it does have a somewhat effective pH of 4, which means it will exfoliate skin. Please see the

The Reviews N

comments above in the introduction for the Glyco Line products as well as the introduction to Natura Bisse regarding AHA concentrations before considering use of this product.

☹ **Glyco-Peeling Plus 50%** *($160 for 12 0.1-ounce ampoules)* is similar to the 25% version above, but supposedly with twice the concentration of AHAs in a pH of 3.5. This amount of AHA in this pH should be of great concern for personal use at home, but I am hoping the concentration percentage is wrong or misrepresented.

NATURA BISSE BRILLIANCE LINE

☺ **$$$ Lightening Milk** *($39 for 6.5 ounces)* is an extremely standard, mineral oil–based, wipe-off cleanser that also contains a small amount of kojic acid and AHAs. The AHAs make up less than 2% of the product's content, and the pH is too high for it to be effective for exfoliation. There is definitely convincing research, both in vitro and in vivo, and also in animal studies, showing that kojic acid is effective for inhibiting melanin production, but kojic acid is an extremely unstable ingredient in cosmetic formulations. Upon exposure to air or sunlight, it can lose its efficacy, and this product's packaging would not help keep it stable.

☹ **Lightening Toner** *($39 for 6.5 ounces)*. Alcohol is the second ingredient listed, which makes this toner too irritating and drying for all skin types, and that doesn't help lighten anything. It does contain kojic acid and AHAs, and the comments for those ingredients in the review for the Lightening Milk above apply here as well.

☺ **$$$ Intensive Lightening Complex** *($120 for 1 ounce)* contains 2% hydroquinone and about 7% AHAs, along with kojic acid. This is a potentially very effective combination for skin lightening, albeit for an absurd price (there are prescription compounds with more active ingredients than this that cost half the price—Tri-Luma, reviewed in this book, is an example). While this product would be an option, the second ingredient is alcohol, and that doesn't help skin in the least.

☺ **$$$ Nourishing Lightening Cream** *($80 for 1.7 ounces)* isn't nourishing in the least; it's just a basic moisturizer with less than 2% AHAs and some kojic acid. The comments for those ingredients in the review for the Lightening Milk above also apply here.

☺ **$$$ Lightening Finishing Mask** *($49 for 2.5 ounces)* is a thicker version of the Nourishing Lightening Cream above, and the same comments apply.

☹ **SPF 15 Protective Lightening Cream** *($80 for 2.5 ounces)* doesn't contain the UVA-protecting ingredients of avobenzone, titanium dioxide, or zinc oxide, and is not recommended.

NATURA BISSE VITAMIN C+C LINE

☺ **$$$ C+C Vitamin Complex Concentrated Serum with Double Vitamin C** *($130 for four 0.2-ounce ampoules)* is an inanely overpriced product that uses ascorbic acid in powder form as the source of vitamin C. You are supposed to mix it into a solution of slip agents, fragrant orange extract, silicone, thymus and placenta extract, more slip agent, more vitamin C, and preservatives. If you're looking for vitamin C this is fine, but lots and lots of products contain it with a lot less cumbersome application process. The thymus and placenta protein are good water-binding agents, but no better than lots of other water-binding agents.

☹ C+C Vitamin Cream Refirming Cream SPF 10 *($80 for 2.5 ounces)* has a dismally low SPF. It also lacks the UVA-protecting ingredients of avobenzone, titanium dioxide, or zinc oxide, and is completely un-firming for skin. It is not recommended.

☹ C+C Vitamin Fluid SPF 10 *($75 for 1.7 ounces)* has the same concerns as the Refirming Cream above, and the same comments apply.

NATURA BISSE CYTOKINES LINE

The Cytokines Line products are supposed to contain "Skin Growth Factors," but there isn't one ingredient in them that functions as, is similar to, or has any relation to any type of growth factor. While these do contain some good water-binding agents and tiny amounts of antioxidants, they are not capable of affecting cellular growth or cellular activity in the way cytokines do. In fact, because two of the products contain mostly alcohol and because the sunscreen has an inadequate SPF and is ineffective for UVA protection, your skin cells will be decreasing, not increasing. And in regard to cytokines, these are not a type of ingredient.

You might be curious as to exactly what cytokines are. Cytokines are diverse, potent, and extremely complex chemical messengers secreted by the cells of the immune system that stimulate the production of other substances to help protect the body. Cytokines encourage cell growth, promote cell activation, direct cellular traffic, and destroy target cells—including cancer cells. Interleukins, transforming growth factor, and interferon are types of cytokines. It is also important to point out that cytokines can also cause unwanted, potentially serious side effects (Sources: http://www.medlineplus.com and the National Cancer Institute, http://www.nci.nih.gov or http://www.cancer.gov). Even the notion that skin-care products can directly affect cytokine production in a way to change the appearance of skin is a scary thought, given that cosmetic ingredients are not tested for safety the way pharmaceuticals or drugs are. There is nothing in these products that can positively affect the skin's immune system or growth structure, but they do contain elements that are not beneficial for skin.

☹ Cytokines Eye Contour Cell Renewal Gel *($68 for 0.8 ounce)* not only can't renew skin, but also contains a good deal of alcohol (the third ingredient), which kills cells; I imagine that would put you back where you began, as well as create irritation and dryness.

☹ Cytokines Top Ten Fluid Cell Renewal Complex *($130 for 0.8 ounce)* is similar to the Eye Contour Cell Renewal Gel above, and the same comments apply.

☹ Cytokines Facial Cell Renewal Day Cream SPF 10 *($72 for 1.7 ounces)* has a substandard SPF and doesn't contain the UVA-protecting ingredients of avobenzone, titanium dioxide, or zinc oxide, and is not recommended.

NATURA BISSE DIAMOND LINE

✔☺ $$$ **Diamond Bio-Lift Eye Contour Cream** *($130 for 0.8 ounce)* is a very good, though exceedingly overpriced, emollient moisturizer that contains an impressive assortment of water-binding agents and antioxidants.

✔☺ $$$ **Diamond Antiaging Bio-Regenerative Cream for Dry Skin** *($235 for 1.7 ounces)* is almost identical to the Bio-Lift Eye Contour Cream above, and the same comments apply.

☺ $$$ **Diamond Antiaging Bio-Regenerative Gel Cream** *($235 for 1.7 ounces)* is similar to the Bio-Lift Eye Contour Cream above, though with alcohol as the fourth ingredient it poses a concern for irritation and dryness.

NATURA BISSE SUN PRODUCTS

Please keep in mind that sunscreens must be applied liberally if you are going to achieve any protection from sun damage. If a sunscreen is so expensive that it prevents you from applying it liberally, you will not be getting the SPF protection indicated on the label.

☺ $$$ **Sensitive Sun Fluid SPF 25** *($45 for 4.2 ounces)* is a very good, though overpriced, titanium dioxide–based sunscreen in an emollient base that contains some good water-binding agents and antioxidants.

☺ $$$ **Extreme Sun Protector SPF 35** *($40 for 4.2 ounces)* is a good, in-part titanium dioxide–based sunscreen. It has an exceptionally mundane moisturizing base that is mostly thickeners, mineral oil, silicone, preservatives, and a teeny amount of antioxidants.

☺ $$$ **Sun Protector SPF 30 Hydrating Sun Block for All Skin Types** *($60 for 4.2 ounces)* is similar to the Extreme Sun version above and the same comments apply.

☹ **Sun Shield SPF 20** *($55 for 4.2 ounces)* doesn't contain the UVA-protecting ingredients of avobenzone, titanium dioxide, or zinc oxide, and is not recommended.

☹ **Sun Body Spray SPF 10** *($38 for 6.8 ounces)* has a substandard SPF and also doesn't contain the UVA-protecting ingredients of avobenzone, titanium dioxide, or zinc oxide, and is not recommended.

☺ **Self Tanning Cream SPF 10 Auto Bronze Cream** *($48 for 4.2 ounces)*. The sunscreen is useless (a too-low SPF and no UVA-protecting ingredients), but this product does contain dihydroxyacetone, the same ingredient all self-tanners use to affect the color of skin.

☺ **After Sun Rehydrating Lotion** *($39 for 8.8 ounces)* is a mediocre moisturizer that is not preferred even a little bit over Cetaphil Lotion or Lubriderm, which are available at the drugstore for a fraction of the price.

NEOSTRATA (SKIN CARE ONLY)

In the world of AHAs, Neostrata is one of only a few lines that offers reliable and effective formulations for exfoliation. Well-formulated AHA products are those that have an effective concentration of AHAs and a base with a pH that allows them to work. The exfoliation they provide reduces the thickness of the skin's outer layer, which in turn can solve many skin problems, including dryness, blemishes, sun damage, and skin discolorations. A good deal of research also shows that AHAs can help increase the thickness of the underlying layers of skin, improve skin structure, increase collagen production, and allow penetration of other skin-care ingredients. Moreover, Neostrata is one of the only companies to sell reliable sunscreens that also contain effective AHA formulations.

Many of Neostrata's products contain glycolic acid, but several also contain polyhydroxy acids (PHAs). PHA refers to gluconolactone or lactobionic acid. According to Neostrata, these PHAs are supposed to be just as effective as AHAs, but less irritating. (Keep in mind that Neostrata is the company that holds the patent for glycolic acid as an antiwrinkle agent, as well as a patent for gluconolactone and lactobionic acid for reducing the appearance of wrinkles.) Gluconolactone and lactobionic acid are chemically and functionally similar to AHAs. The significant difference between them is that gluconolactone and lactobionic acid have much larger molecular structures, which limits their ability to penetrate the skin, resulting in a reduction of irritating side effects. This reduced absorption into the skin supposedly doesn't hamper their effectiveness.

Does that mean gluconolactone and lactobionic acid are better for your skin than AHAs in the form of glycolic acid or lactic acid? Neostrata seems to think so, though there is no other research showing that to be the case. According to an Internet-published class lecture by Dr. Mark G. Rubin (Source: http://128.11.40.183/lasernews/rubin_lecture/21.html), a board-certified dermatologist and assistant clinical professor of dermatology at the University of California, San Diego, research on gluconolactone demonstrated only a "6% decrease in dermal penetration" in comparison to glycolic acid, which "isn't a dramatic improvement." Gluconolactone may be slightly less irritating for some skin types, but this isn't quite the magic bullet for exfoliation that beauty magazines and some cosmetics companies have been extolling. There is no independent research information available about lactobionic acid.

Neostrata products are available only through physicians. Call (800) 628-9904 to find a physician in your area who carries the products. For more information about Neostrata, visit www.neostrata.com.

☺ $$$ **Facial Cleanser PHA** 4 *($22 for 6 ounces)* is a standard, detergent-based, water-soluble cleanser with 4% PHA (or polyhydroxy acid). Even though this doesn't contain much AHA, it is still of concern in a cleanser where it may get into the eye area.

☹ **Solution for Oily and Acne Skin** *($21.50 for 4 ounces)* includes 8% AHAs, but the large amount of alcohol it also contains makes this too irritating and drying for all skin types.

☺ **Face and Body Lotion AHA 15** *($25 for 6.8 ounces)* is a simple moisturizer with 15% AHA. There is concern about using concentrations of AHA over 10% (Source: www.fda.gov); therefore, even though this product would be effective for exfoliation it is not recommended unless your physician recommends it.

☺ **Face Cream Plus AHA 15** *($25 for 1.75 ounces)* is almost identical to the Face and Body Lotion above except for the addition of a plant oil, which makes it better for dry skin. The same basic review applies.

☹ **Gel for Age Spots and Skin Lightening** *($23 for 1.6 ounces)* is a standard 2% hydroquinone skin-lightening product that also contains 10% AHAs. This would be a good product to try on sun-damage spots (also known erroneously as "age" spots), except that the second item on the ingredient list is alcohol, which can be drying and irritating for all skin types.

☹ **Gel Plus AHA 15** *($33 for 4 ounces)* lists alcohol as the second ingredient, and that makes it too drying and irritating for all skin types.

☹ **Oil Control Gel PHA / AHA 8** *($20 for 1 ounce)* lists alcohol as the second ingredient, and that makes it too drying and irritating for all skin types.

☺ **Skin Smoothing Cream AHA 8** *($18.75 for 1.75 ounces)* contains 8% AHAs in a very standard moisturizing cream base. This is a very good, though basic, AHA product for normal to dry skin.

☺ **Skin Smoothing Lotion AHA 10** *($20 for 6.8 ounces)* contains 10% AHAs and is quite similar to the Smoothing Cream above, but in lotion form. This is a good AHA product in an ordinary base for normal to dry skin.

☺ **Bio-Hydrating Cream PHA 15** *($25 for 1.75 ounces)* contains 15% PHA (poly-hydroxy acid) in a standard moisturizing base. It is effective for exfoliation, but it is important to be aware of the concerns about using such a high concentration of PHA (over 10%) given that its long-term effects on skin are unknown.

☺ **$$$ Bionic Face Cream PHA 12** *($40 for 1.75 ounces)* contains 12% PHA (poly-hydroxy acid) in a silicone-based moisturizer that also contains some good plant oils and small amounts of water-binding agents that make it good for normal to dry skin. However, there is concern about using such a high concentration of PHA (over 10%) given that its long-term effects on skin are unknown.

☺ **Bionic Lotion PHA 15** *($22 for 3.4 ounces)* is similar to the Bionic Face Cream above only in lotion form and with slightly more AHAs. The same basic comments apply.

✓☺ **$$$ Bionic Face Serum PHA 10** *($45 for 1 ounce)* contains 10% PHA (poly-hydroxy acid) in a light gel lotion that also contains some good antioxidants. This would work well as an exfoliant for normal to oily skin.

✓☺ **$$$ Eye Cream PHA 4** *($28 for 0.5 ounce)* is a very good 4% PHA (polyhy-droxy acid) product formulated with an emollient base that includes some good plant oils, antioxidants, and tiny amounts of water-binding agents. It would be an option as an exfoliant for dry, sensitive skin.

☺ **$$$ Renewal Cream PHA 12** *($40 for 1.05 ounces)* contains 12% PHA (polyhy-droxy acid) in an emollient moisturizing base that contains tiny amounts of antioxidants and water-binding agents. It does contain fragrance. However, there is concern about using such a high concentration of PHA (over 10%) given that its long-term effects on skin are unknown.

✔☺ **Ultra Moisturizing Face Cream PHA 10** *($27 for 1.75 ounces)* is similar to the Renewal Cream above only with 10% AHA, and this one is preferred for normal to dry skin.

✔☺ **Daytime Protection Cream SPF 15 PHA 4** *($27 for 1.75 ounces)* is a very good sunscreen with titanium dioxide as one of the active UVA-protecting ingredients. It also contains 4% PHA (polyhydroxy acid) in a standard emollient base, and would be an option for normal to dry skin.

✔☺ **Daytime Skin Smoothing Cream SPF 15** *($25 for 1.75 ounces)* is a very good sunscreen with titanium dioxide as one of the active ingredients. It also contains 8% AHA in a standard emollient base, and would be an option for normal to dry skin.

✔☺ **Oil Free Lotion SPF 15 PHA 4** *($28 for 1.75 ounces)* is a very good sunscreen with titanium dioxide as one of the active ingredients. It also contains 4% PHA (polyhydroxy acid) in a matte-finish base that also contains a small amount of antioxidants. It is an option for normal to oily skin.

☺ **Daily Protection Sunscreen SPF 29** *($30 for 3.4 ounces)* is a very good sunscreen with avobenzone as one of the active ingredients in a standard emollient base, and would be an option for normal to dry skin.

☺ $$$ **Lip Conditioner SPF 15** *($6 for 0.14 ounce)* is a very good sunscreen with titanium dioxide and zinc oxide as two of the active ingredients. The emollient base is great for dry lips, though there is a tiny amount of spearmint oil, which can be a skin irritant—hopefully not enough to be a problem for the lips.

NEOSTRATA NEOCEUTICALS

☺ **NeoCeuticals Clarifying Facial Cleanser** *($19.50 for 6 ounces)* is a standard, detergent-based cleanser that also contains 0.3% triclosan, a topical disinfectant. While it does have disinfecting properties there is no research showing triclosan to be effective against the bacterium that causes acne. This would be an option for normal to oily skin.

☹ **NeoCeuticals Acne Spot Treatment Gel** *($11 for 0.5 ounce)* does contain some salicylic acid, but the main ingredient is alcohol and that makes it too drying and irritating for all skin types.

☹ **NeoCeuticals Acne Treatment Solution** *($12 for 2 ounces)* is similar to the Acne Spot Treatment Gel above and the same comments apply.

☹ **NeoCeuticals HQ Skin Lightening Gel** *($25 for 1 ounce)* does contain effective levels of AHA, which can help exfoliate skin, as well as kojic acid, which can help inhibit melanin production, but the second ingredient is alcohol, and that makes it too drying and irritating for skin, results that aren't enlightening in the least.

✔☺ **NeoCeuticals Skin Lightening Cream SPF 15** *($24 for 1.4 ounces)* is a very good sunscreen with titanium dioxide as one of the active ingredients. The standard emollient base also has 8% AHA and 2% hydroquinone, which makes this a unique and potentially very effective all-in-one product for helping to lighten skin discolorations caused by sun damage while protecting skin from more problems.

The Reviews N

☺ **$$$ NeoCeuticals PDS Regular Strength Cream** *($18.50 for 3.4 ounces)* is a Vaseline-based moisturizer that contains about 4% AHA. It also includes small amounts of antioxidants and water-binding agents. The small amount of spearmint oil can be a skin irritant in a product that would otherwise have been an option as an exfoliant for dry sensitive skin.

☺ **$$$ NeoCeuticals PDS Extra Strength Cream** *($18.50 for 3.4 ounces)* is similar to the PDS Regular Strength Cream above only with 6% AHA, and the same basic comments apply.

NEUTROGENA

Neutrogena has been around since 1954, when its first clear amber bar of soap was manufactured. How well I remember discovering it when I was a teenager! It didn't leave quite the same soapy film as most bar soaps, and the amber color seemed different enough to establish the notion that it would work to get rid of blemishes. Of course, that wasn't the case. Bar cleansers of any color can be a problem for breakouts because the ingredients that keep bar cleansers in their bar form can clog pores. Their pH is also typically over 8, and that can make breakouts worse.

Since then, Neutrogena has been sold to Johnson & Johnson and J&J has been busy creating a skin-care line that has some products worth considering for all skin types, including some excellent sunscreens, AHA and BHA products, copper-added moisturizers, and lots and lots of cleansers. If you are looking for some of the latest gimmicks, like retinol, it has those, too, and one of them meets the standards you'd think only the more expensive products would deliver. Although the emphasis here is still on women who worry about breakouts, ironically that is where the products really are a disappointment. One major point of contention: While several of these products are promoted as being noncomedogenic and being good for acne-prone skin, many of them contain either very irritating ingredients or pore-clogging ingredients. However, that's a caution that applies to many products in the world of skin care; that is, many products have ingredients that women with blemish-prone skin always need to be wary of.

It is also important to point out that for all the claims about great skin care and getting rid of wrinkles and acne, this line still sells some poorly formulated sunscreens that do not contain UVA-protecting ingredients. If you're comfortable knowing that this line is largely hit-or-miss, and are still interested in trying it (and there are some beautiful, inexpensive options), pick and choose wisely. For more information about Neutrogena, call (800) 421-6857 or visit www.neutrogena.com. **Note:** All Neutrogena products contain fragrance unless noted otherwise.

NEUTROGENA SKIN CARE

☺ **Fresh Foaming Cleanser Soap-Free Cleanser for Combination Skin** *($5.49 for 5.5 ounces)* is a very good, detergent-based, water-soluble cleanser for most skin types.

☺ **Extra Gentle Cleanser** *($5.49 for 6.7 ounces)* is indeed gentle, using one of the less-irritating detergent cleansing agents in an emollient base. It doesn't remove makeup very well and can leave a slightly greasy film on the skin, but it can be a good option for someone with dry skin. It does contain fragrance.

☺ **Non-Drying Cleanser Lotion** *($6 for 5.5 ounces)* is similar to the Extra Gentle Cleanser above and the same comments apply.

☹ **Alcohol-Free Antiseptic Cleanser, Sensitive Skin Formula** *($3.99 for 8 ounces)*. The number of ingredients in this product that are a problem not just for sensitive skin but also for all skin types is almost shocking. Menthol, peppermint oil, eucalyptus oil, rosemary oil, and camphor are all too irritating for words and make the alcohol-free claim misleading and meaningless.

☹ **Deep Clean Cream Cleanser** *($4.99 for 7 ounces)* contains menthol, a skin irritant, and a small amount of BHA, but the pH isn't low enough for it to be effective as an exfoliant. This product has more problems than benefits.

☹ **Deep Clean for Normal to Oily Skin** *($5.20 for 6 ounces)* contains sodium C14-16 olefin sulfate as the detergent cleansing agent, which is too irritating for all skin types.

☹ **Deep Clean Cleansing Cloths** *($6.99 for 30 cloths)* contain sodium C14-16 olefin sulfate, a fairly drying and potentially irritating detergent cleansing agent.

☺ **Oil-Free Acne Wash Cleansing Wipes** *($6.99 for 30 cloths)* are standard cleansing cloths, and join the ever-growing number of other cleansing cloths crowding drugstore shelves. This version contains 2% salicylic acid (BHA) along with some rather harsh detergent cleansing agents. The pH of this product is too high for the BHA to work as an exfoliant, but the simple act of rubbing these cloths over the skin will provide some exfoliation, about the same as using a washcloth.

☺ **Oil-Free Acne Wash Foam Cleanser** *($5.49 for 5.1 ounces)* is a standard, detergent-based, water-soluble cleanser that contains 2% BHA (salicylic acid). While it would be effective for exfoliation, in a cleanser the BHA is rinsed down the drain before it has a chance to be absorbed into the pores.

☹ **Oil-Free Acne Wash** *($5.49 for 5.1 ounces)* is similar to the Acne Wash Foam Cleanser above only it contains sodium C14-16 olefin sulfate as the detergent cleansing agent, which is too irritating for all skin types.

☹ **Oil-Free Cream Cleanser** *($5.49 for 6.7 ounces)* is similar to the Acne Wash above and the same comments apply.

☺ **Liquid Neutrogena Facial Cleansing Formula Fragrance-Free** *($7.50 for 8 ounces)* is a fairly drying, water-soluble cleanser that can thoroughly clean the face. Even someone with oily skin may find this drying.

☺ **Pore Refining Cleanser** *($5.99 for 6.7 ounces)* adds no new options to the cleansers Neutrogena already has in its lineup. This is a standard, detergent-based, water-soluble cleanser that can be slightly drying. It also contains AHA and BHA, but the pH of the product is too high for them to be effective as exfoliants, which doesn't really matter anyway because in a cleanser they are just washed away.

The Reviews N

☹ **Transparent Facial Bar Acne-Prone Skin Formula** *($2.49 for 3.5 ounces)* is a standard, tallow-based bar cleanser that can be too drying and irritating for all skin types.

☹ **Transparent Facial Bar Dry Skin Formula** (available in **Fragrance** and **Fragrance-Free**) *($2.20 for 3.5 ounces)* is similar to the Acne-Prone Skin Formula bar cleanser above, and the same comments apply.

☹ **Transparent Facial Bar Oily Skin Formula** (available in **Fragrance** and **Fragrance-Free**) *($2.20 for 3.5 ounces)* is similar to the Acne-Prone Skin Formula bar cleanser above, and the same comments apply.

☹ **Transparent Facial Bar Original Formula** (available in **Fragrance** and **Fragrance-Free**) *($2.20 for 3.5 ounces)* is similar to the bar cleansers above, and the same comments apply.

☹ **Extra Gentle Cleansing Bar** *($3.99 for 4.5 ounces)* is similar to Dove soap, and even though it is less drying than many bar cleansers, it is still fairly drying.

☺ **Deep Clean Gentle Scrub** *($5.99 for 4.2 ounces)* is a standard, detergent-based cleanser that uses plastic particles (polyethylene) as the scrub agent. It also contains salicylic acid, but the pH is too high for it to be effective as an exfoliant. This is an option for normal to oily skin.

☺ **Alcohol-Free Toner** *($5.49 for 8 ounces)* has a wafting fragrance that makes it feel more like you're applying cologne than a skin-care product. Aside from that, it is a very average toner with teeny amounts of water-binding agents and nothing else of benefit for skin.

☹ **Clear Pore Oil-Controlling Astringent Salicylic Acid Acne Medication** *($3.99 for 8 ounces)* would be a decent BHA toner except that it is almost 45% alcohol, and that makes it exceedingly drying and overly irritating for all skin types.

☹ **Clear Pore Soothing Gel Astringent** *($4.99 for 4.2 ounces)* contains alcohol and menthol, and that makes it too drying and irritating for all skin types. Plus the pH of 5 means that the 2% salicylic acid in here isn't effective for exfoliation. Calling this soothing is just absurd.

☹ **Deep Clean Astringent Oil-Free** *($4.99 for 6.7 ounces)* is almost identical to the Clear Pore Soothing Gel Astringent above and the same comments apply.

☹ **Pore Refining Toner** *($5.99 for 8.5 ounces)* contains alcohol, eucalyptus, and peppermint—it hurts for me even to write that. This is irritation waiting to happen!

☺ **Clear Pore Shine Control Gel** *($5.99 for 0.3 ounce)* makes the claim that it is "clinically proven to control shine all day while keeping skin clear." I called Neutrogena to ask for information about the study, but I was told it wasn't available. As far as clearing pores goes, both the small amount of salicylic acid (0.5%) here and the pH of 6 make this ineffective as an exfoliant. And if you have even slightly oily skin, you won't find this controlling shine all day, or even for a few hours for that matter. As a lightweight moisturizer under foundation it's an option, but I wouldn't throw away your powder.

☺ **Eye Cream** *($11.99 for 0.5 ounce)* is a lightweight moisturizer with some good antioxidants and small amounts of water-binding agents. It is an option for normal to dry skin.

☺ **Healthy Defense Daily Moisturizer SPF 30** *($11.49 for 1.7 ounces)* is a very good, lightweight moisturizer that features an in-part zinc oxide–based sunscreen; it is available in tinted or untinted versions. The two tinted options are both fine and both colors are extremely sheer. The base formula is nothing exceptional, but it's nevertheless worthwhile for normal to slightly dry or slightly oily skin.

☺ **Healthy Skin Anti-Wrinkle Cream with Retinol** *($10.99 for 1.4 ounces)* climbs aboard the retinol bandwagon and is identical in many ways to Avon's Retinol Recovery Complex or Estee Lauder's Diminish. It can be good as a lightweight, but standard, moisturizer for someone with normal to dry skin, but that's about it. If you're looking for retinol, this is as good a product as any.

☹ **Healthy Skin Anti-Wrinkle Cream SPF 15** *($12.49 for 1.4 ounces)* isn't all that healthy because it doesn't contain the UVA-protecting ingredients of titanium dioxide, zinc oxide, or avobenzone, and thus cannot be recommended. It does contain retinol, but to fight wrinkling, what it really needs is a sunscreen with UVA protection.

☹ **Healthy Skin Face Lotion with SPF 15** *($9.46 for 2.5 ounces)* doesn't contain the UVA-protecting ingredients of titanium dioxide, zinc oxide, or avobenzone, and is not recommended.

☺ **Healthy Skin Anti-Wrinkle Anti-Blemish Clear Skin Cream** *($11.99 for 1 ounce)*. With a pH of 5, this 2% salicylic acid moisturizer won't work as an exfoliant (the optimal pH is 3 to 4, and there are those who would say even a pH of 4 is borderline effective). Aside from that, this is an average moisturizer that is not preferred over Neutrogena's Healthy Skin Anti-Wrinkle Cream with Retinol.

☺ **Healthy Skin Eye Cream** *($11.99 for 0.5 ounce)*. The little bit of glycolic acid in here and the high pH make this a poor choice for an exfoliant. It does contain some good antioxidants and tiny amounts of water-binding agents, which makes it an option for normal to dry skin.

✔☺ **Healthy Skin Face Lotion** *($9.99 for 2.5 ounces)* is a good 8% AHA moisturizer containing glycolic acid in a lightweight moisturizing base that contains some good antioxidants and a tiny amount of a water-binding agent. It is a good option for normal to dry skin.

✔☺ **Healthy Skin Face Lotion Delicate Skin** *($9.99 for 2.5 ounces)* is identical to the original Healthy Skin Face Lotion in almost every way except that the Delicate Skin version contains about a 5% concentration of glycolic acid rather than an 8% concentration. It has a good pH, which makes this an option for a gentler AHA product that still has some effectiveness for exfoliation. It is best for someone with normal to dry skin.

☹ **Intensified Day Moisture SPF 15** *($9.99 for 2.25 ounces)* doesn't contain the UVA-protecting ingredients of titanium dioxide, zinc oxide, or avobenzone, and is not recommended.

☺ **Intensified Eye Moisture 12-Hour Hydration** *($8.99 for 0.5 ounce)* is an OK, though rather ordinary, moisturizer for normal to dry skin. It doesn't contain fragrance.

The Reviews N

☺ **Light Night Cream** *($9.99 for 2.25 ounces)* is an emollient, though very basic, moisturizer for normal to dry skin. It doesn't contain fragrance.

☺ **Moisture Non-Comedogenic Oil Free Facial Moisture Lotion Combination Skin** *($8.99 for 4 ounces)* is a standard, silicone-based moisturizer that is an option for normal to dry skin. Supposedly this moisturizer can "put moisture in dry areas [and] take shine out of oily areas." There is no way this product can hold back its moisturizing agents in dry areas and absorb oil in oily areas—it just deposits the same ingredients all over. It doesn't contain fragrance.

☺ **Moisture Non-Comedogenic Facial Moisturizer for Sensitive Skin** *($9.50 for 2 ounces)* is almost identical to the Light Night Cream above and the same comments apply.

☹ **Moisture Facial Moisturizer SPF 15 Sheer Tint** *($8.99 for 4 ounces)* doesn't contain the UVA-protecting ingredients of titanium dioxide, zinc oxide, or avobenzone, and is not recommended.

☹ **Moisture Facial Moisturizer SPF 15 Untinted** *($9.99 for 4 ounces)* doesn't contain the UVA-protecting ingredients of titanium dioxide, zinc oxide, or avobenzone, and is not recommended.

☺ **Pore Refining Cream** *($11.99 for 1 ounce)* is an AHA-type moisturizer, but I wouldn't recommend it to prevent breakouts or clogged pores. The amount of AHA is about 4% to 5%, which is OK for sensitive skin, but the pH isn't appropriate for it to be an effective exfoliant. It does contain retinol, at the same low percentage as in all retinol products on the market.

☺ **Pore Refining Cream SPF 15** *($13.99 for 1 ounce)* is a good, in-part avobenzone-based sunscreen in a standard moisturizing base. It does contain AHA, but the pH is too high for it to be effective as an exfoliant. It also contains retinol, but that has no effect on pores.

☺ **Skin Clearing Moisturizer** *($9.99 for 1 ounce)* contains 2% salicylic acid in a rather mundane moisturizing base that would be an option for someone with normal to slightly dry skin. The pH of 4.5 makes it minimally passable for reliable exfoliation. It also contains a teeny amount of retinol.

☺ **$$$ Visibly Firm Night Cream, Active Copper Formula** *($19.99 for 1.7 ounces)* and **Visibly Firm Eye Cream Active Copper Formula** *($19.99 for 0.5 ounce)*. As the names clearly indicate, the answer this time is copper tripeptide. (I wonder what Neutrogena expects you to do with their retinol or AHA products that come with the same claims about making skin look firmer, just as this one does?) Neutrogena states that "Since skin's production of collagen and elastin diminish with age, replenishing copper is an effective way to strengthen and regain firmness. However, it is difficult to deliver copper into the skin. Neutrogena's new patented technology, Active Copper, provides an effective solution. Active Copper links copper with a peptide which allows copper to penetrate the skin, replenishing it with this vital ingredient. Active Copper technology works with the skin's natural repair cycle to effectively boost copper levels in the skin's surface, safely and without irritation. It also works to prevent further loss of firmness." I admit this does sound convincing, and it even turns out that there are numerous studies establishing that many forms of copper (including copper tripeptide) are an excellent option for wound healing. But wound healing is unrelated to wrinkles (at least no direct correlation has been established). Just to make one comparison, while stitches can help a deep wound heal, they are useless for wrinkles. Aside from the copper, these two moisturizers are fairly basic products for dry skin, with nothing else of particular interest or uniqueness. It is important to point out that the base for these two products is essentially identical, with the price being the only difference.

✓☺ **Visibly Even Moisturizer SPF 15** *($12.49 for 1 ounce)* is a great, in-part avobenzone-based sunscreen that is lightweight and leaves skin feeling silky. The teeny amounts of ascorbic acid and retinol will not have much effect on uneven skin tone or discolorations, but this is a worthwhile sunscreen for normal to slightly dry skin.

☺ **Visibly Firm Face Lotion SPF 20** *($19.99 for 1.7 ounces)* offers an in-part zinc oxide–based sunscreen with a great SPF. Unfortunately, the base formula is mundane and definitely not capable of firming skin in one week as the ads claim (or even in one decade for that matter). It contains mostly water, glycerin, thickening agents, and silicone. Though this product showcases the same copper tripeptide complex contained in Neutrogena's other Visibly Firm products, it is listed after the preservative in the ingredient list, indicating that it is barely present in any discernible amount, greatly diminishing its potential to offer benefit of any kind. Further, although there are studies that document the effects of copper tripeptide on wound healing and reducing scar formation (Sources: *Federation of European Biochemical Sciences Letter,* October 1988, pages 343–346 and *Archive of Plastic Surgery,* January-March 2001, pages 28–32), those conditions are not related to wrinkles. That means copper's alleged benefit as an antiaging ingredient is still pure speculation.

☹ **Oil-Absorbing Acne Mask Natural Clay Mask** *($5.49 for 2 ounces)* contains 5% benzoyl peroxide, and that's a great way to disinfect blemish-prone skin, but it would be far better in an irritant-free gel or liquid applied twice daily than in a clay mask with menthol used only occasionally.

☺ **Deep Pore Treatment** *($6.29 for 2 ounces)* does contain about 1% salicylic acid (BHA) in a nonirritating gel base, though the pH of 4.5 is borderline for allowing the BHA to exfoliate skin.

☺ **Clear Pore Treatment Nighttime Pore Clarifying Gel Salicylic Acid Acne Treatment** *($6.75 for 2 ounces)* is similar to the Deep Pore Treatment above, only this one contains 2% BHA, and the same comments apply.

☹ **Maximum Strength Oil-Controlling Pads, Salicylic Acid Acne Medication** *($3.80 for 50 pads)* contains almost 50% alcohol, which is too irritating and drying for all skin types.

☺ **Multi-Vitamin Acne Treatment** *($5.99 for 2.5 ounces)* is a lotion that contains 1.5% salicylic acid and 4% to 5% glycolic acid. This would be an interesting combina-

The Reviews N

tion of AHA and BHA to try, given the potential effectiveness of each, though the pH of 4.5 is borderline for allowing them to exfoliate skin. The teeny amounts of vitamins have no effect on acne, though they are antioxidants.

☺ Pore Refining Mattifier *($11.99 for 0.5 ounce)* is primarily a silicone-based, creamy-feeling gel that makes skin look smooth, has a fairly silky texture, and creates a very convincing matte finish. It's worth a try for someone with normal to slightly dry or slightly oily skin, but don't rely on this to hold back an oily feel for very long.

☺ On-the-Spot Acne Treatment Tinted Formula 2.5% Benzoyl Peroxide *($5.49 for 0.75 ounce)* contains benzoyl peroxide, and that's a great way to disinfect blemish-prone skin, but it would be far better in a product that didn't have such a strange, peach-colored tint.

✔☺ On-the-Spot Acne Treatment Vanishing Formula 2.5% Benzoyl Peroxide *($6.75 for 0.75 ounce)* is identical to the Tinted version above, only without the strange color.

☹ On-the-Spot Acne Patch *($5.49 for 27 patches)* contains 2% salicylic acid applied to tiny patches that you stick on skin over blemishes. I'm sure this application gimmick will intrigue teenagers who think that spot-treating blemishes is good for skin, but the patches are coated with film-forming agents to get them to stick to the skin, and that can cause irritation and breakouts.

☹ Pore Refining Mask *($7.99 for 2 ounces)* lists alcohol as the first ingredient, so the claims that this can do anything positive for skin (and also that it is nondrying) are incredibly misleading. Alcohol is drying and irritating, period. This one also contains eucalyptus, peppermint, and menthol! Ouch!

☻ Healthy Defense Oil-Free Sunblock Spray SPF 30 *($8.39 for 4 ounces)* is a good, in-part avobenzone-based sunscreen; however, the second ingredient is alcohol and that can cause skin to be dry and irritated.

☺ Healthy Defense Oil-Free Sunblock Stick SPF 30 *($6.99 for 0.47 ounce)* is oil-free, but this wax-based stick with avobenzone (among other sunscreens) is fairly heavy and emollient, making it best for normal to dry skin. This contains a small amount of antioxidants.

☺ Healthy Defense Oil-Free Sunblock SPF 45 *($8.39 for 4 ounces)* is a very good sunscreen with avobenzone as one of the active ingredients. The somewhat standard moisturizing base also contains a small amount of antioxidants.

☺ Sunblock Lotion with SPF 45 *($8.39 for 4 ounces)* is similar to the Healthy Defense Oil-Free Sunblock SPF 45 above and the same comments apply. This one is fragrance free.

☺ Sensitive Skin UVA/UVB Block SPF 17 *(8.39 for 4 ounces)* and Sensitive Skin UVA/UVB Block SPF 30 *($8.39 for 4 ounces)* are the sunscreens to check out if you have sensitive skin; they have a wonderful smooth feel and would be excellent for normal to dry, sensitive skin. The titanium dioxide (along with zinc oxide) used here has minimal to no chance of causing skin irritation or a sensitizing skin reaction, while other forms of sunscreen ingredients can be a problem for sensitive skin. Both are fragrance free.

☺ **Instant Bronze, Sunless Tanner and Bronzer for the Face** *($8.99 for 2 ounces)*; **Instant Bronze, Sunless Tanner and Bronzer in One** (**Medium** and **Deep**) *($8.99 for 4 ounces)*; **Sunless Tanning Foam, Deep** *($8.99 for 4 ounces)*; **Sunless Tanning Spray** *($8.99 for 3.5 ounces)*; and **Sunless Tanning Lotion** (**Light** and **Medium**) *($8.99 for 4 ounces)* all contain dihydroxyacetone, the ingredient used in all self-tanners to affect the color of skin. These would work as well as any.

NEUTROGENA MAKEUP

The entire staff at Neutrogena had reason to celebrate when competitor Olay announced in 2001 that they were discontinuing their entire makeup line. Olay's makeup was launched in tandem with Neutrogena's, and held a major advantage thanks to the fact that Olay provided testers for almost all of their items. Now that Olay is gone, Neutrogena has done little to stake their claim among such leading drugstore makeup lines as Revlon and Maybelline. Neutrogena's "beautiful and beneficial" pronouncement sounds nice, but other than some excellent foundations with reliable sunscreens, their makeup leaves much to be desired. Each product carries on about the vitamins it contains, yet compared to the leading roles played by cosmetic staples like silicones and thickening agents, the vitamins are cast as extras and as such have little to no impact. The most frustrating aspect of this line is that everything is packaged so you cannot see the color. Several stores I visited had open, used products that were clearly a sign that frustrated women had been trying to find the best shade. Everything was repackaged neatly, but the contents had certainly been compromised. What would truly be beneficial is for Neutrogena to wise up and either offer revealing packaging or provide testers. They need to do something that causes their makeup to stand out, rather than obscuring it and hoping it will sell just by riding on the coattails of their positive skin-care reputation.

FOUNDATION: ✓☺ **Visibly Firm Moisture Makeup SPF 20** *($14.99)*. Calling this a "moisture makeup" is a bit of a misnomer, as no makeup with talc as the fifth ingredient can be much use at moisturizing. Rather, this is a very good liquid makeup for normal to slightly oily skin, with a sunscreen that is pure titanium dioxide, which is excellent. It applies easily, and once blended dries down to a soft matte finish. Coverage is on the light to medium side, and there are 12 shades, although the following colors are too pink or rose for most skin tones: Blushing Ivory, Rose Cream, and Spiced Almond. This foundation does feature Neutrogena's trademarked Active Copper (which is listed way after the preservative on the ingredient list), but the notion that copper of any sort can firm the skin or change a wrinkle is strictly theory and not fact; and in this small amount it is probably strictly hype. ✓☺ **Healthy Defense Sheer Makeup SPF 30** *($10.99)* is a sheer, natural-finish foundation, really more akin to a tinted moisturizer than a traditional makeup base. The great news is that it has an in-part titanium dioxide–based

The Reviews N

sunscreen! This would be an excellent option for normal to dry skin seeking color, sheer coverage, and sun protection all in one. There are five shades, with no options for very light or darker skin tones. Blushing Ivory, Sheer True Beige, and Toasted Honey are slightly peach or pink, but they are so sheer that the color should not be much of an issue.

☺ **Healthy Skin Liquid Makeup SPF 20** *($9.99)* is a standard lightweight liquid foundation that offers sheer to light coverage and a soft matte finish. This does have an excellent titanium dioxide sunscreen, but the number of poor shades among the 16 options is considerable. All of the following are just too peach or pink for most skin tones: Warm Caramel, Spiced Almond, Rose Cream, Real Pecan, Rich Sable, and Soft Mahogany. This would work best for normal to slightly oily skin. **Skin Clearing Makeup Flawless Finish Blemish Treatment** *($11.39)* asks you to believe that getting clear skin from a makeup is possible. Yet the tiny amount of BHA, combined with a high pH, won't clear blemishes or anything else for that matter. This silicone- and talc-based liquid does have a soft feel and blends on evenly with light to medium coverage. It would be best for normal to slightly dry skin, as this does not have a matte finish. There are 12 shades, but Blushing Ivory, Natural Buff, Rose Cream, Spiced Almond, Warm Caramel, and Toasted Honey are too pink or peach for most skin tones. Bronzed Cocoa would be a good choice for dark skin.

☹ **Skin Clearing Oil Free Compact Foundation** *($11.39)* is a thick, creamy-textured cream-to-powder makeup that contains aluminum starch (can be an irritant, though it is a good absorbent) and some thickening agents that just aren't the best for oily skin—and that's precisely the skin type this one is being marketed to. Although it does have a rather dry matte finish that would please someone with oily skin, the 12 shades are all too peach, pink, or orange to recommend, especially without any testers at the store to see if they can blend unseen into your skin tone. The minimal amount of salicylic acid (BHA) comes with the wrong pH and so can have virtually no effect on breakouts. **Healthy Skin Cream Powder Makeup SPF 20** *($11.39)* doesn't have UVA protection, and I have no idea how they could have overlooked that! Another oversight is that each one of the eight colors is either extremely pink, peach, or ash. But wait, there's more: The texture is very thick, and the heavy wax and starch just don't feel great on the skin. Avoid this one at all costs.

<u>CONCEALER:</u> ✓☺ **Visibly Firm Eye Treatment Concealer** *($9.99)* features the big-deal Active Copper and makes dubious claims of firming—but then it goes further, claiming to eliminate dark circles over time, as well as ameliorate puffiness. Sorry, but that is way beyond the means of this silicone-based concealer, and copper has no effect on these common under-eye woes, especially in this scant amount. What this does have going for it is a soft texture and a smooth, even application that can nicely hide dark circles and other blemishes while leaving a natural, crease-free finish. There are four colors and, with the exception of Correcting Yellow, all are decent options.

☺ **Skin Clearing Oil-Free Concealer** *($7.99)* is packaged in a click-pen that feeds the lightweight concealer onto an angled sponge tip. It blends very well (but fast) to a matte finish, and provides excellent coverage. The light, silicone- and clay-based formula is fine for use over blemishes—just don't expect the tiny amount (0.5%) of salicylic acid at this high pH to clear things up. There are four shades, all great except for Correcting Green.

☹ **Under Cover Concealer** *($6.49)* comes in a lipstick-style tube, has four poor flesh-toned colors as well as yellow and mint-green hues, and, due to the greasier texture, easily creases into the lines under the eyes. Overall, this is not worth the trouble of applying it.

POWDER: ✔☺ **Healthy Defense Protective Powder SPF 30** *($9.99)* is a pressed powder with a reliable SPF 30 that contains almost 9% titanium dioxide as the active ingredient. Although this is an excellent product, you need to know that unless you apply a liberal layer of powder (which can look too thick), you will not be getting the stated (or even significant) sun protection. However, this is an excellent idea as a touch-up for makeup as the day goes by to enhance the sun protection you are already wearing (from foundation or moisturizer). The three available shades are fine, but there are no options for darker skin tones.

☺ **Fresh Finish Loose Powder** *($11.39)* and **Fresh Finish Pressed Powder** *($9.99)* have three shades each. Unfortunately, because of the way these products are packaged you can't see the shades. Both formulas are talc-based, with a soft, silky finish. The colors are actually quite attractive, but they are hidden by the packaging, so the chance of getting the wrong shade is fairly high. By the way, the light-diffusing claim these powders make is completely unrealistic.

☹ **Skin Clearing Oil-Free Pressed Powder** *($11.39)* has a dry, smooth texture and an almost too-powdery finish. Plus, the three colors are all too peach for most skin tones. The inclusion of salicylic acid in a powder is never effective, as the very ingredients that compose a powder have too high a pH to allow the BHA to work as an exfoliant.

☺ BLUSH: **Soft Color Blush** *($9.49)* is a powder blush that does have a small amount of shine but also a soft, even finish and an enticing range of nine shades. The hyped vitamins are present in such negligible quantities that you can overlook the inane claim that they are somehow good for the skin.

☺ LIPSTICK: **Lip Boost Intense Moisture Lipstick SPF 20** *($6.79)* would have been a standout if it offered adequate UVA protection, but in the hit-or-miss world of Neutrogena sunscreens, this misses. As a standard, semi-opaque creamy lipstick it works well, but it's hardly distinctive.

☺ MASCARA: **Full Volume Fortifying Mascara** *($6.29)* is supposed to provide "300% fuller lashes," which is statistically impossible. In fact, it's likely you'll not notice lashes that are even 30% fuller. This builds respectable length with very slight thickness and it does not clump or smear, but all other claims are patently absurd. **Weightless Volume Mascara** *($6.79)* is a wax-free mascara that promises full, weightless lashes with no clumps or smudges. It fulfills the latter part of that promise, but is otherwise a lackluster performer, providing debatable length and not a smidgen of thickness. The fact that this is wax-free is fine if you're bothered by waxes. If not, waxes are an essential component of most mascaras, as they add fullness, pliability, and help keep mascara on the lashes.

NEWAYS SKIN CARE

I suspect many of you may have received a slew of spam e-mails back in 1999 with blazing headlines followed by the warning that your cosmetics may be killing you. The message went on to explain why everything from mineral oil to sodium lauryl sulfate, propylene glycol, and even clay (bentonite) were evil and that the cosmetics industry was purposely trying to hurt your skin or at the very least help you to get cancer. I spent quite a bit of time dispelling the myths propagated in that e-mail (as did many other Web sites, of which my favorite is http://urbanlegends.miningco.com). It turned out that from every indication, the information in those e-mails was generated by Neways. The brochure for Neways states: "We recognized years ago that there existed a real need for more healthful alternatives to … mass-produced personal care products.… We were astonished to find that potentially unhealthy, toxic, and damaging chemicals are included in many cosmetics, lotions, and treatments applied day after day to the skin and hair.… Believing that most existing companies were not willing to supply safer, more natural products by sacrificing the exorbitant profits made possible by cheap ingredients, we chose to do so ourselves." So, Neways' claim in essence was that almost everyone else is killing you but Neways.

As is usually the case with companies like Neways that make claims about being "all natural," they warn you about so-called "dangerous" ingredients by taking information out of context, and then conveniently leave out the information about the problematic, completely unnatural ingredients they themselves use. For example, Neways uses sodium C14-16 olefin sulfate in one of its cleansers, which is an extremely irritating ingredient. It also uses the preservatives methylcholorisothiazlinone and methylisothiazolinone (combined to form Kathon CG), which are so potentially irritating they should only be used in rinse-off products due to the problems they can cause if left on the skin. Even more disingenuous is that Neways uses PVP/hexadecane copolymer and polyacrylamide, forms of plastic that couldn't be made much more unnatural if you tried (not to mention "suffocating," something Neways really wants you to worry about from other ingredients—which is all bogus). Another Neways ingredient is perfluoropolymethylisopropyl ether—now doesn't that sound like something natural you'd feel safe putting on a salad? And what about their use of parabens, preservatives that may be linked to concerns about breast cancer? They didn't mention any of those in their fear-tactic advertising. The spin Neways puts on other cosmetics companies' ingredients is clearly not one they pay attention to when it comes to their own products.

I could go on and on about the absurd claims this company propagates (wait until you read about its product that is supposed to help tanning!), but you'll get the gist of it in the reviews below. As usual it's not that Neways products are bad, it's just that their marketing techniques create a false pretense that leads the consumer down a primrose path to a destination that doesn't exist. For more information about Neways, call (800) 326-3051 or visit www.neways.com.

☹ **1st Impression Cleanser/Clear Up Cleanser** *($8.70 for 4 ounces)* contains sodium C14-16 olefin sulfate as the main detergent cleansing agent, which makes it potentially too drying and irritating for most skin types. Several of the plant extracts are also potential skin irritants, including yarrow and papaya, but they would probably be rinsed down the drain before they could have an effect.

☺ **Extra Gentle Cleanser** *($8.70 for 4 ounces)* is a standard, detergent-based, water-soluble cleanser that can be an option for most skin types. It does contain fragrance.

☺ **TLC/Facial Cleansing Lotion** *($6.95 for 4 ounces)* is a wipe-off cleanser that can leave a greasy film on the skin, though it is an option for someone with dry skin. It is actually a better moisturizer than it is a cleanser. It does contain fragrance.

☺ **Milky Cleanser** *($16.15 for 4.2 ounces)* is similar to the Facial Cleansing Lotion above and the same basic comments apply.

☺ **Super Charged Bio-Mist** *($11.90 for 4.2 ounces)* contains lu rong extract, or deer antler velvet, which is the epidermis that covers the inner structure of the growing bone and cartilage that will become deer antlers. Deer antler velvet is marketed as a remedy for a wide range of disorders and health benefits. However, there is a lack of information in the scientific literature to support any of these claims, and there is also a lack of information on any potential toxicity. Areas of potential concern include drug residues, possible deleterious androgenic effects on fetuses and neonates, and allergic reactions (Source: *Veterinary and Human Toxicology,* February 1999, pages 39–41). Further, there is concern about the humane treatment of the animals when the substance is collected.

☺ **Bio-Mist Activator/Moisture Mist** *($8.40 for 4 ounces)* is similar to the Super Charged version above and the same concerns apply.

☺ **Barrier Cream/Protector** *($18.90 for 8.5 ounces)* is a good, though ordinary, emollient moisturizer for normal to dry skin.

☺ **Circles & Lines** *($21 for 1 ounce)* is a lightweight moisturizer for normal to slightly dry skin that contains some very good water-binding agents, but only a minuscule amount of antioxidants.

☺ **Night Science** *($29.95 for 2 ounces)* is a silicone-based moisturizer with a good mix of antioxidants and water-binding agents. It also contains retinol. It is a good option for someone with normal to dry skin.

☺ **$$$ Retention Plus** *($34.60 for 1 ounce)* is a good emollient moisturizer for normal to dry skin, with a good mix of antioxidants and water-binding agents.

☺ **Skin Brightener** *($31.50 for 4.2 ounces)* contains a negligible amount of urea, which is not enough to be effective for exfoliation. It also contains some good antioxidants, but only small amounts of water-binding agents.

☺ **Skin Enhancer Beauty Lotion** *($31.50 for 4 ounces)* is a very good moisturizer for normal to dry skin, with an impressive mix of antioxidants and water-binding agents.

☹ **Snap Back** *($28.80 for 1.7 ounces).* There is nothing in this product that can change sags, bags, or stretch marks anyplace on your body. It's just an OK moisturizer that contains arnica, a skin irritant that should not be applied repeatedly on skin.

☺ **$$$ Wrinkle Drops** *($85 for 0.5 ounce)*. The AHA content isn't more than 2%, which isn't enough to be an effective exfoliant. Other than that, this is just a good, toner-like moisturizer for someone with normal to slightly dry skin. The elastin cannot affect the elastin in your skin. The price is outrageous for what this product contains.

☺ **$$$ Wrinkle Gard** *($37.90 for 1 ounce)* won't prevent one wrinkle, but it is a good emollient moisturizer for normal to dry skin.

☺ **Body Bronzer** *($16.70 for 4.2 ounces)* contains dihydroxyacetone, the same ingredient all self-tanners use to affect the color of skin. This one would work as well as any.

☹ **Great Tan SPF 10** *($14.70 for 1.7 ounces)*. The SPF number of this product is dismally low, and it doesn't contain UVA protection. The dihydroxyacetone is the same ingredient that all self-tanners use, and there are far less expensive versions to consider. Interesting, isn't it, that even Neways doesn't recommend that you rely on this for sun protection—so why include sunscreen in it at all that might mislead some people into using it for that purpose?

☺ **Sunbrero SPF 30** *($11 for 4.2 ounces)* is a very good, in-part zinc oxide–based sunscreen in a standard moisturizing base that would be an option for someone with normal to dry skin.

☺ **Rebound After Sun Lotion** *($29.40 for 4.2 ounces)* is a very good moisturizer for normal to dry skin, with some good water-binding agents and a soothing agent, though nothing in it will reduce the redness and damage from unprotected sun exposure.

☹ **Lightening** *($15.40 for 1 ounce)*. The lemon and sugarcane extract this contains are not AHAs and cannot exfoliate skin, and the teeny amount of citrus extract has no real impact on skin. This also contains minute amounts of mulberry root extract and magnesium ascorbyl phosphate, which have been shown to inhibit melanin production, but not in the small amounts this product contains.

☹ **Tanacity Tanning Accelerator** *($15.70 for 4.2 ounces)*. While this may be a good moisturizer for dry skin, the claims are frightening. "Tanacity may help to prepare your skin for this onslaught of ultra violet rays by enhancing your body's melanin production. This is part of its own protective tanning response. Your skin can be more prepared for exposure of UV rays with Tanacity." Then it goes on to state that it "accelerates the tanning response." This is a dangerous notion, because any and all unprotected sun exposure can lead to sun damage, something Neways mentions several times on their Web site. I can think of no practice in the cosmetics industry that is quite as unethical as a company selling antiwrinkle products side by side with products meant to encourage sun tanning.

☹ **Tanning Oil** *($10 for 4.2 ounces)* doesn't contain the UVA-protecting ingredients of titanium dioxide, zinc oxide, or avobenzone, and is not recommended.

NIVEA VISAGE (SKIN CARE ONLY)

Eucerin, La Prairie, and Nivea Visage are all owned by Beiersdorf, a huge multinational corporation whose product formulation and marketing direction seem to be a response to the mass-market needs of consumers, and whatever it appears they want to buy. Unfortunately, that doesn't always translate into great products. Poorly formulated sunscreens and ho-hum standard ingredients aren't exactly exciting, but the antiwrinkle claims are nonetheless all neatly in place. For more information about Nivea Visage, call (800) 233-2340 or visit www.nivea.com. **Note:** All Nivea Visage products contain fragrance.

☺ **Foaming Facial Cleanser Deep-Cleansing Formula** (*$5.49 for 6 ounces*) is a standard, detergent-based, water-soluble cleanser that can be an option for normal to dry skin. The tiny amount of lanolin has no real impact on skin.

☺ **Oil Control Cleansing Gel Oily Skin** (*$5.99 for 6.8 ounces*) is similar to the Foaming Facial Cleanser above, though this version also contains synthetic scrub particles, which do help exfoliate but can't help control oil. This is an option as a topical scrub for normal to oily skin.

☺ **Refreshing Cleansing Gel, Normal & Combination Skin** (*$5.99 for 6.8 ounces*) is similar to the Foaming Facial Cleanser above except for the addition of some good water-binding agents, though in a cleanser those are just rinsed down the drain before they can be beneficial for skin.

☺ **Gentle Moisturizing Cleanser** (*$6.99 for 6.8 ounces*) is a standard, mineral oil–based cleanser that doesn't rinse off very well and doesn't take off all the makeup without the aid of a washcloth. It can be an option, but only for dry skin.

☺ **Gentle Cleansing Cream Dry & Sensitive Skin** (*$5.99 for 6.8 ounces*) is similar to the Gentle Moisturizing Cleanser above and the same comments apply. There is nothing about this cleanser that makes it better for sensitive skin.

☹ **CoEnzyme Q10 Cleansing Lotion** (*$6.25 for 6.8 ounces*) is similar to the Gentle Cleansing Cream above only with the addition of a minuscule amount of coenzyme Q10. That won't change the appearance of one wrinkle. It's just a wipe-off cleanser that can leave a greasy film on the skin, though it is an option for dry skin.

☺ **Eye Make-Up Remover** (*$4.99 for 2.5 ounces*) is a standard, detergent-based eye-makeup remover with no coloring agents (don't let the blue-colored tube fool you), and it's also fragrance-free, which is great. The lotion form spreads easily with no greasy or sticky after-feel despite the mineral oil content.

☹ **Alcohol-Free Moisturizing Toner** (*$5.79 for 6.8 ounces*) is a reformulation from Nivea and is not much of an improvement over the original. It contains mostly water, glycerin, cleansing agent, preservative, water-binding agents, anti-irritant, slip agent, fragrance, and more preservatives. It would be better if there were more of the anti-irritants and water-binding agents, and if the fragrance weren't so wafting. It does contain niacinamide, the showcase ingredient in Olay's Total Effects, and that product is preferred over this one in that regard.

☹ **Alpha Flavon Perfect Protection SPF 15 Lotion** (*$6.99 for 3.3 ounces*) doesn't contain the UVA-protecting ingredients of titanium dioxide, zinc oxide, or avobenzone, and is not recommended. Alpha Flavon (technically alpha-glucosylrutin) has some studies establishing it as a very good, powerful antioxidant, but those studies were conducted by Beiersdorf, the only company that uses that ingredient. It also contains isoquercitrin, a flavonoid with potent antioxidant properties. Even assuming that these are great antioxidants for skin, they can't help reduce the amount of sun damage that this poorly formulated sunscreen would allow to take place on and in the skin.

☹ **Alpha Flavon Perfect Protection SPF 15 Creme** *($6.99 for 1.7 ounces)* is similar to the SPF 15 Lotion above only in cream form, and the same comments apply.

☹ **ā-Alpha Flavon Perfect Protection SPF 15 Lotion** *($8.99 for 3.3 ounces)* and **a-Alpha Flavon Perfect Protection SPF 15 Creme** *($7.99 for 1.7 ounces)* do not contain the UVA-protecting ingredients of titanium dioxide, zinc oxide, or avobenzone, and are not recommended.

☹ **Anti-Wrinkle and Firming Creme SPF 4** *($8.99 for 1.7 ounces)* has an abysmally low SPF 4 and no UVA-protecting ingredients, which means that if you wear this moisturizer by itself during the day you run the risk of getting wrinkles and sun damage as well.

☹ **CoEnzyme Q10 Wrinkle Control Day SPF 4** *($9.99 for 1.7 ounces)* and **Q10 Wrinkle Control Eye SPF 6** *($9.99 for 0.5 ounce)* both contain coenzyme Q10, but that is not the answer to anyone's wrinkle woes. What is of far more concern is that these products have substandard SPFs and do not contain the UVA-protecting ingredients of titanium dioxide, zinc oxide, or avobenzone. They are absolutely not recommended.

☹ **CoEnzyme Q10 Wrinkle Control Lotion SPF 15** *($9.99 for 3 ounces)* does not contain the UVA-protecting ingredients of titanium dioxide, zinc oxide, or avobenzone, and is not recommended. Even if there were research to support the notion that coenzyme Q10 was good for skin, the sunscreen formulation here would negate any possible benefit because it would allow UVA radiation to damage skin.

☺ **CoEnzyme Q10 Plus Wrinkle Control Night** *($9.99 for 1.7 ounces)* is a good emollient moisturizer for normal to dry skin. Only a handful of studies have shown coenzyme Q10 (CoQ10) to have any effect on skin (Sources: *Biofactors,* September 1999, pages 371–378 and *Zeitschrift für Gerontologie und Geriatrie,* April 1999, pages 83–88). Neither of the sources cited included studies that were double-blind or placebo-controlled, so there is no way to tell whether other formulations could have netted the same results. There is also research showing that sun exposure depletes the presence of CoQ10 in the skin (Source: *Journal of Dermatological Science Supplement,* August 2001, pages 1–4). This isn't surprising, however, because lots of the skin's components become diminished upon exposure to the sun. But whether or not taking CoQ10 supplements orally or applying CoQ10 to skin can stop or alter sun damage is not known. Other than that, this is an OK moisturizer for normal to slightly dry skin, but that's about it.

☹ **Daily Nourishing Creme Essential Daily Moisturizer SPF 4** *($6.49 for 1.7 ounces)* has an embarrassingly low SPF 4, doesn't contain the UVA-protecting ingredients of avobenzone, titanium dioxide, or zinc oxide, and is absolutely not recommended.

☹ **Daily Nourishing Lotion Essential Daily Moisturizer SPF 4** *($6.99 for 3 ounces)* is similar to the Creme Essential version above, and the same comments apply.

☺ **Soothing Eye Gel** *($8.99 for 0.5 ounce)* is a lightweight moisturizer for normal to oily skin that contains a small quantity of water-binding agents.

☹ **Cream** *($3.49 for 2 ounces)* is the original Nivea Cream, and it hasn't changed much over the years. It's incredibly basic, containing mostly Vaseline, mineral oil, and thickeners. It also contains Kathon CG, a preservative that should only be used in rinse-off products.

☹ **Body Silky Shimmer Lotion** *($7.49 for 6.8 ounces)*. Wafting fragrance and a tiny bit of sparkle is about all this moisturizer has to offer. It is about as ordinary a moisturizer for dry skin as you can get and it doesn't even shimmer all that much, which is a disappointment if you were expecting to really glow after applying this well-advertised product. It contains mostly water, glycerin, thickeners, mineral oil, Vaseline, mica (the shine particles), fragrance, and preservatives. Nary an interesting antioxidant or water-binding agent is to be found anywhere in this formulation, not even a token dusting just for effect.

NOEVIR (SKIN CARE ONLY)

Noevir's self-declared claim to fame is its affiliation with the knowledge of Dr. Suzuki (creator of the Noevir product line), who was "one of the few scientists with a PhD in cosmetics research." Actually, the area of cosmetics research is filled with PhDs from all sorts of disciplines—medical, chemical, and cosmetics research. Suzuki hardly stands alone, so that claim is just out of whack. Another quote from the literature: "The medical profession supports Noevir's belief that products with mineral oil and other petroleum-based products are not beneficial to the skin." That could not be further from the truth; plenty of studies have demonstrated that mineral oil and Vaseline are just fine and quite useful for the skin, and I have never seen any studies or data anywhere indicating the opposite.

What is most disturbing about this line of products—which features all kinds of gimmicky ingredients, from plant extracts (many that are potential skin irritants) to umbilical extract—is that Noevir doesn't include a sunscreen as part of its daily skin-care routine. For a skin-care line, such a philosophy is almost prehistoric. In addition, the brochure announces that Noevir products contain no preservatives or fragrances, even though those substances are listed right there on the labels in black and white! In addition, while the water-binding agents in Noevir products are indeed impressive, they are accompanied by lots of alcohol and other problematic ingredients, absurdly high price tags, and clearly untrue marketing claims that are all cause for concern.

Noevir has several different product groupings and a host of specialty items that are very difficult to tell apart because many of the product names (not to mention the formulas) are strikingly identical. Because the individual products are not that different from one another, the main distinctions seem to be price and the quality that the price difference may imply. This system of product classification reminds me strongly of Shiseido, another Japanese line; I imagine Noevir began as a way to compete with Shiseido's successful department-store line. For more information about Noevir, call (800) 872-8888 or visit www.noevirusa.com. **Note:** All Noevir products contain fragrance.

☺ $$$ **Cleansing Crystals** *($25 for 2.4 ounces)* is a detergent-based topical scrub that uses aluminum silicate as the abrasive. It is an option for normal to oily skin, but it can be rough.

☹ **Eye Makeup Remover** *($16 for 3.3 ounces)* is a standard, detergent-based eye-makeup remover, although several of the plant extracts it contains are ill-advised for use in the eye area, or anywhere on the face for that matter.

☹ $$$ **Advanced Moisture Concentrate-EX** *($65 for 0.85 ounce)*. With alcohol listed as the third ingredient, the beneficial water-binding agents and antioxidants in this overpriced gel lotion are just wasted.

☺ $$$ **Extra Moisture Cream** *($40 for 1.2 ounces)* is a very good emollient moisturizer with some good water-binding agents and tiny amounts of antioxidants. However, many of the plant extracts it contains can be skin irritants.

✓☺ $$$ **Eye Treatment Gel** *($65 for 0.52 ounce)* is a very good lightweight gel that has an impressive mix of water-binding agents and antioxidants. It is an option for normal to oily skin.

✓☺ $$$ **Intensive Anti-Wrinkle Treatment** *($35 for 0.6 ounce)* is an emollient moisturizer for normal to dry skin, with some good water-binding agents and antioxidants.

☺ $$$ **Suspension** *($80 for 1 ounce)*. Alcohol is listed as the fourth ingredient, so the water-binding agents this product contains won't have much of a chance to benefit skin.

☺ $$$ **V-Zone Lift** *($60 for 1.3 ounces)* is similar to Suspension above and the same comments apply.

☺ $$$ **Pure Whiteness** *($140 for 1.05 ounces)* does contain kojic acid, which has substantial research showing it can inhibit melanin production. However, there are other products that can do this for skin without costing this kind of money, and they don't contain so much alcohol, either.

✓☺ $$$ **Sun Defense Face SPF 15** *($30 for 1.6 ounces)* is an excellent, titanium dioxide–based sunscreen that contains some good water-binding agents and an antioxidant.

✓☺ $$$ **Sun Defense Body SPF 30+** *($30 for 4.2 ounces)* is an excellent, titanium dioxide– and zinc oxide–based sunscreen that contains some good water-binding agents and an antioxidant.

☹ **Ultimate Peel Off Masque** *($35 for 2.4 ounces)* is mostly water, film-forming agent (polyvinyl alcohol), and alcohol. That will peel off skin, but it offers no benefit and can end up being irritating and drying for skin in the long run. Many of the plant extracts it contains are also skin irritants.

☹ **Clay Masque** *($23 for 3.5 ounces)*. Between the alcohol and the irritating plant extracts this contains, it is a complete no-no for skin.

☺ $$$ **Lip Conditioner** *($9 for 0.12 ounce)* is a good basic emollient balm for lips.

NOEVIR 95

☺ $$$ **95 Herbal Cleansing Massage Cream** *($30 for 3.5 ounces)* is a fairly greasy wipe-off cleanser that is almost identical to several other cleansers in this line. Massaging it around the face may feel good, but you can do that with almost any oil-based moisturizer, most of which cost a lot less. This needs to be wiped off, which can be an option for dry skin, although some of the plant extracts—including coltsfoot, balm mint, yarrow, and sage—can be significant skin irritants.

☺ $$$ 95 **Herbal Facial Cleanser** *($30 for 3.5 ounces)* is a standard, detergent-based, water-soluble cleanser that can be somewhat drying for many skin types. Who thought up these prices for such a basic product? Several of the plant extracts can be significant skin irritants, including coltsfoot, balm mint, yarrow, and sage.

☹ 95 **Herbal Cleansing Rinse** *($20 for 5 ounces)* is a standard, alcohol-based toner that also contains some water-binding agents, but they won't counteract the drying and irritating effects of the alcohol.

☹ 95 **Herbal Skin Balancing Lotion** *($30 for 4 ounces)* is similar to the Cleansing Rinse above and the same comments apply.

☹ 95 **Herbal Enriched Moisturizer** *($36 for 3.3 ounces)* would be a good moisturizer for normal to dry skin except that the second ingredient is alcohol, which has no place in a moisturizer. Several of the plant extracts can also be significant skin irritants, including coltsfoot, balm mint, yarrow, and sage.

☹ 95 **Herbal Skin Cream** *($40 for 1 ounce)*. The third ingredient is potassium hydroxide, which is lye, and that is a significant skin irritant for all skin types when present in this amount. In addition, several of the plant extracts can be significant skin irritants, including coltsfoot, balm mint, yarrow, and sage.

Noevir 105

☹ $$$ 105 **Herbal Cleansing Massage Cream** *($70 for 3.5 ounces)* is virtually identical to many of Noevir's other wipe-off cleansers. Wiping off makeup can leave a greasy film on the skin, but it can be an option for dry skin. However, given the similarity among Noevir's cleansers, choose the least expensive one, because the price for this cleanser is ridiculous. Several of the plant extracts can be significant skin irritants, including fennel, balm mint, and coltsfoot. For this kind of money, those ingredients should not appear here.

☹ $$$ 105 **Herbal Facial Cleanser** *($56 for 3.5 ounces)* is virtually identical to many of Noevir's other detergent-based, water-soluble cleansers. It can be drying for most skin types, and with potassium hydroxide as the fourth ingredient, the skin doesn't stand a chance. That anyone would charge (or spend) this much money for a cleanser (and a poorly formulated one to boot) is just depressing. Also, several of the plant extracts can be significant skin irritants, including fennel, ivy, yarrow, balm mint, and coltsfoot.

☹ 105 **Herbal Cleansing Rinse** *($32 for 4 ounces)* is a standard, alcohol-based toner that is too drying and irritating for all skin types.

☹ 105 **Herbal Skin Balancing Lotion** *($62 for 4 ounces)* is virtually identical to all of Noevir's alcohol-based toners, with the same list of water-binding agents.

☹ **105 Herbal Enriched Moisturizer** *($70 for 2.6 ounces)* is virtually identical to the 95 Herbal Enriched Moisturizer above, and the same comments and concerns apply. Why this one is more expensive is anyone's guess.

☺ **$$$ 105 Herbal Skin Cream** *($70 for 0.7 ounce)* is similar to the 95 Herbal Skin Cream above. This is a good (though ridiculously overpriced) emollient moisturizer for dry skin. Several of the plant extracts can be significant skin irritants, including coltsfoot, balm mint, yarrow, and sage.

NOEVIR 505

☹ **505 Revitalizing Balancing Lotion** *($88 for 5 ounces).* For what is mostly water, glycerin, and alcohol, this is a shocking amount of money. And this product is supposed to be for very dry skin! Several of the plant extracts can be significant skin irritants, including coltsfoot, balm mint, yarrow, and sage. The umbilical extract that's present here cannot make your skin act young, it is just a water-binding agent.

☺ **$$$ 505 Hydrating Emulsion** *($132 for 3.3 ounces)* is incredibly overpriced and incredibly similar to the other moisturizers in this line, and alcohol is the fifth ingredient, making it potentially drying. Other than that, it is just a basic moisturizer with some good water-binding agents and plant oils. That's good, but not for this amount of money.

☺ **$$$ 505 Perfecting Cream** *($220 for 1 ounce).* That is the real price, believe it or not, but there are no words to express how overpriced and overhyped this product is. It is a good emollient moisturizer with some very good water-binding agents, but only a teeny amount of one antioxidant. Several of the plant extracts can be significant skin irritants, including coltsfoot, yarrow, and sage. The umbilical extract cannot make your skin act young, as it is just a water-binding agent, and I don't even want to think about where the umbilical cord came from.

NOEVIR CLEAR CONTROL

☺ **$$$ Clear Control Clean Wash** *($14 for 2.6 ounces)* is a standard, detergent-based, water-soluble cleanser that would work well for most skin types, though it isn't best for dry skin. It does contain a teeny amount of salicylic acid (BHA), but the pH is too high for it to have any effect as an exfoliant.

☹ **Clear Control Toning Lotion** *($16 for 4 ounces)* is an alcohol-based toner that also contains menthol. That makes it too drying and irritating for all skin types.

☹ **Clear Control Blemish Gel** *($16 for 0.7 ounce)* lists alcohol as the second ingredient, and also contains menthol. The BHA in this gel can exfoliate skin, but there are far less irritating (not to mention less expensive) versions.

NOEVIR HERBAL SKINCARE LINE NHS

☹ **Herbal Skincare Line NHS Deep Cleansing Cream** *($27 for 4.2 ounces)* is virtually identical to the 105 Herbal Cleansing Massage Cream above and the same comments apply.

☹ $$$ **Herbal Skincare Line NHS Foaming Cleanser** (*$25 for 4.5 ounces*) is a standard, detergent-based, water-soluble cleanser that lists potassium hydroxide (lye) as the fourth ingredient, which makes it too drying and irritating for all skin types. Several of the plant extracts can also be significant skin irritants, including coltsfoot, balm mint, fennel, and sage.

☹ **Herbal Skincare Line NHS Balancing Lotion** (*$32 for 4 ounces*) is a standard, alcohol-based toner.

☹ **Herbal Skincare Line NHS Enriched Moisture Lotion** (*$36 for 4 ounces*) lists alcohol as the third ingredient, so this otherwise emollient moisturizer for dry skin can have more problems than benefits. Several of the plant extracts can also be significant skin irritants, including coltsfoot, balm mint, yarrow, and sage.

NOEVIR RECOVERY PROGRAM

☹ **Recovery Complex** (*$45 for 1 ounce*). The fruit extracts in this product are not the same thing as AHAs, not to mention that the alcohol is a skin irritant and several of the plant extracts are also potential skin irritants, including yarrow, fennel, sage, balm mint, and thyme.

☹ **Night Recovery Complex** (*$50 for 1 ounce*) lists alcohol as the third ingredient, making this product too potentially irritating and drying for all skin types.

☹ **Quick Recovery Mask** (*$45 for 3.5 ounces*) contains even more potential skin irritants than most of the Noevir products, including menthol and eucalyptus, along with several others. This is not recommended.

NOXZEMA (SKIN CARE ONLY)

Noxzema has been around for as long as I can remember. I wish longevity had meaning when it comes to good skin care, but it doesn't. These formulations haven't changed in more than 40 years and they still either contain irritating ingredients or are just way out of step with any current research about healthy skin. For more information about Noxzema, call (800) 436-4361 or visit www.noxzema.com.

☺ **Triple Clean Antibacterial Lathering Cleanser** (*$4.69 for 6.5 ounces*) is a standard, detergent-based cleanser that uses fairly drying cleansing agents. It does contain triclosan, a topical disinfectant, but there is no research showing that to be effective against the bacterium that causes blemishes.

☹ **H2Foam Cleansing Cloths** (*$6.99 for 30 pads*) is, just as the name describes, a set of cleansing cloths that get sudsy when they're wet. One side of the cloth is abrasive and the other soft, but this is not an improvement over using your own washcloth with a gentle cleanser. The menthol makes it too irritating for all skin types.

☹ **Original Skin Cream** (*$4.99 for 10.75 ounces*) is one of the most irritating skincare products around and it has been for years. It contains lye, camphor, menthol, phenol, clove oil, and eucalyptus oil. It hurts my skin just thinking about it!

☹ **Plus Cleansing Cream** *($2.99 for 10 ounces)* is just as seriously irritating as the Original Skin Cream above.

☹ **Plus Cleansing Lotion** *($3.99 for 10.5 ounces)* is just as irritating as the Cream versions above and is not recommended for any skin type.

☺ **Sensitive Cleansing Cream** *($3.99 for 10.75 ounces)* just isn't a very effective cleanser, but at least they took the irritating ingredients out of this one. It can be an option for cleaning sensitive, dry skin if you aren't wearing makeup, though it can leave a film on the skin.

☺ **Sensitive Cleansing Lotion** *($4.99 for 10.5 ounces)* is similar to the Sensitive Cleansing Cream above, and the same comments apply.

☹ **2-in- Pads Extra Regular Strength** *($2.99 for 60 pads)* contains a host of irritating ingredients that are damaging to skin, including alcohol, camphor, menthol, and eucalyptus.

☹ **2-in-1 Astringent Acne Medication** *($2.99 for 8 ounces)* contains alcohol, menthol, and peppermint, which makes it just too irritating and drying for words. It also has no benefit for blemishes, so this will only make matters worse.

NU SKIN

First, I want to say how impressed I was with Nu Skin's straightforward provision of information to the consumer about its ingredient lists. Without hesitation, the company supplied all the information I requested. I wish all companies made their ingredient lists this accessible, but, alas, only a handful do. In direct contrast to their consumer-thoughtful assistance, however, the Nu Skin salespeople, much like their counterparts at Amway, Shaklee, Jafra, and Neways, were so over-the-top in their presentation that I was left speechless, and for me, that's rare when it comes to the cosmetics industry. During their sales pitch, they not only applied intense pressure to recruit me as a salesperson, but they also tried to convince me Nu Skin was more concerned with curing cancer and AIDS and saving the rain forests than making money.

It is far beyond the scope of this book to investigate every claim this company makes for its products, but at least as far as skin care is concerned, I can assure you Nu Skin is not a miracle, a cure, the total answer, or even part of the answer for every woman's skincare needs. After all, if the products were miraculous for skin care, why did they reformulate and come out with a new line of products making the same claims only with different ingredients? Nevertheless, the people who sell this line want you to believe it can alter your life as well as your skin. Like most of the other lines I've reviewed, this one contains some very good products, some useless ones, and some that are simply overpriced and a waste of money.

When it comes to claims, Nu Skin's brochures state that its products have "all of the good and none of the bad," but that depends on how you define "bad." The line has indeed made major improvements by removing some of the ingredients it previously used in its products, such as peppermint oil, spearmint oil, sulfur, and sulfuric acid. Yet some of the products still contain camphor and alcohol, many contain fragrance, and a few use fairly drying and irritating detergent cleansing agents.

There are some very good products in the line, but they are not the miracles the company would like you to believe they are. For more information about Nu Skin, call (800) 487-1500 or visit www.nuskin.com. **Note:** All Nu Skin products contain fragrance unless noted otherwise.

☺ **Creamy Cleansing Lotion for Normal to Dry Skin** *($15 for 5 ounces)* is an emollient cleanser that needs to be wiped off and can leave a slight greasy feeling on the skin, but it can be an option for dry skin.

☹ **Facial Cleansing Bar** *($10 for 3.5 ounces)* is a standard, detergent-based, water-soluble bar cleanser. It can be drying for most skin types.

☹ **Pure Cleansing Gel, for Combination to Oily Skin** *($14 for 5 ounces)* is a standard, detergent-based, water-soluble cleanser. Some of the plant extracts can be irritating for skin, including fennel and sage.

☺ **Eye Makeup Remover** *($13.15 for 2 ounces)* is a silicone- and plant oil–based wipe-off cleanser that can leave a slight greasy feel on the skin, but it does work to remove makeup.

☺ **Exfoliant Scrub Extra Gentle** *($11.95 for 2.5 ounces)* contains mostly water, aloe, glycerin, seashells (as an abrasive), and thickeners. The seashells can be rough on the skin, so calling this product gentle is a stretch, but it is a good exfoliant for most skin types.

☺ **Facial Scrub** *($11.45 for 2.5 ounces)* is gentler than the Exfoliant Scrub Extra Gentle above, despite the name difference. This one uses walnut-shell powder that does work as a scrub, and it can be good for someone with normal to dry skin.

☹ **MHA Revitalizing Toner** *($11 for 4.2 ounces)* could be considered an option for a lightweight AHA and BHA toner except that it contains camphor, which makes it unnecessarily irritating for all skin types.

✓☺ **NaPCA Moisture Mist** *($10 for 8.4 ounces)* is a lightweight toner of water, slip agent, and water-binding agents. It would be good for most skin types. It does contain about 1% lactic acid, but at that amount, it acts as a water-binding agent, not an exfoliant. The NaPCA in the name refers to a natural component of skin called sodium DL-pyrrolidonecarboxylate; it is a good water-binding agent, but no more so than many other natural components of skin used in skin-care products, ranging from glycerin to cholesterol and glycolipids.

☹ **pH Balance Facial Toner for Combination to Oily Skin** *($10 for 4.2 ounces)*. The witch hazel in this product is mostly alcohol, and that can be irritating and drying for skin. In addition, this includes fennel and boron nitride, which can also be skin irritants.

☹ **pH Balance Facial Toner for Normal to Dry Skin** *($10 for 5 ounces)* is similar to the pH Balance Facial Toner for Combination to Oily Skin above, only this version adds camphor to the mix, an ingredient that is irritating for all skin types, and especially problematic for dry skin.

☺ **Interim MHA Diminishing Gel** *($25 for 1 ounce)* is an exceptionally standard, lightweight moisturizer for slightly dry skin.

☹ **MHA Revitalizing Lotion** *($18 for 1 ounce)* is supposed to be a combination AHA (5% lactic acid) and BHA (0.2% salicylic acid) lotion, but the pH of the lotion is not low enough for them to act as effective exfoliants, and the amount of BHA is insignificant anyway.

☹ **MHA Revitalizing Lotion with SPF 15** *($23 for 1 ounce)* doesn't contain the UVA-protecting ingredients of avobenzone, titanium dioxide, and zinc oxide, and is not recommended.

✓☺ $$$ **Celltrex Skin Hydrating Fluid** *($29 for 0.5 ounce)* is a very good, lightweight moisturizer that contains some very good water-binding agents and antioxidants. This would be an option for normal to dry skin or slightly dry skin.

☺ $$$ **Enhancer Skin Conditioning Gel** *($29 for 2.5 ounces)* is a lightweight gel that contains some good water-binding agents, but only minuscule amounts of antioxidants.

☺ $$$ **HPX Hydrating Gel** *($49 for 1.5 ounces)*. The placenta in this doesn't deserve comment (though it is just a water-binding agent), and the rest of the ingredients, including some very good water-binding agents and antioxidants, just make this a good moisturizer for normal to slightly dry or combination skin.

✓☺ $$$ **Ideal Eyes Vitamins C & A Eye Refining Creme** *($40 for 0.5 ounce)* is a lightweight cream (although it's really more of a serum than a cream) of mostly silicones and slip agents that does contain small amounts of vitamin C (L-ascorbic acid) and vitamin A (retinol). If you're looking for retinol and vitamin C, you will find other, less expensive versions, but this is as good as any, and is in the right kind of packaging to keep the ingredients stable.

☺ $$$ **Intensive Eye Complex Moisturizing Cream** *($36 for 0.75 ounce)* is a very good moisturizer for dry skin. The so-called "barrier repair technology" ingredients are just water-binding agents and antioxidants. They are very good for dry skin, but whatever repair aspect they may have won't change a wrinkle on your face.

✓☺ **Moisture Restore Day Protective Lotion SPF 15 for Normal to Oily Skin** *($30 for 1.7 ounces)* is a very good, in-part, avobenzone-based sunscreen in an emollient moisturizing base with plant oils, water-binding agents, and anti-irritants. This is not the best for normal to oily skin, though it is an option for normal to dry skin.

✓☺ **Moisture Restore Day Protective Lotion SPF 15 for Normal to Dry Skin** *($30 for 1.7 ounces)* is extremely similar to the Moisture Restore for Normal to Oily Skin above only with zinc oxide as one of the active sunscreen ingredients. The same basic comments apply.

☺ **Moisture Restore Intense Moisturizer** *($28 for 2.5 ounces)* is a very good emollient moisturizer for normal to dry skin that contains some good water-binding agents and a tiny amount of antioxidants.

☺ **NaPCA Moisturizer** *($21 for 2.5 ounces)* is a very good lightweight moisturizer for normal to dry skin that contains some good antioxidants and water-binding agents.

☺ **Night Supply Nourishing Cream** *($35 for 1.7 ounces)* is an emollient moisturizer for normal to dry skin that contains some good water-binding agents, anti-irritants, and small amounts of antioxidants.

☺ **Night Supply Nourishing Lotion** *($35 for 1.7 ounces)* is similar to the Night Supply Nourishing Cream above and the same comments apply.

☹ **Rejuvenating Cream** *($28.45 for 2.5 ounces)* won't rejuvenate the skin, although it can be a good moisturizer for normal to dry skin. It's just not as interesting as many other Nu Skin moisturizers. You're supposed to believe that the tiny amounts of royal jelly, algae, and RNA in here can rejuvenate your skin, but they can't, and there is so little of them in this cream that it's almost a bad joke on the consumer.

☹ **$$$ Tru Face Line Corrector** *($39 for 1 ounce)* is a basic, lightweight, silicone-based moisturizer that contains an ingredient called palmitoyl-pentapeptide. It is a good water-binding agent, but the information about it being a miracle ingredient for the skin comes only from the company that manufactures this ingredient and sells it to the cosmetics industry.

☹ **Tru Face Retinol Skin Perfecting Gel** *($49 for 1 ounce)*. Despite the name on the label, this doesn't contain retinol; however, the see-through container it comes in guarantees that almost any antioxidant in it, particularly the retinyl palmitate that it does contain, won't be stable.

☺ **$$$ Clay Pack** *($13 for 2.5 ounces)* is a standard clay mask with small amounts of water-binding agents and antioxidants. This is an option for normal to oily skin.

☹ **$$$ Creamy Hydrating Masque** *($18 for 3.4 ounces)* is more of a simple emollient moisturizer than a mask, and contains more fragrance than anything beneficial for skin.

☹ **Face Lift Powder, Original Formula** *($25 for 2.65 ounces)* and **Lift Activator, Original Formula** *($10 for 4.2 ounces)*. These two formulas are meant to be mixed together and then applied to skin. The Lift Powder contains egg white, cornstarch, and some water-binding agents. The Lift Activator contains water, aloe, and some water-binding agents. This won't lift skin anywhere, and the egg white and cornstarch can be skin irritants. In addition, the cornstarch can promote bacteria growth.

☹ **Face Lift Powder, Sensitive Skin Formula** *($25 for 2.6 ounces)* and **Lift Activator, Sensitive Skin Formula** *($10 for 4.2 ounces)*. These are virtually identical to the Original Formulas above; the only difference is that instead of egg white the Lift Powder uses acacia powder. That is less irritating than egg white for skin, but it still leaves the cornstarch, which can cause irritation and promote bacteria growth.

NU SKIN WHITE

☹ **White Cream** *($28 for 1 ounce)* does contain mulberry extract, which has some value in preventing melanin production, although there is only limited research showing this to be the case. It also contains bearberry extract (containing arbutin), which can also

The Reviews N

inhibit melanin production, though this has only been shown in vitro. Overall, the amounts of these extracts in this skin-care product are unlikely to affect skin or melanin production, but they are a "might make a small difference" option as an alternative to hydroquinone-based skin-lightening products. This also contains some water-binding agents, anti-irritants, and a tiny amount of antioxidant.

☺ **White Essence** *($29 for 1 ounce)* is similar to the White Cream version above, only in lotion form, and the same basic comments apply.

☺ **White Milk Lotion** *($28 for 4.2 ounces)* is similar to the White Cream version above, only in lotion form, and the same basic comments apply.

☺ **White Skin Lotion** *($26 for 4.2 ounces)* is similar to the White Cream version above, only in lotion form, and the same basic comments apply.

☹ **White UV Base** *($28 for 1.7 ounces)* doesn't contain the UVA-protecting ingredients of avobenzone, titanium dioxide, or zinc oxide, and is not recommended.

☹ **White Masque** *($28 for 3.4 ounces)* is a peel-off type mask that uses the film-forming agent polyvinyl alcohol. It contains even smaller amounts of the mulberry and bearberry extracts than the White products above, making it even that much more ineffective for skin lightening.

☺ $$$ **Skin Brightening Complex** *($17.80 for 0.5 ounce)*. This isn't part of the White line but it should be. It uses both mulberry extract and kojic acid to lighten the skin. There is a good deal of research showing that kojic acid is effective for inhibiting melanin production, far better than mulberry extract (which is the only ingredient used in the White products above). Kojic acid can be an unstable ingredient, but this product is an option as an alternative to using hydroquinone-based skin-lightening products.

Nu Skin 180°

Nu Skin 180° is a small group of products that are incredibly overpriced, and that arrive with overhyped claims that they can reprogram your skin by providing the skin with "Barrier Repair Technology." These can't reprogram anything, because if they could that would mean that Nu Skin expected you to only have to buy these products once, use them up, and then your skin would be back to 180 degrees of where it was when you started, meaning younger and less wrinkled. But reprogramming or not, they're just like any other skin-care products—you have to continue using the stuff for it to work. One of the technology breakthroughs for this line is that its AHA product isn't supposed to be as irritating as others on the market. That lower risk of irritation has more to do with the fact that the pH of the product is over 4, while AHAs work best in a pH of 3. That higher pH does indeed mean a decreased chance of irritation, but it also means less effective exfoliation. Although your skin won't do much renewing, these products for the most part would still be quite good, though absurdly expensive, for normal to dry skin. The studies for these products claim that they make skin look better; what a shock! Are there any studies anywhere in the world showing that a cosmetic made skin look bad? Plus, the studies were not done double-blind and they didn't compare the results with the results of other formulations.

For all the glorious claims, it turns out that the ingredients in these products are actually pretty standard, and the products are not nearly as impressive as other Nu Skin formulations with miracle antiwrinkle claims.

☹ **180° Face Wash** *($35 for 4.2 ounces)* is an overpriced, standard, detergent-based cleanser that uses sodium C14-16 olefin sulfate as the cleansing agent, making it potentially too drying and irritating for skin. There are plant oils in it that can cushion some of the dryness, but why use any irritants whatsoever? The vitamin C it contains would be washed away before it had a chance to have any benefit for skin.

☺ $$$ **180° Skin Mist** *($29 for 3.4 ounces)* is an OK toner that contains some good anti-irritants, but lacks antioxidants and water-binding agents. This would be an option for most skin types.

✓☺ $$$ **180° Night Complex** *($64 for 1 ounce)* is an emollient moisturizer that contains an impressive mix of antioxidants and water-binding agents. It is a very good, though very overpriced, option for normal to dry skin.

☹ **180° UV Block Hydrator SPF 18** *($52 for 1 ounce)* doesn't contain the UVA-protecting ingredients of titanium dioxide, zinc oxide, or avobenzone, and is not recommended.

NU SKIN SUN PRODUCTS

☺ **Sunright Body Block SPF 30** *($13 for 3.4 ounces)* is a very good, in-part avobenzone-based sunscreen with a small amount of antioxidants in a matte-finish base that would be an option for normal to oily skin.

☺ **Sunright Body Block SPF 15** *($13 for 3.4 ounces)* is similar to the Body Block SPF 30 above and the same basic comments apply.

☺ **Sunright Lip Balm 15** *($5.65 for 0.25 ounce)* is a very emollient lip balm that has a very good, in-part titanium dioxide–based sunscreen.

NU SKIN MAKEUP

Nu Colour is the name of Nu Skin's makeup, and if you were hoping the "Nu" would translate to "new" as far as product innovation and textural elegance goes, you may want to keep shopping. This makeup has some credible formulas, but completely misses the boat (the entire ocean, for that matter) when it comes to effective sun protection, skin-true colors, and modern application. According to Nu Skin, each item is supposedly skin care masquerading as makeup, and although several items do contain antioxidants and soothing plant extracts or water-binding agents, the amount of these ingredients present in most of the makeup is trivial, and cannot compensate for the uninspired to unbelievably bad products. The only products worth paying attention to are the makeup brushes, the eye and lip pencils, and the lip gloss, but that's only if you're already a Nu Skin fan. Caution: If you decide to attend a Nu Colour makeup presentation, be prepared to listen to enough hyperbole to fill a book of this size!

The Reviews N

☻ **FOUNDATION:** **Skin Beneficial Tinted Moisturizer SPF 15** *($24)* lacks significant UVA protection, which is odd given that Nu Skin's sunscreens contain Parsol 1789 (avobenzone). That's unfortunate, as this has a light, elegant application that blends superbly to a dry matte finish. The five colors tend to get peachier the darker you go, but this is sheer enough so that the peachiness is not an issue. What is an issue (beyond the lack of good UVA protection) is that the base formula lists the irritant witch hazel as the first ingredient, which makes this not worth considering over tinted moisturizers from Bobbi Brown, Aveda, or Neutrogena. **MoisturShade Liquid Finish SPF 15** *($21)* also lacks reliable UVA protection, and is otherwise a moist, light-coverage foundation that comes in 13 noticeably peach, pink, rose, or orange tones. Who thought any of these shades would look convincing on real skin tones? It's a shame these two major faults outweigh an otherwise well-formulated product, but there you have it.

☹ **CONCEALER:** **Skin Beneficial Concealer** *($16)* is a cream concealer with a greasy consistency and far too much slip to cover evenly and stay in place. Did I mention that Nu Skin's proclivity toward peach and rose-toned shades continues here, too? Well, it does. This compact concealer is only beneficial if you avoid it.

☺ $$$ **POWDER:** **Finishing Powder** *($22.50)* is a talc-free, rice starch–based powder, so this has a drier texture that can feel a bit grainy. It comes in one shade, and while Nu Skin claims that it's translucent, this will look too white or ashen on all but fair skin. **Custom Colour MoisturShade Wet/Dry Pressed Powder** *($18 for powder cake, $6.25 for compact)* feels very soft, almost creamy, and blends nicely to a dry, light-coverage finish. However, this mica-based powder has shine, so there goes Nu Skin's "beautiful matte finish" claim. Almost all of the 11 shades have an unattractive peach, pink, or rose cast that's strong enough to matter, especially in daylight. The only possible contenders are Buffed Ivory and Creamy Ivory. **Bronzing Pearls** *($23)* are bronze-colored powder beads that you sweep a brush over and dust on to complete your sheer, shiny tan. The Body Shop has had this type of product for years, and if the concept appeals to you, check out their Brush-On Bronze ($16.50).

☺ $$$ **BLUSH:** **Custom Colour Subtle Effects Blush** *($14 for blush tablet, $5.75 for compact)* is a smooth powder blush with a dry, flaky application that takes patience to apply. If you start sheer and build, this can impart lasting color with just a hint of shine. Given the cost, I can't think of a convincing reason to consider this over powder blushes from Jane, L'Oreal, or (if you like shiny blush) Almay.

☹ **EYESHADOW:** **Desired Effects Eye Shadow** *($9 per color, $5.75 for duo compact)* eyeshadows have an identical formula to the Subtle Effects Blush above, and the same comments apply. Although the powdery blush was tolerable, the flaking from these can really be a nuisance when you're going for a sophisticated eye design and don't want to constantly deal with eyeshadow fallout, which happens with this even when the application is sheer. Every color has at least a soft shine, which only compounds the issues with this problematic eyeshadow.

EYE AND BROW SHAPER: ☺ **Defining Effects Smooth Eye Liner** *($10)* is a standard, creamy pencil that applies easily and holds up surprisingly well. It's no match for a good powder eyeliner, but if you prefer pencils, you could certainly do worse.

☹ **Defining Effects Brow Liner** *($10)* needs to be sharpened and you'll be doing a lot of that if you choose this creamy pencil. The colors go on strong, so achieving a softly defined, natural brow is almost impossible; plus this will smudge before the end of the day, which is hardly a strong selling point.

LIPSTICK AND LIP PENCIL: ☺ **Undeviating Lipstick SPF 15** *($13)* does not list any active ingredients to justify the SPF number, so you cannot count on this for sun protection. This is actually one of the greasiest lipsticks you're likely to use, and while that's great for a moist look, it's trouble for anyone with lines around the mouth.

☺ **DraMATTEics Lip Colour** *($12)* is a thick, standard pencil lipstick that goes on drier than most and has a minimally creamy after-feel. It's not a true matte finish, but it does wear longer than similar pencils. The small color selection favors mauve and rose tones. **Shining Effects Lip Gloss** *($10)* is a syrupy, wand-type gloss that packs a patent leather shine along with a moderately sticky finish. I prefer a smoother gloss, but this is tenacious. **Lip Gloss Pots** *($9)* hold gloss that is less sticky and considerably more emollient than the Shining Effects Lip Gloss and this is worth a try if you don't mind using your fingers or brush for application. **Defining Effects Smooth Lip Liner** *($10)* is nothing unique as far as pencils are concerned, but this sharpen-me tool has a smooth application and a small, but respectable, color collection.

MASCARA: ☺ **Water Resistant Mascara** *($15)* is about as water-resistant as a wet sponge, but it does lengthen and provide enough thickness to satisfy all except those looking for a false eyelashes effect, and without clumping. This also wears well all day without smudging or flaking.

☹ **Nutriol Eyelash** *($25)* is a clear mascara that is supposed to be a conditioning treatment for lashes, complete with a swanky European pedigree. The last time I checked, ingredients like PVP (a film-forming agent typically used in styling gels), butylene glycol, and witch hazel were not conditioning in the least, and these are the backbone of this too-big-for-its-britches formula. Even more offensive is the **Nutriol Mascara** *($25)*, which for a premium price produces negligible length, no thickness, and smears recklessly during application and wear. It's a resounding disappointment.

☺ $$$ **BRUSHES:** The Nu Colour **Brush Collection** *($115)* is the only category of Nu Skin's makeup that did not have inadequacies or problems. This eight-piece set is a handsome, well-constructed group of brushes, each with a practical purpose. They aren't the softest brushes around, but at an average of $14 per brush, this works out to be a fairly good deal, especially if you end up using all of them regularly. For those not inclined to purchase the set, each brush is available separately for $10 to $20.

The Reviews N

NUTRIFIRM ISOMERS

Many women can't help being entranced by infomercials, especially those claiming to get rid of wrinkles. The promises are just too seductive and there is no easy access to information disproving the claims; all you have is the advertisement exclaiming about the miracle products you will miss out on if you don't call now! In the case of Nutrifirm, the Federal Trade Commission (FTC, www.ftc.gov) helped to set the record straight, though it's most likely only a handful of consumers ever saw the truth. According to an FTC news release, July 11, 2001, "ValueVision International, Inc., of Eden Prairie, Minnesota, has agreed to settle Federal Trade Commission charges that it had aired ads for several products with claims that could not be substantiated. ValueVision, now called ShopNBC is the third largest television 'home shopping' network retailer in the United States. The company has agreed not to make unsubstantiated health-related claims about any food, drug, dietary supplement, cellulite-treatment product, or weight-loss program." It also has agreed to offer dissatisfied consumers refunds.

In regard to their skin-care products, what you end up buying are some very good, though overpriced, moisturizers, a poorly formulated sunscreen, and nothing that can live up to the elaborate claims made about these products. For more information about Nutrifirm Isomers, call (800) 884-2212 or visit www.shopnbc.com.

☺ $$$ **NutriBeauty Double Duty Cleanser** *($19.99 for 4 ounces)* is an emollient cleanser that doesn't remove makeup very well, at least not without the help of a washcloth, though it can be an option for normal to dry skin. It does contain salicylic acid, but the pH is too high for it to be effective as an exfoliant.

☺ **Makeup Remover** *($14.99 for 4 ounces)* is just thickening agents and preservatives; there is nothing about this wipe-off cream that makes it preferred over Pond's Cold Cream.

☺ **Moisture Mist** *($19.98 for two 4-ounce bottles)* is a highly fragranced toner with tiny amounts of water-binding agents. The minute amount of lactic acid it contains is too small for it to have any exfoliating properties for skin.

☺ $$$ **Absolute A + C Serum** *($49.99 for 1 ounce)* is a lightweight gel lotion that contains a good water-binding agent and antioxidants. The price is out of line for what you get, but it would be good for normal to oily skin.

☺ $$$ **Absolute A + E Serum** *($59.99 for 1 ounce)* is similar to the A + C Serum above and the same comments apply.

☺ $$$ **Absolute Anti-Redness** *($34.99 for 1 ounce)* is a lightweight gel with a small amount of a water-binding agent, and there is nothing in it that will reduce redness.

☺ $$$ **Absolute Wrinkle Defense Cream** *($39.99 for 3 ounces)* is a very good moisturizer for normal to dry skin that contains an impressive mix of antioxidants and a water-binding agent.

☹ **Day Cream with SPF 15** *($24.50 for 2 ounces)* doesn't contain the UVA-protecting ingredients of titanium dioxide, zinc oxide, or avobenzone, and is not recommended.

☺ **$$$ Enzyme Therapy Treatment Cream** *($39.99 for 2 ounces)* is a good emollient moisturizer that contains a small amount of antioxidant and water-binding agents. It is a good option for normal to dry skin.

☹ **$$$ Fast Lift Eye Serum** *($49.99 for two 1-ounce bottles)* is a lightweight lotion that contains some good water-binding agents, though the rosemary extract it contains can be a skin irritant.

☺ **Gemmotherapy Cream** *($39.99 for 3 ounces)* is a lightweight cream that contains some good water-binding agents and antioxidants. It is a good option for normal to dry skin.

☹ **NutriBeauty Step 3 Perfecting Fluid** *($29.99 for 2 ounces)* contains about 4% lactic acid and 0.5% salicylic acid, though the pH of the lotion is too high for them to be effective as exfoliants. It also contains a teeny amount of kojic acid, but not enough for it to be effective for inhibiting melanin production, and definitely not without the benefit of an effective sunscreen.

☹ **$$$ NutriBeauty Step 4 Hydrafirm Plus** *($29.99 for 4 ounces)* contains arnica, which is a skin irritant. It also contains wild yam extract, which has no hormonal effect when applied topically on skin.

☹ **Pore Minimizer** *($29.89 for 1 ounce)*. This simply contains aloe, mushroom extract, brown algae, and preservatives, none of which can have any effect on pores. To the contrary, brown algae, because of its high iodine content, may trigger blemishes.

☹ **$$$ Purifying Spot Treatment** *($39.95 for 1 ounce)* contains mostly thickener, aloe, cinnamon, water-binding agent, and preservatives. Cinnamon can be a disinfectant, but there is no research showing it to be effective in the treatment of blemishes, nor is it preferred to other readily available topical disinfectants that come without such a high price tag.

☺ **Resurgence Gemmotherapy Nucleus Cream** *($39.95 for 2 ounces)* is a good emollient moisturizer with some very good water-binding agents, antioxidants, and anti-irritants. It is an option for normal to dry skin.

☹ **$$$ Trace Elements Overnight Recovery** *($49.95 for 2 ounces)* is a good emollient moisturizer with some very good antioxidants, but it lacks water-binding agents.

☺ **$$$ Vitamin C Serum** *($39.99 for 1 ounce)*. If you are looking for vitamin C (an antioxidant) and a water-binding agent, this one is as good as any. The wild yam in it, however, has no hormonal properties when applied topically on skin. It is an option for normal to oily skin.

☹ **Vitamin K Serum** *($34.99 for 2 ounces)*. The arnica in this serum can be a skin irritant, and there is no research showing that vitamin K is beneficial for skin.

N.V. PERRICONE, M.D.

I actually don't know where to begin when discussing the nature of Perricone's work. In many ways it embodies some of the worst elements of what is taking place in the world of dermatology (starting with Dr. Murad of infomercial fame), namely using the cloak of medical expertise to promote the sale of skin-care products. The allure of the physician's involvement is seen as giving medical connotations to products that end up not being different in any significant way from other skin-care products being sold from many lines with or without a doctor's endorsement. Even Perricone has admitted how easily women are fooled by all this; he was quoted in the *New York Times* (November 18, 2001, "The Skin Game with New Wrinkles") as saying "Promise them an unlined face, and you can sell them anything."

It's interesting to note that Perricone himself wavers on the issue of what is the "best" skin-care ingredient. His own line has an array of products with disparate groups of ingredients, from vitamin C to tocotrienol (a potent form of vitamin E), alpha lipoic acid, DMAE, olive oil, and glycolic acid.

Perricone's "research," as described in his best-selling book *The Wrinkle Cure*, more often than not refers to his own research or to his own patients' experience as proof for what he states about a particular antiaging treatment (always using his own products by the way). That may sound convincing, but it's not anyone's definition of science.

From a scientific perspective, this is at best problematic territory, though from a profit viewpoint it's good business and looking better all the time. Highlighting how prevalent and serious an issue this is, an article in the August 1999 issue of the *Tufts University Health & Nutrition Letter* stated that the "American Medical Association has issued guidelines advising physicians not to sell health-related products for profit. When a doctor stands to gain from something a patient buys, it creates a conflict of interest." The American College of Physicians–American Society of Internal Medicine issued ethical guidelines for physicians selling products that were reported on in the *Annals of Internal Medicine* (December 7, 1999). The paper stated that sales of cosmetics and vitamins by physicians are "ethically suspect."

Perricone started out proclaiming the importance of the vitamin C (namely ascorbyl palmitate) in his products. But if vitamin C is the best, why bother with these other ingredients and the parade of new products? Plus, none of the ingredients in Perricone's products are proprietary; they are commonly available and are used by many cosmetics companies.

Many of Perricone's products also contain DMAE. What little research there is about DMAE relates to its effect as an oral supplement, and the findings are mixed. DMAE, known chemically as 2-dimethyl-amino-ethanol, has been available in Europe under the product name Deanol for over 30 years. As an oral supplement it is popularly thought to improve mental alertness. Because DMAE is chemically similar to choline, DMAE is thought to stimulate production of acetylcholine. And because acetylcholine is a brain neurotransmitter, it's easy to see how it could be associated with brain function. However, only a handful of studies have studied the use of DMAE for that purpose, and they have not been conclusive in the least, while some have shown that DMAE may be problematic or not very effective (Sources: *Mechanisms of Aging and Development*, February 1988, pages 129–138; *Neuropharmacology*, June 1989, pages, 557–561; and *European Neurology*, 1991, pages 423–425). Despite the lack of evidence supporting DMAE as having any effect on skin, there are hundreds of Web sites claiming that it does. It is possible that DMAE can help protect the cell membrane, and keeping cells intact can have benefit, but so far that appears to be only conjecture, not fact.

Where Perricone and I agree is that inflammation and irritation are a problem for skin and are contributing factors to the skin's wrinkling and aging process. He states, "It is important to emphasize that inflammation is an integral part of the aging process.... Any process that causes inflammation in the cell accelerates the aging process, and prevention of inflammation has the opposite effect." He also writes that "all anti-oxidants act as anti-inflammatories." Again he's right. But his product line is not the only one that can protect skin from this pervasive problem.

It also deserves mention that while reducing already inflamed and irritated skin is nice, it is far better for skin *not* to get inflamed or irritated at all. But many of Perricone's products contain fragrances, which are known skin sensitizers, and others contain alcohol and eucalyptus, which are drying and irritating to skin while offering no balancing benefit. He also uses sodium lauryl sulfate as the main cleansing agent in his cleansers, a known skin irritant. In fact, sodium lauryl sulfate is the standard dermatologic substance against which the comparative irritation levels of other ingredients are tested.

Further, Perricone has completely overlooked the issue of sun exposure or UVA damage for skin. His line doesn't include a facial sunscreen of any kind, and his two body sunscreens don't include UVA-protecting ingredients. It is unbelievable to me that none of Dr. Perricone's sunscreens have UVA-protecting ingredients, and that he doesn't have even one for the face. So much for current or even basic research about skin over the past several years!

So should you run out and buy Perricone's products? I would follow Perricone's own advice, quoted from his published papers and presentations on the issue. He states, The use of antioxidants in the prevention and treatment of ... aging has just begun.... It is simplistic to assume that senescence [aging] is due to one causal factor." By extension, and from my perspective, that also means aging can't be cured by one or even two random ingredients.

Dr. Perricone's products are available at a range of stores, including Nordstrom, Bloomingdale's, and Sephora, as well as through several Web sites. For more information about N.V. Perricone, M.D., call (888) 823-7837 or visit www.nvperriconemd.com. **Note:** All N.V. Perricone, M.D. products contain fragrance unless otherwise noted.

⊗ **Vitamin C Ester Citrus Facial Wash** (*$25 for 6 ounces*) contains sodium lauryl sulfate as the primary cleansing agent (it is the second ingredient), which makes it too irritating and drying for all skin types, and it is not recommended.

☹ **Vitamin C Ester Facial Refresher Splash** *($25 for 6 ounces)* contains eucalyptus and alcohol, and is absolutely not recommended.

☺ **$$$ Vitamin C Ester Amine Complex Face Lift with NTP Complex** *($75 for 2 ounces)* contains a good mix of water-binding agents and antioxidants and is a good moisturizer for normal to dry skin.

☺ **$$$ Vitamin C Ester 15% Concentrated Restorative Cream with NTP Complex** *($90 for 1.86 ounces)* is the one if vitamin C is the goal! Just keep in mind that no one knows how much of it the skin needs, or how long it needs to be on the skin to have an effect. If you do want vitamin C, 15% of an ester sounds good, but from the research, that appears to be meaningless. You would also have to ask yourself: If this has more vitamin C than the other products, why would you need any of the others? It also contains about a 2% concentration of AHA, which isn't enough for it to act as an exfoliant. This is a good moisturizer for normal to dry skin.

☺ **$$$ Vitamin C Ester Eye Area Therapy** *($45 for 1 ounce)* is a good, silicone-based, lightweight lotion that also contains antioxidants and water-binding agents. The fragrant plant extracts can be skin irritants.

☹ **Alpha Lipoic Acid Nutritive Cleanser** *($30 for 6 ounces)* contains sodium lauryl sulfate as the primary cleansing agent (it is the second ingredient) and is not recommended. Even if this weren't the case, there is nothing about this basic, detergent-based, water-soluble cleanser that is worth the absurd price tag. There is a tiny amount of alpha lipoic acid, but even if you did buy the Perricone-promoted hype around this ingredient, this is a cleanser, and any benefit would be rinsed down the drain.

☺ **$$$ Alpha Lipoic Acid Evening Facial Emollient with NTP Complex and Retinol** *($80 for 2 ounces)* contains a good mix of water-binding agents and antioxidants and is a very good moisturizer for normal to dry skin. It's good, and the buzz-worthy ingredients are in here, but the price is part of the gimmick—it has no relation to the actual value of this formulation.

☹ **$$$ Alpha Lipoic Acid Eye Area Therapy with NTP Complex** *($40 for 0.5 ounce)* is an OK lightweight moisturizer for normal to dry skin, but it is not as well formulated as the Evening Facial Emollient above, even though this one costs four times as much.

☺ **$$$ Alpha Lipoic Acid Face Firming Activator with NTP Complex** *($85 for 2 ounces)* contains about a 5% concentration of AHA in a pH of about 3.5. It would work well for exfoliating the skin, and it contains a small amount of water-binding agents, antioxidants, and anti-irritants.

☺ **$$$ Alpha Lipoic Acid Lip Plumper** *($30 for 0.5 ounce)* is similar to many of Perricone's products, and contains the same water-binding agents and antioxidants. It's a good moisturizer, but don't expect fuller lips.

☹ **Alpha Lipoic Acid Body Toning Lotion SPF 15 with NTP Complex** *($60 for 6 ounces)* doesn't contain the UVA-protecting ingredients of titanium dioxide, zinc oxide, or avobenzone, and is not recommended.

☺ **$$$ Alpha Lipoic Acid Anti Spider-Vein Face Treatment with Tocotrienols** *($80 for 1 ounce)* claims it can reduce the appearance of spider veins because it contains alpha lipoic acid and tocotrienols. Alpha lipoic acid is well established as one of many effective antioxidants. It is also an effective anti-inflammatory, but that has very little to do with mitigating spider veins, which are extremely common on sun-damaged skin and extremely stubborn to treat.

Tocotrienols, which are a more potent form of vitamin E (tocopherol), are purported to be better antioxidants. According to the University of California at Berkeley's Web site, *Wellness Guide to Dietary Supplements,* "[Tocotrienol] research in humans is very limited, and the results conflicting." The research that has been carried out has centered on large doses of oral tocotrienols, and the results are being compared and contrasted with what we know about how other tocopherols function in the body. In vitro (test-tube) studies have demonstrated that tocotrienols do have more potent antioxidant capabilities than tocopherol. So how does all of this relate to skin care, and, more to the point, spider veins? Although studies of topical application of tocotrienols have found they can penetrate to the subcutaneous (lower) layer of skin, where they exert their antioxidant properties, there appears to be no association between tocotrienols and treating spider veins. As I have written before about antioxidants, the jury is still out on how much of any topically applied antioxidant is needed for it to be effective. Full-scale clinical studies on humans to assess the benefits of topical tocotrienols have not yet been performed (all of the research on topical use of tocotrienols has been performed on hairless mice), so for now, as is true for all antioxidants, choosing it is a leap of faith, albeit one that is worth taking. There is no research showing topical application of any ingredient, prescription-only, over the counter, or cosmetic, can get rid of spider veins.

This remains a very good, exceedingly overpriced, moisturizer for normal to dry skin. Although it is well-formulated, with good water-binding agents and antioxidants, it is interesting to note that several antioxidants (including the much-ballyhooed tocotrienols) are listed after the preservatives, meaning they are barely present.

☺ **$$$ Phosphatidyl-E Lipid Bi-Layer Repair Face Treatment with Tocotrienols** *($120 for 2 ounces)* contains phosphatidylcholine (PC), which is the most active ingredient found in lecithin. Every cell membrane in the body requires phosphatidylcholine. Nerve and brain cells in particular need large quantities of PC for repair and maintenance. It is also a major source of the neurotransmitter acetylcholine. Acetylcholine is used by the brain in areas that are involved in long-term planning, concentration, and focus. But all of this information is associated with ingesting PC, not putting it on the skin. So how does any of that relate to skin care? PC is considered a very good moisturizing agent and aids in the penetration of other ingredients into the skin. It absorbs well without feeling greasy or heavy, though other ingredients can perform similarly, including glycerin, the third ingredient in this product, and many other water-binding agents this product doesn't contain (such as ceramides and hyaluronic acid). So it is not the be-all and end-all skin-care ingredient (if it were, then shouldn't it be in all Perricone products?). It is just one of many good water-binding agents that show up in skin-care products.

One more interesting ingredient in this moisturizer is tamanu oil. This oil, from a tree native to Polynesia, is reputed to have wondrous wound-healing properties, as well as being a cure-all for almost every skin ailment you can think of, from acne to eczema to psoriasis. Yet all of the miraculous claims are hinged on anecdotal, not scientific, evidence. There's no harm in using this oil in skin care—like most oils, it is composed of phospholipids and glycolipids, and these are good water-binding agents for skin. Tamanu oil also appears to have anti-inflammatory properties, though this has not been proven in any direct research on skin.

Aside from the buzz ingredients, this is an ordinary moisturizer that has most of the antioxidants listed after the preservatives, meaning there isn't much of them. It would be an option for someone with normal to dry skin, although the price is astronomical for what you get. It does contain fragrance.

☺ $$$ **Olive Oil Polyphenols Gentle Cleanser** (*$35 for 6 ounces*) is a standard, gentle cleanser that should be fairly water-soluble even with the added olive oil. However, surrounding all this mildness are potent eye and skin irritants like orange, lemon, grapefruit, geranium, petitgrain, and neroli oils, along with coloring agents, and that makes this cleanser problematic both for the price and for the claims of being superior because of its doctor-associated status.

☺ $$$ **Olive Oil Polyphenols Day Face Treatment** (*$85 for 2 ounces*), if used during the daytime, must be paired with an effective sunscreen. However, you may want to think twice about using such an overpriced moisturizer whose fragrance comes from nothing less than the potentially irritating plant extracts described in the Cleanser above, as well as from comfrey extract. If the lure of olive oil has captured your attention, try turning to plain olive oil instead, which is excellent (though greasy) over very dry skin. This product does contain very good water-binding agents, emollients, antioxidants, film-forming agents, and silicones, but they don't make it any more significant than lots of other products.

☺ $$$ **Olive Oil Polyphenols Night Face Treatment** (*$85 for 2 ounces*) is similar to, but more emollient than, the Day Face Treatment above, and the same comments apply. Contrary to the claim, olive oil is not fine for all skin types, and especially not for those that tend to break out.

☺ $$$ **Olive Oil Polyphenols Face Hydrator** (*$65 for 1.7 ounces*) is similar to the Night Face Treatment above, only this is lighter due to the addition of silicone. The same fragrant plant extracts are present here, too, and the same comments apply.

☹ $$$ **Face Finishing Moisturizer** (*$50 for 1.86 ounces*) is an OK moisturizer for dry skin. It contains small amounts of water-binding agents and tiny amounts of antioxidants.

N.V. PERRICONE ACNE PRODUCTS

☹ $$$ **Pore Refining Cleanser** (*$30 for 6 ounces*) is a standard, detergent-based cleanser that contains about 5% glycolic acid. In a cleanser, the benefit from the AHA would just be rinsed down the drain, but in this case the pH is too high for it to be effective as an exfoliant.

☹ **Pore Refining Toner Pads** *($35 for 60 pads)* lists alcohol as the second ingredient, and also contains some eucalyptus, making this too potentially irritating for all skin types.

☺ $$$ **Acne Treatment Gel Cream** *($55 for 2 ounces)* is a very standard, 2.5% benzoyl peroxide topical disinfectant. While this would definitely be an option for treating blemishes, the price is just out of whack. There are far less expensive versions available at the drugstore and they don't contain the thickening agents that might cause breakouts. This does contain about 4% AHA, but the pH of the base is too high for it to be effective as an exfoliant.

☺ $$$ **Pore Refining Moisturizer** *($55 for 2 ounces)* is a good moisturizer for normal to dry skin, but there is nothing in it that will affect pores.

N.Y.C. (MAKEUP ONLY)

If the N.Y.C. title reminds you of New York City, it should—it's almost the same as the name of this small drugstore makeup line—New York Color. N.Y.C. equates itself with all of the excitement and pulsating action of the Big Apple, but let me assure you it is comparatively tame. In the universe of beguiling makeup descriptions that sound more like *Sex in the City* than *60 Minutes,* N.Y.C. is more like a new Woody Allen film—a few surprises, but predictably familiar in the end. The most appealing part of this line is rock-bottom prices; nothing costs more than $3.99. Although this isn't the cream of the crop for makeup, there are more than enough inexpensive options to make a visit to the land of New York Color worth your while. Just don't expect these products to leave you as pampered and primped as a Park Avenue socialite! For more information about N.Y.C., call (800) 954-5080 or visit www.newyorkcolor.com.

☺ FOUNDATION: **Smooth Skin Liquid Makeup** *($2.99)* is a basic, no-frills liquid foundation that starts out a bit thick but blends out to a soft, sheer finish. This would work well for normal to slightly oily skin, though the three shades are limited to those with a light skin tone. For a color line named after a multicultural melting pot, that's an obvious shortcoming!

☺ CONCEALER: **Cover Stick** *($1.99)* is a lipstick-style cream concealer that has a smooth silicone base. It's still on the thick side and can easily look caked if you overdo, but it stands less chance of creasing than similar, creamier products. The three shades aren't bad either!

☺ POWDER: **Loose Face Powder** *($2.99)* and **Pressed Face Powder** *($1.99)* are both standard, talc-based powders with soft, sheer applications and two color shades, of which Naturally Beige is too peach. The pressed version is very soft, and goes on more like a loose powder. Each version's Translucent color is for fair to light skin tones only.

☹ BLUSH: The **Powder Blush** *($1.99)* is available in a small assortment of matte shades, but the hard, dry texture makes it difficult to pick up color, and what little is deposited on the brush barely registers on the skin, making this a futile product.

☺ <u>EYESHADOW</u>: **Eye Cubes** *($1.99)* have a great, plush texture and a very sheer application. For a soft wash of color, these are an option, though almost all of the shades are shimmery pastels. Autumn Garden is the only matte option. **Eyeshadow Trio** *($3.99)* features the same formula as the Eye Cubes above, and although these trios are well-coordinated, every shade is too shiny for anything but evening wear. **Eye Shimmer** *($1.99)* are small tubes of iridescent, pastel, and metallic colors. They go on sheer and have lots of slip, so don't count on them staying in place for long.

<u>EYE AND BROW SHAPER:</u> ☺ **Eyeliner Duets** *($1.99)* are double-ended standard pencils that feature contrasting colors, one of which is iridescent. As pencils, they'll work as well as any. **Eye Liner Pencil** *(99¢)* is a standard, but good, pencil with an irresistible price. The traditional colors make this one to check out if you prefer pencils to powder. **Liquid Eyeliner** *($1.99)* is excellent if you can tolerate the slow drying. This has a long, thin brush that is surprisingly easy to control, and applies without skipping. Once dry, it stays on quite well without chipping or smearing.

The ☺ **Eyebrow Pencil** *(99¢)* is standard, and a bit greasy, even though it is a bargain.

<u>LIPSTICK AND LIP PENCIL:</u> ☺ **Moisturizing Lipstick** *(99¢)* is a basic creamy lipstick with a soft, glossy finish and minimal stain. Not bad for under a dollar! **Long Wearing Lipstick** *(99 cents)* is certainly less creamy than the one above, but not enough to merit a long-wearing claim. This does apply smoothly and covers evenly, though the colors are not as sophisticated as those from Revlon, for example. **Liquid Lip Shine** *($1.99)* is a very emollient wand-type lip gloss that has an iridescent, sticky finish. It's comparable to many other glosses in all price ranges. ✔☺ **Brush-On Lip Color** *($2.99)* is a sheer, minimally sticky lip gloss with a hint of color. The brush applicator is easy to work with, and this is a gloss lover's find!

✔☺ **Lip Liner Pencil** *(99¢)* needs sharpening, but at this price, you may not mind! It has a smooth texture that glides on and is not overly creamy, and is a liplining steal and a must-try if you find a color you like.

☺ **Fruit Flavored Lip Gloss** *($1.99)* comes in a pot and features sickeningly sweet fruit flavors with a heavy dose of pre-teen appeal. **Roll-On Lip Gloss** *($1.99)* and **Roll-On Fruit Flavored Lip Gloss** *($1.99)* are thick and greasy, able to produce a syrupy-wet shine on the lips, without or with fruity flavor.

☹ **LipForever** *($3.99)* is a poor imitation of Lipfinity. The paint-your-lips, wait for the color to set, and glossy-top-coat directions are the same, but this product comes off easily on cups, tissues, or significant others. What's worse, the remaining color looks spotty.

☺ <u>MASCARA</u>: **Lengthening Mascara** *($1.99)* takes a lot of effort to build noticeable length, and thickness is a foreign concept. At least the price will not leave you disappointed. **Thickening Mascara** *($1.99)* is not much for thickening, but you can achieve decent, clump-free length and subtle definition. I wouldn't choose this over a Maybelline or L'Oreal mascara, but if your budget is extremely tight, this works.

☹ <u>BRUSHES:</u> The **Brush Kit** *($1.99)* is laughable. The tiny, doll-size brushes can't come close to a professional application, and aren't even as nice as the throwaway brushes packaged with most blushes and eyeshadows.

☺ <u>SPECIALTY:</u> **All-Over Body Glitter Gel** *($1.99)* is an inexpensive way to go about adorning yourself in non-sticky, gel-based glitter should the desire or the occasion arise.

OBAGI NU-DERM (SKIN CARE ONLY)

For those of you who aren't familiar with Dr. Zein E. Obagi, he is a dermatologist who created his own skin-care line to be used in conjunction with his Blue Peel and a prescription for Retin-A. His antiaging program took off as dermatologists and plastic surgeons alike started to sell his skin-care products and perform his Blue Peel. Yet the Obagi Nu-Derm products are as far from being "dermatologic" as you can imagine. For the most part, there is nothing in them that cannot be found elsewhere in standard cosmetic or skin-care products for far less money. And the hype is just absurd for such extraordinarily standard products. The products supposedly contain something called Complex 272, which turns out to be nothing more than saponin. Saponin is a carbohydrate produced by plants that can break down cell walls, including human cell walls, among other activities. Saponins can also have water-binding and antioxidant properties for skin, and there is some evidence that they can have antimicrobial benefits. But there is nothing particularly exciting about any of that, and in the teeny amounts found in these products they are inconsequential.

In contrast, the Blue Peel is completely effective, and can be used only by dermatologists. Dr. Obagi's Blue Peel is a standard trichloroacetic acid (TCA) peel of a type that has been performed by dermatologists and plastic surgeons for years. TCA is used for peeling the face, neck, hands, and other exposed areas of the body. It causes fewer pigmentation problems than other doctor-only peels such as phenol, and is considered excellent for "spot" peeling of specific areas. It can be used for medium or light peeling, depending on the concentration and method of application. AHA and BHA peels are considered light peels, and are often done in a series of six. TCA peels are best for fine lines and can be somewhat more effective on deeper wrinkling, but they are performed only once every couple of years. Many of the dermatologists I spoke to believe that a TCA peel is a viable option for many skin types, despite consumers' fascination with AHA peels.

As for the Obagi products, they are sold exclusively through dermatologists' offices and are given the marketing affectation of being "prescribed" by the doctor. However, except for the 4% hydroquinone products in this line, all these items are strictly cosmetic and not prescription-only in the least. There are many reasons why a woman should see a dermatologist. As Obagi states in his brochure, a professionally applied peel, the use of Retin-A or Renova, and an effective skin-lightening product can be the best game plan for reducing the effects of sun damage. The rest of the products, however, are just cosmetics— and are no better or worse than other products being sold today in a wide array of venues.

For more information about Obagi, call (800) 636-SKIN or visit www.obagiskinhealth.com. **Note:** All Obagi Nu-Derm products contain fragrance unless otherwise noted.

☺ $$$ **Nu-Derm Foaming Gel Cleanser** *($29 for 6.7 ounces)* isn't all that gentle, but it is a good, detergent-based, water-soluble cleanser for someone with normal to oily skin. It does contain fragrance and coloring agents.

☺ $$$ **Nu-Derm Gentle Cleanser** *($29 for 6.7 ounces)* is similar to the Foaming Gel above and the same basic comments apply.

☹ **Nu-Derm Toner** *($29 for 6.7 ounces).* The potassium alum in this toner is a potent absorbent and topical disinfectant that can be a skin irritant, and the witch hazel distillate is mostly alcohol, which also can be irritating and drying for skin. Moreover, this product does not return skin to a good pH because the potassium alum has a very high pH, something that is not helpful for skin.

☹ **Nu-Derm Action** *($15 for 2 ounces)* is supposed to "diminish discomfort due to excessive dryness, itching, redness or burning" from the Obagi peel. However, this is just an OK, basic moisturizer for dry skin, with nothing in the formulation to reduce irritation any better or differently than any other moisturizer. It also contains sodium lauryl sulfate as an emulsifier, and in a product meant to reduce irritation, this extremely irritating ingredient is ill advised.

☹ $$$ **Nu-Derm Tolereen** *($40 for 2 ounces)* is a 0.5% hydrocortisone moisturizer. There are many reasons to use a product that contains hydrocortisone—minor irritations, skin rashes, allergic reactions, dermatitis, and some inflammations can be calmed quite effectively with an over-the-counter hydrocortisone lotion or cream. Lanacort and Cortaid, which have a 1% hydrocortisone content (both are available at drugstores for about $6 for 1 ounce), work at least as well as, if not better than, this product because they have a higher concentration. Keep in mind that hydrocortisone is for sporadic, infrequent usage only, because with repeated application it can break down the skin's collagen and elastin. This product also contains sodium lauryl sulfate, a significant skin irritant, which is an ironic ingredient to put in a product meant to reduce skin irritation.

☺ $$$ **Nu-Derm Blender** *($54 for 2 ounces)* is a 4% hydroquinone cream and is only available from a physician. It is absolutely an option when used in conjunction with a good sunscreen because it inhibits melanin production and so reduces the appearance of brown discolorations. However, for the money, Tri-Luma from Galderma (also reviewed in this book under Tri-Luma) is an impressive alternative product for skin lightening.

☹ **Nu-Derm Clear** *($58 for 2 ounces)* is similar to the Blender above except that this contains sodium lauryl sulfate, which adds a significant skin irritant to a product that can already be irritating.

☺ $$$ **Cffectives Eye Contour Serum 5%** *($32.95 for 0.5 ounce)* is a lightweight lotion that contains 5% L-ascorbic acid (vitamin C). If you are looking for vitamin C this is an option, but it ends up being a limited one, as there are no emollients, water-binding agents, or other antioxidants. Obagi's claim that the L-ascorbic acid is the only form of vitamin C that can be used by the body is not true. There is research showing that many other forms of vitamin C, including magnesium ascorbyl phosphate, ascorbic acid, and ascorbyl palmitate, can also be effective for skin.

☺ $$$ Cffectives High Potency Serum 10% ($57.95 for 1 ounce) is similar to the Serum 5% version above and the same comments apply.

☹ $$$ Nu-Derm Eye Cream ($38.50 for 0.5 ounce) is an extremely standard emollient moisturizer that can be OK for dry skin, but it is incredibly overpriced for what you get. It contains minuscule amounts of water-binding agents and antioxidants.

☹ $$$ Nu-Derm Exfoderm ($48 for 2 ounces) is just a moisturizer that lists phytic acid as the third ingredient. Phytic acid is a good antioxidant, but not the only one or the best one. Other than that, this is mostly water and thickeners, which makes it a rather mediocre moisturizer for normal to dry skin.

☺ $$$ Nu-Derm Exfoderm Forte ($48 for 2 ounces) is a good 8% AHA product in an extremely standard moisturizer base, which means it can easily be replaced by AHA products from lots of other lines that provide the same effective exfoliation for far less money.

☺ Nu-Derm Sunblock SPF 25 ($38 for 2 ounces) is a very good, titanium dioxide–and zinc oxide–based sunscreen in a fairly standard moisturizing base. However, there is nothing about this formulation that can't be replaced by less expensive versions from Neutrogena, which is available at the drugstore. Moreover, because sunscreen must be applied liberally to obtain the full SPF benefit, you must take into consideration that using an expensive sunscreen could make you hold back from doing that.

☹ Nu-Derm Sunfader ($50 for 2 ounces) is a 4% hydroquinone product that also contains a sunscreen with an SPF 15. However, this sunscreen doesn't contain the UVA-protecting ingredients of titanium dioxide, zinc oxide, or avobenzone, and, therefore, provides inadequate protection, and that can make skin discolorations worse.

OCEAN POTION

The Ocean Potion line is all about sunscreens, and for the most part the selection is impressive. Unfortunately, they don't list all of their ingredients on the label. Because sunscreens are regulated as over-the-counter drugs, they are not required to list their "other ingredients," only the actives, which Ocean Potion does. That's disappointing, but given that the most important aspect of these products is their SPF, that oversight can be forgiven, a little. What can't be forgiven are the Ocean Potion sunscreens with substandard SPF ratings, the overall lack of UVA-protecting ingredients, and, even more reprehensible, the products that are designed to encourage sun tanning. Ocean Potion lost their way, but hopefully, with time, they will find their path back to offering only reliable and effective products to help protect skin from the serious problems caused by sun damage. For more information about Ocean Potion, call (800) 715-3485 or visit www.opotion.com. **Note:** The FDA's new sunscreen monograph will make sunscreens with SPF ratings over 30 invalid, and they will no longer be allowed to be sold. High SPF numbers can be deceptive because they do not reflect better, more intense protection, only the same level of protection for a longer time, and there just aren't enough daylight hours for SPF numbers greater than 30 to be relevant.

☺ **Antiaging Sunblock SPF 15** *($6.49 for 6 ounces)*; **Antiaging Sunblock SPF 30** *($6.49 for 6 ounces)*; **Antiaging Sunblock SPF 50** *($6.49 for 6 ounces)*; **Kids Sunblock SPF 30** *($6.49 for 6 ounces)*; **Kids Spray Sunblock SPF 30** *($6.99 for 8.5 ounces)*; **Baby Block SPF 50** *($6.99 for 6 ounces)*; **Sport Extreme Sunblock SPF 30** *($6.49 for 6 ounces)*; **Sport Extreme Sunblock Spray SPF 30** *($6.99 for 8.5 ounces)*; **Sport Extreme Sunblock SPF 50** *($6.99 for 6 ounces)*; and **Lip Potion SPF 45** *($1.89 for 0.15 ounce)* are all are very good sunscreens that contain avobenzone as one of the active ingredients. There is no information about what else these products contain.

☺ **Face Potion Clear SPF 45** *($2.99 for 0.5 ounce)* is a very good sunscreen with titanium dioxide and zinc oxide as two of the active ingredients. There is no information about what else this product contains.

☹ **Antiaging Sunscreen SPF 8** *($6.49 for 6 ounces)*; **Extreme Tanning Spray Gel SPF 4** *($6.49 for 8.5 ounces)*; **Extreme Tanning Spray Gel SPF 8** *($6.49 for 8.5 ounces)*; **Extreme Tanning Spray Gel SPF 15** *($6.49 for 8.5 ounces)*; and **Xtreme Amplifier Oil SPF 4** *($6.49 for 8.5 ounces)* all have either abysmally low SPF numbers and/or do not contain the UVA-protecting ingredients of titanium dioxide, zinc oxide, or avobenzone, and are not recommended.

☹ **Xtreme Amplifier Oil** *($6.49 for 8.5 ounces)*; **Xtreme Carrot Oil** *($6.49 for 8.5 ounces)*; **Xtreme Intensifier with Instant Bronzer** *($6.49 for 8.5 ounces)*; and **Stimulating Xcelerator Spray Gel** *($6.49 for 8.5 ounces)* all encourage sun tanning and it's unethical for any skin-care company to sell such products.

☺ **Sunless Potion Streak Free Sunless Tanner** *($6.49 for 6 ounces)* contains dihydroxyacetone, the same ingredient all self-tanners use to affect the color of skin. This one would work as well as any.

OLAY (SKIN CARE ONLY)

Oil of Olay was renamed Olay back in 1999 when it was purchased by its current owner, Procter & Gamble. The name change was a great improvement—after all, there was never a plant, much less any kind of oil, called Olay. Aside from the name change, P&G made other changes at Olay, and some of those have been for the better. Olay now has some great sunscreen formulations, and they have deleted all of the ones that lacked UVA-protecting ingredients, while a few of the cleansers are a great option for skin. Aside from that, though, Olay is just not a particularly exciting line. Most of their moisturizers lack any state-of-the-art moisturizing ingredients such as interesting water-binding agents, plant oils, or antioxidants. In fact, many of these formulations are so boring and dated they seem stuck in a time warp from the '60s. Olay's Age Defying series products do contain salicylic acid (beta hydroxy acid, or BHA), but despite the fact that the original press release for these products discussed the need for a low pH for the BHA to be effective as an exfoliant, only one of the products meets that criterion.

ProVital is a line of skin-care products Olay is aiming at the "mature" woman. Grouping women of a certain age into one grand, indefinite bunch euphemistically called mature is inaccurate, because age does not determine skin type. There are 50-, 60-, and 70-year-old women with all sorts of skin conditions ranging all the way from breakouts, whiteheads, oily skin, and rosacea to sun damage and blackheads. Dry skin is not the only skin type for older women and they should not all be using the same products. Plus, these ProVital products have mediocre, uninspired formulations.

Olay's Total Effects is supposed to be the only product that addresses the "seven signs of aging." I'm not sure how Olay accounted for only "seven" signs, because there are dozens and dozens of changes in the skin that reflect "aging." (Actually, what appears on the surface of skin is only minimally related to aging; it's primarily related to years and years of sun damage.) Total Effects is all about the ingredient niacinamide, a B vitamin that does have some research showing it to be of benefit for skin, and these products do contain more of it than most other products on the market. If you are interested in niacinamide this is the line to consider (refer to Chapter Seven, *Cosmetics Dictionary*, for more detailed information regarding this ingredient). But bear in mind that because of the skin's complexity, one ingredient can't possibly meet all the needs and challenges of sun-damaged skin. For more information about Olay, call (800) 285-5170 or visit www.olay.com. **Note:** All Olay products contain fragrance unless otherwise noted.

☺ **Daily Facials Cleansing Cloths, Normal to Oily** (*$6.99 for 30 cloths*) is basically a detergent-based, water-soluble, wipe-off makeup remover that would be an option if it didn't contain menthol, which adds nothing but irritation to this cleanser. Moreover, the Vaseline in it is not a great option for oily skin types. If the notion of cleansing cloths sounds convenient, Diaparene Baby Wash Cloths, Fragrance-Free ($2.49 for 100 towelettes) or Huggies Baby Wipes Refills, Natural Care, Unscented ($5.29 for 160 towelettes) are far better options than this one and they don't contain fragrance!

☺ **Daily Facials Cleansing Cloths Normal to Dry** (*$6.99 for 30 cloths*) is virtually identical to the Normal to Oily version above and the same comments apply.

☺ **Facial Cleansing Lotion** (*$3.99 for 6.78 ounces*) is a lightweight cleanser that doesn't quite rinse off without the aid of a washcloth, but it is an option for normal to dry skin.

☺ **Foaming Face Wash** (*$3.99 for 6.78 ounces*) is a standard, detergent-based, water-soluble cleanser that cleans the face well and can be good for most skin types.

☺ **Sensitive Skin Foaming Face Wash** (*$3.99 for 6.78 ounces*) is almost identical to the Foaming Face Wash above only without fragrance. That is indeed better for sensitive skin, but it is also better for all skin types.

☹ **Refreshing Toner** (*$3.49 for 7.2 ounces*) contains mostly alcohol, which makes it too irritating and drying for all skin types.

☺ **Active Hydrating Beauty Fluid, Regular** *($9.99 for 6 ounces)* contains mostly water, thickeners, glycerin, mineral oil, Vaseline, silicone, fragrance, preservatives, and, oh, yes, artificial red dye to give it the well-known Olay pink cast. It is an extremely boring, run-of-the-mill, dated formulation for normal to dry skin.

☺ **Active Hydrating Beauty Fluid, Oil-Free** *($9.99 for 6 ounces)* leaves out the Vaseline and mineral oil the Regular version above contains, and still leaves only a handful of waxes, glycerin, some silicones, and preservatives. This is definitely not worthy of becoming part of anyone's skin-care routine.

☺ **Active Hydrating Beauty Fluid, Sensitive Skin** *($9.99 for 6 ounces)* is almost identical to the Regular version above, only minus the fragrance, which doesn't change how dated a formulation this is for skin.

☺ **Active Hydrating Cream, Original** *($6.29 for 2 ounces)* is similar to the Regular version above, only in cream form, and the same basic comments apply.

☺ **Active Hydrating Cream, Oil Free** *($6.29 for 2 ounces)* is similar to the Fluid, Oil-Free version above and the same basic comments apply.

☺ **Active Hydrating Cream, Sensitive Skin** *($6.29 for 2 ounces)* is similar to the Fluid, Sensitive Skin version above and the same comments apply.

☺ **Night of Olay Night Care Cream** *($6.29 for 2 ounces)* is just water, glycerin, thickeners, silicone, and preservatives. It's utterly mundane and a poor option for healthy skin care.

☺ **Complete UV Protective Moisture Lotion SPF 15 (Fragrance and Fragrance Free)** *($7.99 for 4 ounces)* is a very good, in-part zinc oxide–based sunscreen. While the sun protection is impressive, the moisturizing base leaves much to be desired. It contains mostly water and wax and no other interesting water-binding agents or antioxidants. That's not bad, it's just not great. Still, the SPF 15 is what really counts for a daytime product anyway.

☺ **Complete UV Protective Moisture Cream SPF 15 (Fragrance and Fragrance Free)** *($6.99 for 2 ounces)* is similar to the Lotion version above and the same comments apply.

OLAY TOTAL EFFECTS

☹ **Total Effects Daily Cleansing Cloths** *($8.49 for 30 cloths)* is a unique twist on the new fad of cleansing cloths. This one has dry cloths that contain dry ingredients that are mostly detergent cleansing agents, slip agents, Vaseline, film-forming agent, fragrance, preservatives, and menthol (almost identical to the Daily Facials Cleansing Cloths above). You first wet the cloth, lather up, wipe off your makeup, and then discard the cloth. One side of these cloths is soft while the other is slightly abrasive. The soft side is best for all skin types. Although menthol is the last ingredient listed, these do leave a slight tingle on the face and can end up being irritating, especially for the eye area.

☺ **Total Effects Intensive Restoration Treatment** *($19.99 for 1.01 ounces)* contains mostly water, glycerin, niacinamide (vitamin B3), thickeners, silicone, more thickeners, film-forming agent, antioxidants, and preservatives. It would be good for someone with normal to dry skin. There is a small amount of research showing that topical niacinamide is effective in helping repair skin's intercellular matrix (the glue that holds skin cells together), though this was shown only in vitro and not on real human skin (Source: *British Journal of Dermatology*, September 2000, pages 524–531). Extrapolating any of this to wrinkles is a stretch, but it is clearly a good ingredient for skin, it just isn't the only one to show this kind of benefit, though this product from Olay contains more of it than most!

☺ **Total Effects Moisturizing Vitamin Complex (Fragrance and Fragrance Free)** *($19.99 for 1.7 ounces)* is supposed to address all of the issues concerning the "signs of aging." However, this product lacks a sunscreen, and without that, it can't address one of the primary ways to prevent most signs of aging. Aside from that oversight, this is similar to the Restoration Treatment above and the same basic comments apply.

☺ **Total Effects Night Firming Creme for Face and Neck** *($19.99 for 1.7 ounces)* is similar to the Restoration Treatment above and the same comments apply.

☺ **Total Effects Moisturizing Vitamin Complex SPF 15 Fragrance Free** *($8.99 for 1.7 ounces)* is a very good, in-part avobenzone-based sunscreen that comes in a decent, though basic, moisturizing base. Does it fight the "seven signs of aging" Olay has discovered? Basically, the effective sunscreen alone is enough to combat the most noticeable, bothersome signs of "aging," which are really from sun damage and unrelated to aging. It has a similar moisturizing base to the other Total Effects products and those comments apply here as well. This is an option for normal to dry skin.

OLAY AGE DEFYING SERIES

☹ **Age Defying Series Daily Renewal Cleanser** *($4.60 for 6.78 ounces)* contains sodium lauryl sulfate as one of the cleansing agents, which makes it potentially too irritating and drying for all skin types.

☺ **Age Defying Series Daily Renewal Cream** *($9.29 for 2 ounces)* isn't an exciting formula, but it does have a pH low enough to allow the BHA to be an effective exfoliant, though the exact amount of salicylic acid remains a mystery. If you are interested in trying a BHA product instead of an AHA product, this is a reasonable one to consider, though it's best only for someone with normal to dry skin. It comes up short for any other benefit such as antioxidants or water-binding agents.

☺ **Age Defying Series Protective Renewal Lotion Beta Hydroxy Complex SPF 15** *($8.91 for 4 ounces)* is an in-part zinc oxide–based sunscreen that would be fine for daytime use. It does contain BHA, but the pH of this version is too high for it to be effective as an exfoliant.

☹ **Age Defying Series Revitalizing Eye Gel** *($9.92 for 0.5 ounce)* contains witch hazel distillate as the second ingredient, and because that contains a high percentage of alcohol it can be too irritating for any part of the face, especially the eye area.

OLAY PROVITAL

☺ **ProVital Night Cream** *($8.99 for 2 ounces)* is an OK moisturizer with a small quantity of water-binding agents and antioxidants. It is by far a better choice than any of the Active Hydrating Olay products, but it still doesn't add up to much benefit for skin because it lacks a good selection of water-binding agents and antioxidants.

☺ **ProVital Perfecting Cream** *($9.99 for 1.7 ounces)* is simply a more emollient version than the Night Cream above and the same basic comments apply.

☺ **ProVital Protective Moisture Cream SPF 15** *($8.99 for 1.7 ounces)* is a very good, in-part zinc oxide–based sunscreen in a standard emollient base that can be an option for normal to dry skin. It does contain a small amount of antioxidants, but there just isn't much in here to be of any real significance for skin.

☺ **ProVital Protective Moisture Lotion SPF 15** *($8.99 for 4 ounces)* is similar to the Protective Moisture Cream version above, only with a matte finish that is better for normal to slightly dry skin. The same basic comments apply.

OLE HENRIKSEN SKIN CARE

"Facialist to the stars," L.A.'s "number one face man," and "one of Hollywood's hottest facialists" are but a few of the accolades Ole Henriksen has garnered since he first made a name for himself in Los Angeles back in 1974. Henriksen's skin-care philosophy was, and still is, a mix of holistic teachings, common sense, and, as seen in countless other cosmetic lines (though Henriksen was somewhat of a trailblazer here), an affinity for Mother Nature and all she has to offer the skin. He maintains that his products are different because they have "the highest concentration of purest botanicals," although at higher levels, irritating botanicals are a problem for skin and, of course, lots of non-natural ingredients grace these products. Thankfully, aside from a few missteps, the majority of Henriksen's facial-care products contain beneficial plant extracts and oils, though his is certainly not the only line in which such ingredients abound.

Perhaps what's most startling are not the claims made for Ole Henriksen's products, but rather his pronouncements, such as that "sugar is the skin's worst enemy." Consuming too much refined sugar can indeed lead to some health problems such as obesity or cavities, but none of that spells certain doom for your skin. What can and does lead to wrinkles and a host of other complexion woes is unprotected sun exposure, and here Henriksen shamefully missed the boat on effective UVA protection. Even his supposedly client-extolled Herbal Day Creme lacks titanium dioxide, zinc oxide, or avobenzone. Not all the ballyhooed "calming extracts" and "pure botanicals" in the world can stave off one wrinkle without the aid of an effective sunscreen. Omissions like this should make you skeptical of just how expert his advice is.

Henriksen has some fine products to consider, but the overwhelming emphasis on "natural skincare" (which this line definitely is not), in combination with the way the line turns a blind eye to published evidence that many natural extracts are potent skin irritants and allergens, make this a group of products you don't want to view through rose-colored glasses. For more information about Ole Henriksen Skin Care products, call (310) 854-7700 or visit www.olehenriksen.com.

☺ $$$ **Aloe Vera Deep Cleanser** ($28 for 12 ounces) is a decent, though average, detergent-based cleanser that would work well for most skin types except dry skin. It does contain fragrance.

☺ $$$ **Apricot Cleansing Lotion** ($28 for 12 ounces) is a plant oil–based cold cream that can leave a greasy film on the skin. There is little about this product that isn't easily replaced by plain sunflower or sesame oil you can buy at the drugstore.

☺ $$$ **Clear and Gentle Primrose Soap** ($18 for 3.5 ounces) is a pricey bar of soap that holds little advantage over Dove or Cetaphil bar cleansers. It does contain fragrance.

☺ $$$ **On the Go Exhilarating Cleanser** ($28 for 12 ounces) is a standard, detergent-based cleanser that would work well for most skin types except dry skin. It does contain fragrance.

☺ $$$ **Purifying Eye Make-Up Remover** ($18 for 75 pads) is a standard, detergent-based eye-makeup remover that would work as well as any. This one does contain some good antioxidants and water-binding agents, but they are misplaced in a product that is being wiped off the skin along with your makeup. It is fragrance-free and that's a nice touch, since it's intended for use around the eyes.

☹ **Apricot Complexion Scrub** ($22 for 2 ounces) contains sodium lauryl sulfate as the detergent cleansing agent, which can be too irritating and drying for all skin types.

☺ $$$ **New Beginning Skin Smoothing Scrub** ($22 for 2 ounces) is a standard, detergent-based cleanser that contains some plant oils and uses a plant wax as the exfoliant. This could work quite well for someone with normal to dry skin. It does contain fragrance.

☺ **Aromatic Complexion Oil** ($20 for 4 ounces), as the name implies, contains plant oils (sesame seed and almond oil) along with fragrance and fragrant plant extracts. Skip the fragrance and the cost, but if you are interested in such a product, the plain almond or sesame oil at the grocery store will net you the same results.

☹ **Balancing Cucumber Skin Tonic** ($28 for 12 ounces) contains camphor, which makes this problematic for all skin types.

☹ **Grease Relief-Face Tonic** ($28 for 12 ounces) contains alcohol and camphor, which will not relieve skin from anything and can cause dryness and irritation.

☹ **Pick-Me-Up-Face Mist** ($16 for 4 ounces) has an ingredient list that doesn't live up to FDA standards. For example, it lists alpha hydroxy acids and mixed citrus extracts—and that's too vague to meet regulations, which require a label to list specific ingredients, not just categories of ingredients. It also makes it impossible to know exactly what you are buying. Nonetheless, this ends up being little more than water and witch hazel. Witch hazel is mostly alcohol, so this can be problematic for most skin types.

☺ **All Purpose Aloe Vera Gel** *($25 for 3.5 ounces)*, as the name states, is aloe and a gel ingredient along with an anti-irritant and preservatives. Your skin doesn't need the fragrance, so you would do better just getting some pure aloe vera at a health food store.

✓☺ $$$ **Fresh Start Eye Cream** *($35 for 1 ounce)* contains mostly water, plant oils, thickeners, water-binding agents, antioxidants, silicone, and preservatives. This is a very good moisturizer for normal to dry skin.

☹ **Herbal Day Creme SPF 15** *($30 for 2 ounces)* does not contain the UVA-protecting ingredients of titanium dioxide, zinc oxide, or avobenzone, and is not recommended.

☺ $$$ **Invigorating Night Gel** *($30 for 1 ounce)* isn't invigorating, but it is an overly expensive glycolic acid gel. The pH of 6 makes it ineffective as an exfoliant.

☺ $$$ **Nurture Me Replenishing Creme** *($40 for 2 ounces)* is a simple moisturizer of plant oil, thickeners, silicone, vitamin E, fragrance, and coloring agents. The vitamin K in this product can't change spider veins. The only research concerning vitamin K's effectiveness on skin or surfaced spider veins comes from the companies selling the products that contain it. There are no published or peer-reviewed studies that show results you can even remotely count on (Source: *Archives of Dermatology,* December 1998, pages 1512–1514).

☹ **Pure Perfection** *($45 for 2 ounces)* has a confused ingredient label that does not specify which alpha hydroxy acids it contains, plus the pH is too high for the AHAs to be effective as exfoliants, and it is not recommended.

☺ $$$ **Sheer Transformation Crème** *($45 for 2 ounces)* contains several ingredients that may have some ability to inhibit melanin production, including kojic dipalmitate (though this is not as effective as kojic acid) and vitamin C. It also contains some good antioxidants.

☺ $$$ **Truth Serum** *($35 for 1 ounce)* is an interesting name for a product that uses a rather untruthful ingredient list ("natural color" and "natural fragrance" are not terms allowed by the FDA). If the rest of the label is telling the truth, this is a good lightweight moisturizer that contains a small blend of antioxidants and water-binding agents.

☺ $$$ **Ultimate Lift Eye Gel** *($35 for 1 ounce)* is just film-forming agent with some thickeners, water-binding agent, plant extracts, preservatives, and coloring agent. That makes it ultimately boring and uneventful for skin.

☺ $$$ **Vitamin Plus Balancing Crème** *($30 for 2 ounces)* contains an assortment of plant extracts that can be irritants and anti-irritants, which is a waste.

☺ $$$ **Firm Action Pore Refining Mask** *($25 for 2 ounces)* is an average, though good, clay mask that can absorb oil, but it won't change one pore on your face, at least not any more than any other clay mask.

☺ $$$ **Repair Formula Mask** *($25 for 2 ounces)* is just a clay mask with some plant extracts, which would work as well as any clay mask to absorb oil. There is nothing in it that can repair skin.

☺ $$$ **Roll-On Blemish Attack** *($22 for 0.45 ounce)* contains plant extracts that include sugarcane, sugar maple, lemon, and orange extracts, which have no benefit for healing or disinfecting blemishes. The clay in this product can absorb oil, but so can lots of clay masks without the bogus plant extracts. This does contain a teeny amount of tea tree oil, but not enough to have disinfecting properties.

OMBRELLE (SUN CARE ONLY)

The world of sunscreens has changed dramatically over the past two years. Information about UVA protection versus UVB protection has thrown a whole new light on what we need to consider when buying sunscreens. In Chapter Seven, *Cosmetics Dictionary*, I explain why certain UVA-protecting ingredients are essential when considering which sunscreen to buy. L'Oreal-owned Ombrelle is a small line of sunscreen products that includes avobenzone as one of the active ingredients in all of their sunscreen products, and that makes these great options for daily sun protection. For more information about Ombrelle, call (800) 582-8225 or visit www.ombrelle.com.

☺ **Sunscreen Lotion SPF 15** *($7.95 for 4 ounces)* is a very good, in-part avobenzone-based sunscreen in a standard emollient moisturizing base that would be an option for normal to dry skin.

☺ **Sunscreen Lotion SPF 30** *($7.95 for 4 ounces)* is similar to the SPF 15 lotion above only with a higher SPF.

☺ **Sunscreen Lotion Extreme SPF 40** *($7.95 for 4 ounces)* is a very good, in-part avobenzone-based sunscreen in a standard emollient moisturizing base that would be an option for normal to dry skin. The SPF 40 does not indicate better or stronger sun protection, only more hours of the same level of sun protection—but in most parts of the world, there isn't that much daylight. The FDA's new sunscreen regulations will prohibit the use of any SPF numbers over 30.

☺ **Sunscreen Lotion for Kids SPF 44** *($7.95 for 4 ounces)* is virtually identical to the Extreme SPF 40 above and the same comments apply. There is nothing about this formula that makes it preferred for kids other than the name.

☺ **Sunscreen Spray for Kids SPF 28** *($8.69 for 4 ounces)*. If a spray form seems like an easier way to get sunscreen on your kids (or on yourself for that matter), spray away—because this is a very good sunscreen with avobenzone! It also contains other sunscreen agents that might be a bit sensitizing for the eye area so be careful, but for everywhere else, it should be fine. It is a lightweight formula, but it is better for normal to dry skin.

☹ **Spray Mist SPF 15** *($7.95 for 4 ounces)* is an in-part avobenzone-based sunscreen. Unfortunately, it is in an alcohol base, and that can be drying and irritating for the skin when used on a regular basis.

☺ **Sunless Tanning Cream SPF 15** *($7.95 for 2 ounces)*. Along with an in-part avobenzone-based sunscreen, this also contains dihydroxyacetone, the same ingredient used in all self-tanners to affect the color of skin.

☹ **Sunless Tan Spray SPF 12** *($7.95 for 2 ounces)* is similar to the Tanning Cream above only in lotion form, and for some inexplicable reason, a too-low SPF number.

ORIGINS

Estee Lauder created Origins in 1990 to capitalize on the phenomenon of plants as a skin-care panacea that she saw was about to take over the world of cosmetics. Origins uses every plant angle there is to make their products sound like gardens of skin care. Exotic-sounding botanicals, herbs, and oils abound. Never mind that there are also a host of unnatural ingredients that contribute more to the makeup's textures and slip quality than any plant ever could. Origins (like Aveda—which the Lauder corporation purchased in 1997) offers skin-care systems based on "ancient" skin-care treatments, anti-stress formulas, and, of course, aromatherapy, with some of the cutest product names in the industry. The recycling efforts and animal-free testing are praiseworthy examples. However, the "ancient" and "natural" stuff is the real bait that hooks women.

Origins' basic skin-care theory is that all skin wants to act normal, the way it did when we were young. As we grow up, our skin gets confused or behaves badly, not because it wants to, but because it lacks something. If skin is supplied with the correct plants and oil, it can—at least according to Origins' philosophy of "nature's memory"— be retrained so that your skin functions the way all skin wants to function: normally. What an enticing concept! Of course, the ingredients that supposedly retrain your skin are derived from the "ancient science of essential oils," which assumes that people who lived long ago had great skin because of this special knowledge. It does sound convincing, but, alas, that's just not how skin works. If it were, then all of the Estee Lauder companies would sell the same formulations, and they don't. But I have to admit that this is one of the most creative skin-care ploys I've ever seen, and that's saying a lot.

What is most interesting to note is that a relatively new product, Calm Balm Sensitive Skin Eye Creme, doesn't contain any of the myriad irritating plant extracts found in almost every other Origins product. Calm Balm even states on the package that "Irritation ages skin." That is absolutely true, but then why does Origins continue to put irritating plant extracts in almost every other one of their products? For example, Origins is quite fond of using peppermint, menthol, and camphor in many of their products. These are considered counter-irritants (Source: *Archives of Dermatologic Research,* May 1996, pages 245–248), which induce local inflammation to relieve inflammation in deeper or adjacent tissues. In other words, they substitute one kind of inflammation for another. The major function of these types of ingredients is to cause irritation, period. That is never good for skin. Irritation or inflammation, no matter what causes it or how it happens, impairs the skin's immune and healing responses (Source: *Skin Pharmacology and Applied Skin Physiology,* November-December 2000, pages 358–371). And, although your skin may not show it, or doesn't react in an irritated fashion, if you apply irritants to your skin the damage is still taking place and the damage is ongoing and adds up over time (Source: *Skin Research and Technology,* November 2001, pages 227–237). It seems that Lauder's own research as well as basic skin research doesn't jibe with most of what Origins has to offer in the way of skin care. For more information about Origins, call (800)-ORIGINS or visit www.origins.com. **Note:** All Origins products are fragranced unless otherwise noted.

ORIGINS SKIN CARE

☹ **Checks and Balances Frothy Face Wash** *($16.50 for 5 ounces)*. It's a shame the Origins formulas aren't as clever and catchy as their product names. This problematic cleanser not only contains several irritating fragrant oils, but also uses fairly drying cleansing agents that won't balance or help most skin types. It also contains konjac powder to absorb oil. Konjac powder is a dietary fiber that is highly absorbent, but not more so than other food substances (cornstarch for example) or nonfood substances (like talc, magnesium, or other minerals). Although any oil-absorbing substance can be helpful for skin, if you have problems with breakouts, adding absorbents in the form of food ingredients can increase the bacteria content in skin. Thankfully, this product only contains a teensy amount of the powder so it will have little to no impact on skin.

☹ **Get Down Deep-Pore Cleanser** *($16.50 for 5 ounces)* says it "won't irk or irritate" skin, but with peppermint, eucalyptus, sage, and ylang-ylang oils abounding, that's unlikely. This clay-based cleanser is both difficult to rinse off and mildly abrasive. There are far less irritating ways to cleanse and exfoliate the skin than with this poor concoction.

☹ **Chunk of Clay Foaming Cleanser for the Face** *($13.50 for 8.8 ounces)* is a standard, though highly fragranced, bar cleanser. It is a fairly drying way to clean the face and there is nothing about this product other than the clever name that is an improvement over Dove bar cleanser at the drugstore.

☹ **Cream Bar** *($9.50 for 5.2 ounces)* is a standard bar cleanser with fairly drying detergent cleansing agents, but this one also contains some very irritating and sensitizing plant extracts, including clove, wintergreen, and spruce needle.

☹ **Liquid Clay** *($15 for 5 ounces)* is a standard, detergent-based, water-soluble cleanser that also contains a lot of clay, which can leave the skin feeling clean, but that also can be difficult to wash off. The real drawbacks to this product are the eucalyptus, sage, and ylang-ylang, which can cause skin irritation.

☹ **Liquid Crystal Extra Gentle Cleanser** *($16.50 for 6.7 ounces)* contains mostly thickeners and plant oils, which makes it a standard, wipe-off cleanser that can leave a greasy film on the face that still needs to be wiped away. That could be an option for dry skin, but the peppermint is too irritating for any skin type.

☹ **Mint Wash** *($16.50 for 6.7 ounces)*, as the name indicates, includes mint, which is a skin irritant, just like the spearmint, orange zest, and lemon peel that are also in this product.

☹ **Pure Cream Rinseable Cleanser You Can Also Tissue Off** *($16.50 for 6.7 ounces)* contains peppermint, lime, and tangerine oils, which can irritate the skin and eyes.

☹ **Never a Dull Moment Skin Brightening Facial Cleanser with Fruit Extracts** *($16.50 for 5 ounces)*. The irritating ingredients in here will assuredly keep your skin from having any dull moments as it works overtime to fend off the inevitable irritation caused by the grapefruit, eucalyptus, and pine oils. This could have been a great, gentle, water-soluble cleanser, but Origins just can't help using problematic plant extracts in their products, ingredients that unsuspecting consumers would never guess may be hurting their skin.

☹ **Never a Dull Moment Skin Brightening Face Polisher with Fruit Enzymes** *($22.50 for 3.5 ounces)* has a great name, but is just an ordinary, detergent-based cleanser with crushed fruit seeds that also contains eucalyptus, mint, grapefruit, and pine, all significant skin irritants. The tiny amount of papaya is not effective for exfoliation.

☹ **Swept Away Gentle Slougher for All Skins** *($17.50 for 3.4 ounces)* is an abrasive cleanser that also contains peppermint and grapefruit, both useless as skin-care ingredients because they can irritate skin. There is absolutely nothing gentle about this product.

☹ **Swept Clean Special Sloughing for Oily-Acting Skin** *($17.50 for 3.4 ounces)* is almost identical to the Gentle version above except for the addition of menthol and a tiny amount of charcoal. Charcoal can absorb oil, but the irritating ingredients are a problem for oily skin.

☺ **Well-Off Fast and Gentle Eye Makeup Remover** *($11 for 3.4 ounces)* is a standard, detergent-based, water-soluble eye-makeup remover. It works, but there is nothing particularly gentle about it.

☹ **United State Balancing Tonic** *($16 for 5 ounces)*. Great name, poor product! The second ingredient is alcohol, and with fragrance also high up on the ingredient list that makes this completely unbalancing for skin, causing irritation and dryness. This is more like applying cologne to skin than a skin-care product.

☹ **Comforting Solution If Your Skin Acts Sensitive** *($17 for 5.7 ounces)* is supposed to help sensitive skin defend itself against the environment, but the teeny amount of vitamin E in here can't possibly defend against anything. The real drawback is that it contains far too many potentially sensitizing plant extracts to ever be considered reliable for sensitive skin.

☹ **Drenching Solution** *($17 for 5 ounces)* contains far too many potentially sensitizing plant extracts, including eucalyptus, sage, spearmint, and jasmine, to be an option for skin. But what's equally problematic is that it is just an extremely mundane toner with a trace amount of vitamin E.

☹ **Managing Solution** *($17 for 5 ounces)* is a toner that is supposed to normalize oil production, but its ingredients—plant water, essential oils, aloe vera, water-binding agent, vitamin E, slip agents, and preservatives—have no way of affecting oil production. Actually, the fragrant oils and irritating ingredients (including peppermint and lemon) are a problem for all skin types and can make oily skin feel and look irritated and oilier.

☹ **Mending Solution** *($17 for 5 ounces)* is identical to all of Origins' "Solution" toners, only with a change of fragrance. This one is supposed to energize the skin's "look-young systems." No one's skin has "look-young systems." But isn't it amazing that such similar products are supposed to do such disparate things for the skin with only a change of perfume? Plus, irritating the skin hurts its healing process and that can make a mess of skin.

☹ **Oil Refiner Skin Purifying Tonic** *($17 for 5 ounces)* lists alcohol as the second ingredient, and along with the eucalyptus and clove this can make an oil slick on your face worse by making skin irritated and dry.

☹ **Tuning Solution** *($17 for 5 ounces)* is supposed to rebalance the oily and dry areas of your face. It doesn't contain anything capable of doing that, but it does contain lemon and eucalyptus, among other extracts that can be irritating for the skin, and ends up having the same formulation as every other Origins "Solution" product except for a small change in fragrance.

☺ **Sprinkler System** *($13.50 for 6.7 ounces)* is a fragrant toner that also contains a good water-binding agent; that's good, but not great.

☺ **$$$ A Perfect World** *($30 for 1 ounce).* This silicone-based gel lotion does have a silky finish, the same as all silicone-based moisturizers do. Other than the several seriously irritating plant extracts of bergamot, orris, spearmint, and lemon it contains, the only "special" ingredient is the silver tip white tea extract. White tea is the minimally processed buds and leaves of green tea that have a gray, wispy appearance. There is research showing that white and green teas have the highest concentration of antioxidant properties of all teas, and there are several in vitro and animal studies showing that white tea has anticancer and antimutagenic properties. However, even though tea flavonoids are effective antioxidants, it is unclear to what extent they can increase the antioxidant capacity of the human body, and there is no research showing what that means for skin. If anything, there is some question whether the effect of white tea (versus other teas) might simply be related to white tea's higher caffeine level (Source: Oregon State University Linus Pauling Institute, http://lpi.orst.edu). You would be far better off drinking a cup of green or white tea than using this potentially irritating skin-care product.

☺ **Clearance Time** *($22.50 for 1 ounce)* includes sugarcane extract, and because that's not the same as AHAs it can't exfoliate skin. However, this product does contain salicylic acid (BHA, about 1% concentration), and that can exfoliate skin, though the pH of this product is just passable for that purpose. Other than that, this is a very good lightweight moisturizing base for normal to slightly dry skin.

☺ **Starting Over** *($22.50 for 1 ounce)* is supposed to improve cell renewal, and while the sugarcane extract is supposed to make you think you are getting an AHA product, you aren't, because it isn't an effective exfoliant. Even if you were, there isn't enough of the extract and the pH of the moisturizer is too high for it to work as an exfoliant. This is just a very fragrant gel lotion with some good water-binding agents and a small amount of an anti-irritant.

☺ **Balanced Diet Lightweight Moisture Lotion** *($18.50 for 1.7 ounces)* is a reformulation and renaming of Origins former Fine Tuner moisturizer. Aside from being more emollient, not much has changed, and this still contains several irritating fragrant oils such as geranium, spearmint, and bergamot. Perhaps what's most curious is the price tag—because in spite of being an "improved" formula, this now sells for almost four dollars *less* than Fine Tuner, which is almost unheard of in the cosmetics industry. Aside from the plant extracts, this is a bit of a confused formulation, with several emollient ingredients (plant oils and shea butter) along with an absorbent. There are several good water-binding agents and some antioxidants, so this can be an option for normal to dry skin.

✓☺ **$$$ Calm Balm Sensitive Skin Eye Creme** *($25 for 0.5 ounce)* actually admits on the packaging that "Irritation ages skin." How nice of Origins to point out this sobering skin fact while selling dozens of products fraught with well-known skin irritants. It reminds me of one of the best lines from the television series *Friends:* "Hello, Monica? This is the kettle. You're black." It turns out that this product does not contain any of the typically irritating and highly fragrant plant extracts otherwise so abundant in the Origins line. It is actually a very good, fragrance-free moisturizer that contains mostly water, glycerin, film-forming agent, water-binding agents, silicones, antioxidants, more film-forming agents, and thickeners. It is even preservative-free, and would be excellent for sensitive, normal to dry skin.

☺ **Constant Comforter, If Your Skin Acts Sensitive** *($22 for 1.7 ounces)* is a good emollient moisturizer for normal to dry skin, but it won't calm anything; in fact, many of the plant oils and extracts are potential skin sensitizers, including lavender, lemon, lime, and rosemary, similar to those that other fragrant cosmetics contain.

☺ **$$$ Eye Doctor, Moisture Care for Skin Around Eyes** *($25 for 0.5 ounce)* contains a few plant extracts that are problematic for skin, and especially for the eye area, including mint and wintergreen. That's a shame, because this could have been a very good moisturizer for normal to dry skin.

☺ **Fine Tuner, If Your Skin Acts Confused** *($22 for 1.7 ounces)* is supposed to even out combination skin. None of its ingredients can change oily skin, although some of them can make oily skin feel oilier, including plant oils and shea butter, both of which can be a problem for someone with any amount of oily skin. This is a good moisturizer for normal to dry skin, but it's a confused product and many of the plant extracts can be skin irritants.

☺ **Grin from Year to Year Brightening Face Firmer** *($25 for 1.7 ounces)* is supposed to "…firm and tone skin; licorice extract helps block the appearance of brown spots. Used regularly, skin looks and feels fitter, tauter, smoother." The amount of licorice extract in here couldn't change the color of even one skin cell. With a cornucopia of plant extracts woven in between standard synthetic ingredients, this product is another one of the natural-looking cocktails Origins consistently promotes. Though you have to wonder, if these plants are so good, why don't the myriad other Lauder-owned cosmetics companies use them, too? All in all, this adds up to a good moisturizer for normal to dry skin, if you don't have problems or reactions with all the plants in it that range from sage to tangerine, basil, and orange. This one also contains plant extracts that contain arbutin, which can reduce brown spots, but not in the minuscule amounts found here.

☺ **Have a Nice Day Cream SPF 15** *($28.50 for 1.7 ounces)* is a good, in-part titanium dioxide–based sunscreen. The fairly mundane moisturizing base could make this appropriate for someone with normal to dry skin, but the peppermint, lemon, grapefruit, and spearmint extracts mean that it has a strong potential for irritation, and with so many well-formulated sunscreens around these days, why settle for one with any potential risk to your skin?

☺ **Have a Nice Day Lotion SPF 15** *($28.50 for 1.7 ounces)* is similar to the Have a Nice Day Cream above except in lotion form, though the same concerns apply to this one. There are better ways to have a nice day than with this product.

✓☺ **$$$ Line Chaser, Stop Sign for Lines** *($25 for 0.5 ounce)* can't stop wrinkles, but it is a very good lightweight moisturizer for normal to slightly dry skin, and it also omits the irritating plant extracts Origins throws in almost every other product they sell!

☺ **Look Alive Vitality Moisture Cream** *($18.50 for 1.7 ounces)*. If it weren't for the plant extracts you would swear this product is Lauder's Idealist, only for a lot less money. The showcase ingredient is a form of glucosamine (the same as in Lauder's Idealist) that is supposed to work like AHAs only without the irritation (though lots of people can use AHAs without irritation). However, the only research showing that to be the case was carried out by the company selling the ingredient. It is a good moisturizer for normal to dry skin, with several water-binding agents, plant oils, and antioxidants, although some of the plant extracts can be skin irritants.

☺ **Make a Difference** *($30 for 1 ounce)* is supposed to be a "…botanical breakthrough," but I thought that's what all the varying plant extracts in Origins products were, too? I guess they'll have to throw those other ones out if this is the answer. The showcased ingredients are the Rose of Jericho, a plant that can survive after decades of drought; trehalose, a sugar; and sea haricots (sea green beans) to undo dehydration. Whether or not a plant can survive decades of drought has nothing to do with your skin, because after ten days without water a human is no longer living, skin and all. Trehalose is indeed a sugar (carbohydrate), and as is true for a vast number of plant sugars, it is a good water-binding agent, just hardly unique or special. The algae can be good antioxidants, but there is no research about what that means for skin. What Origins doesn't explain is what your skin is supposed to do with the other plant extracts that are potential skin irritants, including lemon, spearmint, and bergamot. This does contain a teeny amount of other water-binding agents and antioxidants, but there is far more fragrance in this product than any of those ingredients.

☺ **Night-A-Mins Cream** *($28.50 for 1.7 ounces)* is named to sound like oral vitamins. Night-A-Mins definitely contains a good group of vitamins that can be helpful as antioxidants, and while that is beneficial for skin, they are not the least bit nutritious. This would be a good moisturizer for someone with normal to dry skin.

☺ **Night-A-Mins Lotion** *(28.50 for 1.7 ounces)* is similar to the Cream version above and the same comments apply.

☹ **Matte Scientist Oil Controlling Lotion** *($18.50 for 1.7 ounces)* is a silicone-based gel lotion that could have been a good option for normal to slightly dry skin, except that the eucalyptus and sage make it too potentially irritating for skin, and there is nothing in it that can control oil production.

☺ **Steady Drencher, If Your Young Skin Acts Dry** *($22.50 for 1.7 ounces)* is a good emollient moisturizer for someone with dry skin. The anti-irritants are wasted because several of the plant extracts can also be irritants, and the effects of the one group cancel out the effects of the others.

☺ **Time Mender, If Your Skin Acts Older Than You'd Like** *($22 for 1.7 ounces)* is a very good moisturizer for dry skin. The company claims that this product can firm the skin, but not all the plant oils and water-binding agents in the world can do that. The anti-irritants in here are wasted because several of the plant extracts can also be irritants.

☺ **Urgent Moisture** *($25 for 1.7 ounces)* is a rather ordinary moisturizer for normal to dry skin. It does contain a minuscule quantity of water-binding agents and soothing agents, but the small amount can have little to no impact on skin. This is not as well formulated as several other Origin moisturizers that have far more impressive antioxidants and water-binding agents.

☺ $$$ **Silent Treatment Instant UV Face Protector SPF 15** *($15 for 1.7 ounces)* is a titanium dioxide–based sunscreen suspended in a simple, though very fragrant, silicone base solution. It is an option for normal to dry skin.

☺ **Summer Vacation, The Natural-Looking Self Tanner** *($17.50 for 5 ounces)*, like all self-tanners, uses dihydroxyacetone to turn the skin brown. This works as well as any.

☺ $$$ **Clear Improvement Active Charcoal Mask to Clear Pores** *($18.50 for 3.4 ounces)* is a standard clay mask. Charcoal has unique absorption and disinfecting properties, but there is so little of it in here that it doesn't have much impact on skin.

☺ $$$ **Drink Up 10 Minute Moisture Mask** *($18.50 for 3.4 ounces)* definitely contains emollient oils, but little else. It should feel nice as a mask if you have dry skin, but no more so than applying a regular moisturizer (say, one better formulated than this).

☺ $$$ **No Puffery** *($20 for 0.64 ounce)* claims it can release trapped fluids and toxins from the skin, but that is not possible. Meanwhile, it does contain plant extracts, including comfrey, ivy, and yarrow, that can cause irritation.

☹ **Out of Trouble** *($17.50 for 3.4 ounces)* is meant to be a way to solve blemish and blackhead problems. I wish it could, but this formulation is what's in trouble. Zinc oxide and titanium dioxide can clog pores and cause breakouts, camphor and sulfur can cause irritation and redness, and there isn't enough BHA (salicylic acid) at the right pH to have an exfoliating impact on the skin.

☹ **Spot Remover to Clear Up Acne Blemishes** *($10 for 0.3 ounce)* is a standard salicylic acid (BHA) and alcohol solution. Without the alcohol, this product may have been an option, but there are far better BHA products to consider for treating blemishes, for less money and in far less irritating bases than this one.

☹ **Zero Oil Instant Matte Finish for Shiny Places** *($10 for 0.64 ounce)* cannot stop oil production, but sodium magnesium silicate can absorb oil, just as most minerals and clays can. However, this product also contains camphor, which can be a skin irritant. This is pretty much a modified version of Phillips' Milk of Magnesia, which can do the same sort of thing, only better. There is no reason to use camphor on skin.

☹ **Lip Remedy** *($10 for 0.17 ounce)* isn't much of a remedy. This lip product contains a long list of thickeners, plant oil, more thickeners, and preservatives, which wouldn't be bad except that it also contains menthol and camphor, which are irritants and not helpful for lips or skin.

☺ **Mind Your Mouth** *($6.50 for 0.15 ounce)* is a very emollient, standard lip gloss. It doesn't contain sunscreen, but it is very good for dry lips any time of year, as long as it isn't daytime.

☹ **Cover Your Mouth Lip Protector SPF 8** *($6.50 for 0.15 ounce)*. I won't even get into how absurd it is for the Lauder Corporation to have a sunscreen product with an SPF 8, but to say the least it would not be smart to rely on this for protecting your lips from sun damage.

ORIGINS MAKEUP

Over the last couple of years Origins' makeup has begun changing—both for the better and, lamentably, for the worse. Gradually, the straightforward matte eyeshadows and blushes started losing space on the Origins Color Wheel, replaced by an overpowering army of iridescent colors with improved textures. While this was transpiring, Origins' Original Skin foundations, which had been with the color line since its debut, were superceded by three new, distinctive formulas. For the most part, these new foundations are marked improvements over the previous formulas. Although Original Skin was hardly problematic, it did have limitations in terms of appealing to (and meeting the needs of) different skin types. Other changes have also been afoot, including reformulated eye and lip pencils, redone pressed powder, new lipsticks, and the launch of even more products that fall in the "cute name, but do I really need this?" category. It's interesting to note that Origins makeup used to have a reliable palette of neutral, natural (and mostly matte) colors that were ostensibly designed to appeal to the all-natural-craving, earthy cosmetics consumer. Yet clearly women who were drawn to Origins by the company's pro-plant position largely ignored the majority of the makeup. Now it's apparent that the company has gotten the message, and has answered with today's collection of shimmer and shine. For those who believe natural beauty means layering on iridescence, you won't leave today's Origins counter empty-handed.

FOUNDATION: ☺ **Reflection Perfection Mattifying Face Makeup** *($15)* is almost identical in every respect to Clinique's Skin Clarifying Makeup ($16.50). Although this foundation contains alcohol as one of the main ingredients (which can be a problem for irritation and dryness), the application is very impressive and the finish is truly matte, offering light to medium coverage. Origins has ten colors with options for very light but not dark skin tones, and the only colors to consider avoiding are Buffy and Fawn—both are too peach for most skin tones.

☺ **Stay Tuned Balancing Face Makeup** *($15)* is a great foundation that is a dead-ringer for Estee Lauder's Equalizer Makeup SPF 10 ($32.50), except for the Equalizer's less-than-preferred sunscreen. You did notice that Stay Tuned costs half as much as the Lauder version, right? Both of these foundations have a silicone-based, ultra-smooth texture that blends beautifully and provides light to medium coverage with a soft matte finish. Stay Tuned comes in 12 excellent shades, including wonderful options for darker skin tones. The following shades are slightly pink or peach, and should be considered carefully: Angel, Eggshell, Fawn, and Buffy. **Original Skin Pressed Makeup** *($22.50)* is a talc-based pressed-powder foundation with a smooth, slightly dry texture and sheer colors that apply easily and blend well. This leaves a great, sheer, matte finish that doesn't look too powdery, and the five colors are all praiseworthy, with Rice being a standout option for very light skin. **Sunny Disposition Liquid Bronzer** *($15)* is a very sheer, pink-bronze tint that would work well on warm or sallow skin tones that want a tanned appearance. ✓☺ **Dew Gooder Moisturizing Face Makeup** *($15)* is a supremely creamy, whipped makeup that should feel great on dry to very dry skin. It blends very well, leaves a soft, dewy (not greasy) finish, and offers light to medium coverage. Of the nine shades, several are slightly pink or peach—but not overwhelmingly so—and this makeup is a must-try for those with dry skin who crave a moisture-rich foundation! Linen, Nude, Bare, and Beach are excellent neutral colors for light to medium skin tones. ✓☺ **Nude and Improved Bare-Face Makeup SPF 15** *($15)* is a beautiful option for light moisture, sheer color, and a smart titanium dioxide sunscreen! Don't expect much coverage from this tinted moisturizer, but do plan to give this a test run if you have normal to dry skin. Almost all of the five shades are perfectly subdued—only Sheer Latte is too peach for most skin tones.

☹ **As Good As It Gets** *($20)* sounds like the ultimate makeup convenience: foundation, concealer, and powder in one. It comes up short on all counts and remains a loose powder that goes on rather thick, with four noticeably shiny, slightly peachy gold shades. If you blend it on well, it can have a sheer to light coverage with a silky finish, but to get all of the extra features, you're supposed to mix it with a moisturizer, which can get messy and streaky. Used alone, it performs much like any standard loose powder with shine, and that is as good as this why-bother foundation gets!

CONCEALER: ☺ **Original Skin Concealer** *($10)* has a smooth, light texture, and some OK colors, but all of the shades are slightly shiny, which isn't best for under the eye when it comes to smoothing out lines or helping the area to look even with the foundation (unless your foundation is also shiny).

☺ **Quick, Hide! Easy Blend Concealer** *($11)* will eventually replace Origins' Original Skin Concealer above, and it is a marked improvement in all respects. This creamy concealer comes in a squeeze tube, is easy to blend, and offers superior coverage with a natural matte finish. One small drawback: It does have a slight tendency to crease, which a light dusting of powder should curtail. There are five mostly excellent shades—Dark is too peach for most skin tones and Neutralizer will be too yellow for lighter skin tones, but is still worth considering.

<u>POWDER:</u> ☺ $$$ **Silk Screen Refining Face Powder** *($22.50)* is a talc-based pressed powder that has a very smooth, slightly dry texture and reasonable coverage—more than you would get from a standard pressed powder. The six available shades are commendable, with only Warm Honey veering ever so slightly toward the orange zone. This would work particularly well for normal to oily skin.

☹ $$$ **Sunny Disposition Powder Bronzer** *($17.50)* is an OK option for bronzing powder if you don't mind the drier, flaky texture and shimmering finish. If this were matte, it would be a slam-dunk, because the tan color is quite realistic.

<u>BLUSH:</u> ☹ $$$ **Brush-On Color** *($16.50)* has a soft, slightly thick texture that blends on easily, providing a hint of shine-infused color. For truly matte powder blush options, you'll need to look elsewhere. But if you like the shine, this is worth a sweep across the cheekbone.

☺ **Pinch Your Cheeks** *($10)* conjures up images of small children running from that too-affectionate aunt who visits once a year! In reality, this is a liquid stain for the cheeks that blends nicely (once you get the hang of it, so be careful), and offers a transparent, berry-pink blush. This works best on normal, small-pored, even-textured skin.

<u>EYESHADOW:</u> Origins ☺ **Eyeshadow** *($12.50)* is now an imposing collection of shiny shades with options ranging from subtle to striking. Nary a matte shade can be found, but Creme Brulee, Vanilla Mousse, and Ballet Class come close. These do have a buttery-smooth texture and very nice application that is neither too sheer nor too intense. If matte eyeshadows aren't important to you, there's much to love here.

☹ **Underwear for Lids** *($12)* is a creamy eyeshadow base that comes in twist-up-stick packaging. Why Origins thought this slightly greasy, crease-prone concealer hybrid would make a good eyeshadow base is a mystery. This does not come close to the long-lasting effect you can achieve using a good matte-finish concealer such as Maybelline's Great Wear or Lancome's MaquiComplet. **Underwear for Lids Delicate Color for Eyes** *($12)* is identical to the regular Underwear for Lids above, only these come in a slew of pastel and neutral iridescent colors. The silicone-based texture makes these easy to apply, but too slick to last without creasing.

<u>EYE AND BROW SHAPER:</u> The ☺ **Brow Pencil** *($11)* is a standard, dry-textured pencil with standard colors. **Just Browsing** *($12)* is a lightweight, softly tinted brow gel with an OK brush that works to add natural color and definition to the eyebrow. All of the shades are great, and although the finish is minimally sticky, it performs well. The Auburn shade is more of a mahogany than a true auburn, and is too dark for most natural redheads. **Brow Fix** *($12)* is basically clear mascara for the brows and, though overpriced, will work to keep them groomed and in place without making them feel sticky.

☺ **Eye Brightening Color Stick** *($12.50)* is a chubby, stout pencil that comes in one shade—a pale, shimmery silver-blue that is intended to be used for lining the inner rims of the eye, a technique that is more theatrical than practical. Also, repeated daily applications put the eye at risk, as cosmetic coloring agents just don't belong next to the cornea. Yes, it can look striking in photographs, but it is not worth doing on a regular (or even infrequent) basis.

☹ **Eye Pencil** *($13.50)* is very slick (almost greasy), with sheer colors that smear at the slightest provocation. You won't even get a chance to use the built-in sponge tip for blending before this sticky-feeling pencil is all over the place!

LIPSTICK AND LIP PENCIL: I find it odd that Origins cannot produce a lipstick that is as good as many of the ones offered by its sister companies, from Estee Lauder to Aveda. ☺ **Creamy Lip Color** *($11)* has a slick, smooth application, but is far too greasy to ever have a prayer of lasting through the morning without a touch-up. If you're prone to lipstick bleeding, this is one to avoid. **Lasting Lip Color** *($12)* is slightly creamier and less greasy than the Creamy Lip Color, but not by much. The "lasting" claim is dubious, as this has minimal stain and a glossy finish that will only "last" if you regularly reapply it. Origins has also added peppermint to flavor the lipstick, and for some this may prove too irritating. What a shame this isn't as elegant as many other lipsticks, as the color selection is super. **Matte, Sheer,** and **Shimmer Sticks** *($12)* are the original "chubby sticks" that many lines now offer. Why these ever caught on is anyone's guess, because they need constant sharpening, and most are too soft to get a controlled lip line. That brings us back to what they really are: a standard, creamy lipstick in pencil form. The Matte Stick is not matte in the least, and is actually rather greasy. The Sheer Stick is even greasier than the Matte version but with less pigment. The Shimmer Stick is just creamy and iridescent. **Bite Your Lips** *($12.50)* are nothing more than sheer, glossy lip tints that tend to slip on and then slide off. For soft sheer color and longer wear, consider Clinique's Almost Lipstick ($13.50).

☺ **Liquid Lip Color** *($11)* is a standard lip gloss with a bit more pigment than usual, which means you'll get a semi-opaque, glossy finish. This has a slightly thick, sticky texture, but a nice selection of gorgeous shades. **Lip Gloss** *($11)* is a fairly standard gloss with a very good light, smooth texture. **Lip Pencil** *($11)* is still a standard pencil that needs sharpening, though the texture is much smoother than the former version and the colors are rich with pigment. There are eight shades, and most are wonderful.

☺ **Underwear for Lips** *($12)* is not really necessary if you have a traditional matte-finish concealer handy. This comes in a tube with a wand applicator, and is similar to BeneFit's Lip Plump ($16). It's designed to smooth the surface of the lips and make it easier to apply lipstick. Although this does have a soft matte finish, the peachy hue is not for everyone and this only works marginally well. Depending on how matte or greasy your lipstick is, this will barely enhance application and will leave you wondering why you bothered. And if this is used with any of Origins greasy lipsticks, expect to be disappointed.

☹ **Rain and Shine SPF 15** *($12)* is almost identical to Clinique's Moisture Sheer Lipstick SPF 15 ($13.50). Both lack adequate UVA protection and are just sheer, glossy lipsticks that impart soft, fleeting color. Origins loses points (and a smiling face) due to the strong presence of peppermint oil. **Transforming Lip Glaze** *($11)* is an opalescent pink lip gloss that imbues the lips with an almost holographic shimmer. Unfortunately, this contains too much mint to make it a safe bet for keeping lips irritant-free.

MASCARA: ☺ **Fringe Benefits Mascara** *($12)* easily builds well-defined, long lashes without smearing or clumping. I wouldn't choose this over less expensive options, but I must admit the name is adorable.

☺ **Underwear for Lashes** *($12)* is described as a "little lash builder" and is nothing more than a semitransparent mascara that adds some length and bulk to lashes prior to applying a regular mascara. It works to add extra impact to lashes, but when so many other mascaras add the oomph without the extra steps (and expense), why not choose one of those instead?

☺ $$$ BRUSHES: Origins' **Brushes** *($15–$50)* are synthetic, which for many animal-rights activists is a strong selling point. What helps even more is that, for synthetics, they are exquisitely soft and yet dense enough to pick up and apply product professionally. What's a detriment is the fact that many of these brushes are too big and full to use with precision and ease when applying eyeshadows, blushes, and powders. They're worth a look if you want good synthetic hair, and the ones to consider include **Powder Eyeliner** *($15),* which can work for a wider line; **Eyeshadow Placement** *($17.50)* and **Eyeshadow Contour** *($15);* the retractable **Lip Brush** *($15);* and, as an extra option, the **Brush On-the-Go** *($25).* For a wider selection of great synthetic brushes, you may also want to look at the offerings from Shu Uemura and Paula Dorf.

ORLANE

Women who buy Orlane products aren't wondering whether they can afford the $500 to $1,000 or more it costs to take care of their skin the Orlane way; they just want what appears to be elegant skin care regardless of cost. Orlane's slick, sapphire-blue packaging with silver letters is stunning. Its opulent, lavish appearance and status-flaunting prices communicate prestige. But there has to be more to skin care than brilliant packaging and hard-to-swallow price tags, right? In Orlane's case, the simple answer is, there isn't much of anything beyond the packaging. Orlane's exterior may look like a BMW 745, but the interior and engine are strictly from a Chevy. The ingredient lists reveal the truth: These are just OK products with a few bells and whistles, but there are no hidden wonders that warrant the price tags or the hype that accompanies every item. There is nothing unique to be found, and not a single product is not easily replaced by better-formulated versions from other lines that are far less expensive.

All of Orlane's brochures feature gushing phrases such as "optimum functioning of the epidermis," "natural molecules called Oxytoners," and "creates the proper environment for the skin." It all sounds so impressive—until you take a closer look and notice that the claims just don't jibe with the information on the ingredient list. No facts, no actual research, no proof is given in anything I've read from the company. Plus, there are no sunscreens for part of the daily skin-care routine, which is a wide-open highway headed straight to more wrinkles from sun damage.

There is little here to extol, and the good products are marred by disproportionate price tags. The competition, from Lauder and Clinique to Neutrogena and Olay, has better options. For more information about Orlane, call (800) 775-2541 or visit www.orlaneparis.com. **Note:** All Orlane products contain fragrance unless otherwise noted.

ORLANE SKIN CARE

☺ **$$$ B21 Vivifying Cleansing Care** *($42.50 for 6.8 ounces)* is an exceedingly ordinary and completely standard, mineral oil– and plant oil–based wipe-off cleanser. It can leave a slight greasy film on the skin, and is an option for dry skin, but this mundane formula is easily replaced by similar versions ranging from Olay to Pond's.

☺ **$$$ B21 Oligo Vit-A-Min, Vitalizing Cleanser for Dry or Sensitive Skin Types** *($35 for 8.4 ounces)* is similar to the Vivifying version above only slightly less greasy. It does have a host of water-binding agents and vitamins, but they are listed well after the preservative and hardly amount to anything. It is an option for dry to very dry skin.

☺ **$$$ B21 Purifying Balancing Gel** *($45 for 6.8 ounces)*. I'm at a loss for words that can fully describe how standard a cleanser this is. This is just a detergent-based, water-soluble cleanser that would be a good option for normal to oily skin, but it could easily be replaced by myriad others with less fragrance for one-fourth the price.

☺ **$$$ Claircilane Hydro Clarifying Cleanser** *($35 for 6.8 ounces)* is a mineral oil–based cleanser with a minuscule amount of arbutin, a skin-lightening agent, though the amount makes it incapable of having any effect on skin. It is an option for dry to very dry skin.

☹ **B21 Gentle Face Scrub** *($50 for 8.4 ounces)* is a mineral oil– and castor oil–based wipe-off cleanser that contains ground-up plastic (polyethylene) as the abrasive. It also contains menthol, citrus, and fragrance, which makes it inappropriate for sensitive skin and every other skin type as well.

☹ **B21 Astringent Purifying Lotion** *($45 for 8.4 ounces)* lists sodium lauryl sulfate as the fifth ingredient, and it also contains menthol, both of which are too potentially irritating and drying for all skin types. The fourth ingredient is a fungus, *Fomes officinalis*, commonly known as brown trunk rot; there is no research showing this to have benefit for skin.

☺ **$$$ B21 Oligo Vit-A-Min Vitalizing Lotion for Dry and Sensitive Skin Types** *($35 for 8.4 ounces)* is merely water, slip agents, aloe, castor oil, preservatives, urea, fragrance, antioxidants, and coloring agents. It is incredibly boring and absolutely not worth the money.

☺ **$$$ B21 Bio-Energic Vivifying Lotion for All Skins** *($42.50 for 6.8 ounces)* is an option for all skin types, but for this kind of money there should be a bevy of antioxidants and anti-irritants (of which there are none), and far more impressive water-binding agents.

☺ **$$$ Claircilane Hydro Clarifying Lotion** *($35 for 6.8 ounces)* contains some good water-binding agents, just not very much of them. It also contains lactic acid and salicylic acid, but the less than 1% concentration makes them ineffective for exfoliation. The fractional amount of arbutin cannot have an impact on skin color.

☺ **$$$ B21 Purete Hydro Matifying Care** *($100 for 1.7 ounces)* contains mostly water, glycerin, coconut oil, silicones, slip agents, mushroom extract, niacinamide, preservatives, anti-irritant, and a teeny amount of antioxidants. This is a good moisturizer for normal to slightly dry skin, but the coconut oil is not the best for "matifying care." Niacinamide is a good ingredient for skin, but this ingredient is found in Olay's Total Effects products at a much higher concentration and for a lot less money. The mushroom extract has no benefit for skin.

☺ **$$$ B21 Bio-Energic Absolute Skin Recovery Care Cream** *($140 for 1 ounce)* is an OK emollient moisturizer for normal to dry skin with a tiny amount of water-binding agents and no antioxidants or anti-irritants anywhere to be found.

☺ **$$$ B21 Bio-Energic Absolute Skin Recovery Care Eye Contour** *($80 for 0.5 ounce)* is an emollient mineral oil– and Vaseline-based moisturizer with some good plant oils and a tiny amount of water-binding agents. It is an option for dry skin, but it is more a waste of money than anything else.

☹ **B21 Absolute Skin Care Recovery Concentrate for the Eyes** *($80 for 10 packets, each 0.07 ounce, and one 0.27-ounce vial)* is a two-part product, and it is absolutely an understatement to say that the whole is less than equal to the sum of its parts. The Gel Energia Water is an OK toner with some good water-binding agents, though several of the plant extracts can be skin irritants. The Compresses contain alcohol and that undoes the benefit of the water-binding agents! It also uses a preservative, Kathon CG, which is not recommended for use in leave-on skin-care products.

☺ **$$$ B21 Bio-Energic Absolute Youth Concentrate, Age Defense Protective Oxytoning System** *($300 for 0.7 ounce)* is a simple gel lotion that contains some good water-binding agents and a small amount of antioxidants. There is nothing "oxytoning" in here, though if there were that would be bad for skin, because giving skin extra oxygen generates more free-radical damage.

☺ **$$$ B21 Bio-Energic Extreme Line-Reducing Care** *($150 for 1.7 ounces)* is a simple emollient moisturizer with a small amount of water-binding agents and an almost undetectable amount of antioxidants.

☺ **$$$ B21 Bio-Energic Intensive Firming Care** *($120 for 1.7 ounces)* is similar to the Line-Reducing Care above and the same comments apply. This does contain a tiny amount of arnica, but probably not enough to be a problem for skin.

☺ $$$ B21 Bio-Energic Intensive Nurturing Care, Nightly Concentrate for Dry and Very Dry Skin ($120 for 1.7 ounces) is a basic emollient moisturizer with a tiny amount of water-binding agents, and I mean really tiny. The minuscule amount of royal jelly in here has no benefit for skin.

☺ $$$ B21 Bio-Energic Morning Recovery Concentrate ($65 for 0.5 ounce) is an OK, lightweight moisturizer for normal to dry skin, but it isn't concentrated in the least, it is just a lotion with some good water-binding agents. The soy protein has no estrogenic properties for skin.

☺ $$$ B21 Bio-Energic Absolute Youth Concentrate Age Defense Protective Oxytoning System for All Skin Types ($300 for 0.7 ounce). If only the price meant you were getting something really concentrated! But there is nothing in this moisturizer that warrants this over-inflated price—instead, it is just a good, emollient moisturizer for normal to dry skin, with impressive water-binding agents, antioxidants, and anti-irritants. There isn't a single element that is unique to this product.

☺ $$$ B21 Bio-Energic Ultra-Light Cream for the Day ($80 for 1.7 ounces) is an emollient moisturizer for normal to dry skin that contains a small amount of water-binding agents and a teeny amount of antioxidants, and without sunscreen it is absolutely not recommended for daytime at any price.

☺ $$$ B21 Bio-Energic Super Moisturizing Concentrate Day and Night ($100 for 1.7 ounces) is an emollient moisturizer for normal to dry skin that contains minuscule amounts of water-binding agents and a teeny amount of antioxidants. The only thing super about this is the price.

☺ $$$ B21 Intensive Firming Serum ($140 for 1 ounce) is a lotion with nothing intense about it, except the lack of anything more than negligible amounts of water-binding agents and antioxidants. You are getting more preservatives and film-forming agent than anything vaguely beneficial for skin.

☺ $$$ B21 Oligo Gentle Soothing Cream for Sensitive Fragile & Allergic Skin Types ($65 for 1.7 ounces) is a very good emollient moisturizer for normal to dry skin that contains some very good water-binding agents and antioxidants. However, there is absolutely nothing about this product that makes it preferred for sensitive or allergy-prone skin.

☺ $$$ B21 Oligo Light Smoothing Cream ($65 for 1.7 ounces) is a good emollient moisturizer with some very good water-binding agents and a small amount of some very good antioxidants.

☺ $$$ Hydro-Climat Moisture Shell Multiprotective Fluid ($60 for 1.7 ounces) doesn't contain sunscreen, and without that there is absolutely nothing multiprotective about it. This is actually a very mundane moisturizer with negligible amounts of water-binding agents and antioxidants. It contains cornstarch high up on the ingredient list, which can be a problem for skin.

☺ $$$ Anti-Wrinkle After Sun Balm for the Face with Vitamin C ($75 for 1.7 ounces). Sun damage cannot be corrected with this or any other moisturizer. This is just a very basic, mineral oil–based moisturizer that contains fractional amounts of water-binding agents and antioxidants.

☺ $$$ B21 Anti-Wrinkle Sun Serum for the Face ($125 for 1 ounce) is a poorly formulated lotion with a dearth of beneficial ingredients, plus it contains PABA, a sunscreen agent almost every other cosmetics line stopped using years ago due to problems of irritation.

☹ B21 Anti-Wrinkle Sun Cream for the Face SPF 15 ($75 for 1.7 ounces) doesn't contain the UVA-protecting ingredients of titanium dioxide, zinc oxide, or avobenzone, and is absolutely not recommended.

☺ $$$ Anti-Wrinkle Sun Cream for the Face and Sensitive Areas SPF 30 ($75 for 1 ounce) is a very good, though exceedingly overpriced, sunscreen with zinc oxide as one of the sunscreen agents. It has a matte-finish base with a tiny amount of antioxidants and water-binding agents and little else. The price is absurd for such an ordinary product that isn't even as well-formulated as many far less expensive options. Keep in mind that sunscreen has to be applied liberally to achieve the SPF benefit, and at this price, liberal application is unlikely.

☹ B21 Anti-Wrinkle Self Tanner for the Face SPF 8 ($75 for 1.7 ounces) fails as a sunscreen. Along with having a substandard SPF number, this doesn't contain the UVA-protecting ingredients of titanium dioxide, zinc oxide, or avobenzone, and is absolutely not recommended. As a self-tanner it is the same as all self-tanners, using dihydroxyacetone as the ingredient to affect the color of skin. There isn't a reason in the world to spend this kind of money on a self-tanner.

☺ $$$ B21 Oligo Vit-A-Min Vitalizing Masque ($32.50 for 1.7 ounces) is a standard, though emollient, clay mask with the tiniest amount imaginable of antioxidants and water-binding agents. It doesn't get much more boring than this, though, as is true for most masks, it will temporarily make the skin feel smoother.

☺ $$$ Claircilane Hydro-Whitening Creme for All Skin Types ($75 for 1.7 ounces) is an ordinary emollient moisturizer with fractional amounts of antioxidants and water-binding agents. It also contains arbutin, a plant extract that has melanin-inhibiting properties, but the amount of it in this product is so minute it isn't able to affect skin color.

☺ $$$ Claircilane Hydro-Whitening Serum for All Skin Types ($100 for 1 ounce) is similar to the Claircilane Whitening Formula above only in a gel lotion form and with a bigger price tag; and the same basic comments apply.

☺ $$$ B21 Bio-Energic Extreme Line Reducing Lip Care ($50 for 0.33 ounce) is an exceptionally ordinary, mineral oil–based moisturizer and there is literally nothing else to say about this absurdly overpriced waste of money.

ORLANE MAKEUP

Orlane's Les Extraordinaires makeup products try to continue the French flair and overblown hype characteristic of its skin-care products (really the focus of this line), but despite the technical names and too-good-to-be-true claims, there is little here to bother with, and the good products (which aren't great by any current standards) are marred by price tags that are out of proportion to any benefit you get.

FOUNDATION: ☺ $$$ B21 Bio-Energetic Teint Absolu Treatment Foundation *($50)* comes in a glass jar and has a moist, silky texture and an impressive natural finish. This would be fine for normal to dry skin seeking light to medium coverage, but of the five shades, three—Dore 21, Beige 23, and Amber Clair 29—are noticeably peach or pink and should be avoided. **Lightening Makeup Base Face & Decollete *($27.50)*** is a basic shimmer lotion for the face and body that feels moist and leaves a sheer veil of shine.

☹ **Satilane *($35)*** is semi-creamy and leaves a minimal matte finish with sheer to light coverage. The five colors are mostly forgettable, with four of them—Porcelaine, Miel Fonce, Topaze, and Biscuit—being too pink, peach, or rose for most skin tones.

☺ $$$ **Dual Compact Cake Foundation *($42.50)*** is a very good, though standard, talc-based powder foundation that has a super-soft and luxurious texture. The satin finish is appropriate for normal to slightly dry skin and the six colors are almost all wonderful. Only Ambre 05, which is too orange, is best avoided. **Ultra Naturel Revealing Ultra-Fluid Foundation *($40)*** is light and creamy, applies easily, and blends perfectly to a soft, sheer finish. The six shades are as neutral as Orlane gets, with the only poor choices being Miel Ambre and Sable Fonce. If you have normal to dry skin and don't mind the cost, this should please. Note: each shade does have a very soft shimmer that's almost imperceptible on the skin.

☺ $$$ **CONCEALER:** **Flash Corrector *($25)*** starts out thick and creamy but blends to a soft matte finish with excellent coverage. The matte finish is in feel only, as this leaves a soft shimmer once it dries, and that can call unwanted attention to wrinkles or blemishes. The three available shades are very good, but only for fair to medium skin.

POWDER: ☺ $$$ **Transparent Loose Powder *($35)*** is a talc-based powder whose texture is silky, but this also has a starchy, dry finish that won't be to everyone's liking. The three available shades are fine for fair skin. **Velvet Pressed Powder *($35)*** has a silky, weightless texture and ultra-fine appearance on the skin. However, two of the four shades are very shiny, which defeats the purpose of using powder. Avoid Perle Blanc and Soleil Blond if you're hoping to get shine control and a matte finish at the same time.

☺ $$$ **Sparkling Loose Powder for Face & Body *($35)*** is a talc-based, ultra-shiny powder that leaves the skin—and (eventually) your clothing, handbag, and coat—sparkling. You get the idea. **Bronzing Pressed Powder *($35)*** comes in a huge, saucer-style compact and has a beautiful texture and believable tan colors—all impaired by iridescence.

☺ $$$ **BLUSH:** **Velvet Blusher *($35)*** has a relatively standard dry, smooth texture, but beware, because almost all of the colors are infused with shiny gold particles. The matte options include Samara and Rose Sensuel.

☹ **EYESHADOW:** **Velvet Eyeshadow *($30 for duos)*** eyeshadows have a wonderful satiny texture that applies and blends well. Yet the majority of these duos feature contrasting colors imbued with shine, and the effect this has on mature eyelids is assuredly not what the women who shop this line are hoping for. **Fluid Eyeshadow** *($25)* is just a creamy, overpriced, ultra-shiny eyeshadow with a slight powder finish. This type of eyeshadow is difficult to work with and is not recommended.

EYE AND BROW SHAPER: ☺ $$$ **Le Crayon Extraordinaire Eyeliner Pencil** *($20)* is a very standard pencil with a creamy texture and a sponge tip. The price is the only thing that's extraordinary about this one. **Extra Liner** *($28)* is a good liquid liner, but it takes excessively long to dry and is not worth this outlandish price tag.

☹ **Crayon Multi-Beaute Lips, Eyes, Cheeks** *($20)* is nothing more than another multipurpose chubby pencil, only this one's texture is slightly sticky and all of the colors speak shine, loud and clear. **Eyebrow Fixing Shine** *($22.50)* is a sheer golden orange brow gel that gives a slightly glossy look to the brows, but it also tends to flake.

☺ $$$ **Brow Definer Pencil** *($18)* is a basic, hard-textured brow pencil that wins points for not being as waxy as most and for offering very good colors.

LIPSTICK AND LIP PENCIL: ☺ $$$ **Treatment Lipstick** *($22.50)* is no more a treatment for your lips than any other opaque, creamy lipstick. This has a sleek, moist texture and wears well, but the same can be said for countless lipsticks sold at the drugstore. **Fluid Lip Color** *($22.50)* is a "liquid" lipstick that applies wet and dries to a natural, slightly greasy finish. The colors are mostly shiny and have enough pigment to last a little longer than usual. One caution: If you have any lines around your lips, this will travel to them easily.

☹ **Rouge Extraordinaire Lipstick** *($20)* has a slick texture and offers moderate, non-staining color, but it just keeps moving on the lips and is not worth the too-frequent touch-ups or the expense.

☺ $$$ **Lip Lining Pencil** *($16.50)* is a boringly standard pencil with typical colors that has very little going for it other than great packaging. **Lip Gloss Lumiere** *($16.50)* is a thick, emollient pot gloss that offers semitransparent and opaque iridescent colors. You've seen this before, and for far less, but it is an option. **Lip Gloss** *($18.50)* is sheer, non-sticky, sparkly, wand-application gloss that has a considerably lighter texture than the one above.

☹ MASCARA: **Lengthening Treatment Mascara** *($25)* is one of the most boring, do-nothing mascaras I have encountered. At this price, I expect to be *im*pressed, not *de*pressed, by the mascara's performance. **Protective Volume-Building Mascara** *($25)* builds no volume, barely any length, no thickness, and almost makes lashes look shorter. The only thing this mascara is good at building is one more cosmetic mistake to sit in the bottom of your makeup drawer.

OSMOTICS

Osmotics wants you to know that they are leaders in the world of skin care, using "breakthrough technology, developed at a leading medical research university." They go on to say that their products are a "revolutionary all-in-one daytime treatment" and that they "conceived and developed the first transdermal patch for treating and preventing lines and wrinkles." You would think every other company was running around just trying to keep up with their advanced formulations. That isn't the case, but it makes for very good advertising copy. All of the Osmotics products contain ingredients that can be found elsewhere and for less money. Their showcased blue copper is available in Neutrogena's Active Copper products. Their kinetin products are not unique either, as both Almay's Kinetin and The Body Shop's Re-Leaf contain the same thing in equally good formulations. Similarly, their vitamin C product is matched by those of other companies, and despite Osmotics' claim that theirs is the only stable option for this vitamin, that isn't what the research shows.

A definite improvement for Osmotics is that they now have sunscreens with UVA-protecting ingredients, something this "advanced, breakthrough" line didn't originally include. What you will still find lacking are products appropriate for blemish-prone or oily skin. There are some good cleansers and very good moisturizers, but that's about it. For more information about Osmotics, call (800) 440-1411 or visit www.osmotics.com. **Note:** All Osmotics products contain fragrance unless otherwise noted.

☺ **$$$ Balancing Cleanser for Normal to Oily Skin** *($27 for 6 ounces)* is a standard, detergent-based, water-soluble cleanser that contains light scrub particles. It is an option for normal to oily skin.

☺ **$$$ Calming Cleansing Milk for Sensitive Skin** *($27 for 6 ounces)* definitely contains several plant extracts that are anti-irritants, and it doesn't contain fragrance (something that would be better for all skin types). Other than that, this is a standard, detergent-based, water-soluble cleanser along with some emollients that make it a good option for normal to dry skin.

☺ **$$$ Hydrating Cleanser for Normal to Dry Skin** *($27 for 6 ounces)* isn't hydrating in the least. It is a standard, detergent-based, water-soluble cleanser similar to many other cleansers available for far less money. It does contain a small amount of water-binding agents, which is nice, but for dry skin they really can't compensate for the drying effect of the cleansing ingredients on the skin. Several of the plant extracts are potential skin irritants, but the amounts are probably too small for them to have a negative impact on skin.

☹ **$$$ Balancing Tonic Facial Mist** *($35 for 6.8 ounces)* would actually be quite good as a toner for most skin types if it weren't for the potentially irritating plant extracts of mint and comfrey.

☺ **$$$ Firming Tonic Facial Mist** *($35 for 6.8 ounces)* is a basic toner that contains some plant extracts, slip agents, water-binding agent, and a minuscule amount of antioxidant. The plant extracts are good anti-irritants.

☺ **$$$ Facial Renewal** *($75 for 1.7 ounces)* definitely contains AHA (glycolic and lactic acids) in about an 8% to 10% concentration in a standard moisturizing base with a tiny amount of antioxidants and water-binding agents. It has the right pH for exfoliation, and would be fine for normal to dry skin. However, be aware that there are many effective AHA products out there for far less money!

☺ $$$ **Antioxidant Eye Therapy** (*$55 for 0.5 ounce*) is an OK lightweight moisturizer that has some antioxidants, but not enough to warrant the name of this product. The balm mint can be a skin irritant.

✔☺ $$$ **Balancing Complex SPF 15** (*$55 for 3.4 ounces*) is a very good, in-part zinc oxide–based sunscreen. It contains some very good water-binding agents and antioxidants and is a good option for normal to dry skin.

☹ $$$ **Daily Eye Protection SPF 15** (*$55 for 0.5 ounce*) lists the only active ingredient as avobenzone. While that is a very good UVA-protecting ingredient, it doesn't protect skin from the range of UVB damage. Either the ingredient listing is in error, or this sunscreen doesn't meet the FDA's regulation for SPF.

✔☺ $$$ **Illuminating Hydrating Complex SPF 15** (*$60 for 3.4 ounces*) is a good, in-part avobenzone-based sunscreen in an emollient base with some very good water-binding agents and antioxidants. A few of the plant extracts in it can be irritants, but the amounts are negligible and it's unlikely they'll have a negative impact on skin.

✔☺ $$$ **Blue Copper Firming Elasticity Repair** (*$98 for 2 ounces*) is an overpriced moisturizer that is described by Osmotics as the answer to every woman's antiwrinkle skin-care need—but that's how Osmotics describes most of their products. Why would you need any of these other products if you could use this? Copper has been shown to be effective in healing serious wounds, but that is unrelated to daily skin care or to preventing wrinkles. It is a good antioxidant, just not *the* answer for skin. This is a very good moisturizer for normal to dry skin with some very good water-binding agents and antioxidants, but the price is over the top for what it contains.

☹ $$$ **Creme de l'Extreme** (*$85 for 2 ounces*) contains mostly water, lanolin, glycerin, silicone, water-binding agents, Vaseline, and vitamin E. It is definitely a good emollient moisturizer for dry skin, but for the money, it should have been loaded with antioxidants and anti-irritants, and more than just a minuscule amount of vitamin E.

✔☺ $$$ **Triceram** (*$30 for 3.4 ounces*) is similar to the Creme de l'Extreme above and actually has more antioxidants, and is a better option for dry to very dry skin.

☺ $$$ **Kinetin Cellular Renewal Serum** (*$78 for 1.7 ounces*) is an OK moisturizer for dry skin that contains lots of ingredients that show up in other skin-care products, such as plant oils and a tiny amount of antioxidants and water-binding agents. It also contains kinetin (the technical name for N6-furfuryladenine). Please refer to Chapter Seven, *Cosmetics Dictionary*, for more information about kinetin. However, if this is the ingredient you are interested in, both The Body Shop's Re-Leaf and Almay's Kinetin line of products contain the same exact item in similar formulations for a fraction of this price.

☺ $$$ **Kinetin Intensive Eye Repair** (*$75 for 0.5 ounce*) is similar to the Kinetin Cellular Renewal Serum above and the same basic comments apply.

☺ **$$$ Intensive Moisture Therapy** (*$65 for 2 ounces*) is a very good emollient moisturizer for dry skin that contains a good amount of antioxidants and some water-binding agents.

☺ **$$$ Protection Extreme Total Body SPF 15** (*$32 for 4.25 ounces*) is a very good, in-part avobenzone- and zinc oxide–based sunscreen in an emollient base that would be an option for someone with normal to dry skin. Because sunscreens must be applied liberally to obtain the SPF benefit, an expensive sunscreen may discourage liberal usage. It takes about one ounce of sunscreen to cover the body adequately.

☺ **Protection Extreme Total Body SPF 25** (*$35 for 4.25 ounces*) is similar to the Total Body SPF 15 above and the same comments apply.

☺ **$$$ Extremely Natural Self Bronzer** (*$28 for 3.7 ounces*) contains dihydroxyacetone, the same ingredient used in all self-tanners, to affect the color of skin. It would work as well as any, but for less money and a similar formulation, there is no reason not to use Neutrogena's or Coppertone's self-tanners instead.

☹ **$$$ Facial Refining Masque** (*$32 for 2 ounces*) is an emollient mask with several plant extracts, most of which can be anti-irritants, though some can be skin irritants. The papaya has no exfoliating properties for skin. This standard group of ingredients can make skin feel smooth, but they won't refine any part of your skin.

☹ **$$$ Antioxidant Skin Care Derms** (*$48 for six treatments*) does have a form of vitamin C that you can patch onto your skin. This is a strange way to apply vitamin C to skin because you can't get it all over. Not to mention that vitamin C is not the most significant skin-care ingredient around and it isn't worthy of this tricky, expensive mode of application.

OXY BALANCE (SKIN CARE ONLY)

In the lineup of acne products at the drugstore, Oxy Balance actually has a few of the better choices, at least when it comes to good topical disinfectants that include benzoyl peroxide. But be careful: You still have to pick and choose to avoid some irritating and drying mistakes. For more information about Oxy Balance, call (800) 245-1040 or visit www.oxyoxygen.com.

☺ **Deep Cleansing Shower Gel for Face and Body** (*$5.25 for 8 ounces*) is a standard, detergent-based cleanser that also contains 2% salicylic acid. The pH of this cleanser is too high for it to have exfoliating properties, but even so, because it's a cleanser, you would risk getting salicylic acid in your eyes.

☹ **Normal Skin Daily Cleansing Pads** (*$5.25 for 55 pads*) contains about 40% alcohol, making this too irritating and drying for all skin types.

☹ **Sensitive Skin Daily Cleansing Pads** (*$5.25 for 55 pads*) contains about 35% alcohol, making this too irritating and drying for all skin types, and this is definitely not appropriate for sensitive skin.

☹ **Maximum Daily Cleansing Pads** *($5.25 for 55 pads)* contains almost 50% alcohol, and that is indeed a maximum amount of irritation and dryness for any skin type.

☺ **Oil-Free Maximum Strength Acne Wash** *($5.25 for 8 ounces)* is a standard, detergent-based, water-soluble cleanser with 10% benzoyl peroxide. While benzoyl peroxide is a great topical disinfectant for blemish-prone skin, in a cleanser the effective ingredients would be washed down the drain before they could go to work. To compensate for that problem, the directions on this cleanser state to "massage gently onto face for 1 to 2 minutes." Even if you had the time to do that, you would be massaging the cleansing agents onto the skin for that length of time, too, which can cause irritation and dryness— and that is not helpful for breakouts.

☹ **Multi-Action Astringent** *($4.25 for 8 ounces)* contains about 40% alcohol, making this too irritating and drying for all skin types.

✔☺ **Sensitive Skin Acne Treatment, Vanishing Formula** *($5.52 for 1 ounce)* is a very good 5% benzoyl peroxide topical disinfectant in a lightweight gel base.

✔☺ **Maximum Acne Treatment, Tinted** *($5.25 for 1 ounce)* is a very good 10% benzoyl peroxide topical disinfectant in a lightweight gel base. This version does have a strange tint to it, but it disappears rather easily once applied.

✔☺ **Maximum Acne Treatment, Vanishing** *($5.25 for 1 ounce)* is identical to the Tinted version above only without the tint, and the same comments apply.

PANOXYL (SKIN CARE ONLY)

This small line of acne products has only one option worth considering, because the two bar cleansers can cause blemish-prone skin more problems. For more information about PanOxyl, call (800) 327-3858.

☹ **PanOxyl Bar Benzoyl Peroxide 5** *($5.11 for 4 ounces)* is a detergent-based bar cleanser that adds 5% benzoyl peroxide to the mix. The ingredients that keep bar cleansers in their bar form can clog pores and this one includes cornstarch and oils, too, which are not the best for skin prone to breakouts. Plus, the benzoyl peroxide in this cleanser is wasted, as it would just be washed down the drain.

☹ **PanOxyl Bar Benzoyl Peroxide 10** *($5.53 for 4 ounces)* is similar to the one above, only this one has 10% benzoyl peroxide, and the same comments apply.

✔☺ **PanOxyl Aqua Gel Treatment** *($9.99 for 1.5 ounces)* is a very good 10% benzoyl peroxide topical disinfectant in a lightweight gel base.

PARTHENA

Parthena is clearly aimed at the burgeoning needs of baby boomers—or "the forgotten woman," as their brochure states, though "forgotten" is hardly the case for women over 40. Given the thousands of antiaging products being sold, the over-40 woman is not only remembered, she is relentlessly pursued and reminded that she is aging and that there are miracles to help her get over that plight!

If you are peri-menopausal or menopausal, Parthena wants you to believe that their products can stop your skin from succumbing to your body's lack of estrogen and progesterone. Part of Parthena's pitch is that some of its products contain wild yam extract. However, there is no research showing that wild yam can have any hormonal effect when applied topically on skin. If anything, the studies that do exist have demonstrated that topical application of wild yam has little to no effect on menopausal symptoms (Source: *Climacteric,* June 2001, pages 144–150). According to *The PDR Family Guide to Natural Medicines & Healing Therapies* and the *American Journal of Obstetrics and Gynecology* (1999, volume 18), as well as the definitive book on the subject from Dr. John Lee, *What Your Doctor May Not Tell You About Menopause: The Breakthrough Book on Natural Progesterone* (Warner Books, 1996), wild yam is used in the production of artificial (synthetic) progesterone, but it will not yield the hormone in the absence of a chemical conversion process that the body can't supply, though it can be created in a laboratory. That means the use of wild yam on skin is a waste of your time and energy, and makes other creams that do contain USP progesterone a far more interesting consideration.

Parthena has a strange mix of good and bad products. Though many products contain an interesting combination of antioxidants and water-binding agents, they are often present in tiny amounts and, therefore, inconsequential for skin. Then there are the problematic ingredients, ranging from irritating and drying cleansing agents to alcohol-based toners. What is a strong point for this line are the more than reasonable prices. It's hard to pass up bargains like this, but if they don't work, even inexpensive products aren't worth the money. For more information about Parthena, call (800) 660-0666 or visit www.parthenacosmetics.com. **Note:** All Parthena products contain fragrance unless otherwise noted.

PARTHENA SKIN CARE

☹ **Multi-Action Marine Cleanser** *($14 for 4 ounces)* lists sodium C14-16 olefin sulfonate as the second ingredient, making this extremely drying and irritating for all skin types.

☺ **2 in 1 Cucumber Cleanser** *($12 for 4 ounces)* is a very standard, detergent-based cleanser that would be an option for someone with normal to oily skin. The teeny amount of cucumber in this cleanser doesn't deserve to be mentioned in the name of the product.

☹ **Resurfacing Enzyme Cleanser** *($16 for 4 ounces).* TEA-lauryl sulfate is the main cleansing agent in this product, and that is too potentially irritating and drying for all skin types.

☺ **Dissolve Eye Makeup Remover** *($9.50 for 2 ounces)* is a standard, plant oil–based makeup remover and it would work as well as any reviewed in this book.

☹ **Confetti Scrub** *($19.50 for 4 ounces)* contains TEA-lauryl sulfate as the main cleansing agent, and that makes it too potentially irritating and drying for all skin types.

☹ **7 Day Mega Peel Serum and Maintain Toner** *($29.95 for 0.5 ounce of the 7 Day Mega Peel and 4 ounces of Maintain)*. This is a two-part product. You are supposed to use the 7 Day Mega Peel for seven days of the month "due to the high percentage of enzyme to literally digest surface skin debris and fine wrinkling" and then the Maintain for the remainder of the month. The 7-Day Mega Peel isn't all that "mega." The bacillus ferment is supposed to be an exfoliant, but the only information showing that to be the case is provided by the company selling this ingredient; there is no other research supporting that claim. Maintain lists dimethyl sulfone as the second ingredient, which is similar in form to dimethyl sulfoxide, DMSO. These are intriguing substances because of their contradictory benefits and problems. Topically, they are potent skin irritants and sensitizers and can cause burning, blistering, drying, and scaling skin. Yet they easily penetrate the skin and facilitate topical penetration of other ingredients. DMSO also has some evidence of having antioxidant properties and can prevent skin from freezing. Given these divergent properties and the well-established risk of skin irritation, it is not recommended to have this as a primary ingredient in skin-care products (Sources: *Natural Medicines Comprehensive Database*, http://www.naturaldatabase.com; *Skin Research and Technology*, May 2001, pages 73–77; and *Contact Dermatitis*, February 1998, pages 90–95 and April 2000, pages 216–221).

☹ **Resurfacer Toner 5%** *($7.95 for 2 ounces)* contains 5% AHAs, but the second ingredient is alcohol, and that makes it too irritating and drying for all skin types.

☹ **Resurfacer Toner 10%** *($7.95 for 2 ounces)* contains 10% AHAs, but the second ingredient is alcohol, and that makes it too irritating and drying for all skin types.

☺ **Custom Formula Rapid Skin Exfoliator Strength 1**, **Strength 2**, and **Strength 3** *($5.95 for 2 ounces each)* would have been three well-formulated glycolic acid– and lactic acid–based AHA products with varying strengths. However, all three of these products have a pH of 5, which makes them ineffective for exfoliation.

☺ **Rapid Skin Exfoliation System for Skin, Eyes, and Lips Strength 1**, **Strength 2**, and **Strength 3** *($9.95 for 1 ounce each)* are virtually identical to the Custom Formula Rapid Skin Exfoliator products above and the same comments apply.

✔☺ **Longevity Daily Line Smoothing Fluid** *($5.95 for 1 ounce)* is a good silky moisturizer for normal to dry skin with a good mix of anti-irritants, water-binding agents, and antioxidants. The tiny amount of wild yam has no hormonal benefit for skin.

☺ **Longevity Resource Cream** *($16 for 1 ounce)* is a very ordinary emollient moisturizer for normal to dry skin. It does contain a tiny amount of wild yam extract. Refer to the introduction for Parthena above and to Chapter 7, *Dictionary*, for more information about wild yam.

✔☺ **Longevity Wonder Serum** *($32.50 for 1 ounce)* is a silicone-based moisturizer with an impressive assortment of water-binding agents, antioxidants, and anti-irritants. It is an option for normal to dry skin.

☺ **Adult Oil Control Gel** *($12.50 for 1.75 ounces)* doesn't contain anything that can control oil. The minuscule amount of salicylic acid and the high pH mean that it can't exfoliate skin.

☺ **Anhydrous Extreme Cream** *($21.50 for 2 ounces)* is an emollient, rather heavy moisturizer that contains a tiny amount of wild yam and a minuscule amount of vitamin E. Wild yam won't affect hormones or menopausal symptoms. For more information about wild yam, refer to the introductory paragraph for Parthena above and to Chapter 7, *Cosmetics Dictionary.*

☺ **Comfort Gel** *($12 for 2 ounces)* isn't all that comforting, it is just a lightweight gel with minuscule amounts of water-binding agents and antioxidants. You're getting far more preservatives in this moisturizer than any beneficial skin-care ingredients.

☺ **Cream International AM** *($16.50 for 2 ounces).* Without sunscreen, there is no reason to consider this an option for daytime. It is just an emollient moisturizer with some good water-binding agents and antioxidants. It does contain retinol, but the jar-type packaging ensures that it won't remain stable once it's opened. The amniotic fluid and placental protein are good water-binding agents, but just because those substances come from animals around the time of their birth doesn't mean they can help your skin be younger.

☺ **Cream International PM** *($16.50 for 2 ounces)* is an emollient moisturizer for normal to dry skin, but it lacks many of the interesting water-binding agents and antioxidants of the International AM version above. This does contain retinol, but the type of packaging means it is unlikely to remain stable once it's opened.

☺ **Daily Support Gel** *($9.95 for 2 ounces)* is a lightweight gel moisturizer that contains plant extracts and yeast. The plant extracts can have antioxidant properties—and in theory so can the yeast—but overall this would be a far better option for skin if the formula had some good water-binding agents. It is an option for slightly dry skin.

☺ **Daisy Gel** *($14.50 for 1 ounce)* is very good, silicone-based gel that also contains some good antioxidants. It is an option for normal to slightly dry skin.

☺ **$$$ Eye Wonder Serum** *($21.50 for 0.5 ounce)* is a good, lightweight lotion that contains some very good water-binding agents and a tiny amount of antioxidants and anti-irritants. It is an option for normal to slightly dry skin.

☹ **Morning Oxygen Duo** *($7.50 for 1 ounce of Detox Cream and 1 ounce of Activator Fluid).* The activator fluid contains sodium C14-16 olefin sulfate, a detergent cleansing agent that can be extremely irritating and drying. It also contains hydrogen peroxide, an ingredient that can generate free-radical damage. The Detox Cream is mostly glycerin, sodium bicarbonate (that's baking soda), and clay. You're supposed to mix these two products together for a morning pick-me-up, but if you really knew what you were putting on your skin, you would probably have to be picked up off the floor.

☺ **Confetti Gel** *($19 for 1 ounce)* does contain some very good antioxidants and water-binding agents, but they appear far after the long list of preservatives, meaning they are barely present and have little to no benefit for skin. This does contain salicylic acid (about 1%), but the pH of 5 is too high for it to have exfoliating properties. The yeast may have antioxidant properties for skin, but there is no research proving that to be the case.

The Reviews P

☺ **$$$ Unwrinkle Serum** *($22 for 0.5 ounce)* won't un-wrinkle skin anymore than any of the other parade of antiwrinkle Parthena products. This is a good, silicone-based moisturizer with a teeny amount of antioxidants, and little else.

☹ **Youthology Multi Facet Lotion** *($21.50 for 1 ounce)* lists alcohol as the second ingredient, and that is a problem for skin. Without that, this would otherwise have been a very good mix of antioxidants and water-binding agents.

☺ **Intercept SPF 30 Spray** *($6.95 for 2 ounces)* is a very good, in-part titanium dioxide–based sunscreen in a very standard, though lightweight, lotion applied via a spray. It would work well for normal to slightly dry skin.

☺ **Spray On Sun Tan Enrichment Spray** *($6.50 for 2 ounces)* contains a tiny amount of tyrosine, an amino acid that in the skin initiates the production of melanin (melanin is the component of skin that gives it "color"). According to information on the FDA's Web site (www.fda.gov), tyrosine's "use is based on the assumption that it penetrates the skin, increases the tyrosine content of the melanocytes, and thus enhances melanin formation. This effect has not been documented in the scientific literature. In fact, an animal study reported a few years ago demonstrated that ingestion or topical application of tyrosine has no effect on melanogenesis [the creation of melanin]."

☺ **Spray On Sun Sunless Tanning Spray** *($6.50 for 2 ounces)* contains dihydroxyacetone, the same ingredient all self-tanners use to affect the color of skin. This one would work as well as any.

☹ **Airless Fading Lotion** *($14.50 for 1.7 ounces)* contains 1.5% hydroquinone, which can inhibit melanin production. The Vaseline-based moisturizing formula is an option for normal to dry skin, but the fifth ingredient is sodium lauryl sulfate and that can be a potent skin irritant.

☺ **$$$ Blanc de Blanc Cream** *($16 for 0.5 ounce)* contains an extract of *Phyllanthus emblica,* a plant that has very good antioxidant properties. Whether or not it can inhibit melanin production is unknown, although that is the contention of the company selling the ingredient. This also contains a tiny amount of mulberry extract, which contains arbutin, another melanin-inhibiting extract from a plant source, but the amount in this product is far below what would be needed to have any effect on skin color. This is a good lightweight moisturizer for normal to slightly dry skin, but don't count on a change in skin color from using this product.

☺ **$$$ Live Cell Derivative Soothing Eye Area Mask** *($9.95 for 0.5 ounce).* There is nothing living in this product, so this is just a good emollient mask that contains film-forming agent and a tiny amount of water-binding agents, antioxidants, and anti-irritants.

☺ **Eyelasticity Line Smoothing Mask** *($16.50 for 1 ounce)* is similar to the Soothing Eye Area Mask above and the same comments apply.

☹ **Hydrating Mask** *($12 for 1 ounce)* is a very ordinary lotion that contains a teeny amount of water-binding agent and minuscule amounts of anti-irritants.

☹ **Deep Pore Cleansing Mask** (*$10 for 4 ounces*) is a basic clay mask. However, it contains menthol (a skin irritant) as well as a preservative, Kathon CG, that is not recommended for use in leave-on skin-care products.

☺ $$$ **Mega Lip Serum** (*$21.50 for 0.5 ounces*) is a standard emollient balm for lips with a tiny amount of antioxidants.

☺ **Cool Off Moisture Magnet Skin Cooling Mist** (*$9.95 for 8 ounces*) contains mostly water, slip agent, wild yam, water-binding agent, anti-irritant, preservatives, and coloring agents. There is nothing in this product that will cool off a hot flash. This is just an OK toner, and spraying it on yourself isn't any more helpful than splashing cool water on your face. For information about wild yam refer to the introduction for Parthena above and to Chapter 7, *Cosmetics Dictionary*.

PARTHENA MAKEUP

For ordinary to downright appalling makeup with fantastical claims, the prize goes to Parthena. Each product is described with brow-raising adjectives such as "revolutionary," "perfect," and "state of the art." Yet almost any other makeup line offers not only better products, but also something Parthena is lacking—choice. Several items come in only one shade, while the rest offer considerably fewer choices than the competition. The couple of good options identified below are indeed worth adding to your list of possibilities, but I wouldn't commit to Parthena before checking out the plethora of recommended products at drugstores and department stores. And if you invest in this line because of your faith in their claims, be prepared for a sobering reality check.

☹ **Anhydrous Healthy Tint Day Cream** (*$9.50*) is "the next generation of sport tint foundation" that allegedly addresses all types of aging and dry skin concerns, but this matte finish, silicone- and clay-based foundation is the wrong choice for addressing even mildly dry skin. This confused product also contains mineral spirits (that's paint thinner) as the fourth ingredient—a significant irritant for all skin types and its inclusion sends this product back to the time when Egyptians used coal to line their eyes! **High Definition Foundation** (*$14*) is a far more modern formulation than the one above, but this highly fragranced, smooth silicone-based foundation comes in only one shade, and it's strongly peach. The coverage is sheer to light, but the pigmentation is dense enough for the unfavorable undertones to show clearly on the skin, and this is not recommended. **High Definition Mascara-Eyeliner Duo** (*$12.50*) is a single tube that gives you mascara on one end and liquid eyeliner on the other. Both formulas show promise, and the mascara thickens instantly, but neither dries completely, and these smear and smudge terribly. **Liquid Pantyhose** (*$12.50*) is a water-resistant body makeup designed to camouflage varicose veins, birthmarks, and other unsightly flaws. The almost comical name was gleaned from the fact that this is an alternative to covering up leg discolorations by wearing support hose. Although the Liquid Pantyhose does hold up in water, you will be disappointed by the surprisingly sheer coverage and unnatural colors.

☺ **Ice Cold Cover Up Concealer** *($8.50)* is a light, water-to-powder stick concealer that contains a good deal of mica, so this leaves a sheer coverage, shiny finish that does little to hide blemishes or discolorations. It does provide a brief cool sensation as it's applied, so if that and the shiny finish are important to you this may be worth a try.

☺ **Play on Lights Light Diffusing Face Color** *($12.50)* comes in a compact that holds five iridescent cream-to-powder colors. Although the sheer colors are workable, with options for eyes and cheeks, this much shine is only for those with smooth, unlined skin. A nice benefit of this product is that it stays in place once it's dry, so the shine stays where you want it. **Mega Lipstick** *($12.50)* is Parthena's alternative to cosmetic surgery for the lips, as they claim this silicone-based lipstick "is a collagen stimulator in a dose-dependent manner." They go on to state that simply using this lipstick will plump up thin lips, stop lipstick bleeding, and reduce lip furrows (lines). All this for fewer than fifteen dollars! You probably know that this simple, slick lipstick does nothing to stimulate collagen, and cosmetic surgeons are not complaining about any decrease in the number of lip-plumping procedures. As a lightweight lipstick that comes in a limited range of colors, this is fine. However, it is slippery enough to migrate easily into any lines around the mouth. **Mega Lipstick Fantasy Duo** *($12.50)* is identical to the Mega Lipstick above, only this offers two iridescent colors (for highlighting or darkening an existing lipstick) in one stick. It's fine if you think you'll ever use it, but this is the stuff impulse buys are made of. **Mega E Stick** *($12.50)* is a clear, emollient lip balm in lipstick form that carries over the same collagen-stimulating claims as the Mega Lipstick. The claims are hot air, but this product does soothe the skin and protect the lips from chapping.

PAULA DORF COSMETICS (MAKEUP ONLY)

Paula Dorf is an in-demand makeup artist whose career has gone from television commercials and music videos to private sessions with top celebrities (Barbara Streisand) and political officials (Hillary Rodham Clinton). Like a number of others, and in addition to her regular behind-the-scenes duties, Dorf has found time to create her own line of cosmetics, and boldly joined the overcrowded makeup artist-turned-entrepreneur arena. Her cosmetics line has many of the same benefits other makeup artist lines have—namely, a superior range of neutral foundations, lush-textured blushes and eyeshadows, and wonderful brushes to pull everything together. Whether or not you think Paula Dorf's products take things a step further than her competitors is really a matter of personal preference. The fact is, almost any line sanctioned by a makeup artist is a boon for cosmetics consumers. The real trick is experimenting with each line's best products (and colors) to discover what's right for you.

One thing you will notice in Dorf's line, unlike those of most of her peers, is a preponderance of unnecessary application tools and products that seem like a good idea but will only become part of every woman's graveyard of impulse cosmetics buys. My suggestion is to ignore these "unique" items unless you can reasonably see yourself using them on a regular basis. Ingenuity and originality are good things, but not when the expense and results don't match one's expectations or the tag line claims on the product itself. That said, there is more than enough here to make this line worth stopping for if you happen to come across a display, which shouldn't be too difficult given the number of department and boutique stores where Paula Dorf products are sold. For more information about Paula Dorf Cosmetics, call (888) 472-8523 or visit www.pauladorf.com.

FOUNDATION: ✓☺ $$$ **Perfect Glo Foundation** *($42)* is a modern twist-on traditional creamy compact-type foundation. It has a slightly greasy, slick texture that glides over the skin and leaves a moist, dewy finish. Coverage can go from sheer to light, and this is tailor-made for normal to dry skin not prone to blemishes. The 12 shades are simply stunning—not a suspect one in the bunch—and there are equally good options for lighter and darker skin tones. This is one of the standout products in Dorf's line.

☺ $$$ **Moisture Foundation Oil-Free** *($34)*. The somewhat confusing combination of "oil-free" and "moisturizing" in the name may leave you wondering exactly who is supposed to use this foundation. It turns out to be a very good, lightweight, matte-finish foundation that is appropriate for someone with normal to oily skin seeking sheer to light coverage. The 13-shade color selection is quite nice. The only colors to consider avoiding are Creme and Cocoa, which can be too peach for most skin tones. There are excellent options for very light and dark skin.

☺ $$$ **Face Tint SPF 15** *($34)* is a very sheer, tinted moisturizer that contains no UVA-protecting ingredients, so it is not recommended for sun protection. Yet if you're willing to wear an effective sunscreen underneath (and have dry skin) the seven colors are decent. Watch out for the too-rose Cannes and the colorless, but shimmery, Just Glow.

☹ **Perfect Primer** *($24)* is one of the few foundation primers that's silicone-free. This very lightweight moisturizer has a watery texture and can feel a bit too stiff and filmy on the skin—not to mention the peppermint that provides a cool feel, along with a dose of irritation.

☹ **CONCEALER: Total Camouflage** *($20)* has two shades of concealer in a single pot. The texture is rather thick and a bit too greasy, while the color combinations are strange. Each duo has one neutral color and a corresponding shade of peach or pink. The emollience of this one ensures that it will fade and crease as the day wears on. Besides, with so many reliable neutral concealer options out there, who wants to waste time blending two separate colors, especially ones that have no relation to skin tone? **Magic Stick** *($15)* is a very greasy, opaque concealer in a lipstick-style tube. The four shades are not as peachy pink as the concealer above, but I strongly disagree with the claim that this is a light-textured product.

POWDER: ✓☺ $$$ **Pressed Powder** *($25)* has a beautiful, smooth, talc-based texture that blends on evenly over the skin. Almost all of the colors are workable, including some excellent matte bronze shades for women of color, though Bronze Glimmer is way too showgirl-shiny to take seriously. This comes with a brush, but it's a bit too firm and scratchy to choose over one of Dorf's own full-size powder brushes.

☺ $$$ **Loose Powder** *($30)* has a soft, sheer, talc-based texture and floats over the skin. A bit strange is the fact that there are only two shades—a "no color" color that will look too white over medium to dark skin tones, and a very shiny version called Glimmer, which could work for evening sparkles.

☹ $$$ **All-Over Glimmer Dust** *($20)* is an even shinier loose powder that comes with either gold or silver pigment. This could work for an evening look, but the small container makes it messy to use and easy to overdo.

BLUSH: ✓☺ $$$ **Cheek Color** *($18)* has a wonderful texture and a soft, dry finish. The colors are a nice range of matte neutrals along with soft pastels with a few token shimmery choices. All of them blend on sheer, allowing you to build on the intensity.

✓☺ $$$ **Cheek Color Cream** *($18)* is a small, but superior, group of cream-to-powder blushes. This dries to a sheer, almost translucent, soft powder finish, and the colors are great. This is best for normal to dry skin, as long as you bear in mind that most of the colors have a touch of shine, though it's not nearly enough to be distracting.

EYESHADOW: ✓☺ $$$ **Eye Color** *($17)* is a range of eyeshadows whose silkiness allows a flawless, even application that wears well. There are fewer matte shades than before, but, if you're interested, the best options in this regard are Cherub, Moonstone, Sea Shell, and Wet Sand. Dorf's shinier shades do go on just as well and tend not to flake.

☺ $$$ **Eye Color Glimmers** *($17)* are a bit more powdery and apply more intensely than the Eye Color above. It's all about shine here, and lots of it. If that's important to you, check these out. Avoid Wild Fire, an iridescent red shade that just doesn't look good near the eye.

☺ $$$ **EyeLite** *($24)* is supposed to be the remedy for dark circles or for one too many late nights. This is a sheer, opalescent pink highlighting cream that is dispensed via a click pen onto a brush applicator. It's fine for highlighting the brow bone if you want shine, but used under the eyes this is shine overload without meaningful coverage.

☹ **Eye Primer** *($20)* is a very thick, waxy eyeshadow base that is completely unnecessary. This will only create a whitish ring around the eye area and, owing to its creaminess, creasing is guaranteed. Paula, what were you thinking?

EYE AND BROW SHAPER: Topping the list of unnecessary makeup products is ☹ **Transformer** *($14)*. This mostly watery substance is supposed to transform eyeshadow to a liquid liner. Funny—tap water does the same thing and it's virtually free, and that's primarily what this product is.

✓☺ **Eye Pencil** *($15)* is a standard pencil, in the sense that it needs sharpening, but this has a dry, powdery finish that does not smudge! Application isn't as carefree as it is with creamier pencils, but the trade-off is worth it.

☺ $$$ **Brow Duet** *($18)* is a dry-textured, almost-matte (a slight shine is visible) brow powder that packages two shades together. There are three duos suited to most brow colors from blonde to black, and they apply softly and easily. Each set's colors are tone-on-tone, so you may find you can use both or, as I suspect will happen for most women, you will prefer one shade over the other. **Perfect Brow** *($14)* is a clear mascara for the lashes or the brows and it does work to keep the brow in place. There are much less expensive options for this kind of look, the least pricey of which is grooming the brows with some hairspray on an old toothbrush. **Brow Tint** *($15)* is a very good brow tint that is identical to the one in my Paula's Select line that sells for half this price, and Dorf's version gives you less product and lacks a dual-sided brush for greater versatility. If you enjoy using this type of product for brow defining and grooming, I'll let you decide whose version makes more sense.

LIPSTICK AND LIP PENCIL: The ☺ **$$$ Lipstick Cream** *($16)* makes the most universal of all lipstick claims—that it is "long-wearing." Well, it might just do that if you reapply it at regular intervals, but otherwise this is a standard, greasy lipstick that has a lot of slip and a glossy finish, though the color range is enticing.

✓☺ **Lip Pencil** *($15)* needs to be sharpened and comes in a nice range of colors. Due to a higher pigment level, these do tend to stain the lips more than usual, so they tend to stay longer than most. The not too creamy but not too dry texture is ideal for a smooth application.

☺ **Lip Gloss** *($15)* is nothing but a standard, fairly sticky gloss in one of the smallest packages I've seen. There is no reason to spend this much on such a very basic product. **Lipsicle** *($17)* is another sticky lip gloss you apply with a wand applicator. The colors are pigment-rich, and if you don't mind the stickiness, this will provide full, glossy color. **Moisture Stick with Vitamin E** *($14)* is a standard waxy lip balm that works as well as any to soothe dry, cracked lips. The vitamin E is only a dusting so it serves little purpose.

☹ **$$$ Lip Color Sheer Tint SPF 15** *($16)* is a standard sheer lipstick that veers slightly toward the greasy side. It's fine for a slick, glossy look and the colors are workable, but it lacks UVA-protecting sunscreens, so don't count on it for broad-spectrum sun protection. Almay and Revlon are the companies to look to if you want lip color with effective sunscreen agents.

☹ **Perfect Illusion** *($18)* is supposed to plump your lips and stop lipstick from feathering. It falls flat on both counts. When tested, it took less than an hour for even a soft matte lipstick to break through into lines, and there was no difference in the size of the lips whatsoever. If this had less oil and emollients and more dry-finish silicone, it would likely perform as intended.

MASCARA: ☺ **Mascara** *($15)* builds nice, long, and clump-free lashes, but it does take some effort to get there. The directions recommend that you apply this ordinary mascara with Dorf's fan brush, but that's completely unnecessary and it does not produce better results than applying it with the brush that comes with it.

☹ **Cake Mascara** *($20)* says on the box it's from "Hollywood's Golden Age," and while that may be true in terms of mascara's history, it by no means makes this anything you should consider today. Why Dorf thought this was a good idea is a mystery. It is awkward and messy to use, builds no length or thickness, and, given the way you have to hold the fan-shaped brush, is very to easy to get in the eye.

☺ **Perfect Lash Lash Thickener** *($14)* is a standard lash
mascara without color. It can add thickness, but the amount is ins
the results from any good thickening mascara (which Dorf's line

BRUSHES: Dorf has a great array of ☺ $$$ **Brushes** *($6–$6*
tional, particularly the eyeshadow and eyelining options. You will f
range of synthetic brushes that are softer and smoother than the no~~~~~ these may be
an option for foundation or concealer and even for shadow application. However, there
are a few to consider avoiding.

☺ $$$ **Foundation Brush** *($35)* is a good choice if you decide to try this type of
brush. Though I feel it doesn't make sense to apply foundation this way, as opposed to a
sponge, there are those who do prefer it. The **Cream Cheek Brush** *($35)* seems superflu-
ous when a sponge or your fingers work just as well, and while the **Cheek Brush** *($40)*
and **Powder Brush** *($60)* are supremely soft, you may not like their lack of density. Still,
they're worth auditioning if your budget allows.

☹ **Mascara Fan Brush** *($16)* is really pointless unless you fall for Dorf's Cake Mas-
cara, while the **Lip Brush** *($17)* is too small for most women's lips, and takes forever to
completely apply color. The **Eye Contour Brush** *($28)* is well-shaped, but too small for
most contouring needs, and the **Eye Blender** *($27)* is too big to be practical, so it tends to
poof on color rather than smooth it on. The **Bronzing Fan** *($28)* is denser than most fan
brushes, but does nothing special during application to make it worth choosing over
other brushes.

☺ **Brush Out Brush** *($12)* is a spray-on brush cleaner that is alcohol-free, so it won't
dry out your brushes. However, this takes a while to dry so it's not ideal for on-the-spot,
need-it-now cleanings. This contains mostly water, slip agent, aloe, detergent cleansing
agent, and film-forming agent.

☺ $$$ **Sweep Away Clean-Up Stick** *($28)* is a wax-and-silicone stick that nicely
removes makeup mistakes without leaving a greasy finish. However, it's way too expensive
to take the place of a cotton swab dipped in regular makeup remover or even in plain water.

PAULA'S CHOICE/PAULA'S SELECT

I created Paula's Choice, my own skin-care line, back in 1995. A few years later, I
added a full makeup line called Paula's Select. Some of you may find that shocking, while
others, about 100,000 of you as this book goes to press, think I have formulated a great,
inexpensive line of skin-care and makeup products. It's not that I haven't had returns—
not everyone's skin can tolerate everything—but for the most part it has been a great
venture, and the feedback and the relationship with the people who purchase my prod-
ucts has been incredibly satisfying.

Some of you may be wondering just why I decided to create a line of skin-care and
makeup products at all. Isn't that like Ralph Nader designing and selling cars? Good ques-
tion. (But personally, I do wish Ralph would come out with a reliable group of automobiles!)

Believe me when I say I did not undertake this endeavor without a great deal of thought. Actually, it's where I started more than 20 years ago, when I owned my own cosmetics stores that included my own skin-care line. If anything, I feel like I've come full circle, except now I know far more than I did back then! After 20 years of analyzing and reviewing hundreds of cosmetics lines and thousands upon thousands of skin-care and makeup products, and after hundreds of readers asked me to create products, it seemed like a natural extension of my work. As you already know, I have been continually frustrated by the endless array of products making claims that are either untrue or misleading. In addition, even when I find products that meet my criteria for performance they often fall short in other ways. For example, many products I otherwise like contain fragrance (a major cause of skin irritation), coloring agents, problematic preservatives, or irritating or sensitizing plant extracts. When it comes to AHA and BHA products, they often have the wrong pH or too low a concentration to be effective—or, more often than not, are just absurdly overpriced.

Paula's Choice is a line of skin-care products that I have formulated to meet my own strict criteria. None of my products contain synthetic coloring agents, fragrance (not even masking fragrances), or any of the irritating ingredients I've been warning about for years, and they aren't tested on animals. I make no exaggerated claims and, better yet, these products are inexpensive—every product is under $18, and they come in comparatively generous-sized containers. Paula's Select is a range of cosmetics that can create a flattering makeup look, one that can go from day to night and work beautifully for women who want to create a sophisticated, professional image. The texture and application of each Paula's Select makeup product is every bit as elegant as what you will find in countless other lines.

A few women have voiced concerns that I would be abandoning my research, as well as my objectivity, in favor of cosmetics sales. This is not my intent. I truly believe that offering inexpensive, high-quality products that live up to my expectations is a service that will not get in the way of my judgment. However, you are the best judges of whether I indeed remain objective. I believe the reviews in this book speak louder than anything I could say directly to you. Clearly, there are plenty of products from other lines that I have no hesitation in recommending. I'm really happy there are many good options that can have a positive effect on skin, because that's what consumers need: choices.

I am committed to maintaining my standards. There will always be great products for me to recommend, and terrible, overpriced products for me to caution you about. My products are one option I've put together from what my research indicates are reliable and effective products and ingredients: nothing more, nothing less.

I debated at length about how to review my own products. After all, this is an area where it is most difficult for me to be impartial. I attempted, as best I could, to review them as if they weren't my own, and decided to just give it a go, trying to be as objective as I could possibly be. I did decide to leave them unrated here (without faces), because I couldn't possibly be *that* impartial (but they do technically meet all of my criteria). Paula's Choice and Paula's Select products are available by calling (800) 831-4088 or (206) 444-1622. You can also order through my Web site at www.PaulasChoice.com.

PAULA'S CHOICE SKIN CARE

One Step Face Cleanser, Normal to Oily/Combination Skin *($11.95 for 8 ounces)* is a standard detergent gel-based cleanser that takes off all makeup without irritating or drying the skin. It rinses easily without causing a dry or tight sensation and leaves the skin feeling soft.

One Step Face Cleanser, Normal to Dry Skin *($11.95 for 8 ounces)* is a standard detergent cleanser that takes off all makeup, including eye makeup, without irritating or drying the skin. It contains glycerin to soften and soothe skin, and has a milkier texture than the Normal to Oily/Combination Skin version above.

Skin Recovery Cleanser, Normal to Very Dry Skin *($11.95 for 8.5 ounces)* is a water-soluble cleanser designed for those with extra dry or more sensitive skin. For those who find my One Step Face Cleanser for Normal to Dry Skin not suitable for their skin type this may be a better option. It still removes eye makeup, doesn't lather, and is extremely gentle, and it also leaves no dry or greasy residue on the skin.

Gentle Touch Makeup Remover *($12.95 for 4 ounces)* is a water- and silicone-based liquid that effectively removes regular and waterproof mascara, long-wearing lipstick, blush, and eye makeup. It contains anti-irritants and is colorant and fragrance-free. Although I have typically not recommended makeup removers as essential, I recognize that many women do prefer this step to make sure every last trace of their makeup is removed.

Final Touch Toner, Normal to Oily/Combination Skin *($9.95 for 8 ounces)* is a nonirritating toner with anti-irritants and water-binding agents. It leaves a clean, soothing feeling on the skin.

Final Touch Toner, Normal to Dry Skin *($9.95 for 8 ounces)* is a nonirritating, moisturizing toner that contains a higher concentration of water-binding agents than the Normal to Oily/Combination Skin version above. It leaves a clean, soothing feeling on the skin.

Essential Non-Greasy Sunscreen SPF 15, Normal to Oily Skin *($12.95 for 6 ounces)* is an avobenzone-based sunscreen in a lightweight lotion base. It contains antioxidants and water-binding agents and leaves a soft matte finish on the skin. Works well on the face and body.

Essential Moisturizing Sunscreen SPF 15, Normal to Dry Skin *($12.95 for 6 ounces)* is a part titanium dioxide–based sunscreen that contains thickeners, plant oil, antioxidants, water-binding agents, and preservatives. This is a good emollient moisturizer for dry skin and can be used on the face and body.

Pure Mineral Sunscreen SPF 15, Normal to Dry or Sensitive Skin *($12.95 for 6 ounces)* uses only titanium dioxide and zinc oxide as the active UVA-protecting sunscreen agents. That makes it a very good option for someone with dry sensitive skin, though it can be effective for any skin type except blemish-prone skin. This does not look or feel greasy on the skin and can be used on the face and body.

Extra Care Moisturizing Sunscreen SPF 30+ with Antioxidants Water-Resistant, Normal to Dry Skin *($12.95 for 6 ounces)* is similar to my Essential Moisturizing Sunscreen SPF 15 above, except that this has slightly more antioxidants and higher SPF protection (it's still part titanium dioxide). It is also water-resistant.

Extra Care Non-Greasy Sunscreen SPF 30+ with Antioxidants Water-Resistant, Normal to Oily Skin *($12.95 for 6 ounces)* is an in-part avobenzone sunscreen that is water-resistant and provides significant sun protection for those who live in sunny climates or who receive more than casual sun exposure. The formula feels light on the skin, is easy to apply, and does not turn thick or sticky on skin.

Completely Non-Greasy Moisturizing Lotion, Normal to Oily Skin *($13.95 for 4 ounces)* is a good, lightweight moisturizer that contains a balanced mix of antioxidants and water-binding agents and is excellent for someone with normal to oily skin with dry areas. It can be used anywhere on the body, as well as around the eyes if that area needs moisturizer.

Skin Balancing Moisture Gel, Normal to Oily Skin *($14.95 for 2 ounces)* is the lightest moisturizer in my line, designed for those with normal to oily skin who have dry patches or want something very light to use around the eyes. Its silicone technology leaves skin feeling smooth, soft, and not at all greasy. This also features a nice combination of antioxidants, water-binding agents, and anti-irritants.

Completely Emollient Moisturizer, Normal to Dry Skin *($13.95 for 4 ounces)* is a good emollient moisturizer for someone with normal to dry skin. It contains a skin-friendly mix of oils, antioxidants, and water-binding agents. It can be used anywhere on the body, as well as around the eye area if that area needs moisturizer.

Extra Emollient Moisturizer, Normal to Extra Dry Skin *($13.95 for 4 ounces)* is richer and a bit thicker than the Completely Emollient Moisturizer above, and is best for someone with dry to very dry skin. It is very emollient and contains many effective water-binding agents and anti-irritants. This can be used anywhere on the body as well as around the eyes.

Skin Recovery Moisturizer, Dry to Very Dry Skin *($13.95 for 4 ounces)* is the most substantial-feeling moisturizer in my line, created for dry to very dry or sensitive skin that needs an emollient, protective feel. It has a thick, creamy feel that softens skin with a blend of plant oil, emollients, silicone, water-binding agents, antioxidants, and anti-irritants. The texture of this is comparable to what many other lines sell as eye creams, and this product can indeed be used around the eyes or anywhere else on the face and body.

Hydrating Treatment Cream, Normal to Dry Skin *($14.95 for 2 ounces)* is a soothing, silky moisturizer with numerous antioxidants, anti-irritants, and water-binding agents. It is a very good option for normal to dry skin. It can be used around the eyes or anywhere on the body.

Remarkable Skin Lightening Lotion, All Skin Types *($13.95 for 4 ounces)* takes into account all of the research indicating that hydroquinone is the most effective choice for inhibiting melanin production when used in conjunction with an effective sunscreen. Strengths with a concentration of 1% to 2% are available over the counter, while 4% to 12% concentrations are available from physicians. My product contains 2% hydroquinone and 7.4% glycolic acid (AHA) in a lightweight moisturizing base with a pH of 3.5 so it works to inhibit melanin production and helps with cell turnover. This product can be used on the face, hands, arms, legs, or neck, and is best for someone with normal to dry skin.

Blemish Fighting Solution, All Skin Types *($13.95 for 4 ounces)* is a 2.5% benzoyl peroxide solution in a lightweight lotion base. It also contains anti-irritants. Benzoyl peroxide is a topical disinfectant, and a 2.5% concentration is a primary consideration in the battle against breakouts. Note: This cannot be used in combination with Retin-A, Renova, or Differin.

Extra Strength Blemish Fighting Solution, All Skin Types *($13.95 for 4 ounces)* combats blemishes by stopping problem-causing bacteria with 5% benzoyl peroxide. It also contains anti-irritants that can reduce redness and irritation. This formulation leaves no residue on the skin. Note: This cannot be used in combination with Retin-A, Renova, or Differin.

8% Alpha Hydroxy Acid Solution, All Skin Types *($13.95 for 4 ounces)* is an 8% glycolic acid gel with a pH of 3.5. It also contains an anti-irritant, water-binding agents, and preservatives. It can be mixed with other moisturizers or used under sunscreens. It is an effective exfoliating product for both the face and the body.

1% Beta Hydroxy Acid Lotion, All Skin Types *($13.95 for 4 ounces)*. This product has a pH of 3.2 and gently exfoliates the skin and unclogs pores without leaving the skin feeling greasy or dry. There are no waxy ingredients to clog pores or make skin feel layered with too many products, and it includes anti-irritants to help soothe the skin. This is best for someone with normal to dry skin and blemishes or blackheads. It can be especially helpful for someone with rosacea. There is anecdotal information that BHA, due to its relationship to aspirin (both are salicylates), can reduce redness and inflammation while gently exfoliating excess skin cells. This can be used with Retin-A, Renova, or Differin.

2% Beta Hydroxy Acid Lotion, All Skin Types *($13.95 for 4 ounces)* is similar to the 1% Beta Hydroxy Acid Lotion, except it has a pH of 3.4, and twice the concentration of salicylic acid. This formula also contains antioxidants, anti-irritants, and water-binding agents to benefit the skin. It works well to reduce blemishes and blackheads while leaving the skin soft and smooth without excess irritation. It can also be used as a topical exfoliant for sun-damaged skin.

2% Beta Hydroxy Acid Liquid Solution, All Skin Types *($13.95 for 4 ounces)* is similar to the 1% Beta Hydroxy Acid Lotion above in terms of pH and performance, but this one is double the strength and in a liquid base. It is better for more persistent blemishes and blackheads.

Super Antioxidant Concentrate, All Skin Types *($17.95 for 1 ounce).* The latest skin-care research indicates that topical application of antioxidants is a powerful tool to help skin stay healthy by reducing free-radical damage. Antioxidants also play a role in soothing skin and reducing inflammation, which is essential to maintaining skin's integrity. This silicone-based, non-aqueous product contains a substantial amount of effective antioxidants and anti-irritants and leaves skin feeling very silky. It can be used once or twice per day alone, or with moisturizer, sunscreen, or under makeup.

Almost the Real Thing Self-Tanning Gel *($12.95 for 6 ounces)* provides a fast, natural-looking tan using dihydroxyacetone, the same ingredient used in almost all self-tanners to affect the color of skin. This is a gel formula that works well for all skin types. It is tinted with caramel coloring so it is easy to see where it has been applied, helping you achieve a more even application.

Protective Lip Balm SPF 15 *($7.95 for 0.5 ounce)* is a very good emollient lip balm, but that isn't so unusual. What is special about this product is that it has an in-part titanium dioxide sunscreen, which provides full-spectrum sun protection and also prevents dry lips.

Moisturizing Lipscreen SPF 15 *($6.95)* is an in-part titanium dioxide–based lip balm in a convenient, twist-up container.

Exfoliating Treatment *($7.95 for 0.5 ounce)* is a unique way to get dry skin off lips, elbows, knees, or heels without irritation. A tiny amount gently massaged over dry skin is all that's needed. Simply keep massaging until the product starts to flake off, taking the dead, dry skin with it. Brush or rinse off what remains, and the skin is left silky-smooth.

Lip & Body Treatment Balm *($7.95 for 0.5 ounce)* is a concentrated blend of skin-compatible emollients, oils, and waxes designed to smooth, soften, and protect dry to very dry lips, knees, elbows, heels, and cuticles. This balm can be used anywhere on the body, and contains anti-irritant and antioxidants.

Oil-Absorbing Facial Mask, Oily/Combination Skin *($10.95 for 6 ounces)* absorbs excess oil from the surface of the skin and from within the pore without irritation or dryness.

All Over Hair & Body Shampoo *($12.95 for 16 ounces)* is an exceptionally gentle, yet effective, shampoo for all hair types (including chemically treated hair). This pH-balanced formula doubles as a gentle body wash and is completely fragrance- and colorant-free. It is ideal for anyone with a sensitive scalp or skin and for children.

Smooth Finish Conditioner *($12.95 for 16 ounces)* is a great everyday conditioner that leaves all hair types feeling soft and silky, looking shiny, and easy to comb through. Even with daily use, this clean-rinsing formula will not make hair feel heavy or greasy. It is completely fragrance-free.

Close Comfort Shave Gel *($10.95 for 6 ounces)* is a non-aerosol, fragrance-free shaving gel designed for both men and women. Both will find that this formula is easy to apply and keeps the skin protected as you shave, yet it rinses cleanly and will not clog your razor. This is tinted with azulene, a natural blue colorant derived from chamomile that also has anti-irritant properties, so you can see where it has been applied.

Skin Relief Treatment *($13.95 for 4 ounces)* contains a stabilized form of aspirin, which is an effective topical agent that can relieve many types of irritation. The formula also has green tea and willowherb—two potent anti-irritants that help to normalize and heal skin. Skin Relief Treatment is in a light liquid base similar to a toner and provides quick post-shaving comfort from head to toe for both men and women. It can also be used to soothe minor skin irritations resulting from insect bites, contact dermatitis, and redness from inflamed blemishes.

PAULA'S SELECT MAKEUP

FOUNDATION: **All Bases Covered Foundation SPF 15 Normal to Dry Skin** *($12.95)* has a light, creamy-smooth texture and is great for normal to dry skin. It offers a soft matte finish with light to medium coverage and excellent blendability in six neutral shades. The long-wearing formula is best for normal to dry skin, but this can be used by combination skin as well. However, if you have oily skin you may not be pleased with it, especially if you've been using a well-formulated matte or ultra-matte foundation. This foundation is fragrance-free and protects skin with a titanium dioxide SPF 15 sunscreen.

Best Face Forward Foundation SPF 15 Normal to Oily Skin *($12.95)*, available in Spring/Summer 2003. Has a light, liquid texture that can provide light to medium coverage. It has a smooth, silken matte finish that holds up well during the day. The sunscreen is a reliable in-part titanium dioxide base and this comes in six beautiful neutral colors.

CONCEALER: **No Slip Concealer** *($7.95)* is a creaseless concealer that you apply with a wand. It blends well, stays put, and each of the four neutral shades has a soft matte finish.

POWDER: **Soft Pressed Powder** *($10.95)* can be used as a talc-based finishing powder over foundation or alone as a powder foundation for all skin types. It can also be used wet or dry. It has a silky-soft texture and six great neutral shades with a light matte finish.

Healthy Finish Pressed Powder SPF 15 *($11.95)* offers the option of shine control and additional sun protection, with a titanium dioxide– and zinc oxide–based sunscreen with an SPF 15. This has a silky, velvety feel and goes on evenly and smoothly without looking chalky or dry on the skin. You'll find this provides light to medium coverage and a soft matte finish in four neutral shades. This can be used as a pressed-powder foundation (best for normal to slightly dry or slightly oily skin), or simply used with a powder brush to set makeup or touch up your sun protection (over sunscreen or foundation with sunscreen) without redoing your makeup. Please keep in mind that I don't recommend relying on *any* SPF-rated pressed powder as your sole source of sun protection because it is unlikely anyone will apply it in a thick enough layer to achieve optimal sun protection. It is best to use an SPF 15 powder in conjunction with a moisturizer or foundation that has an SPF 15 or greater and that contains UVA-protecting ingredients.

Soft Matte Bronzing Powder *($10.95)* is identical to the Soft Pressed Powder above, only this features two soft bronze tones without a hint of shine. Tawny Brown is ideal for fair to light skin tones, while Rich Brown works best on medium skin tones.

<u>BLUSH:</u> **Soft Matte Blush** *($7.95)*. I've chosen blush that has an elegant, velvety, light matte texture and that does not fade or dissipate throughout the day. It goes on smooth and even, and I think you'll find the range of colors are quite workable, and able to blend on soft or dramatic, depending on what you need.

<u>EYESHADOW:</u> **Soft Matte Eyeshadow** *($7.95)* applies without flaking or skipping. These are ultra-silky and easy to blend whether you want sheer shading or all-out drama, and every color is completely matte. Several shades work beautifully to line the eyes and define or fill in the brows.

<u>EYE AND BROW SHAPER:</u> **Brow/Hair Tint** *($8.95)* defines eyebrows with natural-looking color. The brush-on formula is lightweight and flakeproof and the four shades can also be used to touch up gray hair at the roots.

<u>LIPSTICK AND LIP PENCIL:</u> **Soft Matte Lipstick** *($7.95)* is one of the only true matte formulas around. I prefer this type of lipstick for its saturated, opaque colors and notably long wear, yet the non-creamy feel is clearly not universally appealing. True matte lipsticks are a boon to anyone prone to lipstick bleeding into lines around the mouth, or those who do not want to reapply lip color every couple of hours. **Soft Cream Lipstick** *($7.95)* has an emollient, smooth feel with a silky texture and opaque to semi-opaque coverage. **Long-Lasting Anti-Feather Lipliner** *($6.95)* is a standard, automatic lipliner in colors that I chose to coordinate with my lipsticks. These have a smooth application but aren't greasy, and they can help prevent feathering (just like most pencils that have this kind of texture). I've also included a clear Long-Lasting Lipliner that can help keep most lipsticks from bleeding (though it won't stop exceptionally greasy, glossy lipsticks from feathering). **Soft Shine Moisturizing Lip Gloss** *($7.95)* is a lightweight, wand-applicator gloss with an emollient, non-sticky application and requisite glossy finish.

<u>MASCARA:</u> **Lush Mascara** *($7.95)* will create long, thick lashes without clumping, flaking, or smearing, and it will last all day. It's water soluble for easy removal. **Epic Lengths Mascara** *($7.95)* has great lengthening ability without the intense thickening action of the Lush version above. This also wears well and does not flake or smear, yet is easy to remove.

<u>BRUSHES:</u> My brushes are very soft and dense, hold their shape, as well as place color evenly with minimal to no flaking of powder. Most of them come in long- and short-handled versions. The **Powder Brush** *($16.95)*, **Blush Brush** *($13.95)*, two **Eyeshadow Brushes, Small** and **Large** *($10.95 each)*, **Wedge Brow Brush** *($8.95)*, **Eyeliner Brush** *($8.95)*, **Lip Brush** *($7.95)*, **Shadow Softening Brush** *($8.95)*, **Crease Defining Brush** *($8.95)*, **Precision Shadow Brush** *($8.95)*, and **Concealer Brush** *($7.95)* are all professional-style brushes to help you apply makeup using the same tools that most makeup artists rely on. In addition, there is a convenient **Brush Carrying Case** *($12.95; $13.95)*

that can hold up to eight brushes. I also have **Makeup Application Sponges** for applying foundation *($4.95 for ten round Latex-free sponges)*. For those who need to keep excess shine in check, my **Oil-Blotting Papers** *($4.95 for 100 sheets with plastic case)* absorb oil and perspiration without leaving a layer of powder or making skin feel dry.

PERSA-GEL (SEE CLEAN & CLEAR)

PETER THOMAS ROTH
(SKIN CARE ONLY)

Unique in the world of spa and salon specialty lines, Peter Thomas Roth is a rather straightforward line with uncomplicated formulations. Many of the products are quite good and state-of-the-art. Even most of the acne, AHA, BHA, sunscreen, and moisturizing products contain what they should to be effective and helpful for skin. Not surprisingly, many are also redundant, with only minor changes in formulation, but that doesn't make them bad, it just makes this line overcrowded and confusing for the consumer and aesthetician.

Another novel aspect of this line is that there are few (if any) nonsense ingredients. These products conspicuously lack the exotic, potentially irritating, sensitizing, and often unnecessary plant extracts and the irritating, fragrant plant oils that show up in most pricey skin-care lines, especially spa lines. The majority of the products do not contain coloring agents, many don't have fragrance, and they lack the long lists of ingredients that are a clue that you aren't getting much of the special stuff. Even more impressive are the well-formulated cleansers, sunscreens, AHA products, and skin lighteners. And while the moisturizers aren't fancy and won't knock your socks off, they are effective, decent formulations. By and large, this line should be admired for its simplicity and, for the most part, for its well-thought-out formulations.

After all that glowing praise there are a few embarrassing missteps to avoid, such as products that contain hydrogen peroxide, which can generate free-radical damage and hurt skin; irritating acne products; cleansers with some drying and irritating cleansing agents; as well as some preposterous claims for products claiming to get rid of dark circles.

What you will notice immediately is that the prices are somewhat *spa*-tacular and unwarranted for what you're getting, particularly when it comes to the cleansers, toners, and sunscreens. Almost every product in the Peter Thomas Roth line is easily replaced by far less expensive versions. However, this is a line worth looking at, because if you're the type of consumer who is going to overspend on skin care, you may as well choose from well-formulated products that can do something for the skin. For more information about Peter Thomas Roth, call (800) PTR SKIN or visit www.peterthomasroth.com.

☺ **$$$ Chamomile Cleansing Lotion** *($30 for 8 ounces)* is a very standard, detergent-based, water-soluble cleanser that uses a few cleansing agents I wouldn't exactly call gentle. Still, this would be very good for someone with normal to oily skin. The minuscule amount of chamomile is practically nonexistent in this formulation and doesn't warrant being mentioned in the name of the product.

☺ $$$ **Gentle Cleansing Lotion** *($30 for 8 ounces)* is as basic as it gets for a standard, detergent-based cleanser. The tiny amount of safflower oil doesn't help make it gentle. It is a good cleanser for someone with normal to dry skin.

☺ $$$ **Foaming Face Wash** *($30 for 8 ounces)* is similar to the Gentle Cleansing Lotion above, only this version has lemon oil, an unnecessary skin irritant, which does not make this better for oily skin. However, the amount of lemon oil is small enough that it probably doesn't pose much of a problem for skin and it's in here more for fragrance than anything else.

☺ $$$ **Extra Strength Cleansing Gel Oil-Free for Oily, Combination or Problem Skin** *($30 for 8 ounces)* is a very standard, detergent-based, water-soluble cleanser that would be good for someone with normal to oily skin.

☺ $$$ **Sensitive Skin Cleansing Gel** *($30 for 8 ounces)* is similar to the cleansers above, only with a lesser amount of detergent cleansing agents. It would be good for someone with normal to oily skin, but the fragrance it contains is not helpful for someone with sensitive skin.

☺ $$$ **Combination Skin Cleansing Gel** *($30 for 8 ounces)* is similar to the Sensitive Skin version above and the same review applies.

☺ $$$ **Silky Cleansing Cream** *($30 for 8 ounces)* is a standard, emollient, cold cream–like, wipe-off cleanser with a tiny amount of anti-irritants and vitamins. It is an option for normal to dry skin, but it's no better than lots of other similar cleansers at the drugstore.

☺ $$$ **Glycolic Acid 3% Face Wash** *($30 for 8 ounces)* is similar to most of the Peter Thomas Roth cleansers and is a very ordinary, detergent-based cleanser that adds 3% glycolic acid to the formulation. That small an amount of AHA and the high pH of the base make this ineffective as an exfoliant, but it's best not to have any AHA or BHA in a cleanser because it would be a problem if you get it in the eye area.

☺ $$$ **Beta Hydroxy Acid 2% Acne Wash** *($32 for 8 ounces)* is an exceptionally standard, detergent-based, water-soluble cleanser that would be an option for normal to oily skin. The 2% salicylic acid (BHA) is not effective as an exfoliant due to the high pH of the product. It is a problem if you get this in the eye area, so be careful.

☺ $$$ **Anti-Aging Cleansing Gel** *($30 for 8 ounces)* is a standard, detergent-based cleanser that adds some plant extracts and a mix of irritants and anti-irritants, along with less than 1% glycolic acid (not enough to be effective as an exfoliant) and some antioxidants. Even if any of them were helpful to stop aging (they can't, but just hypothetically), they would be washed down the drain before they could have benefit for skin. This is an option for normal to oily skin.

☹ **AHA/BHA Face & Body Polish** *($30 for 8 ounces)* contains sodium C14-16 olefin sulfate as the main detergent cleansing agent (the second ingredient), which is too drying and potentially irritating for all skin types. The amount of AHA in here is not enough to be an exfoliant and the pH is too high for it to have any exfoliating properties even if there were enough AHA.

☹ **Botanical Buffing Beads** *($30 for 8 ounces)* has a fairly gentle abrasive. However, the detergent cleansing agent, sodium C14-16 olefin sulfonate (listed on the label as alpha C14-16 olefin sulfonate) is too drying and irritating for all skin types.

☹ **Pumice Medicated Acne Scrub with 2.5% Benzoyl Peroxide** *($30 for 8 ounces)* contains pumice as the scrub, which can be too abrasive for all skin types. The benzoyl peroxide would be washed off before it had a chance to have a disinfecting effect.

☹ **Silica Face & Body Polish** *($30 for 8 ounces)* uses sodium C14-16 olefin sulfate as the cleansing agent, which is too drying and irritating for all skin types.

☹ **Silica Strawberry Scrub** *($30 for 8 ounces)* uses pumice and ground-up plastic as the scrub particles, but the pumice is too abrasive for most skin types. The strawberry fragrance adds no benefit for skin.

☺ **$$$ Aloe Tonic Mist** *($30 for 8 ounces)* is a rather simple, though nonirritating, toner that contains mostly water, aloe, slip agent, anti-irritant, and a teeny amount of vitamins. It would be an OK option for most skin types. This doesn't contain fragrance.

☺ **$$$ Conditioning Tonic** *($30 for 8 ounces)* is an incredibly simple formulation of water, slip agent, preservative, and about 0.5% BHA, period! The pH is too high for this to be effective as an exfoliant. Clinique has a version that is better than this for half the price.

☹ **Glycolic Acid Clarifying Tonic** *($30 for 8 ounces)* contains a generous amount of alcohol and is not recommended.

☺ **$$$ Oxygen Mist** *($35 for 8 ounces)*. The claim that this product can provide more oxygen to the skin than what is already available in the air is sort of funny, except, of course, to the people who have wasted their money on it. Even if this were a great way to deliver oxygen, it doesn't explain the potential problems associated with the oxidative damage it would cause. Remember, oxygen causes free-radical damage, which is why *anti*oxidants are so important to skin.

☺ **$$$ Power C Firming Spritz** *($35 for 8 ounces)*. If you're looking for a vitamin C product, this one would work well as a toner. Still, I am skeptical that this form of vitamin C is stable in this formulation despite the use of the term "stabilizing complex" on the ingredient label, which is meaningless and doesn't meet the FDA's ingredient labeling regulations.

☺ **$$$ Glycolic Acid 5% Moisturizer** *($40 for 2 ounces)* is a good 5% AHA moisturizer for normal to dry or sensitive skin. While it also contains a tiny amount of antioxidants and water-binding agent, there is nothing this product can do that can't be done by any of Alpha Hydrox's AHA products at the drugstore.

☺ **$$$ Glycolic Acid 10% Moisturizer** *($40 for 2 ounces)* is similar to the 5% Moisturizer above, and the same comments above apply. This would be a very good 10% AHA moisturizer for someone with normal to dry skin.

The Reviews P

☺ $$$ **Glycolic Acid 10% Hydrating Gel** *($45 for 2 ounces)* is quite similar to Alpha Hydrox's oil-free AHA version (available at the drugstore), which costs about $10 for 1.7 ounces. This one is definitely a good AHA formula for someone with normal to oily skin and it does have a teeny amount of good water-binding agents and vitamins, but the price is out of line for what you get.

☹ **Glycolic Acid 10% Clarifying Gel** *($45 for 2 ounces)* contains both BHA and AHA, but it also contains a large amount of alcohol, and is not recommended.

☺ $$$ **AHA 12% Hydrating Ceramide Repair Gel** *($45 for 2 ounces)* is a good, lightweight 12% AHA exfoliant containing primarily glycolic and lactic acids, although it also contains citric, malic, and tartaric acids. The additional AHA ingredients are unnecessary because they don't work as well as the glycolic or lactic acid, but this would still be a good AHA product for someone with normal to oily skin, and the tiny amount of water-binding agents is helpful for skin.

☺ $$$ **Glycolic Acid 3% Eye Complex** *($48 for 0.75 ounce)* is a good emollient moisturizer for dry skin, but the 3% AHA isn't enough to exfoliate skin, and the pH isn't low enough to have that effect even if there were more of it.

☺ $$$ **AHA/Kojic Acid Under Eye Brightener** *($48 for 0.75 ounce)* is an OK, emollient moisturizer for dry skin similar to the Glycolic Acid 3% Eye Complex above, except that this one also contains kojic acid. Kojic acid can have some effect on reducing melanin content, but it is not a stable ingredient and, therefore, is less effective than hydroquinone for skin lightening.

☹ **Oxygen Eye Relief** *($50 for 0.75 ounce)* contains hydrogen peroxide, a significant oxidizing agent that generates free-radical damage. Because of the cumulative problems that can arise from impacting the skin with a substance like this that is known to generate free-radical damage, impair the skin's healing process, cause cellular destruction, and reduce optimal cell functioning, it is better to avoid its use (Sources: *Carcinogenesis,* March 2002, pages 469–475 and *Anticancer Research,* July-August 2001, pages 2719–2724).

☹ **Co-Oxygen Q-10 Wrinkle Repair** *($110 for 2.3 ounces)* is an incredibly confused product. On the one hand, it is a very standard, basic, Vaseline-based moisturizer with thickeners and glycerin (which is just fine for dry skin, but Lubriderm would be just as good if not better for that). It also contains hydrogen peroxide, and the comments for that ingredient in the review for the Oxygen Eye Relief above apply here. The other issue is that while the coenzyme Q10 this contains is a good antioxidant, the hydrogen peroxide releases oxygen, so they would at best cancel each other out. Finally, there is also a minuscule amount of BHA, but the pH is too high for it to be effective as an exfoliant. If you're looking for a coenzyme Q10 product, Nivea's version is far less confused and far better formulated than this one, though neither can repair a wrinkle.

☹ **Oxygen Detoxifying Masque** *($45 for 4.5 ounces)* contains hydrogen peroxide, and the same comments for this ingredient in the review above for the Oxygen Eye Relief apply here as well.

☺ **All Day Moisture Defense Cream SPF 20** *($30 for 1.7 ounces)* is a very good, in-part titanium dioxide–based sunscreen in a standard emollient base that contains a small amount of antioxidants and water-binding agents.

☺ $$$ **Max All Daily Moisture Defense Moisture Cream SPF 30** *($37 for 1.7 ounces)* is almost identical to the Defense Cream SPF 20 above except with an SPF 30. The same basic comments apply.

☺ $$$ **Ceramide Moisture Renewal** *($45 for 2 ounces)* is a very good emollient moisturizer for dry skin that contains good water-binding agents and antioxidants. Ceramide is a good water-binding agent, but it is no more a must-have ingredient for skin than dozens of other good water-binding agents.

☺ $$$ **Ceramide Ultra-Rich Night Renewal** *($55 for 2 ounces)* is similar to the Ceramide Moisture Renewal above, only with more plant oils and emollients, which makes it better for someone with dry to very dry skin.

☺ $$$ **Ceramide Eye Complex** *($48 for 0.75 ounce)* is similar to the Ceramide Moisture Renewal above and the same comments apply.

☺ **Environmental Repair Hydrating Gel** *($35 for 2 ounces)* won't repair anything, but it is a good, lightweight moisturizer for normal to slightly dry skin.

☹ $$$ **Oil-Free Moisturizer** *($40 for 2 ounces)*. The interesting ingredients (which are only vitamins A and E) are barely present here, which makes this a very basic, mundane moisturizer for someone with normal to slightly dry skin.

☺ $$$ **Power C 10 Serum Liquid** *($75 for 1 ounce)* contains 10% L-ascorbic acid, along with slip agents, antioxidant, water-binding agent, and preservatives. If you want a vitamin C toner, this is good, though it's an absurdly expensive option for most skin types, and dry skin would still need an emollient moisturizer over it.

☺ $$$ **Power C 10 Anti-Oxidant Serum Gel** *($80 for 1 ounce)* is similar to the Serum Liquid above only in lotion form, and the same basic comments apply.

☺ $$$ **Power C 20 Anti-Oxidant Serum Gel** *($80 for 1 ounce)* is similar to the Serum Gel above only with more of the vitamin C.

☺ $$$ **Power C Eye Complex** *($48 for 0.75 ounce)* is a good moisturizer for normal to dry skin that contains a few good antioxidants and water-binding agents. The vitamin C is present as a small amount of magnesium ascorbyl phosphate, which makes it a lower "power C" than the other versions above.

☺ $$$ **Power C Souffle** *($85 for 1.5 ounces)* is similar to the Power C Eye Complex above and the same comments apply.

☹ $$$ **Power C Instant Glow** *($110 for 0.8 ounce)* contains 10% ascorbyl palmitate in a standard group of thickening agents and preservatives. Ascorbyl palmitate is a good antioxidant, and 10% is a nice amount, but the price tag is bizarre when you consider that the benefit to skin is more theoretical than factual. This won't change a wrinkle, and if you have dry skin, you will still need a moisturizer over it.

☺ $$$ **Power C Ultra Lite Skin Luminizer** *($110 for 1 ounce)* is similar to the Instant Glow above, only with about a 5% concentration of ascorbyl palmitate in a slightly more emollient base.

☺ $$$ **Power K Eye Rescue** *($100 for 0.5 ounce)*. The primary claim for vitamin K's use in cosmetics is to reduce the appearance of dark circles and reduce the appearance of surfaced capillaries. Yet there is no independent research showing vitamin K to be effective for any aspect of skin care. The study that is cited as proof that it works was carried out by the patent holder and the company that sells vitamin K products. This is a good moisturizer with good water-binding agents and antioxidants, which is great for dry skin, but it's not worth this price tag. It does contain magnesium ascorbyl phosphate, which can inhibit melanin production in a concentration of 3% or greater, but this doesn't even have a 1% concentration. It also contains kojic acid, which can inhibit melanin production, but the amount is so small as to have little benefit for skin. This also contains arnica, a skin irritant, but the amount is probably too small for it to be a problem for skin.

☺ $$$ **Power K Skin Brightener** *($110 for 1 ounce)* is similar to the Power K Eye Rescue version above, and the same comments apply.

☹ $$$ **Retinolique Forte II** *($85 for 1 ounce)* claims to contain 5% retinol (vitamin A), which I strongly doubt. At that amount, there would be a risk of toxic effects, which is why even the prescription drugs Retin-A and Renova only contain a 0.5% to 0.1% concentration of tretinoin (the acid form of vitamin A).

✓☺ $$$ **Potent Botanical Skin Brightening Gel Complex** *($45 for 2 ounces)* contains 2% hydroquinone as well as azelaic acid and kojic acid, all of which have melanin-inhibiting properties, though hydroquinone is the most reliable and well-documented ingredient for improving skin discoloration.

☺ $$$ **Ultra Gentle Botanical Skin Lightening Gel Complex** *($45 for 2 ounces)* contains azelaic acid and kojic acid, which have melanin-inhibiting properties, though kojic acid is considered a very unstable ingredient in cosmetic formulations. It also contains salicylic acid, but the overall pH is too high for it to have exfoliating properties.

☺ $$$ **Potent Botanical Skin Brightening Lotion Complex** *($45 for 2 ounces)* is similar to the Ultra Gentle version above, only this contains about 10% glycolic acid. That's a good amount, though the pH is just passable for it to be effective for exfoliation.

☹ **AHA/BHA Acne Clearing Gel** *($45 for 2 ounces)* contains alcohol, which is too drying and irritating for all skin types.

✓☺ **BPO Gel 2.5%** *($20 for 3 ounces)* is a very good benzoyl peroxide product in a lightweight gel base for disinfecting areas of skin that tend to break out.

✓☺ **BPO Gel 5%** *($22 for 3 ounces)* is similar to the 2.5% version above only with a stronger concentration, and the same comments apply.

✓☺ $$$ **BPO Gel 10%** *($24 for 3 ounces)* is similar to the 5% version above only with a stronger concentration, and the same comments apply.

☹ **BPO Gel 10% and Sulfur** *($30 for 3 ounces)*. Adding sulfur to this benzoyl peroxide product only makes it harder on skin, causing redness, irritation, and flaky skin.

☹ **Therapeutic Sulfur Masque** *($40 for 5 ounces)* contains 10% sulfur, along with clay, thickening agents, and preservatives. Sulfur is a topical disinfectant, but it can be quite irritating and drying for skin, while the high pH that results can actually increase bacteria growth in skin.

☹ **Sulfur Cooling Masque** *($40 for 5 ounces)* has the same problems as the Therapeutic Sulfur Masque above, plus this one also contains eucalyptus. Ouch!

☺ **Oil-Free Sunblock SPF 20** *($25 for 4 ounces)* is a very good, in-part titanium dioxide–based sunscreen in a very ordinary emollient base. The emollient wax thickeners in this product aren't oil, but they may not make someone with oily skin happy.

☺ **Oil-Free Sunblock SPF 30** *($25 for 4 ounces)* is almost identical to the SPF 20 version above only with an SPF 30, and the same basic comments apply.

☺ **Water Resistant Sunblock SPF 20** *($25 for 4 ounces)* is similar to the Oil-Free Sunblock versions above, only with a water-resistant formula. This basic formulation is easily replaced by many similar and far less pricey versions at the drugstore.

☺ **Water Resistant Sunblock SPF 30** *($25 for 4 ounces)* is similar to the Water Resistant SPF 20 version above and the same comments apply.

☹ **Oil-Free Hydrating Sunscreen Gel SPF 20** *($25 for 4 ounces)* does not contain the UVA-protecting ingredients of titanium dioxide, zinc oxide, or avobenzone, but it does contain alcohol, and it is absolutely not recommended.

☺ **$$$ Max Sheer All-Day Moisture Defense Lotion SPF 30** *($37 for 1.7 ounces)* is a good, in-part avobenzone-based sunscreen in a standard moisturizing base that includes a small quantity of water-binding agents and vitamin A.

☺ **$$$ Max Tinted Protective Day Cream SPF 30** *($40 for 2.3 ounces)* has a color that isn't for everyone, but it disappears well into the skin so it doesn't have much effect. Other than that, it is a very good sunscreen with titanium dioxide and zinc oxide as the active sunscreen agents. A few of the plant extracts can be skin irritants, but the amount present in this product is probably too small for them to have much, if any, impact on skin.

☺ **Titanium Dioxide Sunblock SPF 15** *($25 for 4 ounces)* is a very good, but very ordinary, pure titanium dioxide–based sunscreen that is almost identical to Neutrogena's Sensitive Skin UVA/UVB Block SPF 17 that costs $8.39 for 4 ounces.

☺ **Titanium Dioxide Sunblock SPF 30** *($25 for 4 ounces)* is similar to the SPF 15 version above, and the same comments apply, although keep in mind that Neutrogena's Sensitive Skin UVA/UVB Block SPF 30 ($8.39 for 4 ounces) easily replaces this version for a lot less money and an almost identical formulation.

☺ **Ultra Lite Oil-Free Sunblock SPF 30** *($25 for 4 ounces)* is a very good sunscreen with in-part avobenzone and titanium dioxide as active ingredients. The name for this product implies it would be good for oily skin, but it is not. It is rather emollient and creamy and so would be far better for someone with normal to dry skin.

☹ **Cucumber Gel Masque** (*$40 for 4.5 ounces*) contains several irritating ingredients, including pineapple, orange, and lemon, and is not recommended.

☺ **$$$ Hydrating Nutrient Masque** (*$40 for 5 ounces*) is a standard clay mask with several thickeners and a small amount of plant oil, plus teeny amounts of water-binding agents and vitamins. It isn't hydrating, but it is a good, albeit ordinary, clay mask.

☺ **Aloe-Cort Cream** (*$25 for 2 ounces*) is a very standard 1% hydrocortisone cream, which makes it virtually identical to Lanacort or Cortaid available at the drugstore for half the price. Cortisone must be used infrequently, however, because it can break down collagen in the skin with repeated, long-term application.

☺ **Post-Peel Healing Balm** (*$25 for 0.8 ounce*) is almost identical to the Aloe-Cort above and the same comments apply.

☺ **$$$ Soothing Repair Ointment** (*$45 for 2 ounces*) contains 2% lidocaine. Lidocaine is synthesized from cocaine and is a popular and very effective anesthetic. It can also be a skin irritant or sensitizer, not to mention that there are far cheaper versions at the drugstore.

PEVONIA BOTANICA SKIN CARE

Pevonia is a spa/salon line of skin-care products. Its vast range of products showcases just about every hyped marketing angle the cosmetics industry has to offer. From plants and DNA to oxygen and vitamins, there is a little bit of everything here, along with products to reduce thighs, plump up breasts, and, of course, get rid of wrinkles, de-puff eyes, cure acne, and leave you spiritually elevated.

"Experience a realm of skin care far beyond the norm. Each and every pore is drenched with nature's most selective, unadulterated plant extracts; every sensitizer and photosensitizer has been meticulously eliminated." That's quite a claim, but then, one might wonder, how does Pevonia rationalize the use of diazolidinyl urea (a formaldehyde-releasing preservative), triethanolamine, tetrasodium EDTA, camphor, lemon oil, arnica, and sodium C14-16 olefin sulfate in its products?

As is true for most companies with a natural bent, Pevonia brags that its products "contain no mineral oil [and] no lanolin." With so many companies picking up on the absurd, unsubstantiated myth that these two ingredients are somehow bad for skin, it's possible it will be just a matter of time before the entire industry starts leaving these ingredients out of their formulations. Lanolin, an animal derivative, might pose a problem of principle for vegans, but other than that it is an excellent moisturizer for very dehydrated, parched skin. It can be an allergen for some sensitive skin types, but it is not a "bad" or "evil" ingredient. Likewise, mineral oil is an exceptional ingredient for dry skin and its demise in skin-care products would be sad to see.

What gets lost in all the marketing mumbo jumbo and foolishness is the one definite and rather poignant strength of this line: Pevonia's rather simple, but elegant, formulations. Forget the far-fetched, distorted claims, and you'll see that there are some interesting ingredient combinations in this line's products. If you are going to spend money on expensive skin care, it is far better to consider a line that has state-of-the-art combinations of water-binding agents, antioxidants, emollients, and (especially) sunscreens with effective UVA protection. Pevonia is definitely more interesting than some of the other overpriced spa and prestige lines I've reviewed, such as Decleor Paris, Guinot, Givenchy, Yon Ka Paris, and Phytomer, among others, which don't have anywhere near the impressive formulations that Pevonia has. For a nice change, some of these products are indeed well-formulated and not a complete waste of money. For more information about Pevonia Botanica Skin Care, call (800) PEVONIA or visit www.pevonia.com. **Note:** All Pevonia Botanica Skin Care,products contain fragrance unless otherwise noted.

PEVONIA DRY SKIN LINE—LIGNE SEVACTIVE

☺ **Dry Skin Cleanser** *($23 for 6.8 ounces)* is a plant oil–based cold cream that can leave a greasy film on the skin and needs to be wiped off. It also contains arnica and ivy, which are skin-irritating plant extracts.

☺ **Dry Skin Toning Lotion** *($22 for 6.8 ounces)* is a very simple toner that is more like applying fragrance to the skin than anything else. It also contains a minuscule amount of lettuce extract, which can be an anti-irritant, but has no real impact on skin when present in such a small amount. The lactic acid is less than 1%, which makes it ineffective for exfoliation.

☺ **Dry Skin Care Cream** *($33 for 1.7 ounces)*. Other than the plant extracts of pine needle, rosemary, and orange, which can be skin irritants, this is just an OK, extremely ordinary moisturizer for dry skin.

☺ $$$ **Dry Skin Mask** *($33.50 for 1.7 ounces)* is a simple emollient mask with teeny amounts of water-binding agents and antioxidants. It would be an option for dry skin, although the arnica, a plant extract, is a skin irritant.

☺ **Dry Skin Face Oil "Jouvence"** *($31 for 1 ounce)* is just hazelnut oil with fragrance and a teeny amount of vitamin E. Skip the fragrance, which can be a skin sensitizer, and just mix a vitamin E capsule into some pure hazelnut oil, all for far less money.

PEVONIA SENSITIVE SKIN LINE—LIGNE LAVANDOU

☺ $$$ **Sensitive Skin Cleanser** *($23 for 6.8 ounces)* is almost identical to the Dry Skin Cleanser above, only this leaves out the potentially irritating plant extracts. This can be a good option for dry to very dry skin.

☺ **Sensitive Skin Toning Lotion** *($22 for 6.8 ounces)* is a very simple toner that contains mostly water, glycerin, anti-irritants, water-binding agents, and preservatives. The tiny amount of lactic acid has no exfoliating properties. This can be an OK toner for most skin types.

☺ $$$ **Sensitive Skin Care Cream** *($40 for 1.7 ounces)* is a good, though ordinary, moisturizer for very dry skin.

☺ $$$ **Sensitive Skin Mask** *($35 for 1.7 ounces)* is an emollient mask with some plant oils and a tiny amount of anti-irritants. It can be an option for normal to dry skin, and amazingly, this is one of the only Pevonia products that doesn't contain fragrance.

☺ **$$$ Propolis Concentrate** (*$46 for 1 ounce*) does contain propolis, with some water, thickeners, fragrance, and preservative. Propolis is a brownish resinous material collected by bees that they then use to build the hive. It has antibacterial and anti-inflammatory properties for skin. The belief that this is a miracle skin-care ingredient is myth and not based on any research or data.

☺ **Face Oil "Douceur"** (*$28 for 1 ounce*) is just hazelnut oil with fragrance and a teeny amount of vitamin. Skip the fragrance, which can be a skin sensitizer, and just use some pure hazelnut oil that you buy at the grocery store for far less money.

PEVONIA NORMAL TO COMBINATION SKIN LINE —LIGNE FONDAMENTALE

☹ **Combination Skin Cleanser** (*$23 for 6.8 ounces*) is an emollient, plant oil–based cleanser that is inappropriate for combination skin, plus the grapefruit oil and pine and lemon extracts can cause irritation.

☹ **Combination Skin Toning Lotion** (*$22 for 6.8 ounces*). This standard toner contains witch hazel distillate, which is primarily alcohol, and it can be irritating and drying for skin. It does contain lactic acid, but the amount is so tiny it is not effective as an exfoliant.

☹ **Combination Skin Care Cream** (*$33 for 1.7 ounces*) is too emollient for combination skin and the arnica extract is potentially irritating for all skin types.

☺ **$$$ Combination Skin Mask** (*$32 for 1.7 ounces*) is a standard clay mask. It doesn't get more basic than this, though the plant oils aren't the best for combination skin. Still this is a decent mask for normal to slightly oily skin.

☺ **$$$ Face Oil "Harmonie"** (*$31 for 1 ounce*) is just fragrant oils and a tiny amount of vitamin E. Fragrant oils are not helpful for skin and definitely not for combination skin. This is more like applying perfume than a skin-care product.

PEVONIA OILY SKIN LINE—LIGNE PURILYS

☹ **Phyto-Gel Cleanser** (*$26.50 for 6.8 ounces*) contains sodium C14-16 olefin sulfate as the main cleansing agent, which makes it too drying for most skin types. It also contains lemon, ivy, sage, and pine extracts, which only add to the irritation.

☹ **Oily Skin Toning Lotion** (*$22 for 6.8 ounces*). Except for the change in fragrance, this is almost identical to the Combination Skin Toning Lotion above, and the same comments apply.

☹ **Oily Skin Care Cream** (*$33 for 1.7 ounces*) is a simple gel moisturizer that contains pine, lemon, and grapefruit, all of which are skin irritants and have no effect on oil production. It also contains plant oil, which isn't the best for oily skin!

☺ **$$$ Oily Skin Mask** (*$33.50 for 1.7 ounces*) is a very standard clay mask for oily skin that contains a good deal of fragrance.

PEVONIA RS2 LINE—LIGNE ROSE (ROSACEA AND SENSITIVE SKIN)

☺ **$$$ RS2 Gentle Cleanser** (*$26 for 6.8 ounces*) is a standard, detergent-based, water-soluble cleanser that would work well for most skin types. However, the notion that this or any of the products in the RS2 line is appropriate for sensitive skin of any kind, particularly for someone with rosacea, is nonsense. The basic rule for anyone with sensitive skin is not to use products that contain irritants, and because fragrance is a potent skin irritant (and it's something all these products contain), these can be a problem for the very skin type they're aimed at. What is particularly disappointing is that all these products contain good anti-irritants, yet all they would be combating here are the irritating effects of the fragrance, instead of helping your skin.

☹ $$$ RS2 Gentle Toning Lotion *($22 for 6.8 ounces)*. The irritating fragrance present in the RS2 Gentle Cleanser above is also present here. It doesn't help that the guarana extract—from a plant that contains two and a half times more caffeine than coffee—can have constricting properties on skin, and can therefore be a potent skin irritant. Overall, that makes this problematic for anyone with sensitive skin or rosacea.

☺ $$$ RS2 Concentrate *($50 for 1.7 ounces)* still contains fragrance, but if that isn't a problem for you, this is an OK gel lotion that contains some good anti-irritants, but lacks water-binding agents and antioxidants.

☺ $$$ RS2 Care Cream *($50 for 1.7 ounces)* is a very emollient, though basic, moisturizer for someone with normal to dry skin. This is easily replaced with Lubriderm or Cetaphil moisturizers available at the drugstore, and then you wouldn't have to worry about either the fragrance or the price.

PEVONIA EYE LINE—LIGNE YEUX

☹ Eye Make-up Remover Lotion, Ligne Yeux *($22 for 6.8 ounces)* doesn't remove makeup very well. This product also contains arnica, which is just bizarre to put in a product meant to be used around the eye, as arnica is not supposed to come into contact with mucous membranes.

☺ $$$ Evolutive Eye Gel *($42 for 0.7 ounce)* is a good lightweight moisturizer for slightly dry skin. The orange extract (rather high up on the ingredient list) can be an irritant for sensitive skin, particularly around the eyes, but this does contain some good water-binding agents and a small amount of antioxidant.

☺ $$$ Evolutive Eye Cream *($36 for 0.7 ounce)* is a very good moisturizer for dry skin with a good mix of water-binding agents and antioxidants.

PEVONIA OXYGENATING LINE—SOIN OPTIMALE

This group of products from Pevonia borders on the ludicrous, not because the products aren't well formulated, but rather because the company (or the people who name the products or write the brochure) are extremely confused about what antioxidants are supposed to do for skin. None of the Oxygenating Line of products contains any form of oxygen, which is good news for skin because increased oxygen would generate free-radical damage and that's bad for skin. What these products do contain are some very good antioxidants. Note the prefix "anti," meaning these are "against" oxygen, and are intended to stop it from impacting the skin. One of the showcased ingredients in these products is superoxide dismutase, which Pevonia describes as being able to "oxygenate and heal." But what makes superoxide dismutase a good skin-care ingredient is that it is an effective *anti*oxidant. Of course, you can't stop free-radical damage from taking place, but theoretically slowing it down even a little can be helpful for skin.

☺ $$$ **O2ptimale C Complexe Concentrate** *($69 for 1 ounce)* is just water, fragrant plant extract, water-binding agent, thickener, plant oil, a form of vitamin C, water-binding agent, and preservatives. Vitamin C can be a good antioxidant, but the amount of it in this pricey product is negligible.

☺ $$$ **O2ptimale Combination Skin Care Cream** *($49 for 1.7 ounces)* is an overpriced moisturizer that would be a problem for combination skin, though it would be a good choice for dry skin.

☺ $$$ **O2ptimale Dry Skin Care Cream** *($56 for 1.7 ounces)* is an OK, emollient moisturizer for dry skin. It is almost identical to the O2ptimale Combination Skin Care Cream above, and the same comments apply. It also contains algae, propolis, and royal bee jelly, but on skin these only work as anti-irritants—they don't have any rare or miraculous skin benefits.

☺ $$$ **O2ptimale Sensitive Skin Care Cream** *($50 for 1.7 ounces)* is an emollient moisturizer for dry skin, though the arnica makes this inappropriate for sensitive skin. It does contain celandine, a plant extract that can have antiviral properties, though it has no known benefit for skin.

PEVONIA LIGHTENING LINE—LIGNE RADIANCE

✓☺ $$$ **Lightening Gel** *($38 for 1 ounce)* is a very good skin-lightening gel that contains mostly water, azelaic acid, AHA, kojic acid, arbutin, glycerin, thickener, and preservatives. Kojic acid, azelaic acid, and arbutin can all have a positive effect on inhibiting melanin production, but keep in mind that without the use of a reliable sunscreen, skin-lightening products are ineffective (because unprotected sun exposure stimulates melanin production, causing skin discolorations).

☹ **Lightening Fluid** *($38 for 1 ounce)* contains small amounts of AHA and BHA, but the amounts are too small and the pH is too high for them to be effective as exfoliants. Nor does this contain any skin-lightening (melanin-inhibiting) ingredients. The sulfur can be a skin irritant.

☺ $$$ **Lightening Mask** *($29.75 for 1.7 ounces)* is a standard clay mask that contains a small amount of AHA and BHA. The pH of this mask isn't low enough for the AHA or BHA to have any effect as exfoliants. It also does not contain any skin-lightening (melanin-inhibiting) ingredients.

☺ $$$ **Glycocides Cream** *($46 for 1.7 ounces)* is a good 10% to 12% AHA cream that would be good for dry skin, though this is easily replaced by Alpha Hydrox's AHA products available at the drugstore for far less. AHAs exfoliate skin, and that's helpful and definitely can improve the appearance of skin, but it takes more to inhibit the production of brown skin discolorations. It is also essential to use an effective sunscreen (SPF 15 or greater with UVA-protecting ingredients) to really make a difference in brown discolorations, something this group of products leaves out.

PEVONIA ACNE/PROBLEMATIC SKIN LINE—LIGNE CLARIFYL

☹ **Clarigel Exfoliating Cleanser** *($29 for 6.8 ounces)* uses sodium C14-16 olefin sulfate, which is an extremely irritating and drying detergent cleansing agent.

☹ **Clarifyl Toning Lotion** *($23 for 6.8 ounces)* contains camphor, which is a completely unnecessary skin irritant, and this is not recommended.

☹ **Problematic Skin Care Cream** *($39 for 2.5 ounces)*. The pH of this lightweight moisturizer is too high for the small amount of glycolic acid to be effective as an exfoliant, and that is definitely a problem.

☹ **Problematic Skin Purifying Mask** *($39 for 2.5 ounces)* is a standard clay mask that contains sulfur and camphor, which are unnecessary irritants for all skin types. Sulfur can have disinfecting properties, but there are far less irritating ways to disinfect against breakouts.

☹ **Clarifyl Spot Treatment** *($39 for 1 ounce)* contains camphor, and that is too irritating for skin. It also contains hydrogen peroxide. Refer to the comments above for the Oxygenating Line for specifics of why that ingredient is a significant problem for skin.

PEVONIA SPECIAL LINE—LIGNE SPECIALE

☺ **$$$ Gentle Exfoliating Cleanser** *($25.50 for 5 ounces)* is a standard, detergent-based cleanser that uses jojoba beads as the scrub agent. This is fairly gentle and would be a good option for normal to oily or normal to dry skin.

☹ **Enzymo-Spherides Peeling Cream** *($31.50 for 1.7 ounces)* contains sodium C14-16 olefin sulfonate as the main cleansing agent, making this too irritating and drying for all skin types.

☺ **$$$ Reactive Skin Care Cream** *($41 for 1.7 ounces)* is simply an ordinary emollient moisturizer for dry skin with no interesting water-binding agents or antioxidants.

PEVONIA SUN LINE—CHEMICAL-FREE SUNSCREENS—LIGNE SOLEIL

✓☺ **Sunblock Dry to Sensitive Skin SPF 15** *($31 for 2.5 ounces)* is a good, titanium dioxide–based sunscreen that would indeed work well for dry skin. It contains some good water-binding agents and antioxidants, too.

✓☺ **Sunblock Combination to Oily Skin SPF 15** *($31 for 2.5 ounces)* is almost identical to the Dry to Sensitive Skin SPF 15 version above and, while it would be a problem for combination or oily skin, it is an option for normal to dry skin.

✓☺ **Sunblock Body Milk SPF 15** *($29.25 for 5 ounces)* is similar to the sunblocks above, and the same basic comments apply.

☺ **$$$ Phyto-Aromatic Mist** *($22.25 for 8.5 ounces)* is just a basic toner in a spray container. This would be a good, irritant-free toner, but it serves no purpose in a sun-care lineup. It contains nothing that would help reduce or change sun damage.

☺ **Self-Tanning Emulsion Spray** *($33 for 5 ounces)* contains dihydroxyacetone, the same ingredient in all self-tanners that affects the color of skin. This would work as well as any, though there is no reason to spend this kind of money when Coppertone and Bain de Soleil have excellent self-tanners for far less.

PEVONIA POWER REPAIR LINE—LIGNE POWER REPAIR

✔☺ $$$ **Collastin Eye Fluid** *($52 for 1 ounce)* is a very good emollient lotion for normal to dry skin that contains mostly water, water-binding agents, plant oils, anti-irritant, vitamin E, AHA, silicone, and preservatives. This does not contain fragrance. The amount of AHAs is less than 1% and, therefore, will not be effective for exfoliation. The collagen and elastin are good water-binding agents, but that's it; they have no ability to affect the collagen and elastin in skin.

☺ $$$ **Firm-Active Concentrate** *($50 for 1 ounce)*. The only reason to buy this is if you "buy" the claim that amniotic fluid has a youthful impact on skin. It can't. Amniotic fluid is merely a water-binding agent. The connection between young and old skin may be compelling, but it's one that amounts to little more than wishful thinking.

☺ $$$ **Liposomes Gel Concentrate** *($62 for 1 ounce)* is similar to the Firm-Active Concentrate above, only with collagen and thymus extract, and the same basic review applies.

☺ $$$ **Marine Collagen Cream** *($50 for 1.7 ounces)* is similar to the Collastin Eye Fluid above, only in cream form, and the same basic comments apply. This does contain a tiny amount of arnica, which can be a skin irritant, but there's probably not enough of it to have any impact on skin.

☺ $$$ **Marine Elastin Cream** *($51 for 1.7 ounces)* is virtually identical to the Marine Collagen Cream above, only this contains elastin instead of collagen. The same basic comments apply.

☺ $$$ **Marine Collagen Concentrate** *($48 for 1 ounce)* is similar to the Firm-Active Concentrate above, only this contains collagen. The same basic comments apply.

☺ $$$ **Marine Elastin Concentrate** *($48 for 1 ounce)* is similar to the Firm-Active Concentrate above only with elastin. The same basic comments apply.

☺ $$$ **Marine DNA Cream** *($53 for 1.7 ounces)*. There is no research showing that DNA (the genetic material of cells) in a cosmetic can affect any aspect of skin or cellular function. This is merely water, plant oils, DNA, glycerin, thickeners, vitamin E, anti-irritant, water-binding agent, silicone, fragrance, and preservatives. It's a good moisturizer for normal to dry skin, but showcasing the DNA is misleading, and it is not helpful for skin.

☺ $$$ **Marine DNA Concentrate** *($50 for 1 ounce)* is similar to the Firm-Active Concentrate above, only with DNA as the showcase ingredient. If you were to choose this, you would be banking on a false concept that DNA can be helpful for skin, because that is the only interesting, though useless, ingredient in here.

✔☺ $$$ **Youthful Lip Cream** *($40 for 0.7 ounce)* is a basic, but good, emollient balm for lips that includes some good water-binding agents, vitamin E, azelaic acid, and retinol. That can be great for skin, but it won't bring youth back to your lips.

✓☺ **$$$ Youthful Lip Serum** *($36 for 0.5 ounce)* contains water, retinol, thickeners, and preservatives. For a retinol-only moisturizer this is an option, but there are other far less expensive versions to consider from Neutrogena to L'Oreal and Cetaphil.

PHARMAGEL

What's in a name? In this case, just about everything, because there is very little inside these products that constitutes good skin care. Pharmagel's name is meant to evoke images of a pharmaceutical company involved in making superior skin-care products. I can't imagine a woman that wouldn't hear this company's name and think to herself—these aren't cosmetics, they're pharmaceuticals, and therefore, more like prescription-strength products than just regular products at the drugstore or the cosmetics counters. Yet, nothing could be further from the truth. The claim that Pharmagel's products are unique in any way is nothing more than sheer fantasy and marketing hype. There are so many problems with these products I don't know where to begin. The sunscreens either don't contain UVA-protecting ingredients or the SPF is substandard. The toner is mostly fragrance, the eye treatment contains mostly alcohol, and the moisturizers are in packaging that won't keep the good ingredients stable. Even the AHA products are ineffective for exfoliation. The few good products are not anything to run out and buy. For more information about Pharmagel, call (800) 882-4889 or visit www.pharmagel.net. **Note:** All Pharmagel products contain fragrance.

☹ **Fleur 5 Cleansing Bar** *($7.50 for 3.5 ounces)* is a standard bar cleanser that is similar in many ways to Dove bar cleanser at the drugstore; however, this version contains menthol, and that can be irritating for skin.

☺ **Hydra Cleanse Foaming Gel** *($14.95 for 8 ounces)* is a standard detergent-based cleanser with some algae extracts. Even if algae had some special benefit for skin, in a cleanser that benefit would all be rinsed down the drain.

☹ **Enzyme Ex-Cell Natural and Gentle Exfoliating Scrub** *($15.95 for 6 ounces)* is a standard detergent-based cleanser that uses ground-up walnut shell as the exfoliant. This also contains menthol, which is too irritating for all skin types. The papaya and papain cannot exfoliate skin and the small amount of salicylic acid is ineffective for exfoliation because the product has a pH of 5.5.

☹ **Botanical Tonique Facial Toner** *($14.95 for 8 ounces)* is more like applying fragrance than anything beneficial to skin. Several of the plant extracts, including arnica, bergamot, and comfrey, are potent skin irritants, and this product lacks any amount of water-binding agents and antioxidants.

☹ **HydrO2xy-10 Lifting and Firming Concentrate with Stabilized Oxygen** *($17.95 for 8 ounces)*. Assuming the company is accurate and this product does actually contain "stabilized oxygen," that would be a significant problem for skin, because when an oxygen molecule comes into contact with skin it generates free-radical damage (Sources: *Human and Experimental Toxicology,* February 2002, pages 61–62; *Journal of Clinical*

The Reviews P

Pathology, March 2001, pages 176–186; and *Drugs and Aging,* 2001, volume 18, number 9, pages 685–716.

☹ **Glyco-8 Facial Firming Complex with 8% AHA** *($26.95 for 2 ounces)* doesn't contain 8% AHA. At best, this contains about a 3% concentration and that isn't enough to be effective for exfoliation. It is an emollient moisturizer with a minute amount of antioxidants and water-binding agent.

☹ **DermaFade Lightening and Fading Creme SPF 15** *($24.95 for 2 ounces)* doesn't contain the UVA-protecting ingredients of titanium dioxide, zinc oxide, or avobenzone, and is not recommended.

☺ **Aloe FirmaDerm Fast Action Age Defying Skin Treatment with Retinol-A and Vitamins C and E** *($11.95 for 7 ounces)* is a good emollient moisturizer with some very good antioxidants and water-binding agents. It does contain retinol at a good concentration, but the less-than-air-tight packaging prevents the retinol from remaining stable once the container is opened. It is still an option for normal to dry skin.

☹ **Complexe Eye Beaute Puffy Eye Treatment** *($17.95 for 60 pads)*. This contains more alcohol (part of the second ingredient and the entire third ingredient) than it does any beneficial ingredients for skin, plus a few of the plant extracts are potential skin irritants. This product is not recommended.

☺ **Complexe Eye Firme Firming Eye Gel** *($18.95 for 1 ounce)* is a light weight gel with some good water-binding agents and antioxidants. There is nothing in here that will firm skin, but it is a good moisturizer for normal to slightly dry skin.

☺ **DN-24 Hydracreme Intensive Vitamin Facial Treatment** *($18.95 for 2 ounces)* does contain a good amount of retinol, but the jar packaging means it will not remain stable once the product is opened. This is an emollient moisturizer with some good plant oils and antioxidants, and is an option for normal to dry skin. You would expect that a so-called pharmaceutical line would know that jar packaging is a problem for the stability of antioxidants.

☺ **Pharma C Serum Vitamin C Facial Treatment** *($29.95 for 1 ounce)* contains a good amount of vitamin C in a lightweight lotion that would be an option for normal to slightly dry skin. It also contains a small amount of water-binding agents and other antioxidants. The yeast in this product has no rare properties for skin; it is just an antioxidant with no research about its efficacy on skin.

☺ **Bio A Concentrate Anti Aging Resurfacing Serum** *($29.95 for 1 ounce)* is an emollient moisturizer that contains a small amount of antioxidants. It also contains retinol, but the clear packaging is unlikely to keep it stable because retinol breaks down in the presence of sunlight.

☹ **Beta C Dual Action Facial Refirmer SPF 6** *($24.95 for 2 ounces)*. The SPF 6 is embarrassing and in total disregard of the SPF 15 standard set by the American Academy of Dermatology and the Skin Cancer Foundation. It does contain salicylic acid, but the pH of 5 makes it ineffective for exfoliation.

☺ **C Nutra-Lift Facial Firming Mask** (*$16.95 for 6 ounces*) is a standard, extremely ordinary clay mask with a tiny amount of vitamin E and water-binding agents. It does contain a tiny amount of AHAs (about 1%), but that isn't enough to be effective for exfoliation.

philosophy

philosophy has an upscale, department-store élan, with a touch of Zen, family values, and a heavy dose of twenty-something attitude thrown into the mix. It's hard to tell if you are shopping a cosmetics line or looking for a new religious experience. philosophy's philosophy is clearly to capture the attention of women in all age ranges, but chiefly those between 18 and 30, as evidenced by the large number of acne products as opposed to wrinkle creams. Younger women who are not yet fighting off the unwanted advance of time seem to want more from life than just beauty. They also want meaning and fun. philosophy meets that need with a brochure that looks more like a volume of poetry than a sales catalog. The only graphics are a series of photographs, circa 1950 and up, of children, parents, and grandparents on outings or just enjoying life. No glamour shots to be found anywhere. Unbelievable!

Skin care is philosophy's real raison d'être, and its line is more entertaining than anything else. The company preaches about cause and effect, offering the product it says you need to create the effect, and gives it a fetching name. It's hard not to be curious about something named "hope and a prayer" (philosophy likes to use lowercase letters for product names). philosophy has similar statements that appear on each and every product. Its sunscreen with SPF 15 is called "the naked truth," and the label reads "philosophy: if withholding the truth is an act of love, then is telling the truth only an act of courage?" Wow. Heavy. What that has to do with sunscreen is anyone's guess, but it's a great marketing gimmick. The eyeshadows are romantically called "windows of the soul." The rest of the label reads, "philosophy: to know the true story of the soul, look deeply into the eyes"—presumably past the eyeshadow. I've never seen products with such riveting copy. For more information about philosophy, call (800) 568-3151 or visit www.philosophy.com.

philosophy SKIN CARE

☹ **on a clear day, super wash for oily skin** (*$15 for 4 ounces*) contains sodium lauryl sulfate as the main cleansing agent (it is actually the second ingredient). Sodium lauryl sulfate is a potent skin irritant for all skin types and this product is not recommended.

☺ **real purity cleanser, one step facial cleanser** (*$20 for 8 ounces*) is a standard, detergent-based, water-soluble cleanser that would work well for most skin types. It does contain several fragrant plant oils that can be potential skin irritants, as well as black pepper seed extract.

☺ **the health bar, oatmeal cleansing bar** (*$9 for 3.2 ounces*) is a standard bar soap with oatmeal, and while oatmeal can have anti-irritant properties and exfoliate skin as a gentle abrasive, the cleansing agents in this soap can be fairly drying.

☺ **change me, make-up remover** *($12 for 4 ounces)* is a standard, detergent-based makeup remover that would work as well as any. The sage extract can be a skin irritant.

☹ **the great awakening, two step exfoliant** *($25 for 1 ounce of gel and 2 ounces of foam)* might better be called a rude awakening. It's supposed to be a two-part facial: The gel is a cleanser to prepare the skin, and the foam is meant to bring oxygen to the skin. How does it do that? With hydrogen peroxide. And that's not good for skin, because hydrogen peroxide is a significant oxidizing agent that generates free-radical damage, which can impair the skin's healing process, cause cellular destruction, and reduce optimal cell functioning (Sources: *Carcinogenesis,* March 2002, pages 469–475 and *Anticancer Research,* July-August 2001, pages 2719–2724).

☺ $$$ **the greatest love, hydrating microdermabrasion scrub** *($25 for 3 ounces)* is "formulated to mimic the action of microdermabrasion crystals," but you would have to use this quite aggressively to even get close to what millions of aluminum oxide crystals shot at the skin and vacuumed back up during microdermabrasion can do. When microdermabrasion is done carefully, the results can be positive, but not what I would call impressive, at least compared to results from peels or lasers. But the notion that this scrub is akin to microdermabrasion is truly a great fiction.

☺ $$$ **the great mystery one-minute daily facial** *($20 for 3.3 ounces)* is basically glycerin, water, sea salt, and thickeners, along with some token marine plant extracts and a tiny amount of lavender oil. Salt can be a problem for skin. It does work as a scrub, but for that purpose baking soda with a cleanser works far better.

☺ **under your skin, face and body scrub** *($21 for 8 ounces)* is a detergent-based scrub in a gel form that uses crushed rock as the abrasive. It does work without being too abrasive, but this is extremely standard and doesn't work any better than baking soda mixed with Cetaphil Gentle Skin Cleanser. The minuscule amount of plant extracts that sound like they are related to AHAs are not and have no exfoliating properties.

☺ $$$ **eye believe, eye cream** *($27.50 for 0.5 ounce)* is a good moisturizer for dry skin, with several very good water-binding agents and a small amount of antioxidants. The plant extracts it contains are meant to sound like AHAs, but have no ability to exfoliate skin.

☺ **hope in a bottle, oil-free moisturizer normal to oily skin** *($32.50 for 2 ounces)* is a 2% BHA product in a rather ordinary, lightweight moisturizing base. It is an option for exfoliating for most skin types.

☺ **hope in a jar, for all skin types** *($35 for 2 ounces)* is about a 6% AHA in an OK moisturizing base, though the pH isn't low enough for it to exfoliate the skin.

☺ $$$ **hope and a prayer, topical vitamin C powder & solvent** *($45 for 1 ounce)* is philosophy's attempt to keep abreast of the vitamin C craze. The gimmick here is that you mix this product up every time you use it. The kit comes with a bottle of vitamin C powder along with some water-binding agents, plus a bottle of toner that also contains some antioxidants. Vitamin C is a good antioxidant, although there are lots of good antioxidant products for skin that don't require going through this rigmarole.

☺ **$$$ hope in a jar, high density eye and lip contour cream** *($30 for 0.5 ounce)* contains mostly water, plant oil, mineral oil, glycerin, thickeners, Vaseline, slip agents, vitamin E, anti-irritant, preservatives, and silicone. This is a good, but fairly basic, moisturizer that is easily replaced by far less expensive and more impressive formulations available at the drugstore or from Clinique. I think you could easily be more hopeful than this.

☺ **hope in a jar for dry, sensitive skin** *($35 for 2 ounces)* contains mostly water, glycerin, plant oil, thickeners, vitamin E, water-binding agents, slip agent, plant extracts, fragrant plant extracts, and preservatives. This is a good, though not great, moisturizer for normal to dry skin. The claim about this being good for sensitive skin would be far more acceptable if the fragrant extracts weren't included.

☺ **$$$ dark shadows, eye balm** *($27.50 for 0.5 ounce)* is a very good moisturizer for dry skin that contains mostly water, slip agent, silicones, film-forming agent, thickeners, plant oils, plant extracts, vitamins (antioxidants), and preservatives. Although these ingredients are great for dry skin, they will not do anything to fade or change dark circles. The small amount of coffee and vitamin K in this product (which show up in lots of eye moisturizers these days) will not improve or alter dark circles in the least (Source: *Archives of Dermatology*, December 1998, "Snake Oil for the 21st Century"); the only "evidence" to the contrary comes from the companies selling products that contain these ingredients.

☹ **the present, oil-free moisturizer sensitive skin** *($20 for 2 ounces)* is just thickeners and silicone, and that's nice for normal to slightly dry skin, but it is really basic and ordinary. The lavender oil doesn't make this the best for sensitive skin types.

☹ **$$$ between the lines topical vitamin A** *($35 for 0.5 ounce)* is an ordinary, silicone-based moisturizer with a teeny amount of retinyl palmitate. If vitamin A is your goal, which is the only benefit this product offers, there are many far less expensive versions to consider.

☺ **$$$ help me, retinol night cream** *($45 for 1.05 ounces)* does contain retinol and a few other antioxidants, but there is nothing about this product that is an improvement over L'Oreal's Line Eraser, which is available for a quarter of the price.

☺ **the healthy tan, self tanning gel** *($16 for 3.3 ounces)* is a standard self-tanner that uses dihydroxyacetone, the same ingredient all self-tanners contain to affect the color of skin. This one would work as well as any.

☺ **shelter, moisturizing SPF 15 facial sunblock** *($16 for 2 ounces)* contains avobenzone as one of the active sunscreen ingredients, which makes it a very good option for sun protection for normal to oily skin. It is overly fragranced and lacks any other beneficial skin-care ingredients, but it will work as a sunscreen.

☹ **$$$ a pigment of your imagination, eye gel** *($27.50 for 0.5 ounce)* is a simple, emollient moisturizer that contains a small amount of vitamin K and even less vitamin C. There is no independent research showing vitamin K to have any benefit for skin when applied topically, and the amount of vitamin C is unlikely to have any effect on skin, much less be able to affect skin color.

The Reviews P

☹ **a pigment of your imagination, skin lightening gel** (*$22 for 1 ounce*) could have been a good, hydroquinone-based skin-lightening product, but the second ingredient is alcohol and that makes it too drying and irritating for all skin types.

☺ **hope in a jar super hydrating mask** (*$25 for 2 ounces*) is an OK emollient mask with plant oils and a tiny amount of antioxidants.

☹ **on a clear day blemish gel for adult acne** (*$20 for 1 ounce*). Alcohol is listed as the first ingredient, meaning that this is clearly an irritation waiting to happen.

☹ **on a clear day botanical blemish cream** (*$15 for 1 ounce*) contains camphor and sulfur, which are potent skin irritants. Camphor has no benefit for skin, and though sulfur can be a topical disinfectant, the irritation it can cause creates more problems for skin in the long run.

☺ **on a clear day non drying surface oil control** (*$12.50 for 1 ounce*) is just water, slip agent, absorbent, fragrance, and preservatives. The plant extracts are problematic for skin, particularly the peppermint. There is little benefit to be gained by using this product versus applying a pressed powder over your makeup.

☺ **$$$ kiss me lip balm** (*$10 for 0.5 ounce*) is little more than Vaseline and lanolin in a pot. It's fine for dry lips.

☺ **$$$ kiss me red lip balm** (*$10 for 0.5 ounce*) is the same as the kiss me lip balm above, only in an intense red shade.

philosophy MAKEUP

It seems that philosophy's makeup sells better when it is sold in sets, as only a smattering of products are now sold separately. In a way, this downsizing puts philosophy makeup right back where it started, which was offering preselected shades of blushes, eyeshadows, pencils, lipsticks, and makeup brushes in a "book." This is a clever alternative to buying makeup piece by piece, but more often than not it isn't the best way to be certain you'll really use all the products and like all the colors you get. It's unfortunate that philosophy has done away with selling its terrific blush and eyeshadow colors separately. Although today's philosophy is leaning more toward facial and body-care products, the makeup still has some contenders that you shouldn't overlook. Just watch out for the more ordinary offerings that have eclipsed the main attractions.

☺ **$$$ FOUNDATION: complete me SPF 15** (*$30*) is a loose, "mineral powder" foundation that's quite similar to Origins' As Good As It Gets, only the nine shades here are much more neutral. The sunscreen is zinc oxide, but even with that plus, this is not an easy or convenient way to apply foundation, and the high mineral content may be irritating to drier skin types. Since this is a powder, it has a dry texture, yet you are left with more of a sheen than a matte finish. If this still sounds appealing to you and you have normal to slightly oily skin, you may want to check this one out.

☺ **CONCEALER: trust me SPF 15** (*$15*) has a great, titanium dioxide–based sunscreen, but the consistency is heavy and so creamy it will crease by the time you are done applying your makeup! What a shame, because the colors are excellent. If you aren't worried about creasing and you have dry skin, it is a consideration.

☺ $$$ <u>BLUSH:</u> **the supernatural lip & cheek tint** *($15)* is a liquid stain that can go from sheer to an intense reddish pink. The sponge-tip applicator allows you to dot on the color, but blending must be swift or this will dry in place. The effect is akin to the effect of other liquid blushes, and this type of product is best for normal, even-textured skin.

<u>LIPSTICK AND LIP PENCIL:</u> ☺ **the supernatural lipstick** *($15)*, also known as **word of mouth** lipstick, is available in a matte or cream formula. The mattes are smooth and softly matte, which is great, while the creamy formula tends to be quite glossy and doesn't hold up well. **the supernatural coloring crayon** *($12.50)* is a small collection of standard lip and eye pencils that have good pigmentation. These are not supernatural, but they will do for real-world application!

☹ **the supernatural lipstick SPF 15** *($15)*, also known as **word of mouth lipstick SPF 15**, is very greasy, and the sunscreen offers no reliable UVA protection. **the supernatural lip gloss** *($15)* is a very emollient, slightly sticky wand-type gloss that comes in standard and not-so-standard colors. It's OK for what it is, it's just not great.

☹ <u>MASCARA:</u> **the supernatural lash darkener** *($15)* is sort of a mascara hybrid; it does almost no lengthening or thickening to speak of, but does darken the lashes. If you love the lashes you were born with but want a little extra depth, it's worth a try.

<u>BRUSHES:</u> philosophy has a small band of ☹ **brushes** *($10–$25)* that are satin-soft and nicely tapered. However, most of them are inferior in shape and density when compared to those from such neighboring lines as Trish McEvoy, Bobbi Brown, Stila, M.A.C., and others. The only ones to take seriously are the **blush** *($25)* and **shadow** *($20)* brushes— both are acceptable and correctly sized.

☹ $$$ **the workbook** *($120)* gets you seven philosophy brushes in a microfiber pouch, while **the pocketbook** *($47.50)* provides three brushes in a smaller, tri-fold case. The ergonomics of both brush cases are great—it's the overpriced brushes inside that are the problem.

<u>SPECIALTY:</u> philosophy established its color line with an all-in-one kit known as ☹ $$$ **the coloring book studio** *($160)*. It comprises ten eyeshadows, four blushes, two lipsticks, and two eye/lip pencils, along with a set of brushes, and I imagine it seemed utterly practical at first glance, but may now be collecting dust next to that unread copy of *War and Peace*. If you happen to like all of the colors in this kit and aren't fussy about your brushes, this has merit. As an impulse buy, it will likely turn into an expensive misstep. **the coloring book supercool** or **superneutral** *($140)* are scaled-down versions of the coloring book studio. You get fewer makeup brushes, no pencils, and eight blush/ eyeshadow colors instead of ten. This seems like a safer bet, but if the concept appeals to you why not pay a bit extra for a more comprehensive set? **deluxe pocketbook** *($110)* comprises one little black book (see below) along with three brushes, a lipstick, and lip gloss. Considering the price and how singularly practical the little black book is, why pay almost three times as much for a carrying case and the few extra pieces of makeup?

✓☺ $$$ **the little black book** *($37.50)* is the reason to pay attention to philosophy makeup, for here is where the best of this line resides. These sleek, pocket-sized palettes contain powder eyeshadows (with at least one suitable color for brows or eye lining) and/or powder blushes. A few of the sets feature odd colors or the occasional shiny shade, but the majority of the color combinations are foolproof and the products have superior textures that blend well and last. The best of the bunch are the superbasics and superneutrals sets, but platinum has some great colors too.

PHISODERM (SKIN CARE ONLY)

For years pHisoDerm has been about acne, and for years it has fallen short in that arena. This line lacks an effective topical disinfectant and the exfoliants are not in a base where they can be effective for that purpose. Even the information on pHisoDerm's Web site about acne is a bit out of whack. They answer the question, "What causes acne?" correctly: "It's a combination of factors, actually, which can depend on hormones, heredity and bacteria on and in the skin's pores. When a buildup of dead skin cells and oil stick together in the pores, it creates a disorder in the follicles. Bacteria then feed off this mixture, which can lead to inflamed acne." But then when they pose the question "What triggers acne?" They answer: "Lifestyle: Inadequate sleep, drug and/or alcohol use" or a high salt intake. That isn't true in the least, and there is no research showing that any of those things trigger breakouts. The one thing pHisoDerm does really well are cleansers, and for that they have several very good options. For more information about pHisoDerm, call (800) 745-2429 or visit www.phisoderm.com.

☺ **Deep Cleaning Cleanser, Normal to Dry Skin** *($3.99 for 8 ounces)* is a very good, though very basic, detergent-based, water-soluble cleanser that would work well for normal to dry skin. The mineral oil in this product is a good buffer for the cleansing agents. It does contain fragrance.

☺ **Deep Cleaning Cleanser, Normal to Oily Skin** *($3.99 for 8 ounces)* is almost identical to the Deep Cleaning version above only with less mineral oil, though the same basic comments apply.

☺ **Deep Cleaning Cleanser, Sensitive Skin** *($3.99 for 8 ounces)* is similar to the Deep Cleaning Cleanser, Normal to Oily Skin above, but it includes two somewhat gentler detergent cleansing agents and excludes the fragrance, which makes this better for all skin types!

☺ **Gentle Skin Cleanser for Baby** *($3.99 for 8 ounces)* is similar to the Deep Cleaning Cleanser, Sensitive Skin above, and the same basic comments apply. There is nothing in this product that makes it more appropriate for a baby's skin. If anything, the Sensitive Skin version above would be far better because it doesn't include fragrance.

☹ **Clear Confidence Acne Facial Wash** *($3.99 for 6 ounces)*. The main cleansing agent listed is sodium C14-16 olefin sulfate, which makes this too potentially irritating and drying for all skin types. It also contains 2% salicylic acid, but the pH of the cleanser is too high for it to be effective for exfoliation.

☹ **Sensitive Skin Cleansing Bar** *($2.49 for 3.3 ounces)* is a standard, tallow-based bar cleanser that includes Vaseline and lanolin. Tallow and lanolin are a problem for blemish-prone skin.

☺ **Clear Confidence Blemish Masque** *($5.99 for 6 ounces)* is a very standard clay mask that can absorb some amount of oil. The 2% salicylic acid it includes is not effective as an exfoliant because the pH of the product is too high.

☺ **Clear Confidence Clear Swab** *($5.50 for 24 swabs)* comes packaged with cotton-tip swabs soaked with a simple solution that contains 2% salicylic acid. The pH of 4.5 is just above the limit that makes it effective for exfoliation, and the inclusion of menthol is a hindrance. Plus, the application directions for these swabs suggest that they should be used only to treat an individual blemish. If you break out all over or are struggling with blackheads, this becomes a cumbersome and time-consuming way to deal with an overall blemish problem.

☺ **Blemish Patch** *($6.95 for 24 patches)* are patches meant to be placed over blemishes to help reduce their appearance. That is unlikely. These patches are coated with a film-forming agent (like those used in hairspray) and that's not great for blemished skin. They do contain a tiny amount of salicylic acid, but not enough to be effective for exfoliation. Plus, if you tend to break out all over, an effective salicylic acid lotion, gel, or toner would be far more effective than dotting these things all over your face.

PHYSICIAN'S CHOICE

This Arizona-based skin-care company states that "Your physician is the natural choice for guidance when it comes to your skin-care regimen. As a medical expert, your doctor wants to be sure your home skin-care program will support your clinical care. For this reason, Physician's Choice products are available only through caring physicians." Does that mean any physician not selling these products is uncaring? They go on to say, "The Physician's Choice family of products are all natural. They are free of dyes, color additives, fragrances, comedogenic oils, waxes, and other ingredients that are known to cause irritation or other sensitive reactions." While it's true these products are free of color additives, the rest is blatantly false information. Jasmine alcohol (gardenia alcohol) is absolutely a fragrant additive, and one of the products actually lists "fragrance" on the label; if that isn't "fragrance," I don't know what is! Several ingredients in these products can be irritants, including sodium C14-16 olefin sulfonate, sulfur, pumpkin wine (that's just alcohol, and that's drying and irritating in any form), as well as citrus. There are also thickening agents in Physician's Choice products, ranging from isopropyl palmitate to fatty acids that can trigger breakouts. One of the "natural" products even contains polyethylene, a plastic. There is almost nothing "all natural" about these products save for a few plant extracts.

Some of the Physician's Choice products are indeed worthy of consideration, but overall none of them stand out over lots of other options from Neutrogena to Persa-Gel or other physician-oriented lines from BioMedic to Glyderm. For more information about Physician's Choice, call (800) 758-8185 or visit www.physchoiceaz.com or www.drugstore.com.

☹ **pHaze 1 Facial Wash** *($14.95 for 6 ounces)* is an extremely standard, detergent-based, water-soluble cleanser. One of the cleansing agents is sodium C14-16 olefin sulfonate, which can be too drying and irritating for all skin types.

☹ **pHaze 1 Facial Wash, Oily/Problem Skin** *($14.95 for 6 ounces)* is almost identical to the pHaze 1 above, and the same basic comments apply.

☺ $$$ **pHaze Haze 10 Psor-Ecz Bar** *($19.95 for 4 ounces)* is a fairly standard bar cleanser that also contains salicylic acid and resorcinol. The pH of this bar is too high for the salicylic acid to work as an exfoliant. The resorcinol can work as an antimicrobial agent, but it is considered extremely irritating to skin and is therefore rarely used in cosmetics anymore.

☹ **pHaze 13 Pigment Bar** *($24 for 4 ounces)* is a standard bar cleanser that contains a small amount of kojic acid, which has melanin-inhibiting properties. Kojic acid is an exceptionally unstable ingredient and does not maintain its efficacy when exposed to light or air, which makes it especially unreliable in this product. Even if it were stable, it would be rinsed off the skin before it had a chance to have any impact on skin color.

☺ **pHaze 31 BPO 5% Cleanser** *($14 for 6 ounces)* is a standard, detergent-based, water-soluble cleanser that also contains 5% benzoyl peroxide. Benzoyl peroxide is a good topical disinfectant for blemishes, but in a cleanser any benefit from it would just be rinsed down the drain. The surfactant in this product is succinic acid sulfate, which can be too drying and irritating for most skin types, while the shea butter can be too emollient for those struggling with breakouts. It does contain fragrance.

☺ **Beta-C Gentle Eye Makeup Remover** *($10 for 2 ounces)* is an exceptionally standard, detergent-based eye-makeup remover that would work as well as any. The pumpkin wine in it can be drying and irritating for the eye area.

☺ **pHaze 2 Smoothing Toner** *($16 for 6 ounces)* is basically aloe vera gel with AHAs. The pH of 5 makes this 10% AHA product not the best for exfoliation.

☹ **pHaze 5 Nutrient Toner** *($34 for 6 ounces)* lists the second ingredient as pumpkin wine, which is mostly alcohol, and that is too drying and irritating for all skin types.

☺ $$$ **pHaze 3 The Peel** *($39.95 for 1 ounce)* is supposed to be a high concentration of AHA, but after confirming the ingredient label, the amount of AHA (less than 1%), and the pH with the company, it's clear that this product can't "peel" skin. Both the small amount of AHA and the pH of 5 make it incapable of exfoliation.

☺ **pHaze 4 Gentle Exfoliant** *($14.95 for 6 ounces)* uses ground-up pieces of plastic (polyethylene) as the exfoliant in a standard cream base. That does make it an option as a topical scrub for normal to dry sensitive skin.

☺ **pHaze 6 Collagen Hydrator** *($24 for 2 ounces)* is an OK moisturizer for dry skin, though collagen is nothing more than a water-binding agent; it will not have any effect on the collagen in your skin.

☺ $$$ **pHaze 6+ Hydrator Plus SPF 15** *($26.95 for 2 ounces)* is a very good, avobenzone-based sunscreen in a moisturizing base that contains mostly water, aloe, thickeners, glycerin, silicone, vitamins, water-binding agents, and preservatives. This would work well for someone with normal to dry skin, if the price doesn't "phase" you!

☺ $$$ **pHaze 7 Protecting Hydrator SPF 15** *($25 for 2 ounces)* is almost identical to the Hydrator Plus above, only this one excludes the water-binding agents. If you want hydration, that makes this a poorer option than the one above.

✓☺ **pHaze 8 Face & Body Hydrator SPF 15** *($12.95 for 12 ounces)* takes the best of what the two SPF 15s above contain, including the avobenzone, vitamins (antioxidants), and water-binding agent, and then also adds titanium dioxide, boosting the UVA protection. Yet the price is a fraction of what the others cost. Sigh. Pricing in the world of cosmetics is completely unrelated to efficacy or quality! The quality is here, and there would be no reason to buy any of the other sunscreens in this line over this one.

☺ $$$ **pHaze 12 Eye Wrinkle Cream** *($25 for 0.5 ounce)* contains aloe water, Vaseline, slip agent, water-binding agent, thickeners, silicone, vitamins, plant oil, water-binding agents, and preservatives. This is a good moisturizer for someone with normal to dry skin.

☹ $$$ **pHaze 15 Serum C** *($36.95 for 0.5 ounce)* contains a citrus blend, but that does not get you a form of vitamin C your skin can use. The research involving vitamin C has involved magnesium ascorbyl phosphate, ascorbyl palmitate, and L-ascorbic acid, not orange juice—plus this product contains ivy, which can be a skin irritant.

☹ $$$ **pHaze 15+ C Quench** *($46 for 1 ounce)* lists witch hazel distillate as the second ingredient, and that makes this product too irritating and drying for most skin types. The ingredient list also shows phtyoalexin. Phytoalexins are antimicrobial substances that are produced by a plant in response to infection by fungi or bacteria and that help to defend the plant by inhibiting the growth of invading microbes. Phytoalexins can also be potent antioxidants, and the combination of those two properties is thought to have benefit for skin, particularly for wound healing (Sources: *Free Radical Research,* June 2002, pages 621–631 and *Biochemical Pharmacology,* January 2002, pages 99–104). How that relates to daily skin care or wrinkles is unknown, but it is probably a good antioxidant for skin.

☺ $$$ **pHaze 16 C-Cream** *($36 for 1 ounce).* The citrus water in this cream may make you think of vitamin C, but it does not have the same effect on skin, though it can be a skin irritant. There are also several plant extracts that are potential irritants, including sage, rosemary, and watercress. Finally, this product does contain a form of vitamin C that is known to be of help to skin, magnesium ascorbyl phosphate, but the amount is so tiny that with the other problems here this adds up to a real "Why bother?"

The Revie

☺ **pHaze 17 Rebalance** *($26.95 for 2 ounces)* is a basic moisturizer for normal to dry skin that contains mostly water, aloe vera, thickeners, plant oils, water-binding agent, and preservatives. The borage oil and evening primrose oil may be beneficial in reducing irritation and for some types of dermatitis, but all of the published research showing these two ingredients to be of help used pure concentrates alone. If your goal is to try alternatives for dealing with dermatitis or irritation, a pure concentrate of borage oil or evening primrose oil, like those found at most health food stores, would be a far better option to net you a positive result.

☺ **pHaze 20 Silkcoat** *($17.95 for 4 ounces)* is just Vaseline, wax, mineral oil and film-forming agent. This is an option for dry skin, but there is no real reason to use this over plain old Vaseline.

✓☺ $$$ **pHaze 13 Light Block Pigment Cream SPF 25** *($33.95 for 1 ounce)* is a very good, though overpriced, sunscreen with an in-part titanium dioxide base. It does contain hydroquinone (about 1%) in an amount that is somewhat effective for inhibiting melanin production.

☺ $$$ **pHaze 13 Pigment Gel** *($35.50 for 1 ounce)*. The claim that this product "bleaches" skin is misleading. The active ingredients, 2% hydroquinone and about 2% kojic acid, really just help to inhibit melanin production, which is not a bleaching action. This product also contains a small amount of witch hazel distillate, which can be a skin irritant due to its alcohol content. The amount of AHAs is not enough for them to be effective for exfoliation.

☺ $$$ **pHaze 13 Pigment Gel Forte HQ Free** *($39.95 for 1 ounce)* is similar to the pHaze 13 Pigment Gel above, minus the hydroquinone, and the same concerns apply for this product as well. However, it is an option for someone who is allergic or sensitive to hydroquinone. Keep in mind that kojic acid is a light- and air-sensitive ingredient and does not remain stable for very long (though the 1 ounce of this you get will be gone in no time).

☺ $$$ **pHaze 13 Pigment Gel HQ Free** *($35.95 for 1 ounce)* is similar to the Gel Forte above, only with a lower concentration of kojic acid.

☹ **pHaze 18 Clearskin** *($19.95 for 2 ounces)* is a basic moisturizer with some thickening agents that can be a problem for those with blemish-prone skin. It does contain some plant extracts that can be good anti-irritants, but it also contains sulfur, and that can be a skin irritant. There is nothing in this product that is helpful for reducing blemishes or clogged pores.

☹ **pHaze 32 Acne Bar** *($13.95 for 2 ounces)* is a bar cleanser that contains sulfur, eucalyptus, and pine tree oil, which are all extremely irritating for all skin types. It also contains salicylic acid, but the pH is too high for it to be effective as an exfoliant.

☹ **pHaze 33 Acne Cream** *($14.95 for 1 ounce)*. As a topical disinfectant with 5% benzoyl peroxide this may be an option, but the castor oil in it can leave a tacky feel on skin and the cream base can be too emollient for those with breakouts. The lemon oil and jasmine make this product a poor choice for sensitive skin. It also contains 5% lactic acid (an AHA), but the pH of the product isn't low enough for it to be effective as an exfoliant.

☹ **pHaze 34 Acne Gel** *($14 for 1 ounce)* contains 10% benzoyl peroxide and 4% sulfur. Sulfur can be very irritating for skin, and I would strongly suggest avoiding this option, or at least trying a 10% (or lower) benzoyl peroxide concentration in a product without additional irritants (Persa-Gel comes to mind) before even considering this one. The castor oil in here can leave a slight tacky feel on skin. It does contain fragrance.

☹ **pHaze 35 Acne Gel with 2% Salicylic Acid** *($16 for 1 ounce)* is almost identical to the pHaze 34 above, only this one contains 2% salicylic acid. The pH of this product is too high for it to be effective as an exfoliant.

☺ **pHaze 11 Apres Peel** *($16.95 for 2 ounces)* is a 0.5% hydrocortisone cream in an emollient, moisturizing base that would be an option for someone with normal to dry skin who has irritation or minor dermatitis. However, Lanacort and Cortaid, available at drugstores, have identical efficacy, and cost only a fraction of this price. Caution: Repeated use of a cortisone cream can cause thinning and premature aging of the skin.

PHYSICIANS FORMULA

There aren't really any doctors at Physicians Formula (the founder of the company was an allergist, Dr. Frank Crandell, but that was back in 1937), and no physicians currently sell or endorse it either. The company asserts that "The term hypoallergenic is more than just a cosmetic claim for Physicians Formula. It is the basis for every product that is created. Physicians Formula honors this claim through stringent product testing and quality control. In fact, Physicians Formula products are formulated without 132 known irritating ingredients still found in many cosmetics on the market today. Physicians Formula was born of a steadfast pledge to purity. A promise never to allow fragrance … into anything we make." This is one of the more inexcusable, disingenuous claims the cosmetics industry has to offer. Perhaps Physicians Formula hasn't looked at their product formulations, which list fragrance prominently right on the labels. While the line doesn't list the "132 known irritating ingredients" that they claim not to use, what they do use, and that are notorious for causing irritation and skin sensitivity, are sodium lauryl sulfate, camphor, menthol, coloring agents, and formaldehyde-releasing preservatives. And as if that weren't bad enough, almost every single one of the sunscreen products lacks UVA-protecting ingredients—an oversight that is assuredly *not* what the doctor ordered! If you are at the drugstore shopping for cosmetics, this is one line to hurry quickly past. For more information about Physicians Formula, call (800) 227-0333 or visit www.physiciansformula.com. **Note:** All Physicians Formula skin-care products contain fragrance unless otherwise noted.

PHYSICIANS FORMULA SKIN CARE

☺ **Enriched Cleansing Concentrate for Dry to Very Dry Skin** *($5.95 for 4 ounces)* is an exceptionally basic, mineral oil–based, cold cream–style cleanser that is an option for dry to very dry skin.

☺ **Gentle Cleansing Cream for Dry to Very Dry Skin** *($5.95 for 4 ounces)* is similar to the Enriched version above only with more mineral oil and Vaseline. The same basic comments apply.

☺ **Gentle Cleansing Lotion for Normal to Dry Skin** *($7.25 for 8 ounces)* is similar to the Enriched version above only with more Vaseline. The same basic comments apply.

☺ **Deep Pore Cleansing Gel for Normal to Oily Skin** *($6.95 for 8 ounces)* is a standard, detergent-based cleanser that would be a good option for normal to oily skin.

☺ **Eye Makeup Remover Lotion for Normal to Dry Skin** *($4.75 for 2 ounces)* is a standard, detergent-based makeup remover, similar to almost every other product of this type, and it would work as well as any.

☹ **Eye Makeup Remover Pads for Normal to Dry Skin** *($5.75 for 60 pads)* lists its third ingredient as witch hazel distillate, whose main component is alcohol, and that makes this too drying and irritating for all skin types.

☹ **Oil Free Eye Makeup Remover Pads for Normal to Oily Skin** *($5.75 for 60 pads)* contains ivy extract, a potential skin irritant, high up on the ingredient list. This is a formulation best left on the shelf.

☺ **Vital Lash Oil Free Eye Makeup Remover for Normal to Oily Skin** *($4.75 for 2 ounces)* is just mineral oil and some thickeners, along with preservatives. There is little benefit to using this over plain mineral oil, and although this will remove makeup, it can leave a greasy film on skin.

☺ **Gentle Refreshing Toner for Dry to Very Dry Skin** *($6.95 for 8 ounces)* is just water, glycerin, water-binding agents, preservatives, and coloring agents. It is an OK toner for most skin types.

☹ **Conditioning Skin Toner for Normal to Oily Skin** *($6.95 for 8 ounces)* contains alcohol, camphor, and menthol, which add up to serious irritation and dryness for all skin types.

☹ **Pore Refining Skin Freshener for Normal to Dry Skin** *($6.95 for 8 ounces)* is just water, alcohol, glycerin, fragrance, and coloring agents. This is a useless, if not problematic, toner for all skin types.

☺ **Beauty Spiral Brightening Moisturizer** *($8.95 for 1 ounce)* is an emollient, though basic, moisturizer for normal to dry skin that contains more shine (mica) than it does any beneficial ingredients for skin. The teeny amounts of water-binding agents and antioxidants are not going to do anything for beauty.

☺ **Mood Swirls Mood Setting Moisturizers** (comes in ZENsation/Relaxing, Cyber/Energizing, Seducer/Sensual, and Globe-trotter/Refreshing) *($8.95 for 2 ounces)*. The only difference between these basic moisturizers is the fragrance (that this line supposedly doesn't contain). This is just water, slip agent, mineral oil, talc, thickeners, small amounts of antioxidants and water-binding agents, shine (mica), fragrance, and preservatives. This is an OK moisturizer for normal to slightly dry skin if the fragrance doesn't bother you.

☺ **Collagen Cream Concentrate for Dry to Very Dry Skin** *($8.95 for 2 ounces)* is an ordinary emollient moisturizer that contains a small amount of water-binding agents and a minuscule amount of antioxidants. It is an OK option for normal to dry skin.

☺ **Deep Moisture Cream for Normal to Dry Skin** *($8.50 for 4 ounces)* is a mediocre moisturizer for normal to dry skin that is just thickeners, mineral oil, Vaseline, and plant oil.

☹ **Elastin/Collagen Moisture Lotion for Normal to Dry Skin** *($8.50 for 4 ounces)* is similar to the Collagen Cream Concentrate above, only this version contains sodium lauryl sulfate rather high up on the ingredient list, a substance that is a skin irritant and a problem, especially in a leave-on formulation.

☺ **Enriched Dry Skin Concentrate for Dry to Very Dry Skin** *($8.50 for 4 ounces)* is just plant oils, Vaseline, lanolin, and fragrance. It's emollient, but a completely dated formulation.

☺ **Extra Rich Rehydrating Moisturizer for Normal to Dry Skin** *($8.50 for 4 ounces)* is a mediocre moisturizer for normal to dry skin that is just thickeners and mineral oil.

☺ **Nourishing Night Cream for Dry to Very Dry Skin** *($5.95 for 1 ounce)* is similar to the Enriched Dry Skin Concentrate above, and the same comments apply.

☺ **Oil Control Oil Free Moisturizer for Normal to Oily Skin** *($8.50 for 4 ounces)* is oil-free, but it still contains several ingredients that can be a problem for oily skin. It also lacks any beneficial ingredients, such as water-binding agents, antioxidants, or anti-irritants.

☹ **Self Defense Color Corrective Moisturizing Lotion SPF 15** *($7.50 for 2 ounces)* doesn't contain the UVA-protecting ingredients of avobenzone, titanium dioxide, or zinc oxide, and is not recommended.

☹ **Sun Shield for Faces Formula SPF 20** *($8.50 for 2 ounces)* doesn't contain the UVA-protecting ingredients of avobenzone, titanium dioxide, or zinc oxide, and is not recommended.

☹ **Sun Shield Sunless Tanning SPF 20 Light/Medium** and **Medium/Dark** *($8.50 for 4 ounces)* doesn't contain the UVA-protecting ingredients of avobenzone, titanium dioxide, or zinc oxide, and is not recommended.

☹ **Sun Shield Moisture Formula SPF 20** *($8.50 for 4 ounces)* doesn't contain the UVA-protecting ingredients of avobenzone, titanium dioxide, or zinc oxide, and is not recommended.

☹ **Sun Shield Oil Free Formula SPF 20** *($8.50 for 4 ounces)* doesn't contain the UVA-protecting ingredients of avobenzone, titanium dioxide, or zinc oxide, and is not recommended.

☹ **Sun Shield for Faces Extra Sensitive Skin Formula SPF 15** *($8.50 for 2 ounces)* doesn't contain the UVA-protecting ingredients of avobenzone, titanium dioxide, or zinc oxide, and is not recommended.

☹ **Sun Shield Sport Non-Stick Lotion SPF 15** *($8.50 for 5 ounces)* doesn't contain the UVA-protecting ingredients of avobenzone, titanium dioxide, or zinc oxide, and is not recommended.

☹ **Sun Shield Sport Team Two-in-One Sun Spray and Lip Care SPF 15** *($10.95 for 4 ounces)* doesn't contain the UVA-protecting ingredients of avobenzone, titanium dioxide, or zinc oxide, and is not recommended.

☺ **Sun Shield Lip Care SPF 15** *($2.50 for 0.15 ounce)* is a very good, titanium dioxide–based sunscreen in a standard but emollient base. I don't know what finally possessed this company to make a good sunscreen, but here it is.

PHYSICIANS FORMULA MAKEUP

Does this line have what the doctor ordered? When it comes to makeup, not unless your doctor advocates off-color foundations, greasy, thick concealers, and a glittery metallic finish for almost everything else. In just a few short years, Physicians Formula has gone from offering several viable, inexpensive makeup options to a display of contrived products that are the cosmetic equivalent of all talk, no action. Reading the claims on the back of each package, you would swear that no safer, more pure, or more stringently tested makeup could exist. Yet few of the products contain anything exceptional, while many add out-of-line ingredients that contradict proclamations like "safe for sensitive skin" and "non-comedogenic." The only reason to pay attention to this makeup is one good mascara and the superior quad eyeshadow sets. Among drugstore lines, these shadows are a standout for their application and matte finish. The rest of the line has too many faults that are disguised in unusual packaging or glossed over with an eye-catching design—don't fall for it and you'll avoid disappointment.

FOUNDATION: Physicians Formula's foundations leave me frustrated. On the one hand, many of them have reliable SPF 15 protection, which is great. Yet at the same time most of these offer some of the poorest colors and dated textures around.

☹ **Le Velvet Film Makeup SPF 15** *($5.14 refill, $3.69 for compact)* is an ordinary cream-to-powder foundation that goes on surprisingly moist and creamy and can be blended out fairly sheer. The SPF is part titanium dioxide, which is great, but the finish is somewhat chalky. Even if testers were available, most of the shades are just too pink, peach, or orange to recommend. If you're willing to settle for what's left, Buff is an OK option. **Le Velvet Powder Finish Makeup SPF 15** *($5.14 refill, $3.69 for compact)* is similar to the one above, including the in-part titanium dioxide sunscreen, only this has a lighter, smoother texture (it's silicone based) that looks somewhat more natural on the skin. The colors are all a problem, though, with strong rose or peach tones prevailing. **Sun Shield Liquid Makeup SPF 15** *($5.19)* is a standard, almost antiquated liquid foundation whose sunscreen does not offer UVA-protecting ingredients. None of the six shades come close to resembling real skin tones. **Beauty Spiral Skin Brightening Liquid Foundation** *($9.89)* is a sheer, light-textured foundation that has an uneven, slightly pasty finish due to the high amount of titanium dioxide it contains. The four shades are passable, but nothing this chalky can have any sort of brightening effect. **Beauty Spiral Brightening Compact Foundation** *($9.89)* is a cream-to-powder makeup that "spirals" two colors together. It's eye-catching, but that's all this substandard foundation has going for it. The thick texture offers sheer coverage and a dry, powdery finish that just doesn't feel great on the skin. The four colors are passable, but there are far more elegant cream-to-powder foundations in the other racks at the drugstore.

☺ **Virtual Foundation Multi-Reflective Luminous Makeup** *($9.89)* is not only Physicians Formula's most elegant-feeling foundation, but it also features four almost-neutral shades that would be OK options for light to medium skin tones. The luminous part is just pink iridescence, and it's quite obvious despite this makeup's natural finish and smooth, light coverage. The Revlon SkinLights line has products that surpass this by providing superior sun protection right along with a low-key shine that is decidedly more beguiling—rather than blatantly obvious. **Pearls of Perfection Multi-Colored Face Tint** *($12.89)* is a sheer, gel-based face tint that has a lightly creamy texture and subtle sparkly finish. This is fine for a very soft wash of all-over color, but the only acceptable colors are Translucent Glow and Bronzer.

☹ **CONCEALER:** Few if any companies have such a broad variety of color-correcting concealers (there are 11 options here). Yet all these really do is place a strange and far from natural color on the skin (in this case, yellow or lime green), and their texture ensures a less than subtle finish. **AquaCover Cooling Concealer Stick** *($6.89)* has a cool, water-to-powder feel and sets nicely to a solid matte finish. However, the cooling sensation continues even after it dries, thanks to the menthyl lactate (a form of menthol) in here. This is not recommended for use anywhere near the eye, unless you want the tears to flow! **Gentle Cover Concealer Stick** *($4.89)* is a lipstick-style concealer that is very creamy, feels heavy, and is hard to blend on the skin. The flesh-toned shades are too peachy pink, and the color correctors should just be avoided. **Gentle Cover Cream Concealer SPF 10** *($4.89)* is a mineral oil– and wax-based concealer with a wand applicator and a titanium dioxide sunscreen. This formula will easily crease into any lines around the eye. The colors are the same as those of the Gentle Cover Concealer Stick, and the same comments apply. **Concealer Twins 2-in-1 Correct and Cover Concealer Stick SPF 15** *($5.89)* are dual-sided, lipstick-style concealers whose color combinations and textures are simply awful. The SPF is great, but cannot save this terrible product. **Concealer Twins 2-in-1 Correct and Cover Concealer Pencil** *($6.89)* are dual-ended greasy pencils that have a thick, waxy texture and really bad colors. **Concealer Twins 2-in-1 Correct and Cover Cream Concealer SPF 10** *($7.89)* has a decent (though not quite high enough) titanium dioxide sunscreen, but an otherwise lackluster creamy texture. You get a flesh-toned color on one end and a yellow or green hue on the other, but both leave much to be desired. Rounding up the twin series are **Concealer Twins Correct and Cover Duo 2-in-1 Stick** and **Cream Concealer SPF 10** *($7.89)*, which share the same sunscreen as the 2-in-1 options above. *This* version gets you a creamy liquid concealer on one end and a pencil concealer on the other, for those who like their concealers bad *and* terrible. **Powder Finish Concealer Stick SPF 15** *($4.89)* is another creamy stick concealer with titanium dioxide as one of the active ingredients for sun protection, which is nice, but the only flesh-toned shade is too pink to look natural, and the powder finish is minimal—it tends to stay creamy and can easily crease. **Beauty Spiral Perfecting Concealer** *($6.89)* comes in the typically bad assortment of colors, just like the rest of the Physicians Formula concealers, meaning one substandard flesh tone and two color-correcting shades (yellow and green). This one has an unusually dry, powdery finish, yet still manages to slip into lines, and looks chalky on the skin. **Beauty Spiral Perfecting Cream Concealer** *($6.89)* is identical to the Beauty Spiral Brightening Liquid Foundation above, and the same comments apply. As a concealer, the chalky finish does little to deal with dark circles or anything else you may want to hide. **Neutralizer Color Corrective Primer SPF 15** *($4.89)* comes through with a great titanium dioxide sunscreen, but what good is that when you have to put up with the yellow and green colors? Neither shade looks natural on the skin, no matter how much you blend.

POWDER: ☹ **Powder Palette Multi-Colored Pressed Powder/Corrector** *($11.89)* is a kaleidoscopic arrangement of different colors that all come off as the same color on the skin, as it should be. The colors are a strange lot—you'll find neutral bronze tones along with greens, whites, and, believe it or not, grays! The only one worth recommending is the Translucent version, which would be a good, talc-based powder for lighter skin tones that are normal to dry. **Pearls of Perfection Multi-Colored Face Powder** *($11.89)* are large pots of colored powder beads, available in bronze, flesh, and shiny highlighting shades. They're fun in concept, but the execution is messy and not worth the effort. **Les Botaniques Botanical Highlighter**, **Face Powder**, and **Bronzer** *($11.89)* are all talc-based pressed powders embossed with cutesy designs like flowers and the blazing sun. Each design incorporates different colors, such as pink, white, and yellow, but on the skin they show up as just one color. Which shade you end up with depends on which design you choose, but this eye candy is not worth more than a passing glance. **Skinsitive Ultra-Gentle Face Powder** *($11.89)* is hailed as "a revolutionary powder to protect, respect, and smooth even the most sensitive skin," but this talc-based pressed powder holds no particular advantage over any other powder. In fact, the inclusion of aluminum starch as the second ingredient is a disadvantage for those with sensitive skin, as aluminum starch is known to cause contact dermatitis.

☺ **Retro Glow Illuminating Face Powder** *($11.89)* is supposed to be a return to the heritage of Physicians Formula, when Dr. Crandall's wife was the emblem for the brand. These talc-based powders contain aluminum starch, so they have a slightly grainy feel and dry finish, replete with shine. The shine is described as "imperceptible," but one application will prove what a laughable claim that is. If you're seeking a shiny powder, the two shades are surprisingly neutral. **Jungle Fever** and **Summer Eclipse Bronzing & Shimmery Face Powder** *($11.89)* are pressed-powder bronzers, each with an embossed picture stamped in the middle of the powder. The tan colors are realistically soft, but the shine is way too intense to look convincing during daylight hours. **Aqua Powder Cooling Loose**

Powder *($11.89)* is strikingly similar to Prescriptives' very successful Magic Liquid Powder ($32.50). Now all of you who were wondering when a less expensive option would be available can consider this—another wet-feeling, cooling powder that leaves behind a not-so-subtle shiny finish. This version is a touch shinier than the Magic Liquid Powder, but not by much, and the three color options are a mixed bag. If you decide to try this, stick with Translucent, as it's more akin to the Magic version anyway.

☺ BLUSH: **Blush Palette Multi-Colored Blusher** *($9.89)* comes in either mauve or brown tones, each with five shades arranged (without dividers) in one compact. These just end up as one color when applied on the skin, and the center color is quite shiny, which makes these fun to admire, but impractical to wear because the shine doesn't get applied evenly over the cheek. **Planet Blush 2-in-1 Blush and Face Powder** *($10.89)* features a split compact with a shiny pressed powder on one side and a softly shiny blush tone on the other. The domed top is there to allow a tiny blush brush to stand upright in the center of the compact, but its rough texture and extremely short handle make it impractical to use. This is another gimmicky product that makes you long for the days when blush was just called "blush." **AquaCheeks Cooling Blush Stick** *($7.89)* is a very sheer, water-to-powder blush stick that contains menthyl lactate to prolong the cooling sensation, which isn't helpful for skin and can trigger unnecessary irritation. This has a soft, shimmery finish.

EYESHADOW: ✔☺ **Quad Eye Shadow** *($6.49)* has some of the best neutral color combinations around, with a completely matte texture that applies and blends beautifully. How this marvelous product ended up in a line fraught with missteps and atrocious colors is anyone's guess!

☺ **Eyebrightener Multi-Colored Eyelighter** *($7.89)* is definitely eye-catching. Unfortunately, this variegated display of colors ends up placing a sweep of intense, metallic shine on the eyelid, which will undoubtedly have teen appeal. **Virtual Eyes Multi-Reflective Eye Gloss** *($6.89)* is a water-and-silicone based eye gel that you apply with a built-in brush. The effect is strong, semi-opaque iridescence rather a wet-look gloss, though this does stay slightly moist. Applying this evenly is very difficult, so you basically need to settle for a smudge of glistening shine. **Planet Eyes Quad Eye Shadow** *($5.89)* is a compact of five colors with no dividers, so application can be tricky. Although these feel smooth and apply easily, the color pales in comparison to the shiny finish.

☹ **Virtual Eyes Multi-Reflective Loose Eyelighter** *($7.89)* is just small vials of loose, metallic shine powders to use anywhere you want potent shine. This is especially messy because the powder has a hard time clinging to the skin. **Pearls of Perfection Multi-Colored Eye Shadow Pearls** *($6.89)* are shiny beads of color housed in a small, clear plastic jar. What a misguided, unsophisticated way to apply eyeshadow!

EYE AND BROW SHAPER: ☺ **Virtual Eyes Eye Pencil** *($6.89)* are wider than usual, but are still standard creamy pencils whose iridescence is the main attraction, if you're drawn to that sort of thing. **Virtual Eyes Liquid Eyeliner** *(6.89)* is actually a very good liquid eyeliner if you don't mind the garish metallic colors. **Eyebrightener Brightening Liquid Eyeliner** *($6.49)* is a standard liquid eyeliner with a good, firm brush and a sheer application that dries to a metallic finish. The consistency is not the best, and this is not the most attractive look I can think of, but for an interesting evening look, it's an option. Please humor me and avoid the Gold and Silver shades. **Eyebrightener Pencil Duo** *($5.89)* is a standard, dual-ended pencil with two color combinations, shiny black and shiny white, or metallic bronze and black. For an iridescent lashline, they'll work as well as any other pencil. **FineLine Brow Pencil** *($4.19)* comes in four decent shades and has a standard, dry texture. If you're keen on brow pencils, this is one of the least expensive reliable options. **Brow Corrector** *($5.89)* is a standard, sticky brow gel available in Clear or with a very sheer tint. This is an OK option for grooming and minimally—and I mean minimally—coloring the brows, and the price is more than reasonable.

☹ **Eye Definer Automatic Eye Pencil** *($4.99)* is a twist-up eye pencil that is greasier than most, which means it can smear and smudge easily.

MASCARA: ☺ **To Any Lengths Lash Extending Mascara** *($4.89)* is excellent for length and clean, clump-free definition. Don't expect any thickness from this, but as a lengthening formula this wins high marks, and it no longer smears!

☺ **Month 2 Month Mascara Thickening Formula** *($6.49)* and ☹ **Month 2 Month Mascara Lengthening Formula** *($6.49)* both have two mascaras packaged together rather than just one, which is intended to provide a "freshness system." You note the date when you start one of the tubes and after a month you dispose of it and start the next one. The ophthalmologists I spoke to said they had never heard of mascara going bad in a month, and instead recommended (as I do) discarding mascara after three to four months. One month just seems wasteful, and if this practice is so vital, why don't all the Physicians Formula mascaras utilize it? As for the formulas, the Thickening version thickens admirably with only a slight tendency to smear. The Lengthening version builds hardly any length, and smears terribly. **AquaWear Mascara** *($6.49)* will build some length, but no thickness, and is fairly waterproof. Contrary to the claim here, no waterproof mascara can condition lashes, nor do lashes need conditioning. **LipLash Splash 2-in-1 Clear Mascara and Lip Gloss** *($7.89)* is a dual-ended product with an iridescent, peppermint-flavored gloss on one end and a shiny, clear mascara on the other. Gloss and mascara together? Why?

☹ **Eyebrightener Mascara** *($7.89)* is blah all the way around, doing little of anything except making lashes feel especially brittle. This does not curl lashes nor does it make eyes look any brighter. **Eyebrightener Waterproof Mascara** *($7.89)* would be the centerpiece on display if there were a Boring Mascara Hall of Fame. The only thing this has going for it is the fact that it's waterproof. **PlentiFull Thickening Mascara** *($4.59)* is a boring, minimalist mascara that builds no thickness whatsoever and tends to smudge.

☺ **SPECIALTY:** **Refill Sponges** *($2.50)* are both for the Le Velvet makeups, but can work well with any foundation and are superior to the wedge-shaped sponges normally sold at the drugstore.

PHYTOMER (SKIN CARE ONLY)

When it comes to fantastic claims versus extremely unimpressive ingredient formulations, Phytomer is one of the less responsible cosmetics companies around. What I find even more startling is the way a cosmetics line can carry on about its superior formulations, remarkable ingredients, and unequaled ability to erase wrinkles, and yet not include one sunscreen product as part of a daily skin-care routine. In fact, of the sunscreens Phytomer does carry, most lack UVA-protecting ingredients, though what is even more outrageous is that this line is irresponsible enough to sell sunscreens with SPFs of 2, 4, and 8, which is tantamount to an oncologist who specializes in lung cancer selling cigarettes. Their information about sun protection is actually scary. "The protection index is not linked to the length of exposure…. Good protection is always the recipe for even tanning." They even attribute antiaging properties to their products that encourage tanning! How frightening. None of that is accurate or even remotely true in the least (please refer to Chapter Seven, *Cosmetics Dictionary*, for specifics about SPF, UVA, and free-radical damage). Abundant research has shown that unprotected sun exposure is dangerous for skin, and that tanning of any kind is the road to serious wrinkling and possibly skin cancer.

Phytomer's claim to fame is the ocean, or to be more precise, algae and seawater. In fact, different kinds of algae extracts show up in almost every one of the Phytomer products. Algae is unquestionably a stylish ingredient these days. Does the sea offer any special advantage for skin? Do salt water and sea plants repair skin? I guess you would have to go on faith with this one, because while there is indeed research indicating some algae derivatives can have anti-inflammatory and anti-irritant benefit for skin, as well as water-binding properties, the studies about what they can do for skin are limited (after all there are thousands of species of algae). Moreover, these aren't the only ingredients that have such properties. Seawater is great to swim in, but it is not automatically helpful to skin and, if anything, needs to be rinsed off after you're done swimming to prevent dry skin and dry hair.

Aside from the algae and seawater, Phytomer also uses the same plant extracts, plant oils, thickening agents, water-binding agents, and other standard ingredients found throughout the cosmetics industry, and many of the nonalgae plant extracts used are skin irritants (which would seem to negate the benefit of the algae). What Phytomer leaves out of their products that many other skin-care lines do include are any significant amounts of water-binding agents, antioxidants, or anti-irritants. You may not notice this omission, as Phytomer is busy elaborating about their completely natural contents. Yet none of these natural claims could be further from the truth. These products contain a sea of "unnatural" ingredients, including synthetic coloring agents, acrylates (a form of plastic), sodium lauryl sulfate, triethanolamine, dipropylene glycol, nonoxynol-9, polyethylene glycol, polyisobutene, artificial fragrance, and on and on.

Phytomer's claims are mostly about fantasy and fiction, with little factual information. If you are looking for expensive, so-called spa skin-care products, you would be far better off checking out lines like Jan Marini, BioMedic, or Pevonia than this collection of inadequate formulations. For more information about Phytomer, call (800) 227-8051 or visit www.phytomer.com.

☹ **Gentle Cleansing Cream** *($25 for 5 ounces)* is a standard, detergent-based, water-soluble cleanser clearly similar to Cetaphil Gentle Skin Cleanser. In fact, it is almost identical except that this one contains menthol, a completely unnecessary skin irritant. That makes the Cetaphil product not only far more reasonably priced, but also far gentler on the skin.

☺ $$$ **Gentle Cleansing Milk** *($25 for 6.8 ounces)* is a standard emollient, cold cream–style cleanser and it is an option for normal to dry skin. But there is no reason to choose this cleanser over Neutrogena's Extra Gentle Cleanser (the formulations are incredibly similar) for one-fourth the price. Note: It does contain fragrance.

☺ $$$ **Neutralizing Cleanser** *($34 for 6.8 ounces)* is almost identical to the Gentle Cleansing Milk above except for a minuscule amount of yeast and algae extract. This product can't neutralize anything—it is merely a wipe-off cleanser, nothing more, nothing less, though it is an option for normal to dry skin.

☺ $$$ **Purifying Cleansing Gel** *($26 for 5 ounces)* is a standard, detergent-based, water-soluble cleanser with a minute amount of algae. Again, the faith in the benefit of algae is up to you, because that would be the only reason to consider spending this kind of money on such an exceptionally standard cleanser that is easily replaced at the drugstore for a fraction of the price.

☹ $$$ **Phormidiane Cleanser-Toner** *($26 for 6.8 ounces)* is a standard, rather boring toner. The negligible amount of algae is unlikely to have any benefit for skin.

☹ $$$ **Purifying Gommage Exfoliant** *($28 for 1.7 ounces)*. The bits of clay can feel slightly abrasive, but this is pretty waxy stuff, and several of the plant extracts can be skin irritants, including yarrow, coltsfoot, and birch.

☹ $$$ **Vegetal Exfoliant with Natural Enzymes** *($28 for 1.7 ounces)*. The natural enzyme in this product is a minuscule amount of papain, which has no research showing it to be effective for exfoliation.

☹ $$$ **Refreshing Seawater Spray** *($31 for 4.25 ounces)*. At least the name is clear—this is regular water and seawater. Charging this much money for water out of the ocean is amazing, but if you are looking for salt water (though I can't imagine why), here it is.

☹ $$$ **Rosee Visage Face Dew** *($25 for 8.5 ounces)* is basically water, rosewater (glycerin and fragrance), slip agents, preservatives, fragrance, and salt water. This has none of the water-binding agents, antioxidants, or soothing agents that would make this product interesting for skin care.

☹ **Eau Marine Lotion** *($34.50 for 8.5 ounces)* includes the tiniest amount of seawater, which is good news, because salt can be a skin irritant. It also contains arnica and ivy, which are also potential skin irritants. All in all, this product would provide you with more preservatives and slip agents than anything of benefit for skin.

☺ $$$ **Beauty Restoring Treatment Cream** *($56 for 1.05 ounces)*. This ordinary moisturizer is all about algae, but there is no research showing that it can be restoring in any way for skin.

☺ $$$ **Extended Youth Day Cream** *($46.50 for 1.7 ounces)*. Without sunscreen, this should not be worn for daytime. This is a simple moisturizer with insignificant amounts of vitamin E and algae.

☺ $$$ **Extended Youth Night Cream** *($87.50 for 1.7 ounces)* is almost identical to the Extended Youth Day Cream above and the same basic comments apply. There is no reason to spend the extra money on this "night" version because the only real difference is in the name.

☺ $$$ **Extreme Climate Skin Cream** *($62 for 1.7 ounces)* is an emollient moisturizer for normal to dry skin that contains fractional amounts of water-binding agents and an antioxidant.

☺ $$$ **Eye Contour Cream** *($23.50 for 1 ounce)* is just water, thickeners, plant oil, algae, and preservatives. It doesn't get much more ordinary than this.

☺ $$$ **Hydrating Moisture Base Skin Cream** *($30 for 1.7 ounces)* is an OK moisturizer for normal to dry skin, but it is unimpressive and ordinary, with only a small amount of water-binding agents and some good plant oils. This is a better formulation for less money than the Extreme Climate version above, though that isn't really saying much.

☺ $$$ **Hydration Reinforcement Moisture Supplement Cream** *($54 for 1.7 ounces)* is a simple moisturizer formulation with water, wax, and less than a dusting of algae and vitamin E. This is neither hydrating, reinforcing, nor supplemental in any way.

☺ $$$ **Intensive Hydrating Formula Skin Cream Anti-Pollution** *($50 for 1.7 ounces)* is a simple moisturizer for normal to dry skin, and a rather ordinary one at that.

☺ $$$ **Lift Contour Replenishing Formula** *($43.50 for 0.5 ounce)* is an emollient moisturizer for normal to dry skin, but this expensive Replenishing Formula is all about algae and there is no research indicating that it can lift or replenish skin in any way.

☺ $$$ **Neutralizing Cream** *($49 for 1.7 ounces)* is almost identical to many of Phytomer's moisturizers, containing mostly water, plant oils, thickeners, slip agent, preservatives, fragrance, and algae. The tiny amount of yeast in this product can have no impact on skin.

☺ $$$ **OligoForce Contouring Enforcement Serum** *($34 for 0.5 ounce)* is an emollient lotion of thickeners, silicone, algae, plant oil, preservatives, sea salt, and coloring agent (blue, of course). The only thing being enforced here is mediocrity.

☺ $$$ **OligoForce Purifying Enforcement Serum** *($34 for 0.5 ounce)* is virtually identical to the Contouring Enforcement Serum above except for the addition of a minute amount of tea tree oil, but in such a small quantity that it can have no benefit for skin.

☺ $$$ **OligoForce Moisturizing Enforcement Serum** *($34 for 0.5 ounce)* is virtually identical to the Contouring Enforcement Serum above, only with slightly more algae.

☺ $$$ **OligoForce Replenishing Enforcement Serum** *($34 for 0.5 ounce)* is an emollient moisturizer for normal to dry skin, but is not worth the cost or the effort of applying it.

☺ $$$ **OligoForce Soothing Enforcement Serum** *($34 for 0.5 ounce)* is virtually identical to the Contouring Enforcement Serum above, only with a minute amount of yeast added, even though it can't do anything.

☹ **Purifying Emulsion** *($30 for 1.7 ounces)* contains several plant oils that can be a problem for oily skin, plus it contains arnica and orris root, which are skin irritants. There isn't enough tea tree oil in this product to work as a disinfectant for breakouts, and the minute amount of zinc and vitamin A would have no effect on skin.

☺ $$$ **Soothing Eye Contour Gel** *($43.50 for 1 ounce)* is just water, fragrant water, thickeners, plant oil, algae, and preservatives. It is another boring moisturizer for normal to dry skin.

☺ $$$ **Soothing Skin Cream for Sensitive and Blotchy Skin** *($59 for 1.7 ounces)* is a simple emollient moisturizer for normal to dry skin with minute amounts of algae. The small amount of plant extracts can act as anti-irritants, but this is a lot of money for such a narrow benefit when this product could have offered so much more.

☺ $$$ **Toning Serum** *($74.50 for 1 ounce)* is an emollient moisturizer with slightly more water-binding agents and antioxidant than the other Phytomer moisturizers. However, that still only warrants a barely passable rating.

☺ $$$ **Urban Protection Moisturizing Cream** *($51 for 1.7 ounces)* is an ordinary moisturizer for normal to dry skin that can't protect one iota of skin from any urban or non-urban environment.

☹ **Acnigel** *($30 for 1.7 ounces)* contains several plant oils that would be inappropriate for blemish-prone skin. It actually lacks any ingredients (disinfectants or exfoliants) that can be of benefit to stop blemishes.

☺ $$$ **Comedogel** *($26 for 1 ounce)* does contain a tiny amount of tea tree oil (less than 0.1%), which is not enough for it to be effective as a topical disinfectant. The minute amount of bromelain does not have exfoliating properties for skin.

☹ **Corrigel** *($26 for 1 ounce)* is similar to the Acnigel above and the same comments apply.

☺ $$$ **Desensitizing Mask** *($29 for 1.7 ounces)* is just emollients and thickening agents and, of course, a fractional amount of algae. It's OK for dry skin, but this is little more than a poorly formulated moisturizer.

☺ $$$ **Gentle Mask for Sensitive Skin** *($28 for 1.7 ounces)* is an extremely standard clay mask. Fragrance in products for sensitive skin is always problematic, but this could be a good mask for someone with normal to slightly dry skin.

☺ $$$ **Hydrating Seaweed Facial Mask** *($26 for 1.7 ounces)* is similar to the Gentle Mask above, minus some of the emollients. It would be OK for someone with normal to oily skin.

☹ **Purifying Facial Mask** *($23.50 for 1.7 ounces)* is a standard clay mask that also contains several ingredients that are problematic for oily skin, including plant oils and rice starch, plus skin irritants like arnica and peppermint.

☹ **Revitalizing Mask** *($39.50 for 1.7 ounces)* lists sodium hydroxide (lye) as the fifth ingredient, which means this product leaves much to be desired for skin.

☺ $$$ **Whitening Cleansing Milk** *($24 for 6.8 ounces)* is almost identical to the Gentle Cleansing Milk above except for the addition of a minute amount of algae and mallow extract, although neither of those can have any effect, in any amount, on skin color.

☺ $$$ **Whitening Day Cream** *($41 for 1.7 ounces)* does contain some of the more popular "natural" ingredients for inhibiting melanin production, including kojic acid, licorice extract, and mulberry extract. In the amount they are used in this formula, however, it is doubtful they would have any effect on skin. Regardless, no whitening product can produce positive results without an effective sunscreen, and Phytomer doesn't have anything to offer in that regard.

☺ $$$ **Whitening Night Cream** *($52 for 1.7 ounces)* is similar to the Whitening Day Cream and the same review applies.

☺ $$$ **Whitening Mask** *($57 for seven treatments)*. There are no melanin-inhibiting ingredients in this mask, which makes it useless for the purpose of lightening skin. Other than that, it is merely citric acid with baking soda, titanium dioxide, and algae. Titanium dioxide can make the skin *look* white, but it can't do anything to the color of skin itself.

☺ **After-Sun Reconditioning Cream, for Face and Body** *($26 for 4.4 ounces)* is an emollient moisturizer for normal to dry skin. It contains a small amount of tyrosine, which cannot stimulate melanin production in skin. There is nothing in this product that will repair skin from the damage caused by unprotected sun exposure.

☺ **After Sun Soothing Lotion** *($33 for 4.2 ounces)* is just water, salt water, glycerin, slip agent, preservatives, castor oil, fragrance, and algae. Your skin would be far better off with just some aloe you buy from the health food store than with this ordinary, do-nothing toner.

☺ $$$ **Intensive Self-Tanning Spray** *($33.50 for 4.23 ounces)* contains dihydroxy-acetone, the same ingredient all self-tanners use to affect the color of skin. This one would work as well as any.

☺ $$$ **Rapid Self-Tanning Gel** *($31 for 1.7 ounces)* contains dihydroxyacetone, the same ingredient all self-tanners use to affect the color of skin. This version contains a higher concentration than most, which creates a rapid tan.

☹ $$$ **Absolute Solar Protection SPF 30** *($33.50 for 2 ounces)* is an in-part tita-nium dioxide–based sunscreen in an ordinary emollient base. However, this also contains Kathon CG, a preservative not recommended for use in leave-on skin-care products.

☹ $$$ **High Protection Lotion SPF 15** *($32.50 for 4.2 ounces)* is similar to the Absolute Solar version above, only with an SPF 15, though the same comments apply.

☹ **Moisturizing Sun Lotion SPF 7** *($33 for 4.25 ounces).* No one really thinks an SPF 8 is appropriate anymore, right? SPF 15 is the standard for any kind of sun product, so this one is substandard and a problem for skin.

☹ **Intensive Tanning Gel SPF 2** *($28 for 4.25 ounces)* is a product that encourages intensely tanning the skin. They've got to be kidding! This is one of the more unconscionable skin-care products in this book.

☹ **Intensive Tanning Oil SPF 4** *($33 for 4.25 ounces)* is equally as offensive as the SPF 2 Gel above and the same comments apply.

POLA

This Japanese cosmetics company was established in 1929, and started by selling a handful of products door-to-door. If you're wondering about the name, it pays homage to the silent film star Pola Negri, who, according to the International Movie Database, played earthy, exotic, strong women. Her reported romances with such prominent stars as Charlie Chaplin and Rudolph Valentino made her the Madonna of her day.

Today, Pola is Japan's top cosmetics manufacturer in the direct sales industry. (In 1998 the top Japanese cosmetics companies by market share in Japan were Shiseido 22%, Kanebo 20.2%, Kose 17%, Pola Cosmetics 10.2%, Max Factor 10%, and Kao 8.2%, with the remaining brands totaling 12.4%.) As would be true for almost any international company, Pola is interested in tackling the desirable U.S. market, much the way Shiseido and other Japanese cosmetics companies are, though Shiseido is definitely at the front of the game.

What does Pola have to offer? What you will find in this line is really a mix. There are some poorly formulated products (some with SPFs of under 15 and others with a complete lack of sun protection, alcohol-based toners, and lye-based cleansers), ordinary products (mineral oil–based wipe-off cleansers), and some very standard, almost boring, moisturizers—but all with prices that will knock you over for what you get. Some of the showcased plant extracts and hyped ingredients include algae, vitamin P (hesperidin), carrot oil, royal jelly, ginseng, placenta protein, and angelica. I've discussed the pros and cons of many of these ingredients before, but all of them are present in such minute amounts in these products that they are hardly worth mentioning, as the benefits or risks to skin are barely present. One area where Pola does have some interesting options is skin-lightening products, because they have a few products that offer interesting alternatives to the typical ones using hydroquinone or arbutin extract to reduce melanin production.

Keep in mind that as far as the cosmetics industry is concerned there isn't a plant that can't perform some kind of miracle for skin, even when it makes up less than 1% of the product. This line is no exception to the rule, and their promises are nothing less than monumental when it comes to ingredients that are barely there in these formulations. It is the other 99% of the content they never discuss—but then I guess that's my job. For more information about Pola, call 800-POLA-USA or visit www.pola.com. **Note:** All

Pola products contain fragrance unless otherwise noted. In the United States, Pola is sold primarily at specialty boutique stores, salons, and on the Internet.

POLA PLENNA LINE

☺ $$$ **Pure Skin Cleanser** *($22 for 3.5 ounces)* lists its first ingredient as mineral oil, followed by thickeners, preservatives, and fragrance. This is little more than an over-priced cold cream, and it can leave a slight greasy film on the skin, though it is an option for normal to dry skin.

☹ **Pure Clear Wash** *($22 for 4.2 ounces)* is a very run-of-the-mill, detergent-based, water-soluble cleanser that can be drying for some skin types due to the presence of potassium hydroxide (lye), which is listed as the fifth ingredient.

☹ **Pure Moist Lotion** *($24 for 5 ounces)* is a toner that lists alcohol as the third ingredient, which makes it anything but a pure moist toner; it can be drying and irritating to skin.

☹ **Freshener** *($20 for 6 ounces)* is a toner that is mostly alcohol, and that is a problem for skin.

☹ **Pure Moisturizer Day SPF 10** *($26 for 3.3 ounces)* has an SPF of 10, which does not meet the standard of SPF 15 for sun protection set by the American Academy of Dermatology and the Skin Cancer Foundation, and it is not recommended.

☺ **Pure Moisturizer Night** *($26 for 3.3 ounces)* is a mediocre moisturizer for normal to dry skin. The teeny—and I mean really teeny—amounts of algae and water-binding agents are hardly worth mentioning.

☺ $$$ **Revitalizing Essence** *($35 for 0.9 ounce)* is a basic, lightweight, silicone-based moisturizer that would be OK for someone with normal to dry skin. The minuscule amounts of plant extracts and water-binding agents are hardly detectable and will have minimal impact on skin.

☺ $$$ **Revitalizing Cream** *($28 for 1.4 ounces)* is similar to the Pure Moisturizer above, but this one does contain a small amount of vitamin C (in the form of magnesium L-ascorbic acid phosphate). That's a good antioxidant, but it is not revitalizing, nor is it enough for good skin health. Other than that, the same basic comments for the Pure Moisturizer above apply here.

☺ $$$ **Massage Mask** *($24 for 3.5 ounces)* is just mineral oil, slip agents, thickeners, preservatives, plant extracts, and fragrant plant extracts. Several of the plant extracts can be skin irritants, but just like the more soothing extracts, they are present in negligible amounts, and neither would probably have any impact on skin.

POLA VITAX LINE

☺ $$$ **Deep Clear Cleanser** *($44 for 3.5 ounces)* lists mineral oil as the first ingredient, followed by thickeners, preservatives, and fragrance. That makes this little more than an overpriced cold cream, and it can leave a slight greasy film on the skin. The handful of interesting water-binding agents and anti-irritants is nice, but the amounts are almost negligible. This can be an option for someone with dry skin.

☹ **Double Clear Wash** *($44 for 5.2 ounces)* is a very run-of-the-mill, detergent-based, water-soluble cleanser that can be drying for skin due to the presence of potassium hydroxide (lye) as the cleansing agent, which is listed high up on the ingredient list.

☺ $$$ **Smooth Up Toner Normal to Dry Skin** *($50 for 5 ounces)* is a standard toner that contains teeny amounts of some very good water-binding agents and antioxidants. You would be getting far more preservatives with this than any beneficial ingredients for your skin.

☹ **Smooth Up Toner Normal to Oily Skin** *($50 for 5 ounces)* lists alcohol as its second ingredient, which won't make skin smooth, and it can be drying and irritating on skin.

☺ $$$ **Smooth Up Milk Normal to Dry Skin** *($56 for 3.3 ounces)* is a good moisturizer for normal to dry skin. A lot of the good stuff in here (and the hyped items like royal jelly) is listed well after the preservatives in the ingredient list. That makes them barely present, though at least there are several of them, which is better than many of the products in the Pola line.

☺ $$$ **Smooth Up Milk Normal to Oily Skin** *($56 for 3.3 ounces)* is almost identical to the Smooth Up Milk Normal to Dry Skin above except this one leaves out the Vaseline, which makes it better for normal to slightly dry skin. This one would be a problem and completely unnecessary for someone with oily skin.

☺ $$$ **Vitax Balancing Essence** *($70 for 1.3 ounces)*. It would only take one application for you to notice that this product won't control oil (the silicone polymer can leave a matte feel on the skin, but that's about it). The only ingredient in this product that may affect skin discolorations is dipotassium glycyrrhizinate, but the amount is trifling and therefore it's not really capable of having an effect. Other than that, with its share of silicones (dry-finish ones) and water-binding agents, this is a good, lightweight, extremely overpriced moisturizer for someone with normal to oily skin.

☺ $$$ **Deep Moisture Essence** *($70 for 1.3 ounces)* lists quince extract as the second ingredient. Quince extract is a creamy, viscous substance that has thickening properties and some emollient properties, but because it also has some antibacterial properties it can be a skin irritant. This is a basic lightweight moisturizer with negligible amounts of water-binding and soothing agents.

☺ $$$ **Vita-Force Cream** *($68 for 1 ounce)* is an OK, though extremely overpriced, moisturizer for dry skin. It contains mostly water, slip agents, thickeners, water-binding agents, silicone, preservatives, plant extracts, and a minute amount of antioxidants.

POLA BOTANEX LINE

☺ $$$ **Wash-Off Cleanser** *($33 for 4.4 ounces)* is a very run-of-the-mill, detergent-based, water-soluble cleanser that can be drying for some skin types. It is almost identical to all the other cleansers in the varying Pola product groupings that include potassium hydroxide (lye) as one of the main cleansing agents.

The Reviews P

☺ **$$$ Cleansing Cream** *($33 for 3.5 ounces)* is similar to all the other mineral oil–based cleansers in the Pola lines. This one can leave a greasy film on the skin, but may be an option for someone with dry skin.

☹ **Toning Lotion S** *($34 for 5 ounces)* lists alcohol as the second ingredient, which makes it too drying and irritating for all skin types.

☹ **Toning Lotion R** *($34 for 5 ounces)* lists alcohol as the second ingredient, which makes it too drying and irritating for all skin types.

☺ **$$$ Extra Rich Lotion** *($37 for 5 ounces)* is not extra rich in the least. It is an extremely mundane, relatively irritant-free toner that contains water, slip agent, glycerin, plant extract, preservatives, film-forming agent, fragrance, vitamin E, and water-binding agent.

☺ **$$$ Moisture Lotion R** *($37 for 3.3 ounces)* is a good, but very standard, moisturizer for dry skin.

☺ **$$$ Moisture Lotion S** *($37 for 3.3 ounces)* is similar to the Moisture Lotion R above and the same comments apply.

☹ **Hydrating Essence** *($44 for 0.9 ounce)* lists alcohol as its third ingredient, which hardly makes this hydrating.

☺ **$$$ Emollient Cream** *($40 for 1.1 ounces)* is an OK, though extremely ordinary, moisturizer for dry skin. The handful of specialty ingredients, such as vitamin P and carrot oil, are present in such minute amounts as to be inconsequential for skin. By the way, vitamin P is a name given to hesperidin, a bioflavinoid that has antioxidant and water-binding properties for skin.

☺ **$$$ Extra Rich Cream** *($44 for 1 ounce)* is similar to the Emollient Cream above, only with plant oil and Vaseline, which does make it better for normal to dry skin and very dry skin.

☺ **$$$ Eye Cream** *($44 for 0.67 ounce)* is almost identical to the Extra Rich Cream above and the same comments apply.

☺ **$$$ Oil-Absorbing Clay Mask** *($33 for 3.5 ounces)* is a basic clay mask that would work as well as any to absorb oil. The tiny amounts of alcohol and witch hazel are unlikely to cause irritation or dryness.

☹ **Botanex Peel-Off Mask** *($38 for 3.5 ounces)* is a layer of plastic, polyvinyl alcohol, and alcohol, along with some thickeners. The teeny amounts of copper, peach kernel extract, and royal jelly make them inconsequential for skin, but the generous amount of alcohol ensures irritation and dryness.

☺ **$$$ Massage Cream** *($35 for 2.6 ounces)* is mostly just water, mineral oil, thickeners, Vaseline, water-binding agents, fragrance, and preservatives. That makes it only slightly better to consider for a massage than just plain mineral oil.

POLA LUMIERA WHITISSIMO LINE

Pola's skin-lightening products deserve some discussion. These products contain two interesting ingredients for reducing the production of melanin (the pigment agent in skin that causes brown spots). One is vitamin C, in the form of magnesium L-ascorbic acid phosphate, and the other is calcium d-pantetheine-s-sulfonate. Vitamin C is only considered effective in concentrations of more than 5%, an amount these products don't contain, and calcium d-pantetheine-s-sulfonate has only been researched in vitro (*Pigment Cell Research,* June 2000). There is no research information about how much calcium d-pantetheine-s-sulfonate is required to be effective. Because of the limited research about whether or not these ingredients work, the decision to try these products is up to you in terms of cost and value for skin. To say the least, there are other far less expensive products for skin lightening than these. And remember, even the benefits of effective skin lighteners will be cancelled out without the diligent application of sunscreen.

☹ **Cleansing Clear** (*$48 for 4.2 ounces*) is a mineral oil–based, cold cream–style cleanser that is an option for dry skin. It contains many of the ingredients mentioned above for skin lightening. However, it also contains peppermint, an unnecessary skin irritant.

☹ **Wash Clear** (*$48 for 4.2 ounces*) is almost identical to all the other cleansers in the varying Pola product groupings, as it includes potassium hydroxide (lye) as one of the main cleansing agents. It is too drying and irritating for all skin types, and this version also contains peppermint, which adds even more irritation to the mix.

☹ **Milky White Day** (*$66 for 2 ounces*) does not have an SPF rating, although it does contain sunscreen ingredients. Without an SPF number there is no way you can rely on this for sun care of any kind, and it is not recommended.

☺ **$$$ Milky White Night** (*$72 for 2 ounces*) contains magnesium L-ascorbic acid and calcium d-pantetheine-s-sulfonate in an emollient base, which gives it the potential for reducing brown skin discolorations.

☺ **$$$ Cream White** (*$132 for 1 ounce*) contains magnesium L-ascorbic acid and calcium d-pantetheine-s-sulfonate in an emollient base, which give it the potential for reducing brown skin discolorations. Given that the Milky White Night moisturizer above has the same ingredients for skin lightening with no other significant differences, why spend the money on this one?

☺ **$$$ Essence White** (*$132 for 0.8 ounce*) contains magnesium L-ascorbic acid and calcium d-pantetheine-s-sulfonate in an emollient base, which gives it the potential for reducing brown skin discolorations. Given that the Milky White Night moisturizer above has the same ingredients for skin lightening, with no other significant differences, why spend the money on this one?

☹ **Lotion White** (*$59 for 5 ounces*) lists alcohol as the second ingredient, and that makes this too drying and irritating for all skin types.

☹ **Lotion White Extra** (*$116 for 3 ounces*) is similar to the Lotion White above and the same comments apply.

☹ **Pack White** (*$66 for 3.5 ounces*) is a mask that lists "plastic" as its second ingredient and alcohol as the fourth ingredient. The titanium dioxide in this product is what gives it its white appearance. As a basic, peel-off mask it will work as well as any, but it can be irritating to skin and that won't help skin color.

☹ **White Shot** *($175 for 0.9 ounce).* If the price tag didn't make you choke, you will have another chance when you realize that this product doesn't even contain any of the potentially effective ingredients for lightening brown discolorations that the other products in this group do! In addition, the third ingredient in this product is alcohol, which makes this more a shot of dryness and irritation than anything else.

POLA 1/F LINE

☹ **1/f White Wash** *($30 for 4.2 ounces)* is almost identical to the other detergent-based cleansers in the other Pola product groupings because it contains a significant amount of lye as one of the cleansing agents. It can be drying for most skin types.

☹ **1/ f White Lotion** *($38 for 5 ounces)* lists alcohol as its second ingredient; that won't control oil and it can cause dryness and irritation.

☹ **1/f White Sheet Essence** *($48 for 60 sheets)* lists alcohol as its third ingredient, which can cause dryness and irritation. It contains no ingredients known to reduce skin discolorations.

☺ **$$$ 1/f Sunscreen Face SPF 30** *($24 for 1 ounce)* is a very good, pure titanium dioxide–based sunscreen in a rather basic, lightweight moisturizing base that would be good for normal to slightly dry skin.

☺ **$$$ 1/f Suncut Milk SPF 30** *($24 for 1 ounce)* is a very good, in-part titanium dioxide– and zinc oxide–based sunscreen in a very ordinary moisturizing base.

☺ **$$$ 1/f White Gel Cream** *($48 for 1.4 ounces).* While this is a good, though basic, moisturizer for dry skin, it only contains a form of vitamin C with little to no research showing it to be effective for skin discolorations.

☺ **$$$ 1/f White Moisturizer** *($40 for 3.3 ounces)* is similar to the Gel Cream above, only this one contains mineral oil and silicone, which makes it better for dry to very dry skin. The other comments above about lack of skin lighteners apply here as well.

☹ **1/f White Mask** *($40 for 3.5 ounces)* is a standard plastic peel-off mask. Polyvinyl alcohol is the plastic that is used, and this also contains menthol, and none of that is helpful for skin. Except for a minuscule amount of vitamin C, this doesn't contain anything that can lighten skin.

POLA ALL LIFT LINE

☹ **$$$ Ex Essence** *($132 for 0.7 ounce)* is a lightweight lotion with some plant oil and tiny amounts of water-binding agents and antioxidants. For the money, this should be totally overflowing with antioxidants, water-binding agents, and anti-irritants, but it ends up shortchanging skin on all accounts.

☹ **$$$ Ex Lotion** *($75 for 2.7 ounces)* lists alcohol as the third ingredient, and that makes it too potentially irritating and drying for all skin types.

☹ **Ex Firming Cream** *($76 for 2.9 ounces).* The fourth ingredient listed is witch hazel distillate, and that contains a good deal of alcohol. Aside from that, this is an ordinary mix of silicones, slip agents, thickeners, preservatives, film-forming agents, and a shocking number of potentially irritating plant extracts, including eucalyptus, fennel, ivy, coltsfoot, yarrow, and menthol.

☺ $$$ **Ex Massage** *($107 for 2.8 ounces)* contains mostly mineral oil, waxes, preservatives, and fragrance. This just about wins the prize for the most overpriced bottle of mineral oil you will ever find. The minuscule amounts of vitamin E and ginseng are more of a joke on the consumer than anything capable of benefiting skin.

POLA ESTINA LINE

☹ **Clear Mild Cleansing** *($72 for 3.5 ounces)* is an overpriced, mineral oil–based cleanser that is more of a cold cream than anything else. There isn't a single ingredient in it that warrants even a fraction of this product's price tag, though the peppermint can be a skin irritant.

☹ **Clear Mild Wash** *($69 for 4.2 ounces)* is identical to almost all of Pola's detergent-based cleansers. It lists potassium hydroxide as the fifth ingredient, and that makes it too potentially irritating and drying for all skin types.

☺ $$$ **Bright Up Lotion I** *($76 for 4 ounces)* contains mostly water, glycerin, slip agents, preservatives, castor oil, water-binding agents, and plant extracts. Any potentially interesting ingredients are scarcely present and can have little to no benefit for skin.

☺ $$$ **Bright Up Lotion II** *($76 for 4 ounces)* is almost identical to the Bright Up Lotion above only minus the castor oil, and the same basic comments apply.

☺ $$$ **Bright Up Cream** *($89 for 1 ounce)* is an emollient, though exceptionally ordinary, moisturizer for normal to dry skin. It does contain some good water-binding agents, but only a minuscule amount of one antioxidant. This is hardly worth the trouble, even if it were free.

☺ $$$ **Bright Up Essence** *($119 for 0.8 ounces)* contains mostly water, glycerin, slip agents, film-forming agent, preservatives, and water-binding agents. The bovine gland extract won't brighten up skin or benefit skin in any way beyond being an OK water-binding agent.

☺ $$$ **Bright Up Milk I** *($85 for 2.7 ounces)* is an emollient, though basic, moisturizer that contains mostly water, slip agent, plant oils, thickeners, Vaseline, fragrance, more thickeners, film-forming agents, water-binding agents, and vitamin E. It's an option for dry skin, but not worth the cost.

☺ $$$ **Bright Up Milk II** *($85 for 2.7 ounces)* is similar to the Bright Up Milk I above except that it contains more Vaseline, making it better for dry skin—but it is still just a fairly ordinary moisturizer.

☺ $$$ **Bright Up Massage** *($76 for 3.5 ounces)* is similar to the Bright Up Milk I above and the same basic comments apply. However, this does contain a small amount of peppermint, which can be irritating for skin.

☹ **Mild Freshener** *($32 for 6 ounces)* lists alcohol as its second ingredient, and that is too irritating and drying for all skin types.

☹ **Bright Up Pack** *($119 for 3.5 ounces).* The third ingredient is quince, which can be a skin irritant. Other than that, this is just a basic moisturizer lacking any significant amounts of water-binding agents or antioxidants.

POLA POLISSIMA LINE

☹ **Aqua Clean** *($77 for 4.2 ounces)* is a standard, detergent-based cleanser similar to almost every single other Pola cleanser. Potassium hydroxide is one of the main cleansing agents, making this potentially too irritating and drying for all skin types.

☺ **$$$ Cleansing Cream** *($77 for 3.5 ounces)* is a plant oil–based cold cream that contains a small amount of mink oil. There is no special benefit for skin from using mink oil versus any other animal oil. This also contains a teeny amount of placental extract, which can be a water-binding agent for skin, but it holds no other special property despite its allusion to youth.

☹ **Facial Freshener, Mild** *($40 for 6 ounces)* lists alcohol as the second ingredient, and that makes this too drying and irritating for all skin types.

☹ **Toning Lotion R** *($77 for 4 ounces)* lists alcohol as the second ingredient, and that makes this too drying and irritating for all skin types. Even without the alcohol, there is nothing in this product to warrant the price tag. All of the interesting anti-irritants and water-binding agents in the ingredient list come well after the fragrance and preservatives, so you know they amount to only a minuscule percentage of this product.

☹ **Toning Lotion S** *($77 for 4 ounces)* is similar to the Toning Lotion R above and the same comments apply.

☺ **$$$ Cold Cream N** *($77 for 2.4 ounces)* is as, the name states, a standard cold cream made of plant oils and lanolin. It is an option for normal to dry skin, but the price is absurd for such a simple formula. The teeny amounts of water-binding agents and antioxidants are barely even detectable.

☺ **$$$ Emollient Cream R** *($90 for 1 ounce)* is a very emollient moisturizer for very dry skin, but the price is ludicrous for such a basic formulation. Mink oil holds no special moisturizing properties for skin.

☺ **$$$ Emollient Cream S** *($90 for 1 ounce)* is similar to the Emollient Cream R above and the same comments apply.

☺ **$$$ Moisture Milk R** *($90 for 3 ounces)* is similar to the Emollient Cream R above, only without the mink oil. The same basic comments apply.

☺ **$$$ Moisture Milk S** *($90 for 3 ounces)* is an OK moisturizer for normal to dry skin, but there is nothing in it that makes it worth the expense.

☹ **Creamy Pack** *($90 for 3.5 ounces)* is creamy, but it is also just an ordinary moisturizer with a tiny amount of placental protein, garlic, vitamin E, and anti-irritant. Unfortunately, this product lists quince seed extract high up on the ingredient list, and that can be a skin irritant.

The Reviews P

POLA BA BIO ACTIVE

☺ $$$ **Cream B.A.** *($382 for 1 ounce)* contains mostly water, mineral oil, thickeners, water-binding agents, plant extracts, preservatives, silicones, fragrance, antioxidant (vitamin E), and film-forming agent. The plant extracts are mulberry and barley. Mulberry may have some skin-lightening properties, but probably not when present in such a small amount. Barley extract has no research showing it to have benefit for skin. Then there's a small amount of yeast protein (it can be a water-binding agent) and birch bark (which can be a skin irritant). It also contains the skin-lightening agent calcium-pantetheine-sulfonate, but the amount is so minute as to be insignificant for skin. The colossal price tag ends up being the most impressive thing about this otherwise OK moisturizer for dry skin.

☺ $$$ **Eye Moist B.A.** *($165 for 0.5 ounce)* lists alcohol as the fourth ingredient, and that does not mean moisture for skin. Other than that, it has merely a dusting of several water-binding agents and antioxidants. It has more Vaseline and sodium hydroxide (that's lye) than it does any beneficial ingredients.

POLA PRESSED POWDER

☺ $$$ **SunPowder SPF 15** *($40)* is a standard pressed powder that comes in only one color, Translucent—and it is fairly translucent. It does have an in-part titanium dioxide–based sunscreen, which is good, too, but for the money Neutrogena's SPF 30 Pressed Powder ($14.29), with a pure titanium dioxide–based sunscreen, is a far better option.

POND'S (SKIN CARE ONLY)

Pond's has been around since 1846, when Theron T. Pond founded the firm. Pond's Cold Cream was created in 1918, and it hasn't changed much since then—even today most cold creams still follow that original basic formula. Unilever bought Chesebrough Pond's in 1987. Since then, Pond's has launched a mixed bag of products, but it is a contender in some areas, particularly cleansers and lightweight moisturizers. Where it falls down is with several irritating products for blemish-prone skin, poorly formulated sunscreens, and some dated moisturizers that seem to be stuck in a time warp. For more information about Pond's, call (800) 743-8640 or visit www.ponds.com. **Note:** All Pond's products contain fragrance.

☺ **Cleansing and Make-Up Remover Towelettes** *($5.99 for 30 towelettes)* are towelettes with a cleansing agent, some anti-irritants, fragrance, and preservatives. These will remove makeup and work as well as any of the wipe-off cleansers being sold.

☺ **Age Defying Cleansing Towelettes** *($6.99 for 30 towelettes)*. As a facial cleanser these towelettes leave much to be desired. They place a somewhat sticky residue on the skin, which is not the best idea for a cleanser. They do have a good concentration of glycolic acid (AHA), so the claim that this product contains alpha hydroxy acids is true (though Pond's uses the term "alpha hydroxy," leaving off the word "acid" so as not to worry its consumer base that they're putting acid on their face). However, in a cleanser with a pH of 5 the glycolic acid is not effective as an exfoliant, which is what AHAs are all about. This product does contain a small amount of retinol, other antioxidants, and some good anti-irritants, but they will not remain stable for long in this kind of packaging.

☺ **Clear Cold Cream** *($4.99 for 4 ounces)* is a clear, thick version of regular opaque, white cold cream. Neither the clear nor the white version can be rinsed away; they need to be wiped off and can leave a slight residue on the skin. This can be an option for dry skin.

☺ **Cold Cream Deep Cleanser** *($5.49 for 6.1 ounces)* is a classic cold cream of mineral oil and waxes. It is emollient and can leave a slight greasy residue, but it can be an option for very dry skin.

☹ **Clear Solutions Deep Pore Foaming Cleanser Normal to Oily Skin** *($5.99 for 6 ounces)* is a standard, detergent-based, water-soluble cleanser that uses sodium C14-16 olefin sulfate as one of the main cleansing agents, which is far too drying and irritating for the skin.

☹ **Fresh Start Daily Wash** *($5.99 for 5 ounces)* contains menthol, and the red scrubber beads that it contains can feel irritating on skin.

☺ **Foaming Cleanser & Toner in One Normal to Oily Skin** *($4.69 for 4 ounces)* is a good, though standard, detergent-based, water-soluble cleanser that can take off all your makeup without causing irritation. It is a good option for normal to oily skin.

☺ **Cleansing Lotion & Moisturizer in One Normal to Dry Skin** *($3.99 for 4 ounces)* is a water-soluble cleanser that doesn't remove makeup all that well without the help of a washcloth, though it can be good when you aren't wearing makeup, or for someone with dry skin.

☺ **Clear Solutions Deep Pore Scrub** *($5.69 for 3 ounces)* is a standard, detergent-based, water-soluble cleanser that uses ground-up plastic (polyethylene) as the scrub material. It is an option for topical exfoliation for normal to oily skin.

☹ **Clear Solutions Pore Clarifying Astringent** *($4.39 for 7 ounces)* is a problem waiting to happen. It contains mostly water, alcohol, witch hazel distillate, menthol, and eucalyptus oil. Ouch!

☺ **Age Defying Complex Cream** *($10.99 for 2 ounces)* is a very good, 8% glycolic acid (AHA) exfoliant in a standard emollient base that would be an option for normal to dry skin. It does contain several forms of vitamin A, including retinol, but they are not stable in the jar-type packaging this comes in.

☺ **Age Defying Complex Cream for Delicate Skin** *($10.49 for 2 ounces)* is a good AHA product similar to the Age Defying Complex Cream above, only this one contains about 4% AHA. This version does contain sunscreen ingredients, but the SPF is only about 4 and there are no UVA-protecting ingredients.

☺ **Age Defying Lotion** *($10.99 for 3 ounces)* is similar to the Age Defying Complex Cream above only in lotion form and with 4% AHA. The same basic comments apply.

☺ **Age Defying Lotion for Delicate Skin** *($12.49 for 3 ounces)* is similar to the Complex Cream for Delicate Skin above, only in lotion form, and with about 4% AHA. The same comments apply.

☹ **Age Defying Eye Cream SPF 8** *($10.29 for 0.5 ounce)* contains about 2% to 3% glycolic acid in a very lightweight, standard moisturizing base, but the sunscreen agent has a too-low SPF rating and lacks UVA-protecting ingredients.

☹ **Prevent and Correct Cream Age Defying System SPF 15** *($13.69 for two products, totaling 2.5 ounces)* is simply a repackaging of the Age Defying Complex AHA cream and a sunscreen. The sunscreen part is called Prevent, but it doesn't contain the UVA-protecting ingredients of avobenzone, zinc oxide, or titanium dioxide, and is not recommended. You can buy a good SPF 15 sunscreen and buy the Age Defying Complex individually for less, and get more of both.

☹ **Prevent and Correct Lotion Age Defying System SPF 15** *($13.69 for 4.25 ounces)* is identical to the Prevent and Correct Cream version above, only in lotion form.

☺ **Clear Solutions Combination Skin Moisturizer** *($6.99 for 4 ounces)*. As a combination AHA (about 4% to 5% lactic acid) and BHA (about 0.5%) product, this is a good option. Some of the plant extracts can be skin irritants, but it also contains some good water-binding agents and antioxidants.

☺ **Dramatic Results Advanced Anti-Aging Care Active Face & Neck Moisturizer** *($13.24 for 1.7 ounces)* is a well-formulated, 8% to 10% glycolic acid product in a matte-finish base that would be best for someone with normal to slightly dry or slightly oily skin. The pH of 3.5 and the concentration of AHA ensures that you will get the exfoliation this kind of product is supposed to provide but often doesn't. It does contain a small amount of antioxidants (including retinol), which is nice, but the matte finish is most appropriate for normal to slightly dry or slightly oily skin.

☺ **Dramatic Results Anti-Wrinkle Cream** *($14.99 for 1.25 ounces)* is similar to the Dramatic Results Advanced Anti-Aging version above, and the same comments apply.

☺ **Dry Skin Cream, Extra Rich Skin Cream** *($3.99 for 3.3 ounces)* is a standard, mineral oil– and Vaseline-based moisturizer with thickeners and preservatives. It would be good for dry skin, but its ingredients are very ordinary and dated for any product that calls itself moisturizing.

☺ **Nourishing Moisturizer Cream** *($5.99 for 2 ounces)* can't nourish the skin and it definitely isn't oil-free, but it is a good moisturizer for normal to dry skin. The teeny amounts of vitamins and water-binding agents are barely worth mentioning.

☺ **Nourishing Moisturizer Lotion** *($4.69 for 4 ounces)* is similar to the Cream version above only in lotion form, and the same comments apply.

☺ **Nourishing Moisture Lotion with SPF 15** *($5.99 for 2.5 ounces)* won't nourish anyone's skin, but it does contain a good, in-part titanium dioxide–based sunscreen with an SPF of 15 in a lightweight moisturizing base with a tiny amount of antioxidants and water-binding agents for normal to dry skin.

☺ **Overnight Replenishing Cream** *($5.99 for 2 ounces)* is similar to the Nourishing Moisturizer Cream above, and the same comments apply.

☺ **$$$ Revitalizing Eye Capsules for Delicate Eye Area** *($10.99 for 20 capsules totaling 0.26 ounce)* are capsules that contain silicones, slip agents, antioxidants, and a small amount of water-binding agent. If you want a lightweight silky moisturizer for slightly dry skin, this one is a fine option.

☺ **$$$ Skin Smoothing Capsules** *($10.99 for 26 capsules totaling 0.33 ounce)* is similar to the Revitalizing Eye Capsules above and the same comments apply.

☹ **Revitalizing Eye Gel with Vitamin E** *($4.69 for 0.5 ounce)*. Witch hazel distillate is the second ingredient, and it contains a lot of alcohol, making this drying and irritating for skin, particularly around the eyes.

☺ **Soothing Cucumber Eye Treatments** *($8.99 for 24 pads)* is a very lightweight gel with a tiny amount of cucumber extract and other plant extracts that have anti-irritant properties. It also contains some good antioxidants. The tiny amount of orange peel is more for fragrance than anything else. This isn't the most convenient way to apply a lightweight moisturizer, but these pads are an option for normal to slightly dry skin.

☹ **Clear Solutions Overnight Blemish Reducers** *($5.99 for 24 dots)* are patches coated with film-forming agent (a hairspray-like ingredient), 0.5% BHA and about the same quantity of AHA, as well as some plant extracts, tea tree oil, and slip agents. The AHA and BHA are useless as exfoliants because the pH is too high (not to mention that 0.5% is too small an amount for BHA to have any effectiveness). Tea tree oil can be an alternative to benzoyl peroxide as a disinfectant, but probably not at such a low concentration. Plus, the film-forming agent can be problematic for skin. There are far better ways to treat acne, but I imagine teenagers will find this product way too tempting to pass up.

☺ **Clear Solutions Clear Pore Strips, Assorted** *($8.99 for 12 strips)* and **Clear Solutions Clear Pore Strips, Nose** *($4.99 for 6 strips)* are Pond's version of Biore Strips and they work about the same, which isn't great. The strip material has a sticky substance on one side, and that's what you press on your skin, wait a few minutes, and then rip it off. Along with some amount of skin, blackheads are supposed to stick to it and come right out of the skin on your nose. The main ingredient is a film-forming agent, a type of hairspray ingredient. These strips are accompanied by a strong warning not to use them over any area other than the nose and not to use them over inflamed, swollen, sunburned, or excessively dry skin. Can this product be helpful? Only momentarily, but if you use the Pond's Pore Strips regularly, the film-forming agent can get into the pores and possibly cause irritation.

POSNER (MAKEUP ONLY)

Posner is a line of cosmetics designed for women of color. My original impression of this line when I first saw it years ago was unfavorable. Moreover the line was poorly distributed, at least when compared to front-runners like Black Opal. It turns out my initial impression was fairly accurate, because this ranks as one of the most disappointing, poorly formulated makeup lines, regardless of skin tone or ethnicity. Almost without exception, product after product left me bemoaning the sorry state of affairs that reigns in so many lines aimed at women with darker skin tones or, specifically, at African-American women. The bottom line is that despite Posner's assertions, there is nothing about their makeup that is better for women of color. If you happen to be in a drugstore that carries Posner and Black Opal, a quick comparison of the colors right in front of you will speak volumes about why Posner is a line to avoid. However, although the outlook sounds bleak, there are a few possibilities, and the prices are exceedingly low. Think of shopping Posner for some good accessories, but not a whole makeup wardrobe. For more information about Posner, call Carson Consumer Affairs at (800) 442-4643.

FOUNDATION: ☹ **Cream Foundation Stick** *($5.39)* is packaged so that you cannot see the colors, and even though there are some OK options, the formula is a confused mix of emollients, waxes, and absorbents. What this amounts to is an overall greasy-feeling foundation that has a slightly grainy matte finish. Elizabeth Arden and Estee Lauder have far better stick foundations that feature colors for darker skin. **Cream-to-Powder Makeup for All Skin Types** *($5.89)* has a better texture, application, and finish than the Foundation Stick above, but the colors! Posner should be ashamed of providing African-American skin tones with such peachy orange hues that make a woman with golden brown skin look like she has overdosed on vitamin A. Golden Bronze is the only realistic option to consider. **Cream Foundation** *($5.39)* is exceptionally greasy and only for those with dry skin who can find a potential shade among the five unworthy, coppery red options. Again, Golden Bronze is the only salvageable color.

☺ **100% Oil-Free Makeup** *($4.39)* starts out fluid and light, and blends down to a fairly dry matte finish. This provides sheer to light coverage and is available in nine mostly unimpressive shades. Avoid Toffee, Nut Brown, Tender Tan, and Golden Bronze. Copper Sand is slightly peach, but sheer enough to work for tan skin tones. Toasted Almond and Bare Tan are considerably light for a line that caters to darker skin tones.

POWDER: ☺ **Finishing Touch Pressed Powder for All Skin Types** *($4.39)* has a lovely soft, talc-based texture and sheer application, along with some surprisingly excellent colors, each laced with a small amount of sparkles. Why these need random sparkles is beyond me, but they're not too distracting. Of the nine shades, avoid Fresh Apricot, Hot Chocolate, Red Amaretto, and Copper Tan.

☺ **Finishing Touch Translucent Pressed Powder** *($4.39)* is also talc-based and noticeably shinier than the powder above. The colors are attractive, though Deep is too red for most dark skin tones. You can find textures that are more elegant available from lines like Clinique and Black Opal, but this is a consideration. **Maximum Coverage Powder** *($4.99)* is just as shiny as the Translucent Pressed Powder, but this talc- and cornstarch-based pressed powder has a drier, more powdery texture. Within the four shades, only Light/Medium and Medium are workable options. **Finishing Touch Translucent Loose**

Powder *($4.95)* is a talc- and mineral oil–based powder that feels very soft but does little to hold back excess oil. There are two shades, and Medium/Deep is too rosy red for most dark skin tones.

☺ BLUSH: **Natural Blush** *($4.95)* comes in a limited selection of colors, but is an acceptable powder blush with a smooth application and a few matte shades. Avoid the overtly shiny Golden Ginger.

☹ EYESHADOW: **Eye Shadow Collection** *($3.99)* eyeshadows have a slick, waxy feel and, except for the shine, don't show up as strongly on dark skin tones as they should. NARS, Prescriptives, and Trish McEvoy shadows cost more, but their performance and pigmentation far surpass this.

☺ EYE AND BROW SHAPER: **Eye Pencil** *($1.99)* is your everyday needs-sharpening pencil, but this one has a distinctly attractive price and competes nicely in the realm of creamy pencils.

☺ LIPSTICK AND LIP PENCIL: **Moisturizing Lipstick** *($3.99)* showcases some rich, bold colors, but this is quite the greasy lipstick that tends to slide around and will definitely migrate into lines around the mouth. I would suggest Revlon or L'Oreal full-coverage formulas before this one, unless you prefer overly greasy lipstick. **Plexi Shine Lips** *($4.50)* is fine and, dare I say, cheap for a moist, moderately sticky lip gloss. It's not as smooth as many others, but does the job when it comes to adding gleaming iridescence to lips. **Lip Pencil** *($2.99)* needs regular sharpening and has a rather dry texture and mediocre colors that don't fully complement the selection of Posner lipsticks.

☹ MASCARA: **Lash Supreme Mascara** *($3.99)* is an all-out dud, and seriously misnamed. This provides little in the way of lash enhancement regardless of your prerequisites.

PRADA BEAUTY

Only a few names in the fashion industry automatically command widely recognized status and elan, and Prada is one of them. Whether it is a calfskin handbag costing $650, or four-inch high-heeled leather boots for $780, or a suede belt for $280, the Prada image is one of extravagance, sleek elegance, and haute couture, and the logo exudes the glamour of wearing fashion accessories costing almost as much as a mortgage payment. Prada is an Italian designer line that has entered the world of skin care with a certain panache that is practically a stand-alone in the cosmetics industry. But leave it to a fashion house to be more concerned about packaging (what's on the outside) than content (what's on the inside).

Under the guise that skin-care products need to travel well and be hygienic, Prada Beauty products are packaged primarily in individual capsules, tiny tubes, and small packets for single-use application. The idea was to offer high-tech packaging that mimics the pharmaceutical industry, with unit dose applications secured in airtight containers. As clever as that sounds, the packaging ends up being far less user friendly than you can ever imagine. Having to open these packages every time you want to use a product is time consuming and wasteful. Plus, if you don't use the product up, there is no way to easily save it because the packaging doesn't roll up or store well, if at all. Finally, these hermetically sealed containers must offer no other freshness benefit, because Prada uses the same preservatives in the same percentages as the rest of the industry. It's also hard to believe that Prada came up with packaging that is actually quite unattractive.

Apart from the packaging, there isn't much to discuss about these overpriced, rather basic formulations. There are some good moisturizers to consider, but the price is out of line for what you get. Most surprising is that several of the products contain significant skin irritants. On a more serious note, the sunscreens are beyond expensive, which means most people would not be applying them liberally and that would result in not getting the protection indicated by the SPF number on the label, which is dangerous for skin. It is an understatement to say that there are far less expensive skin-care products available that are better formulated than these. Even if money is no object, there are other fully as expensive and better-formulated skin-care products than these. For more information about Prada Beauty, visit www.neimanmarcus.com. (As this book went to press the Web site www.prada.com was still under construction.) **Note:** All Prada Beauty skin-care products contain fragrance.

☺ **$$$ Purifying Gel/Face** *($50 for 3.4 ounces)* is a standard, detergent-based cleanser that is an option for normal to oily skin, but there isn't a single aspect about this product that warrants the accompanying price tag.

☹ **$$$ Purifying Milk/Face** *($60 for 5 ounces)* is a mineral oil–based cleanser that also contains some plant oil, Vaseline, and lanolin. This is an exceedingly average cold cream–style cleanser that can be an option for normal to dry skin.

☹ **Purifying Toner/Face** *($60 for 5 ounces)* lists alcohol as both the second and third ingredients! That's just shocking! Plus this contains peppermint, menthol, and camphor, which are all seriously irritating and drying for skin.

☹ **Soothing Concentrate/Face** *($130 for 15 packets each containing 0.1 ounce for a total of 1.5 ounces)*. With alcohol as the third ingredient, this spray-on toner is not soothing in the least. It is one of the most boring and absurdly expensive products I've reviewed in this entire book. It lacks any water-binding agents or antioxidants and would be a waste of money and time at any price.

☹ **$$$ Reviving Balm/Eye/Neck** *($95 for 6 packets each containing 0.04 ounce for a total of 0.24 ounce)* contains mostly lanolin, Vaseline, castor oil, plant oils, a teeny amount of antioxidants, and preservatives. This is an emollient balm for dry skin, but it is almost mind-numbing how ordinary a moisturizer this is.

☹ **$$$ Reviving Concentrate/Face** *($130 for 15 packages each containing 0.04 ounce for a total of 0.6 ounce)* contains mostly thickener, silicones, Vaseline, and antioxidants. This is an OK moisturizer for normal to dry skin, but it is easily replaced with formulations from a number of lines that are far more impressive.

☺ **$$$ Reviving Cream/Eye** *($95 for 36 packages each containing 0.001 ounce for a total of 0.08 ounce)* is an OK moisturizer for dry skin that contains mostly water, castor oil, glycerin, thickeners, silicone, slip agent, plant oil, water-binding agent, preservatives, a minute amount of antioxidants, and more preservatives. The tiny amount of lactic acid has no exfoliating properties. When you do the math this product ends up costing about $1,140 for about 1 ounce. This wins as the most expensive, ordinary product that the cosmetics industry has launched to date.

☹ **$$$ Reviving Bio-Firm Moisture SPF 15/Face** *($95 for 1.7 ounces)* is a good, in-part avobenzone-based sunscreen, but the third ingredient is alcohol, and that makes it too potentially drying and irritating for all skin types, especially for the face. It does contain some very good water-binding agents and antioxidants, but that can't make up for what the alcohol will do to the skin.

☹ **Shielding Concentrate SPF 12/Face** *($90 for 15 packets each containing 0.04 ounce for a total of 0.6 ounce).* Not only does this have a substandard SPF of 12, but the second ingredient is alcohol, and that is too irritating and drying for all skin types. It would take more than one packet to apply this liberally enough to even achieve the protection of the SPF on the label.

☺ **$$$ Soothing Cream/Face** *($90 for 20 packets each containing 0.04 ounce for a total of 0.8 ounce)* is an exceedingly ordinary moisturizer for normal to dry skin.

☹ **Soothing Gel/Eye** *($95 for 36 packets each containing 0.013 ounce for a total of 0.468 ounce).* With alcohol as the fourth ingredient and a minimal amount of water-binding agents, this is a complete waste of money.

☺ **$$$ Hydrating Cream/Face** *($90 for 1.7 ounces)* is an ordinary moisturizer for normal to dry skin with minute amounts of water-binding agents and antioxidants.

☹ **Hydrating Gel Cream/Face** *($90 for 1.7 ounces).* The first ingredient is alcohol! Calling this product hydrating is just unbelievable.

☺ **$$$ Hydrating Serum/Face** *($90 for 1.7 ounces)* is a lightweight lotion that contains some very good water-binding agents, though it lacks any antioxidants. It turns out that this is the best Prada has to offer, and it is just above average.

☹ **Exfoliating Concentrate/Face** *($130 for 15 packets each containing 0.04 ounce for a total of 0.6 ounce)* lists alcohol as the second ingredient, making this too irritating and drying for all skin types. Aside from the alcohol, all you are getting is water, glycerin, AHAs, thickener, fragrance, and coloring agents, which are hardly unique or special. It is understating it to say that there are far better-formulated AHA products than this for a fraction of the price.

☹ **Lightening Gel/Face** *($90 for 30 packets each containing 0.04 ounce for a total of 1.2 ounces).* The third ingredient is alcohol, and that can be drying and irritating for skin.

☹ **Lightening Concentrate/Face** *($130 for 15 packets each containing 0.06 ounce for a total of 0.9 ounce)* is similar to the Lightening Gel/Face above and the same comments apply.

922 Don't Go to the Cosmetics Counter Without Me

☺ **$$$ Lightening Serum/Eye** *($95 for 30 packets each containing 0.01 ounce for a total of 0.3 ounce).* At least this one left out the alcohol—but it also leaves out the plant extracts that have melanin-inhibiting properties. All you're left with is a small amount of vitamin C and some emollients. That isn't bad, but it ends up being just an OK moisturizer for normal to dry skin.

☺ **$$$ Exfoliating Mask/Face** *($85 for 15 packets each containing 0.1 ounce for a total of 1.5 ounces)* is a standard clay mask that also contains some talc, emu oil, thickeners, plant oil, water-binding agent, preservatives, and BHA. This is an option for oily skin, but for the most part it is just a waste of money. The salicylic acid is present in too tiny an amount to have exfoliating properties, and the emu oil does not impart special properties for skin.

☺ **$$$ Reviving Mask/Face** *($85 for 15 packets each containing 0.01 ounce for a total of 1.5 ounces)* is a basic emollient mask with a tiny amount of vitamins and soybean protein. That won't revive anyone, but it is OK for normal to dry skin.

☺ **$$$ Shielding Pack/Face** *($85 for 15 packets each containing 0.01 ounce for a total of 1.5 ounces)* is an emollient, Vaseline-based mask with a minute amount of vitamins. It is OK for dry skin, but is void of any significant or interesting ingredients for skin. It is shockingly basic and completely not worth the money.

☺ **$$$ Soothing Mask/Face** *($85 for 15 packets each containing 0.01 ounce for a total of 1.5 ounces)* is a good emollient mask for dry skin that contains some good anti-irritants, plant oils, water-binding agents, and a small amount of vitamin E.

☺ **$$$ Shielding Balm SPF 15** *($60 for 30 packets each containing 0.05 ounce for a total of 1.5 ounces)* is a good, in-part avobenzone-based sunscreen in an emollient balm that contains mostly lanolin oil, emollients, plant oils, and a teeny amount of vitamin E. It is incredibly easy to replace this with far less expensive versions, which are probably safer for skin in the long run. Because sunscreen must be applied liberally to obtain the benefit of the SPF specified on the label, you have to ask yourself how liberally you are going to apply this overly expensive sunscreen. Anything less than liberal application puts skin at risk for sun damage, no matter how good the formulation.

☺ **$$$ Shielding Balm SPF 15/Lip Tint** *($38 for 10 packets each containing 0.05 ounce for a total of 0.5 ounce)* is virtually identical to the Shielding Balm above, except that this one contains color, and the same basic comments apply, though for the lips this is easily replaced by many less expensive versions reviewed in this book that are of equal or better quality.

☹ **Shielding Cream SPF 12 Sunscreen/Lip** *($55 for 90 packets each containing 0.013 ounce for a total of 1.17 ounces)* does contain in-part avobenzone in a simple emollient moisturizing base, but the menthol it contains is a problem for the lips and can cause dryness and irritation.

PRESCRIPTIVES

Prescriptives is owned by Estee Lauder, which also owns Clinique, Origins, and many other lines that range from Bobbi Brown, M.A.C., Stila, Creme de la Mer, and Aveda to Jane at the drugstore. So where does Prescriptives appear on the map of cosmetics niche marketing? While Estee Lauder certainly appeals to the upscale baby-boomers-and-up crowd, Clinique is about the teenager to young adult, and Origins is for the plant-obsessed crowd in their twenties and thirties. That brings us to Prescriptives, which aims for the thirty-something urban sophisticate who needs a bit more scientific convincing and a slicker image. Just think of what comes to mind when you hear the name "Prescriptives." A physician's prescription, maybe? Even some of the packaging has a medical or clinical appearance, and all of the products are labeled with a Px, looking suspiciously similar to a doctor's Rx. What a great gimmick!

In terms of skin care, you'll find a mixed assortment of options, with the strong points being the same ones as those for most of the Estee Lauder companies: great moisturizers, good sunscreens, a mixed group of cleansers, toners with irritants, and a complete lack of products appropriate for blemish-prone skin. For more information about Prescriptives, call (888) 550-4567 or visit www.prescriptives.com.

PRESCRIPTIVES SKIN CARE

☺ **All Clean Fresh Foaming Cleanser** *($21 for 6.7 ounces)* is a standard, detergent-based cleanser that can be somewhat drying, but that can also work well for someone with normal to oily skin. The plant extracts are included for fragrance.

☹ **All Clean Rich Cream Cleanser** *($21 for 6.7 ounces)* is a standard, wipe-off cleanser that can leave a greasy film on the skin, though it is an option for someone with dry skin.

☹ **All Clean Sparkling Gel** *($21 for 6.7 ounces)* is a standard, detergent-based, water-soluble cleanser that contains small amounts of grapefruit, lemon oil, and spearmint oil, which can irritate the skin and eye area.

☺ **Quick Remover for Face Makeup** *($18.50 for 4.2 ounces)* is a standard, detergent-based makeup remover that would work as well as any. This does not contain fragrance.

☹ **Px Purifying Scrub** *($18.50 for 3.4 ounces)* is really more of a standard clay mask (which is one of the uses recommended) than a scrub. It also contains menthol, which can be a skin irritant.

☺ **$$$ Vibrant Scrub** *($19 for 3.4 ounces)* uses synthetic scrub particles in an emollient base that would be an option for normal to dry skin. It is also fully loaded with antioxidants, anti-irritants, melanin-inhibiting ingredients, and water-binding agents. What a shame all of that would be rinsed down the drain before they could have an effect on skin.

☹ **Flight Mist** *($20 for 4.2 ounces)* could have been a great toner with its array of water-binding agents, antioxidants, and anti-irritants, but this also contains eucalyptus, peppermint, spearmint, and grapefruit, among other irritating plant extracts that are a flight risk for skin.

☹ **Immediate Matte Skin Conditioning Tonic** *($18.50 for 6.7 ounces)* contains alcohol and peppermint, which are drying and irritating for all skin types. The only thing immediate about this product is the decision not to use it.

☹ **Immediate Glow Skin Conditioning Tonic** *($18.50 for 6.7 ounces).* Menthol can give the skin a glow, but it's also an irritant; other than that, this is just an ordinary toner.

☺ **All You Need Action Moisturizer for Dry Skin** *($40 for 1.7 ounces)* doesn't have an SPF rating, so it isn't all you need for daytime. It would be fine as a nighttime moisturizer for someone with normal to somewhat dry skin, but it's nothing exceptional. This is Prescriptives' attempt at an AHA/BHA combination product, though the pH of the base isn't low enough and the AHA/BHA concentration is too low for them to be effective as exfoliants.

☺ $$$ **All You Need Action Moisturizer for Normal Skin** *($40 for 1.7 ounces)* is similar to the Dry Skin version above, only more emollient, but the same basic review applies.

☺ $$$ **All You Need Action Moisturizer Oil-Free** *($40 for 1.7 ounces)* is similar to the Moisturizer for Normal Skin above, only this one includes more AHAs and BHA, and the pH is still too high for it to be very effective for exfoliation. It contains some very good water-binding agents and a tiny amount of an antioxidant.

✓☺ $$$ **All You Need Broad Spectrum Moisture Lotion SPF 15** *($40 for 1.7 ounces).* Finally, in 2002, Prescriptives added a sunscreen to their All You Need line of moisturizers. However, this still isn't all you need (you wouldn't want to wear sunscreen as your moisturizer for nighttime), but they have plenty of options for that "need," too. For daytime this is a very good, in-part avobenzone-based sunscreen in a lightweight, silicone-based moisturizer that would work well for normal to slightly dry skin or oily skin. It contains a very good mix of antioxidants, anti-irritants, and water-binding agents. It also contains fragrance and some plant extracts that are potential skin irritants. A rather unique ingredient in this formula is nordihydroguaiaretic acid, which is a component of some plants. There is a good amount of research showing that this substance not only has anticancer properties for skin, but also provides protection from sun damage (Sources: *British Journal of Cancer,* April 2002, pages 1188–1196; *Molecular Carcinogenesis,* June 2002, pages 102–111; and *Biochemical Pharmacology,* March 2002, pages 1165–1176). Of course, this research did not use low concentrations, such as what is included in this moisturizer, or in any cosmetic formulation for that matter, but it is nonetheless an intriguing addition.

✓☺ $$$ **All You Need Broad Spectrum Moisture Cream SPF 15** *($40 for 1.7 ounces)* is similar to the Lotion SPF 15 version above except that this one uses in-part titanium dioxide as the UVA-protecting sunscreen ingredient. It is also more emollient than the lotion and, therefore, including the titanium dioxide, is far better for dry skin. The other comments for the Lotion SPF 15 above apply here as well.

✓☺ **Px Comfort Lotion** (*$35 for 1.7 ounces*) would be a very good moisturizer for normal to dry skin that contains a good mix of water-binding agents, antioxidants, and anti-irritants.

☺ **$$$ Px Comfort Cream 24 Hour Care for Sensitive Skin** (*$37.50 for 1.7 ounces*) is a good moisturizer for someone with dry skin. Fragrant plant extracts always pose a particular irritation potential for someone with sensitive skin, but aside from that, this is a very good moisturizer for normal to dry skin, and it's brimming with water-binding agents, antioxidants, and anti-irritants.

☹ **Px Super Flight Cream** (*$35 for 1.7 ounces*) is supposed to help skin when it's subjected to the rigors of flying conditions. It is an OK, standard moisturizer for dry skin, but it contains a surprising number of potentially irritating plant extracts, including colts-foot, sage, rosemary, peppermint, spearmint, eucalyptus, and grapefruit. Ouch!

☺ **$$$ Px Retinol LSW** (*$50 for 1 ounce*) is, as the name states, a moisturizer that contains retinol. If you are interested in retinol, this would be an option, though L'Oreal's Line Eraser ($12 for 1 ounce) also contains it, and for a fraction of the price.

☺ **$$$ Px Uplift Active Firming Cream** (*$45 for 1 ounce*) is a lightweight cream with the proclaimed virtue of actively firming the skin, instantly and for the long term. Wow! That's a lot to accomplish for some pretty standard cosmetic ingredients. Despite the claims about firming and long-term moisturization, you are supposed to wear it in conjunction with Prescriptives' Super Line Preventor or All You Need Action Moisturizer, and that still leaves you without sun protection. Uplift isn't all that uplifting, but it is a good lightweight moisturizer for someone with normal to slightly dry skin.

☺ **$$$ Px Uplift Firming Eye Cream** (*$35 for 0.5 ounce*) is an OK emollient moisturizer for normal to dry skin with some good water-binding agents.

☹ **Px Blemish Specialist Fast Acting Lotion, Spot Treatment for Acne** (*$17 for 1 ounce*) is just another alcohol-based blemish product with a small amount of salicylic acid. The alcohol is too irritating and drying for skin, and that isn't helpful for any skin type.

✓☺ **$$$ Px Insulation Anti-Oxidant Vitamin Cream with SPF 15** (*$40 for 1.7 ounces*) is a very good, in-part titanium dioxide–based sunscreen in a moisturizing base for normal to dry skin that has some good water-binding agents and antioxidants.

☺ **$$$ Super Line Preventor** (*$45 for 1 ounce*) is a good moisturizer for normal to slightly dry skin, but that's about it.

☺ **$$$ Vibrant Instant Eye Brightener** (*$37.50 for 0.5 ounce*) is just a standard, lightweight moisturizer for normal to dry skin with a small amount of water-binding agents.

☺ **$$$ Vibrant Vitamin Infuser for Dull, Stressed Skin, Lotion** or **Cream** (*$45 for 1.7 ounces*) are good moisturizers for dry skin, but neither infuses the skin with anything that you won't find in lots and lots of other products. They both contain a tiny amount of mulberry root extract, which is backed by some research demonstrating it can inhibit melanin production, but not when present in such a small amount. These do contain some good water-binding agents and antioxidants, just not enough to make them an exciting pick.

PRESCRIPTIVES MAKEUP

If you're at all familiar with Prescriptives makeup, then you know their raison d'être is foundation. They were one of the first department-store lines to develop a distinctive method for determining one's exact foundation shade, using a process (since copied by other companies) called colorprinting. This technique of striping various foundation undertones on a customer's jawline supposedly allows the salesperson to determine the foundation shade that exactly matches your skin. While that is ultimately the goal, colorprinting does not replace the need to check how the foundation color looks on your skin in daylight. And figuring out which color is best only addresses one part (albeit a crucial part) of shopping for foundation. From there, you will still need to examine Prescriptives' many foundation formulas to choose the texture, application, coverage level, and finish that suit your needs and desires. The good news is that all of their foundations tip the scales toward the positive side of things. You still need to watch out for a fair number of unnatural colors, and the fact that four of the six foundations with sunscreen lack UVA protection, but otherwise there is little doubt you will be impressed. Prescriptives also excels in offering a huge selection of mostly admirable eyeshadows, blushes, and lipsticks. The color displays are well organized into what Prescriptives has termed "color families," though the products themselves are not well-organized in their "families," which can be confusing. One other distinctive feature of Prescriptives makeup is the hocus-pocus assertions within their Magic line. Agreeing with even half of what you're likely to hear about these alleged marvels may mean that you are prone to serious suspension of disbelief. More than many other makeup lines, Prescriptives prides itself on the science and technology that goes into their color. Although they have a right to be proud, you have the right to know what works and what doesn't when it comes to cosmetics trickery.

FOUNDATION: ☺ $$$ **Traceless Skin Responsive Tint SPF 8** *($32.50)*. According to the ad copy for this alleged makeup marvel, "Traceless reflects a perfect balance of light to neutralize imperfections for an undetectable finish," and is described as being "intuitive, interactive, individual." Wow factors aside, this is merely a smooth-textured foundation that blends imperceptibly into the skin, creating an extremely sheer, ultra-natural finish. That means any imperfections you were hoping to hide will simply be glossed over, so if you have a noticeably uneven skin tone or anything more than minor discolorations, you will need a more substantial foundation. The sunscreen is meager and lacks adequate UVA-protecting ingredients. A slightly shiny finish is also left on the skin, courtesy of the mica this product contains. There are only 6 shades, which is strange, as Prescriptives prides itself on its bountiful selection of foundation colors—but these neutral tones are so sheer, it's easy to see why they introduced 6 instead of 16. All of the shades will work for more than one skin tone, although this product is only for those whose skin is almost perfect. ✓☺ **Virtual Skin Super Natural Finish SPF 10** *($32.50)* has sun protection that lacks significant UVA protection and has an SPF rating that's far below par. Yet despite that downside, this is one of the most natural-looking foundations available, and the elegantly light texture blends wonderfully. The 30+ shade range is impressive, and this goes from sheer to light coverage. The only colors to avoid are Real Cameo (very pink), Real Bisque, Real Peach, and Real Fawn (all slightly peach to orange), along with Real Camellia, Real Petal, and Real Blush. (noticeably pink). ✓☺ **Photochrome Light Adjusting Compact Makeup SPF 15** *($37)* is a slick, cream-to-powder foundation with a good, titanium dioxide–based sunscreen. The claims about this one having "self-adjusting, photochromatic pigments" don't hold up in any light, but this is still a superior option for someone with normal to slightly dry skin wanting medium coverage and a short-lived powder finish. This formula blends very well, but dries quickly, calling for a deft hand when it comes to application. It is also transfer-resistant, and really holds up well throughout the day. Among the 16 shades, avoid Warm Ivory (slightly pink), Cool Desert (too rosy), and Warm Ginger (slightly orange, but may work if blended on sheer). ✓☺ **Exact Matchstick Foundation SPF 15** *($37)* is a great stick foundation that has come out ahead of many others, since this has a reliable titanium dioxide sunscreen and an SPF of 15 and a beautifully neutral range of shades. It is still only best for someone with slightly dry to slightly oily skin, as the very ingredients that keep this in solid form may clog pores. The coverage can go from sheer to full, but keep in mind that if this is blended on too sheer, the sun-protection benefit may be compromised. This dries quickly to a soft powdery finish, but tends to let a lot of shine show through on oilier areas. Of the 13 shades, watch out for Cool Shell (slightly pink), Warm Vellum and Warm Ivory (both slightly peach), and Cool Desert (peach).

☺ $$$ **100% Oil Free Matte Finish SPF 15** *($32.50)* is a traditional, true-matte finish makeup, and Prescriptives' heaviest makeup in terms of feel and coverage. However, this isn't too thick to not try it if you have oily skin and prefer medium to full coverage. A significant drawback (especially for oily skin) is the lack of adequate UVA protection. That means using a separate effective sunscreen underneath, and that will compromise this matte makeup's best qualities. Considering the plethora of shades, the colors to steer clear of include Fresh Ivory, Fresh Antelope (starts out well, but can turn orange), Fresh Fawn, Fresh Petal, Fresh Cameo, Fresh Blush, and Fresh Porcelain (slightly pink, but may be OK for some light skin tones). There are some excellent shades here for very fair skin. **Custom Blend Foundation Oil Free** *($55)* has a soft, moist feel that is similar to, but more emollient than, Prescriptives' Luxe Makeup. This is best for normal to dry skin, because, despite its name, the texture of this would not make someone with oily skin happy. **Custom Blend Foundation Moisturizing Formula** *($55)* would be great for a normal to dry skin needing light to medium coverage and it does have a creamy, moist feel on the skin. Both Custom Blend formulations are great alternatives if you are having trouble finding the ideal color out there in the world of foundations. But be patient and don't rush the process, and be sure you find a salesperson who has been doing this procedure for a while. While this may just be the best match in a foundation you've ever found, you still need to check the color in the daylight and it may take several tries until you get the shade you want. Prescriptives will reblend the color at no charge until you are satisfied with the result. In addition to creating a custom color, you can also choose additives for either formula, such as adding iridescence ("Candlelight"), or using colorless fillers to make the formula more sheer. However, this catering comes at a price.

☺ $$$ **Luxe Soft Glow Moisture Makeup SPF 15** *($32.50)* is quite similar to M.A.C.'s Hyper Real Foundation ($24) and Clinique's Gentle Light Makeup ($22.50) in that all of them are lightweight, natural-finish foundations that leave behind a subtle layer of pink or gold iridescence. The same "light-reflecting" and "makes-skin-glow-from-within" claims are attached to Luxe, but no matter how you slice it, shine is shine, and even though this is soft, it can look glaring in daylight. The sunscreen is without UVA protection so you can ignore this makeup's youthfulness claims. Among the glistening shades, consider avoiding Rich Peach, Rich Fawn, Rich Petal, Rich Cameo, Rich Blush, Rich Camellia, and Rich Rose. There are few options for very dark skin. Although this is recommended for normal to dry skin, the high talc content (it's the fifth ingredient) makes it a better option for normal to slightly dry or slightly oily skin—but think twice about adding this much shine to your routine, not to mention paying top dollar for what Prescriptives offers. **Sunsheen Bronzing Gel** *($25)* is a sheer, lotion-like bronzer laced with lots of gold sparkles for that artificially shimmering tan look that's sweeping the nation's cosmetics counters. There is no reason to consider this over similar (often seasonal) options from Revlon, Almay, or even Wet 'n' Wild.

CONCEALER: ✓☺ $$$ **Camouflage Cream** *($16.50)* has a creamy, smooth application and only a slight chance of creasing. It is definitely one of the better concealers at the department store, and it allows plenty of playtime before it dries into place. The numerous shades are divided into color families that correspond with the foundations, and each group has its weak shades. The following colors are too peach, pink, or rose to look convincing on most skin tones: Yellow/Orange Medium, Blue/Red Medium, Blue/Red Dark, Red Medium, and Red/Orange Dark. There are some excellent dark shades available that do not turn copper or ash.

☺ $$$ **Camouflage Kit Full Coverage Concealer** *($27)*. Leave it to Prescriptives to expand on the notion of putting concealer and powder together in one package. These kits contain two complementary concealers along with a thin strip of pressed powder and a couple of too-small-to-be-workable brushes. The concept of blending two shades of concealer to create a custom shade is intriguing, but most women will find this step tedious and/or unnecessary. The real question is how to deal with such thick, greasy concealers. Yes, they do cover well, but that's about all they have going for them. All of the six trios have drawbacks, whether it's at least one poor color, or else two great colors that turn ashy or too white when the pressed powder is brushed over them. If you're curious to test this yourself, the best sets are Level 1, Level 3, and Level 4.

POWDER: ☺ $$$ **All-Skins Loose Powder** *($26)* is a standard, talc-free powder with a small amount of shine, and the same loose powder Prescriptives has sold for years.

It has a smooth feel with a dry finish. The shimmer won't help you re
your skin if that's the reason you are looking for a loose powder, though t.
and sheer. **Sunsheen Bronzing Powder** *($25)* is a pressed-powder bronze
one matte and one shimmery shade in one split-pan container. The applicati
and even, but the shine is too intense to make this look real.

✓☺ $$$ **Virtual Skin Pressed Powder** *($25)* is an overpriced, but good, talc-free pressed powder with a slightly heavier application than most and a great range of six colors. This would work well as a powder foundation if you prefer light rather than medium coverage.

☺ $$$ **Powderful Adjustable Coverage Pressed Powder** *($28)* is undeniably smooth. This talc-based powder claims to have "smart microspheres" that "absorb oil and release moisture where needed to custom balance the skin." Even if these "smart" microspheres had a PhD in skin physiology they wouldn't be able to overcome the absorbent properties of talc (the main ingredient). Powderful is indeed a great pressed powder, and it comes with a dual-sided sponge that allows for sheer or more significant coverage in one stroke, but it's still just a powder. Be careful of the shine—it is subtle, but still visible in daylight, and not the best idea if you're using powder to temper shine. All six colors are beautiful.

☺ $$$ **BLUSH:** Powder Cheekcolor *($16.50 for blush tablet; $6 for refillable compact)* comes in beautiful shades, though most have visible shine. Some of the colors tend to go on quite sheer, so you'll need to layer this to get much impact. **Mystick Swivel Cheekcolor** *($25)* is an aptly named product with a small color selection that features both sheer and vivid tones. The texture is somewhat dry, making this harder to blend than a creamy-finish version, but for nearly flawless skin, this is an option. Racy and Woman are the non-shiny blush tones to consider first.

EYESHADOW: ☺ $$$ **Pick 2 Eyeshadow** *($13 each, $3 for refillable duo compact)* is a great concept that allows you to choose two colors out of a sea of choices. This almost always ensures you will end up using both shades, and there are some wonderful matte colors available. Many shiny shades have crept back into the fray, but that choice is up to you. All of the colors have a soft texture and blend on evenly, although the pigmentation is on the lighter side (just like the Blush above), so some fading may be apparent at day's end. Each color goes on softer than it looks, which is nice for novices or for those who want to gradually build color. **Eyepaints Wet/Dry Eyeshadow** *($20)* are much tamer than they used to be when it comes to colors. These preselected powder eyeshadow duos have a texture that's a bit silkier than the Pick 2 version above, but you have to be OK with having one very shiny shade in each set. These work well (and are more intense) when used wet.

☹ $$$ **Eyelights Shadow Tint** *($16)* are cream-to-powder eye colors in a tube. These go on quite smoothly and tend not to crease, but every color is extremely shiny. Adding this to your routine will be for the shine, not for the very sheer, almost transparent color this imparts.

EYE AND BROW SHAPER: ☺ **Eyecoloring Pencil** *($14)* is a standard pencil with a decent color selection. The application is on the greasy side, and stays that way. There are dozens of better pencils available for a fraction of the cost. **Softlining Pencil** *($15)* is a powdery eyeliner in pencil form with an effortless application (sans sharpening!). This is almost too creamy, and could easily smudge or fade, but that seems to be intentional since you would use this for a smoky eye design. **Automatic Eye Pencil** *($13)* is exactly that: A pencil that doesn't need sharpening. This is great, but very standard and hardly unique, as lines from Almay to Revlon have identical versions for far less. **Browshaping Pencil** *($15)* comes in some workable colors, but has a rather dry, hard texture and is not the best for an even application.

☺ $$$ **Brow Shaping Kit** *($25)* is more or less a carbon copy of Hard Candy's Training Brow Kit ($28). You get two complementary, slightly shiny brow powders along with a cream-colored underbrow highlighter (which is absent from the Hard Candy kit) and throwaway mini tweezers, along with a scratchy brow brush. The brow colors apply well, but few women really need two colors, and the effect of defined brows can be had for far less money.

☹ **Inklings Liquid Eyeliner** *($16.50)* has a poor brush that tends to overapply color, and the smear-prone formula takes too long to dry. Other Lauder-owned companies seem to be able to get liquid liner right, but not Prescriptives. **Colorclick Eye Stick** *($15)* is a slick cream eyeshadow that moves easily and is only for those who want a short-term eye design that's shiny and high maintenance.

LIPSTICK AND LIP PENCIL: Prescriptives lipsticks are frustratingly organized on their tester unit by color family, not by formula. Therefore, trying to find a specific formula requires a salesperson's assistance or good old trial and error. The ✓☺ $$$ **Soft Suede Lipstick** *($17.50)* offers great colors and an unusually smooth, semi-matte finish. This feels plush and rich on the lips, wears well, and comes in several excellent full-coverage colors. This is a must-try if you don't mind the price. ✓☺ $$$ **Paints Liquid Lipcolor** *($20)* are dual-ended liquid lipsticks that come in an attractive but small range of colors. The matte side is not matte in the least, though the color is opaque, while the satin side is more sheer and glossy. These go on with a wand applicator, are non-sticky, and the colors coordinate nicely with each other. All that adds up to create a winner whose only drawback is a steep price. ✓☺ $$$ **Deluxe Lip Pencil** *($17.50)* is a very smooth, automatic and retractable lip pencil that features a brush on one end for blending. It's an attractive package—although the price is a bit out of line for what amounts to just another pencil. The color selection is very nice, and this is comfortably creamy without being greasy. If you need a lip pencil and have room to splurge, this would be a great way to do it.

☺ $$$ **Lavish Lipstick SPF 15** *($17.50)* has a great name and a veritable kaleidoscope of colors. The application is smooth and light, with a greasy finish. The claim of long wear may have something to do with the fact that these are quite pigmented, but the "anti-feathering" claim is contradicted by the slick application. Still, this is more comfortable than the Incredible Lipcolor below. **Sheer Lipstick** *($15)* is pretty standard and nothing exceptional. **Potent Lipstick** *($16)* is Prescriptives' ultra-matte lipstick. It is not as matte as many others, though it does nicely stain the lips and tends to not roll or chip off. This is worth a look if you've had challenges in the past with a matte lipstick. **Lip Shine** *($16.50)* is a fine choice for a standard, semi-sticky lip gloss, if you don't mind the price tag. The bright, but sheer, iridescent colors are worth a peek if you're looking for an impulse buy next time you're shopping the cosmetics counters. **Lip Gloss** *($12.50)* is a standard wand-applicator gloss with a nice selection of colors. **Lip Lacquer** *($15)* offers a creamier, more opaque formula with a non-sticky, "wet" finish.

☺ $$$ **Swirled Lippity Split** *($20)* is a lot of money for a split pan of lip gloss, one side of which is sticky while the other is smooth. Used together, this is a very goopy-feeling way to get glossed. **Incredible Lipcolor** *($17.50)* sounds indulgent, but is ultimately disappointing, and not as impressive as Estee Lauder's Sumptuous or Go Pout lipsticks. Instead of the creamy-smooth texture of most other Lauder-owned lipsticks, this one has a thicker, very emollient texture that feels slightly sticky on the lips. The colors are awesome, with some traffic-stopping reds and other playful hues, but that's not enough to earn a full-fledged smiling face given the rather unappealing texture. **Lip Polish** *($14)* is the ultimate rich, sticky gloss, and unless you like stickiness, this should be far down on your list of gloss choices. **Colorclick Lipstick** *($14)* is a thick lipstick pencil that you can attach (the "click" portion of the name) to the Colorclick Eye Stick above. This is high-pigment lip color that goes the distance and is creamy, but you get very little product and the regular sharpening can't help but increase the use-up rate. **Lipcoloring Pencil** *($14)* is nothing to get excited about—it's a standard, twist-up pencil with OK colors. This one tends to drag at the lips and go on unevenly.

<u>MASCARA:</u> ☺ **Intensified Mascara** *($15)* and **Dramatic Mascara** *($15)* perform nearly identically, despite the different names. Both remain decent mascaras that don't clump or smear, but neither goes beyond good to great.

☺ $$$ **False Eyelashes Plush Mascara** *($17.50)* doesn't come close to mimicking false lashes. Although it certainly provides good length, it takes time to get there. Thickness is minimal to none, and the formula tends to smear a bit too easily. The packaging is impressive, though it's too bad the rather large, thick container doesn't translate to large, thick lashes. For a real false-lashes effect without the adhesive glue, consider Lancome's Amplicils or L'Oreal's Lash Architect mascaras.

<u>BRUSHES:</u> The makeup ☺ $$$ **Brushes** *($16–$50)* for the most part have a satiny-soft feel. Most of the shapes are quite workable, while others are not for everyone. The eyeshadow and eyeliner brushes are particularly great, with good density and shapes. If you're curious about them, the **Foundation Brush** *($30)* is one of the better ones out there. The only ones to consider avoiding are the ☺ $$$ **Powder Brush** *($35)* and **Finishing Brush** *($50)*, which are too floppy and/or big for most faces; the **Buff Brush**

($45), both unnecessary and cumbersome; the **Lip Brush** *($16)*, which is very pointed and would take forever to apply lip color evenly; and the **Fan Brush** *($20)*, which is denser than most but still an unnecessary brush for day-to-day makeup application. The **Cheek Shaper Brush** *($45)* is OK, but should be denser given the considerable price.

PRESCRIPTIVES MAGIC

Magic is a brilliant name for a collection of products that claim to optically change the face, fool the eye, and cause any skin imperfection (most often lines and wrinkles) to vanish. The positioning is definitely over-the-top, but given the price, this mostly amounts to more low-glow, shimmering makeup.

✓☺ $$$ **Illuminating Liquid Potion** *($30)* gets a stellar rating for being one of the best sheer, liquid-shimmer products available. A little goes a long way, which is a nice benefit when you're spending this much on soft shine. It edges out many others because of the way it melds with the skin, creating a shine that, while noticeable, is never intrusive or glittery. The claims for this are as exaggerated as it gets at the cosmetics counters, but what else would you expect from a "magic potion."

☺ $$$ **Invisible Line Smoother** *($35 for 0.5 ounce)* is a thick silicone cream that is virtually identical to M.A.C.'s Matte Creme Matifiance *($16.50 for 0.75 ounce)*, with the same matte-cream texture that is reminiscent of a sheer, soft spackle. It definitely can give the appearance of smoother skin, but the effect is temporary, lasting only a few hours depending on what you wear over it and how much you move your face. **Liquid Powder** *($32.50)* is, as the name implies, a powder with a wet finish that dries to a sheer powder feel. It works well, and the cool feel is nice. This is an intriguing product to test, but don't count on anything even vaguely magical (wait until you hear the claims the salesperson will bestow on it at the counter!). There are several colors available, but avoid the Red Neutralizer (too *Goldfinger*-yellow). **Soft Powder** *($28)* is a pressed-powder version of the Magic Liquid Powder, although getting it to stay pressed means the liquid content is all but gone. As a softly shiny highlighting powder, this works well if you don't mind the price. Avoid Red Neutralizer.

☺ $$$ **Illuminating Cream Potion** *($35)* is a cream-to-powder compact makeup in a soft pink shade that has a shiny effect (OK, OK, luminescent, not glitter) with a sheer finish. This slips around considerably more than the Liquid Potion above. **Concealing Wand Corrector/Concealer** *($25)* are a collection of half-size pencils that you can interlock at the base with a second pencil. The idea is to choose one creamy pencil shade to conceal and another to correct discolored areas (blue under-eye circles, red patches) and "optically retouch the skin." A highlighting pencil is also available. The best thing about this customizable duo is that the pencils do blend exceptionally well, though the formula is creamy enough to crease into lines under the eye. Coverage is somewhat sparse even when this is layered, so to achieve the promise of flawless skin will take several applications before you're satisfied. Despite some strong points, I can't justify using this two-part product over one reliable, neutral-toned concealer—and you won't have to deal with sharpening! **Diffusion Liner** *($18)* is a standard pencil that comes in three flesh-toned colors and has an iridescent finish. Prescriptives recommends these for optically altering the shape of eyebrows and lips, or for filling in wrinkles, but that would be a mistake because shine draws attention to problems—it doesn't hide, blur, or downplay them. What's truly magical is how many women fall for the notion that shine is a cure-all for any and all flaws. **Highlight** *($15)* is one more shimmery liquid than this collection needed, but the three shades are enticing for low-wattage glimmer.

PRESCRIPTIVES BLUE

Prescriptives Blue is a spin-off of Prescriptives Magic, and essentially offers the same products, but with an ethereal bluish-pink glow that can look ghastly on the wrong skin tone. This was a larger collection that has been whittled down to only those items that remain popular.

☺ **$$$ Soft Powder Phosphorescent** *($28)* is a very sheer, pale mauve powder blush that has a subtle, but still noticeable, shine. The dry texture is not the best for this type of product, but if shiny blush is what you are looking for, there are countless less expensive options to be found. **Phosphorescent Lighting Wand** *($25)* comes in a pen that contains a silicone-based, semi-opaque gel that is fed into a brush tip when you click the base of the product. It's a clever, but unnecessary, delivery system for something that is just a very sheer, almost translucent highlighter. The shine is present, but barely discernible, making this worth considering for a subtle, and I mean really, really subtle, highlight (which Prescriptives refers to as a "halo"!).

PRESTIGE COSMETICS (MAKEUP ONLY)

Prestige is a bold name for a cosmetics line that is sold in mass market outlets and drugstores at prices that any self-respecting makeup snob would scoff at. Yet that would be a mistake, because there are some undeniably good products, especially pencils and lipsticks. The quality of these items exceeds the reasonable price, and is a prime example of why expensive does not equate with being better. There are limitations among the average concealers and the pared-down selection of matte blushes and eyeshadows, but Prestige should be proud of its products. The packaging and display units are much sleeker and look right at home among heavy hitters like Cover Girl and L'Oreal, proving that Prestige is aiming to have their image match their name. For more information about Prestige Cosmetics, call (800) 722-7488 or visit www.prestigecosmetics.com.

CONCEALER: ☹ **Extreme Cover Concealer Creme** *($6.49)* is extremely thick and feels heavy on the skin. It covers well, but be prepared for creasing and a cakey appearance from the eight mostly poor colors.

☺ **Correctives Concealer** *($4.49)* is a standard, lipstick-style concealer with coverage that is almost identical to the one above. Unfortunately, it also has the same problems—though this has more slip and is easier to blend. If your eye area is unlined, the colors make this worth a try—but stay away from the yellow, mauve, and mint green color-correcting shades.

☺ **BLUSH:** The **Blush** *($3.89)* is mixed in with the eyeshadow colors at the store, and the number of suitable matte shades has plummeted. Still, if you want a shiny blush, this does apply smoothly and blends well.

☺ **EYESHADOW:** Prestige **Shadows** *($3.89)* have gone from a collection of muted neutrals to an expanded array of bright and pastel tones, most full of iridescence. The silky, sheer texture allows a soft application, but don't expect much pigment. If you decide to give these a go, the matte options are Camel, Sandstone, Coffee Bean, Sandalwood, Ivory, and Blanc. I wish I could say the **Shadow Quads** *($5.99)* were great, but the majority of them are quite shiny and the color combinations are mostly unworkable. If you have a yen for shine, though, there are some neutral quads to consider (such as Velvet or Naked), and the texture is soft and sheer. Avoid Sea Breeze and Safari.

EYE AND BROW SHAPER: ✔☺ **Liquid Eyeliner** *($4.89)* comes in an inkwell package and has a great, firm, but not-too-stiff brush that lays down a thin or thick line. It's dramatic, but for the most part this is an excellent liquid liner that dries quickly and doesn't chip. Of the six shades, stick with Black-Brown and Black unless you want a strong metallic finish. ✔☺ **Eye Liner** *($3.29)* is a standard pencil that has a superior soft, but dry, texture that does not smudge easily. There are more than a few wild colors, enough to keep an experimental artist happy for hours.

☺ **Waterproof Automatic Eye Liner** *($4.99)* are similar to the pencils above that need sharpening, though these are creamier. Avoid Smokey Green, Bronze, and Midnight Blue. These are no more waterproof than most pencils. **Waterproof Eyeliner** *($4.99)* is a standard pencil that has a soft, silky application that tends not to smudge, but it does remain tacky to the touch. It is waterproof, if that's a selling point that intrigues you. **Browliner** *($3.29)* is nothing more than your basic brow pencil with a dry finish and a soft application. What's great for brow-pencil lovers is the incredibly reasonable price! There is a mini brow brush on the cap, which is a nice little extra.

LIPSTICK AND LIP PENCIL: ✔☺ **Moisture Intense Lipcolor** *($3.99)* is a brilliant creamy lipstick that strikes the perfect balance of smoothness without greasiness. The 70+ shades represent one of the best selections of creamy lipsticks at the drugstore, and these last as long as a good cream lipstick should.

☺ **Vinylwear High Shine Lip Gloss** *($3.89)* is a thick, sticky gloss that comes in a tube with a wand applicator. The color selection is decent, with all shades offering sheer to medium coverage. What's really problematic is the incredibly strong fragrance wafting from this product! If that is not a concern, this is a consideration for an inexpensive lip gloss with lots of shine. **Jetstream Twist-Up Lipcolor** *($5.89)* is another click-pen, brush-applicator gloss, available in Sheer or Full color options. For extra-thick, goopy lip gloss that shines intensely, this should top your list. **Lipliner** *($3.29)* pencils come in a good assortment of colors (including some original hues) and are overall standard, but very affordable, pencils for those who don't mind sharpening. **Waterproof Lip Liner** *($4.99)* is identical to the Waterproof Eyeliner above. The colors go on creamy, stay well, and are waterproof, but not anymore so than your average pencil. **Waterproof Automatic Lip Liner** *($4.99)* are nonretractable pencils you don't have to sharpen, but their coverage isn't any more waterproof than most lip pencils. The color selection is small, and includes three shades (Leather, Raw Sugar, and Penny) that are too brown for most women's lips. **Aromatherapy Lip Gloss** *($3.19)* is a pot of standard, sparkly lip gloss with a fairly intense fragrance that not everyone will find all that therapeutic, but it is still a good basic gloss.

☺ <u>BRUSHES:</u> Prestige's **Makeup Brushes** *($2.49–$12.99)* are an unexpected surprise. They are soft and relatively firm, with good flexibility. If you're in need of brushes and on a budget, the best of the bunch include the **109 Powder** *($12.99)*, **105 Mini Blush** *($7.49)*, **103 Shadow Crease** *($5.49)*, **102 Shadow Contour** *($5.49)*, and **110 Mini Powder** *($11.99)*. The remaining brushes have their drawbacks (such as being too sparse), but are still functional.

PRINCIPAL SECRET

Is there something about acting talent or being beautiful that is equal to knowledge? I guess there must be, because having celebrities endorse products is big business the world over. It is simply amazing to me that Victoria Principal can convince women that they can have great skin like she does by using her skin-care routine. In fact, Victoria Principal's infomercial is one of the most successful ever.

Victoria Principal's skin-care products were formulated and manufactured by Aida Thibiant, a Beverly Hills aesthetician who has run a successful skin-care boutique and cosmetics manufacturing business there for years. Because the Guthy Renker Corporation that markets and distributes the line felt they no longer needed Thibiant to establish Principal's credentials, they severed ties with her in 1995. That isn't good or bad, it just means it isn't Principal's own skin-care genius behind these products.

This is a line with deals, or at least that's what they appear to be on the surface. Look a little deeper and these are just expensive products, and the deals are smoke and mirrors. You can buy groups of products for what appears to be a much-reduced price, but if you really don't need all those products, or if some of them are poorly formulated (like many of the sunscreens, products for blemish-prone skin, and moisturizers) you would be wasting your money, and that's no bargain.

I should mention that several of these products aren't bad, and a few are actually quite nice, specifically for someone with normal to dry skin. But no one needs six to ten different products to take care of her face and body, and many of the claims for these products are grossly exaggerated. For more information about Principal Secret, call (800) 545-5595 or visit www.principalsecret.com or www.qvc.com. **Note:** All Principal Secret products contain fragrance.

The Reviews P

PRINCIPAL SECRET SKIN CARE

☺ $$$ **Advanced Gentle 4-in-1 Cleanser** *($19 for 6 ounces)*. There is nothing advanced about this standard, detergent-based, water-soluble cleanser. The teeny amount of vitamins and water-binding agents would just be washed away before they could have an effect on skin. It would work fine for normal to oily or slightly dry skin.

☺ $$$ **Gentle Deep Cleanser** *($17.25 for 6 ounces)* is almost identical to the Advanced version above only minus the trace amounts of vitamins and water-binding agents, and the same basic comments apply.

☺ $$$ **Gentle Exfoliating Scrub** *($16.75 for 4 ounces)* is a standard, detergent-based, water-soluble cleanser that uses ground-up plastic as the scrub agent. It would work well for most skin types.

☹ $$$ **Gentle Deep Revitalizing Scrub** *($21.50 for 4 ounces)* is a standard, detergent-based, water-soluble cleanser that uses pumice as the scrub agent; it works, but this can be too rough on skin. It does contain some good antioxidants and water-binding agents, but these would be rinsed away before they had much chance to have any benefit for skin.

☺ $$$ **AHA Booster Complex** *($45 for 1 ounce)* includes a handful of exotic-sounding ingredients, but because they are at the very end of the ingredient list, it means they're almost nonexistent. However, this is a good, though absurdly overpriced, 4% AHA product for exfoliation. It would be good for someone with sensitive skin, but it is almost indistinguishable from Pond's Age Defying Cream for Sensitive Skin, which costs one-fourth as much.

☹ $$$ **Intensive Serum with AHA** *($48.25 for 0.5 ounce)*. There is nothing intense about this product except the price. The plant extracts are not true AHAs and they cannot exfoliate the skin. This product also contains urea, which can be an exfoliant, but not when present in such a teeny amount.

✓☺ $$$ **Advanced Continuous Lift Serum** *($40 for 0.5 ounce)* is a good moisturizer for normal to dry skin that contains a good mix of antioxidants, water-binding agents, and anti-irritants. The vitamin K cannot affect surfaced capillaries and no aspect of this serum will lift skin anywhere.

☹ **Advanced Continuous Moisture with SPF 8** *($31.50 for 2 ounces)* has a dismal SPF and no UVA-protecting ingredients of titanium dioxide, zinc oxide, or avobenzone, and is not recommended.

☺ $$$ **Advanced Eye Conditioner** *($34.50 for 0.5 ounce)* is a very good, silicone-based moisturizer for normal to dry skin that contains a very decent mix of water-binding agents and antioxidants.

☺ $$$ **Advanced EyeSaver Gel** *($27 for 0.5 ounce)* is a good, lightweight moisturizer for normal to dry skin with good water-binding agents and antioxidants. The vitamin K has no effect on surfaced capillaries or dark circles.

✓☺ $$$ **Advanced Nighttime Treatment** *($35 for 1 ounce)* is an emollient moisturizer with an impressive mix of antioxidants and water-binding agents. It is a very good option for normal to dry skin.

☹ **Advanced Gentle Enzyme Treatment** *($49 for 1 ounce)* lists the second ingredient as aluminum starch (octenylsuccinate), which isn't gentle—it's an absorbent that can be a skin irritant. The teeny amount of papain is not effective as an exfoliant.

☺ $$$ **Booster Complex** *($46 for 1 ounce)* isn't much of a booster. It contains about 3% AHA in a pH of 5, which makes it ineffective for exfoliation.

☺ **Extra Nurturing Cream** *($32 for 2 ounces)* is an OK, basic moisturizer for dry skin, but it isn't as well formulated with state-of-the-art ingredients as several of the other Principal Secret products.

☺ **Eye Relief** *($26 for 0.5 ounce)* is a light gel with a tiny amount of water-binding agents. It would be an OK option for normal to slightly dry skin.

☹ **Oil-Control Hydrator with SPF 8** *($35 for 2 ounces)* only has an SPF of 8, and with so many good SPF 15s around, why even think about this one? It does contain in-part titanium dioxide, but that is only part of what makes a good sunscreen.

☹ **Time Release Moisture with SPF 8** *($29.75 for 2 ounces)* has a dismal SPF and no UVA-protecting ingredients of titanium dioxide, zinc oxide, or avobenzone, and is not recommended.

☺ $$$ **Sun Secret Tan Sustainer SPF 15** *($18.25 for 4 ounces)* is a good, in-part avobenzone-based sunscreen in a lightweight moisturizing base with some good antioxidants and water-binding agents. It would be good for someone with normal to slightly dry skin. It contains erythrulose, a substance chemically similar to the self-tanning agent dihydroxyacetone. Depending on your skin color, there can be a difference in the color effect of erythrulose. However, dihydroxyacetone completely changes the color of skin within two to six hours, while erythrulose needs about two to three days for the skin to show a color change.

☺ $$$ **Advanced Eye Conditioner Pads** *($24.50 for 40 pads)* lists lemon water as the first ingredient, and that can be a skin irritant, which is not conditioning in the least for eyes. That's a disappointment, because everything else about this product makes it a good lightweight moisturizer.

☺ $$$ **Advanced Pore Minimizing Detox Mask** *($21.75 for 2.5 ounces)* contains mostly water and olive oil, and that is a problem for oily or blemish-prone skin. The other emollients it contains would also be problematic for such skin. It does contain an abrasive, but there are better ways to exfoliate skin. Besides, nothing in this or any other product can affect the size of pores.

☹ **Advanced Clear Pore Liquid Strips** *($16.75 for 1.5 ounces)* contains mostly plastic and alcohol. That isn't advanced, but it is potentially drying and irritating for skin.

☹ **Blemish Buster Solution** *($20 for 0.5 ounce)* is just alcohol, sulfur, and zinc. It can irritate the skin and, more important, like many other much less expensive acne products with the same ingredients, it won't get rid of acne. Sulfur can be a disinfectant, but there are far gentler ones to try, and with prices that aren't so out of line.

☺ $$$ **Invisible Toning Masque** *($23 for 2 ounces)* is a moisturizing mask that won't tone anything and that contains a minimum of interesting ingredients for skin.

☹ **Rosemary Mint Hydrating Mask** *($24.50 for 6 ounces)* is a standard clay mask with some peppermint, and that isn't the best for any skin type.

COLOR PRINCIPAL MAKEUP

Once you've been antiaged, smoothed, and soothed with Principal Secret skin care, you may want to see what the Color Principal is all about. With the mantra of what "looks good, feels good, is good," Ms. Principal proudly carries on about how her cosmetics are formulated with the best ingredients, including the usual words that cause consumers to perk up their ears, such as "natural," "vitamins," and "sensitive skin." But these state-of-the-art additives end up sidetracked when you consider the inconsequential amounts present in every product, not to mention the discouraging fact that all but one of the makeup items with sunscreen have no reliable UVA protection. Few things look or feel as good as healthy skin, but using this makeup will not help you attain it any more than using most other makeups, and in some cases Color Principal falls flat on its proverbial face with some unacceptable products. You will find a few nice surprises, but unless you can't imagine being disloyal to the Color Principal club, there's no need to have any of these items rushed to your door—not when there are plenty of stellar, less expensive options that are easy to obtain. For some reason the Color Principal makeup is not featured on the Principal Secret Web site. If you want the makeup, you need to order directly from QVC.

FOUNDATION: ☺ $$$ **Liquid Foundation SPF 15** *($30)* comes in four shades, and they are all a substantial improvement over the colors from the Cream Foundation reviewed below. This has a lightly creamy texture that blends very well and dries to a smooth matte finish that would be fine for normal to slightly oily skin seeking light coverage. However, the sunscreen falls short of offering good UVA protection, so this will require a separate sunscreen underneath.

☺ $$$ **Time Release Tinted Moisture Plus SPF 15** *($25)* at least has a good UVA-protecting ingredient in the form of avobenzone, but why this one has it and not the others is a mystery. Count on this as a fairly emollient, tinted moisturizer whose colors leave much to be desired. Of the four shades, only Sheer Beige looks like skin. The others are incredibly peachy or rose, and although this is sheer, it's noticeable enough to matter.

☹ **Cream Foundation SPF 15** *($26.75)* is a standard cream-to-powder makeup that calls itself "a wonder of science." Well, so is Silly Putty, and you wouldn't want to smear that on your face! There are four compacts that contain two shades each, with the idea being to mix the two shades (if need be) to exactly match your skin. Yet all of the four duos have a slight to strong peachy tint that is unflattering to most skin tones. Plus, having to mix the right portions of foundation every morning is not the most convenient method of applying makeup. Add the fact that the sunscreen is still without significant UVA protection and this one is easy to ignore.

<u>CONCEALER:</u> ☺ **Perfect Concealer SPF 8** *($14)* has no UVA-protecting ingredients and the SPF 8 is inadequate for daylong protection, but for a creamy, smooth concealer with good coverage and only a minimal chance of creasing into lines, this one is an option, and the three shades are great.

☹ $$$ **Concealer Duo SPF 15** *($21.25)* is a new spin on concealers. A single stick houses a too-sheer liquid concealer along with a twist-up full-coverage stick concealer. Both options contain inadequate UVA sunscreen, which is disappointing. I'm not sure what to make of this, as having two concealing options in one package is not necessary for most women, and the differences between the night and day coverage are perplexing. If you're intrigued, the only duo to stay away from is Medium.

<u>POWDER:</u> ☹ **Pressed Powder SPF 8** *($21)* does not have UVA-protecting ingredients, and even if it did, getting SPF protection from a powder takes opaque coverage, just a light dusting won't do it. This is a talc-free formula that has a silky, though fairly powdery application and a slight amount of shine with each of the four colors. If powdering to increase shine appeals to you, this will do nicely, but it's a real "Why bother?" and doesn't begin to compare to Neutrogena's titanium dioxide–based SPF 30 pressed powder, available at almost half this price and with a much higher SPF.

☺ $$$ **Loose Face Powder** *($23)* arrives packaged in a petite Lucite container, which holds the tiniest amount of loose powder around. Still, this has a luscious texture and leaves a beautifully smooth, satiny finish on the skin, and the talc-free formula's four shades are suitably neutral.

☹ $$$ <u>BLUSH:</u> **Blush Duo** *($22.25)* comes in an attractive black case with two shades of blush, one matte and the other shiny. They have a silky-soft feel and go on even and smooth, but so do lots of other blushes for far less money and without the shine. **All in One Cream Color** *($19.50)* is a multipurpose cream designed for eyes, lips, and cheeks. There are two formulas, and both are emollient and feel thick on the skin. This is an option for dry skin, but really no different from using your lipstick as blush and lip color. Using a product this moist on the eyes just begs for creasing.

☺ $$$ <u>EYESHADOW:</u> **Eye Shadow Quad** *($25)* is a set of four eyeshadow shades that are coordinated nicely, are surprisingly matte, and have a soft, even application—but $25 for such tiny amounts? These aren't *that* nice.

☹ <u>EYE AND BROW SHAPER:</u> **Dual Sided Defining Eye Liner** *($11.25)* is just a standard, two-ended eye pencil with a smooth, slightly creamy finish. **Golden Shimmer Eyeliner** *($11)* is a creamy, twist-up pencil that colors your eye area a pale, shiny golden color that will accentuate any wrinkles or lines you have. For those who are wrinkle-free, this is a fairly standard highlighter for the brow bone.

<u>LIPSTICK AND LIP PENCIL:</u> ☹ **Extra Rich Lipstick SPF 15** *($16.25)* is only rich in the creamy, almost greasy feel it leaves on the lips. The semi-opaque colors have a

limited selection, and once again a good SPF number shows up without reliable UVA protection. A major problem for these lipsticks is the container—either the swivel-up mechanism is too loose, which causes the lipstick to wind down as you use it, or the lipstick itself breaks apart from the base.

☺ **LipTensive Lip Tint SPF 15** *($16.25)* is nearly identical to the Extra Rich Lipstick above, only the colors are sheer. They also share the same packaging issues, so buyer beware. **Golden Shimmer Lipstick** *($15)* is "the Midas touch for lips," which is a fancy way of saying this shimmery lipstick adds a golden gleam whether used alone or over other colors. This would be recommended as a fun lipstick add-on if the packaging were more stable. As it is, this breaks off too easily.

☺ **Natural Gloss** *($15)* is a very good, wand-type lip gloss that offers soft, light-coverage colors and a slick feel that is only a problem if you have lines around the mouth. Otherwise, gloss fans should check this out if the price is acceptable. **Defining Lip Liner** *($11.25)* is a standard, two-ended lipliner. The limited colors are fine and the application is creamy but not greasy. **LipTensive Lip Liner** *($12.25)* is another standard, creamy lip pencil but with a larger color selection than the Defining Lip Liner. It works well, but for the money you'd be wise to explore lip pencils from almost any drugstore line.

☹ **MASCARA: Eye Mazing Dual Mascara** *($20)* is an updated version of the Double Duty Mascara, but other than the name change I couldn't tell much difference. This is a two-brush mascara that does little to impress, tends to flake, and can smear during application. Considering that, the price tag is way out of line.

☹ **BRUSHES:** The **Color Principal 6-Piece Brush Set** *($39.75)* is a substandard brush set that has too many weaknesses to make this a good investment. The only really good brush is the Powder—the rest are too sparse, floppy, or stiff. The case is nice, but it's what's inside that counts, and this set is a letdown. A **7-Piece Brush Set** *($44.50)* is also available, and it's identical to the one above except for the inclusion of an average foundation brush.

☺ **$$$ SPECIALTY:** For those who can't be "Principal-ed" enough, Victoria offers her **Deluxe Color Principal Collection** *($99.75)*, which is a 13-piece kit containing everything from foundation to mascara. There are three separate kits available, so you can choose between three looks: natural (soft earth tones), daytime (pale peaches and corals), or nighttime (intense berry tones). The pigeonholed color logic is a bit limiting, and it's up to you to weigh the pros and cons of every item in the total package.

PROACTIV (SKIN CARE ONLY)

ProActiv is a small group of products aimed at those with breakouts. It was created and endorsed by two dermatologists, Dr. Katie Rodan and Dr. Kathy Fields, who market these products via infomercials and on their Web site. Their promises of results are so overexaggerated that someone should take these doctors to task for their unmedical hype and hyperbole. While I don't doubt their dermatologic expertise, the notion that their products are the be-all and end-all for acne is at best misleading and, coming from physicians, shockingly inappropriate; but so many doctors are into the skin-care game it's hard to be shocked by this anymore. Some percentage of people will benefit from this routine (it contains the basics that are necessary for over-the-counter treatment of acne), but it's definitely not for everyone, and every dermatologist knows this (just check out the American Academy of Dermatology Web site at www.aad.com, for example, on their recommendations for battling blemishes). It also goes without saying that other lines offer many less expensive versions of all the ProActiv products.

Some of the ProActiv products are very good, while some of their other product formulations are problematic for some skin types. Plus, many of the products contain fragrance, which is a particularly egregious oversight from a so-called dermatologic line. Finally, the prices are steep for what you get, unless of course you join their club. In order to get your first order at the discount price ($39.95 plus shipping), you need to agree to automatic shipments of the same four products for $39.95 plus shipping every two months. If you want to pick and choose which products work best for you, the price goes up considerably. My constant reminder to all of you who are trying to take good care of your skin is to pick and choose carefully, and to remember that battling blemishes takes experimenting to find the products that work for you. For more information about ProActiv, call (800) 950-4695 or visit www.proactiv.com.

☺ **$$$ Renewing Cleanser** *($16 for 4 ounces)* contains 2.5% benzoyl peroxide. Though benzoyl peroxide is an effective disinfectant for breakouts, putting it in a cleanser doesn't make much sense. You not only risk getting the disinfectant in your eyes but you also rinse the effective ingredient down the drain before it can work. To counter that issue, the directions suggest massaging your face with the cleanser for 1 to 2 minutes. Even assuming you have the time to do this, leaving the cleansing agent base on your skin for that long can be irritating to skin. There are other ways to get the benefits of benzoyl peroxide than in a cleanser. This contains ground-up plastic (polyethylene) as the abrasive material.

☺ **$$$ Revitalizing Toner** *($16 for 4 ounces)* is a good 6% AHA liquid. However, when it comes to most kinds of breakouts, research indicates that BHA (salicylic acid) rather than AHA is the best way to exfoliate for breakout prevention. Salicylic acid can exfoliate on the surface of skin as well as within the pore because it is lipid soluble (meaning it can penetrate oil). AHAs exfoliate primarily on the surface of skin because they are water soluble and can't work inside the pore lining.

☺ **$$$ Oil Free Moisture with SPF 15** *($25 for 1.7 ounces)* is a good, in-part titanium dioxide–based sunscreen in an ordinary moisturizing base. This is pricey for such an exceptionally basic sunscreen that lacks any antioxidants or water-binding agents. It does have a fairly matte finish, but the titanium dioxide can be a problem for someone with breakouts.

✓☺ **Repairing Lotion** *($21.75 for 2 ounces)* contains 2.5% benzoyl peroxide. This is a fine benzoyl peroxide product, but it doesn't repair anything in the skin; it only disinfects. Keep in mind there's nothing special or unique about this benzoyl peroxide lotion; you can find several products just like it in the acne section at your local drugstore.

☹ **Advanced Blemish Treatment** *($17 for 0.33 ounce)* is a 6% benzoyl peroxide solution. However, the fourth ingredient is alcohol, which makes this unnecessarily drying and irritating. There are far more gentle 5% and 10% benzoyl peroxide products at the drugstore for a fraction of this price.

☹ **Daily Oil Control** *($18 for 1.7 ounces)* contains mostly alcohol and a form of aluminum starch found in deodorants. There are better ways to deal with oil than this irritating combination.

☹ **Refining Mask** *($20 for 2.5 ounces)* is a standard clay mask that also contains at least 6% pure sulfur. Sulfur can be a good, mild antibacterial agent, but it is also a pretty good skin irritant. There are better ways to disinfect skin than this.

✓☺ **Skin Lightening Lotion** *($22 for 1 ounce)* is a very good, 2% hydroquinone skin-lightening lotion. It also contains about 4% AHA and kojic acid, which can both have a beneficial impact on skin discolorations.

PROPAPH (SKIN CARE ONLY)

I remember this line of acne products from when I was a kid, and it hasn't changed since way back then. They are just as irritating and problematic for skin today as they were in the '70s! For more information about PropapH, call (800) 954-5080 or visit www.propaph.com.

☹ **Foaming Face Wash** *($3.79 for 8 ounces)* is a detergent-based, water-soluble cleanser, but this one contains menthol and peppermint, which are too irritating, and the salicylic acid is wasted in a cleanser where it would just be rinsed down the drain. The fruit acids it lists are not the same thing as alpha hydroxy acids and have no exfoliating benefits for skin.

☹ **Astringent Cleanser Maximum Strength** *($3.79 for 10 ounces)* contains salicylic acid, which would have made this a nice product if it didn't also contain menthol, peppermint, and alcohol. This is a burn for the skin, causing more problems than it could ever hope to help.

☹ **Astringent Cleanser Acne Medication and Moisturizer Normal to Sensitive Skin** *($3.79 for 12 ounces)* is almost identical to the Maximum Strength version above, and the same review applies.

☹ **Peel-Off Acne Mask Acne Treatment and Moisturizer** *($4.21 for 2.66 ounces)* doesn't contain unnecessary irritants, but the pH of this part-salicylic acid–, part-AHA–based product isn't low enough for it to be an effective exfoliant.

PURPOSE (SKIN CARE ONLY)

The Purpose line of skin-care products is owned by Johnson & Johnson, a company that, prior to 1987, was better known for baby care and Band-Aids than for skin-care products. That has changed. These days Johnson & Johnson has become well known for its prescription-only wrinkle treatments Retin-A and Renova. Leaving no stone unturned,

Johnson & Johnson made great strides convincing physicians that a prescription for Retin-A and Renova should be accompanied by the Purpose line of products. Along with Purpose, J&J has also added the Neutrogena, RoC, Aveeno, and Clean & Clear lines of skin-care products. Your face could easily live without most of the Purpose products, although one sunscreen is a consideration for daily sun protection. For more information about Purpose, call (800) 526-3967 or visit www.jnj.com.

☹ **Gentle Cleansing Bar** *($3.17 for 6 ounces)* is just a standard bar cleanser that contains tallow and a strong detergent cleansing agent. They added a little glycerin, but that won't counteract the drying effect of the soap.

☺ **Gentle Cleansing Wash** *($5.29 for 6 ounces)* is a standard, but good, detergent-based, water-soluble cleanser. It is an option for someone with normal to oily skin.

☺ **Moisturizing Foaming Cleanser** *($5.49 for 6 ounces)* isn't moisturizing in the least, it is just a standard, detergent-based, water-soluble cleanser for normal to oily skin. This is fragrance-free.

☹ **Alpha Hydroxy Moisture Lotion with SPF 15** *($10.29 for 4 ounces)* doesn't contain the UVA-protecting ingredients of titanium dioxide, zinc oxide, or avobenzone, and is not recommended.

☹ **Dual Treatment Moisturizer with SPF 15 Protection** *($7.89 for 4 ounces)* is a good, in-part titanium dioxide–based sunscreen in a rather mediocre moisturizing base that would be an option for someone with normal to slightly dry skin. The problem is that it contains Kathon CG, a preservative that should only be used in rinse-off products.

☺ **Intensive Daily Moisturizer SPF 15 Protection** *($8.49 for 4 ounces)* is a good, in-part avobenzone-based sunscreen in an ordinary, mediocre moisturizing base that would be an option for someone with normal to slightly dry skin.

QUO COSMETICS (MAKEUP ONLY)
(CANADA ONLY)

After nearly 20 years of reviewing thousands upon thousands of skin-care and makeup products, it's safe to say it takes a lot to impress me. More often than not, I find myself marveling at the crazy repetitiveness of the cosmetics industry, and the various marketing hooks that serve as bait for unsuspecting consumers. However, on a recent trip to our northern neighbor, Canada, I found myself amid displays of several products that were the exception to the rule, all from a relative newbie named Quo. This small but comprehensive makeup line is sold exclusively at Shoppers Drug Mart in Canada, and is rightly one of their star performers. The impetus behind this simply packaged line was the need to bring makeup artist–applauded cosmetics into a mainstream drugstore, complete with velvety, smooth textures, even application, and a fair selection of matte blushes and eyeshadows that go the distance. Also on hand are a suitable range of neutral foundations, standard pencils, creamy lipsticks, and a remarkable selection of realistically priced makeup brushes.

The Reviews Q

I'm not enamored of everything Quo has to offer, but the few items that didn't thrill me were primarily due to taste and style preferences—and your criteria may rightfully differ from mine. Either way, Canadian shoppers (and visitors) truly have an ace in the hole with Quo. For more information about Quo Cosmetics, visit www.shoppersdrugmart.ca. and click on "exclusive brands." **Note:** All prices for Quo Cosmetics products are in Canadian dollars.

FOUNDATION: ✓☺ **$$$ Wet and Dry Foundation** *($21)* is a talc-based, pressed-powder foundation that has an amazing silky texture that applies smoothly and practically looks like a second skin. This is not a tightly pressed powder, so you need to be careful you don't overapply, but it blends so readily it's easy to correct mistakes. It also has a natural matte finish and light coverage. The selection of nine shades features predominantly neutral colors that are best for fair to medium skin. Watch out for Beige 4 and Bronze 1, which can be too peach for most skin tones.

☺ **$$$ Face Erotica Foundation Primer** *($21)* is a standard, silicone-based fluid that is more liquidy than any other I have seen. That can make this tricky to use, but with a little effort you can still get decent smooth results. Although this won't make a huge difference in how long your makeup lasts, it will make application smoother and will lightly hydrate the skin. **Face Erotica 1** and **2** *($21)* are fluid, lightweight shimmer lotions that add a soft shine to the skin. They're fine for evening wear, but can look too sparkly in broad daylight.

CONCEALER: Quo's ☺ **Concealer** *($12)* comes in a squeeze tube and is a bit runny. However, the smooth cream texture blends well and has a natural finish. This doesn't provide ample coverage, and is best for minor discolorations or blemishes. The two shades are fine, though #2 may be too peach for some skin tones.

☺ **$$$ Bags Away** *($18)* is a creamy compact concealer that features three different tones that can be used alone or blended for a custom shade. Makeup artists may get a kick out of these, but most consumers will be turned off by the thick texture and heavy appearance this has on the skin, though it does cover well!

☹ **Corrector** *($12)* supposedly allows you to say "bye, bye, blotchy skin!" but the light-coverage formula and green or pale yellow colors do little (if anything) to camouflage blotchiness. Despite the blendable texture, these are best avoided by most skin tones.

☺ **$$$ POWDER: Mosaic Perfecting Powder** *($18)*, **Mosaic Bronzer** *($18)*, and **Mosaic Highlighter** *($18)* are all talc-based pressed powders that feature various colored "squares within a square" that look artsy, but come off as one color on the skin. The Perfecting Powder is a great pressed powder for light skin, the Bronzer is a soft tan color with a hint of shine, and the Highlighter is a soft, pale yellow shade that would work on fair skin. The regular **Bronzing Powder** *($19)* is a talc-based pressed powder that comes in two suitably bronze shades and has a wonderfully smooth texture. I wish both shades didn't have noticeable shine, but you can't win them all!

<u>BLUSH:</u> The ✔☺ **Blush** *($16)* is a pleasure to apply, since it goes on without a hitch and remains color-true. The small selection of matte shades has a superlative texture, and each one, though understated, has an intensity that allows all-day wear without fading.

<u>EYESHADOW:</u> Quo's ✔☺ **Eye Shadow** *($12)* has an astonishingly silky texture that feels almost decadent. What's surprising is how well this "creamy"-feeling formula lasts without creasing or fading. There are even a handful of good matte shades, including Jealousy, Soft, Delicate, Placid, Blur, Sensible, and Tone. The ✔☺ **Eyeshadow Quads** *($20)* don't offer a lot of color combinations, but what's available is choice and the shades are expertly coordinated and include all-matte options.

☺ **Eye Primer** *($12)* is identical to the Concealer above, despite its name. This comes in a gorgeous neutral shade, but if you're looking for something to enhance eyeshadow application and wear, a true, matte-finish concealer (or foundation) would be preferred.

<u>EYE AND BROW SHAPER:</u> ☺ **Automatic Eye Liner** *($11)* is a great standard eye pencil that applies smoothly and comes with a built-in smudger to soften the line. I wouldn't choose this over a powder eyeshadow, but it's fine for pencil fans. The traditional, standard **Eye Pencils** *($11)* feature a soft, dry texture that has a nice slip and is relatively impervious to smudging. Definitely worth a test run if you prefer pencils.

<u>LIPSTICK AND LIP PENCIL:</u> Quo's ✔☺ **Lipstick** *($14.50)* features three different formulas, though these are not designated on the tester unit (they are indicated on the lipstick's shade label). The **Creams**, which comprise the bulk of the color palette, are smooth and opaque, with just the right balance of emolliency and creaminess. The **Sheer** formula is glossier than the Creams, and the colors are transparent. The **Mattes** only come in a handful of shades, and although they're not true mattes, they are noticeably "drier" than the Creams.

☺ **Lip Gloss** *($13.50)* is a straightforward wand gloss that's minimally sticky and otherwise everything you'd expect from a basic lip gloss. **Lipstick/Lip Gloss** *($15)* presents a split compact of lipstick and lip gloss. The colors are complementary and this comes with brushes for on-the-go, hands-free application. **Automatic Lip Pencil** *($11.50)* has an agreeable, soft texture that's still firm enough to draw a precise line. True to its name, this doesn't need sharpening. **Tinted and Minted** *($14.50)* is a standard lipstick that comes in a transparent pink tone and has an emollient feel. There is a small amount of mint for flavor, but it's barely noticeable and likely it's present in too low a concentration to be of concern as an irritant. **Lip Moisture Stick** *($10)* is a glossy, colorless lip balm in lipstick form. Dry, chapped lips will be happy to meet this rather standard product.

☺ **Lip Primer** *($12)* is a silicone-based cream that has a frothy texture and initially applies white, and then dries to a transparent, dry finish. It's supposed to make lipstick wear longer, but this formula isn't strong enough to add staying power to most oil- and wax-based lipsticks. However, it can give an extra nudge of longevity to matte or ultra-matte lipsticks. **Lip Scrub** *($12)* is a fairly abrasive scrub that uses synthetic plastic beads as the scrub particles. This comes in a creamy base, but the lips don't need this type of aggressive exfoliant.

The Reviews Q

A soft, baby-type toothbrush or a damp cotton washcloth would be gentler, yet effective, options. This "lip" product *would* work well to exfoliate dry knees, heels and elbows!

MASCARA: ✓☺ **Lush Mascara** *($12)* allows you to build full, long lashes and enough thickness to satisfy all but the most demanding dramatic lash divas. Best of all, it does this without clumps or globs while separating each lash for maximum effect.

BRUSHES: The brush collection from Quo is not to be missed. It is doubtful Canadians will find anywhere else such an admirable collection of professional brushes at such reasonable prices. The best ones are the ✓☺ **Crease Brush** *($12)*, ✓☺ **All Over Shadow Brush** *($12)*, ✓☺ **Definer Shadow Brush** *($12)*, regular and retractable ✓☺ **Lip Brushes** *($15 and $12)*, ✓☺ **Liner/Brow Brush** *($12)*, and ✓☺ **Retractable Powder/Blush Brush** *($20)*. The ☺ **Powder Brush** *($20)* is a bit too large and floppy for controlled application and the **Blush Brush** *($16)* is soft and dense, but too full for most women's cheeks. It would make a better powder brush. Last, the **Brush Wallet** *($12)* holds all the makeup brushes you'll need to transform yourself, and it's made of a durable synthetic fabric.

RACHEL PERRY (SKIN CARE ONLY)

Health food stores have been selling Rachel Perry products for years. This is one of the original "natural" cosmetics lines, and it is now also available at some large drugstore chains. Rachel Perry products contain many, if not more, of the same natural-sounding ingredients included in more highbrow natural-product lines such as Aveda, Clarins, and Origins. For the consumer on a budget who is interested in the ballyhoo surrounding botanical skin-care products, this line could satisfy that curiosity without hurting the pocketbook. But watch out for your skin, because there are skin irritants and allergens lurking everywhere in these products. And with ingredients like TEA cocoyl glutamate, butylene glycol, polyisobutene, triethanolamine, carbomer, formaldehyde-releasing preservatives, and a form of plastic, there are lots and lots of unnatural ingredients in these products. For more information about Rachel Perry, call (800) 966-8888 or visit www.rachelperry.net. **Note:** All Rachel Perry products contain fragrance.

☹ **Citrus-Aloe Cleanser and Face Wash, for Normal to Dry Skin** *($13 for 4 ounces)*. The oils make this more of a wipe-off product than a face wash, and it can leave a greasy residue on the skin. The reason for the rating is that several of the plant extracts, including arnica, sage, and clary, are potent skin irritants.

☹ **Tangerine Dream Foaming Facial Cleanser** *($13 for 6 ounces)* is a standard, detergent-based, water-soluble cleanser that contains about 3% AHAs. At only 3%, they wouldn't be effective as an exfoliant, but even if they were, AHAs are wasted in a cleanser because they are rinsed down the drain before they can have an effect. Plus, several of the plant extracts and the menthol in this product can be skin irritants.

☹ **Peach & Papaya Gentle Facial Scrub** *($12 for 2 ounces)* contains menthol, lemon peel, balm mint, and several other potentially irritating ingredients. Papaya is not effective for exfoliation.

☺ $$$ **Sea Kelp-Herbal Facial Scrub** *($12 for 2.5 ounces)* uses cornmeal, walnut shell, and sea salt as the scrubbers. It will exfoliate skin, but it can be fairly abrasive for some skin types. Food products should also not be used on blemish-prone skin as they can encourage bacteria growth.

☹ **Lemon Mint Astringent, for Normal to Oily Skin** *($12 for 8 ounces)* has more than its share of irritating ingredients, including mint, lemongrass, peppermint, and witch hazel.

☹ **Perfectly Clear Herbal Antiseptic, for Oily or Acne Prone Skin** *($10.50 for 8 ounces)* is mostly alcohol, but contains a host of even more irritating ingredients, including camphor, eucalyptus oil, menthol, peppermint oil, and clove oil. This is nothing less than a perfectly irritating product with no benefit of any kind for skin.

☹ **Violet Rose Skin Toner** *($12 for 8 ounces)*. Several of the plant extracts this contains, including arnica, yarrow, coltsfoot, and juniper, are skin irritants.

☺ **Visible Transition 10% Alpha-Hydroxy Serum** *($27.50 for 1.1 ounces)* has a good concentration of AHAs, but the pH is too high for them to be effective as an exfoliant.

☺ **Bee Pollen-Jojoba Maximum Moisture Cream** *($15 for 2 ounces)*. This rather basic moisturizer contains several potentially irritating plant extracts, including arnica and juniper.

☺ **Calendula-Cucumber Oil Free Moisturizer** *($13.50 for 4 ounces)* might be oil-free, but this basic moisturizing formula is still better for normal to slightly dry skin than for someone with oily skin. The product does list information about sun protection, but it doesn't indicate an SPF and doesn't contain UVA-protecting ingredients, so it should not be relied on in any way for sun protection.

☺ **Elastin and Collagen Firming Treatment** *($20 for 2 ounces)*. The collagen and elastin this contains won't firm anything, but the yarrow, ivy, and comfrey can cause irritation.

✓☺ **Environmental Skin Protector SPF 18** *($27 for 4 ounces)* is a very good, in-part zinc oxide–based sunscreen in an emollient base with some very good antioxidants. It is an excellent option for normal to dry skin.

☺ **Ginseng and Collagen Wrinkle Treatment** *($20 for 2 ounces)*. The vitamins are way down on the list, but they can provide some antioxidant benefit. This would be a good moisturizer for dry skin, but several of the plant extracts, including arnica and comfrey, can be skin irritants.

☺ **Hi Potency "E" Special Treatment Line Control** *($14.50 for 2 ounces)*. This product lists the vitamin E content at 16,000 IU. While that number may sound impressive, it ends up being less than 0.33 ounce, and the 50,000 IU of vitamin A is only 0.000529 ounce. None of that is particularly potent or special, and it is powerless to control lines. This is an OK emollient moisturizer for normal to dry skin with a tiny amount of antioxidants, but that's about it.

The Reviews R

☺ $$$ **Immediately Visible Eye Renewal Gel-Cream with Liposomes** *($27 for 0.5 ounce)* includes bee pollen, and while that can be a good antioxidant it can also be an allergen. The algae can work as a good antioxidant and anti-irritant, but it won't change a wrinkle on your face. Still, this is a very good moisturizer for dry skin that contains some very good water-binding agents and antioxidants.

☹ **Lecithin-Aloe Moisture Retention Cream for Normal-Combination Skin** *($12.50 for 2 ounces)* includes enough oil so that it isn't good for combination skin, and the amount of sunscreen is minimal and doesn't provide UVA protection. It also contains arnica and balm mint, which are both skin irritants.

☹ **Clay and Ginseng Texturizing Mask** *($12 for 2 ounces)* is a standard clay mask that also contains mint, balm mint, and eucalyptus, which makes it too irritating for all skin types.

☺ **Color Therapy** *($35 for 12 ounces of toner and a corresponding colored light bulb)*. This is a standard toner of water, sea salt, algae, plant extracts (that impart color), fragrance, and preservatives combined with a matching-colored light bulb, and together it is supposed to impart the benefits of "The Ancient Art and Practice of Color Therapy." Skin care and balanced energy is the sales pitch here. According to Rachel Perry, "Studies done at UCLA and hundreds of other research facilities, world-wide, have shown the validity of using Color Therapy." I beg to differ: There aren't hundreds of studies. Perry's Web site doesn't include even one reference. A medical search pulls up only about 21 studies and none of them indicates efficacy, and definitely not in relation to skin care. If colors can affect your energy, you don't need to spend $35 for some grape juice–colored seawater to get it. However, if you want to believe these products supply your "depleted Energy Center with the color needed to balance the Electromagnetic Field (also called the "Aura") surrounding the body," then it's a cheap fix.

☺ **Lip Lover** *($3.50 for 0.2 ounce)* is a good, emollient, and even tasty group of lip balms in a host of flavors.

RE VIVE (SKIN CARE ONLY)

There is no doubt that the founder of Re Vive, Dr. Greg Brown, has some impressive credentials. According to his curriculum vitae, he is a board-certified general and plastic surgeon who trained at Vanderbilt, Harvard, and Emory Universities, and received his medical degree from the University of Louisville where he is currently a clinical professor of plastic surgery. Given this estimable medical background and the products he is marketing, he joins the ranks of Dr. Howard Murad (of Murad infomercial fame), Dr. Sheldon Pinnell (of SkinCeuticals), and Dr. N.V. Perricone (with products bearing his name) as a physician-turned-skin-care-salesperson. Now there is one more doctor telling you that his research is the way to go for the fountain of youth, and it will cost you a pretty penny (in fact, lots of pretty pennies) if you decide this one's got the answer.

Brown says that the solution to "rejuvenated, young-looking skin is bioengineered products." The Web site for Re Vive products mentions Brown's "experiments using human Epidermal Growing [sic] Factor (EGF) to stimulate wounds to heal faster" and quotes him as saying "'I saw evidence of absolute [healing] acceleration the first day and I became impassioned.'" This statement appears to be based on Brown's wound healing research that was done on 12 subjects in 1989 (Source: *New England Journal of Medicine*, July 1989, pages 76-79). So, is EFG the answer for your wrinkles?

Growth factors are produced by the body to regulate various types of cell division. EGF (epidermal growth factor) stimulates cell division, and primarily cell division of skin cells. There is research showing EGF to be helpful for wound and burn healing (Sources: *Journal of Burn Care and Rehabilitation*, March-April 2002, pages 116–125 and *Journal of Dermatologic Surgery and Oncology*, July 1992, pages 604–606). However, there is also research showing that its effect is no different from that of a placebo, and that it may not be effective at all (Sources: *Wounds*, 2001, volume 13, number 2, pages 53–58 and *Plastic and Reconstructive Surgery*, August 1995, pages 251–254) or on closed wounds (Source: *Journal Watch*, July 1989). One study showed it to have anti-inflammatory properties when applied to skin (Source: *Skin Pharmacology and Applied Skin Physiology*, January-April 1999, pages 79–84), though it has also been noted that it may promote tumor growth (Source:–*Journal of Surgical Research*, April 2002, pages 175–182; and–*Cell Growth and Differentiation*, November 1995, pages 1447-1455).

You have to wonder what happens when you put EGF on skin over time. Unfortunately, all of the research that does exist on EGF has looked primarily at short-term use for wound healing. Re Vive's products aren't about wound healing or short-term use, but rather ongoing application for wrinkles. Brown purports that EGF "stimulates skin cells to revert to their adolescent renewal pattern." This is quite a statement, given there are no studies showing this to be the true. Though theoretically he may be right, after all skin cells slowing down is one of the things that happen with age and sun damage. Technically, EGF's should increase cell division.

What I suspect to be the case is that these products can't do what they claim, despite the inclusion of EGF in the ingredient labels. EGF is a very large molecule and probably cannot penetrate intact skin. Further, the amount of EGF in these products is very tiny, no more then 0.2 micrograms.'

If you do decide to consider EGF, you don't need to use this entire line. Only one of the products containing EGF is necessary. The other products are standard with only the price tag being the exceptional part.

Incidentally, aside from all the purported benefit of EGF, Brown appears to be less aware about sun protection issues. Of his three SPF products, only one includes UVA-protecting ingredients. For more information about Re Vive, call (888) 704-3440 or visit www.revivecosmetics.com. **Note:** All Re Vive products contain fragrance.

☺ **$$$ Cleanser Agressif for Normal to Oily** *($65 for 16 ounces)* is an exceedingly ordinary, detergent-based cleanser that is absurdly overpriced. The negligible amount of water-binding agents and small amount of plant extracts, including *Melia azadirachta* leaf extract (neem extract, which may have unwanted side effects on skin) and *Arctium lappa* root extract (which may have some anti-inflammatory properties), are not unique to this product or unusual in any way. Lots of products for a fraction of this price have similar ingredients.

☺ **$$$ Cleanser Gentil for Normal to Dry** *($65 for 16 ounces)* is similar to the Normal to Oily version above only with slightly more gentle detergent cleansing agents. One of the plant extracts is an antioxidant, but there is also one that can be phototoxic (can cause negative skin reactions when exposed to sunlight). However, the amounts of both are so small they probably have no effect on skin.

☹ **$$$ Arrete Booster de Nuit** *($300 for 0.5 ounce)* simply contains silicones, vitamin C, vitamin E, glycine, soybean oil, retinol, and preservatives. The claims that this is in any way unique or even vaguely worth the inexcusable price tag (which comes to $9,600 per pound) border on the ridiculous. (There are lots of products that contain similar formulations for a lot less.) This doesn't even contain the EGF that is supposed to be the cornerstone of this line and that is supposed to make it worth the expense. If you really want a boost, feel proud that you didn't fall for this ordinary product!

☹ **$$$ Eye Renewal Cream** *($85 for 0.5 ounce)* is a decent moisturizer with some good water-binding agents and a tiny amount of antioxidants. The only reason to consider this product is if you accept the notion that Brown's EGF is a good ingredient for skin care.

☹ **$$$ Lip and Perioral Renewal Cream** *($105 for 0.5 ounce)*. This is a nice, silky-soft moisturizer (due to the high content of silicone). The decision about whether or not to spend this kind of money to get the EGF it contains is up to you. There really is no other reason to choose this over many other ordinary lip moisturizers.

☹ **$$$ Moisturizing Renewal Cream** *($120 for 2 ounces)* contains about 4% to 5% AHA (glycolic acid) and the pH is around 4. That makes it a good AHA exfoliant in a very good moisturizing base. However, if you're spending this kind of money on an AHA product it is only because it contains the showcased EGF.

☹ **$$$ Sensitif Cellular Repair Cream SPF 15** *($165 for 2 ounces)* is a very good, in-part avobenzone-based sunscreen in a very good moisturizing base with some good antioxidants and water-binding agents. It does contain EGF, and that would be the only reason to consider wasting money on this sunscreen. Keep in mind that sunscreens must be applied liberally to obtain the SPF benefit on the label; and it's unlikely that most people are going to apply a product that is this expensive liberally enough, and that would be dangerous for skin.

☹ **Fermitif Neck Renewal Cream SPF 15** *($105 for 2.5 ounces)* does not contain UVA-protecting ingredients and is not recommended.

☹ **Sensitif Cellular Repair Cream SPF 15** *($165 for 2 ounces)* does not contain UVA-protecting ingredients and is not recommended.

REJUVENESS (SKIN CARE ONLY)

You may have noticed ads in fashion magazines for a product called Rejuveness, claiming that it can magically heal scars. ☺ **Rejuveness** *($39.50 to $150, depending on the size ordered),* and other products like it, are nothing more than pliable sheets of silicone. Silicone is used in over 80% of all skin-care and hair-care products due to its flexibility, texture, and water-binding properties. Topical silicone sheets have been used for more than 20 years to help reduce the size of hypertrophic (raised) scars and keloids (thickened scars). Their clinical efficacy and safety are well established, and they have even been shown to help prevent hypertrophic scars and keloids after surgery (Sources: *Dermatologic Surgery,* July 2001, pages 641–644 and *Annals of Plastic Surgery,* October 1996, pages 345–348).

It is not clear how these sheets of silicone work. Some theorize that they increase the amount of water in the scar, and continuous hydration may soften the tissue, making it more elastic and pliable, resulting in a flattening process. No one is sure if that's true, but silicone sheets do work, and rather successfully (although I use the word "successfully" with caution).

As effective as this may be, there are disadvantages. Users purchase one relatively inexpensive sheet of silicone that is worn over and over again. You have to wear these sheets of silicone over the scar for prolonged periods of time, which means that you might not want to wear one on your face or other exposed parts of your body, at least not during the day. You need to keep the sheet clean, too, which requires some amount of care and maintenance time. Also, the silicone sheet can stick to the skin and clothing (wearing camisoles or T-shirts can help), and skin reactions such as rashes or irritation can occur.

What's even more difficult and uncomfortable is that you have to wear the covering for long periods—for hours at a time, over a span of at least two to nine months—in order to see a difference. But patience pays off: the longer you wear it, the more likely it is that the scar will dissipate to some extent. Of course, these sheets work best over new scars, but they also can make a difference with old ones. Be aware that the word "reduce" can be a suspect term. Do not give these a try if you are hoping for extraordinary results, of the kind that the advertising implies. Dr. Loren Engrav, associate director and chief of plastic surgery for the University of Washington burn unit at Harborview Medical Center, Seattle, Washington, explains that the "silicone strips are standard treatment for helping dissipate scars, and though the results may be good, they are absolutely not a miracle."

Some women buy the sheets to use over stretch marks, but there is no clinical evidence that this product will have any effect on them whatsoever, and the Rejuveness company will not guarantee its product for this use. These sheets use a flattening process, not a raising process, which would be required for stretch marks. For raised scars this isn't for everyone, but if you are willing to be persistent, it is absolutely worth a try. For more information about Rejuveness, call (800) 588-7455 or visit www.rejuveness.com.

REJUVENIQUE

With Linda Evans as its spokesperson, Rejuvenique has gotten some attention for its claims of ridding the face of wrinkles. As beautiful and captivating as Evans is, her appearance is not the result of these products. The fact that her beautiful features have been surgically altered and the photos of her visage have been nicely retouched are what accounts for the way this woman appears.

What is Rejuvenique? It is a set of skin-care products packaged with a face machine costing $99.99 that's sold at Target and via infomercials. The skin-care products are ordinary enough, although they carry the same amazing claims as most other skin-care products being sold. What makes this system unique is the Rejuvenique Mask. This Halloween-looking mask is worn as you would wear any mask, only this one has electric pulsations being sent through 26 metal contact points that press against the skin. These electrical pulses are meant to achieve "a smooth, toned, radiant look without undergoing time consuming procedures, harsh chemicals or other expensive invasive measures." What you end up getting is passive muscle stimulation. However, muscle strength has nothing to do with how the face wrinkles or sags. For example, the efficacy of Botox is due to its effect of *preventing* any muscle movement, which creates a perfectly smooth forehead or eliminates frown lines between the brows. Further, given that the muscles of the face are already the ones we use the most (due to facial expressions), making them firmer won't affect the way the face appears. In other words, wrinkles and sagging skin are not only the result of sun damage but also the result of muscles stretching and changing positions, not muscles that have become less strong. A firmer muscle in the wrong place on the face won't make it look better.

Aside from the lack of information indicating that strengthening facial muscles has any effect on wrinkles or sagging, my concern is that the electrical pulses from this mask generates may stimulate circulation and increase the risk of creating surfaced capillaries. There is an interesting disclaimer in the booklet that comes with the Rejuvenique products and mask. It says, "It is not intended [for] any permanent physical changes." Well, at least that's honest—but that information wasn't easy to find, and every other claim made sounds different from that one small well-hidden statement. For more information about Rejuvenique, call (800) 934-7455 or visit www.facetone.com. However, I don't recommend that you call or even think about surfing in that direction.

☻ **Facial Toning System** *[$99.99; includes Rejuvenique Mask, Purifying Cleanser (4 ounces), Vitamin C Serum (1 ounce), Eye Toner (1 ounce), Facial Moisturizer (2 ounces), Toning Gel (2 ounces), and Body Lotion (not reviewed)].*

☹ **Rejuvenique Mask** *($49.99)*. See the introductory section for Rejuvenique above for a discussion of this mask.

☺ **$$$ Purifying Cleanser** *($18.50 for 4 ounces)* is a very standard, detergent-based, water-soluble cleanser that would work well enough.

☺ **Vitamin C Serum** *($50 for 1 ounce)*. If you're looking for a vitamin C product this is one to look at, but that would be the only reason to consider this, because the skin needs more than that; vitamin C alone is not the answer to your skin-care woes. However you look at it, Avon's version is similar and it's available for less than half this price.

☺ **Eye Toner** *($22 for 1 ounce)* is an OK moisturizer for normal to slightly dry skin, and this amount of film-forming agent (it's the first ingredient) can make things look "tighter" for a brief period of time, although producing that effect doesn't make for good skin care. This contains only a minute amount of water-binding agent and antioxidant.

☺ **Facial Moisturizer** *($24 for 2 ounces)* is an OK moisturizer for normal to dry skin with minimal water-binding agents and an insignificant amount of an antioxidant.

☺ **Enriched Toning Gel** *($5 for 4 ounces)* is "a conductive gel" that helps transmit the electrical shock of the mask to your skin. The gel is just the same "gel-like" thickening agent used in all clear products of this nature, similar to what they use to administer an EKG or do an ultrasound. It is not enriched in any way, containing only a negligible amount of vitamins.

☺ **Neck Recovery Cream** *($30 for 4 ounces)* is similar to the Facial Moisturizer above and the same comments apply.

☺ **Retinol Evening Recovery** *($50 for 2 ounces)* doesn't contain retinol, but it does contain a fractional amount of retinyl palmitate, another form of vitamin A. It is a good antioxidant, but in this minute amount, it is unlikely to have any effect on skin. This ordinary lotion contains very little of benefit for skin. In fact, there is more preservative than vitamins.

REMEDE

Owned by Bliss Spa, Remede is their upscale line with price tags that are meant to give an instant impression of elite quality and superiority. What else are you supposed to think about a line that sells $40 cleansers and $135 moisturizers? Well, Remede is marketed as a line with "patented technology delivering more of what your skin needs—vitamins, botanicals, hydration and oxygen—for daily reparative rejuvenation." If there is something patented in these formulations or rejuvenating about them in any way, it is not evident in the ingredient lists. These are some of the most ordinary, standard formulations I've seen, not to mention that there are no sunscreens to be found. That isn't "reparative rejuvenation," rather it is the main road straight to wrinkles and skin damage. And the prices! If you're wondering whether or not any of these products are worth the flagrantly out-of-line price tags they carry, the answer, in one word, is NO. Most of these products wouldn't be worth the trouble for half the price, and others wouldn't be worth it

The Reviews R

even if they were free. Many aspects of these products are either potentially too irritating for skin or are accompanied by outlandish and distorted claims that are flagrantly misleading or just plain wrong. For more information about Remede, call (888) 243-8825 or visit www.blissout.com.

Note: All Remede products contain fragrance. Also, several of the Remede products mention that they contain something called SR-38, which is the trade name for the ingredient decyloxazolidinone. This ingredient is a film-forming agent (plasticizing agent similar to hair-spray ingredients) and it has some emollient properties. It is a good water-binding agent, but it is not a must-have ingredient for skin, nor is it worth the price tag on these products.

☺ $$$ **Convertible Cleanser All Skin Types** ($40 for 6.7 ounces) is more of a toner than a cleanser. That would be an option for normal to slightly oily skin, but it doesn't remove makeup very well. There is nothing about this cleanser that isn't easily replaced by far less pricey versions from other lines.

☺ $$$ **Convertible Cleanser Mature Fatigued Skin** ($40 for 6.7 ounces) is a mineral oil–based cleanser that is about as standard a cold cream–type formula as you can get. The minuscule amount of vitamins in this product makes them useless for skin. This formula is what ends up being fatigued, not your skin.

☹ **Convertible Cleanser Oily Active Skin** ($40 for 6.7 ounces) lists mineral oil as the first ingredient and corn oil as the fourth, along with some irritating plant extracts. Aside from the irritating plant extracts, this formula is almost identical to the Cleanser Mature above and the Cleanser Sensitive and Dry Dehydrated below. This product is an insult to those with oily skin.

☺ $$$ **Convertible Cleanser Sensitive Delicate Skin** ($40 for 6.7 ounces). The fragrance in this product makes this inappropriate for sensitive skin. The formula is just a cold cream, and there is nothing about this that makes it preferred over Olay or Neutrogena cleansers available at the drugstore.

☺ $$$ **Convertible Cleanser Dry Dehydrated Skin** ($40 for 6.7 ounces) is almost identical to the Cleanser Sensitive above and the same comments apply.

☺ $$$ **Cleanser Converter** ($24 for 6.7 ounces) is meant to be used with any of Remede's thick, heavy, oily cleansers (what they call condensed) to convert them into a washing option. This is a waste of time and effort. Rather than having to buy two cleansers to create one, why not just find one great cleanser that washes off and leaves the face clean but not greasy or dry, all in one step. (I recommend many such cleansers in Chapter Eight of this book.)

☺ $$$ **Dissolve** ($33 for 6.7 ounces) is an exceptionally standard, detergent-based makeup remover containing the most basic ingredient list imaginable. It works as well as any of this ilk.

☺ $$$ **Sweep** ($44 for 2.5 ounces). It takes a great deal of marketing know-how to convince women that a scrub containing mostly water, calcium carbonate (the ingredient in Tums, similar to baking soda—sodium bicarbonate), talc, some thickeners, clay, and preservatives is worth this kind of money. There is nothing about this product that isn't easily replaced by just plain baking soda and water.

☺ $$$ **Primer Mature Fatigued Skin** *($38 for 6.7 ounces)* is a standard toner that contains a tiny amount of water-binding agents and antioxidant. For this kind of money you would expect it to be overflowing with beneficial ingredients, but it comes up lacking on all fronts.

☹ **Primer Oily Active Skin** *($38 for 6.7 ounces)* lists alcohol as the second ingredient, and it also contains peppermint. Both are bad for your skin, and this price is bad for your budget.

☹ **Primer Sensitive Delicate Skin** *($38 for 6.7 ounces)* contains more fragrance than beneficial skin-care ingredients, because the insignificant amounts of green tea, aloe, and vitamin E in here are barely worth mentioning. This is little more than applying cologne to skin.

☺ $$$ **Primer Dry Dehydrated Skin** *($38 for 6.7 ounces)*. The myrtle extract in this product can be a problem for skin. It also contains mostly water, honey, slip agent, castor oil, silicone, preservatives, water-binding agents, and preservatives. You are getting more preservatives in this product than you are beneficial ingredients for skin, and at this price that is really disappointing.

☺ $$$ **Anti Wrinkle Intensive Cream Line Softening Anti Fatigue Formula with Retinol Derivative and SR-38** *($135 for 1.7 ounces)* doesn't contain retinol; rather, it contains a fractional amount of retinyl palmitate, which is too minute to have benefit for skin.

☺ $$$ **Alchemy** *($72 for 1.7 ounces)* is a good moisturizer for normal to dry skin that contains a small amount of some very good water-binding agents and antioxidants. But the only part of this that's like alchemy is that a woman would actually spend this amount of money for a product that is easily replaced (and improved on) by much less expensive options. Now that's magic.

☺ $$$ **Brightening Active Booster** *($65 for 1 ounce)*. The only ingredient in this product that has any hope of improving the color of skin is kojic acid, but it contains less than 0.1% of it and that isn't enough to be effective in any way for inhibiting melanin production. It also contains about 2% AHA, which is not even close to enough to be effective for exfoliation. The fractional amount of vitamin C is just a waste.

☺ $$$ **Complete Treatment with SR-38 Dry Dehydrated Skin** *($95 for 1.7 ounces)* is an emollient moisturizer for normal to dry skin that contains some good plant oils. The trivial amounts of water-binding agents and antioxidants make it completely overpriced.

☺ $$$ **Complete Treatment Mature Fatigued Skin** *($95 for 1.7 ounces)* is an emollient moisturizer that contains far more fragrance than beneficial ingredients for skin. It has an insignificant amount of antioxidants and water-binding agents, and that is really tiring when you consider how much you're spending on this product.

☺ **$$$ Complete Treatment Sensitive Delicate** *($95 for 1.7 ounces)* is an ordinary emollient moisturizer for dry skin that contains some good antioxidants and water-binding agents. Some of the plant extracts are good anti-irritants, but there are also some plant extracts that can be problematic for skin. The fragrance doesn't help sensitive skin.

☺ **$$$ Hydrating Treatment Cream Complex Day, Dry Dehydrated Skin** *($125 for 1.7 ounces)* is a standard emollient moisturizer for dry skin that contains the tiniest amount of antioxidants and water-binding agents imaginable. Without sunscreen, this is inappropriate for daytime.

☺ **$$$ Moisture Intensive Cream Dry Dehydrated Skin Saturating Formula with SR-38 Night** *($135 for 1.7 ounces)* is an emollient moisturizer for normal to dry skin that contains minute amounts of antioxidants and water-binding agents.

☹ **Complete Treatment with SR-38 Oily Active** *($95 for 1.7 ounces)* contains several ingredients that are problematic for oily skin, including caprylic/capric triglyceride, shea butter, and plant oil. Several of the plant extracts are skin irritants, too.

☹ **Purifying Intensive Cream Oily Active Skin Control Formula with SR-38** *($135 for 1.7 ounces)* is similar to the Complete Treatment above and the same basic comments apply.

☹ **Purifying Active Amplifier Intensive Regulating Serum Day Night** *($70 for 1 ounce)* lists alcohol as the second ingredient, which makes this too drying and irritating for skin. It also contains a tiny amount of tea tree oil, but not enough to be effective for disinfection.

☹ **Matifying Treatment Cream Complex Oily Active Skin** *($125 for 1.7 ounces)* offers little benefit for dry skin. It is a silicone-based moisturizer with emollient ingredients that are a problem for oily skin, as are several of the plant extracts. The minute amount of retinyl palmitate can have no beneficial impact on skin.

☺ **$$$ Neck Specific Lift Serum** *($65 for 1 ounce)* is an emollient lotion that doesn't contain one ingredient that is in any way special for the neck, or capable of lifting skin anywhere. It is just an OK moisturizer for normal to dry skin.

☺ **$$$ Firming Active Amplifier Intensive Reinforcing Serum with SR-38 Day Night** *($75 for 1 ounce)* is similar to the Neck Specific Lift Serum above and the same comments apply.

☺ **$$$ Night Eye Contour Barrier Balm Intensive Treatment Creme with SR-38** *($80 for 0.5 ounce)* is a good emollient moisturizer for normal to dry skin that contains some good antioxidants and water-binding agents, just not very much of them.

☺ **$$$ Sensitive Intensive Cream Soothing Skin Formula with SR-38 Night** *($135 for 1.7 ounces)* is similar to the Night Eye Contour Barrier Balm above and the same basic comments apply. There is nothing in this product that makes it preferred for sensitive skin.

☺ **$$$ Soothing Treatment Creme Complex Sensitive Delicate Skin Day** *($125 for 1.7 ounces)* is similar to the Night Eye Contour Barrier Balm above and the same basic comments apply. There is nothing in this product that makes it preferred for sensitive skin. And without sunscreen, it is not to be worn during the day.

☺ $$$ **Wrinkle Diffusion Treatment Cream Complex Mature Fatigued Skin with SR-38 Day** *($125 for 1.7 ounces)* is a plant oil– and lanolin-based moisturizer for dry to very dry skin. It contains tiny amounts of water-binding agents and antioxidants, but these are just trace amounts and, therefore, will not impart much, if any, benefit to the skin.

☹ **Oxygenating Active Amplifier Intensive Energizing Serum Day or Night** *($70 for 1 ounce)* contains hydrogen peroxide, a significant oxidizing agent that generates free-radical damage. There's plenty of research detailing the cumulative problems that can stem from impacting the skin with a substance that is known to generate free-radical damage, impair the skin's healing process, cause cellular destruction, and reduce optimal cell functioning (Sources: *Carcinogenesis,* March 2002, pages 469–475 and *Anticancer Research,* July-August 2001, pages 2719–2724). More oxygen is not what you want—that's why most good skin-care products include *anti*oxidants in their formulations.

☹ **Double Oxygenating Active Amplifier Intensive Serum for Control of Oily/ Active Skin** *($65 for 1 ounce)* is similar to the Oxygenating Active Amplifier Intensive Energizing version above and the same comments apply.

☺ $$$ **Retexturizing Active Amplifier Intensive Exfoliating Serum for Night** *($70 for 1 ounce)* contains about 4% AHA, but the pH isn't low enough for it to be effective for exfoliation. This is even more unimpressive than any of the other Remede products (there's nary a water-binding agent or antioxidant in sight), which make this a substandard formulation. For AHAs you would be far better off with any of the AHA products from Alpha Hydrox at the drugstore.

☺ $$$ **Line Softening Active Amplifier Intensive Wrinkle Refining Serum with Retinol Derivative and SR-38 for Night** *($75 for 1 ounce)* doesn't contain retinol, but it does contain a fractional amount of retinyl palmitate. There is more preservative content in this product than any beneficial ingredients for skin.

☺ $$$ **Clarifying Active Amplifier Intensive Brightening Serum with SR-38 Night** *($70 for 1 ounce)* is similar to the Line Softening version above and the same comments apply, only this doesn't contain retinyl palmitate.

☺ $$$ **Soft Focusing Lotion Light Diffusing Luminizing Topcoat Oil Free Day** *($38 for 1 ounce)* is a silicone-based serum that has some oil-absorbing properties, but there are no water-binding agents, antioxidants, or anti-irritants in this somewhat shimmery lotion. There is little benefit to skin from using this.

☹ **Skin Exacting Mask** *($88 for 1.7 ounces)* contains peppermint, eucalyptus, and coriander, which make this too irritating for all skin types.

☺ $$$ **Creme Converter All Skin Types Oil Free** *($44 for 1.7 ounces)* is just silicone (similar to hair serums you buy at the drugstore). You're supposed to mix this into your moisturizer to increase its "barrier protection." It will do that, but it would have been better just to include more silicone in the moisturizer in the first place.

The Reviews R

☹ **Lotionizer All Skin Types** *($27 for 1.7 ounces)* is supposed to be a gel you mix in with other cream moisturizers to make them lighter weight. This will do the job, but it doesn't add one interesting or beneficial ingredient to the mix and could end up diluting the efficacy of an otherwise well-formulated product. Of course, given the lack of well-formulated products in this line that shouldn't be a problem.

☺ **$$$ Translucent UV Coat Tinted SPF 30** *($36)* has a fluid, slippery texture that is a bit difficult to control, but is nevertheless a lightweight, moist-finish option for someone with normal to dry skin seeking ultra-light coverage and excellent sun protection. This features an in-part titanium dioxide sunscreen and three very sheer colors. Price-wise, you may want to consider the tinted-moisturizer options from Aveda, Bobbi Brown, and Clinique before this one.

REVERSA (CANADA ONLY)

This Canadian-based skin-care company is, as the name implies, all about reversing the signs of aging. It can't do that, though there are some products that can definitely make skin look better and that do offer good sun protection. What these products are really about are alpha hydroxy acids (AHAs). Most of them contain glycolic acid, one of the more effective forms of AHA, in formulations with pH levels that make them good options for exfoliation. Another strong point for this small line of products is their well-designed sunscreens. But even the sunscreens contain AHA, and if you are using them in combination with some of the other AHA-containing products, that can end up being too much AHA for one face. The skin only needs one effective AHA product to help improve cell turnover and exfoliation, and it doesn't necessarily need to be applied twice a day; often once a day, at night, is plenty. More important, the skin needs more than AHAs and sunscreen to help combat the onslaught of sun damage and the passing of time. Moisturizers or toners with good concentrations of antioxidants, water-binding agents, and anti-irritants should be part of the game plan, and in that area this line comes up short. For more information about Reversa, call (800) 465-8383 or visit www.reversa.ca. **Note:** Prices are in Canadian dollars.

☺ **3 in 1 Mild Gel Cleanser** *($17.99 for 130 ml)* is a standard, detergent-based, water-soluble cleanser that contains a tiny amount of water-binding agents. This is an option for normal to dry skin.

☹ **Solution for Oily to Acne-Prone Skin** *($26.99 for 60 ml)* is an alcohol-based 8% AHA product, which makes it too irritating and drying for all skin types.

☺ **$$$ Eye Contour Cream** *($23.99 for 15 ml)* is about a 3% glycolic acid–based moisturizer with a pH of 4. The pH makes it effective for exfoliation, although the amount of AHA is on the low side. The ordinary emollient base has a minuscule amount of a water-binding agent and an antioxidant. For a gentle and basic AHA product, this is an option for normal to dry skin, but for the money it is easily replaced by AHA products from Alpha Hydrox at the drugstore.

☺ **Skin Smoothing Cream 5%** *($26.99 for 60 ml)* is similar to the Eye Contour Cream above with a 5% AHA concentration. The same basic comments apply, but this is more effective for exfoliation due to the increased amount of AHA. It is an option for normal to dry skin.

☺ **Skin Smoothing Cream 8%** *($26.99 for 60 ml)* is similar to the Skin Smoothing Cream above only with an 8% concentration of AHA, and the same basic comments apply.

☺ **Corrective Night Cream** *($26.99 for 50 ml)* is a 4% AHA product with an effective pH of 4. It contains a small amount of antioxidants and a water-binding agent.

☺ **UV Ultra Vigilance Restorative Skin Tone Cream SPF 15** *($25.99 for 50 ml)* is a very good, in-part avobenzone-based sunscreen that also contains about 4% AHA in an ordinary moisturizing base that would be OK for someone with normal to dry skin. The pH of 4 makes this effective for exfoliation. However, for daytime wear, your skin would be far better off with a sunscreen loaded with water-binding agents and antioxidants, something this product contains almost none of. Still, for an effective combined AHA and sunscreen product, this is one of the few well-formulated ones being sold.

☺ **UV Ultra Vigilance Anti-Wrinkle Cream SPF 15** *($25.99 for 60 ml)* is almost identical to the Restorative Skin Tone Cream above and the same basic comments apply. This contains about an 8% AHA concentration and is an option for normal to dry skin.

☺ **UV Anti-Wrinkle Fluid SPF 15** *($25.99 for 50 ml)* is almost identical to the Restorative Skin Tone Cream above and the same basic comments apply. This contains about an 8% AHA concentration and is an option for normal to dry skin.

☺ **$$$ UV Anti Wrinkle Eye Contour Cream SPF 15** *($25.99 for 15 ml)* is almost identical to the Restorative Skin Tone Cream above and the same basic comments apply. This contains about an 8% AHA concentration and is an option for normal to dry skin.

☺ **Self Tanning Spray** *($13.49 for 125 ml)* contains dihydroxyacetone, the same ingredient that all self-tanners use to affect the color of skin. This would work as well as any. It also contains mixed fruit acids, but they aren't the same as AHAs, nor is the pH of this product effective for exfoliation. That's actually good news, because if it were effective as an exfoliant you would be exfoliating away the very tan you were applying.

☺ **UV Moisturizing Lip Balm SPF 15** *($5.99 for 15 ml)* is a very good, in-part avobenzone-based sunscreen in a very ordinary, Vaseline-based balm that is an option for dry lips and sun protection. It contains about a 2% AHA concentration, which isn't enough to make this effective for exfoliation.

REVLON

As one of the leading mass-market cosmetics lines in the world, Revlon has done an excellent job with product innovation as well as with keeping abreast of the industry when it comes to makeup products. When it comes to skin care, however, Revlon's products are not well diversified or particularly creative. Revlon's Eterna '27' is still around and remains unchanged after decades on the market. In an attempt to improve their skin-care line Revlon launched Age-Defying products, but those never took off. Now they have Vitamin C Absolutes, which are less about vitamin C and more about wafting fragrance that smells like oranges. Hopefully, consumers are aware that the fragrance is not indicative of how much vitamin C a product contains. There are some well-formulated sunscreens, but the limited choices aren't the best for a range of skin care needs. When it comes to skin care, Revlon-owned Almay has far more effective options. For more information about Revlon, call (800) 4-REVLON or visit www.revlon.com.

REVLON SKIN CARE

☺ **Age Defying Performance Skin Care Face Cream SPF 15** *($12.61 for 1.75 ounces)* and **Age Defying Performance Skin Care Oil-Free Face Lotion SPF 15** *($12.61 for 1.7 ounces)* are very good, in-part avobenzone-based sunscreens in ordinary moisturizing bases that contain a small amount of antioxidants. These do contain a tiny amount of salicylic acid, but not enough for it to be effective for exfoliation.

☺ **Eterna '27' All Day Moisture Lotion** *($12.99 for 2 ounces)* is an emollient moisturizer for normal to dry skin that contains some good water-binding agents.

☺ **Eterna '27' All Day Moisture Cream** *($12.99 for 1 ounce)* is very similar to the Lotion above, but with still more thickeners and mineral oil. It would be good for dry to very dry skin.

☺ **Eterna '27' with Exclusive Progenitin** *($13.99 for 2 ounces)* contains pregnenolone acetate, often derived from animal urine. Pregnenolone acetate is a precursor to other hormones and can, when taken orally, affect levels of progesterone and estrogen in the body. When applied topically to skin it may work as a water-binding agent. There is no information on whether absorption through skin is possible.

REVLON VITAMIN C ABSOLUTES

The orange-colored products and the color of the packaging speak volumes about these skin-care products. The name and color, along with a wafting citrus aroma, are the clinchers for getting across the marketing message these products want you to hear. This is about vitamin C being great for skin. But for skin care, ignore the orange fruit water, which is useless for skin and, if anything, can be a skin irritant (ever get real orange juice on a cut?). What these products do contain is magnesium ascorbyl phosphate (MAP), a very stable and good form of vitamin C. While MAP is a good skin-care ingredient, acting as an antioxidant and potential melanin inhibitor, the amount of it in these products is minuscule and not of much benefit for skin. If they didn't have such a pungent aroma, I would be more excited about recommending what appear to be some well-formulated products. As far as formulation is concerned, there are some very good water-binding agents, anti-irritants, and antioxidants in this group, along with reliable sunscreens, and that is what really feels good for skin.

☺ **Vitamin C Reviving Cleanser** *($7.69 for 6.6 ounces)* is a standard, detergent-based cleanser that would actually work well for most skin types, that is if you can get beyond the smell and coloring agents.

☹ **Vitamin C Absolutes Refreshing Tonic** *($7.69 for 6.7 ounces)*. Between the alcohol and orange water, this is far more irritating than refreshing. It does contain magnesium ascorbyl phosphate, a stable form of vitamin C, but the alcohol makes this formula more of a problem than a benefit.

☹ **Vitamin C Absolutes Radiant Skin Scrub** *($7.69 for 3.2 ounces)* is a standard scrub that uses ground-up plastic (polyethylene) as the abrasive agent. This also contains sodium lauryl sulfate as one of the main ingredients, which would make this otherwise OK scrub a problem for most skin types due to the risk of irritation and dryness.

✓☺ **Vitamin C Absolutes Overnight Renewal Cream** *($14.89 for 1.6 ounces)* is a very good moisturizer for dry skin that contains an incredibly long list of ingredients—the "everything but the kitchen sink" approach is used here, including vitamins A, E, C, and several other antioxidants, as well as water-binding agents. None of these will firm the skin, but they can certainly make dry skin look and feel smoother and softer. This does contain fragrance.

✓☺ **Eye Contour Radiance Cream** *($14.89 for 0.45 ounce)* is far more emollient than the Renewal Cream above, although it contains many of the same other assets that warrant a good rating.

✓☺ **Daily Radiance Cream SPF 15** *($12.99 for 1.6 ounces)* is a good, avobenzone-based sunscreen with several antioxidants that would work well for normal to dry skin. The fragrance can be overpowering, but the formulation is still good for dry skin. The radiance comes from the slight bit of shimmer that the mica imparts.

✓☺ **Oil-Free Radiance Lotion SPF 15** *($14.89 for 1.6 ounces)* is similar to the Cream version above, only in lotion form, and the same basic comments apply.

REVLON MAKEUP

The mainstay of Revlon's makeup over the past several years has been its two major color lines, Age Defying (for the 35 and over crowd) and ColorStay (for the under-35, oily-skin crowd). Both age groups are served well, as these lines offer excellent options. Age Defying is best for normal to very dry skin, while ColorStay, whose namesake lip color spawned a new generation of lipstick consistency that is both ultra-matte and dry, is great for oily to very oily skin. New Complexion is more for normal to oily skin, and is sort of a go-between for those too oily (or young) for Age Defying and too dry for ColorStay. Recent additions that have caused a resurgence of interest in Revlon are the shine-all-the-time Skinlights and High Dimension lines. The weakest spot in this enormous line are the mascaras, most of which just aren't in the same league (or even the same sport) when measured against L'Oreal and Maybelline mascaras. Still, Revlon has earned its reputation for its superior products, and that helps offset these deficiencies. You can't go wrong

The Reviews R

if you pay attention to their mostly awesome foundations, concealers, Absolutely Fabulous LipCream SPF 15, and many of the eye pencils. Until the new management team accomplishes their lofty goals, Revlon, for all its strong points, will have to concede as runner-up to L'Oreal when it comes to the best makeup line at the drugstore. But stay tuned, because the competition will undoubtedly become more heated as the perpetual one-upmanship continues.

<u>FOUNDATION:</u> Revlon seldom has testers for its foundations, but many stores do sell sample packs with three shades so you can try the colors for a minimal investment.

☺ **Age Defying Makeup with SPF 10** *($11.49)* is best for someone with normal to dry skin (the formula contains oil) and provides light to almost medium coverage. The SPF is titanium dioxide–based, although the number is marginally low. However, if you're willing to wear an SPF 15 underneath, the makeup's texture, soft matte finish, and 12 shades are quite good. The only shades to view with caution are Cool Beige, Medium Beige, and Sand Beige.

✓☺ **Age Defying Makeup and Concealer Compact SPF 20** *($13.89)* is an excellent option for foundation and sunscreen in one product. The active ingredients are titanium dioxide and zinc oxide, which provide the required broad-spectrum protection. The foundation portion is a cream-to-powder makeup that has a smooth, even finish and some great colors, though nothing for very light or very dark skin tones. The concealer portion has the same SPF, but is fairly greasy and can easily crease into lines under the eyes. Medium skin tones may find that some of the concealer colors are too dark to cover circles under the eye, yet these shortcomings are minor compared to the strong positives, and this would work well for normal to dry skin. There are eight shades, but Honey Beige and Medium Beige are too peachy pink, while Natural Beige is borderline peach. ✓☺ **Age Defying All Day Lifting Foundation SPF 20** *($12.49)* won't lift your skin anywhere. However, it is a luxurious, emollient foundation for normal to dry skin that blends impeccably and can provide medium to almost full coverage. It also has a brilliant SPF, with titanium dioxide and zinc oxide as the active ingredients. There are ten shades to consider, but none for very light or very dark skin tones, which is disappointing. Avoid Honey Beige, Cool Beige, and Natural Beige, which are too pink or peach for most skin tones. ✓☺ **ColorStay Lite Makeup SPF 15** *($11.29)* is simply the best ultra-matte foundation with sunscreen available. Before I delve into a description, let me say that (as of this writing) this foundation *has not* been discontinued. Revlon has done away with the six darkest colors, and some drugstores have stopped carrying it in favor of Revlon's Skin Mattifying Makeup, but Revlon repeatedly confirmed that it is still available. The six remaining shades are great for fair to medium skin, and only Ivory is slightly pink, though it can still work for some fair skin tones. These shades apply lighter than they look, which can make choosing the right one even trickier. ColorStay Lite has a smooth, fluid texture and provides medium to full coverage that dries quickly to a solid, long-wearing ultra-matte finish. It is best to blend this systematically, because any mistakes that dry will require removal and reapplication—this isn't a makeup you can easily smooth out if it's not applied right the first time. Yet if you have oily to very oily skin, the trade-offs and shine control are worth it. The SPF is pure titanium dioxide, and some women may find that exacerbates breakouts, yet that's the paradox and agony of using sunscreen when you have oily skin. The packaging isn't the smartest choice for this liquidy formula, but if you're cautious, it shouldn't be too much of a problem. ✔☺ **ColorStay Stick Makeup SPF 15** *($11.29)* glides on smooth and slightly creamy, and then dries to a soft, translucent finish. It can have light to medium coverage, comes in ten mostly great colors, and the SPF is part titanium dioxide and part zinc oxide. The noncomedogenic claim is bogus, but this is absolutely worth a try if you want a soft, matte, slightly powdery finish. However, please be aware that while this can be great for someone with normal to slightly dry or slightly oily skin, it doesn't have the staying power of the other ColorStay foundations. It can slip and let oil show through like most stick foundations do. Avoid Natural Beige, and be careful with Caramel, which may be too orange for darker skin tones. ✔☺ **New Complexion One Step Compact Makeup SPF 15** *($12.79)* is a cream-to-powder foundation with titanium dioxide as the only sunscreen agent. This one is surprisingly similar to Clinique's City Base Compact Foundation SPF 15 ($20). I simply could not tell the difference in a side-by-side face test of the two products. They applied, felt, looked, and wore the same. Revlon has 12 shades (Clinique has 10), and they are, for the most part, fairly neutral, although the range of tones is strange. The selection of lighter shades is extremely limited for Revlon, and the darker colors are all a bit coppery. If you have a more medium skin tone, you're in luck, and if you have normal to slightly dry skin you'll do well if you prefer this type of product. Avoid Natural Beige, Cool Beige, Warm Beige, and Sun Beige. Tender Peach is fairly true to its name, but may work for some light skin tones.

☺ **ColorStay Makeup SPF 6** *($11.29)* is beyond matte, beyond no shine, and far beyond the claim of "it won't rub off." In fact, it won't rub (or wash) off even when you want it to! This is one of the most stubborn makeups I have ever tested. Get it on right the first time, because once it dries, it won't budge. If you get even the slightest wrong color it can look like a chalky mask, and removing it at night takes a great deal of effort, including several attempts with your cleanser and washcloth. Therefore, this is only appropriate for someone with truly oily skin and a deft hand at blending who is looking for medium to heavy coverage. Revlon has expanded the number of shades to 16, but all of the deeper shades, from Rich Tan through Mocha, are way too copper, orange, or red for darker skin tones. Also, the deeper colors are without sun protection, but the SPF 6 (titanium dioxide–based) is really far too low to count on anyway. The remaining shades for light to medium skin tones fare better, but watch out for Ivory and Natural Beige— both are slightly pink. Medium skin tones have the best selection of neutral colors with this one. **New Complexion Makeup SPF 4** *($11.79)* has an embarrassingly low titanium dioxide–based SPF, but it does have a very light texture that blends evenly and dries to a natural, light-coverage finish. Of the nine shades, the only good options are Sand Beige,

The Reviews R

Medium Beige, and Sun Beige. The rest are too pink, orange, or peach. **Shine Control Mattifying Makeup SPF 15** *($10.99)* definitely wins points for having an excellent titanium dioxide– and zinc oxide–based sunscreen, along with a fluid, light texture that applies quite well and dries (almost instantly) to a sheer, solid-matte finish. What's disappointing is the addition of SD-alcohol (it's the third ingredient), which makes this unnecessarily irritating for all skin types, not to mention the subtle alcohol odor. In addition, the 12 colors are a mixed bag. The lighter shades all lean toward being too peach to work well for most skin tones. The darker shades fare better, and the ones to consider are Honey Beige, Natural Tan, Caramel, and Cappuccino. So how does this compare to ColorStay Lite? It's assuredly lighter in texture, and has an even thinner consistency that offers less coverage. It's also not transfer-resistant, but it does stay on well, and although it is not being billed as an ultra-matte foundation, it's extremely matte finish may make you think otherwise! **New Complexion Even Out Makeup Oil-Free SPF 20** *($11.79)* is an amalgam of traits that tries to be a little bit of everything and comes up far too short in most departments and way ahead in others. The sunscreen is excellent, containing both zinc oxide and titanium dioxide. Yet the color selection, with many of the nine shades being too peach, pink, or ash, is disappointing. The consistency is rather light and moist, which is great for a sheer finish if you have dry skin. However, this also contains salicylic acid (BHA), which is a waste in a foundation, where the pH is too high for it to be effective. All in all, there are more problems than positives with this one, and I wouldn't choose it over Revlon's New Complexion One Step Compact Makeup reviewed above. If you want to brave the odds, the only colors that look like skin are Sand Beige, Caramel, Nude Beige, and Natural Tan. **Wet/Dry Foundation SPF 10** *($13.89)* is not an impressive foundation in the least, especially when weighed against Revlon's top-notch foundations. This is a basic pressed powder–type foundation, and includes an in-part titanium dioxide sunscreen whose SPF number is far below the recommended standard of SPF 15. The talc-based texture is not as silky-smooth as many powder foundations, the finish is slightly chalky, and, when used dry, it is hard to blend into the skin. Ironically, this tends to go on better when used wet, though like all wet/dry powders, streaking will be apparent unless you blend very well. What's more, six of the nine shades are too peach or pink for most skin tones. The only colors worth considering are Ivory Beige (slight pink), Sand Beige, and Natural Tan.

<u>CONCEALER:</u> ✔☺ **ColorStay Concealer SPF 6** *($9.69)* is awesome and ranks up there with the best of them. It absolutely doesn't crease, stays on very well, isn't nearly as heavy or thick as the ColorStay original foundation, and comes in three very good neutral colors. It does provide opaque coverage and can be a problem if you want to hide, instead of accentuate, lines under the eyes, but it takes good care of dark circles all day long. If the finish seems too matte, try mixing it with a drop of moisturizer.

☺ **Age Defying All Day Lifting Concealer SPF 20** *($8.89)* is an ideal, creamy, compact-type concealer that covers well and blends evenly without being too slippery.

True to the nature of cream concealers, this will crease unless it is set with powder. Unfortunately, that's not the best look if you have prominent lines around the eye. However, for facial discolorations in wrinkle-free zones, this works well, and the titanium dioxide/zinc oxide sunscreen is gravy!

POWDER: ☹ **Love Pat Moisturizing Powder** *($9.49)* is still around and all the colors are still too pink or peach for most skin tones.

☺ **New Complexion Powder Normal to Oily Skin** *($11.69)* is a standard, talc-based powder with a decent color selection, but nothing about this powder will control oil—it's just a good, standard, dry-finish powder. It blends on smooth and soft and comes in a decent assortment of shades. Avoid Warm Beige and Even Out, which is a color-correcting shade of yellow. **New Complexion Bronzing Powder** *($11.99)* is a talc-based, pressed-powder bronzer that comes in a very natural-looking tan shade with minimal shine. It would work best on light to medium skin tones.

☺ **Age Defying Pressed Loose Powder** *($12.59)* is a puzzle. Pressed loose powder is a contradiction in terms, isn't it? This is a lightweight, talc-based pressed powder that applies rather sheer but also slightly chalky. It feels silky and the three colors are fine, but I wouldn't choose this over pressed powders from L'Oreal or Clinique. **Age Defying Smoothing Powder** *($12.59)* is also talc-based and leaves a slightly chalky finish, but it's OK if dusted on with a brush. The six shades offer some good colors, but you'll want to steer clear of Medium Beige and Honey Beige. **New Complexion Shine Control Mattifying Powder SPF 8** *($8.19)* is a talc-based pressed powder that has a somewhat thick, dry texture and a slightly heavy-feeling, but sheer, matte finish. The sunscreen is in-part titanium dioxide, and although the SPF is too low, this can still be a good addition if used with a reliable foundation with adequate sunscreen. Of the six shades, half are worth a look if you have light to medium skin. The colors to avoid are Sheer Mattifyer (too yellow) and Light-Medium and Medium (both too peach, especially for oily skin).

☺ BLUSH: **Sleek Cheeks Creme Blush Duo** *($9.49)* offers a sheer, shiny cream-to-powder blush along with a luminescent highlighter. These apply moist and are surprisingly easy to blend to a soft powder finish. Each of the six duos has a subtle amount of shine, but it's not really enough to be distracting. The highlighter shade is shinier, and this would be more appropriate for an evening look. Overall, the colors are beautiful and this is worth checking out if you prefer this type of blush and want it to shine. Because it contains waxes, this is not recommended for blemish-prone skin. **Smooth-On Blush** *($8.89)* is a powder blush with a luscious, silky texture and a soft, sheer finish. The original colors weren't much for depth or brightness, and they're deceptively shiny, but this has since been merged with Revlon's former Naturally Glamorous Blush-On, and it now offers some beautiful matte options. Check out Wine with Everything, Berry Rich, and Tawny Blush.

EYESHADOW: ☹ **Wet/Dry Eyeshadows** *($4.19 singles; $4.49 duos; $5.89 quads)* are all shiny and have a texture that just doesn't wear well, wet or dry. The notion of applying eyeshadows wet for a more intense, opaque effect is interesting, but opaque shine often leads to flaking, and this formula doesn't rise above that common side effect. As an option, there is one matte quad set, called In the Buff, as well as a matte duo, Raisin Rage, whose colors are nicely coordinated. The rest just have too much shine and won't look as foolproof and elegant as they do in Revlon's ads. **ColorStay Powder Shadow** *($7.69)* comes in a tube, which is not my favorite way of applying eyeshadow, since blendability is essential and that isn't easy with such a dry, unmovable eye color. All of these colors are about as stubborn as they come; they "grab" onto the skin before you can blend them. And forget about adding more than one color or applying it again, because once this formula sets, any efforts to blend result in clumps and eyeshadow fingerprints! The only positive is that they will definitely last throughout the day without fading. **ColorStay Powder Shadow** *($7.69)* comes in a tube and offers two shiny colors in one stick. Try this if you're one of the few people who might possibly want a stubborn, difficult-to-blend eyeshadow that grabs onto the skin, sets far too soon, and then won't budge. The only plus is that it lasts and lasts—but with the way it looks, do you really want that?

 ✓☺ **Illuminance Creme Eyeshadow** *($6.29)* offers four shades of cream-to-powder eyeshadow in a sleek compact. Although I am not a fan of cream eyeshadows, as they tend to crease and can be troublesome to blend with other colors, these hold up quite well and go on softly. The color palette is limited, especially if you prefer neutral tones, but those who enjoy cream eyeshadows should strongly consider these. The best sets are Not Just Nudes, Pink Petals, and Wild Orchids (although Wild Orchids can be too purple for some of those with fair skin tones).

 <u>EYE AND BROW SHAPER:</u> ✓☺ **Softstroke Powderliner** *($6.79)* has a great powdery texture and a matte finish that has great staying power, and it glides on effortlessly. The only drawback is the frequent sharpening that it needs.

 ☺ **TimeLiner for Eyes** *($6.79)* are very good, standard pencils that apply and blend easily. They have a very soft tip, so be wary of applying too much pressure. **Wet/Dry Eyeliner** *($6.49)* is a standard pencil that is slightly creamy and that can smudge if used dry. Wet application dries to a more solid finish, but also gives a more dramatic look. Pure Pearl is a shiny white that can look too stark against most skin colors. **ColorStay Brow Color** *($8.19)* is a two-ended product: one end is a mascara-like wand with color to stroke on the brow, and the other end is a pencil. In some ways, this is the best of both worlds—particularly if you already use a brow pencil and a brow groomer to thicken and tint the brow. This one's tinted brow gel goes on easily and stays well, while the pencil is just a pencil, nothing special, and it doesn't stay around any better than other pencils.

 ☺ **ColorStay Eyeliner** *($7.19)* is a standard pencil that comes in a twist-up container. It eventually sets and stays put, but it may still smear and go on somewhat choppy. **Brow Maker** *($5.99)* presents a matte brow powder along with a clear, lightweight brow wax. The accompanying (very small) brush is used to apply the slightly waxy powder, and then you simply add a dab of the clear wax to hold brows in place. The concept is fine, but this can feel somewhat sticky and is really no substitute for the mascara-type brow tints available from Bobbi Brown, Origins, and my own line, to name a few. Still, if your brows are annoyingly unruly, this is worth a look.

☹ **ColorStay Liquid Liner** *($7.19)* still has a strange, hard applicator that scratches at the eyelid as you put it on. Why Revlon hasn't changed this yet is beyond me. It does stay well, but applying it is a less than ideal process. **High Dimension Eyeliner** *($7.49)* is nothing more than a standard, creamy pencil that is infused with sparkle and applies easily. It tends to smear, and the sparkles can separate and fall onto surrounding skin, making this even more frustrating to use than the average pencil!

<u>LIPSTICK AND LIP PENCIL:</u> ☺ Most of the **Moon Drops Moisture Creme** and **Frosts** *($8.69)* and **Super Lustrous Creme** and **Frosts** *($8.69)* have great colors (including some one-of-a-kind vivids) and an emollient, creamy texture. When it comes to lipstick, it doesn't get any more traditional than this, and the latest colors are fragrance-free. **Lip Conditioner** *($8.69)* is your everyday colorless lipstick designed as a lip balm. It works as well as any, and the price is realistic. **ColorStay Lip Liner** *($7.89)* is undeniably tenacious and far less greasy than most. This retractable, twist-up pencil really holds up against greasy lipsticks! **TimeLiner for Lips** *($6.79)* is as standard a lip pencil as it gets, but the price is right. **Line and Shine** *($9.69)* is a two-in-one product that has a standard lip pencil on one end and a liquid lip color on the other. The Shine portion is just semi-opaque lip gloss, and in the end you get a little convenience in exchange for a tiny amount of each product.

✓☺ **Absolutely Fabulous Lip Cream SPF 15** *($6.99)* is pretty close to fabulous in every sense of the word! This has a luscious, creamy, opaque texture and an in-part avobenzone sunscreen, so the lips will be beautifully protected from the sun. This is highly recommended as one of the better creamy lipsticks available, with reliable sunscreen to boot, and the color selection is superb. ✓☺ **LipGlide Color Gloss** *($9.49)* is an innovative combination of deeply pigmented gloss and packaging. By turning the base at its mid-point, the lip color is slowly fed onto an angled sponge tip, which allows you to easily control how much product comes up. This is actually easier to work with than most of the click-pen/lip-brush products sold by other companies. It applies smoothly and evenly, though the texture is sticky. However, if that doesn't bother you, LipGlide is something you should check out.

☺ **ColorStay Lipstick** *($9.69)* is slightly less ultra-matte than the original version, but still peels off from the inside out, and that's not a pretty picture. There have been numerous knockoffs of this ultra-matte finish, but without adding extra oils or emollients (the very things that make lipstick fleeting) to prevent the peeling, the ultra-matte paradox lived on—until Max Factor shook up the lipstick world with their almost-perfect Lipfinity, which all but solves the problems inherent to ultra-matte lipsticks. **ColorStay Liquid Lip** *($8.99)* is supposed to be a transfer-resistant lip gloss that comes in a tube with a wand applicator. It applies fairly emolliently and then, after what seems like several minutes, it slightly—"sets." However, the finish stays moist, is not transfer-resistant in the least, and can tend to roll off. Do not expect this to be the sheer, moist stain the ads proclaim. **ColorStay Lip Shine** *($10.19)* is a dual-ended product with one end being a liquid lipstick and the other a silicone-based gloss. You're supposed to apply the lipcolor, wait three minutes for it to set, and then apply the wet-looking gloss. You could wait an hour for this creamy lipstick to set, and miss getting to work on time, and it still feels creamy. It lasts well by itself and isn't anywhere near as greasy as true lip gloss, but once you apply the glossy component, the color tends to slip and bleed and you're right back with the same old problem. That's progress?

    MASCARA: ☺ **ColorStay Lash Color** *($6.49)* quickly lengthens, and with repeated effort will add some thickness. This has a slight tendency to clump, but not nearly as much as it has in the past. And it really does stay—removing it will take more than a once-over with a water-soluble cleanser. **ColorStay Extra Thick Lashes Mascara** *($6.49)* takes awhile to build any length, but with patience you do get relatively long, thick, separated lashes without clumping or smearing. The jumbo brush isn't an advantage and has a tendency to feel scratchy if you get it too close to the rim of the eye. **ColorStay Extra Thick Lashes Mascara Waterproof** *($6.49)* is far and away Revlon's best waterproof mascara. It adds enough length, thickness, and clean definition to make it a top choice for those times when you need waterproof mascara. The oversized brush poses the same concern as the brush that comes with the original Extra Thick Lashes Mascara above.

    ☺ **Everylash Mascara** *($6.49)* is virtually identical in look and performance to Almay's Stay Smooth Mascara, and remains just an OK lengthening mascara with a gimmicky, built-in comb you're unlikely to use more than once. **Everylash Mascara Curling** *($6.49)* does little as far as adding curl, and is otherwise identical to the original Everylash Mascara, though the curved brush lends itself to minor clumping. **Everylash Mascara Waterproof** *($6.49)* meets basic expectations in terms of length, but it takes some effort for this to just be a standard, sufficiently waterproof mascara. Again, you'll have little use for the built-in lash comb. **ColorStay Waterproof Mascara** *($6.49)* is waterproof, but that's about all this ordinary mascara has up its sleeve. Length and thickness are slow-going, and not nearly as impressive as many of Maybelline's waterproof mascaras.

    ☹ **High Dimension Lash-Lengthening Mascara** *($7.49)* supposedly contains "new light interplay technology for soft-lit lashes" that "goes beyond basic black" to "spark a subtle glint with every flutter of your lashes." I can guarantee you will be doing lots of lash-fluttering, but that's not because of any new technology. Rather, this mascara contains lots of iridescent particles that tend to flake off and end up getting into your eye—not exactly the image this product's description begs you to conjure up. This mascara also builds no length or thickness. In fact, it takes a lot of effort just to look like you have any on. **ColorStay Overtime Lash Tint** *($8.99)* is horrible. I need to say that again: this is *horrible*. This is not mascara per se, but a lash tint that goes on a bit too wet and tends to stick lashes together. Carefully working the wand through will net you adequate lash separation, but once (and whichever way) this dries, you're stuck with that result for three days. That's right, the supposed benefit of this product is it gives you "up to 3 days of dark, defined lashes with no smudges, flakes, or clumps." I wore this for two days and had had enough. There was mild flaking, but otherwise this did not budge, even after a full night's sleep and shower. The major problem with this formula is how it tends to stick lashes together and becomes increasingly uncomfortable the longer it's worn. And removing it is akin to sandblasting your lashes—nothing gets through this (not even oil, as Revlon suggests), and you end up chipping the tint off lash by lash.

☺ <u>BRUSHES:</u> **Beauty Shapers Brushes** *($5.99–$7.99)* are a small collection of decent, workable brushes. The **Shadow Brush Plus** *($5.99)* is a reliable, soft, eye-contouring brush, and one end has a pointed rubber tip for blending eyeliner. The **Powder Brush** and **Travel Face Brush** *($7.99 each)* are options as well. Both are soft, reasonably full, and have a good shape. The only "maybe" in the bunch is the **Blush Brush** *($5.99)*, which tends to flare out a bit too much for a controlled application of powder blush.

REVLON SKINLIGHTS MAKEUP

Skinlights is designed to "instantly brighten skin, boost luminosity, and soften flaws." But aside from the addition of some trace minerals, all of these products use the same standard, shiny pigments the rest of the industry uses, namely, mica, ultramarines (mineral-based coloring agents), and iron oxides. Still, the Skinlights product line was Revlon's most successful launch of 2001, with sales of over $20 million in the United States alone (Source: *The Rose Sheet*, November 5, 2001). Not surprisingly, Revlon quickly added more products to keep the sales momentum going and inspire even more women to "Come play with the power of light …" which you can read as "add as much shine to your makeup routine as possible!" The majority of the Skinlights products offer a subtle, low-wattage shine (glow), but in natural light you can still plainly see bits of sparkles wherever the product was used—and also wherever it has migrated. Yet if you do want to incorporate shine into your makeup routine, the majority of these products have a contemporary edge that competes strongly with similar offerings from department-store lines.

☺ **Skinlights Face Illuminator SPF 15** *($10.99)* is a sheer tint for the skin that offers reliable UVA-protecting ingredients, and the SPF was wisely bumped up from a 10 to the standard SPF 15. The formula has a lightweight, softly creamy texture that does not feel heavy or greasy, though the illuminating effect you may have been hoping for is achieved with iridescent particles that are hard to blend away, soften, or control, and they can spread to places where you didn't intend them to go. Seven tints are available and, as sheer colors, all are acceptable except Golden Light, which is too orange for most skin tones. Bronze Light is quite dark, and will look too coppery over fair or light skin tones. If you're a fan of shiny, sheer foundations like M.A.C.'s HyperReal ($24), you may want to check this out—you'll get the same effect, but Revlon's offers great sun protection and a better price point. Otherwise, this type of product is best as an adjunct to foundation or used alone for an evening look. **Skinlights Diffusing Tint SPF 15** *($12.29)* has an excellent, in-part titanium dioxide– and zinc oxide–based sunscreen and a soft, slightly creamy texture that can feel somewhat thick when applied, though it blends down to a smooth, natural finish. Of all the Skinlights products, this one has the least amount of visible shine, and it's a decent, sheer-coverage option for daytime wear. There are six colors, with no choices for very light or very dark skin tones. Only Nude is a bit too peach to work for most skin tones—the other colors are beautiful. It does contain rather strong fragrance. **Skinlights Color Lighting for Eyes/Cheeks** *($7.89)* is a collection of five sheer, iridescent cream-to-powder compacts with colors that are a breeze to apply and blend. However, the shine is intense enough to be distracting, and while these are options for nighttime eye makeup, you may want to reconsider applying this much shine to your cheeks. The colors, though limited, are great. **Skinlights Illusion Wand SPF 12** *($7.89)* is a very good concealer that comes in a pen-style container with a brush tip. Like others of its ilk, you need to click the base of the container to feed product into the brush tip. This sounds better than it really is because it's quite easy to click up too much product, and then there's no putting it back. Nevertheless, this has a light, smooth texture that is easy to work with, and the finish (at least in "feel") is matte, with only the faintest hint of shine. The two flesh-toned shades are fine, but are best for light to medium skin tones Luminous Touch is a pale pink highlighting shade that's not as attractive as the others. Finally, although the sunscreen is a winning combination of titanium dioxide and zinc oxide, Revlon knows better than to stop at SPF 12. **Skinlights Glosslights for Lips** *($7.89)* are standard tube glosses that are a bit slicker than most, thanks to the inclusion of mineral oil as one of the main ingredients. Don't expect much longevity from them, but for an emollient, very sparkly lip gloss, these work well.

☺ **Skinlights Face Illuminator Loose Powder** *($10.99)* is a standard, talc-based powder with a silicone-enhanced silky feel and a fair amount of shine. Why anyone would want to dust this much iridescence onto their skin is beyond me, but if that floats your boat, the five available colors are all fine, though Bronze Light is too coppery for all but dark skin. A nice change of pace with this product is the packaging—the cap has a flip-top that houses a small, but workable, brush, a clever touch that eliminates the mess of storing a puff or brush inside the powder itself. **Skinlights Face Illuminator Stick SPF 10** *($10.99)* is a sheer highlighter/cream blush that goes on cool and slightly wet, then dries to a slightly moist finish as you blend. The sunscreen is all titanium dioxide, but SPF 15 would have really been illuminating. The colors are a bit more vibrant than those for the other Skinlights items, and the shine is at its most intense here, too. There are some great options for creating a warm, sun-kissed look, but the shine is almost intrusive, and is about as natural-looking as Styrofoam.

RIMMEL (MAKEUP ONLY)

Rimmel is a London-based company under the ownership of Coty, which explains why the Coty line of makeup disappeared; it has been replaced by this import. According to the press release surrounding the U.S. launch of Rimmel, it is reported to be the top-selling makeup line in England. How this English import ended up being exclusive to the Wal-Mart chain is anyone's guess, but that's the only place you'll find it stateside. Given the very low price point and several good products (though nothing groundbreaking), that report may indeed be true. What's worth paying attention to if you happen to come across this line are the blushes, mascaras, and powders. The foundations and concealers are worth a look as well, but without testers, it's always a guessing game as to which color would be best for you, though Rimmel has made some notable color improvements since the previous edition of this book. Even so, the prices are so low it may not be a bad idea to buy two or three shades and experiment. The pencils are basic but worth a look, and there are dozens of nail polishes to consider, not to mention the lipstick selection. In fact, you'll be surprised that such inexpensive lipsticks and glosses feel so elegant and offer such fashion-forward and classic colors.

My only significant complaint about Rimmel is the packaging. The tops to the blushes and eyeshadows are awkward and tricky to remove. However, these are small technicalities that are easy enough to live with, especially at these prices! For more information about Rimmel, visit www.rimmellondon.com. **Note:** Over a dozen Rimmel products featured on their Web site are not available in the United States. The products reviewed below reflect what is consistently found at Wal-Mart stores nationwide.

<u>FOUNDATION:</u> All of Rimmel's foundations are packaged in squeeze tubes, which can take some getting used to when it comes to controlling how much is dispensed. ☹ **Stay Matte Foundation** *($3.97)* is recommended for normal to oily skin, but the moist texture and slightly creamy finish would be more suitable for normal to dry skin. This comes in a tube, provides light to medium coverage, and blends evenly. There are six shades, three of which—Sand, Soft Beige, and Warm Honey—are too pink or peach for most skin tones. Porcelain is slightly pink, but may work for lighter skin tones.

☺ **Natural Sensation All Day Natural Smooth Finish Makeup** *($4.97)* is a water-less, silicone-based foundation that is very thick, but it blends out surprisingly sheer and light, leaving a smooth, satiny finish. The six shades present some great neutral options, but Natural Nude and Soft Tan are too peach and should be avoided. This would be fine for normal to dry skin, but beware—this has an overpowering baby-powder scent. **Hydrasense Flawless Hydrating Makeup** *($4.97)* is indeed hydrating, and best for dry skin. This makeup starts creamy and blends to a sheer coverage, moist finish. All of the six shades are great except Warm Honey.

<u>CONCEALER:</u> ☺ **Hide the Blemish Concealer** *($2.97)* is a very greasy, lipstick-style concealer that doesn't cover that well, though it does have three very good colors. A concealer like this is the last thing you would want to place over a blemish, at least if the goal is to not make them worse! If you prefer this type of concealer, it would be OK over non-blemished areas, but if you're using it under the eye, creasing is inevitable.

☺ **Hydrasense Flawless Concealer** *($3.97)* is excellent as a sheer to light coverage liquid concealer. This blends wonderfully and sets to a natural matte finish that poses little to no risk of creasing. Of the three colors, avoid the peachy Deep Beige.

☺ <u>POWDER:</u> **Stay Matte Pressed Powder** *($2.97)* is talc-based and has a light, silky texture that goes on smooth, even though it doesn't have quite as dry a finish as the name implies. Oilier skin types may see shine before too long, but normal to dry skin should enjoy the feel of this one. There are three shades, with no options for darker skin tones.

<u>BLUSH:</u> Rimmel's powder-based ☺ **Blush** *($2.97)* comes in a small compact and features predominantly warm-toned shades, all with a softly shiny finish. If only these were matte, they would be a steal, as the texture and blendability are wonderful.

☺ **Colour to Go Cream Blush** *($2.97)* imparts next to no color, but does leave behind a soft layer of shine. This works best over a regular blush for those times when you want a low-wattage glow.

<u>EYESHADOW:</u> ☺ **Special Eyes Eyeshadow** *($1.97)* has a silky, slightly powdery (it can be a bit messy to apply), but easy-to-blend texture, and some worthwhile matte options among many pastel blue or shiny colors. The matte shades to consider are Moonstone, Matte White, and Daylight.

☺ **Special Eyes Duos** *($2.97)* and **Trios** *($2.97)* have the same texture as the Special Eyes Eyeshadow above, but most of the colors are shiny. The trios are easy to pass up, with lots of iridescence and hard-to-combine colors. Orchid and Spice are the matte duos, and are worth a look. **Metallic Eye Gloss** *($2.97)* is a cream-to-powder, crease-prone shiny eyeshadow whose colors are sheer even though the shine is far from subtle. **WaterCool Shadow** *($3.97)* is a water-to-powder shadow that has an initial cool feel and then sets to a solid matte (in feel) finish. The array of colors is similar to the shimmery pastels and jewel tones of Maybelline's preferred Cool Effects Cooling Cream Eyecolor.

<u>EYE AND BROW SHAPER:</u> ☺ **Special Eyes Eye Liner Pencil** *($1.97)*, **Soft Kohl Kajal Pencil** *($1.97)*, and **Professional Eyebrow Pencil** *($1.97)* are standard in every sense of the word. They need to be sharpened and they have a dry finish, which can mean less smudging. The Eyebrow Pencil includes a brush on the cap, which can come in handy.

✓☺ **Exaggerate Full Colour Eye Definer** *($1.97)* is a superior automatic eye pencil that's also retractable. This applies well, but it takes a few strokes to build intensity. It sets to a soft powder finish that has a low risk of smudging or smearing. The colored tip on the pencil's package is a good indicator of how the color will look on the skin.

☺ **Shade & Define Two Tone Eye Pencil** *($3.97)* is another dual-ended thick pencil, similar to the ones in many other lines. Rimmel's are just as standard, but the color combinations (one for shadow, the other for lining) mostly go together like oil and water in terms of compatibility.

☹ **Liquid Eye Liner** *($1.97)* is a standard liquid liner that comes with a long, skinny brush that can be hard to control over the lash line. Although some may prefer this type of brush, this formula takes too long to dry (even when applied lightly) and smears easily.

<u>LIPSTICK AND LIP PENCIL:</u> ✓☺ **Lasting Finish Lipstick** *($3.97)* feels wonderful and glides on with a soft, creamy texture and slightly glossy finish. ✓☺ **Rich Moisture Lipstick** *($3.97)* is a very good, creamy lipstick that goes on smoothly and is less slippery than the Lasting Finish. ✓☺ **Exaggerate HydraColor Lipstick** *($3.97)* improves even further on the two lipsticks above by offering a weightless, moist application and a soft glossy finish from each of its beautiful colors.

☺ **Lasting Finish Sheer Finish Lipstick** *($3.97)* is a sheer tint for the lips that provides the expected glossy finish. This one won't last as long as Rimmel's other lipsticks. **Vinyl Lip Lipgloss** *($3.97)* has a bit of a tacky feel, but is still a good, semi-opaque lip gloss that provides a gleaming finish. The colors coordinate well with the lipstick shades.

☹ **1000 Kisses Stay On Lipstick** *($3.97)* is Rimmel's take on an ultra-matte lipstick and it is slightly matte, with a texture that tends to ball up and chip off over time, like most other ultra-matte lipsticks. This is not an improvement over the original ultra-matte lipstick introduced by Revlon. **1000 Kisses Stay On Lip Liner Pencil** *($1.97)* is a standard pencil that needs to be sharpened. It has a smooth and comfortably creamy texture and stays on as well as most other pencils. **Exaggerate Fineline Retractable Lip Liner** *($3.97)* is an automatic, retractable lip pencil that is creamy without veering into greasiness. It stays on quite well, and the colors are rich with pigment. It doesn't apply as smoothly as others, but for the money, this is a safe bet.

<u>MASCARA:</u> ☺ **Extra Super Lash Mascara** *($3.97)* is supposed to give "extra definition and super separation" to lashes, and it does, but not as gloriously as the label indicates. This is a reliable lengthening mascara that applies clump-free and tends to not flake or chip.

✓☺ **Exaggerate Extra Volume Mascara** *($3.97)* is the one to choose for a quick, clean application with lots of length and decent thickness without clumps or smears. I wouldn't say it triples lash volume (as it claims), but this is still impressive mascara! ✓☺ **Curly Mascara** *($3.97)* will have you crying tears of joy over how easily this magnifies lashes to their fullest, longest potential—all with a fringed curl. If you feel jaded by mascaras that over-promise and under-deliver, this one will reaffirm your hopes.

☹ **Endless Lash Mascara** *($2.97)* takes a seemingly endless amount of time to build what amounts to unimpressive length and not a bit of thickness. What a letdown after the stellar performance of the mascaras above.

☺ **100% Waterproof Mascara** *($3.97)* builds so-so length that is actually less than most other waterproof mascaras. It does hold its own in the rain or pool, but it's also difficult to remove.

ROC (SKIN CARE ONLY)

Johnson & Johnson, owner of Purpose, Neutrogena, Clean & Clear, and the prescription-only drugs Retin-A and Renova, also own RoC, a line whose image is designed to align itself with the notion of pharmaceutical-oriented skin care. The mortar and pestle in the logo are meant to convey the idea that these are more than just the usual cosmetic

The Reviews R

products, and hold to a higher medical standard. But image is not fact you are not buying anything even remotely medical by investing in this relatively pricey drugstore line of skin-care products. What you would be purchasing are relatively gentle, skin-care products that have some decent formulations. Although there are a handful of exceptions, RoC products generally contain far fewer irritating ingredients than many cosmetics lines, and for the most part RoC's simple formulations are distinctive for their concern about preventing skin irritation or skin sensitivity. The product line as a whole is definitely a consideration for sensitive and dry skin types, though if you have oily or blemish-prone skin there are few, if any, options among RoC products.

Note: RoC in the United States makes some products that are available only in Canada; the reviews of these products follow the first section of reviews, which includes products available in both the United States and Canada. For more information about RoC in Canada, call (519) 836-6500; in the United States, call (800) 526-3967 or visit www.roc.com.

☺ **Cleanser + Toner in One** (*$7.99 for 6.76 ounces*) isn't much of a toner or cleanser. It is more of a wipe-off cleanser and it doesn't tone a thing. It could be good for someone with dry skin, but it doesn't take off makeup very well without a lot of wiping. [In Canada this product is called **Cleanser and Refresher for Face and Eyes 2 in 1** (*$16 for 200 ml*).]

☺ **Deep Action Facial Wash with Beta Hydroxy** (*$6.99 for 5.07 ounces*) is a standard, detergent-based cleanser that contains a small amount of salicylic acid (BHA), but the pH of the cleanser makes the BHA ineffective for exfoliation. This is an option for someone with normal to oily skin.

☺ **Protient Lift Daily Firming Cleanser** (*$7.79 for 5 ounces*) won't lift skin anywhere; it's just an extremely standard, detergent-based cleanser that is an option for normal to oily skin. Protient is supposed to be "a natural firming nutrient, which helps support the skin's natural ability to fight the appearance of sagging skin." Yet there is not one unique or unusual ingredient in this product, and there is no ingredient called "Protient" in it either.

☺ **Retinol Actif Pur Anti-Wrinkle Cleansing Lotion** (*$8.99 for 4.2 ounces*) is an emollient cleanser that is an option for normal to dry skin, though it doesn't rinse off very well without the aid of a washcloth. It contains a minute amount of retinol, but in a product like this any efficacy it would have is rinsed down the drain before it has a chance to be of benefit for skin.

☺ $$$ **Hydra + Effet Reservoir for Normal Skin SPF 15** (*$13.99 for 1.35 ounces*) is a very good, in-part avobenzone-based sunscreen in an emollient, though fairly standard, moisturizer for normal to slightly dry skin. [In Canada this is called **Hydra + Effet Réservoir Light Texture** (*$24.50 for 40 ml*).]

☺ $$$ **Hydra + Effet Reservoir for Dry Skin SPF 15** (*$13.99 for 1.35 ounces*) is almost identical to the Normal Skin version above and the same basic comments apply. [In Canada this is called **Hydra + Effet Réservoir Enriched Texture** (*$24.50 for 40 ml*).]

☺ **Melibiose Active Firming Treatment for Dry Skin** *($13.99 for 1.35 ounces)* does contain melibiose, a sugar that has a small amount of research (all done in a test tube) showing that it protects other skin substances from breaking down (Source: *Mechanisms of Ageing and Development,* January 1999, pages 241–260). That's nice, but it's not enough to rely on as the only way to take care of skin. Especially because, aside from its basic emollient formula, that's the only special ingredient in this product. [In Canada this is called **Melibiose Anti-Ageing Action-Enriched Texture** *($30 for 40 ml)*.]

✔☺ **Retinol Actif Pur Anti-Wrinkle Treatment, Day, SPF 15** *($16.99 for 1.01 ounces)* is a very good, in-part avobenzone-based sunscreen in a standard moisturizing base with a matte finish. It has a small quantity of water-binding agents and an antioxidant. There is a negligible amount of retinol as well. [In Canada this is called **Rétinol Actif Pur Jour, Moisturizing Anti-Wrinkle Day Care** *($32.75 for 30 ml)*.]

☺ **Retinol Actif Pur Skin Refining Treatment** *($17.99 for 1.35 ounces)* is a basic, though good, retinol product that is an option if you are looking for retinol in your moisturizer.

☺ **Retinol Actif Pur Anti-Wrinkle Treatment, for Night** *($18.69 for 1.01 ounces)* does contain retinol (about 0.1%), with water and thickening agents. This also contains about 3% to 4% AHA, though the product's pH of 5 means it will be ineffective for exfoliation.

☺ **$$$ Retinol Actif Pur, Eye Contour Cream** *($16.99 for 0.51 ounce)*. If you are looking for a retinol product, this one contains it, but that's about it, as there is no other special benefit to buying this basic moisturizing formula. [In Canada this is called **Rétinol Actif Pur Eye and Lip Contour** *($28.75 for 15 ml)*.]

RoC (CANADA ONLY)

Note: The following RoC products are available only in Canada. Refer to the above RoC reviews for products that are available in both the United States and Canada. All prices listed below are in Canadian dollars.

☺ **Endrial Dermo Calming Cleanser** *($14.50 for 200 ml)* is a basic emollient cleanser that is an option for normal to dry skin.

☺ **Cleansing Milk Normal to Combination Skin** *($14.50 for 200 ml)*. Despite the claim that this can unblock pores, it contains problematic ingredients that are known for blocking pores. This product is not recommended for combination skin, though it is an option as a cleanser for normal to dry skin.

☺ **Cleansing Milk Dry Skin, Extra Gentle** *($14.50 for 200 ml)* is an emollient cleanser containing lanolin oil, and that does make it appropriate for dry to very dry skin, although it can leave a slight greasy film.

☹ **Foaming Facial Cleanser** *($14.50 for 150 ml)* lists the second ingredient as sodium lauryl sulfate, a cleansing agent that is a potent irritant and also extremely drying and sensitizing. This is not recommended.

☺ **Eye Makeup Remover Lotion** *($14.50 for 125 ml)* is a standard, detergent-based, water-soluble, wipe-off cleanser; it would work as well as any.

☺ **Gentle Exfoliating Cream** *($14 for 50 ml)* is a mineral oil–based scrub that can leave a greasy film on the skin, although it is an option for dry skin.

☹ **Skin Toner Normal to Combination Skin** *($14.50 for 200 ml)* lists alcohol as the second ingredient, and that's a skin irritant. This is not recommended for any skin type.

☺ **Skin Toner, Dry Skin** *($14.50 for 200 ml)* is a standard, detergent-based toner that contains a teeny amount of water-binding agent. It has little benefit for skin other than as an extra step to remove traces of makeup.

☺ **Nutri + Protect, Amino Moisturizing Cream, Dry Skin** *($23 for 50 ml)* is a very emollient, though ordinary, moisturizer for dry skin that contains only water, plant oil, mineral oil, thickeners, lanolin, and preservatives.

☺ **ChronoBlock Daily Moisturizing Care SPF 15** *($32 for 40 ml)* is a very good, in-part avobenzone-based sunscreen in a very ordinary, moisturizing base that is good for normal to dry skin.

☺ $$$ **ChronoBlock Yeux (for Eyes) SPF 15** *($25 for 15 ml)* is almost identical to the Moisturizing Care SPF 15 version above, only RoC gives you less product and charges more.

☺ **Protient Lift Jour (day)** *($38 for 40 ml)*. Without sunscreen this should not be worn for daytime, though regardless of the time of day it won't lift skin anywhere. This is just a basic moisturizer with about 2% AHA, which isn't enough for it to be effective as an exfoliant. Protient is supposed to be "a natural firming nutrient, which helps support the skin's natural ability to fight the appearance of sagging skin." Yet there is not one unique or unusual ingredient in this product and no ingredient called "Protient" is listed either. It does contain tyrosine, an amino acid that is supposed to stimulate melanin production, but according to the FDA and Health Canada, it can't do that when applied topically on skin.

☺ $$$ **Protient Lift Eye** *($30 for 15 ml)* is similar to the Protient Lift Jour version above except that it contains more tyrosine. Even if that ingredient could stimulate melanin production, why would anyone want more dark color in the area under their eyes?

☺ $$$ **Melibiose Anti-Ageing Action Eye Contour** *($24 for 15 ml)* is almost identical to the Melibiose Active Firming Treatment for Normal Skin reviewed in the RoC section above.

☺ **Revitalizing Night Cream** *($30 for 40 ml)* is a good moisturizer for someone with dry skin; it has a small amount of water-binding agents and antioxidant.

☺ **Retinol A+C+E Triple Action Day/Night** *($38 for 30 ml)* is an emollient moisturizer with some good antioxidants and a small amount of water-binding agents.

☺ **Hydra + Mat, for Combination Skins** *($24.50 for 40 ml)* is a simple, matte-finish moisturizer that includes sunscreen ingredients on the label but does not make any SPF claims. Therefore, it cannot be relied on for sun protection.

☺ **Hydra + Teint Tinted Moisturizing Cream: Clair, Hale, Dore** *($24.50 for 40 ml)* comes in colors that are all a strange shade of peach, and are not recommended.

☹ **Hydra + Masque Moisturizing Mask** *($20 for 40 ml)* is just some emollient and a tiny amount of clay, making it a boring, do-nothing mask for someone with normal to dry skin.

☹ **Rétinol Actif Pur Radiance Anti-Wrinkle Mask** *($25 for 40 ml)* contains only a negligible amount of retinol, so even if retinol could make a difference in the skin, it couldn't do so here. This is just glycerin, thickeners, and a small amount of a water-binding agent; boring, but OK for normal to dry skin.

☹ **$$$ Nutri + Lips, Lip Protector** *($7.25 for 3 grams)* is a good, but basic, emollient for dry skin. The teeny amount of vitamin E has no impact on skin.

☺ **Minesol High Protection Sun Cream SPF 25** *($16 for 118 ml)* is a titanium dioxide–based sunscreen, but because it doesn't list any other ingredients there is no way to know what else you might be putting on your face. As a sunscreen, this is a very good option for dry or sensitive skin.

☺ **Minesol Mineral Sunblock Cream Very High Protection SPF 40** *($16 for 50 ml)* is similar to the SPF 25 version above only with zinc oxide and titanium dioxide, and the same basic comments apply.

☺ **$$$ Minesol High Protection Lipstick SPF 20** *($10 for 3 grams)* is an avobenzone-based sunscreen for the lips, but because it doesn't list any other ingredients there is no way to know what else you might be applying. As a sunscreen, this is a good option.

☹ **Minesol Tan Prolonging Lotion** *($18 for 200 ml)* is a good moisturizer for dry skin, although the tiny amount of tyrosine cannot encourage melanin production.

☺ **Auto Bronzant Self-Tanner** *($18 for 100 ml)* contains dihydroxyacetone, the same ingredient all self-tanners use to affect the color of skin. This one would work as well as any.

SEA BREEZE (SKIN CARE ONLY)

Like so many product lines aimed at those struggling with breakouts, Shiseido-owned Sea Breeze adds the most absurd combinations of irritating, skin-damaging ingredients to its products. I suspect all these companies think consumers who have oily or acne-prone skin want a cool, tingling feel from their skin-care products. While that may or may not be true, the truth is that cool and tingling means irritating and skin-damaging, qualities that hurt the skin's healing process and can encourage bacteria growth. Not to mention that irritation causes the skin to be redder, which only makes acne more noticeable. For more information about Sea Breeze, call (800) 831-2684 or visit www.seabreezezone.com.

☺ **Foaming Face Wash for Sensitive Skin** *($3.99 for 6 ounces)* is a standard, detergent-based, water-soluble cleanser that would be an option for someone with oily skin.

☹ **Exfoliating Facial Scrub** *($3.99 for 3.5 ounces)* would have been an OK synthetic scrub, but I guess they just had to add camphor to it so it would irritate the skin.

☹ **Alcohol-Free Toner** *($3.99 for 10 ounces)* would have been an OK toner for most skin types, but the wafting fragrance from the orange and tangerine oil makes this a problem for blemish-prone skin.

☹ **Original Astringent** *($3.99 for 10 ounces)* would be the product for you if you want red, irritated skin; it contains an amazing list of extremely irritating ingredients, including alcohol, camphor, clove, eucalyptus, and peppermint.

☹ **Oily Skin Astringent** *($3.99 for 10 ounces)* is similar to the Original version above and is absolutely not recommended.

☹ **Sensitive Skin Astringent** *($3.99 for 16 ounces)* is similar to the Original version above, and the same review applies. Calling this "sensitive" is completely misleading and insensitive.

SENSE USANA SKIN CARE

Sense Usana is a line of products sold much the way Shaklee, Amway, Jafra, and Mary Kay products are sold. And, as with them, part of the business involves getting others to sell the products, too. That probably explains why I receive so many questions asking if these products are as good as they say, because people want to know if they should buy them or start selling them. My response is that while there are definitely some very good products in the Usana line, their exaggerated claims are hard to swallow. What is a little on the eerie side is the cultlike, enthusiastic following of the believers who sell the stuff. All of this zeal is understandable, thanks to the enticement of "Usana's Business Plan…" that claims it can help "…people create perpetual, long-term wealth." Who wouldn't want to obtain wealth and get rid of wrinkles at the same time?

The good news is that this line contains some excellent sunscreen formulations and some decent moisturizers with good water-binding agents and anti-irritants. The disappointing news is that they all contain fragrance and a few problematic plant extracts. One noticeable shortcoming is that there are no options for blemish-prone or oily skin, and there are inadequate sunscreen options for those with normal to oily skin.

Another claim the company makes (like many cosmetics companies) that is just irksome is the notion that they have independent research demonstrating how remarkable their product line is. The research they cite is not from published studies, was not done double-blind, and was not independent—it was paid for by Usana. These aren't products to be dismissed, but I wouldn't exactly encourage anyone to give up their day job to sell these products. For more information about Usana, call (888) 950-9595 or visit www.usana-nutritionals.com. **Note:** All Sense Usana products contain fragrance.

☺ **Gentle Daily Cleanser** *($20 for 6 ounces).* The antioxidants in this product (including magnesium ascorbyl phosphate, a form of vitamin C) are nice, but any benefit from them would be rinsed down the drain in a cleanser. Other than that, this is a standard, detergent-based cleanser that would be an option for most skin types, though a few of the plant extracts can be skin irritants.

☺ **Rice Bran Polisher** *($17 for 3.7 ounces)* is a scrub that uses rice bran as the abrasive. That can help exfoliate skin, but the emollients and thickening agents make this appropriate only for normal to dry skin. The teeny amount of papain (an enzyme) doesn't have much effect as an exfoliant. The product does contain BHA, but the pH is too high for it to be effective as an exfoliant. A few of the plant extracts can be skin irritants, but hopefully they are present in such a small amount that they won't have an effect on skin.

☺ **Hydrating Toner** *($18 for 6 ounces)* would have been a very good option as a toner for most skin types if it weren't for a handful of potentially irritating plant extracts. The water-binding agents, vitamin C, and anti-irritants are impressive, but the grapefruit, rosemary, and orange peel extracts can be problematic. This does contain fragrance.

✓☺ **Daytime Protective Emulsion SPF 15** *($28.45 for 1.7 ounces)* is a very good, in-part avobenzone-based sunscreen that would work well for normal to dry skin. It contains some very good antioxidants and water-binding agents. This does contain salicylic acid, but the pH is not low enough to make it effective as an exfoliant.

✓☺ **Night Renewal** *($36 for 1.7 ounces)*. Thankfully, Sense Usana left out almost all of the problematic plant extracts, which makes this a very good moisturizer for normal to dry skin. It contains mostly water, thickeners, silicones, vitamins (antioxidants), water-binding agents, anti-irritants, preservatives, and fragrance.

☹ **Serum Intensive** *($39 for 1 ounce)* is a product that does contain AHA and BHA, but the second ingredient listed is alcohol, and that is too drying and irritating for all skin types. There are many AHA and BHA products at the drugstore and in other lines that are effective as exfoliants without the unnecessary addition of such a problematic ingredient as alcohol.

☺ **Eye Nourisher** *($16.50 for 0.5 ounce)* is a very good moisturizer for dry skin. There are tiny amounts of balm mint and grapefruit extract, but probably not enough to be a problem for skin.

✓☺ **$$$ Perfecting Essence** *($45 for 1 ounce)* is an emollient moisturizer for dry skin that contains some very good antioxidants and water-binding agents. It also contains some plant extracts that can have melanin-inhibiting properties, but probably not at this minute amount. The vitamin C may be more effective for that purpose.

☺ **$$$ Nutritious Creme Masque** *($16.95 for 3.7 ounces)* is a standard clay mask that would work as well as any. It can't draw anything out of the skin, but like most masks it can leave skin feeling smooth. The emollients make this better for normal to slightly dry skin.

☺ **Body Sunblock Lotion SPF 15** *($12.95 for 4 ounces)* is a very good sunscreen with an in-part zinc oxide formulation in a standard emollient base. It would be a good option for someone with normal to dry skin.

☺ **Body Sunblock Lotion SPF 30** *($16.50 for 4 ounces)* is similar to the SPF 15 version above, and the same comments apply.

SEPHORA

Considering the fact that Sephora is a cosmetics boutique whose fame was built on the trendy and established brands they proffer, it seems strange that they have also launched their own makeup line. Even more peculiar is the fact that Sephora's makeup is attractively priced, with many products costing substantially less than similar options the next aisle over. Although the mainstream and fringe lines are tempting reasons to visit Sephora, don't overlook Sephora's own brand, for you'll find not only some great products but also some real bargains. Every color of each item has a tester, and the display includes built-in shelves stocked with makeup remover and cotton pads, along with a receptacle to dispose of them, which is inviting and smart. The colors are laid out by their respective undertone and finish (such as Cream or Gloss) and arranged from light to dark on the unit, so choosing from the color group you prefer is efficient and easy. Sephora also has quite a few professional brushes that win high marks for their shape, density, and performance.

Of course, not everything comes up roses with any line, and Sephora is no exception. It seems Sephora hasn't mastered the ability to make shiny powders that don't feel grainy, as all of their shiniest powders have this characteristic. There are also some color missteps and a preponderance of wild, unusual shades that likely won't become your (or anyone's) makeup staples anytime soon. However, as long as Sephora continues to offer a decent selection of traditional colors for sophisticated makeup design, I'm not complaining. And when you compare Sephora's top makeup products to those from competing lines under the same roof, it's doubtful you'll have anything to complain about either!

For skin care, Sephora has a tiny selection that is easily overlooked as you move quickly to the products they do best—makeup. For more information about Sephora, call (877)-SEPHORA or visit www.sephora.com.

SEPHORA SKIN CARE

☺ **Cleansing Gel for Face & Eyes** *($6 for 3.3 ounces)* is a very simple, standard, detergent-based cleanser that would work well for most skin types.

☹ **Makeup Remover Towelettes** *($10 for pack of 25)* uses Kathon CG, a preservative that is recommended for use only in rinse-off skin-care products. Because some of the product is left on the skin with this kind of makeup remover, it is best to avoid this product.

☺ **Express Waterproof Eye Makeup Remover with Vitamin E** *($8.50 for 5 ounces)* is a standard, silicone-based makeup remover, but it contains witch hazel distillate. Because that contains a good deal of alcohol, this isn't the best for skin anywhere on the face.

☺ **Soothing Eye Makeup Remover** *($8 for 4.9 ounces)* is a standard, detergent-based eye-makeup remover that would work as well as any.

☺ **Deep Cleansing Facial Scrub** *($8 for 3.3 ounces)* is a detergent-based cleanser that uses ground-up plastic (polyethylene) as the abrasive. It is an option for normal to oily skin.

☹ **Operation Smile Lip Baume SPF 15** *($5 for 0.5 ounce)* doesn't contain the UVA-protecting ingredients of titanium dioxide, zinc oxide, or avobenzone, and is not recommended.

SEPHORA MAKEUP

<u>POWDER, BLUSH, AND EYESHADOW:</u> ☺ **All Over Skins** *($12)* are talc- and cornstarch-based pressed powders that feel smooth and offer a dry, powdery finish. The cornstarch it contains makes this best for oily skin that's not prone to blemishes. Of the eight shades, two are shiny **Bronzing Powders** *($12)*, while the rest are matte. Unfortunately, most of the six other colors are too peach, pink, or ash. The only shades to consider are No. 1 and No. 2.

☺ **Sun Discs** *($18)* are identical to the All Over Skins formula above, but this is a pressed bronzing powder that comes in an oversized compact. The colors are fairly light compared to most bronzers, but will still work for fair skin if you don't mind shine.

The ☺ **All Over Colors** *($9)* are a dizzying array of pressed-powder compacts that come in almost every color imaginable. There are flesh-toned shades to use as pressed powder, blush tones to use on cheeks, and all manner of eyeshadow shades. You can choose Sheer, Cream, or Matte finishes, though these distinctions apply in name only, since almost all of the shades have a slight to glaring shine. The true matte shades have the best texture and smoothest application, and include some attractive, workable colors. Although there is a huge number of shades, the majority are variations on blue, green, orange, yellow, and purple, and are only for those going for shock value or creating a fantasy makeup look.

☺ **Glitter** *($8)* is precisely that, and it's available both in large flecks that barely stick to the skin (they should be mixed with a moisturizer prior to use) and in finely milled, ultra-shiny powders. Each color is loose and packaged in a small container without a sifter, so the messiness is considerable.

☹ **Glitter All Over Color** *($9)* are ultra-shiny pressed powders available in the standard selection of highlighting shades, along with a few deeper hues. This is way too grainy to pass muster given the abundance of smooth-textured shiny powders from other lines.

✓☺ **Aqua Tints** *($14)* are Sephora's take on BeneFit's BeneTint *($26)* and you'll be hard-pressed to find a difference between them. Since Sephora owns BeneFit, there'll be no love lost if you opt for this less expensive version—and you'll be able to choose from several great colors. BeneTint seems to have a bit more pigment, but judging the difference is splitting hairs and barely worth mentioning.

<u>PENCILS:</u> Along with their seemingly endless supply of lipsticks, Sephora offers dozens upon dozens of needs-sharpening ☺ **Pencils** *($4)* that can be used for eyes, brows, and lips depending on the shade you choose. Of course, many of the colors are best reserved for theatrical makeup or a production of *Cirque de Soleil,* but you will find that the colors in the Browns and Black/White/Gray are competitive with (and less costly

than) pencils from most other lines. These aren't the smoothest-applying pencils, but they have a dry finish that stays on without smudging.

☺ **Jumbo Crayon** *($5)* is a thick, standard pencil that is much creamier than the pencil above, and the colors go on softly. The creaminess may facilitate application, but also makes these crayons prone to smudging.

☺ LIPSTICK: With over 250 colors available, even the most particular person is bound to find a Sephora **Lipstick** *($10)* to love. There are five types available. The **Satins** are smooth and creamy with a good stain, the **Mattes** are not true matte but rather a semi-matte with opaque coverage and striking colors, and the **Gloss** is sheer, glossy, and fruit-scented. The colors are excellent, too! **Glitter** is creamy with a slightly rough edge due to the flecks of glitter in the formula, and **Metallic** has a great creamy feel and comes in bold, full-coverage colors with a metallic finish. **Lip Gloss** *($12)* is a light-textured, slightly sticky wand-type gloss. It's fine for a sheer standard gloss, but it is highly fragranced. **Lip Lacquer** *($15)* is yet another click-pen liquid lipstick you apply with a built-in brush. This one has a smooth, non-sticky texture and is comparable to similar, pricier versions from Stila. The color selection is fine, though surprisingly small for Sephora.

☺ MASCARA: The very basic **Mascara** *($6)* is available in Black or Clear, and neither wins any sort of bragging rights. They're both rather boring, and no match for drugstore mascaras in this price range.

BRUSHES: Sephora's ✔☺ **Brushes** *($4–$42)* present some prime choices, especially for applying eyeshadow and blush. There are over a dozen brushes available, with the best ones being the **Foundation Brush** *($20)*, **Round Blush Brush** *($42)*, **Beveled Blush Brush** *($40)*, **Large Eyeshadow Brush** *($14)*, and **Concealer Brush** *($16)*. The **Professional 5 Essential Brushes in a Pouch** *($38)* is a sensible set that includes travel-sized brushes for powder, blush, eyeshadow, and lipstick, all in a foldout case. Check this out if you're in the market for a basic brush set.

The other brushes have their strong points too, but you may want to avoid the overpriced ☹ **Fan Brush** *($28)* and the **Slanted Blush Brush** *($20)*, which is too sparse for precise application.

The ☺ **Powder Brush** *($22)* comes in both a short- and long-handled version and works well, but it isn't as soft and elegant as it could be.

SPECIALTY: ✔☺ $$$ You will not be disappointed by Sephora's vast selection of **Makeup Bags** *($4–$38)* and **Train Cases** *($65–$98)*. The variety is astounding, especially for the makeup bags, and although the train cases are not the sturdiest around they'll make elegant, ready-to-travel makeup organizers (unless you'll be carting them around everywhere the way a working makeup artist would).

SERIOUS SKIN CARE

Serious Skin Care has changed a lot since it was first launched as a line featuring a small group of acne products. Its successful infomercial has generated a significant number of additional products, and the original three- to four-step regimen has become vastly more complicated, and, of course, the claims more overblown. It's not that there aren't some good products in this line, because there are, it's just that several of them are still fairly serious when it comes to irritation, while others can clog pores, and still others fall short for sun protection or effective exfoliation. There are some excellent products to consider, so just be sure to choose carefully. For more information about Serious Skin Care, call (800) 540-8662 or visit www.hsn.com or www.seriousskincare.com.

SERIOUS SKIN CARE OILY-COMBINATION LINE

☺ $$$ **Super Hydrate Oil Free Mist** *($19.95 for 4 ounces)* is a good toner that would work well for most skin types. It contains some good water-binding agents. The tiny amount of willow bark it contains has no exfoliating properties for skin.

☹ **Balance Glycolic Toning Spray** *($22 for two 4-ounce bottles)* lists alcohol as the second ingredient, and it also contains eucalyptus, making it completely un-balancing for skin.

☺ **Unplugged Pore Purifying Spray** *($29.95 for two 2-ounce bottles)* contains no ingredients that can unplug, much less purify, pores in any way. This is just an OK, basic toner with water, slip agent, water-binding agent, and preservatives.

☺ **A-Copper Oil Control Serum** *($21 for 1 ounce)* is a lightweight lotion for normal to slightly oily skin. However, the zinc sulfate can be a skin irritant, and there is no research showing it to be effective for oily or blemish-prone skin. Copper PCA is a good water-binding agent, and may help with wound healing, but in this minute amount there is no research as to its benefit for skin. Due to the product's high pH, the salicylic acid it contains will not be effective for exfoliation.

☺ **A-Copper Oil Control Cream** *($24.50 for 1 ounce)* is an emollient moisturizer for normal to dry skin. It contains a tiny amount of water-binding agents and antioxidants. The salicylic acid it contains cannot exfoliate skin because the pH of the product is too high, and the zinc sulfate can be a skin irritant (plus there is no research showing it to be effective for blemish-prone skin).

SERIOUS SKIN CARE CONTINUOUSLY CLEAR LINE

☹ **Clear Wash Specialized Target Cleanser** *($16.50 for 4.2 ounces)* is a standard, detergent-based cleanser. This contains peppermint oil, which is too irritating for all skin types and a problem for the eye area. It also contains salicylic acid, although the pH is too high for it to be effective as an exfoliant. Even if the pH were right, when salicylic acid is added to a cleanser it is just rinsed down the drain before it can deliver a benefit.

☺ **Daily Ritual Acne Medication Cleanser** *($21 for 4 ounces)* is a standard, detergent-based cleanser. It contains 2% salicylic acid, although the pH is too high for it to be effective as an exfoliant. Even if the pH were right, in a cleanser any potential benefits would just be rinsed down the drain. It also contains a small amount of ground-up plastic for a topical scrub. It is an option for normal to oily skin.

The Reviews S

☹ **Clear Pads** *($19.95 for 45 pads)*. Alcohol is the second ingredient, making the Clear Pads too irritating and drying for all skin types. The tiny amount of tea tree oil is not enough to be effective as a topical disinfectant.

☺ **Clarify Clarifying Treatment** *($17.50 for 2 ounces)* is a simple 2% BHA in a lotion with a pH of 4, which makes it effective for exfoliation.

☺ **Continuously Clear Acne Medication Moisture Replenishing Cream** *($26.50 for 4 ounces)* is an emollient-base moisturizer that contains 0.5% BHA and less than 0.1% AHA, which are tiny amounts, but the pH is 5 anyway, which would make them ineffective as exfoliants. The small amount of antioxidants and water-binding agents are worth a consideration for dry skin. It does contain fragrance.

☹ **Unmasked Sulfur Mask** *($22 for 2.5 ounces)* contains 8% sulfur. Sulfur is a topical disinfectant, though it is also a potent skin irritant due to its high pH, so this is best avoided.

✔☺ **Clearz-it Daytime Blemish Preventor** *($17.50 for 2 ounces)* is a very good lightweight lotion that contains both 5% benzoyl peroxide and about 2% tea tree oil. It also contains some good water-binding agents. It is an option as a topical disinfectant for blemish-prone skin.

☹ **Dry Lo Spot Treatment** *($22.50 for 1 ounce)* lists alcohol as the second ingredient, and it also contains camphor, making this too irritating and drying for all skin types.

SERIOUS SKIN CARE C-NO WRINKLE LINE

☺ **$$$ C-Clean Vitamin C Cleanser** *($19.95 for 4 ounces)* is a standard, detergent-based cleanser that would work well for normal to oily skin. The helpful antioxidants it contains would just be rinsed down the drain before they had a chance to have any benefit for skin.

☹ **C-Mist Vitamin C Refresher** *($16.50 for 4 ounces)* lists witch hazel distillate as the second ingredient. That's primarily alcohol and makes this too drying and irritating for all skin types.

☺ **C-Cream Protective Moisturizer with SPF 15** *($24.50 for 2 ounces)* is a very good, in-part titanium dioxide–based sunscreen in a matte-finish lotion. The cornstarch it contains can be a problem for skin. It does contain some good antioxidants though, and that is a plus.

✔☺ **C-Repair Vitamin C Moisturizing Night Cream** *($22.50 for 2 ounces)* is a mineral oil–based, emollient moisturizer with some good antioxidants, and if you are looking for a vitamin C cream for normal to dry skin, this is an option.

☺ **$$$ C-Eye Vitamin C Eye Beauty Treatment** *($19.50 for 0.5 ounce)* is a lightweight lotion that contains a good amount of vitamin C and a tiny amount of water-binding agents and vitamin E. It is an option for slightly dry skin or for an extra shot of vitamin C.

☺ **C-Serum Vitamin C Skin Conditioner** *($26.50 for 1 ounce)* is similar to the C-Eye version above and the same basic comments apply.

☺ **C-Mask Vitamin C Conditioning Mask** *($21 for 3 ounces)* is a standard clay mask that is a good option for normal to oily skin.

SERIOUS SKIN CARE A-DEFIANCE LINE

☹ **A-Force Vitamin A Serum Double Strength** *($25 for 1 ounce)* lists alcohol as the third ingredient, and that makes it too drying and irritating for all skin types.

☹ **Pucker Up Vitamin A Lip Exfoliator** *($15 for 0.25 ounce)* contains several potentially irritating plant oils as well as the preservative Kathon CG, which is recommended for use only in rinse-off products. Other than that, this is just a wax you rub over your lips that helps exfoliate skin. There are definitely better options available.

☹ **A-Force Vitamin A Serum with Retinol** *($28.50 for 1 ounce)* lists alcohol as the third ingredient, and that makes this too drying and irritating for all skin types. There are many gentler ways to get vitamin A on the skin.

☺ **1 Million I.U. Vitamin A Cream** *($29.95 for 2 ounces)* contains 1 million International Units (IU) of retinyl palmitate, an ester of vitamin A. While 1 million is an impressive number, that ends up being less than a tenth (0.1) of an ounce of retinyl palmitate, not exactly as exciting as that big number would lead a consumer to believe. But that's good news, because if it was really as high a concentration of vitamin A as the name implies, it could be toxic (Source: www.teratology.org/pubs/vitamina.htm). Retinyl palmitate is a good antioxidant, but that is all this product contains, and not very much of it. Other than that, this is a fairly ordinary Vaseline-based moisturizer.

☺ **Two Million I.U. Vitamin A Cream Double Strength** *($26.50 for 2 ounces)* is similar to the 1 Million I.U. version above, meaning there's still not very much retinyl palmitate (far less than 1 ounce) in it, and the same basic comments apply.

☺ **$$$ A-Eye Vitamin A Eye Cream with Retinol** *($21 for 0.5 ounce)*. If you are looking for a retinol product this is one to consider. It also contains a small amount of additional antioxidants, a teeny amount of water-binding agent, and some good anti-irritants.

☺ **A-Good Night Beta-Carotene Night Cream** *($26.50 for 1 ounce)* is an emollient moisturizer that contains a tiny amount of antioxidants and no water-binding agents. It is an option for normal to dry skin. It also contains tea tree oil, but not enough to be effective as a topical disinfectant. The jar packaging is not the best for keeping the antioxidants stable.

☹ **A-Facial Meringue Exfoliating Mask** *($22.50 for 1 ounce)* is more of a cleanser than a mask and because the second ingredient is a detergent cleansing agent, it should not be left on the skin for any length of time; otherwise, it can be too drying and irritating.

☹ **Lip A-llure Vitamin A Lip Conditioner** *($15 for 0.5 ounce)* contains peppermint oil, which can be drying and irritating for the lips.

SERIOUS SKIN CARE REVERSE LIFT LINE

☺ **Quick Lift Firming Facial Mist** *($21 for 2 ounces)* is an overly fragranced toner that contains a large amount of film-forming agent. That can place a layer of plastic-like

The Reviews S

material over the skin, but it isn't lifting in the least. It also contains wild yam extract and pregnenolone acetate. (Refer to Chapter Seven, *Cosmetics Dictionary* for information on why those ingredients don't have benefit for skin.)

☺ $$$ I-Refirm Quick & Temporary Lifting & Firming Eye Gel *($21 for 0.5 ounce)* contains only water, magnesium aluminum silicate (an absorbent), sodium silicate (a buffering agent), slip agent, and preservatives. This may be quick, but it is also useless for the skin around the eyes, containing not a single beneficial ingredient.

☺ $$$ I-Finish Sealing Eye Gel *($18.50 for 0.5 ounce)* contains mostly film-forming agent and boron nitride, which gives it a matte finish. It is meant to lock in the benefits of the I-Refirm above, only the I-Refirm doesn't have any benefits worth locking. This version does contain some good antioxidants, emollients, and water-binding agents, but how well this works under the eye area as a moisturizer or for any purpose is questionable, and it definitely doesn't help to use it with the I-Refirm.

☹ Face Refirm Instant & Temporary Lifting & Firming Serum *($24 for 1 ounce)* lists witch hazel distillate as the third ingredient. That consists mostly of alcohol, and it means this isn't firming, though it is irritating. Adding to the problem are the menthol and camphor this contains.

☹ Reverse Lift Firming Facial Cream *($26.50 for 2 ounces)*. The hyped ingredients in this product include wild yam extract. According to the *American Journal of Obstetrics and Gynecology* (1999, volume 18), "Wild yam is used in the production of artificial [synthetic] progesterone but it will not yield the hormone in the absence of a chemical conversion process that the body can't supply, though it can be created in a laboratory." It also contains pregnenolone acetate, a precursor to other hormones that can affect levels of progesterone and estrogen in the body when taken orally. When applied to skin it may work as a water-binding agent; there is no information about whether absorption through skin is possible. This also contains royal jelly, which may have an antibacterial benefit, but in this amount it has no real impact on skin at all. And the menthol this product contains just adds irritation and a misleading sensation that something is happening to the skin.

☺ Neck Refirm Neck & Decollete Firming Lotion *($24.50 for 4 ounces)* is an exceptionally ordinary moisturizer that lacks any of the water-binding agents and antioxidants that are present in many other moisturizers in this line. This product is boring for any and all parts of the body or face. It does contain a small amount of menthol, which can be a skin irritant.

SERIOUS SKIN CARE GLUCOSAMINE LINE

The claims for these products revolve around the notion that glucosamine replaces the need for AHAs, a theory that is clearly showcased by the product names. Given that Serious Skin Care has several AHA products, I wonder why they are taking the "acid-free" slant, but here it is, and clearly they want you to think these products are more gentle than their other products for the purposes of "renewing skin." Technically, glucosamine is a constituent of hyaluronic acid. Hyaluronic acid, among many other natural components of the skin's structure, makes a good skin-care ingredient to prevent moisture loss and to shore up the skin's own structure, so it can definitely have benefit, especially for dry skin. But that doesn't make glucosamine all that special or any kind of a wonder ingredient, and there is no independent research showing it to have exfoliating properties—which are the primary function and benefit of a well-formulated AHA product.

☹ **Acid-Free Skin Resurfacing Cleanser** *($21 for 5 ounces)*. The main detergent cleansing agent in this product is sodium lauryl sulfate, which is too potentially drying and irritating for all skin types.

☺ **$$$ Phyto-Pumpkin Scrub Acid-Free** *($21 for 2 ounces)* is an emollient scrub-type cleanser that includes plant oils and an abrasive (ground-up plastic). The tiny amount of pumpkin is really irrelevant, though it does have antioxidant properties. This is an option as a topical scrub for normal to dry skin.

☺ **$$$ Hydrating Facial Mist Acid Free** *($18 for 4 ounces)* is just water, acetyl glucosamine, slip agent, sunscreen agent, preservative, fragrance, and coloring agent. Mainly, it is just a basic toner, though if you are looking for acetyl glucosamine, this would be a good option for that purpose.

✓☺ **Acid-Free Skin Resurfacing Moisturizer** *($22 for 4 ounces)* is a very good emollient moisturizer for normal to dry skin with some good water-binding agents and antioxidants.

✓☺ **Acid-Free Skin Resurfacing Serum** *($26.50 for 1 ounce)* is similar to the Resurfacing Moisturizer above only in lotion form, and would be a good option for normal to slightly dry skin.

✓☺ **$$$ Eye Firming Gel Acid-Free** *($19.50 for 0.5 ounce)* is a very good, lightweight moisturizer for normal to slightly dry skin with some good water-binding agents and antioxidants.

SERIOUS SKIN CARE SUN PRODUCTS

☺ **Instant Bronze Sunless Tanning Lotion** *($16.50 for 4 ounces)* contains dihydroxyacetone, the same ingredient in all self-tanners that affects the color of skin. This would work as well as any.

☹ **Serious Shade SPF 15** *($16.50 for 4 ounces)* doesn't contain the UVA-protecting ingredients of titanium dioxide, zinc oxide, or avobenzone, and is not recommended.

☹ **Sun Chill After Sun Cooling Gel** *($16.50 for 4 ounces)* lists witch hazel distillate as the second ingredient, and that contains alcohol as its major component, making this too irritating and drying for all skin types.

SERIOUS SKIN CARE LIGHTEN-UP LINE

☺ **Fading Cream Skin Lightening Formula** *($24.50 for 2 ounces)* is just a 2% hydroquinone-based skin lightener in a very standard moisturizing base. It also contains about 5% AHA in a pH of 4 that makes it effective for exfoliation. There is only a teeny amount of kojic acid, which means that the hydroquinone will be what makes this effective for inhibiting melanin production.

☺ $$$ **Phase Out** *($19.95 for 0.5 ounce)* is supposed to be "specifically for the problem of dark circles underneath the eyes," yet there is nothing in it that is unique or special for dark circles. Some vitamin K is included, but that has no effect on dark circles. It also contains arnica, which is an irritant that should not be used repeatedly on skin.

☹ **Lite-Guard Brightening Moisturizer with SPF 15** *($16.50 for 2 ounces)* doesn't contain the UVA-protecting ingredients of titanium dioxide, zinc oxide, or avobenzone, and is not recommended.

☺ **Fading Mask Skin Lightening Formula with 2% Hydroquinone** *($22.50 for 2 ounces)* is a 2% hydroquinone-based facial mask that peels off the skin. It can leave the face feeling smooth, but as far as skin lightening, you are better off with one effective skin lightener and a well-formulated sunscreen than these extra bells and whistles that offer nothing more for skin.

☺ **Fading Pads Skin Lightening Formula with 2% Hydroquinone** *($24.50 for 30 pads)* is a very good 2% hydroquinone-based skin lightener with about 1% BHA, though the pH of the product is too high for it to be effective for exfoliation.

SERIOUS SKIN CARE DAILY ESSENTIALS LINE

☺ **Glycolic Cleanser Thorough Cleansing Formula** *($36.50 for 12 ounces)* is a standard, detergent-based cleanser that contains about 4% AHA, though the pH of this cleanser is too high for it to be effective for exfoliation, not to mention that in a cleanser the AHA would be rinsed down the drain before it had much chance to affect the skin at all.

☺ $$$ **Buff Polish Facial Exfoliation Treatment** *($21 for 4 ounces)* is a standard, detergent-based cleanser that contains ground-up plastic (polyethylene) as the abrasive. It is an option for normal to oily skin. The small amount of AHA isn't enough to be effective for exfoliation. This also contains several plant extracts that can be skin irritants.

☹ **Glycolic Kleen Deep Pore Cleansing Cloths** *($16.50 for 25 cloths)* lists alcohol as the second ingredient, and that makes these too drying and irritating for all skin types.

☺ **Renewal Gel Glycolic Skin Perfector** *($20 for 4 ounces)* is a good gel/liquid 8% AHA (glycolic acid) product with about 0.5% BHA (salicylic acid). This is a good option for exfoliation for someone with normal to oily or combination skin. However, the sound-alike AHA plant extracts it contains have no exfoliating properties.

☺ **Glycolic 3 Cleansing, Exfoliating, and Tightening Mask** *($29.50 for two 5-ounce jars)* is a standard clay mask with less than 2% AHA, which isn't enough to have exfoliating properties for skin.

☺ **Haven Stabilizing Serum for All Skin Types** *($26.50 for 2 ounces)* is supposed to precondition the skin so you can use the supposedly more potent products that Serious Skin Care sells. There is nothing in this product that can stabilize skin or prepare it for other products. It is a good moisturizer for normal to dry skin, with small quantities of water-binding agents and antioxidants, but that's about it.

☺ **Megamins Multi Vitamin Beauty Serum** *($28 for 1 ounce)* is a lightweight lotion with some good antioxidants, but it just isn't all that "mega." It is a lightweight moisturizer option for all skin types.

☺ **$$$ Home Spa Facial Peel Six Week Facial Peel Program** *($19 for 6 towelettes)* is a good 10% AHA product that would work well for exfoliation, especially for someone with oily skin. Keep in mind that you only need one exfoliating skin-care product, any more than that is overkill and can cause problems.

SERIOUS SKIN CARE MISCELLANEOUS PRODUCTS

☺ **Emu & Aloe Soothing Cream** *($29.95 for two 2-ounce jars)* is an OK, though exceptionally standard, moisturizer for dry skin. If you want emu oil, this product has it, but that's about all it has.

☹ **$$$ Eye Help Moisture & Correct Eye Cream** *($19.95 for 0.5 ounce)* is an extremely simple, silicone-based moisturizer that contains a small amount of plant extracts that can be good anti-irritants, but that's about it. This won't correct any problems you're having around the eye area.

☺ **$$$ Vitamin A Moisture Stick** *($15.75 for 0.17 ounce)* includes a teeny amount of retinyl palmitate, but it's barely detectable. This is just an emollient clear lipstick with small amounts of water-binding agents and antioxidants that make it a good option for dry lips.

SERIOUS SKIN CARE LIQUID LASER LINE

☺ **Face Laser** *($16.50 for 2 ounces)* is a clever name for what ends up being nothing more than a depilatory that uses calcium thioglycolate to "eat" or dissolve hair. There is nothing about this product that makes it related in any remote way to the laser hair-removal systems performed in a doctor's office. Instead, it is similar in all respects to any depilatory you may find at the drugstore for a lot less money, such as Surgi-Cream ($4.95 for 1 ounce).

☺ **Liquid Laser** *($26.50 for 8 ounces)* is similar to the Face Laser version above and the same comments apply.

☺ **Post Laser** *($21 for 4 ounces)* is supposed to inhibit hair growth, but there is nothing in this product capable of inhibiting anything, other than the facts.

SHADE UVA-GUARD (SEE COPPERTONE)

SHAKLEE (SKIN CARE ONLY)

Shaklee's line of skin-care products is called Enfuselle, and its claims portray these products as nothing less than outstanding. Statements about patented formulations and substantial research (said to be published) from two independent labs are the basis of its primary marketing push. The Shaklee brochure states, "In collaboration with physicians from the Dermatology Division of the Scripps Clinic and Research Foundation, Enfuselle products have been clinically tested at the independent laboratories of the California Skin Research Institute for safety and performance." In fact, the studies were never published—well, at least not other than in the Shaklee brochure, and were sent to other cosmetics chemists working in the industry—and without documentation of the actual study, the reliability of the research cited by a company that paid for its own study is limited. It is no more accurate than a child relating the results of his or her report card and, as any parent knows, you need to see it yourself to get the real story. It may sound impressive to have patented formulations, but patents never ever indicate efficacy; patents are concerned with a product's content or use, not about its effectiveness on skin.

The way the Shaklee tests were performed also renders the information useless. The Shaklee brochure even states as much: "The results of the Enfuselle clinical tests dramatically reflect the difference between one side of the face being untreated and exposed to changing climatic conditions, and the other side of the face being treated with Enfuselle under the same climatic conditions." That isn't much of a test. If the skin is dry, and you leave one side of the face without any moisturizer, it's going to look dry and dehydrated (which will emphasize any wrinkles), and the side you treat with a moisturizer, any decent moisturizer, is going to look a thousand percent better.

While the claims for these products are as exaggerated and overblown as any in the cosmetics industry, a lot of Shaklee salespeople definitely believe this is the gospel (of course, they also felt that way about the products the Enfuselle line has replaced). However, I haven't said the products are bad, at least not all of them, because many are impressive, at least as far as moisturizers go. But given that all of the ingredients found in the Shaklee products show up in lots and lots of other skin-care products, these simply can't live up to their claims about getting rid of wrinkles or stopping the skin from aging, and they are definitely not any better than a host of other products with similar to identical formulations.

Shaklee is very proud of the antioxidants it uses in its products, and that seems to be the reality behind the brouhaha about them, because they all do contain antioxidants. Antioxidants are theoretically beneficial for skin, and most skin-care products contain them; however, there is no research anywhere proving that they can affect or stop aging or change one wrinkle on your face, much less that one particular form or combination of them is better than another. As a group, all antioxidants have potential merit for skin.

As it turns out, nothing in the Shaklee products makes them unique in any way, and a few have serious problems that you need to be aware of. Several products contain potentially irritating ingredients that are just bad for skin and completely unnecessary. Further, for all the patented ingredients and "serious scientific" research that is supposed to be supporting the claims, whoever these scientists are, they don't have any information about UVA sun protection, because none of the sun products contain the UVA-protecting ingredients of avobenzone, zinc oxide, or titanium dioxide (Sources: *International Journal of Pharmaceutics,* June 2002, pages 85–94; *Photodermatology, Photoimmunology, Photomedicine,* August 2000, pages 147–155, and http://www.photodermatology.com/sunprotection.htm; and *Skin Therapy Letter,* 1997, volume 2, number 5). As a footnote, one Shaklee representative told me that the sun products were tested and approved by the FDA for UVA protection, yet according to the FDA (http://www.fda.gov) no such standard, testing, or approval for UVA exists. For more information about Shaklee, call (800) 742-5533 or visit www.enfuselle.com. **Note:** All Shaklee products contain fragrance.

☹ **Gentle Action Cleansing Bar** *($16.80 for 4.5 ounces)* is a standard bar cleanser that can be drying to the skin. It does contain some good antioxidants, but in a bar cleanser they wouldn't remain stable (antioxidants deteriorate when exposed to light or air), though even if that weren't a problem, they would be rinsed down the drain before they could have benefit for skin.

☺ **Hydrating Cleansing Lotion** *($18.15 for 6 ounces)* is a standard, creamy cleanser that is meant to be rinsed off, but comes off better when you use a washcloth. It can be an option for normal to dry skin. It also contains antioxidants, but they would be rinsed away before they had much benefit for skin.

☺ **Purifying Cleansing Gel** *($16.50 for 6 ounces)* is a good, detergent-based, water-soluble cleanser for most skin types. There are a handful of antioxidants in this formula, just as in most of the Enfuselle products, but even if these could somehow be effective in fighting wrinkles, in a cleanser such as this they would simply be rinsed down the drain before having any effect.

☺ **Eye Makeup Remover** *($9.15 for 2 ounces)* is an extremely standard, detergent-based eye-makeup remover. It works as well as any reviewed in this book.

☹ **Refining Polisher** *($16.50 for 2.5 ounces)* contains menthol and alcohol, which are too irritating for all skin types. It does contain bilberry fruit extract, but that is not an AHA and it has no exfoliating properties.

☹ **Hydrating Toner** *($14.05 for 6 ounces)* contains witch hazel distillate, which is mostly alcohol. It also contains menthol, and those two ingredients combine to make this too irritating and drying for all skin types.

☹ **Purifying Toner** *($14.05 for 6 ounces)* is almost identical to the Hydrating Toner above, and the same comments apply.

✓☺ **Balancing Moisturizer** *($22 for 2 ounces)* is a good moisturizer for normal to dry skin that contains some very good antioxidants and water-binding agents.

✓☺ $$$ **Eye Treatment** *($22 for 0.5 ounce)* is similar to the Balancing Moisturizer above, and the same comments apply.

✓☺ **Hydrating Moisturizer** *($22 for 1.7 ounces)* is similar to the Balancing Moisturizer above, and the same comments apply.

☹ **Time Repair A.M. SPF 15** *($49.50 for 2 ounces)* doesn't contain the UVA-protecting ingredients of avobenzone, titanium dioxide, or zinc oxide, and is not recommended.

The Reviews S

☹ **SPF 15 for Body** *($16.50 for 4 ounces)* doesn't contain the UVA-protecting ingredients of avobenzone, titanium dioxide, or zinc oxide, and is not recommended.

☹ **SPF 30 for Body** *($16.50 for 4 ounces)* doesn't contain the UVA-protecting ingredients of avobenzone, titanium dioxide, or zinc oxide, and is not recommended.

☹ **Lip Treatment SPF 15 for Body** *($7.45 for 0.15 ounce)* doesn't contain the UVA-protecting ingredients of avobenzone, titanium dioxide, or zinc oxide, and is not recommended.

☺ **$$$ Calming Complex** *($45 for 2 ounces)* is an OK lightweight moisturizer for normal to slightly dry skin, but it doesn't contain the same impressive array of antioxidants and water-binding agents as the other moisturizers in the Shaklee lineup.

☺ **$$$ C+E Repair P.M.** *($45 for 1 ounce)* contains mostly silicone and vitamins. Silicones leave a nice silky feel on the skin, but that's about it. If you're looking for this group of antioxidants (vitamins A, C, and E) this is an option.

☺ **$$$ Infusing Mineral Masque** *($16.50 for 2.5 ounces)* is a standard clay mask with a tiny amount of BHA (salicylic acid); however, the pH is too high for it to work as an exfoliant. It also contains menthol, which is a completely unnecessary skin irritant, and the cornstarch can be a problem for skin.

☹ **Acne Clearing Complex** *($16.45 for 4 ounces)* lists alcohol as the second ingredient, which makes this 0.5% BHA lotion too drying and irritating for all skin types.

SHISEIDO

Shiseido is the largest and one of the oldest cosmetics companies in Japan. Because of its prowess and marketing adroitness, Shiseido has been able to successfully enter other markets, particularly the United States, where it is found in most major, upscale department stores. The claims made about the company's products run the gamut from the benefits of natural ingredients to almost every antiaging trick in the book, and the prices reflect the high-end appeal Shiseido strives for.

In 2000, Shiseido launched a line called <u>The</u> Skin Care, which added another group of products to its already existing lines (Benefiance, D-Program for Sensitive Skin, Pureness, Whitening, and Bio-Performance), available at Shiseido counters in department stores. I have only one question to sum all this up: What in the world are all these products for? It is difficult to understand why there should be so much blatant redundancy, along with endlessly repetitive claims about getting rid of wrinkles and curing what ails skin, all attached to formulations that product after product are shockingly ordinary or poorly formulated. It's almost impossible to address all the premises behind Shiseido's assertions for this cumbersome array of unnecessary products.

What most consumers aren't aware of is that the Shiseido-owned line Cle de Peau, which sells skin-care products at prices ranging from $60 for a cleanser to $400 for a skin-lightening product, contains formulations identical to its counterparts at the regular Shiseido counter. Even though this is a line you could easily pass up, there are of course some items to consider—but ignore the scientific-sounding claims, they are over the top and without a supportive leg to stand on. For more information about Shiseido, call (800) 354-2160 or (212) 805-2300 or visit www.shiseido.com. **Note:** All Shiseido products contain fragrance except their D Program for Sensitive line.

SHISEIDO SKIN CARE

SHISEIDO BENEFIANCE

☺ $$$ **Benefiance Creamy Cleansing Emulsion** *($29.50 for 6.7 ounces)* is a very standard, mineral oil– and Vaseline-based wipe-off cleanser that also contains a small amount of detergent cleansing agent. It can leave a slight greasy residue on the skin, though it may be an option for someone with dry skin.

☹ $$$ **Benefiance Creamy Cleansing Foam** *($29.50 for 4.4 ounces)* is a very standard, detergent-based, water-soluble cleanser that can be drying for most skin types due to its high alkaline content.

☺ $$$ **Benefiance Balancing Softener** *($35 for 5 ounces)* is an OK, though extremely mundane, irritant-free toner. There are some water-binding agents, but they're at the very end of the ingredient list, which makes them completely irrelevant for skin.

☹ **Benefiance Enriched Balancing Softener** *($35 for 5 ounces)* is similar to the Enriched version above, except that it contains alcohol, which can irritate and dry the skin.

☹ **Benefiance Daytime Protective Emulsion SPF 8** *($38 for 2.5 ounces)*, besides having a substandard SPF 8, doesn't contain the UVA-protecting ingredients of avobenzone, zinc oxide, or titanium dioxide, and is absolutely not recommended.

☹ **Benefiance Daytime Protective Cream SPF 8** *($38 for 1.4 ounces)* is similar to the Emulsion SPF 8 version above and the same comments apply.

☺ $$$ **Luminizing Day Essence SPF 24** *($50 for 1.4 ounces)*. This product indicates that Shiseido has finally realized the need for a reliable SPF with UVA-protecting ingredients, so why still sell the poorly formulated versions above? This one is a very good, in-part titanium dioxide–based sunscreen in an ordinary silicone-based moisturizer that has minute amounts of water-binding agents and antioxidants.

☺ $$$ **Luminizing Night Essence** *($75 for 1.3 ounces)* is an alcohol-based lotion that contains a good concentration of arbutin (a plant extract), an ingredient that can have melanin-inhibiting properties, though this has only been established in animal and test-tube research. Other than that, it includes a small quantity of water-binding agents and antioxidants. As intriguing an option as arbutin is, the alcohol in this product is bound to make this one problematic.

☺ $$$ **Benefiance Revitalizing Eye Cream** *($42 for 0.51 ounce)* is mostly plant oil, mineral oil, and Vaseline, along with a small amount of water-binding agents and a tiny amount of antioxidants. It is an OK, though ordinary, emollient moisturizer for normal to dry skin.

The Reviews S

☺ $$$ **Benefiance Revitalizing Emulsion** *($42 for 2.5 ounces)* is similar to the Revitalizing Eye Cream above, though it is even less endowed with ingredients significant for skin care.

☺ $$$ **Benefiance Revitalizing Cream** *($40 for 1.3 ounces)* is similar to the Revitalizing Eye Cream above and the same comments apply.

☺ $$$ **Facial Lifting Complex** *($50 for 1.7 ounces)* won't lift the skin anywhere. It is a silicone-based lotion with a lot of alcohol (alcohol is the fourth ingredient). It has minute amounts of beneficial ingredients and altogether that isn't uplifting in the least. This also contains a small amount of menthol, which can be a skin irritant.

☺ $$$ **Benefiance Eye Treatment Mask** *($35 for 10 packettes)* is mostly water, thickeners, film-forming agent, alcohol, and trace amounts of antioxidants and water-binding agents. This has more problems for the eye area than benefits.

☺ $$$ **Benefiance Firming Massage Mask** *($39 for 1.9 ounces)*. Massaging the skin is nice, but it doesn't take this non-firming, ordinary moisturizing formulation to do it.

☹ **Benefiance Energizing Essence** *($49 for 1 ounce)* is an alcohol-based serum, and that makes it potentially irritating to skin; it is not recommended.

☹ **Benefiance Neck Firming Cream** *($43 for 1.8 ounces)* is meant for the neck, but what makes it special for this area is not reflected in the ingredient listing. However, what isn't a mystery is that this cream contains alcohol and menthol, which are irritating and drying for every part of the body.

D PROGRAM FOR SENSITIVE SKIN

These products are far more simply formulated than any of the others Shiseido sells. The good thing is they lack the fragrance, alcohol, and problematic plant extracts that show up too frequently in the other Shiseido lines. However, these also lack any beneficial ingredients such as antioxidants and water-binding agents, which are essential for all skin types, even though almost all of those types of ingredients pose no problems of irritation or sensitizing reactions for skin.

☺ $$$ **Make Up Cleansing Gel** *($23 for 4.4 ounces)* is a fairly gentle, rinseable cleanser with a small amount of detergent cleansing agent. This is a good option for normal to dry skin.

☺ $$$ **Cleansing Foam** *($23 for 4.9 ounces)* is far gentler than almost every other detergent-based cleanser by Shiseido. This would be an option for normal to dry skin.

☺ $$$ **Cleansing Water** *($23 for 4.2 ounces)* is a detergent-based cleanser that would work well for most skin types, except for very dry skin—though, for some unknown reason, this does contain fragrance.

☺ **Soap** *($12 for 3.5 ounces)* is a standard bar cleanser with fairly drying detergent cleansing agents. It is not as gentle for skin as, say, Dove Bar Cleanser would be.

☺ $$$ **Mist QQ** *($16 for 1.6 ounces)* is an ordinary toner with nothing more than water, slip agents, humectant, and preservatives.

☺ $$$ **Lotion I** *($32 for 4.2 ounces)* is an exceedingly ordinary lotion, formulated with little more than water, slip agents, and humectants.

☺ $$$ **Lotion II** *($32 for 4.2 ounces)* is similar to the Lotion I above, only this one contains some detergent cleansing agents, which doesn't add any benefit for skin.

☺ **Emulsion I** *($34 for 3.3 ounces)* is an exceedingly ordinary moisturizing lotion that lacks any beneficial ingredients for skin. It is just water, slip agent, humectants, silicone, preservatives, and thickeners.

☺ **Emulsion II** *($34 for 3.3 ounces)* is almost identical to the Emulsion I above, only with the addition of plant oil. That doesn't make it any more helpful for state-of-the-art skin care; it only makes it a boring moisturizer for normal to dry skin.

☺ **Emulsion III** *($34 for 3.3 ounces)* is similar to the Emulsion II above, only with more plant oils. Again, that is better for drier skin, but this is still a mundane option.

☺ **Lotion AC** *($32 for 4.2 ounces)* is almost identical to the Emulsion I above and the same comments apply.

☺ **Essence AC** *($36 for 1.6 ounces)* is almost identical to the Emulsion I above and the same comments apply.

☺ **Lotion AD** *($32 for 4.2 ounces)* is almost identical to the Emulsion I above and the same comments apply. There are minute amounts of plant extracts in this lotion (rosemary and mugwort), but they are completely inconsequential when it comes to having an effect on skin.

☹ **Essence AD** *($36 for 1.6 ounces)* is similar to the Lotion AD above and the same basic comments apply.

☺ $$$ **Cream AD** *($23 for 0.52 ounce)* is an emollient moisturizer for normal to dry skin, and while it does contain some good plant oils, it lacks any water-binding agents and contains only a trace amount of vitamin E.

☺ $$$ **Treatment Spots AC** *($23 for 0.52 ounce)* is mostly water, silicones, talc, water-binding agents, and preservatives. It contains a minute amount of a plant extract that may have antibacterial properties, but at such a low concentration that it is unlikely to have any effect. None of this is helpful for any kind of spots.

☺ $$$ **Lip Care** *($23 for 1 ounce)* is an OK, emollient lip balm, but it's incredibly overpriced for what is little more than Chap Stick, which you can find at the drugstore for a fraction of the cost.

SHISEIDO PURENESS

☹ **Pureness Deep Cleansing Foam** *($18 for 3.7 ounces)* is almost identical to the Benefiance Creamy Cleansing Foam above and the same basic comments apply. It also contains a small amount of menthol, which can be a skin irritant and does not help blemish-prone skin.

☺ **Pureness Foaming Cleansing Fluid** *($18 for 5 ounces)* is similar to the Benefiance Creamy Cleansing Foam above and the same basic comments apply.

The Reviews S

☺ **Pureness Refreshing Cleansing Water** *($18 for 5 ounces)* is a very simple, irritant-free toner containing mostly water, slip agents, and detergent cleansing agents. It's OK for most skin types, but really very ordinary and more of a do-nothing kind of product.

☺ **Pureness Refreshing Cleansing Sheets** *($18 for 5 ounces)* is identical to the Refreshing Cleansing Water above, only the cloths are supplied for you.

☺ **Pureness Balancing Softener Alcohol Free** *($20 for 5 ounces)* can't balance anything. It is just a very simple toner of slip agents and a small amount of detergent cleansing agents. It provides little benefit for skin.

☺ **Pureness Matifying Moisturizer Oil Free** *($29 for 1.6 ounces)* lists alcohol as the fourth ingredient, which is a problem for skin. It is just a simple, silicone-based lotion that has little to no ability to absorb oil. It will go on matte, but it offers no other benefit for skin.

☹ **Pureness Matifying Stick Oil Free** *($23 for 0.14 ounce)* contains several problematic waxes (including ceresin and carnauba) that someone with oily or blemish-prone skin would want to avoid putting on their face. It also lacks beneficial ingredients that would be helpful for any skin type.

☺ **Pureness Moisturizing Gel-Cream** *($29 for 1.4 ounces)* is similar to the Matifying Moisturizer above and the same basic comments apply.

☹ **Pureness Blemish Clearing Gel** *($16 for 0.5 ounce)* lists alcohol as the first ingredient, which makes this too irritating and drying for all skin types, and that won't help clear up blemishes. The 0.5% concentration of BHA (salicylic acid) is too low and the basic pH too high for it to be of any help for exfoliation.

☺ **Pureness Oil-Blotting Paper** *($13.50 for 100 sheets)* is just what the name implies. You press these small sheets over your face to help absorb oil during the day. The sheets are coated with a light layer of clay that can absorb oil.

SHISEIDO BIO-PERFORMANCE

☺ **$$$ Bio-Performance Advanced Super Revitalizer Cream** *($66 for 1.7 ounces)* is a very standard moisturizer for someone with dry skin. The minuscule amounts of antioxidants and water-binding agents are almost funny.

☹ **Bio-Performance Advanced Super Revitalizer Whitening Formula** *($90 for 1.7 ounces)* contains none of the ingredients that research shows will lighten skin, such as hydroquinone, magnesium ascorbyl palmitate, azelaic acid, or kojic acid, or even Shiseido's own patented ingredient for skin lightening, arbutin, which makes this product a complete waste of time and money.

☺ **$$$ Bio-Performance Intensive Clarifying Essence** *($65 for 1.3 ounces)*. The good stuff in this product is listed well after the preservatives, and so adds up to only a negligible, relatively useless amount. If you're going to splurge on a moisturizer for normal to dry skin, this is not the one to consider.

☺ **$$$ Bio-Performance Revitalizing Cream** *($135 for 1.4 ounces)* is a shockingly ordinary moisturizer of mostly water, plant oil, mineral oil, thickeners, water-binding agents, fragrance, vitamin E, and preservatives. For this amount of money, the water-binding agents and antioxidants should be abundant and in packaging that ensures their stability (which they are not). The minute amount of placenta extract in this product has no unique properties for skin.

SHISEIDO SUN PROTECTION

☹ **Ultimate Cleansing Gel for Sunscreen** *($21 for 3.5 ounces)* is the ultimate unnecessary product. It is just a silicone-based makeup remover that also contains a good amount of alcohol. This doesn't add any benefit to cleaning the skin or removing sunscreen.

☺ $$$ **Ultimate Sun Block Lotion SPF 50** *($35 for 3.3 ounces)* is a very good, in-part zinc oxide–based sunscreen in an ordinary moisturizing base. This would be an option for someone with normal to dry skin. According to the FDA, the SPF 50 is actually not an acceptable rating; sunscreens cannot be labeled over an SPF 30. SPF ratings indicate only how long you can stay in the sun without burning, and you would rarely find 16 hours of daylight (which is how long an SPF 50 would protect your skin) anywhere in the world.

☺ **Gentle Sun Block Cream SPF 22** *($20 for 3.8 ounces)* is a very good, pure titanium dioxide–based sunscreen in a slightly matte base that includes talc. It is an option for normal to slightly oily skin.

☺ $$$ **Sun Block Compact SPF 32** *($25 for 0.42 ounce)* is a very good, in-part titanium dioxide–based sunscreen for someone with dry skin, but it has a rather ordinary, Vaseline-based moisturizing formulation. This may be convenient to apply but keep in mind that you must apply sunscreen liberally, and that makes this a one-application product if you are using it over your entire body and not just on your lips.

☺ $$$ **Sun Block Face Cream SPF 35** *($24 for 1.7 ounces)* is a very good, in-part titanium dioxide–based sunscreen for someone with dry skin, but the rather ordinary moisturizing base isn't the most exciting.

☹ **Sun Block Lip Treatment, SPF 15** *($17 for 1 ounce)* doesn't contain the UVA-protecting ingredients of avobenzone, titanium dioxide, or zinc oxide, and is not recommended.

☺ $$$ **Sun Block Stick SPF 35** *($21 for 0.31 ounce)* is a very good, in-part titanium dioxide–based sunscreen with a small amount of tint for someone with dry skin. Unfortunately, the amount you get in this package wouldn't last you more than a day if you were to use it properly.

☺ $$$ **Translucent Sun Block Stick SPF 30** *($21 for 0.31 ounce)* is similar to the Sun Block Stick SPF 35 above and the same comments apply.

☹ **Sun Protection Emulsion SPF 8 Waterproof** *($16 for 5 ounces)* has a paltry, low SPF 8 (SPF 15 is the minimum according to the American Academy of Dermatology and the Skin Cancer Foundation), and it doesn't contain the UVA-protecting ingredients of avobenzone, zinc oxide, or titanium dioxide. It is not recommended.

☺ **Ultra Light Sun Block Lotion SPF 30** *($27 for 3.3 ounces)* is a very good, in-part titanium dioxide–based sunscreen in a matte-finish base that includes a good amount of talc. It would be best for someone with normal to oily skin.

☹ **Self-Tanning Moisturizing Gel** *($20 for 5 ounces)* contains too much alcohol, and that can be drying to the skin; nevertheless, it does contain dihydroxyacetone, the same ingredient all self-tanners use to turn the skin brown.

SHISEIDO UV WHITE

According to the Shiseido brochure for its "specialty" line of skin-lightening products, "Pore Cell Clarifying actually removes excess keratin containing melanin, thereby enhancing the saturation of clarifying agents deep within the skin's inner layers." That sounds great, but it's merely a fancy way to suggest that these products exfoliate the skin and then deliver ingredients that Shiseido claims inhibit melanin production. The only unique ingredients in these products are lempuyang extract, hypotaurine, and rehmannia. Lempuyang extract is a form of ginger that, according to Shiseido, can inhibit melanin production; but there is no independent research substantiating this claim, and it is important to note that these products contain only minuscule amounts of the extract, so even if it could possibly have an effect on skin, it is doubtful the amount it contains would be effective. Hypotaurine is a moisturizing ingredient and has no benefit for skin lightening. Some of the products also contain rehmannia, a Chinese herb with no research about its effect when applied topically on the skin. What is perhaps the most inadequate part of this line are the sunscreens, which do not contain the UVA-protecting ingredients that are of primary importance if any skin lightening is to take place. On a positive note, these products do contain ascorbyl glucoside, a form of vitamin C that is potentially stable and a good antioxidant, though again there is no research about its effect as a skin lightener.

One of the products does contain arbutin, a Shiseido-patented ingredient for skin lightening. There are some in vitro studies that show arbutin to be effective for inhibiting melanin production, but that's about it. It is interesting to note that an almost identical product in Shiseido's Cle de Peau line sells for four times more than this version.

With no hydroquinone, magnesium ascorbyl palmitate, or even such plant extracts as bearberry and mulberry, which have been shown to inhibit melanin production (in vitro), to be found in any of these products there is little reason to accept the notion that your skin will change color one iota if you use Shiseido's UV White Line. There is research supporting the conclusion that hydroquinone, as well as magnesium ascorbyl palmitate, bearberry, and mulberry, are effective for inhibiting melanin production (Sources: *Cosmetics & Toiletries,* January 2000, pages 20–25; *Cosmetic Dermatology,* June 1998, pages 16–18, and March 2000, pages 13–18; and *Fourth International Symposium on Cosmetic Efficacy,* page 26).

☺ **Clarifying Cleansing Cream** *($32 for 4.1 ounces)* is a very basic, Vaseline-based, wipe-off cleanser that can leave a greasy film on the skin.

☺ $$$ **Clarifying Cleansing Foam I** *($27 for 4.5 ounces)* is similar to many of the Shiseido cleanser formulations that use potassium myristate as the cleansing agent. This one includes synthetic scrub particles, which makes it an option for exfoliation, though it can be more drying than necessary for some skin types, not to mention unnecessarily expensive.

☺ $$$ **Clarifying Cleansing Foam II** *($27 for 4.5 ounces)* is almost identical to the Cleansing Foam I above, only without the scrub particles.

☺ $$$ **Whitening Softener I** *($43 for 5 ounces)* is a good toner that contains some good water-binding agents and antioxidants. It is an option as an irritant-free toner for all skin types, but it is unlikely to have any effect on the color of skin.

☹ **Whitening Softener II** *($43 for 5 ounces)* is an alcohol-based toner that can be too drying and irritating for all skin types.

☹ **Whitening Massage Essence** *($48 for 1.6 ounces)* lists alcohol as the third ingredient, which makes this too drying and irritating for all skin types.

☹ **Whitening Toner** *($43 for 5 ounces)* is an alcohol-based toner that can be too drying and irritating for all skin types.

☹ **Whitening Protective Moisturizer I SPF 15** *($35 for 2.5 ounces)* does not contain the UVA-protecting ingredients of titanium dioxide, zinc oxide, or avobenzone, and is absolutely not recommended.

☹ **Whitening Protective Moisturizer II SPF 15** *($35 for 2.5 ounces)* does not contain the UVA-protecting ingredients of titanium dioxide, zinc oxide, or avobenzone, and is absolutely not recommended.

☺ $$$ **Whitening Moisturizer I** *($43 for 3.3 ounces)* is a decent moisturizer for dry skin, but there is nothing in it that can alter skin color. The minuscule amount of water-binding agents makes this a relatively unexciting moisturizer, unless the plant extracts have you convinced to give this a try.

☺ $$$ **Whitening Revitalizer Cream** *($48 for 1 ounce)* contains mostly water, slip agent, plant oils, glycerin, silicones, vitamin C, thickeners, preservatives, fragrance, and plant extracts. Not bad for a moisturizer, but abysmal if the goal is skin-lightening.

☺ $$$ **Refining Emulsion** *($43 for 1 ounce)* is a good, though standard, emollient moisturizer for normal to dry skin.

☺ $$$ **Whitess Intensive Skin Brightener** *($120 for 1.4 ounces)* is an absurdly overpriced skin-lightening product that contains a high concentration of arbutin to inhibit melanin production. Arbutin is a constituent of cranberries, bearberries, and blueberries, among other fruits. Although arbutin has been shown to have the same skin-lightening capability as hydroquinone, this has only been established in vitro or in animal studies. Still, it might be worth the price to see if this amount of arbutin, as an alternative to hydroquinone, can have an effect on skin. It is interesting to note that an almost identical product in Shiseido's Cle de Peau line sells for four times more than this version. The alcohol and menthol in this serum-type moisturizer make it potentially irritating for all skin types.

☹ **Intensive Whitening Treatment** *($55 for 0.4 ounce of Essence and 12 patches)*. The Essence part of this product is mostly alcohol, and that is certainly intense, but only intensely drying and potentially irritating for all skin types. The Mask part is a simple formulation of water, glycerin, film-forming agent, slip agents, silicone, preservatives, and fragrance. The teeny amount of vitamin E and royal jelly is almost a joke. None of this will affect the color of skin.

SHISEIDO THE SKIN CARE

The products from The Skin Care are based on Shiseido's "Basement membrane and Epidermal communication Skincare Treatment Theory [B.E.S.T] ... skincare for the 21st century and beyond...." Shiseido claims to have an ingredient in these products called "phyto-vitalizing factor" that is supposed to promote restoration of the skin's "basement membrane." Phyto-vitalizing factor sounds impressive, but the only unique ingredient in a few of these products is thiotaurine, an antioxidant. Taurine is an amino acid that has great antioxidant properties, and there is a lot of research showing that taurine is an excellent dietary supplement for many human body functions (and also particularly for cats), ranging from the heart (taurine was found to be superior to coenzyme Q10 in some studies) to the bile ducts. If you take taurine orally, that's great—but how that translates to skin is unknown. There is no research demonstrating that thiotaurine is better or preferred over lots of other antioxidants used in cosmetics these days. And even if this was the be-all and end-all of antioxidants, the notion that thiotaurine, in the truly minute amounts used in these products, could change cell production is a stretch of reality. It is also questionable to find Shiseido making claims about repairing skin when several sunscreen products in this line (considering that sun is one of the major reasons skin gets damaged in the first place) have a dismal SPF 10. **Note:** All Shiseido The Skin Care products contain fragrance unless noted otherwise.

☹ **Gentle Cleansing Cream** *($25 for 4.3 ounces)* lists alcohol as the third ingredient, and that doesn't make it gentle—it makes it problematic for causing dry or irritated skin.

☺ $$$ **Gentle Cleansing Soap** (**with case**) *($21 for 3.2 ounces)* is a standard bar cleanser; it can be too drying for most skin types.

☺ $$$ **Gentle Cleansing Foam** *($25 for 4.8 ounces)* is a standard, detergent-based cleanser that can be drying for most skin types, though it may be an option for someone with oily skin.

☹ **Gentle Cleansing Lotion** *($25 for 5 ounces)* is a toner with some detergent cleansing agents, but it lists alcohol as the fourth ingredient, and that makes it too drying and irritating for all skin types. It also lacks any beneficial ingredients for skin.

☺ $$$ **Eye & Lip Makeup Remover** *($19 for 2.5 ounces)* is an extremely standard, but good, silicone-based eye-makeup remover. It would work as well as any of the ones reviewed in this book, of which there are many.

☹ **Hydro Refining Softener** *($30 for 5 ounces)* lists alcohol as the second ingredient, which makes this too irritating and drying for all skin types.

☺ $$$ **Soothing Spray** *($20 for 2.5 ounces)* contains mostly water, slip agents and preservatives, which makes this a very ordinary, do-nothing-except-get-you-wet kind of product.

☹ **Day Essential Moisturizer SPF 10** *($35 for 2.5 ounces)* is a sunscreen that does contain avobenzone for UVA protection, but at SPF 10 it's just a waste. With all the many great SPF 15 products available (and that's the standard recommended by the American Academy of Dermatology and the Skin Cancer Foundation), an SPF 10 is inadequate for basic healthy skin care. If it's going to be essential, it should at least meet the basic criterion for sun-damage protection. Further, this lacks any significant amount of water-binding agents and has no antioxidants.

☹ **Day Essential Moisturizer, Enriched SPF 10** *($35 for 2.5 ounces)* is similar to the Day Essential Moisturizer SPF 10 above and the same comments apply.

☹ **Day Essential Moisturizer, Light SPF 10** *($35 for 2.5 ounces)* is similar to the Day Essential Moisturizer SPF 10 above, but the second ingredient is alcohol, and that makes this product even less desirable than the ones above.

☺ **Day Protective Moisturizer SPF 15** *($30 for 1.4 ounces)* is a very good, titanium dioxide–based sunscreen in an ordinary moisturizing base. The price is completely unwarranted for what you get (Neutrogena has similar products for far less). It would work well for someone with normal to slightly dry or slightly oily skin.

☺ **Essential Tinted Moisturizer SPF 15** *($30 for 1.4 ounces)* is similar to the Day Protective Moisturizer above, only with a slight tint that disappears into the skin, so the color is actually rather irrelevant.

☺ **Night Essential Moisturizer** *($37 for 2.5 ounces)* is about as boring a moisturizer as you can find, with a mere dusting of interesting water-binding agents. Why bother? It does contain thiotaurine, a good antioxidant, but the amount is so negligible as to make it barely present, and there are lots of other great antioxidants—this is not the only one.

☺ **Night Essential Moisturizer, Enriched** *($37 for 2.5 ounces)* is similar to the Night Essential Moisturizer above, only this version contains Vaseline. This does make it better for dry skin, but there isn't much reason to bother with this ordinary formulation.

☹ **Night Essential Moisturizer, Light** *($37 for 2.5 ounces)* is a standard moisturizer that lists alcohol fairly high up on the ingredient list, and that doesn't make it light. This lacks any significant amounts of water-binding agents or antioxidants.

☹ **Multi Energizing Cream** *($40 for 1.7 ounces)*. By any name, you still end up with a moisturizer that is very similar to the Night Essential Moisturizer above, and the same comments apply.

☺ **$$$ Eye Revitalizer** *($35 for 0.53 ounce)* is a good basic moisturizer for normal to dry skin, but there is nothing in this product that is special for the eye area; it is simply a standard moisturizer with the same formulation as most of the face moisturizers in this group of products.

☺ **$$$ Moisture Relaxing Mask** *($30 for 1.7 ounces)* is a standard, plasticizing-type mask. Other than the plastic-type ingredients, this mask is virtually identical in formulation to the various moisturizers in this line.

☹ **Purifying Mask** *($25 for 3.2 ounces)*. The alcohol and eucalyptus in this standard clay mask make it anything but purifying—rather it is a risk for irritation and dryness.

☹ **T-Zone Balancing Gel** *($25 for 1 ounce)* lists alcohol as the second ingredient, and it also contains menthol. That won't balance anything, but it will cause irritated, red, flaky skin. The third ingredient is cornstarch, which can be a problem for clogging pores.

☺ **$$$ Protective Lip Conditioner SPF 10** *($20 for 0.14 ounce)*. This does contain in-part avobenzone as one of the sunscreen ingredients, but the low SPF 10 is a strange oversight. There are more reliable, less expensive lip products to consider than this.

SHISEIDO MAKEUP

SHISEIDO THE MAKEUP

It is not often that a well-established cosmetics line looks at its *entire* makeup collection and basically scraps it in favor of new formulas and colors. Yet that is almost exactly what Shiseido did in the spring of 2001. Along with a whole battery of reformulated products and sleek, metallic packaging come new claims about their makeup featuring "light-controlling pigments, Advanced Luminous Technology, and Multi-Nutrient Factor"—ad copy that is so overinflated that P. T. Barnum would bow in deference! You won't see any light shows on your face here, and none of these products are nourishing in the least. What *has* taken place is Shiseido's attempt to modernize their color line.

The main and most impressive improvement is in the foundations. For the most part, they have silky textures and every one has adequate sun protection (at least an SPF 15 with UVA-protecting ingredients!). Aside from that, however, there is very little to praise. While the foundations sport mostly great textures, the color selection still has problems with unnatural-looking shades. The lipsticks are average, the concealers are almost all lacking, the mascaras are a mixed bag, and the eye, lip, and brow pencils leave much to be desired. The Makeup is not The best overall.

FOUNDATION: ✓☺ **$$$ Stick Foundation SPF 15** *($32)* is much less emollient than Shiseido's former Stick Foundation, and has a wonderfully smooth, light texture and a titanium dioxide sunscreen. This applies and blends with ease, can go from sheer to almost full coverage, and dries to a soft powder finish. Like most stick foundations, this is best for someone with normal to slightly dry or slightly oily skin—as there are several waxes in it that can be problematic for those with breakouts and/or oily skin. Fifteen shades are available, including a Color Control shade, which is a greenish yellow tint most often apparent on someone who is seasick! The other shades to avoid are Natural Light Beige, Natural Fair Beige, Natural Deep Beige, Deep Beige, and Very Deep Ochre.

☺ **$$$ Cream Foundation SPF 16** *($32)* starts out thick and creamy, but once blended dries to a soft, natural finish that is best suited for normal to combination skin—not dry skin as the name implies. Coverage can go from light to medium, and of the 14 shades the following 7 are too peach, pink, or orange for most skin tones: Natural Fair Ivory, Natural Deep Ivory, Natural Light Beige, Natural Fair Beige, Deep Beige, Deep Ochre, and Natural Deep Bronze (I swear this is the color of the original "Man Tan" lotion that turned skin orange!). The sunscreen is all titanium dioxide, which is right on for daytime protection. **Fluid Foundation SPF 15** *($32)* sounds like a good option for normal to oily skin, but the formula is actually ideal for those with normal to dry skin seeking sheer to light coverage. This foundation has an all–titanium dioxide sunscreen and a moist, creamy texture that blends very well and sets to a satin finish. Of the 14 shades, the following 7 are too peach, pink, or orange for most skin tones: Natural Fair Ivory, Natural Light Beige, Natural Fair Beige, Natural Deep Beige, Deep Ochre 080, Deep Ochre 100, and Natural Deep Bronze. **Powdery Foundation SPF 15** *($26 for powder cake, $6 for compact)* is almost identical to the Compact Foundation below (including a great sunscreen), except for two points: the texture and feel of this are slightly lighter, and the 14 colors are a vast improvement over the Compact Foundation. The only shades to consider avoiding are Deep Beige and Deep Ochre. **Benefiance Enriched Revitalizing Foundation SPF 15** *($42)* is a good sheer foundation that blends evenly, leaving a soft matte finish. It also uses in-part titanium dioxide as one of the active sunscreen ingredients. There are 13 great shades, with only 2 to avoid: B2 and B4 are either too pink or too peach. In many ways, this product is similar to Neutrogena's Healthy Finish Liquid Makeup SPF 20 ($9.99), basically a liquid foundation with talc. Shiseido recommends this for dry or combination skin, but it is not appropriate for dry skin.

☺ $$$ **Compact Foundation SPF 15** *($26 for powder cake, $6 for compact)* has an in-part titanium dioxide sunscreen and a very soft, silky texture. For a wet/dry powder foundation, it applies more sheer than most—it is not too thick or cakey, which makes this easy to work with. The major drawback is the colors—of the 13, almost all are noticeably peach, pink, or orange. The only options in the bunch are Natural Fair Ochre, Natural Light Ochre, Natural Deep Ochre, and Very Deep Ochre (a good shade for dark skin tones). **Hydro-Liquid Compact Foundation SPF 15** *($36)* isn't liquid at all, but rather a very dry-finish, cream-to-powder foundation. The SPF 15 with titanium dioxide is excellent. All that would make this a foundation to consider if the colors weren't so blatantly peachy pink. The only shades that look like real skin color are 00, 02, and 04!

<u>CONCEALER:</u> ☹ **Optimal Cover Concealer** *($20)* has an extremely thick, heavy-feeling texture. This ultra-creamy concealer is pigment-rich, so full coverage is ensured, but the finish can look heavy and obvious, and the more it is blended, the more coverage is lost. There are nine shades available, five of which are designated as **Base Color** and four of which are **Control Colors** that can be mixed as needed with the Base Colors. Both options have several undesirable colors that are too rose or peach for most skin tones. The Control Color group includes some truly strange shades that have no practical use—how does mixing bright yellow or pink with concealers that are already unrelated to skin tone result in any kind of improvement? There is truly nothing optimal about this concealer—if anything the texture is a step backward compared to the latest concealers by everyone from Almay to Lancome. **Corrector Pencil** *($15)* is a standard, dry-finish pencil that comes in three fairly peach or pink colors. This provides good coverage, but application is an issue and it looks quite obvious on the skin.

☺ $$$ **Concealer** *($17)* has a formula that is much more workable than the ones above. The texture is very smooth, and it blends well, but do it quickly, before this dries to a soft matte finish. There are four shades, of which Medium is too peach, while Light Enhancer has a subtle iridescence that can look obvious (and unattractive) under the eyes, so consider using it elsewhere on the face for highlighting.

POWDER: ☹ **Luminizing Color Powder** *($20 for powder, $10 for compact)* is a talc-based pressed powder that features three colors in one powder cake, one of which is quite shiny. The color selection ranges from pure white iridescence to glittery bronze, and none of them would help set makeup or reduce shine. If adding shine (or non-skin-related colors) is what you want in a powder, this is an option. **Loose Powder** *($30)* is talc-based and has a soft, dry, light-as-air texture. Regrettably, the two colors are slightly pink and sparkly. What did Shiseido think this was supposed to do for skin?

☺ $$$ **Pressed Powder** *($20 for powder cake, $6 for compact)* is superb. This talc-based powder is ultra-soft, applies easily, and looks natural and not at all powdery. Normal to dry skin will appreciate this sheer coverage powder, and of the three shades, only Deep is too peach to consider.

BLUSH: ☺ $$$ **Blush Duo** *($26)*. These blushes feature one wearable but shiny blush tone along with a very shiny highlighter color. The texture is quite nice, but don't you think there's already enough shine out there so you don't need to add it to the only blush option in your makeup line? ☹ **Creamy Blush** *($27)* is a very sheer cream-to-powder blush that has a minimal powder finish. Each of the four shades has some amount of shine, which would be tolerable if you actually got some decent color. At this price, such a sheer payoff is insulting.

☹ **EYESHADOW:** **Eye Shadow Duos** *($24)* have an exquisite sheer texture, being almost creamy and blending remarkably well. Unfortunately, all of the colors are shiny, and feature some odd combinations of greens, blues, and violets that will compete with the eye, instead of enhancing it. **Silky Eye Shadow Duos** *($25)* have an even finer texture than the one above, but this one tends to be too flaky despite its smooth application. These are also even shinier than the original Duos.

EYE AND BROW SHAPER: ☺ **Eyeliner Pencil** *($15)* is completely standard and slightly creamy, so smearing and fading are imminent risks. **Eyebrow Pencil** *($15)* is fine, but not worth the price tag since the formula and application are utterly standard.

☺ $$$ **Translucent Eyebrow Shaper** *($22)* is one of the most expensive brow gels around, and let me be the first to tell you how indistinguishable this is from the under-four-dollar version from Cover Girl.

☹ **Eyebrow and Eyeliner Compact** *($27)* is a wet/dry pressed powder for filling in brows or lining the eyes, and for some inexplicable reason Shiseido has made these shiny, too. The tiny wedge brush that accompanies this is too stiff and scratchy for comfortable use. **Liquid Eyeliner** *($20)* is miserable. Talk about asking for trouble! This has an over-sized brush that lays down a thicker than usual line, and the formula stays (and stays) wet and feels heavy. Once it dries, it tends to smear. **Fine Eyeliner** *($27)* is another liquid eyeliner with a brush that is only capable of applying a thick line. The color is seeped into the brush much like a fountain pen, making it hard to control how much comes out at once. Watch out for Soft Black, which is really olive green.

LIPSTICK AND LIP PENCIL: Shiseido's lipstick selection has been streamlined, and is an unbalanced mix of atypical and standard shades. ☺ **$$$ Lipstick** *($18)* has a slick texture, opaque coverage, and a glossy finish that will be an exercise in futility for anyone prone to lipstick feathering! **Matte Lipstick** *($18)* is far from most people's definition of matte, offering a creamy texture and smooth, opaque colors that have a good amount of pigment—so the color will last longer than usual, but not as long as a true matte lipstick would. **Sheer Gloss Lipstick** *($18)* wins a prize for a name that says it all! The color selection is certainly worth a look if you prefer this type of lipstick. **Translucent Gloss Lipstick** *($20)* is a colorless, emollient lip balm that leaves a glossy finish and helps prevent chapping, just like countless other less expensive lip balms.

✓☺ **$$$ Lip Gloss** *($19)* makes a wonderfully non-sticky, lightweight gloss if you aren't put off by the price. Shiseido's lip color selection tends to run hot and cold, but these shades definitely sizzle.

☹ **Staying Power Moisturizing Lipstick** *($20)* is not a bad lipstick, but gets a sad face due to its duplicitous name and utterly false claims. This slick, light-to-medium-coverage formula has far too much slip and a greasy finish that has about as much staying power as snow in the summer sun. **Lip Liner Pencil** *($15)* is a standard pencil—which is fine—but this one has a formula that is too creamy to last long and the color fades quickly with little effort. For the money, these have nothing over almost every other lip pencil at the drugstore.

MASCARA: ☺ **$$$ Curl Mascara** *($18)* doesn't really do much as far as curling lashes, and it offers no length, but it holds up great under water. For waterproof mascara, this is fine, but for the money, L'Oreal's Le Grand Curl Waterproof ($7.39) is a far better option.

☺ **$$$ Volume Mascara** *($18)* is a great lengthening and thickening mascara that won't smear or flake during the day. It can go on slightly clumpy but not enough to take away the positive rating. **Distinguish Mascara** *($19)* doesn't distinguish itself from lots of other mascaras that can produce equally impressive length with a hint of fullness. This is a very good mascara, but considering the name and price, the very first use ought to give you the impression that it will rise above the rest, and that just doesn't happen. It is waterproof, but takes extra effort to remove.

☺ **$$$ BRUSHES:** The straightforward collection of **Brushes** *($25–40)* is lackadaisical and definitely not worth purchasing when compared with similarly priced brushes from M.A.C., Stila, or Laura Mercier. The **Powder** *($40)* and **Blush** *($35)* brushes are very soft, but not as dense as they should be to hold and deposit color evenly. Actually, the only acceptable brushes are the **Concealer** *($37)* and **Eye Shadow** *($24)*, and even they have drawbacks compared to the options in most other lines.

☺ **SPECIALTY: Paper Powder** *($9 for 75 sheets)* is standard oil-blotting paper that contains kaolin and several mineral pigments that are not the best at absorbing excess oil.

They can work, but there are less expensive options. **Eraser Pencil** *($15)* is a wax-based pencil (like almost all other needs-sharpening pencils) that is colorless and designed to remove makeup mistakes, such as those from mascara or eye pencils. You swipe the pencil over the makeup and it wipes off cleanly. This is nice to have on hand, but not an essential unless you're using substandard makeup or tend to be heavy-handed in your application.

SHISEIDO UV WHITE MAKEUP

The only logical reason to consider these makeup items is for the outstanding sun protection they offer. None have an SPF of less than 25, and every sunscreen features titanium dioxide for effective UVA protection. UV White makeup is sold to create a "naturally fair look." Regardless of a foundation's best attributes, if you choose a color that is too light or ashy it will not look right, and the pickings here are slim. I know it is particularly hard for Asian women to accept their olive to golden skin tones, but since the goal is natural-looking makeup that matches the skin, it just doesn't make sense to use makeup that causes skin to appear whiter or lighter than it is. Think twice about why you're wearing makeup if you find yourself leaning toward colors that are too pale and that mask your natural skin tone.

☹ UV White Whitening Compact SPF 25 *($45, $35 for refills)* is a talc-free powder foundation that contains a large amount of titanium dioxide for broad-spectrum sun protection. Unfortunately, the titanium dioxide gives the foundation a thick, dry texture, which, unless applied sparingly (which will compromise the sun protection), leaves the skin looking chalky. Rather than using trustworthy talc, Shiseido opted to create this powder using barium sulfate, an earth mineral used as a whitening agent that is known to cause frequent skin reactions. Despite the high SPF, this has too many drawbacks to recommend, including some poor colors.

☺ $$$ UV White Control & Protect Base Cream SPF 25 *($35)* is a very good titanium dioxide–based sunscreen in an ordinary silicone-based moisturizer that has a fairly matte finish. The colors are meant to cover skin discolorations, but neither of these is an appealing choice, and foundation does that just fine without layering more products over skin. Some good sunscreens that are less expensive than this include Clinique's Super City Block SPF 25 ($16.50) and Neutrogena's Sensitive Skin SPF 30 ($8.39 for 4 ounces).

☺ $$$ UV White Whitening Pre-Makeup Stick SPF 25 *($30)* is a smooth stick-type concealer that has an excellent sunscreen and provides light coverage. Calling this a "treatment that helps render spots and freckles invisible" is a fancy way of saying "this is a concealer." Although there is only one shade, it is a good neutral option for light skin.

SHU UEMURA

Shu Uemura began as a Hollywood makeup artist and started his skin-care line back in 1960, with the makeup collection debuting a decade later. His Tokyo-based line has been available in the United States for quite a few years. It isn't widely known, but that has been slowly changing since L'Oreal acquired a 35% share in the company in 2000—a move that puts Shu Uemura on the fast track to international expansion, plus gives it access to L'Oreal's formidable research and development facilities, which have generated a range of new products. In the United States, the Shu Uemura line is sold at select upscale department stores such as Barneys New York and Nordstrom. Shu Uemura has boutiques in Los Angeles and New York, and this is where you should visit if you're intent on seeing everything Shu Uemura has up his sleeve. The line has an exclusive yet simple flair; the products are plainly packaged and the descriptions are straightforward and refreshingly uncomplicated. Unfortunately, I can't say the same for the prices, which scream prestige much louder than the less than impressive skin-care formulas should allow them to. Plus, the skin-care lineup is void of sunscreen. For this skin essential you'll need to look to Uemura's foundations. Any claims that these products can benefit skin or reduce environmental damage are a joke, with what ends up being a potentially risky oversight for skin. For more information about Shu Uemura, call (800) 743-8205 or visit www.shu-uemura.co.jp.

SHU UEMURA SKIN CARE

☹ **Acnormal Wash** *($15 for 2 ounces)* is a fairly drying and potentially irritating skin cleanser. The third ingredient is potassium hydroxide, and this also contains menthol, and none of that is helpful for any skin type.

☺ **$$$ Cleansing Beauty Oil Balancer** *($40 for 8.4 ounces)* is a lot of money for mineral oil and corn oil, which is most of what this product contains. It will cut through makeup as you wipe it off, but you could just use pure mineral oil and save lots of money and get the same results. It is supposed to be washed off, but why do two steps when a gentle, water-soluble cleanser can do it all in one?

☺ **$$$ Cleansing Beauty Oil Freshener** *($40 for 8.4 ounces)* is almost identical to the Cleansing Beauty Oil Balancer above, and the same review applies.

☺ **$$$ Cleansing Water** *($30 for 8.4 ounces)* is a detergent-based, water-soluble gel cleanser that is an option for most skin types.

☹ **Acnormal Lotion** *($20 for 5 ounces)*. The second ingredient is alcohol, and that makes this too drying and irritating for all skin types. There is nothing in this that can normalize skin or have any beneficial impact on breakouts.

☺ **$$$ Moisture Lotion** *($35 for 8.4 ounces)* is a good toner for most skin types that contains a decent amount of water-binding agents, though only a tiny amount of antioxidants.

☺ **$$$ Refreshing Lotion** *($35 for 8.4 ounces)* is similar to the Moisture Lotion above, and the same comments apply.

☺ **$$$ Whitening Lotion** *($33 for 5 ounces)* is a toner that contains nothing that can affect skin color. It does contain some good water-binding agents and a small amount of anti-irritants and antioxidants, but that's about it. It is an option as a toner for most skin types.

The Reviews S

☺ $$$ **Absolute Cream** *($42 for 1.05 ounces)* is an OK, emollient moisturizer for normal to dry skin that contains some good water-binding agents, but only a minute amount of antioxidants.

☺ $$$ **Moisture Fluid** *($42 for 1.6 ounces)* is similar to the Absolute Cream above only in lotion form, and the same basic review applies.

☹ $$$ **Moisture Essence** *($55 for 1 ounce)* is similar to the Moisture Fluid above, only this lists alcohol as the fourth ingredient, which in any amount shouldn't be the essence of a moisturizer.

☹ $$$ **AID Oil** *($58 for 0.8 ounce)* is an exceedingly ordinary, and I mean *really* ordinary, blend of mineral oil, thickeners, and plant oils. It is shocking how overpriced this is—what a truly waste-of-time product. You could easily apply plain mineral oil or plant oil, such as the safflower oil this product contains, for pennies and get the same benefit.

☹ $$$ **B-G Emulsion** *($60 for 1 ounce)* is an emollient moisturizer for normal to dry skin that contains some good water-binding agents, but only the teeniest amount of antioxidants. This is overpriced for what you get.

☹ $$$ **Principe 21 Bio-Energizing Concentrate** *($60 for 1 ounce)* is supposed to contain revolutionary ingredients to increase cell production (the cosmetics industry has more "revolutionary" ingredients than the world of medicine). It contains some good water-binding agents and a tiny amount of vitamin E. This is hardly revolutionary, but it is an OK moisturizer for normal to dry skin.

☹ $$$ **Principe Eye Zone Complex** *($42 for 0.5 ounce)* is not as well formulated as the Principe 21 above, though it is slightly more emollient. For some reason this product contains tea tree oil, a topical disinfectant. Putting that in an eye product is just strange.

☹ $$$ **Principe Lip Serum** *($21 for 0.33 ounce)* is a good emollient moisturizing fluid with a small amount of water-binding agents and antioxidant. This can be a good option for lips, but the claims around the benefits are overblown and ludicrous.

☺ $$$ **Regenerate Accelerator** *($60 for 0.6 ounce)* contains mostly mineral oil, plant oils, thickeners, vitamin E, water-binding agents, and fragrance. This is an emollient moisturizer for dry skin, but it won't generate even one skin cell.

☹ $$$ **Regenerate Cream** *($60 for 1 ounce)* is an emollient moisturizer with a small amount of water-binding agents and a teeny amount of antioxidants.

☹ $$$ **Regenerate Smoothing Lotion** *($45 for 6.7 ounces)* is an OK toner for most skin types, with a tiny amount of water-binding agents and minute amount of vitamin E.

☹ $$$ **Regenerate Hydrator** *($60 for 0.6 ounce)* is an OK emollient moisturizer with some good water-binding agents, but only a teeny amount of antioxidants, and for this amount of money you would expect much, much more. Actually, this product contains more alcohol than any beneficial ingredients!

☹ **Regenerate Regulator** *($60 for 0.6 ounce)* lists alcohol as the third ingredient, and that doesn't help regulate anything, although it can cause irritation and dry skin.

☺ **$$$ Regenerate Regenerator** *($60 for 0.6 ounce)*. With all these Regenerate products I thought it funny that they actually needed a product to regenerate the regenerator. Talk about product redundancy! This is a good moisturizer for normal to dry skin with some very good water-binding agents, but it lacks antioxidants, so I guess we should stay tuned for another generation of regenerators!

☹ **Moisture Eyezone Mask** *($38 for 12 packets)* contains more alcohol than any beneficial ingredients, and alcohol can be drying and irritating for the eye area. The water-binding agents are nice, but this product doesn't benefit the skin in any way over a well-formulated moisturizer and ends up being a waste of time.

☹ **Moisture Face Mask** *($55 for 8 packets)* is almost identical to the Eyezone Mask above. Why this is more expensive is sheer marketing caprice.

☺ **$$$ Balancing Mask** *($33 for 2.2 ounces)* is supposed to be ideal for oily skin, but the thickening agents and plant oils would be a problem, leaving the face more oily and running the risk of clogging pores. It could be good for someone with dry skin.

☺ **$$$ Whitening Essence** *($60 for 1 ounce)* is an emollient lotion that may be an OK moisturizer for normal to dry skin, although the ingredients it contains won't help lighten skin. Placenta extract has no research showing it to be effective for inhibiting melanin production.

☹ **Whitening Lotion** *($35 for 5 ounces)* lists alcohol as the third ingredient, which makes this too irritating and potentially drying for all skin types. It contains ascorbyl glucoside, a form of vitamin C, but that has no research showing it to be effective for inhibiting melanin production, though it is most likely a good antioxidant.

✓☺ **$$$ Whitening Lipo** *($67 for 0.11 ounce)* is mostly thickener with a good amount of magnesium ascorbyl phosphate. There is research showing that this ingredient in this amount can potentially be effective for inhibiting melanin production.

☺ **$$$ Lip Fix** *($15 for 0.6 ounce)*. This won't fix anyone's lips. This is little more than Chap Stick, containing mostly waxes and plant oils. It's OK, but overpriced for what you're buying.

SHU UEMURA MAKEUP

The sumptuous eyeshadows, blushes, and brushes are the best reasons to pay attention to this line. Although many of the colors aren't much to look at, the textures are some of the most exquisite around. It is worth the trouble to check out the application of these shades just to see how creamy, smooth, and evenly they cover. The makeup brushes are also worth a test run, and the choices are practically limitless (though so are the prices). For more information about Shu Uemura, call (800) 743-8205 or visit www.shu-uemura.co.jp.

FOUNDATION: Shu Uemura's foundations are quite good overall, with formulas that offer something for every skin type. However, the color range is inconsistent, with some formulas having almost too many shades and others not enough, plus the SPF numbers for some of these are far less than they should be. A safe bet in any of the foundation formulas below is to avoid the shades labeled as Pink Tone or Peach Tone, for self-explanatory reasons. Not surprisingly, the shades designated as Neutral and Beige Tone sell the best and look the most natural on skin.

☺ $$$ **Fluid S Foundation SPF 8** *($30)* is a titanium dioxide–based sunscreen. However, the SPF would be far better if it were an SPF 15, because as it is you can't rely on this for adequate daily sun protection. Otherwise, it is an excellent sheer-coverage foundation whose moist finish is great for normal to dry skin. There are some off colors among the selection of nine shades, but even the pink- and peach-toned shades like #130, #165, and #355 are so sheer as to be inconsequential for most skin colors. **Fluid N Foundation SPF 8** *($30)* is a liquid foundation that is not as moist or sheer as the Fluid S above. It's a good choice for normal to slightly dry or dry skin seeking light coverage and a natural finish. The SPF is titanium dioxide–based, but the SPF is disappointing and means this cannot be relied on for daily protection. There are 30 shades, with equally good options for all skin tones. The colors to avoid are: #145, #155, #175, #185, #325, which are slightly pink, and #375 and #775, which are too yellow for most skin tones. **UV Powder Foundation SPF 26** *($32.50)*. This smooth, sheer, talc-free powder has four workable colors, and lists titanium dioxide as the active sunscreen agent. Keep in mind that with powder-type makeup it takes a liberal application to get the SPF protection indicated on the label; a light dusting will not provide adequate sun protection. By the way, Neutrogena's Healthy Defense Protective Powder SPF 30 ($9.49) is available for about one-third of this price, and has even better all-day protection. **UV Cream Foundation SPF 31** *($32.50)* is an in-part titanium dioxide–based compact foundation. It has a smooth, but greasy, cream-to-powder finish and a small range of five colors, of which two are best avoided. Pink 130 and Beige 290 are just too pink for most skin tones. This would be best for someone with normal to dry skin who doesn't want a solid powder finish. **UV Liquid Foundation SPF 21** *($32.50)* has a great in-part titanium dioxide–based sunscreen and a light, fluid texture that dries to a matte finish. This is appropriate for those with normal to oily skin who prefer medium coverage and have the knack for blending this systematically—the formula spreads well and dries quickly. Of the seven colors, the following three should be avoided: #375 and #565, and #323 (can turn copper).

☺ $$$ **UV Underbase SPF 17** *($30)* is a mousse makeup that has an expectedly light, airy texture and dries to a soft matte finish. This contains titanium dioxide, and is a unique, lightweight consideration for normal to oily skin. UV Underbase comes in only one sheer, slightly pink shade, but it could work under any other foundation as a super-light sunscreen.

☺ **Nobara Cream Foundation** *($22)* is said to be a "worldwide professional makeup artist choice." It's a compact cream-to-powder makeup that comes in some beautiful colors, and although it is also a bit greasy going on it dries to an opaque, powdery finish. However, the finish is short-lived, as the emollients and waxes in this formula show through quickly, making this a poor choice for oily skin. The main issue with this formula is coverage—it provides almost full coverage instantly, and is a bit difficult to soften if that's not the look you're going for. This is a worthwhile option as a concealer, though it can slip into lines around the eyes and look caked unless blending is meticulous. Among the 18 light-to-dark shades, the following colors are too peach, copper, or rose for most skin tones: #314, #365, #524 (slightly rose), and #554. Numbers 513 and 523 are excellent options for darker skin, and if you have fair to light skin the choices are numerous.

☹ **Base Control** *($26)* is a group of color correctors with a mineral oil base that go on extremely sheer but add a strange color to the skin that does nothing to minimize color flaws, though almost all of the colors create their own "discoloration." It just adds another layer to the skin, and if you have any skin type other than dry, this is going to feel greasy.

CONCEALER: ☹ **Cover Crayon** *($20)* is a two-ended pencil concealer with a thick, greasy texture. Both ends of the pencils and all four shades are too peach or pink for most skin tones—there are far more modern formulations available than this.

☺ $$$ **Mark Cealer** *($20)* comes in a tube with a wand applicator and has a smooth, but very opaque, texture and dry finish. This is potent stuff and very easy to overdo, and then it just looks heavy. There are three shades, and the only one to avoid is Pink 5. If you can get this blended on well, it expertly covers dark circles and discolorations.

POWDER: ☺ $$$ **Face Powder** *($30)* is a standard, talc-based loose powder with a soft, dry translucent finish. Most of the colors are excellent, but avoid Peach, Purple, Pink 100 (ashy), Pink 200, Pink 300, and Pink 5. Brown 14 is an excellent shade for dark skin tones. If you're of Asian descent and think a pink powder will give you porcelain skin, think again and learn to love your naturally warm skin tone. **Compact Powder M** *($30)* is billed as "a super velvet pressed powder" infused with moisture for dry, sensitive skin. However, nothing that's talc-based can moisturize skin, as the nature of talc (and talc substitutes) is absorbent. Nevertheless, this is indeed velvety, and leaves a soft finish on the skin that isn't as dry as many powders. The four colors are all superb, though Colorless has a faint pink cast.

☺ $$$ **Face Paper** *($12 for 30 sheets)* are microscopically thin sheets coated with rice powder. These will absorb oil and leave a powder finish on the skin, but compared to options from Maybelline and Shiseido (and my line), these are outrageously expensive.

☺ $$$ **Compact Powder** *($30)* feels light and goes on softly, but half of the colors are a strange lot. Of the eight shades, the real-skin tones to consider are Colorless, Beige 4, and Beige 6.

BLUSH: ✓☺ $$$ **Glow On Blush** *($22)* has an ultra-sheer, soft finish and a luscious texture. There's a huge range of colors, including some excellent matte shades. The shiny ones are clearly identified as "metallic," while the others shades are labeled "pearl."

☺ $$$ **Luminizer** *($21)* is a sheer and creamy twist-up highlighter stick that can be used anywhere. It leaves a shiny finish and blends readily on the skin, but will eventually appear greasy and doesn't have great staying potential.

EYESHADOW: ✓☺ $$$ **Pressed Eyeshadows** *($18)* have an extraordinary silky-smooth texture, and they go on beautifully, without streaking or flaking. Most powders this smooth have a difficult time clinging evenly, but not these. The color selection features nearly 80 shades, half of which are matte! The remaining shiny shades are labeled Iridescent, Pearl, or Metallic. Just be wary of the many colors in intense shades of peacock blue, taxicab yellow, orange, and green. The best neutral matte shades are Pink 102M, Orange 206M, Beige 802M, Beige 804M, Brown 862M, and Brown 871M.

☺ **Etincell** *($18)* is finely milled loose shiny powder for eyes that comes in small pots. For intense, deeply pigmented shine, they'll work, but this is a messy way to put shine on. **Eye Shimmer** *($15)* is a small group of sheer, shimmery eyeshadows that are OK for shine, but leave a glossy finish that can shorten the life of any other eye makeup used with them, including mascara.

<u>EYE AND BROW SHAPER:</u> The price for these ordinary pencils is just beyond belief; I had to check the numbers twice just to be sure I wasn't seeing things. The pencils are decent, but the prices are completely indecent. ☺ **$$$ Retractable Pencil Eyeliner** *($30, $15 for refill)* and **Retractable Eyebrow Pencil** *($37, $15 for refill)* are standard, twist-up pencils with a smooth application and minimal tendency to smudge. **Hard Formula Eyebrow Pencil** *($20)* is hugely popular with Shu Uemura's Asian clientele, and the counter people extol the special sharpening/shaving technique they use as essential to getting this undeniably hard-textured pencil to perform at its best. If you're set in your preference for using this product, nothing I can say will convince you to switch to something different. I advise the uninitiated to stay away, as almost any brow pencil, gel, powder, or wax is easier to use than this—though it does stay put. **Liquid Eyeliner** *($35, $15 for refill)* has a great soft-but-firm brush and performs well, but I can't in good conscience recommend this when L'Oreal and Almay have equally great liquid eyeliners for one-fifth the price. **Eyebrow Manicure** *($30)* is a tinted brow gel that comes in six very good colors. It's moist, barely sticky texture makes it easy to use for natural brow enhancement, but I would seriously consider the less expensive, drier-finish options from Bobbi Brown and Borghese before this.

☹ **Eyebrow Pencil** *($15)* is a very standard pencil that goes on almost the same as the Retractable version. **Kajal** *($15)* is for eyelining and comes in two shades. It's a noticeably greasy pencil, which means it can easily smear and smudge.

<u>LIPSTICK AND LIP PENCIL:</u> ☺ **$$$ Lip Rouge SPF 8** *($18)* has three types of finishes: **Sheer**, which isn't all that sheer but does have a good creamy, slightly glossy finish; **Matte**, which is fairly creamy, opaque, and not really matte; and **Neutral**, which is a standard, creamy lipstick with medium coverage. The color range is staggering, with the Neutrals offering the most hues, followed closely by the Mattes. This lipstick collection has one of the best selections of pinks and reds you'll ever see. Finally, the sunscreen, though too low, is pure titanium dioxide.

☺ **$$$ Liquid Lip Rouge** *($20)* is overpriced but still one of the smoothest, nongoopy lip glosses out there. The colors provide medium coverage and are imbued with sparkles for a striking, glass-like shine. Unfortunately, the glitter particles tend to stick around long after the color has worn (or been wiped) off.

☺ **$$$ Lip Gloss** *($20)* is a group of standard, incredibly overpriced pot glosses that have a slightly sticky texture. **Lipliner Pencil** *($18.50)* and **$$$ Retractable Lipliner Pencil** *($30, $15 for refill)* are almost identical. Both are very standard lip pencils with smooth applications, but the extremely overpriced one you don't have to sharpen is by far easier to use.

☺ **$$$ Lip Fix** *($16.50)* is a standard, wax-based emollient lip balm that claims to prevent smearing and extend the life of any lip color—but it is no more capable of that than rain is of not feeling wet! As a clear, overpriced lip balm, it works as well as any.

<u>MASCARA:</u> ☺ **$$$ Mascara Basic** *($27)* is wildly overpriced, but does go on evenly and quickly. It builds lots of clump-free length but very little thickness, and it lasts all day.

☹ **$$$ Mascara Color** *($25)* comes in circus-clown colors that have little appeal, unless having green or turquoise eyelashes excites you. The brown shade is misleading— it's actually a coppery red!

<u>BRUSHES:</u> ✓☺ **$$$** Shu Uemura's reputation for superior **Brushes** *($5–$260)* is well deserved. Few lines offer such an extensive (at times eclectic) assortment of brushes, with all manner of natural hair and synthetics. Although the prices on many of them are out of line, for sheer variety (there are more than 70) this brush collection is hard to beat. The most useful brushes are priced competitively with those from other artistry-driven lines such as M.A.C. and Bobbi Brown. You'll get the most bang for your buck if you stick with the **Handy Brush** collection (natural hair) or the **IS collection** (synthetic). Avoid the limited, tiny **Brush Set** *($30)*.

☺ **$$$ SPECIALTY:** Shu Uemura also excels when it comes to accessories. From **Sponges** and **Powder Puffs** *($2–$4.50)* to refillable, customized **Palettes** *($8–$50)* and top-of-the-line **Makeup Boxes** *($225–$700)*, the professional makeup artist and makeup-savvy consumer will appreciate these options, though they're not for everyone.

SISLEY

I often wonder what it would be like to be a fly on the wall at a meeting of Sisley marketing executives when they sit down to establish the prices for their products. I imagine it going something like this: "Let's see, this product is really similar to a drugstore moisturizer that costs $9 for 6 ounces, but if we package it in an elegant box, put it in a matching jar with a shiny gold cap, play up the European know-how angle with French words and accents on the label, and stick in some exotic-sounding plant extracts and oils, we can probably charge $145 for 2 ounces. Women just love that kind of foolishness and fall for it every time." Even if that isn't exactly what they are saying behind closed doors, it comes through loud and clear on the product label and in the brochures. What is perhaps most distressing is that the Sisley formulations are some of the most embarrassingly ordinary, yet outrageously and insultingly overpriced, I've seen. I can emphatically state that there is nothing in these products you can't find at the drugstore from lines such as Nivea, Pond's, Neutrogena, Eucerin, and L'Oreal; and actually, those lines have products with far more interesting formulations than this one does.

When it comes to reliable skin-care information, Sisley's is best described as spurious. For example, it states that "oily skin, which is thicker [there is no research anywhere showing this to be true] ... is very well protected and ages less quickly than other skin types." That myth was put to rest years ago with the research about sun damage and genetic aging. Oily skin prevents dry skin, but dry skin is unrelated to skin's wrinkling or to the processes involved in aging. For more information about Sisley, call (214) 528-8006 or visit www.sisley-cosmetics.com. **Note:** All Sisley products contain fragrance unless otherwise noted.

SISLEY SKIN CARE

☺ **$$$ Botanical Cleansing Milk with Hawthorn for Dry/Sensitive Skin** *($65 for 8.4 ounces)* is an exceptionally mundane, mineral oil–based cold cream. It can leave a greasy film on the skin, and if you are of a mind to waste this kind of money on a product that has more in common with Pond's Cold Cream than anything else, go right ahead if you have dry skin. The hawthorne extract can have antioxidant properties, but that would be wiped away with the cleanser.

☹ **Botanical Cleansing Milk with Sage for Combination/Oily Skin** *($65 for 8.4 ounces)* is similar to the Hawthorn product above except that this one contains sage, a skin irritant. Everything about this product is unacceptable for someone with oily skin.

☹ **Botanical Soapless Foaming Cleanser for All Skin Types** *($70 for 4 ounces)* is indeed soapless, but it does contain several very drying and potentially irritating standard detergent cleansing agents, including sodium lauryl sulfate (the second ingredient)!

☹ **Soapless Facial Cleansing Bar with Tropical Resins** *($71 for 4.4 ounces).* The first ingredient is sodium lauryl sulfate, one of the most irritating and drying detergent cleansers especially when used in such an amount.

☺ **$$$ Creamy Mousse Cleanser** *($65 for 4.2 ounces)* is a standard, detergent-based cleanser that is an option for most skin types; that is, if the price doesn't make you break out. There is nothing about this cleanser that isn't easily replaced by a wide variety of cleansers available at the drugstore for a fraction of this price.

☺ **$$$ Buff and Wash Botanical Facial Gel for Daily Use** *($74 for 3.5 ounces)* contains standard synthetic scrub particles (ground-up plastic) in a base of thickening agents and castor oil and some water-binding agents. It also contains a good amount of lemon, and that can be a skin irritant. For this price, the sheer mediocrity of this standard scrub for dry skin is just shocking.

☺ **$$$ Gentle Facial Buffing Cream for All Skin Types** *($60 for 1.3 ounces)* contains standard synthetic scrub particles (ground-up plastic) in a base of wax and clay. This is not suitable for all skin types, but it is an OK topical scrub for someone with normal to slightly oily skin. The price is just inane for such an unimpressive, tedious formulation.

☺ **$$$ Eye and Lip Special Cleansing Lotion** *($50 for 4.2 ounces)* is a standard, detergent-based makeup remover, and when I say standard, I mean very standard!

☹ **Botanical Floral Spray Mist** *($61 for 4.2 ounces)* is as ordinary and do-nothing a toner as I've seen for the most absurd amount of money. It is just fragrance and witch hazel. Witch hazel contains mostly alcohol, so this can also be drying and irritating for all skin types.

☹ **Botanical Floral Toning Lotion for Dry/Sensitive Skin** *($60 for 8.4 ounces)* is similar to the Floral Spray Mist above, and the same review applies.

☹ **Botanical Grapefruit Toning Lotion, for Combination/Oily Skin** *($61 for 8.4 ounces)* contains alcohol and grapefruit, both of which are useless for oily skin. These two ingredients can also leave skin feeling irritated, dry, and red.

☹ **Botanical Lotion with Tropical Resins for Combination/Oily Skin** *($56 for 4.2 ounces)* contains too much alcohol to be recommended for any skin type. The tropical resins are just standard plant extracts; some are irritants while others are anti-irritants.

☺ **$$$ Hydra-Flash with Beta-Hydroxy Acid and Natural Plant Extracts for All Skin Types** *($160 for 2.1 ounces)* contains no beta hydroxy acid of any kind! This is just an extremely overpriced, standard, emollient moisturizer for dry skin that contains a teeny amount of water-binding agents and antioxidants.

☹ **Botanical Day Cream with Lily for Normal to Oily Skin** *($115 for 1.6 ounces)* lists isopropyl myristate as the second ingredient, and the fifth is mineral oil. Why anyone with oily skin would want to spend this kind of money on ingredients known to make oily skin look and feel worse is anyone's guess. This mundane moisturizer that lacks any real beneficial ingredients for skin is made still more absurd by its price tag.

☹ **Tropical Resins Complex Oil Free** *($127 for 1.7 ounces)* is similar to the Botanical Day Cream above and the same comments apply.

☺ **$$$ Botanical Intensive Day Cream** *($220 for 1.7 ounces)* isn't even remotely intensive, and as a day cream it is actually a problem because it has no sunscreen. It is an emollient moisturizer for normal to dry skin with a tiny amount of water-binding agents and anti-irritants and a mere dusting of an antioxidant. If you can get over the price—but wait, there is no reason to get over this price.

☺ **$$$ Botanical Intensive Night Cream for All Skin Types** *($248 for 1.6 ounces)*. I don't have any good words for how out-of-date and beyond dull this moisturizer is. The price would be laughable if there weren't women out there wasting their hard-earned money on this do-nothing product.

☺ **$$$ Botanical Moisturizer with Cucumber** *($115 for 1.5 ounces)* is a standard, mineral oil–based moisturizer with absolutely nothing else of any consequence. Cucumber extract and some thickening agents do not add up to good skin care or skin care of any kind.

☺ **$$$ Botanical Night Cream with Collagen and Woodmallow** *($137 for 1.6 ounces)* is a mineral oil– and lanolin-based moisturizer. It would be good for dry skin, but the price is painful for this below-average formula. The teeny amount of collagen has no impact on skin. Mallow can be an anti-inflammatory, but it can have little effect when present in such a minuscule amount.

☺ $$$ **Botanical Restorative Facial Cream with Shea Butter for Day and Night** *($137 for 1.6 ounces)* is similar to the Botanical Night Cream above with the addition of shea butter. That is a good emollient, but it's hardly unique to this product, and this still lacks antioxidants and water-binding agents.

☺ $$$ **Botanical Tensor Immediate Lift** *($143 for 1.05 ounces)*. The plant extracts in this product won't lift your skin anywhere. In fact some of them can be skin irritants—for example, the witch hazel distillate contains mostly alcohol, and none of that is helpful for skin in the least. This is a standard moisturizer for dry skin that is priced as if it contained something special. It doesn't.

☺ $$$ **Botanical Throat Cream** *($127 for 1.5 ounces)* is a mineral oil–based moisturizer with thickeners, plant oil, fragrance, and preservatives. It does contain a small amount of antioxidants and water-binding agents, but nothing out of the ordinary or worthy of this price tag.

☺ $$$ **Ecological Compound Day and Night for All Skin Types** *($176 for 4.2 ounces)* is a mineral oil–based moisturizer with just thickening agents, fragrance, preservatives, and a tiny amount of plant extracts, which are a mix of irritants and anti-irritants. It lacks water-binding agents and antioxidants.

☹ $$$ **Botanical Tinted Moisturizer for All Skin Types** *($78 for 1.4 ounces)* has a tint that isn't for everyone. Otherwise, it's just water, mineral oil, plant oil, preservatives, and fragrance. Gee, I didn't think it could get more boring, but it just did.

☺ $$$ **Sisleya** *($300 for 1.7 ounces)*. It's up to the consumer to decide if minuscule amounts of algae, some plant extracts, and a minute amount of vitamin E are worth this kind of money (because most of these ingredients show up in other skin-care products for a fraction of this price). The plant extracts can have an anti-inflammatory effect on skin, but the ones in this product are not the only ones that can do this. The vitamins are barely present and can have no effect whatsoever on skin.

☹ $$$ **Sisleya Eye and Lip Contour Cream** *($150 for 0.53 ounce)* is similar to the Sisleya above and the same comments apply. This contains far more fragrance than anything beneficial for skin.

☹ $$$ **Sisleya Elixer** *($350 for 4 vials each containing 0.18 ounce)* is supposed to be an intensive renewing and restructuring treatment. The only thing it can restructure is your budget. This lightweight lotion contains a small amount of water-binding agents, a minute amount of antioxidants, and some plant extracts that can be anti-irritants. That's good, but not great, and it's definitely not worth this expense.

☹ **Botanical Facial Sun Cream SPF 8** *($154 for 2 ounces)* is sun damage waiting to happen. Not only is the SPF inadequate for daily wear, it does not contain the UVA-protecting ingredients of titanium dioxide, zinc oxide, or avobenzone, and is not recommended. Moreover, because sunscreens must be applied liberally, chances are that at this price no one is going to apply this appropriately.

☺ $$$ **Botanical Facial Sun Cream SPF 15** *($100 for 1.4 ounces)* is a very good, in-part avobenzone-based sunscreen in an emollient, though extremely standard, moisturizing base. It is an option for normal to dry skin, but the price is likely to prevent liberal application, and that would negate the benefit of the SPF.

☺ **$$$ Broad Spectrum Sun Protection SPF 25** *($100 for 2.1 ounces)* is a very good, in-part titanium dioxide–based sunscreen in an emollient, though exceedingly standard, moisturizing base. It is an option for normal to dry skin, but the price is likely to prevent liberal application and that would mean you would not get the benefit of the SPF.

☺ **$$$ Botanical Sun Block SPF 20** *($100 for 1.5 ounces)* is a good, though incredibly overpriced, in-part titanium dioxide–based sunscreen. To suggest that there are equally good sunscreens at the drugstore for a fraction of the price is a huge understatement.

☹ **$$$ Botanical Self Tanning Gel** *($93 for 2.7 ounces)*, like all self-tanners, uses dihydroxyacetone to turn the skin brown. Unlike other self-tanners, this one is the most expensive one I've reviewed and the most ordinary for the money.

☹ **$$$ Botanical Facial Mask, with Tropical Resins for Combination/Oily Skins** *($71 for 1.5 ounces)* is a standard clay mask that contains several ingredients, including isopropyl myristate, that are problematic for someone with oily skin. The plant extracts are a mix of irritants (frankincense and myrrh) and anti-irritants, like burdock.

☹ **$$$ Express Flower Gel** *($88 for 2.15 ounces)* is just fragrant water, silicone, thickeners, and plant oil. None of that is worth the time or expense of buying or applying this product.

☹ **$$$ Radiant Glow Mask** *($71 for 2.15 ounces)* is just water, wax, and clay. It is a very standard, boring clay mask that would be an option for normal to dry skin, but I just can't imagine why anyone would want to spend this kind of money on such uselessness.

☹ **$$$ Botanical Eye and Lip Contour Complex** *($137 for 0.5 ounce)* is just thickeners and plant oil, with a minuscule amount of vitamin E. What a waste of money for an ordinary lightweight moisturizer.

☹ **$$$ Botanical Eye and Lip Contour Balm** *($93 for 1 ounce)*. You really do have to sit down for this one. This contains water, witch hazel, tomato extract, thickeners, and preservatives. Honest! How this line has the effrontery to charge this kind of money for this kind of nonsense is just astounding.

SISLEY MAKEUP

Sisley's makeup, complete with the tag line "A profusion of colours, a wide choice of advanced formulas ... all this, and skin care too" is a bit more straightforward than its skin care, at least in terms of exaggerated claims. However, the shockingly high prices are still intact and made all the more insulting by makeup that barely makes it across the finish line in terms of texture, color choice, and performance. Let me assure you that there is absolutely nothing in Sisley's makeup line that is worth the imposing price tags. It is more or less an adjunct to an expertly packaged, slickly marketed skin-care line that, if you dig beneath the polished-to-perfection surface, is just good old-fashioned smoke and mirrors.

FOUNDATION: ☺ $$$ **Transmat Cucumber Makeup Cream** *($66)* is a light-weight, but creamy, foundation with a natural, sheer finish. The seven shades leave very light and darker skin tones without a choice, but given the ludicrous price for this very basic makeup, that's not so bad. Avoid #1 and #5, both of which are too peach for most skin tones. ☹ $$$ **Tinted Foundation Compact** *($68)* is an OK powder foundation that has a very soft texture and merely OK colors. It can't hold a candle to products like M.A.C.'s Studio Fix Powder Plus Foundation or Lancôme's Dual Finish, and both of these cost less than half of what Sisley is asking.

☹ **Botanical Tinted Moisturizer** *($78)* also has a creamy texture and leaves a moist finish. The four shades are quite pink or peachy, and at this price it is absolutely not recommended.

☹ **CONCEALER:** **Phytocernes Botanical Concealer** *($61)* has a price that is insulting. Are there really women buying this stuff? It has a greasy, easy-to-crease texture and three just barely OK colors.

☹ **POWDER:** **Pressed Powder Compact** *($71)* is nothing more than standard pressed powder. It feels silky and nice, but why tempt yourself with this when those features are so easily obtained from almost every powder in my *Best Products* list at a small fraction of the price? Not to mention that the two shades are poor contenders for most skin tones. **Translucent Loose Face Powder** *($56)* also feels great, but of the three colors only #1 is an option, and only then if you have money to burn. **Sun Glow Pressed Powder** *($71)* is the same sparkly, orange-toned bronzing powder seen in dozens of other lines that wouldn't have the audacity to charge this much money for such a mediocre product.

☺ $$$ **BLUSH:** **Double Blush** *($56)* is a bargain by Sisley's standards—you get two blush tones (although one is more for highlighting) in one compact. These have a dry, soft texture and a few are noticeably shiny, but they work well.

☺ $$$ **EYESHADOW:** **Eye Shadow Singles** *($20)* have a very nice texture and apply darker than they look, but almost every one of them is shiny. What a perfect way to play up any lines around the eyes that you had hoped to alleviate with one of Sisley's $100+ eye creams. For a similar line-emphasizing effect, Sisley has **Golden Touch**, **Copper Touch**, and **Silver Touch** *($25 each)*, three cream-to-powder highlighters for eyes, cheeks, or wherever you want to artificially shine or enhance wrinkles.

☹ **EYE AND BROW SHAPER:** **Eye Liner** *($34)* and the **Brow Pencil** *($34)* are hopelessly ordinary and greasy enough to smear or smudge shortly after you apply them.

LIPSTICK AND LIP PENCIL: The regular ☹ $$$ **Lipstick** *($34)* and **Long Lasting Lipstick** *($34)* are practically indistinguishable. Both have a very greasy texture with full-coverage color and a slippery finish that would test even the most lenient definition of "long lasting." The regular Lipstick apparently offers some matte colors, but none of the colors I saw came even close to that description.

☺ $$$ **Phyto Brilliant Lip Gloss** *($25)* is a standard lip gloss in a tube. It offers minimal stickiness, fine colors, and a maximum price. **Glossy Gloss** *($34)* proves not even Sisley is immune to the lure of glitter-infused products, as this semi-opaque, sticky gloss attests. Do I really have to tell you that you've seen this type of gloss at your local drugstore for under $7?

☺ $$$ **Lip Liner** *($34)* is a standard pencil with a built-in brush that leans to the greasy side of creamy, but it does have a good stain. Contrary to the claim, these won't do much to help stop feathering.

☹ **MASCARA: Phyto-Protein Mascara** *($44)* is, without a doubt, one of the most expensive mascaras I've ever purchased. It absolutely created long, thick lashes without clumping, but it takes longer than usual to dry, so some smearing is highly possible. This held up much better throughout the day than it has in the past, but suffice it to say you can buy four to six tubes of mascaras from L'Oreal or Maybelline for what one tube of this will cost you.

☺ $$$ **BRUSHES:** Sisley offers a small group of good **Brushes** *($30–$44)* that are nicely shaped and properly sized. There is nothing too exceptional, but if you simply must have Sisley brushes, you won't be disappointed. The **Velvet Powder Puff** *($22)* is not worth the luxury price tag, not to mention that using a puff to apply powder is antiquated and a great way to place too much powder on the skin.

SKINCEUTICALS (SKIN CARE ONLY)

SkinCeuticals is the line Dr. Sheldon Pinnell started after his falling out with the skin-care company Cellex-C. The Cellex-C line of skin-care products originated around a $70-an-ounce product containing a form of vitamin C called L-ascorbic acid that was researched by Dr. Pinnell, although Duke University holds the patent for that ingredient. According to Dr. Pinnell, Cellex-C products use an unstable form of L-ascorbic acid; and of course, Dr. Pinnell's line contains the stable good form. Aside from the disagreement between these two companies, L-ascorbic acid is considered a potent antioxidant and anti-inflammatory (Sources: *Bioelectrochemistry and Bioenergetics,* May 1999, pages 453–461; and *International Journal of Radiation Biology,* June 1999, pages 747–755), but claims that it can eliminate or prevent wrinkles when applied topically are not substantiated in any published studies. In addition, it is stable only in a formulation with a low pH, and that is potentially irritating for skin (Source: *Dermatologic Surgery,* February 2001, pages 137–142).

What is absolutely clear is that there are no published studies showing that vitamin C in any form is paramount or of any vital importance on human skin, much less in the fight against wrinkles. The propaganda about this ingredient, or any "must-have" cosmetic ingredient, is intended to sell skin-care products, not to offer women truly viable options for addressing the health of their skin. There are lots of good antioxidants, and vitamin C in any or all of its forms is not the only one, though Dr. N.V. Perricone has made a success of his line of vitamin C products using ascorbyl palmitate.

The Reviews S

Keep in mind that the entire arena of antioxidants is new, and that as yet there are no definitive findings to warrant the high cost or intense hype. Antioxidants won't get rid of wrinkles or replace sunscreen. They can offer increased sun protection, and in theory can help the skin to defend itself from free-radical damage while maintaining its integrity. Yet that doesn't stop companies from making claims about reversing aging, building collagen, and feeding the skin. For more information about SkinCeuticals, call (800) 811-1660 or visit www.skinceuticals.com. **Note:** All SkinCeuticals products contain fragrance.

☺ **Delicate Cleanser** *($24 for 8 ounces)* isn't all that delicate—it is just an overpriced cold cream–type cleanser for dry skin that can leave a slightly greasy film on the skin. The plant extracts, including yarrow and comfrey, can be skin irritants.

☺ **Simply Clean** *($24 for 8 ounces)* is a standard, detergent-based cleanser that would work for normal to oily skin. It contains a tiny amount of something called fruit acids. "Fruit acid" is a term with no official or regulated definition, and thus it means nothing, because you don't really know what you are applying to your skin.

☺ **Foaming Cleanser** *($24.50 for 6.7 ounces)* is a standard, detergent-based cleanser that contains several potentially irritating plant extracts, including arnica and lime.

☺ **Equalizing Toner** *($22 for 8 ounces).* If there were information as to what the mixed fruit acids in this product really were (the term "fruit acids" is not legal for an ingredient label), this might be a decent liquid AHA. But without specifics, you have no idea what you are putting on your skin, and the pH is too high for this to be an effective exfoliant anyway.

☺ **Revitalizing Toner** *($22 for 8 ounces)* is similar to the Equalizing Toner above and the same comments apply.

☺ $$$ **Daily Moisture** *($49.50 for 2 ounces)* does not contain sunscreen, so using this during the day can present a problem. The algae it contains is not a miracle for skin, though it may have some water-binding properties. This does contain a tiny amount of antioxidants, but it also contains plant extracts that can be skin irritants, including cinnamon and thyme. Overall, this is not a stellar moisturizer to consider, for day or for night.

☺ $$$ **Emollience** *($49.50 for 2 ounces)* is similar to the Daily Moisture version above, only this one contains more plant oils and some very good antioxidants. It lacks water-binding agents, and several of the plant extracts can be skin irritants, and that's disappointing for what would otherwise be a well-formulated (and higher-rated) moisturizer.

✓☺ $$$ **Eye Cream** *($53 for 0.67 ounce)* is a good moisturizer for dry skin with some good antioxidants and water-binding agents. If you are a believer in the vitamin C craze, this product will give you what you are looking for.

✓☺ $$$ **SkinC Serum 10** *($60 for 1 ounce)* is a lightweight lotion that is good for slightly dry skin. It is almost identical to the SkinCeuticals Primacy Serum, but for some reason costs half the money. It contains some very good antioxidants and a water-binding agent.

✓☺ **$$$ SkinC Serum 15** *($75 for 1 ounce)* is almost identical to the Serum 10 above except that this one contains more ascorbic acid. Given that no specific amount of vitamin C has been established as being most effective for skin, this is as good a guess as the one above.

✓☺ **$$$ Eye Gel** *($42 for 0.5 ounce)* is almost identical to the SkinC Serum above only in gel form. The same basic comments apply.

☺ **Eye Renewal Gel** *($27 for 1 ounce)* is a lightweight moisturizer for slightly dry skin, but the vague "mixed fruit acid" is useless for skin, especially as the pH of this product isn't low enough for it to be effective as an exfoliant—even if it could be. This lacks any of the interesting antioxidants or water-binding agents used in other SkinCeuticals products.

☺ **Renew Overnight, Oily** *($45 for 2 ounces)* lists mixed fruit acid as the second ingredient, and so has the same problem as the products above that include "mixed fruit acids" on their ingredient lists. Besides, how many AHA, or even more accurately, pseudo-AHA, products does one face need? Even if the fruit acids were known to act as AHAs or BHA, the pH isn't low enough for them to make this an effective exfoliant. Other than that, while this is an OK moisturizer for normal to dry skin, several ingredients make it problematic for oily skin.

☺ **$$$ Renew Overnight, Dry** *($45 for 2 ounces)* is similar to the Renew Overnight, Oily version above and the same comments apply.

☺ **$$$ Hydrating B5 Gel** *($55 for 1 ounce)* is a good lightweight moisturizer, but vitamin B5 (pantothenic acid) offers nothing that's any more special for skin than lots of other vitamins that show up in skin-care products that cost far less. The claim is that this product is essential for use with the vitamin C products in this line. Now that's confusing! Does that mean that L-ascorbic acid (vitamin C) isn't the big deal, but that you need to layer products to get the miracle results? One more thing: This product is supposed to restore hyaluronic acid, "your skin's natural moisturizer." The skin has dozens and dozens of substances that act as "natural" moisturizers, ranging from glycerin and cholesterol to amino acids, ceramides, saccharides, and on and on. There is nothing about hyaluronic acid alone that makes it superior to lots of other water-binding agents.

☺ **$$$ Intense Line Defense** *($50 for 1 ounce)*. This simple group of ingredients is similar to those in the Hydrating B5 Gel above and the same basic comments apply. You have to decide if the water-binding agent this contains, a form of hyaluronic acid, is the answer for your wrinkles, because that is all it really contains. The "mixed fruit extract" on the ingredient list is an invalid term and, therefore, there is no way to know what you are really putting on your skin.

☺ **$$$ Phyto Corrective Gel** *($45 for 1 ounce)* contains water-binding agents, plant extracts, and a tiny amount of antioxidants. One of the plant extracts, bearberry, has minimal impact for inhibiting melanin production. This is a good lightweight moisturizer for normal to slightly dry skin.

☺ $$$ **Skin Firming Cream** *($85 for 1.67 ounces)* is a very good moisturizer for normal to dry skin, with a good mix of water-binding agents and antioxidants.

☺ $$$ **Daily Sun Defense SPF 20** *($28 for 3 ounces)* is a good, in-part zinc oxide sunscreen. It would work well for normal to dry skin. Aside from that, this product's standard ingredient list does not warrant its price tag. In fact, Olay's Complete UV Protection Moisture Lotion SPF 15 ($9.99 for 6 ounces) contains 3% zinc oxide and works equally well for dry skin. Moreover, because you are more likely to use the correct amount (that is, a liberal amount) of sunscreen with a less expensive product, the Olay is ultimately the better choice. Keep in mind that sunscreens must be applied liberally to get the full benefit of the SPF, so if this price tag keeps you from slathering it on you would be hurting your skin.

☺ $$$ **Ultimate UV Defense SPF 30** *($34 for 3 ounces)* is a good, in-part zinc oxide sunscreen in an ordinary moisturizing base. It would work well for normal to slightly dry skin. The standard ingredient list does not warrant the price tag, and Eucerin with SPF 25 will provide you with close to the same protection and the same zinc oxide active ingredient for UVA protection. The comments about liberal application for the SPF 20 version above apply here, too.

☺ $$$ **Ultimate UV Defense SPF 45** *($34 for 3 ounces)* is similar to the SPF 30 above and the same basic comments apply.

☺ $$$ **Sans Soleil** *($28 for 4 ounces)* contains dihydroxyacetone, the same ingredient in all self-tanners that affects the color of skin. This one would work as well as any, and there is no reason to consider this over versions from Coppertone or Bain de Soleil at the drugstore for far less money.

☹ $$$ **Clarifying Clay Masque** *($33 for 2 ounces)* is an exceptionally standard clay mask. It does contain fruit acids, but they are useless for anything other than looking interesting and sounding natural on an ingredient list.

☺ $$$ **Antioxidant Lip Repair** *($30 for 0.3 ounce)* is a Vaseline-based lip balm with some good water-binding agents and antioxidants, but none of that will repair anything on or around your lips.

PRIMACY BY SKINCEUTICALS

Primacy is a group of four exceedingly overpriced products that chiefly claim to be the best at preventing free-radical damage. While the zinc sulfate, vitamin C, and vitamin E may indeed be great antioxidants (though this has not been established for application on human skin; it is all strictly theoretical), there is no research establishing whether or not these can change or prevent one wrinkle.

☺ $$$ **C + AHA** *($115 for 1 ounce)*. The pH of 3 allows the glycolic acid and lactic acid to be effective exfoliants, but the belief that the zinc and vitamin C in this product are the be-all and end-all for skin care is up to you and your pocketbook.

☹ **C + E** *($115 for 1 ounce)* lists alcohol as the third ingredient, which makes this product too irritating and drying for all skin types. One of the concepts about skin aging that is fairly uncontroversial and well established is that inflammation and irritation are damaging to skin, so why it would ever be a wise option to include unnecessary and irritating ingredients in a skin-care product is beyond me.

☺ **$$$ Serum 20** *($95 for 1 ounce)*. For all intents and purposes, this is the original mixture Dr. Pinnell tested on the backs of hairless pigs and found that it reduced the incidence of sunburn. Subsequent research has shown that to be true for many antioxidants and it works on human skin, too.

☺ **$$$ Phyto +** *($65 for 1 ounce)* contains kojic acid and arbutin, and both are supposed to be effective for inhibiting melanin production to reduce the appearance of brown discolorations on skin. Kojic acid can inhibit melanin production, but it is a highly unstable ingredient, and is not as effective as hydroquinone. Arbutin is a naturally occurring form of hydroquinone, and can suppress melanin production. However, arbutin's effectiveness has only been shown in vitro, unlike the huge body of research demonstrating hydroquinone's effect on skin. This product also contains bearberry, a plant that contains arbutin. There are some good antioxidants in here, but some of the plant extracts can be skin irritants.

☺ **$$$ Primacy Eye Balm with Triple Age Defense Technology** *($68 for 0.5 ounce)* is an emollient moisturizer for normal to dry skin that contains some good antioxidants and water-binding agents. However, there is nothing in this worth the extreme price.

✓☺ **$$$ Primacy Face Cream with Triple Age Defense Technology** *($128 for 1.67 ounces)* is similar to the Primacy Eye Balm above, and the same comments apply.

smashbox

Perhaps the most interesting things about smashbox are that its name refers to the early, accordion-style cameras and that smashbox is first and foremost a Hollywood-based photography studio. How smashbox's makeup got launched is a question worth asking, because there is very little that is exciting about the products and they are ridiculously overpriced. The company's creators, Dean and Davis Factor, have their heritage in makeup—their great-grandfather was legendary makeup artist Max Factor. However, this seems to be a case where the proverbial apple fell too far from the tree. It is apparent that Dean and Davis are better at their respective careers as CEO and photographer than at creating a cosmetics line. The makeup, which debuted in 1996, has changed little since the previous edition of this book. The pencils are still incredibly standard, the selection of powder blushes remains almost too soft to show depth on darker skin tones, the eyeshadow singles and duos are almost all shiny, and the newer products are more or less "me too" contributions to what other makeup companies have done, and done better. If anything, smashbox's reputation as a premier photography studio should mean that the makeup produced and (ostensibly) used for photo shoots should be top-notch and work for a wide variety of skin tones. Alas, that is not the case. It turns out that smashbox isn't so smashing after all, and its products pale in comparison to those of other artistry-driven lines like M.A.C., Bobbi Brown, Stila, Trish McEvoy, and Laura Mercier. All the cleverly named products and the familial legacy of makeup innovator Max Factor don't count for much when what sounds so promising ends up being such an overall expensive disappointment. On the plus side, for those in the mood to play with some good foundations (and a parade of iridescence), the tester unit is nicely set up for experimentation. As for their lackluster skin care, don't get me started. For more information about smashbox, call (888) 558-1490 or visit their interactive Web site at www.smashbox.com.

smashbox SKIN CARE

☺ $$$ **Cleanser** *($26 for 3.5 ounces)* is a mostly ineffective cleanser that is more of a cold cream than anything else, but it doesn't even succeed well in that category.

☺ $$$ **Eye Makeup Remover** *($14 for 4 ounces)* is standard, detergent-based eye-makeup remover that is about as ordinary as it gets.

☺ $$$ **Moisturizer** *($34 for 3.5 ounces)* is a moisturizer that barely deserves comment. It is an ordinary mix of water and thickening agents with the most minuscule amount of vitamin E imaginable.

smashbox MAKEUP

FOUNDATION: smashbox's main strengths lie with its foundations. The colors and textures are a bit dated, but worth a look, although there are few options for very light and darker skin tones.

☺ $$$ **PhotoFinish Foundation Primer** *($36)* is a standard, silicone-based serum that has little going for it other than being a decent lightweight mattifier that makes the skin feel smooth, and that can, to a mild extent, temporarily fill in large pores and ensure a matte finish. For a similar, considerably less expensive product, consider Neutrogena's Pore Refining Mattifier ($11.99 for 0.5 ounce). **Artificial Light Luminizing Lotion** *($28)* has a very silky, fluid feel and produces a subtle, non-glittery glow on the skin. It's an OK option for soft shine, but the price is prohibitive considering the wide assortment of similar products at the drugstore. **Studio Matte Oil-Free Foundation SPF 15** *($28)* would've been a slam dunk for normal to oily skin craving a matte-finish, lightweight foundation, but this one lacks significant UVA protection. If you insist on smashbox, and you're willing to wear a separate sunscreen underneath, you will find eight neutral colors, but no options for darker skin tones.

☺ $$$ **Anti-Shine Foundation** *($26)* is an intriguing product. It is mostly water and magnesium with a hint of color. Magnesium (as in Phillips' Milk of Magnesia) absorbs oil very well and does not feel as heavy on the skin as clays do. This formula goes on extremely matte and dry and has great staying power. The colors (or lack thereof) can be a problem, but they go on sheer, and clearly this product is more about shine control than coverage. I wouldn't bet on this for a true foundation, but for those who need an oil-controlling product with some longevity, this is a definite option. **Studio**

Seamless Liquid Foundation *($28)* is a water-based foundation containing a small amount of oil, making it best for someone with normal to dry skin. It blends on evenly, allowing for light to medium coverage, and has a silky-soft finish. Of the nine shades, the only one to avoid is Sand. Ivory and Bisque 1.5 are excellent shades for fair skin. **Foundation Stick** *($28)* has a creamy, mineral oil– and wax-based texture that can blend out sheer and soft, though it takes some patience to get it to do that. It is similar to (but not as modern as) most cream-to-powder makeups, making it ideal for normal skin— those with breakout-prone skin, both dry and oily, should look elsewhere. There are seven shades, and the ones to avoid are Ivory (can be slightly pink) and Sand and Warm Beige (both slight peach). **Wet/Dry Foundation** *($32)* is a talc-based pressed-powder foundation that is much better used dry than wet. It has a smooth, slightly dry texture with natural coverage and five mostly neutral shades—only Sand is too peach for most skin tones.

☹ **CONCEALER: Retouch** *($12)* is a thick pencil concealer that goes on creamy and heavy, and will definitely crease into any lines around the eyes. Of the five shades, only numbers 1 and 1.5 are neutral and would work for fair to light skin tones.

☺ **$$$ POWDER: Flash Powder** *($28)* is talc-based and has a soft, powdered-sugar texture that goes on soft and light. There is only one color available, and although it is neutral, its lightness makes it appropriate only for fair to light skin tones. **Pressed Powder** *($26)* is also talc-based and offers one more shade than the Flash Powder, with a sheer, silky texture and a soft finish. Again, the limited shades make this an option only for very light skin.

☹ **$$$ Compact Anti-Shine** *($26)* is a dry-textured, colorless powder that is meant to absorb excess shine, but it can look whitish on the skin unless it is applied sparingly— and that may not be sufficient for shine control. This is an OK option for fair skin, but it isn't as impressive as the Anti-Shine Foundation above. **Reflectors** *($16)* are just small pots of very sparkly loose powder that are messy to use. There are easier ways to add sparkles to the face or body.

BLUSH: ☹ **$$$ Blush Compact** *($24)* is comparable to several other blushes that sell for far less. Otherwise, there are some beautiful colors that all have a very sheer application that does not show up well on darker skin tones, let alone under the hot photographic lights that are no doubt present at the smashbox studio. Cost aside, this is an option for lighter skin tones, though unless you want shiny cheeks stay away from Golden Beige. **Soft Lights** *($26)* is a small collection of large-pan blushes (similar to M.A.C.'s) that offer more color intensity than the Blush Compact above, but still not enough for dark skin tones. All of the colors are slightly shiny.

☹ **Skin Tint** *($28)* is a water-based stick blush that offers a very soft application of translucent color. Unfortunately, this also has a greasy texture and slightly glossy finish, which means it can undermine carefully applied foundation and can make cheeks look like an oil slick in no time.

☺ $$$ <u>EYESHADOWS</u>: **Single Eye Shadow** *($16)* offers a soft texture that applies evenly, but sheer, so building intensity takes some effort. Most of the 28 colors available are shiny. **Eye Shadow Duos** *($24)* shares the same comments as the Single Eye Shadow above, except that some of the pairings are strange (shiny pink and purple, shiny black and white) and hard to work with. For fantasy makeup, these are contenders, but you'll still have to put up with sheer colors that don't cover well. The following matte duos are good pairings: Bare/Reflection and Smashing/Profile. **Eyelights** *($32)* presents three eyeshadows in a compact. Each color has mega-watt shine, but otherwise this is similar to the Singles and Duos. **Highlighters** *($24)* are cream-to-powder shine with a slippery texture for any area that needs enlightenment.

☺ $$$ <u>EYE AND BROW SHAPER</u>: **Eye Pencil** *($14)* is a standard pencil that comes in a handful of good colors. The texture and application are drier than most, so this isn't the easiest to apply, but it does decrease the chance of smearing and enhances wearing time. **Cream Eye Liner** *($22)* is an interesting notion that sounds better than it is. On the one hand, these do go on very smoothly and intensely. However, they tend to fade, smear, and run with the slightest excuse, which makes them not worth the effort, especially at this price. For a superior version of this product, consider Bobbi Brown's Long Wear Gel Eyeliner ($18). **Key Lights** *($14)* are standard thick pencils that are supposed to put the wearer in their "key light" (photographer's jargon for finding a subject's perfect lighting). What a clever way to describe what amounts to a shiny, chunky pencil. **Brow Tech** *($22)* is named to sound as if it is a revolutionary product for brows. It's merely a split-pan compact with a matte brow powder that you mix with the other half, which is a clear wax. The effect is billed as "the answer to anyone's prayers," but the same look can be achieved with any good brow pencil (where the waxes and pigments are premixed) or a matte eyeshadow set with brow gel or, for a glossy look, a dab of Vaseline.

<u>LIPSTICK AND LIP PENCIL</u>: ☺ $$$ **Lipstick** *($16)* is a standard creamy formula that leans toward the greasy side of creamy, although almost half of the colors are frosted. These do provide full coverage, but if you're prone to lipstick feathering into lines around the mouth, this will quickly migrate there. **Lip Gloss** *($14)* is standard gloss in a tube that has a non-sticky feel and all iridescent colors. For a lacquered-look gloss, it's as good as any. **Lip Brilliance** *($26)* includes three-color lip palettes that proclaim "the coverage of a lipstick, the smooth feel of a gloss," and this turns out to be partially true. Although this lipstick/gloss hybrid offers full coverage, the texture is thick and sticky, and for the money this is not preferred to using a standard gloss over a good creamy lipstick. **Lip Pencil** *($14)* includes standard pencils with a creamy, but firm, texture and a dry finish. They'll work as well as most other pencils in all price ranges, but if you fall in love with one of smashbox's colors, these are worth a try.

☹ **Limitless Lip Stain** *($24)* has serious limitations. It starts out splendidly as an intense lip stain you apply with a sponge-tip wand. Once the color sets, you apply a coat of clear lip gloss, which comes packaged with the stain in one unit. However, for some reason the gloss undoes the stain, immediately causing a blotchy, une... doesn't matter if you let the stain "set" (no directions accompany the... minutes—once the gloss goes on, the stain breaks down. For the mo... performance, Max Factor's Lipfinity wins again.

☺ $$$ <u>MASCARA:</u> smashbox's **Mascara** *($16)* takes some effort, but eventually builds impressive length and stays on well. It is no more water-resistant than other water-soluble mascaras, so don't be fooled into thinking you can go for a swim while wearing this!

☹ $$$ <u>BRUSHES:</u> The assortment of **Brushes** *($18–$42)* is more realistically priced than those of other artistry-based lines, and there are some options to consider. However, most of these are either too soft, too large, or their usage is too limited to warrant spending the extra money. The ones to consider are the #3 **Blending** *($30)*, #12 **Angle Brow** *($19)*, #15 **Crease Definer** *($28)*, and #9 **Shadow Liner** *($18)*, which is one of the better types of this brush around. It is thin enough to use for both upper and lower lashlines and you can make the line as thin or thick as you like using almost any eyeshadow. For those so inclined, smashbox's #13 **Foundation Brush** *($32)* is one of the better brushes of its type available, and the price is comparable to those of most other lines.

SONIA KASHUK (MAKEUP ONLY)

Although Target stores seemed like an odd place for internationally renowned makeup artist Sonia Kashuk to launch her line, the exclusivity has meshed well with Target's latest fashion-conscious marketing strategies. The fact that Kashuk has found a niche here has no doubt paved the way for noted fashion designers like Mossimo and Todd Oldham to also ink deals with this Marshall Field's–owned retailer. The combination of exclusive high-fashion names and practical makeup sold at value-driven prices is great bait for savvy consumers. Shopping for makeup from Sonia Kashuk is a wise decision in many respects—you'll find great products in every category, with quality to spare, and a well-edited assortment of contemporary and classic colors.

Perhaps the only drawbacks with this line, which has many more strong points than weak points, are that its display doesn't include testers and that the packaging, though attractive (a shiny, slick, silver-plastic casing that has a great mirrorlike surface), doesn't let you see the colors. What a shame, because all the neighboring product lines have far more enticing "see me, feel me" displays. What's worse, Target does not allow returns or exchanges on cosmetics, which is a disadvantage you may not want to live with if you happen to choose the wrong color. Still, if you know exactly what you're after or are willing to gamble, this is a relatively safe line to place your bets on. For more information about Sonia Kashuk, visit www.target.com.

<u>FOUNDATION:</u> ☺ **Perfecting Liquid Foundation** *($9.99)* is a very sheer-to-light coverage liquid foundation for someone with normal to dry skin, and thanks to the significant amount of silicone and mineral oil it contains it has a great soft texture. However, the price is not as reasonable as it may appear. There is only 0.6 ounce of foundation in

The Rev

the package, while most other foundations sold at drugstores and department stores contain at least a full ounce or more, and that makes Kashuk's one of the more expensive mass market options. Five shades are available, but the packaging makes it almost impossible to see the real color. However, all of them are nicely neutral and worth considering by light to medium skin tones.

✓☺ **Dual Coverage Powder Foundation** *($9.99)* is a great option for a light-coverage, silky-smooth, pressed-powder foundation. The formula is talc-based and blends superbly. The five shades are all winners, but good luck choosing your best one based on the way this is packaged and the lack of testers.

☺ **CONCEALER: Confidential Concealer** *($4.99)* has a soft, creamy texture that you may find has a bit too much slip, which means you'll get only sheer to light coverage. It does eventually blend well and has a satiny finish, but it can crease, and keep creasing—so if you have lines, be warned. There are only two colors, which seems strange for a makeup artist's line, and while Light is great, Medium is too peach for most skin tones.

POWDER: ✓☺ **Bare Minimum Pressed Powder** *($7.99)* is almost indistinguishable from the Dual Coverage Powder Foundation above, save for being a bit more sheer, but otherwise the same comments apply. There are three neutral shades available. ✓☺ **Barely There Loose Powder** *($7.99)* is probably the most elegant, gossamer loose powder you'll find in this price range. This finely milled, silky powder blends beautifully on skin and comes in two very good colors, best for fair to light skin tones. One caveat: This contains cornstarch, which can (in theory) feed the bacteria that cause blemishes.

BLUSH: ☺ **Beautifying Blush** *($7.99)* has a great silky feel and goes on quite smooth, but almost too sheer. The colors are not visible through the packaging so picking which one of the five shades that will be best for you is a guessing game. Still, blush is hard to get wrong, unless you have an extremely sallow (olive) or ruddy (red) skin tone. **Luminous Creme Blush** *($7.99)* is indeed luminous, but read that to mean slightly shiny. This is an excellent sheer cream blush that applies and blends wonderfully and leaves a dewy finish. Although only two shades are available, they are both excellent and worth a look if you prefer cream blush and are not too picky about color choice! ✓☺ **Illuminating Color Stick** *($7.99)* has been a big hit for Sonia Kashuk, but is this product worth your attention? Well, if you're into products like The Multiple ($32) from NARS, this is almost identical and considerably less expensive (and less greasy). It's an easy-to-apply, sheer wash of color and very subtle shimmer in stick form, and can make for a very attractive evening look when softly blended onto collarbone, brow bone, or cheeks.

☺ **Sheer Bliss Lip & Cheek Tint** *($8.69)* is another rose-colored sheer liquid tint reminiscent of the tint that started this trend, BeneFit's BeneTint. This comes in a small vial, and you're supposed to apply the color with the built-in brush. That could work well for the lips, but it isn't so great for the cheeks. Blending can be tricky, and the end result (a very soft, fuchsia-rose tone) is almost not worth the extra effort. If this look appeals to you L'Oreal's Translucide Gel Blush ($9.49) is much easier to work with.

EYESHADOW: ☺ **Enhance Eye Color** *($4.99)* shares the same packaging problem as the rest of the line, making it hard to view the colors. That's a disappointment, because several of these eyeshadows are matte and go on quite softly. There are now 22 shades, including several neutral tones, but be prepared to open boxes to sneak a peek at the actual color. **Eyeshadow Palette** *($12.99)* provides eight eyeshadows (in Neutrals or Colors) in one sleek silver compact. This is a veritable bargain if the included shades entice you, though the shades are predominantly shiny.

☺ **Enlighten Eye Cream** *($5.99)* consists of small tubes of exceedingly iridescent eyeshadow. These have a cream-to-powder texture that lays down opaque shine that tends to easily crease into the fold of the eye. Maybelline's Cool Effect Cooling Cream Eyecolor *($5.59)* gives you oodles of shine without the creasing.

EYE AND BROW SHAPER: ☺ **Eye Definer** *($4.99)* is a standard, fairly greasy pencil that requires sharpening. This can easily smear if you are lining under the eye, but can work decently if it's set with powder eyeshadow. **Smudge Pencil** *($4.99)* is a standard pencil that is almost indistinguishable from the Eye Definer except for a slightly thicker application. The name is appropriate for what this pencil will do in short order on its own.

☺ **Brow Gel** *($5.99)* is another basic brow gel that works as well as any other, only this one won't break the bank!

LIPSTICK AND LIP PENCIL: ☺ **Luxury Lip Color** *($5.99)* is a good cross between a gloss and an opaque lipstick. It gives good coverage but has a very slippery, greasy finish. Again, the (mostly attractive) shades are hidden, but the color swatches are a fair representation of what's inside. **Lip Sheers** *($5.99)* are nice, but nothing exceptional. They are standard sheer and glossy lipsticks that come in a small, but superior, range of shades. For a soft look, they work just as well as Clinique's Almost Lipstick, which costs twice as much. **Lip Glossing** *($5.99)* provides a smooth application and a light, non-sticky feel that leaves a soft, glossy finish. The colors have good intensity, so you can almost consider this a liquid lipstick rather than a standard sheer gloss. **Lip Palette** *($14.99)* gets you eight lip colors plus one clear lip balm, all housed in a single compact. The lip brush needs to go, but this is otherwise a fine assortment of colors that encourages you to mix and match the well-coordinated shades.

☺ **Lip Pencil** *($4.99)* is identical to the Eye Definer, but the somewhat greasy application is not a problem for the lips, unless you have a problem with lipstick feathering. The four shades are attractive and the color representation on the tip is rather accurate.

MASCARA: ✓☺ **Lashify Mascara** *($5.99)* is a very good mascara that builds reasonable length and some thickness without clumping or smearing. With a little effort it can make lashes really long and thick, and it wears all day without a hitch. You did notice the great price, right?

BRUSHES: Sonia Kashuk offers ten professional makeup ☺ **Brushes** *($1.99–$9.99)*. Their feel isn't as soft and velvety as some of the more expensive brushes you may find,

The Reviews S

but for the money they are a consideration. The **Powder** *($9.99)* and **Blush** *($9.99)* brushes are fine, and the various eyeshadow and liner versions allow you to experiment with different types of eye brushes without sabotaging your budget. There is also a ☺ 4-**Piece Travel Set** *($12.99)* that includes a substandard mini-blush brush along with two good eyeshadow brushes and a traditional brow/lash comb. Not bad for travel, but don't expect seamless results.

SPECIALTY: The well-assembled ✔☺ **Face Palette** *($19.99)* is one of the few all-in-one products that lives up to its name of being a complete palette for the face. What you'll find, housed in a large, flat silver compact, are three eyeshadows, three lip colors, two shades of cream concealer (a creamier version of Kashuk's original concealer, and one that provides better coverage), one neutral pressed powder, and two workable brush applicators. Two different sets are available, and Kashuk occasionally offers seasonal or holiday palettes. Both sets are smartly coordinated and feature a fair mix of matte and soft shimmer shades.

SOTHYS PARIS (SKIN CARE ONLY)

It would take an entire book unto itself to deal with all of the exaggerated claims attributed to Sothys Paris's relatively ordinary, overly hyped, and often poorly formulated products. Sothys Paris has the same élan and prestige that are associated with other high-end French lines, but unlike Chanel and Lancome, this line relies strictly on prestige and has very little to offer in product content. As is typical for many cosmetics lines that for some unknown reason don't yet know about the insidious risk of sun damage, Sothys Paris makes recommendations for your daily skin-care routine that do not include the use of a reliable sunscreen. No matter how many dozens of moisturizers you choose, the lack of even one UVA-protecting SPF 15 product in Sothys Paris's daily skin-care regimens means your face is just asking for more wrinkles. There are also many other areas where Sothys Paris falls short. The blemish products either contain useless irritants or pore-clogging ingredients, but no disinfectant or effective exfoliant; the cleansers contain cleansing agents known for their irritation or are little more than expensive cold creams; and the AHA products are poorly formulated and completely ineffective for exfoliation. The large number of moisturizers are redundant, with few differences among them, not to mention that the claims made for them are out of proportion for such basic formulations. Many contain some state-of-the art water-binding agents (albeit only in small amounts), yet most of them lack any significant amount of antioxidants.

Suffice it to say there are far better and less expensive products. If you're looking for pricey skin-care products to splurge on, this is not the line to shop. For more information about Sothy Paris, call (800) 325-0503 or visit www.sothys.com. **Note:** All Sothys Paris products contain fragrance.

☹ **Blanc Perfecting Cleansing Cream** *($24 for 4.2 ounces)* contains sodium lauryl sulfate as the main cleansing agent, which is a leading ingredient for causing irritation and dryness. This cleanser is not recommended.

☹ **Desquacreme Emulsion for a Deeply Cleansed Radiant Skin** *($26 for 1.7 ounces)* is a standard, detergent-based cleanser, though it does include sodium lauryl sulfate as one of the primary cleansing agents, and that makes it a problem for all skin types.

☹ **Nettoyant du Matin Morning Cleanser Face Wash** *($24 for 4.2 ounces)* is similar to the Desquacreme above, and the same comments apply.

☺ **Lait Demaquillant Comfort Soothing Beauty Milk for Sensitive Skins** *($26 for 6.7 ounces)* is an emollient, cold cream–style, wipe-off cleanser that can be an option for dry skin.

☺ **Lait Demaquillant Douceur Softening Beauty Milk for Dry Skin** *($21 for 6.7 ounces)* is a standard, detergent-based cleanser that is fairly gentle and can be an option for someone with normal to dry skin.

☹ **Lait Demaquillant Satine Normalizing Beauty Milk, for Normal or Combination Skin** *($26 for 6.7 ounces)* contains several ingredients that would be a problem for combination skin, including coconut oil and acetylated lanolin.

☹ **Lait Demaquillant Purifiant Purifying Beauty Milk, for Oily Skin** *($22 for 6.7 ounces)* contains several ingredients that are problematic for oily skin, including acetylated lanolin.

☺ **Purifying Foaming Gel** *($23 for 4.2 ounces)* is a standard, detergent-based, water-soluble cleanser that is an option for most skin types.

☺ **Biological Skin Peeling** *($23 for 1.7 ounces)* contains a fairly gentle oat- and wax-based exfoliant that makes this an option for someone with normal to dry skin.

☹ **Eye Makeup Remover Gel** *($20 for 2.5 ounces)* is an emollient makeup remover that contains the preservative Kathon CG, which is not recommended for use in leave-on products and should not be used even short-term in the eye area.

☹ **Peau Normal Normalizing Lotion for Normal or Combination Skin** *($20 for 6.7 ounces)* contains the preservative Kathon CG, which is not recommended for use in leave-on skin-care products. Moreover, this lacks any beneficial skin-care ingredients. It is a completely mediocre formulation.

☹ **Peau Grasse Skin Lotion for Problem Skin** *($26 for 6.7 ounces)* contains camphor, which is a real problem for all skin types, plus this lacks any beneficial ingredients for skin.

☺ **Soothing Skin Lotion for Dry Skin** *($21 for 6.7 ounces)* is just water, slip agent, castor oil, fragrance, and preservatives, adding up to a do-nothing toner that isn't worth using at any price.

☹ **Soothing Skin Lotion for Sensitive Skin** *($21 for 6.7 ounces)* contains the preservative Kathon CG, which is not recommended for use in leave-on skin-care products, and it is definitely not acceptable for sensitive skin.

☺ **$$$ Active Contour Creme Anti-Rides Age-Defying Cream** *($34 for 0.5 ounce)* is an OK emollient moisturizer with fractional amounts of water-binding agents and antioxidants.

☹ **Active Creme, Nourishing Creme for Oily Skin** *($34 for 1.7 ounces)* contains several ingredients that are problematic for oily skin, including acetylated lanolin. This also contains the preservative Kathon CG, which is not recommended for use in leave-on skin-care products.

☺ $$$ **Active Contour Tensor Gel** *($38 for 0.5 ounce)* is an exceptionally ordinary and overpriced moisturizer for normal to slightly dry skin. The small amount of algae has no miracle properties for skin.

☹ **Bio-Relaxing Eye Contour Gel** *($27 for 0.5 ounce)* contains several potentially irritating plant extracts and although it contains a good water-binding agent, it lacks any antioxidants. It also contains the preservative Kathon CG, which is not recommended for use in leave-on skin-care products.

☹ **Blanc Perfect Fluid SPF 8** *($51 for 1.7 ounces)* has an SPF that is far below the standard SPF 15 set by the American Academy of Dermatology and the Skin Cancer Foundation, plus this doesn't contain the UVA-protecting ingredients of titanium dioxide, zinc oxide, or avobenzone. It is absolutely not recommended.

☺ $$$ **Blanc Perfect Serum** *($52 for 4 vials, each containing 0.17 ounce)* includes a good amount of magnesium ascorbyl phosphate, a form of vitamin C that can have melanin-inhibiting properties. It also contains some good water-binding agents and anti-irritants. This is one of the better-formulated Sothys Paris products.

☹ **Capital Fermete Light Texture** *($50 for 1.7 ounces)* is an emollient moisturizer for normal to dry skin that contains a good mix of water-binding agents and a small amount of antioxidants. However, it contains the preservative Kathon CG, which is not recommended for use in leave-on skin-care products, and is not recommended.

☹ **Capital Fermete Comfort Texture** *($57 for 1.7 ounces)* is similar to the Capital Light Texture above and the same basic comments apply.

☹ **Creme de Jour, Day Creme for Normal or Combination Skins** *($29 for 1.7 ounces)* contains only a modicum of water-binding agents and little else of benefit to skin. It also contains the preservative Kathon CG, which is not recommended for use in leave-on skin-care products.

☹ **Creme de Nuit, Night Creme for Normal or Combination Skins** *($39 for 1.7 ounces)* is similar to the Creme de Jour above and the same basic comments apply.

☹ **Creme Speciale, Special Cream for Dry Skin** *($34 for 1.7 ounces)* is similar to the Creme de Jour above and the same basic comments apply.

☹ **Creme Toutes Peaux, Cream for All Skin Types** *($37 for 1.7 ounces)* is similar to the Creme de Jour above and the same basic comments apply.

☺ $$$ **Hydra-Matt Fluid for Oily Skin** *($27 for 1.7 ounces)* is an OK, lightweight moisturizer for normal to slightly dry skin that contains a small amount of water-binding agents and a teeny amount of antioxidant.

☺ $$$ **Hydro-Protective Cream** *($33 for 1.7 ounces)* is just water, thickening agents, shea butter, a teeny amount of antioxidant, and preservatives. This is just an ordinary moisturizer for normal to dry skin.

☺ **$$$ Hydra-Protective Softening Emulsion** *($31 for 1.7 ounces)* is an emollient lotion for normal to dry skin that has a small amount of water-binding agents and a minute amount of antioxidant.

☺ **$$$ Hydrobase Light Moisture Base** *($33 for 1.7 ounces)* is an exceedingly ordinary moisturizer for normal to dry skin that contains the most minute dusting of antioxidant and water-binding agent imaginable. The less than 1% concentration of lactic acid makes it ineffective as an exfoliant.

☹ **Hydroptimale Creme for Dehydrated Skin** *($49 for 1.7 ounces)* is an OK moisturizer for dry skin that contains the preservative Kathon CG, which is not recommended for use in leave-on skin-care products.

☹ **Hydroptimale Gel for Normal Skin** *($46 for 1.7 ounces)* is similar to the Hydroptimale Creme above, and the same comments apply.

✓☺ **$$$ Immunisience Cream for Sensitive Skin** *($32 for 1.7 ounces)* is an emollient moisturizer with some good water-binding agents and antioxidants. It is an option for someone with normal to dry skin.

✓☺ **$$$ Immunisience Fluid for Ultra-Sensitive Skin** *($32 for 1.7 ounces)* is similar to the Immunisience Cream above, and the same basic comments apply.

☹ **Lift Defense Enriched Cream** *($50 for 1.7 ounces)* is an OK moisturizer for normal to dry skin, but it contains the preservative Kathon CG, which is not recommended for use in leave-on skin-care products.

☹ **Lift Defense Enriched Silky Cream** *($50 for 1.7 ounces)* is an OK moisturizer for normal to dry skin, but it contains the preservative Kathon CG, which is not recommended for use in leave-on skin-care products.

☺ **$$$ Moisturizing Intensive Care Liposomes Hydrogel** *($62 for 1.7 ounces)* is a good, emollient moisturizer for normal to dry skin that contains a small amount of water-binding agents and some good antioxidants in the form of olive oil.

☹ **Nutrithys Day Creme for Dry Skin** *($32 for 1.7 ounces)* is an OK moisturizer for normal to dry skin, but it contains the preservative Kathon CG, which is not recommended for use in leave-on skin-care products.

☹ **Nutrithys Creme for Ultra-Dry Skin** *($33 for 1.7 ounces)* is an OK, ordinary moisturizer for normal to dry skin (not ultra-dry skin), but it contains the preservative Kathon CG, which is not recommended for use in leave-on skin-care products.

☺ **$$$ Nutrithys Nourishing Serum for Dry Skin** *($45 for 1 ounce)* is a good, emollient moisturizer for normal to dry skin that contains a small amount of water-binding agent and a teeny amount of antioxidants.

☺ **$$$ Source de Radiance Oxygenating Serum** *($55 for 1 ounce)*. The good news is that, despite the name, there is nothing in this product that can provide extra oxygen to the skin, because if it could that would only generate free-radical damage. Other than that it contains a small amount of water-binding agents and antioxidants. Regrettably, the plant extracts are a mix of irritants and anti-irritants.

☹ **Oxyliance Creme for Normal/Dry Skin** *($52 for 1.7 ounces)* is similar to the Oxygenating Serum above, except that this version contains the preservative Kathon CG, which is not recommended for use in leave-on skin-care products.

☹ **Oxyliance Fluid for Combination Skin** *($52 for 1.7 ounces)* is an OK moisturizer for normal to dry skin, but it contains the preservative Kathon CG, which is not recommended for use in leave-on skin-care products.

☹ **Placentyl Cell Renewal Cream, with Vegetable Protein** *($33 for 1.7 ounces)* is an exceptionally mundane moisturizer that contains mostly water and thickening agents; it lacks any ingredients of benefit to skin. It also contains the preservative Kathon CG, which is not recommended for use in leave-on skin-care products.

☺ **$$$ Retinol 15** *($48 for 1.05 ounces)* does contain retinol, as well as small amounts of vitamins E and C, in a standard emollient base that is an option for normal to dry skin. However, there is nothing about this formulation that makes it better than less expensive versions from L'Oreal and Cetaphil that also contain retinol and are available for one-fourth the price.

☺ **$$$ Secrets de Sothys** *($120 for 1.7 ounces)*. The only secret about this product is why someone would be willing to spend this much money on such an ordinary moisturizer. It is emollient and would be an OK option for normal to dry skin, although the amount of water-binding agents and antioxidants is so minute it's almost funny.

☹ **Serum Clarte, Clearness Serum, Fragile Capillaries Line** *($50 for 1 ounce)* contains the preservative Kathon CG, which is not recommended for use in leave-on skin-care products. It also contains arnica, which is a potent skin irritant.

☹ **Serum Purifiant, Purifying Serum for Oily Skin** *($50 for 1 ounce)* lists alcohol as the second ingredient, which makes this potentially too drying and irritating for all skin types. It does contain a small amount of triclosan, a topical disinfectant, but there is no research showing that to be effective against the bacteria that cause blemishes.

☹ **Time Interceptor Night Cream** *($50 for 1.7 ounces)* contains about 3% AHAs, but the pH of this product is too high for them to be effective for exfoliation. This is an emollient moisturizer with some good water-binding agents but only a minuscule amount of antioxidants. Unfortunately, it also contains the preservative Kathon CG, which is not recommended for use in leave-on skin-care products.

☺ **High Protection Cream SPF 15** *($21 for 2.5 ounces)* is a very good, in-part titanium dioxide–based sunscreen in an ordinary moisturizing base. This does contain some good water-binding agents, but the amount is so minuscule they are completely inconsequential for skin.

☺ **Sunblock for Exposed Areas SPF 30** *($16.50 for 0.8 ounce)*. The name of this product is strange, because why would you apply sunscreen to any part of your body covered by clothing? This is similar to the misnamed High Protection version above, because an SPF 30 product provides longer sun protection than an SPF 15 product.

☺ **SPF 25 Sunblock** *($23 for 2.5 ounces)* is similar to the High Protection version above, and the same comments apply.

☹ **Intense Sun Spray SPF 4** *($21 for 5 ounces)*. A skin-care company selling a product meant to encourage tanning is like an oncologist encouraging someone to smoke cigarettes. This is an offensive product and it is not recommended.

☹ **Tanning Activator SPF 4** *($21 for 5 ounces)* is similar to the Intense Sun Spray above and the same comments apply.

☹ **Hydrating Tanning Lotion SPF 8** *($21 for 5.1 ounces)* is similar to the Intense Sun Spray above and the same comments apply.

☹ **Protecting Tanning Spray SPF 12** *($21 for 5 ounces)* has an SPF 12, which is less than the standard SPF 15 recommended by the American Academy of Dermatology and the Skin Cancer Foundation. More important, it doesn't contain the UVA-protecting ingredients of titanium dioxide, zinc oxide, or avobenzone, and it is not recommended.

☺ **Illuminating Express Self-Tanner** *($21 for 4.2 ounces)* contains dihydroxyacetone, the same ingredient all self-tanners use to affect the color of skin. This one would work as well as any.

☹ **Absorbent Mask for Oily Skin** *($25 for 1.7 ounces)* is an exceedingly standard clay mask with some thickening agents that may be a problem for oily skin. It also contains menthol, which can be a skin irritant and is not helpful for any skin type.

☺ **$$$ Active-Contour Destressing Mask** *($30 for 1 ounce)* contains nothing that can "de-stress" skin. It is just a very simple moisturizer with a tiny amount of water-binding agents and that's about it. The plant extracts are a mix of irritants and anti-irritants.

☺ **$$$ Hydroptimale Mask** *($29 for 1.7 ounces)* is an emollient moisturizer for dry skin that has little benefit as a mask. It contains some good plant oils, but lacks antioxidants and significant water-binding agents.

☺ **$$$ Hydra-Protective Vitality Mask** *($25 for 1.7 ounces)* is a standard clay mask that also contains some plant oils. This can be an option for normal to slightly oily or dry skin. The yeast offers no special benefits for skin, though it may have some minor antioxidant properties.

☹ **Immuniscience Mask** *($30 for 1.7 ounces)* is a standard clay mask with some plant oil and a tiny amount of water-binding agents. The arnica can be a skin irritant.

☺ **$$$ Refirming Mask** *($28 for 1.7 ounces)* contains nothing that can firm skin in the least, though that should not be a surprise. It simply contains water, water-binding agent, slip agent, thickeners, and preservatives. It isn't even a very good moisturizer.

☺ **$$$ Time Interceptor Mask with AHA** *($32 for 1.7 ounces)* is nothing more than an ordinary, emollient moisturizer for dry skin with a tiny amount of AHAs. The concentration of AHAs is too low for it to be effective for exfoliation, and the pH of this product is too high for that anyway.

ST. IVES (SKIN CARE ONLY)

With few notable exceptions, this Los Angeles–made pseudo–spa line with its "high on the mountaintops of Switzerland" allure is one of the most mundane at the drugstore. The prices are very reasonable, but considering the number of Swiss-themed products fraught with potent irritants, you would be wise to look past most of these products and focus on the skin-friendly offerings from Neutrogena, Olay, Pond's, and well, just about everyone else crowding the shelves. For more information about St. Ives, call (800) 333-0005 or visit www.stives.com. **Note:** All St. Ives products contain fragrance unless otherwise noted.

☺ **Cream Cleanser with Soothing Chamomile** *($2.79 for 6 ounces)* is a mineral oil–based, wipe-off makeup remover that also contains lanolin oil and plant oil. It is an option for dry to very dry skin.

☺ **Age-Defying Hydroxy Cleanser** *($3.99 for 12 ounces)* is a standard, mineral oil–based, wipe-off cleanser that can leave a greasy film on the skin. It can be an option for someone with dry skin. This does contain about a 2% concentration of AHAs and about 0.5% BHA, but in these small amounts, and given the high pH of this product, they are ineffective as exfoliants.

☺ **Foaming Facial Apricot Cleanser** *($3.99 for 10 ounces)* is a standard, detergent-based cleanser that can be an option for someone with normal to oily skin.

☺ **Peaches and Cream Renewal Wash** *($4.09 for 12 ounces)* is a standard, detergent-based, water-soluble cleanser that would be an option for someone with normal to oily skin. It does contain about 1% BHA, but that is a problem in a cleanser because it can get in the eyes, even though the pH of this product is too high for the BHA to be effective as an exfoliant. Besides, BHA works better when its effect isn't just washed down the drain.

☹ **Purifying Clear Pore Cleanser** *($4.09 for 12 ounces)* is similar to the Cream Renewal Wash above and the same basic comments apply, although this version adds eucalyptus, lemon, thyme, and bergamot to the mix, making this too irritating for all skin types.

☺ **Apricot Exfoliating Cleansing Cloths** *($5.99 for 30 cloths)* contains standard detergent cleansing agents soaked on cloths. These would work as well as any.

☹ **Medicated Apricot Scrub with Soothing Elder Flower** *($2.99 for 6 ounces)* includes sodium lauryl sulfate among the cleansing agents, which makes it too potentially irritating for all skin types. It also contains lanolin oil, making it a problem for oily or blemish-prone skin.

☹ **Invigorating Apricot Scrub with Soothing Elder Flower** *($2.99 for 6 ounces)* is almost identical to the Medicated Apricot Scrub above and the same basic comments apply.

☺ **Ultra Gentle Apricot Scrub Sensitive Skin** *($3.99 for 6 ounces)* is a standard, detergent-based cleanser that uses plant wax as the scrub agent, and that means this would be better for someone with normal to dry skin.

☹ **Shine Control Refreshing Toner** *($3.99 for 12 ounces)* lists alcohol as the second ingredient, which doesn't make this refreshing in the least, though it does make it drying and irritating for all skin types. It also contains eucalyptus, lemon, thyme, and tangerine, which just add fuel to the fire.

☺ **Age-Defying Hydroxy Moisture Lotion** *($2.32 for 6 ounces)* contains about 5% AHA and 1% BHA in a moisturizing base. While this would have been a good combination AHA and BHA product, the pH is too high for it to be effective as an exfoliant. It is still an option, but only as a good moisturizer if you have dry skin.

☺ **Multi-Vitamin Retinol Anti-Wrinkle Cream** *($8.99 for 1.05 ounces)* is an emollient moisturizer that contains retinol. This is as good a retinol product as any, and the packaging is the type that will help keep it stable.

☺ **Vitamin A Anti-Wrinkle Serum** *($6.99 for 14 0.16-ounce capsules)* has no advantage over the Cream version above. The capsules don't help ensure stability any better than the kind of aluminum packaging many lines use (and also how the Cream above is packaged). This is still a good lightweight moisturizer with retinol, but it's just not worth the trouble to break open a capsule every night.

☺ **Vitamin K Dark Circle Diminisher Under Eye Treatment** *($8.99 for 0.5 ounce).* The only research showing vitamin K to be effective for dark circles comes from the company that sells this ingredient and the physician who holds the patent for it. There is no independent research showing vitamin K to be effective for any aspect of skin care. This also contains retinol in an emollient base similar to the Multi-Vitamin Retinol Anti-Wrinkle Cream reviewed above.

☺ **Extra Relief Collagen Elastin Lotion** *($1.99 for 3 ounces)* is a very ordinary, emollient moisturizer for dry skin that contains a teeny amount of water-binding agents (including elastin) and a minute amount of vitamin E.

☺ **Collagen-Elastin Essential Moisturizer** *($3.19 for 18 ounces)* is similar to the Extra Relief version above and the same basic comments apply. The vitamins are present in such a teeny concentration as to be completely inconsequential for skin, and collagen and elastin in a skin-care product cannot affect the collagen or elastin in your skin.

☹ **Protective Nourishing Moisturizer with Vitamins and SPF 15** *($2.79 for 4 ounces)* does not contain the UVA-protecting ingredients of titanium dioxide, zinc oxide, or avobenzone, and is not recommended.

✓☺ **Dark Spot Fade Cream with Vitamins E & A** *($8.99 for 1 ounce)* is a very good 2% hydroquinone-based emollient moisturizer. This also contains a good amount of retinol and other antioxidants. This product has the potential to effectively reduce skin discolorations, and this is definitely an option to consider.

☺ **Hypo-Allergenic Oil-Free Moisturizer** *($2.99 for 4 ounces)* doesn't contain fragrance, and that has benefit for all skin types. However, "hypoallergenic" is not a regulated term so the claim is meaningless. This is a good moisturizer for normal to dry skin that has a good mix of antioxidants and a small amount of water-binding agents.

The Reviews S

☹ **Alpha Hydroxy Exfoliating Peel-Off Masque** *($3.49 for 6 ounces)* lists alcohol as the second ingredient, which makes this too irritating and drying for all skin types.

☺ **Cucumber & Elastin Eye & Face Stress Gel** *($2.79 for 4 ounces).* This is a good lightweight gel moisturizer for normal to slightly dry skin that contains a small amount of antioxidants and water-binding agent.

☺ **Coenzyme Q10 Eye Cream** *($8.99 for 0.5 ounce)* is a rather standard, ordinary moisturizer for normal to dry skin that contains a teeny amount of coenzyme Q10. Coenzyme Q10 can be a good antioxidant for skin, but it is neither the one best antioxidant for skin care nor a miracle ingredient for wrinkles.

☹ **Coenzyme Q10 Wrinkle Corrector with SPF 15** *($8.99 for 2 ounces)* does not contain the UVA-protecting ingredients of titanium dioxide, zinc oxide, or avobenzone, and is not recommended.

STILA (MAKEUP ONLY)

Out of the entire group of makeup artist–branded lines, the most successful and prolific are Bobbi Brown, M.A.C., and Stila. All are Lauder-owned companies that entered the mainstream as independents and eventually found themselves expanding rapidly once under Lauder's corporate wing. Compared to the Bobbi Brown and M.A.C. lines, Stila is the youngest, and when it comes to successfully merging cuteness with chic Stila definitely corners the market. When Stila came on the scene with their shiny aluminum tubes, recycled cardboard packaging, and icon-ready Stila girl, consumers noticed. Makeup artist Jeanine Lobell has been at the helm of Stila since its inception in 1994, and her creations have become the unofficial benchmark for innovation and appealing, feminine packaging. Of course, this innovation is not without its price, and you will find some rather ordinary products where the packaging is the only thing that's exciting. Where Lobell struck gold is with her superlative collection of foundations. I've examined hundreds of makeup lines for this and previous editions of this book, and I can say unequivocally that (as of this writing) Stila has the best collection of truly neutral foundation colors. For anyone confused about what I mean by "neutral tones," you need look no further. I wish the prices weren't so high, but it's critical to get foundation right, and that may mean splurging. The rest of Stila offers a mostly excellent combination of what most makeup artist–driven lines do so well, such as attractive blush and eyeshadow options, neutral powders, and expertly designed brushes. You will also find Stila to be a great line to shop if you're interested in assembling a makeup palette. They sell several versions, and you can choose which colors to fill them with, which is always a plus. It's not surprising that this line has taken off and remains a favorite among cosmetics-savvy shoppers. Stila's unique-looking products and easygoing feminine flair stir curiosity, and once you're at the counter and know where to focus your attention, you will find this line is a pleasure to use and, dare I say, fun. For more information about Stila, call (888) 550-4567 or visit www.stilacosmetics.com.

FOUNDATION: ✓☺ $$$ **Complete Coverage** *($40)* is housed in an aluminum tube. The name is a bit misleading, as this elegantly smooth, easy-to-blend foundation provides medium coverage at most. The lightly creamy formula is best for normal to dry skin. Almost all of the ten pigment-dense shades are gorgeous and truly neutral. The only ones to avoid are shade H (though this may work for some dark skin tones) and the too-orange shade I. ✓☺ $$$ **Liquid Makeup** *($30)* is preferred to the one above if you desire a sheer-to-light-coverage foundation that is slightly creamy and dries to a natural, sheer finish. The colors are superior—there's not a bad one in the bunch—making this excellent for normal to slightly dry or slightly oily skin types. ✓☺ $$$ **Illuminating Powder Foundation SPF 12** *($23 for powder; $20 for compact)* now lists titanium dioxide as an active ingredient, so you can rely on this for sun protection, though SPF 15 would be preferred. This talc-based powder foundation is inordinately silky and applies seamlessly, offering light, nonpowdery coverage and a barely-there shiny finish. The nine shades are breathtaking and not to be missed if you prefer this type of foundation and don't mind the initially high price. ✓☺ $$$ **Illuminating Liquid Foundation** *($35)* is the fluid counterpart to the Illuminating Powder Foundation. This creamy, mineral oil–based makeup is a treat for normal to dry skin seeking light to medium coverage with a satin-smooth, shiny finish. The shine is more noticeable than in the powder version, but with a sheer powder dusted over it, this can lend a radiant glow to the skin. Of the ten shades, the only one to avoid is 70 Watts.

CONCEALER: ☹ $$$ **Eye Concealer** *($16)* comes in a round glass pot and is a rather thick, dry concealer that provides great coverage and a slightly powdery finish. This is drier than it has been in the past, and talc is now the first ingredient. Unless you're very careful with the application it can look heavy and appear too chalky. If you can master the application and find a good color, this does cover dark circles quite well. Avoid Dark, which is too peach for most skin tones.

☺ $$$ **Cover-Up Stick** *($17)* is a roll-up stick concealer. Alas, this has a creamy texture that will easily lend itself to creasing under the eye. However, this is fine to use if you need heavier coverage over birthmarks or broken capillaries, as the colors are almost all excellent, although this is not a matte-finish concealer, as stated. Shade F is an iffy color that may be too orange for its intended skin tone, but the other deeper shades are great.

POWDER: ☺ $$$ **Loose Powder** *($27)* has a velvety-soft texture and a smooth, dry finish, which is exactly what a good powder should have. The color selection is limited, and the container (saltshaker style) is not my favorite, but if that and the high price don't bother you, it's worth purchasing. Avoid Fair, which is pure white; if white is what you want, save your money and use plain baby powder instead. **Pressed Powder** *($17 for powder cake, $15 for refillable compact)* has a nice, but dry, texture and a smooth application that blends evenly. The color selection has been expanded in both lighter and darker directions. Avoid the pure white Fair, and use caution with the slightly peach Warm. **Illuminating Pressed Powder** *($35)* has a lush, talc-based texture that meshes well with skin. This dual-sided powder puts matte and shiny versions of the same color side by side, and ironically, the shiny version is smoother. Although this defeats the purpose of powdering to dust down shine, the five colors (save for Fair) are fine options. **Sun** *($36)* is an overpriced bronzing powder that has a soft shine but almost irresistible colors, particularly the golden brown Sun 2.

☺ $$$ **All Over Shimmer Powder** *($30)* is a very shiny talc-based pressed powder that works for highlighting, but is hard to control and is a bit flaky. Shiny powders abound for a lot less money than this.

BLUSH: Stila features a good selection of ☺ $$$ **Blush** *($16)* colors that have a slightly dry texture, which can make blending difficult. There are some choice matte shades and the in-demand shiny colors, but these go on sheer, and the lack of smoothness is disappointing.

☺ $$$ **Convertible Color Dual Lip and Cheek Cream** *($28)* is a find for dry skin. This is basically a sheer, emollient blush that feels more like a lipstick in compact form. This is intended for use on lips and cheeks for a simple, easy, "finger-painted" look. The texture is creamy bordering on greasy (akin to traditional lipstick), and the large color range is exceptional, with a few eye-catching sheer, but bright, hues.

EYESHADOW: Stila's ✔☺ $$$ **Eyeshadows** *($16)*, in contrast to the blush, have a gorgeous, smooth texture that blends very well. Shine rules the roost here, but at least these apply easily and cling well. The matte options include Bouquet, Chinois, Dune, Eden, Fog, Toffee, and Urchin.

☺ **Eye Rouge** *($15)* offers two pale, pastel colors that leave a shiny finish. The dance-themed names are almost too cute to pass up, but the shine is too much for daytime.

☺ $$$ **Eye Glaze** *($24)* is a relatively creaseproof sheer liquid eyeshadow that is cleverly dispensed from a pen-style applicator. You get an incredibly small amount of product for your money, and all of the colors are slightly to very shiny, but these do have potential for an evening look. Caution: The sponge tip will dry out and stiffen if you leave this uncapped. **Convertible Eye Color** *($28)* is a dual-ended product that gives you an automatic, retractable eye pencil along with an iridescent powder eyeshadow dispensed from a sponge tip. This can be a fun product if you like shine, but Clinique's Quick Eyes is nearly identical (though you have to sharpen the pencil) for almost half the price.

☺ **EYE AND BROW SHAPER: Brow Set** *($15)* offers two slightly shiny brown shades in one pan for lining the eyes and shaping the brows, but the two colors will not work for everyone. It's an option, but the price is steep for what you get. If this price range is acceptable, consider Bobbi Brown's brow-defining options instead.

☺ $$$ **LIPSTICK AND LIP PENCIL:** The small selection of **Lipstick** *($16.50)* colors are available in four finishes, none of which are designated on the tester unit, which is frustrating. There are **Creams**, which are traditionally creamy with a thick, glossy finish, and **Mattes**, which are more creamy than matte but definitely opaque. The **Sheers** are identical in texture to the Creams, only with less color, and the **Velvets** are indistinguishable from the Mattes. With the exception of the Sheers, all have a good amount of stain that helps keep the color on the lips. **Lip Gloss** *($17)* comes in a squeeze tube with a slightly sticky feel; and there's a wide range of colors. L'Oreal's Glass Shine Lip Gloss is nearly identical to this for half the price. **Demi Creme** *($24)* is packaged just like the Lip Polish and Lip Glaze below, but this delivers an elegant, creamy lip color that feels smooth and moist while imparting opaque, glossy color. If you have money to burn, you'll get more bang for your buck with this one's handsome payoff. The **Lip Pencil** *($14)* used to be made of recycled paper, but is now very similar to most other standard pencils. The colors are surprisingly muted, but a few are nicely versatile. **Lip Rouge** *($26)* claims to be a magic marker for the lips. I wouldn't call it indelible, but it has some excellent staying power, just not as much as you would expect for the money. (This is similar to Lip Ink, which is also reviewed in this edition.) Inside a fountain pen–style package, a very pigmented liquid is fed into a brush tip, which is applied to the lips; it then sets into a long-lasting, feel-like-nothing stain. One word of warning: It dries up easily and the hard brush tip makes application almost painful.

☺ **$$$ Lip Polish** *($24)* is a lip gloss in a self-dispensing brush applicator, for more money than this clever packaging is really worth. A few clicks at the base release a flow of gloss onto the lip-brush applicator. It's nifty and convenient, but it is just a gloss, and an unbearably sticky one at that. **Lip Glaze** *($24)* has the same container as the Lip Polish, but this is a group of sheer, fruit-and-berry flavored glosses that are way too sticky for someone who doesn't want the fact that they're wearing gloss to be a constant, irksome reminder. **Lip Glaze Palette** *($45)* is for those who can't decide which color or flavor to purchase. You get ten Lip Glaze colors housed in split pans in a slim compact. This is certainly worth a look if you flip over this overpriced product. **Pocket Palette** *($36)* is more sticky lip gloss (four shades to be exact). These are just small amounts of lip gloss in a compact, and the amount of each is so small the price is out of line.

☹ **MASCARA:** The **Mascara** *($16)* goes on too wet, and never really achieves any length or thickness without creating a clumpy, smear-prone mess. It's almost shocking that this has not changed or been retooled after four years, especially given Lauder's (and almost everyone else's) tendency to launch new mascaras.

BRUSHES: Stila provides several great ✓☺ **$$$ Brushes** *($15–$58)*, most with a soft but firm feel and excellent shapes. There are even a few dual-sided and retractable options, and almost every brush is available in long- or short-handled versions. Stop by and check these out if you are shopping for brushes, but try to avoid the ☹ **#4 Precision Liner** *($15)*, which is too thick and soft to create a fine line; the **#7 Precision Crease** *($17)*, which is too floppy for detailed crease work, and the too small, incomplete **Brush Set** *($75)*. The ☺ **$$$ Brow Brush** *($17)* is too thin for a softly defined brow, but works well for eyelining. The **Blush Brush** *($25)* is not as soft as it could be, but is still an option.

SPECIALTY: ☺ **$$$ All Over Shimmer** *($28)* is a slick cream that feels somewhat powdery, but never quite dries and doesn't stay in place. It is easy to rub off or smear even after you think it has been absorbed. The colors are loaded with shine, and they will do nicely to add glistening glow to the skin, but this can also flake while you're wearing it.

☺ $$$ **All Over Shimmer Body** *($28)* is easier to work with and is a diluted, lotion version of the regular All Over Shimmer above. The two shades offer warm (gold) or cool (silver) shimmer, and this is a decent option for evening body glamour. **Flaunt** *($35)* is a large container of shimmery, fragranced body powder. For those times when you feel like shining from head to toe and want a whiff of scent, too, throw common sense out the window and flaunt!

✔☺ $$$ **4-Pan Compact** *($12)* is a sturdy cardboard compact that you can fill with the eyeshadow and blush tins of your choice. These are a great option if you're stuck on Stila. ☺ $$$ **5-Pan Compact** *($28),* **6-Pan Compact** *($26),* and **8-Pan Compact** *($38)* are metal palettes that magnetically hold powder blush, eyeshadow, and brow color pans. This allows you to customize a makeup kit and it's convenient for travel or vanity use. Each mirrored palette includes a brush that's worth keeping, and these certainly hold up better over time than the 4-Pan cardboard compacts. Stila also offers practical, functional **Accessory Bags** and **Train Cases** *($18–$50).*

STILA SPORT MAKEUP

Stila is known for its standout packaging and "Why didn't anyone else think of that?" products. Though the products themselves are rarely unique, their original packaging and dispensing methods are distinctive. Most manage to be quite fetchingly feminine and high tech (the aluminum packaging is attractive) at the same time. This image continues with Stila Sport Makeup, a small collection of products featuring irrefutably sporty names and multipurpose benefits. The concept is intriguing, but the actual products break no new ground in terms of texture or performance. If anything, these colors are so sheer and soft you'll be lucky if they hold up through a standard aerobic workout!

☺ $$$ **Skin Visor SPF 30** *($22 for 2.5 ounces)* is a very good, in-part titanium dioxide–based sunscreen in an ordinary moisturizing base that contains a teeny amount of water-binding agents and antioxidants.

☺ $$$ **H₂O Off** *($18 for 40 cloths)* is a standard, detergent-based cleanser soaked onto fairly soft cloths. These work and are fragrance free!

✔☺ $$$ **Pivotal Skin Foundation SPF 8** *($25)* is a unique, modernized foundation that features a sponge (secured to the inside compartment) soaked with a silicone-based makeup. You apply the foundation with your fingers (as Stila recommends) or with your own sponge. The makeup itself has a semi-fluid, lightweight, and slippery texture that applies easily and blends well, leaving sheer coverage and a very soft matte finish. The titanium dioxide–based sunscreen has an SPF that's too low for recommended daily protection, but will nicely augment a sunscreen worn underneath this foundation. There are ten shades, and that includes some great sheer colors for darker skin tones! Shade I is the only disappointment in an otherwise stellar roster.

☺ **$$$ Pivotal Sun Bronzing Tint** *($25)* is similar in concept and identical in execution to the Pivotal Skin Foundation above. The main differences with this formula are the absence of sunscreen and the addition of a soft shimmer finish. The two bronze tones are great, but very sheer, so successive applications will be necessary for a noticeable tan look.

☺ **$$$ Color Push-Ups All Over Color** *($20)* is a sheer cream blush that comes in solid form and is housed in a deodorant-style container. It applies and blends reasonably well, and leaves a slightly moist finish. The colors are beautiful, and this would be an option for those with dry skin who prefer a moist finish and soft application. It's a good thing that the concept of a little goes a long way applies here, as this is pricey for blush.

☹ **Clear Color SPF 8** *($12)* offers a too-low SPF without any UVA protection, which makes this an otherwise completely standard, sheer lipstick with a glossy, slippery finish and pretty colors. The only new feature is the incredibly small package, and only half of that is actual product.

☹ **Color Courier** *($20)* is a creamy, oversized, standard pencil that can be used on lips and cheeks. This version glides on well, but the slick, creamy texture won't last long, especially if you have anything sporty planned.

✓☺ **$$$ Lash Visor Waterproof Mascara** *($16)* is a vast improvement over Stila's regular mascara. As is the case for most waterproof mascaras, this is not much for thickness. However, it does lengthen nicely and applies easily, with no clumps or flaking. Bottom line: You can expect long wear and it is most definitely waterproof.

STRI-DEX (SKIN CARE ONLY)

What do you get when you take the most useless, terribly irritating ingredients for acne (or any skin condition, for that matter) and dress them up in colorful boxes with teen-appeal zit-zapper lingo? None other than Stri-Dex, a problematic line that has been masquerading as a sensible purveyor of anti-acne products for far too long. There is not a single product in this line that can be of genuine help to anyone with blemishes or blackheads, and the fact that it has lasted this long means too many consumers have continued to needlessly suffer through red, irritated skin while hoping their blemishes would heal using Stri-Dex. What a shame. For more information about Stri-Dex, call (800) 761-1078 or visit www.stridex.com.

☹ **Antibacterial Foam Wash, Herbal** *($4.89 for 6 ounces)* is a standard, detergent-based cleanser that also contains 1% triclosan, a topical disinfectant. However, there is no research showing this to be effective against the bacteria that cause acne.

☹ **Anti-Bacterial Foaming Wash, Cooling** *($4.99 for 6 ounces)* contains both peppermint and menthol, and while that may feel cooling it is also a problem for causing irritation and redness, and that isn't helpful for any skin type. This does contain 1% triclosan, a topical disinfectant, but there is no research showing it to be effective against the bacteria that cause acne.

☹ **Facewipes to Go** (*$5.49 for 32 cloths*) contain menthol, as well as alcohol, high up on the ingredient list, making this a problem for all skin types. There is nothing beneficial about irritating skin; if anything, it can hurt the skin's immune response, making it harder for blemishes to heal.

☺ **Day & Night Acne Medication** (*$7.49 for one set of the Day Gel and Night Gel*). The Day Gel contains alcohol and witch hazel distillate (which is also mostly alcohol) and that makes it too potentially drying and irritating for all skin types. That is disappointing, because the 2% concentration of salicylic acid it contains would be effective for exfoliation. The Night Gel is a very good 2.5% benzoyl peroxide lotion. What a shame they don't sell these separately, because the Night Gel is a good option as a topical disinfectant for blemishes.

☹ **Dual Textured Maximum Strength Acne Medication Pads** (*$3.49 for 32 pads*) contain both alcohol and menthol, and that makes a BHA product like this too irritating to even think of using.

☹ **Triple Action Acne Medicated Pads, Maximum Strength Pads** (*$3.44 for 55 pads*) don't contain alcohol, but do include menthol. This also contains some fairly irritating detergent cleansing agents. That is truly disappointing because this 2% salicylic acid product has an effective pH for exfoliation.

☹ **Triple Action Medicated Pads, Sensitive Skin** (*$3.99 for 55 pads*). These contain menthol, which is a problem for all skin types, but especially for someone with sensitive skin. They also contain some problematic detergent cleansing agents.

☹ **Triple Action Medication Pads, Regular Strength** (*$3.49 for 55 pads*) contain menthol and alcohol, which makes this way too irritating for all skin types.

☹ **Triple Action Medicated Pads, Super Scrub Oil Fighting Formula** (*$3.44 for 55 pads*) is almost identical to the Regular Strength version above, and the same comments apply.

SUAVE (SKIN CARE ONLY)

More often than not, I'm a big fan of inexpensive skin-care and makeup products. If the same thing is available for less money, and you can't live without the image and packaging, there is no reason to spend extra cash. I was hoping that concept would hold up for the Suave line of skin-care products, but, alas, it doesn't. That's too bad, because the prices of these products are great. Two of the cleansers are an option for some durable skin types, but they leave a bad taste if you accidentally get any in your mouth and cause slight irritation when used over the eyes. The moisturizers are dated, pointless formulations, and there is no effective sunscreen. For more information about Suave, call (800) 621-2013 or visit www.suave.com.

☺ **Balancing Facial Cleansing Gel** (*$2.75 for 8 ounces*) is supposed to gently clean and maintain the skin's moisture balance. It does clean, but it doesn't maintain any moisture balance, though this standard, detergent-based cleanser can be an option for someone with normal to oily skin.

☺ **Foaming Face Wash** *($2.75 for 8 ounces)* is similar to the Cleansing Gel above, and the same basic comments apply.

☹ **Deep Cleansing Cream** *($3.99 for 7 ounces)* contains menthol, and that makes it potentially irritating for all skin types.

☹ **Deep Cleansing Gel** *($3.99 for 6.7 ounces)* contains sodium C14-16 olefin sulfonate as one of the main detergent cleansing agents, which makes it too drying and irritating for all skin types.

☺ **Water Rinsable Cold Cream** *($1.99 for 4 ounces)* is a standard, wipe-off cold cream made with mineral oil and wax that is not rinseable, as it can leave a slightly greasy film on the skin. However, this can be an OK option for someone with dry skin.

☹ **Transparent Facial Bar** *($1.99 for 3.5 ounces)* is a standard bar cleanser that can be too drying and irritating for all skin types.

☹ **Refreshing Facial Astringent** *($1.99 for 10 ounces)* is mainly water and alcohol, plus menthol and eucalyptus. Ouch!

☺ **Revitalizing Anti-Wrinkle Cream** *($4.99 for 2 ounces)* contains about 8% glycolic acid (AHA) in an ordinary moisturizing base of thickening agents and slip agents. However, the pH of this product is too high for the AHA to be effective for exfoliation.

☹ **Hydrating Beauty Cream** *($4.99 for 2 ounces)* is an extremely poor and dated moisturizer that contains little more than water and thickening agents. This isn't beautiful; if anything, it's rather pathetic.

☹ **Hydrating Beauty Lotion** *($4.99 for 4 ounces)* is similar to the Hydrating Beauty Cream above, and the same comments apply.

☹ **Hydrating Overnight Cream** *($3.99 for 2 ounces)* is similar to the Hydrating Beauty Cream above, and the same comments apply.

☹ **UV Protective Moisture Lotion SPF 15** *($3.99 for 4 ounces)* doesn't contain the UVA-protecting ingredients of titanium dioxide, zinc oxide, or avobenzone, and is not recommended.

SUE DEVITT STUDIO MAKEUP

As if the onslaught of American-based makeup lines weren't enough, we now have the Australian import Sue Devitt Studio as one more option in this once-a-niche category of the cosmetics world. According to www.suedevittstudio.com, "Devitt first received recognition in the industry at NARS, where she worked as creative assistant to Francois Nars for two years. Being the youngest makeup artist in history to be awarded an international product development contract for the Japanese and U.S. markets, Sue was responsible for the creation of the extensive color line AWAKE, receiving praise for her work and securing a nomination as one of the world's top cosmetic forecasters." Apparently, lines like M.A.C., Bobbi Brown, and Stila were not meeting the needs of Australian cosmetics consumers, as Devitt maintains that "…the Australian market was not adequately serviced at a premium level, especially in terms of the colours and textures being created for our climate and lifestyle." I am not certain what she means by premium service, but her line is only available in Australia via mail order, while it is expanding rapidly at the retail level in the United States. Furthermore, if she is referring to elegant, modern, and functional products, almost every makeup artist–driven line has this in spades, including Devitt's. And nothing in particular about Devitt's makeup is better suited to Australia's temperate, often sun-drenched climate. If anything, the fact that none of Devitt's foundations offer significant sun protection is a serious problem for those who live in Australia and anywhere else. When asked if her foundations contain sun protection, Devitt replied "Yes, SPF 10. I prefer not to increase that coverage as it thickens the formulations and they can appear heavy and old-fashioned. I prefer to offer women a lightweight, modern coverage and leave it up to them as individuals to increase or decrease their sunscreen coverage." I understand the logic behind avoiding a foundation that feels heavy, but if other cosmetics companies can produce lightweight foundations with effective sunscreens, then so can Devitt, especially since she claims to have "an incredible team of private chemists" working with her. To be fair, only one of Devitt's foundations advertises a sunscreen, but without any active ingredients listed, it cannot be relied on for daily sun protection.

Inaccurate and debatable claims aside, is this line from Down Under worth checking out? For the most part, the answer is yes. This line excels with its foundations, powders, blushes, and eyeshadows, all of which have exemplary textures that make working with them effortless and rewarding. The rest of the makeup offers some acceptable options, but nothing extraordinary, especially at these prices. The makeup brushes are beautiful, but the prices are on the very high end when you consider similar brushes from such artistry lines as Lorac, Laura Mercier, and others. You can find Sue Devitt Studio products at select Sephora, Nordstrom, and Barneys New York stores—but ironically, you'd be hard-pressed to find this line in its native Australia! For more information about Sue Devitt Studio Makeup, call (212) 673-7104.

☺ $$$ <u>FOUNDATION:</u> **Balanced Foundation SPF 10** *($36)* does not list any active ingredients for the sunscreen, which means it cannot be relied on for sun protection even though titanium dioxide is the third ingredient. If you have normal to dry skin and are willing to wear a separate sunscreen underneath this, this foundation's dewy but light texture, natural moist finish, and sheer coverage will delight you. The six shades are all excellent, with options for light and darker skin, though the medium shades are very slightly peach. **70% Triple Seaweed Gel Foundation** *($36)* comes in a pump bottle that tends to squirt out too much product, but if that doesn't bother you, this has a smooth, airy texture that floats over the skin and blends beautifully to a soft matte finish. Coverage runs from sheer to light, and the six mostly neutral shades are top-notch—only Summer Monsoon is too peach for most skin tones. The "70%" label refers to the amount of water in this formula. Although it might seem impressive, lots of foundations contain the same amount of water but simply choose not to spotlight such an ordinary, albeit necessary, ingredient. This does contain seaweed, which can be a good antioxidant.

✓☺ **$$$ Triple C-Weed Whipped Foundation** *($39)* is Devitt's richest foundation, and is a good choice for someone with dry skin who prefers a light but noticeably creamy makeup. This blends exceptionally well, provides sheer to light coverage, and leaves a moist finish. The form of vitamin C this contains is sodium ascorbyl phosphate (also known as L-ascorbic acid), which is a good antioxidant and anti-inflammatory agent. Seaweed is present as well, and functions as an antioxidant. This also features six very good colors that present options for light and dark skin tones, though Nullarbor Plain is too peach for most skin tones.

☹ <u>CONCEALER:</u> **Automatic Camouflage Concealer** *($20)* is a roll-up stick concealer that has a creamy, crease-prone texture and reasonably opaque coverage that tends to dissipate quickly. Compared to the foundation colors, the five shades are disappointingly peach or pink.

<u>POWDER:</u> ✓☺ **$$$ Triple C-Weed Loose Powder** *($29)* is a talc-based powder that has a superlative, ultra-light texture that would change even the most militant antipowder person's mind. It's pricey, but if you feel like splurging, you will find six superior shades. This is also easier to use than many loose powders because it comes in a sturdy tub with a sifter so powder doesn't fly everywhere once the container is opened.

☺ **$$$ Silky Pressed Powder** *($26)* is also talc-based and has a slightly drier texture than the Loose Powder above. Although the finish leaves a slight sheen on the skin, this is not sparkly and is worth a look if you don't mind the price. The six shades are excellent. **Gold Coast Bronzing Powder** *($28)* has a texture similar to the Silky Pressed Powder and comes in one color—a sheer tan shade with a slight red cast. This does have a subtle shimmer, so check it out in daylight before making a final decision.

<u>BLUSH:</u> ✓☺ **$$$ Silky Blush** *($20)* has an awesome silky texture and a smooth, even application. There is an interesting mix of splashy vivid colors and muted tones, and each shade is quite pigmented, so these tend to last well on the skin. The only shiny shade to watch out for is Koh Samui.

☺ **$$$ <u>EYESHADOW:</u> Silky Matte** and **Silky Sheen Eyeshadows** *(both $18)* have a very smooth texture and suitable dry finish. These go on intensely, but blend well. Despite the Matte and Sheen name distinctions, most of the colors are shiny. The few truly matte shades offer some great earthy brown tones.

<u>EYE AND BROW SHAPER:</u> ☺ **$$$ Eye Intensifier Pencil** *($20)* is a standard chunky pencil that claims it is smudgeproof and water-resistant, but ends up being neither. This comes with a sponge tip for blending, and these types of pencils tend to work best for a deliberately smudged or smoky look.

☹ **Eyebrow Pencil** *($18)* is a standard pencil with a stiff, dry texture that isn't worth the effort or the expense.

<u>LIPSTICK AND LIP PENCIL:</u> ☺ **$$$ Balanced Lipstick** *($20)* is available in two formulas. **Balanced Matte** claims it is "groundbreaking," but if this standard creamy, opaque lipstick with a slightly glossy finish is progress, then we may as well go back to

dial-up modems. This is not a bad lipstick by any means—it's just very ordinary and not matte in the least. **Balanced Sheer** is simply a greasy lipstick with the requisite sheer colors and glossy finish. The color range for both of these formulas focuses on brighter hues and reds. **Starbrights** *($35)* features three sheer, slightly greasy lip or cheek colors in a compact. Each shade has some iridescence and these are too slippery to have much longevity.

☺ $$$ **Mini Lip Gloss** *($18)* is fine as a sheer, shiny (and sticky) gloss, yet offers nothing that you can't find in dozens of other lines for a lot less money. **Long-Lasting Lipliner** *($20)* is a standard pencil that features a lip brush for blending the color or applying lipstick. Even though this is overpriced, it does have a smooth, easy-glide texture and great colors.

☹ $$$ <u>MASCARA:</u> **Water-Resistant Mascara** *($28)* applies well with no clumping, but is just average in terms of building length and thickness. This can smear a bit if you're not careful, but it wears well. It's definitely not worth the extra expense considering the superior mascaras available at the drugstore.

☺ $$$ <u>BRUSHES:</u> Sue Devitt Studio **Brushes** *($15–$70)* offer some beautiful natural-hair options, and are available in regular and what Devitt refers to as mini-travel sizes. The **Powder Brush** *($45)* is the size of a standard blush brush, and too sparse for concise application of powder, while the **Blush Brush** *($50)* is sized like a powder brush but is also too sparse for its task. The various **Eye Base Brushes** *($45–$70)* and **Lashline Definer** *($55)* are excellent, but way overpriced. Finally, the **Mini Travel Lip Brush** *($30)* is as standard as they come, and with no cap or retractability, this is one expensive inconvenience.

T. LE CLERC

Theophile Le Clerc, a French pharmacist, was fond of creating makeup at his Paris drugstore, and his best-known "invention" turned out to be loose powder. Apparently, it was quite a hit at the turn of the nineteenth century. The present-day resurgence of this standard, very overpriced, talc-based powder has been the key to open the gates for this small company's expansion into the United States. A complete makeup line now complements the original loose powders, and T. Le Clerc has been quick to capitalize on the powder's alleged status with celebrities. The hype surrounding this line makes it seem very tempting, but let me assure you there is nothing here that is at all deserving of such steep price tags. The powders are mostly talc and rice starch, along with a touch of zinc oxide for coverage (but not for sun protection). Rice starch lends a light, dry feel to powders but it's hardly unique, and can actually cause problems for those with sensitive skin or a tendency toward breakouts. There are dozens and dozens of powders that perform just as well as these, at prices from $5 to $30. The add-on makeup items deliver little to extol, with the exception of one incredible mascara. If you're dying to test these for yourself, that's easy enough to do—but before you purchase, make sure you can confidently say to yourself, "I am willingly paying top dollar for a remarkably ordinary product." If that sits well with you, nothing in the reviews below is likely to dissuade you. For more information about T. Le Clerc, call (800) 788-4731. **Note:** All T. Le Clerc products contain fragrance.

T. Le Clerc Skin Care

☺ **$$$ Gentle Cleansing Milk** *($27.50 for 6.7 ounces)* is indeed gentle, containing one of the less irritating detergent cleansing agents in an emollient base. It doesn't remove makeup very well and can leave a slightly greasy film on the skin, but it can be a good option for someone with dry skin. However, for the money, it is virtually identical to Neutrogena's Extra Gentle Cleanser ($5.49 for 6.7 ounces).

☺ **$$$ Purifying Gel Cleanser** *($25 for 4.16 ounces)* is a standard, but good, detergent-based cleanser that would work well for someone with normal to oily skin. However, there is nothing about this formulation to make it preferred over far less pricey versions at the drugstore.

☺ **Lip and Eye Make-Up Remover** *($19 for 4.16 ounces)* is a standard, detergent-based makeup remover similar to almost every other one reviewed in this book.

☹ **Gentle Toning Lotion** *($22.50 for 6.7 ounces)* is an OK toner for most skin types, containing mostly water, slip agents, aloe, water-binding agents, preservatives, and fragrance.

☹ **$$$ Moisture Soothe Serum** *($50 for 1 ounce)* is an OK, though ordinary, moisturizer for normal to dry skin that contains a tiny amount of antioxidants and even fewer water-binding agents.

☹ **Oil Control Serum** *($45 for 1 ounce)* lists alcohol as the second ingredient. That doesn't control oil, but it can cause dryness and irritation for all skin types.

☹ **$$$ Total Hydration Creme** *($50 for 2 ounces)* is an emollient moisturizer that contains an impressive mix of water-binding agents but no antioxidants.

☹ **$$$ Total Hydration Fluid** *($45 for 1.7 ounces)* is similar to the Total Hydration Creme above only in lotion form, and the same basic comments apply.

☹ **$$$ Wrinkle Control Creme 901** *($70 for 1.7 ounces)*. Nothing in this can control wrinkles in the least—it is just an emollient moisturizer that contains a good mix of water-binding agents, but only the teeniest amount of antioxidants.

T. Le Clerc Makeup

FOUNDATION: ☹ **$$$ Matte Fluid Foundation** *($37)* has a thick, slightly dry texture and a natural matte finish. This provides medium to full coverage that may feel (and look) heavy. The six colors are acceptable, though Rose, Ochre, and Beige can be too pink or peach for most skin tones.

☺ **$$$ Powder Compact Foundation** *($45)* is a standard, pressed powder–type foundation that has a very soft texture and a satin finish with a small amount of shine. The formula is talc-free and all six colors are worthwhile. The only drawback is the steep price.

☺ $$$ <u>CONCEALER:</u> T. Le Clerc's **Concealer** *($19)* is similar in feel, application, and finish to the foundation above. This can look heavy and cake under the eye unless it is used sparingly. Of the four shades, the only possible options are Banane and Beige.

☺ $$$ <u>POWDER:</u> **Loose Powder** *($45)* is a talc-based powder that also contains a small amount of rice starch. It has a very fine, dry texture and will work as well as any powder, price notwithstanding. The 20 shades may seem like a real bonus, but most of them are unusually impractical, being all manner of pink, rose, peach, green, lavender, and so on. If you're intent on trying this one, the most realistic skin-tone shades are Translucide, Bistre, Bronze, Nacre, Camelia, Chair Rosee, Cannelle, Chair Ocree, and Rose The. Several of the aforementioned shades look much softer on the skin than they do in the container. **Pressed Powder** *($45)* has the same talc-based texture and matte finish as the Powder Compact Foundation above, save for a slight graininess, and is available in 15 colors. There are several options for fair to medium skin tones, but avoid Dore Soleil, Banane, Orchidee, Tilleul, and Bronze.

☺ $$$ <u>BLUSH:</u> **Powder Blush** *($25)* has a wonderfully silky texture, and the densely pigmented colors are great for darker skin tones. Deplorably, almost all of them have a slight to intense shine that is too obvious for daytime wear.

<u>EYESHADOW:</u> ☺ $$$ **Mono Eye Shadow** *($23)* is sold as tonally similar duos, with no divider between the colors, which makes selecting just one of the colors almost impossible, as the brush will likely pick up both shades. The texture is dry and powdery, but blends better than you might expect. All the "mono" eye shadows are intensely shiny, and while they may work for an evening look, they're not well-suited for the light of day. **Duo-Eyeshadows** *($23)* are identical to the Mono Shadows, except that they have distinctive light and dark colors positioned side by side in one compact, with most of them being highly contrasting.

☹ **Powder Eyeshimmer** *($20)* is one of the priciest cream-to-powder eyeshadows around, especially considering that the proof is not in the pudding with this one. In fact, this is a mess of flaky shine that's leagues below many other shadows.

<u>EYE AND BROW SHAPER:</u> ☺ **Eye Pencil** *($15)* is a standard pencil that has a creamy, easy-glide texture and a dry finish. It's tricky to get a thin line with this one, but there are several colors to consider.

☹ **Eyebrow Pencil** *($17)* has an impossibly hard, dry texture that is painful to apply and not worth the bother or expense. **All Over Glitter Pencil** *($22.50)* is a thick pencil infused with large flecks of glitter. It's messy to use and the glitter tends to stick just where you don't want it.

☺ $$$ <u>LIPSTICK AND LIP PENCIL:</u> **Satin Lipsticks** *($20)* are creamy lipsticks with an opulent, glossy finish. The color range is stunning, with some great reds. Still, dollar for dollar, I wouldn't choose this formula over creamy lipsticks from Revlon or M.A.C. **Matte Lipstick** *($23)* is definitely not matte, but actually creamy and slick, with a slightly greasy finish. The small selection of colors has a nice stain, so these do wear moderately well. **Liquid Matte Lipstick** *($23)* is a full-coverage lip gloss that's definitely not matte, but it doesn't provide a wet, glossy look either. This product is available exclusively online, but you can find similar products that sell for one-third the price from Revlon or L'Oreal. **Lip Gloss** *($19)* features a small selection of sheer, iridescent colors with a light, non-sticky texture. The price is way out of line for gloss, despite the positives. **Lip Pencil** *($15)* is utterly standard, and any other pencil at the drugstore would perform as well as this.

MASCARA: ✔☺ $$$ **Mascara** *($19)* goes on well, building great length and some thickness with only minimal clumping, and it lasts all day without smudging or flaking. Forget the overhyped powders and try this instead!

☹ **Glitter Mascara** *($19)* is almost bad enough to make you forget about the excellent original mascara, but if you avoid using this flake-prone mess, you won't have the same problems I did!

☹ **BRUSHES:** The three makeup brushes *($25 and $35)* are too large and poorly constructed to recommend for practical, everyday use. If you're going to spend over $40 on powder (though for the life of me I cannot understand why), you may as well splurge on a luxurious powder brush from Laura Mercier, M.A.C., or Stila.

THALGO

Since 1976 Thalgo has been touting the benefit of their "marine algae and plant based cosmetics." Their brochures and Web site are decidedly about the sea and its advantages for skin. "Thalgo treatments draw their richness and efficiency from the marine universe. Our scientific team have developed a unique know-how in harnessing the powerful riches of the sea for aesthetic use." As far as marine ingredients go, small to minuscule amounts of algae extracts and even lesser amounts of sea salt show up in most Thalgo products. Is any of that beneficial for skin? That depends on your perspective. Algae are very simple organisms that have over 20,000 different known species and countless more extracts on top of that. A number of these have been used for drugs, where they work as anticoagulants, antibiotics, antihypertensive agents, blood cholesterol reducers, dilatory agents, insecticides, and anti-tumorigenic agents. In cosmetics, algae are used as thickening agents, water-binding agents, and antioxidants. On the other hand, some algae are also potential skin irritants. For example, the phycocyanin found in blue-green algae has been suspected of allergenicity and of causing dermatitis on the basis of patch tests (Source: *Current Issues in Molecular Biology*, January 2002, pages 1–11). Other forms of algae, such as Irish moss and carrageenan, contain proteins, vitamin A, sugar, starch, vitamin B1, iron, sodium, phosphorus, magnesium, copper, and calcium, which are all useful as sources for skin care, either as emollients or antioxidants (Source: *Journal of Agricultural Food Chemistry*, February 2002, pages 840–845).

However, the claims that algae can stop or eliminate wrinkling, heal skin, cure acne, or provide other elaborate benefits are completely unsubstantiated. Plus, algae extracts are hardly miracles, at least not any more than other vitamins, minerals, plant extracts, antioxidants, and myriad water-binding agents. Perhaps what is most surprising about this overpriced spa line of skin-care products is that they are distinctly unnatural (except for the algae and sea salt) and not exactly overflowing with current state-of-the-art skin-care ingredients. Most of the moisturizers are mineral oil– or Vaseline-based, with nothing more than standard thickening agents, slip agents, and lanolin. There are some good water-binding agents that show up, but that's about it. This line is, almost without exception, about the belief in algae and sea salt meeting all your skin-care needs. Talk about a leap of faith!

One more point: the marine contribution of sea salt in these products is not the best for skin. Salt absorbs moisture and can be a skin irritant. Adding sea salt may conjure up images of the tranquil ocean, but that isn't helpful for skin. For more information about Thalgo, call (800) 228-4254 or visit www.thalgo.com or www.nordstroms.com. **Note:** All Thalgo products contain fragrance.

☹ **Marine Algae Cleansing Bar** *($14 for 3.5 ounces)* is a standard bar cleanser that can be drying for most skin types. It does contain a small amount of algae, but even if algae had benefit for skin, in a cleanser they would just be rinsed down the drain before they could have an effect.

☹ **Delicate Cleansing Milk** *($30 for 10 ounces)* is a mineral oil–based cleanser that also contains sodium lauryl sulfate as the detergent cleansing agent. None of that is gentle and none of that is appropriate for delicate skin.

☹ **Marine Cleansing Milk with AHA** *($30 for 10 ounces)* is similar to the Delicate Cleansing Milk above and the same comments apply. The minute amount of algae has no benefit for skin.

☹ **Combination Skin Cleansing Milk** *($28 for 10.14 ounces)* is similar to the Delicate Cleansing Milk above and the same comments apply. The minute amount of sea salt has no benefit for skin.

☺ $$$ **Silky Cleansing Cream** *($30 for 5.07 ounces)* is a good, but exceptionally standard, detergent-based cleanser that would be an option for normal to oily skin. The addition of sea salt doesn't relate to taking a swim in the ocean or offer any benefit for skin.

☺ $$$ **Thalgodermyl Cleansing Gel** *($24 for 1.7 ounces)* is a standard, and overpriced detergent-based cleanser. It would work well for normal to oily skin but so would lots of cleansers found at the drugstore for a fraction of this price, such as Cetaphil Daily Facial Cleanser for Normal to Oily Skin ($5.99 for 8 ounces). Plus, the Thalgo version doesn't even contain the algae or sea salt that is supposed to make these products worth the cost.

☺ $$$ **Double Action Cleanser and Toner** *($32 for 10.14 ounces)* is an exceedingly basic makeup remover that contains mostly a gentle detergent cleansing agent, aloe, sea salt, and preservatives. It works, but is so completely overpriced for a rote formulation that costs only pennies.

☺ **$$$ Cleansing Lotion for Eyes and Lips** *($18 for 4.2 ounces)* is similar to the Double Action version above only with the addition of two plant extracts that can be anti-irritants.

☹ **Marine Tonic Lotion with AHA** *($28 for 10 ounces)* does not contain AHA. The third ingredient is lime fruit extract, and that is not an AHA. It also contains lemon oil and that isn't an AHA either. Both lemon and lime can be significant skin irritants.

☺ **$$$ Tonifying Lotion Sensitive Skin** *($30 for 10.14 ounces)* is just water, slip agent, plant extracts, detergent-cleansing agent, and preservatives. The plant extracts are good anti-irritants, but this lacks water-binding agents and antioxidants.

☹ **$$$ Tonic Lotion with Marine Nutrients** *($26 for 10.14 ounces)*. The small amount of algae and sea salt in this product doesn't add any nutrients to skin. The algae may have some water-binding or antioxidant benefit for skin, but the sea salt can be a skin irritant.

☹ **$$$ Protective Cream** *($36 for 1.7 ounces)* is an ordinary, mineral oil–based moisturizer with not one interesting water-binding agent or antioxidant.

☹ **$$$ Marine Fluid Exfoliant Cream** *($50 for 1.7 ounces)* is an almost shockingly ordinary moisturizer with a minute amount of sugarcane extract, which does not have any exfoliating properties, and a microscopic amount of green tea and algae.

☺ **$$$ Marine Replenishing Serum with BHA** *($120 for 1 ounce)* does not contain BHA, but this is one of the few Thalgo products that does contain some good water-binding agents and antioxidants. However, there is nothing in this formulation worth the price tag, and it is easily replaced by numerous less pricey alternatives from Neutrogena to Clinique.

☹ **$$$ Marine Night Cream** *($64 for 1.7 ounces)* is an exceptionally ordinary, though emollient, mineral oil– and Vaseline-based moisturizer that contains a small amount of water-binding agents and a minuscule amount of algae. It is an OK option for normal to dry skin.

☹ **$$$ Bio Marine Cream** *($50 for 1.7 ounces)* is similar to the Marine Night Cream above and the same basic comments apply.

☹ **$$$ Essential Moisture Cream** *($64 for 1.69 ounces)* is an OK moisturizer for normal to dry skin that contains some very good water-binding agents.

☹ **$$$ Moisturizing Cream with Micro-Nutrients** *($32 for 1.69 ounces)* is a standard, mineral oil–based moisturizer that contains a small amount of good water-binding agents. It is an option for normal to dry skin.

☹ **$$$ Nourishing Cream with Marine Nutrients** *($32 for 1.69 ounces)* contains far more mineral oil, Vaseline, lanolin, and thickening agents than it does any marine life. The minute amount of algae is inconsequential and wouldn't nourish even one skin cell.

☹ **$$$ Oxygenating, Hydrating Day Cream** *($62 for 1.69 ounces)* is a standard moisturizer composed mostly of water and thickening agents and a tiny amount of algae and plant oils. Thankfully, this does not supply one molecule of oxygen to the skin, because that would generate free-radical damage.

☹ **Eye Contour Cream** *($30 for 0.5 ounce)* contains sodium lauryl sulfate rather high up on the ingredient list, making this too potentially irritating for all skin types.

☹ **Tri-Active Restoring Cream** *($54 for 1.7 ounces)* is similar to the Eye Contour Cream above and the same comments apply.

☺ **$$$ La Creme Day Moisturizer** *($70 for 1.7 ounces)* is a good moisturizer for normal to dry skin that contains a decent mix of water-binding agents and a tiny amount of antioxidant.

☺ **$$$ L'Emulsion Night Moisturizer** *($60 for 1.7 ounces)* is a standard, mineral oil–based moisturizer that contains some good emollients, but only a tiny amount of water-binding agents and antioxidants.

☺ **$$$ Marine Elastin Cream** *($40 for 1.7 ounces)* is a standard, extremely ordinary, mineral oil–based moisturizer that contains a tiny amount of elastin; that is helpful as a water-binding agent but it can't affect the elastin in skin.

☺ **$$$ Marine Collagen Cream** *($44 for 1.7 ounces)* is almost identical to the Elastin version above only with collagen instead, and the same basic comments apply. One quick point, even if collagen and elastin were both essential for skin care, why not put them together in one product rather than in two separate ones as most companies showcasing these ingredients do?

☺ **$$$ Reviviscent Serum** *($82 for 1 ounce)* is just slip agent and thickeners, along with a small amount of fish, algae, and mussel extracts, which adds up to minimal benefit for skin. None of that is worth the price tag of this product.

☺ **$$$ Perfect Contour Facial Gel Serum** *($100 for 1 ounce)* has some decent water-binding agents and a tiny amount of antioxidant in a lightweight lotion that can be OK for normal to slightly dry skin, but the price tag will hurt you more than this product will help your skin.

☹ **L'Serum** *($84 for 1 ounce)*. The fourth ingredient is balm mint, and that can be a skin irritant. Other than thickening agents and slip agents the only notable ingredients are pea and soybean extracts, both of which may have antioxidant properties, but there is little research indicating that these extracts have this benefit when applied topically.

☹ **Rebalancing Cream** *($30 for 1.7 ounces)* contains several potentially irritating and problematic ingredients for skin, including sodium lauryl sulfate and peppermint oil. Plus the lanolin and wheat germ oil are not the best for oily or combination skin.

☺ **$$$ Thalgo Moisture T-Zone Gel** *($52 for .5 ounces)* is an OK lightweight moisturizer for normal to slightly dry skin that contains some very good water-binding agents, but regrettably, it lacks antioxidants.

☺ **$$$ Delicate Moisture Veil for Eyes and Lips** *($22 for 0.17 ounce)* contains two good water-binding agents in a lightweight lotion and a minuscule amount of sea salt, which is good news for the eye area. This is an OK moisturizer for normal to slightly dry skin, but there is nothing that is particularly beneficial for eyes or lips.

☹ **Satiny Bronzing Oil for Body and Hair SPF 4** *($25 for 4.2 ounces)*. If you're looking to damage your hair or skin, then using this product is the way to go because it cannot protect from sun exposure. The SPF is pathetic and it does not contain UVA-protecting ingredients.

☹ **Protective Refreshing Emulsion SPF 8** *($28 for 4.2 ounces)*. While this does contain in-part avobenzone, the SPF 8 is far below the standard of SPF 15 set by the American Academy of Dermatology and the Skin Cancer Institute.

☺ $$$ **Hydra Protective Emulsion SPF 15** *($28 for 4.2 ounces)* is a very good, in-part titanium dioxide–based sunscreen in an exceptionally standard moisturizing base. It is an option for normal to dry skin, but there is nothing about this sun protection product that is not easily replaced with a far less pricey version at the drugstore.

☺ $$$ **Sun Shield Cream SPF 30** *($30 for 1.7 ounces)* is similar to the Hydra Protective version above and the same comments apply. This version does contain a dusting of vitamin E, but the negligible amount is not helpful for skin.

☺ $$$ **Sun Shield Emulsion SPF 25** *($30 for 3.4 ounces)* is similar to the Hydra Protective version above and the same comments apply.

☺ $$$ **Sublime Self Tanning Spray** *($28 for 4.2 ounces)* contains dihydroxyacetone, the same ingredient all self-tanners use to affect the color of skin. This one would work as well as any.

☺ $$$ **Scintillating Gel** *($28 for 1.7 ounces)* contains dihydroxyacetone, the same ingredient all self-tanners use to affect the color of skin. This one would work as well as any.

☹ **Bronzing Activator** *($28 for 4.2 ounces)* is designed to enhance the tanning process when sun bathing. That is equivalent to an oncologist selling cigarettes.

☺ $$$ **Sun Repair Cream Mask** *($28 for 1.7 ounces)*. This is a good emollient moisturizer that contains some good plant oils and water-binding agents, and algae, but none of that will repair any of the damage caused by inadequate protection from sun exposure.

☺ $$$ **Youthful Look Patch-Mask** *($40 for 20 patches)* contains mostly water, slip agents, water-binding agents, and preservatives. That's OK for normal to slightly dry skin, but it won't give back one minute of youthfulness to your skin.

☹ **Smoothing Cream Mask** *($32 for 1.69 ounces)* contains menthol, a potential skin irritant, and almost nothing of benefit for skin.

☺ $$$ **Delicate Facial Peel** *($26 for 1.7 ounces)* contains only water, cornstarch, thickeners, and mineral oil. This is then rubbed over the skin, which can help eliminate dead skin, but the rubbing isn't the best for a "delicate" peel. It's an option, but nothing that you can't duplicate with some water and cornstarch.

☹ **Descomask Pumicing Cream** *($32 for 1.7 ounces)* contains camphor, menthol, and sodium lauryl sulfate, which adds up to the potential for a lot of irritation.

☹ **Skin Lustre Mask** *($32 for 1.7 ounces)* lists alcohol as the second ingredient, which makes this too drying and irritating for all skin types.

☺ $$$ **Nourishing Cream Mask with Marine Nutrients** *($30 for 1.7 ounces)* is an exceptionally standard, but good, clay mask with a minute amount of sea salt and an extract from beeswax.

☹ **Radiance Mask for Eyes and Lips** *($36 for 1.7 ounces)* contains sodium lauryl sulfate high up on the ingredient list, which can be a significant skin irritant.

☺ $$$ **Thalgo Essential Moisture Mask** *($48 for 1.7 ounces)* is a silicone-based moisturizer with some good water-binding agents, but that's about it.

☹ **Re-Balancing Mask Oily Skin** *($32 for 1.69 ounces)* is an exceptionally standard clay mask with a tiny amount of algae. It also contains sodium lauryl sulfate, which makes this too potentially irritating for all skin types.

☺ $$$ **Unizones Skin Lightener** *($58 for 1 ounce)* doesn't contain one ingredient capable of affecting the color of skin. The second ingredient is yeast, and there is no research showing that to have an impact on skin discolorations.

☺ $$$ **Unizone Protective Day Cream SPF 15** *($58 for 1 ounce)* is a good, in-part titanium dioxide–based sunscreen in a rather ordinary moisturizing base that contains only a small amount of anti-irritants and an antioxidant. That's good, but the price is out of line for what you get, and this is easily surpassed by many less pricey options.

THREE CUSTOM COLOR (MAKEUP ONLY)

The number in this line's name refers to the three people who started and continue to manage this unique line. Three Custom Color specializes (and excels) in what they have dubbed a Custom Blending Service. Send them a color swatch or the last sliver of a favorite discontinued lipstick, or a drop of a beloved nail polish shade that you cannot find a perfect lip color match for, and they will duplicate it so accurately you will be stunned, and perhaps even overjoyed, that you and a favorite color are together again. And guess what? Their custom blending, color-matching services now extend from **Lip Color** *($50 for two tubes)* to **Cream to Powder Blush** *($37.50)*, **Powder Blush** *($34)*, **Powder Eyeshadow/Eyeliner** *($34)*, **Brow Powder** *($34)*, and **Creme Concealer** *($36.50)*. Available in 2003 will be loose or pressed **Face Powder**, among other items.

I'm the first to admit these customized options are pricey, but you do get an attractively reduced price for duplicates of the same color, which is of particular advantage with items you'll use up quickly, such as lipstick. The personalization for every product below is beautifully executed, right down to the postage-paid envelope you receive to send in a remnant or piece of fabric that represents your ideal color. You can even choose the texture and finish for several of the items. It's a remarkable service that is made even sweeter by the attention to detail and enthusiasm the Three Custom Color team shares. Furthermore, all custom colors are 100% guaranteed, and will be redone (at no additional charge) in the unlikely event that they don't get it just right the first time. For more information about Three Custom Color, call (888) 262-7714 or visit www.threecustom.com.

In addition to their Custom Color menu, you can also choose from a range of several other makeup essentials, featuring a combined total of over 140, never-to-be-discontinued **Ready to Wear** colors *($12.50–$20.50)* that are as follows:

☺ $$$ **Creme Concealer** *($19.50, $15 for refill)* is indeed creamy, yet it is also very concentrated and melts into the skin, providing good, even coverage. The range of ten shades is very good, but unless you're certain of which color to purchase it is best to contact the company for descriptions—otherwise, you're left to guess from color swatches online, and that's always tricky. As is true for any creamy concealer, this has a tendency to crease if not set with powder. However, this version fares quite well in that department. For makeup artists, a **Professional Concealer Palette** *($58)* offers a concealer brush and all ten shades to use alone or mix as needed for the ideal shade. **Creme to Powder Blush** *($20.50)* is aluminum starch–based, so this sets quickly to a soft powder finish. If you're adept at the dab-and-blend application this type of blush requires, you will be thrilled by the colors. These are pigment-rich, so use them sparingly for best results and build color from there. **Brow Powder** *($17.50, $12.50 for refill)* is a talc-based brow powder that is a great choice for softly defined brows, and the six colors run the gamut from blonde to raven. This also works as a true matte eyeshadow, but is not as supremely smooth as the Eyeshadow Singles below. **Lip Liner** *($12.50)* has been improved, and it shows. This is still a needs-sharpening pencil, but it is creamier and applies better than the previous version. The deeper hues are brilliant for women of color.

✔☺ $$$ **Eyeshadow Singles** *($17, $12.50 for refill)* comes in a huge range of colors, including some avant-garde shades that can be a fun departure from the norm. Still, it's the wealth of neutral earth tones and sophisticated charcoal hues that you'll want to focus on, and the texture of these is sublime. Even the extremely shiny shades blend on effortlessly without flaking, which is quite a feat. ✔☺ **Lipstick** *($15, $18.50 for Special Shades)* is marvelously creamy without feeling too slick or greasy. The full-coverage colors were my favorite, but the **Special Shades** are intriguing as well, since these are custom or "themed" colors that have made their way into the line's regular rotation. There are also sheer options, and many of these ready-made shades have matching lip glosses. The actual ✔☺ **Lip Gloss** *($15)* is ultra-emollient and has a texture that is quite unlike almost all other glosses. It reminds me of a creamy lipstick that has softened in the sun. It has a rich, buttery smoothness that is absolutely not sticky or thick and very wearable. Don't be tempted by this if you're prone to lip colors bleeding because (just like any gloss) this will move, but otherwise it is a superior choice! Various **Lip Gloss Palettes** *($53)* are also available, and include a synthetic lip brush.

☺ $$$ **Refillable Trio Compact** *($13.50)* is sold separately and includes a dual-sided brush. It's a wise investment if you routinely use three colors, and the compact will hold shadows or blushes from other lines, too.

☺ **Eye Liner** *($12.50)* is a fairly standard pencil that glides on but is creamy enough to smudge. I wouldn't choose this for lining over one of the Three Custom Color shadows, but it's fine for pencil lovers.

The Three Custom Color line is nicely rounded out by a beautiful collection of professional ✔☺ $$$ **Brushes** *($3.50–$55)* that feature elegant, long-handled options for applying color. The only brushes that you may want to think twice about are the ☺ **Retractable Lip Brush** *($12.50)*, which is too small for most women's lips, and the **Spoolie** *($8)*, which is just a mascara wand that is easily replaced by an old, clean wand from your previous mascara.

TONY & TINA

Tony & Tina definitely have found a distinctive approach that sets this line apart from the rest because their "intention is to expand the use and understanding of Vibrational Remedies." The company's earnest belief is that all living things give off energy, which in turn can be influenced or controlled by certain colors, aromas, and herbs. Whether or not it is plausible that applying a certain shade of lipstick or blush can enable one to obtain "conscious evolution," or "positively manipulate energy," or "discover … endless potential" is a matter for discussion, but it is important to keep in mind that we're talking about makeup here, not a religious epiphany. However, for those who subscribe to the notion of cosmic energy and color therapy, either can certainly be enjoyed and practiced with or without Tony & Tina. Once you get past the embellishments, there is not much here to meditate on, unless your preference is for all manner of shine and sparkle (does conscious evolution require glitter?). Besides, I wonder how long it took Tony & Tina to visualize that a 75% share of their company would be sold to the international cosmetics firm Wella in 2002. It seems that befriending "the silent space in which evolution will naturally occur" must have a lot to do with expansion and commerce.

Viewed in person, the packaging is artful and the counter displays are nicely accessible—you are free to play and achieve all the bliss you can handle. The nail polishes are this line's original attention-getters, and they do dazzle, but Tony & Tina's notion that "each color has both physical and metaphysical therapeutic qualities" is pretty much at the outer limits of reality. Regardless, you'll find colors both subdued and shocking in every product group. The skin-care products appear to be nothing more than a poorly meditated afterthought. This small group of products is uninteresting and something you can quickly pass over to get to the colorful Vibrational Remedies. For more information about Tony & Tina, call (212) 226-3992 or visit www.tonytina.com.

TONY & TINA SKIN CARE

☹ **Herbal Aromatherapy Cleanser, Normal to Dry** *($24 for 8 ounces)* contains some fairly irritating plant extracts, including lemon and eucalyptus. This is just an emollient cleanser that is more of a cold cream than anything else. Remember that aromatherapy is great for the nose, but a problem for the skin.

☺ **Herbal Aromatherapy Make-Up Remover** *($18 for 6 ounces)* is actually better as a moisturizer than as a makeup remover. It contains some very good water-binding agents and antioxidants. It would be a shame to wipe this stuff off, except for the fragrance, which is really wafting.

☺ $$$ **Herbal Skin Refiner with Apple Seed Enzyme** *($32 for 1.15 ounces)* contains far more fragrance than it does ingredients that are beneficial for skin. Although the interesting antioxidants and water-binding agents are in short supply, the musk and lavender pour forth.

☺ $$$ **Herbal Eye Refiner** *($36 for 0.61 ounce)* is similar to the Herbal Skin Refiner above and the same comments apply.

TONY & TINA MAKEUP

☺ $$$ **FOUNDATION: Environmental Rescue** *($28)* claims to not only cover up imperfections, but also to save skin from pollution and fight off acne and the signs of aging. It's a wonder that this do-it-all foundation is not in every woman's makeup bag! All claims and kidding aside, this is a standard, light-textured liquid foundation that spreads well and affords sheer-to-light coverage that can feel a bit sticky. The eight shades aren't the best around, but a few of the colors are worth a look. Avoid Aphrodite, Ri, and Eos.

☺ $$$ **CONCEALER: Therapeutic Eye Base** *($22)* has changed from a cream-to-powder compact to a liquidy concealer packaged in a tube. This now has a sheer-coverage, soft-matte finish and comes in four reasonably neutral shades. The antiaging claim is linked to apple seed enzyme, and even if this were a miracle ingredient (it's not—enzymes are notoriously unstable exfoliants on skin), there isn't enough of it in this product to work for better or worse.

☺ $$$ **POWDER: Herbal Environmental Protector Pressed Powder** *($28)* is a drier-than-usual talc-based pressed powder that can seem thick, but blends out quite sheer. The two shades are good, but only for fair to light skin; the Color Corrector is slightly yellow, but still worth considering if you buy into Tony & Tina's belief that this cosmetic can protect your skin from harsh pollutants.

BLUSH AND EYESHADOW: ✓☺ **Herbal Cheek Gel** *($15)* is one of the better stains for cheeks, and the least liquidy, so blending is more easily controlled. This comes in a pump bottle that tends to dispense more product than you need to create a flushed appearance, but it's otherwise recommended if you have smooth, even-textured skin.

☺ **Universal Color Dust** *($15)* is, on the surface, another shiny loose powder. However, this one does hold an advantage for those who want this type of product, as it is well packaged and considerably less messy than other versions. This also clings well and the dimensional shine in it changes color depending on what direction the light hits it. I'm sure that has something to do with our bodies' vibrational energy, but I can't think what.

☺ $$$ **Cosmetic** *($24)* is a small pot of highly iridescent loose powder. It's not a terrible option if the messy application doesn't faze you, but is still not preferred to the Universal Color Dust above. **Aura Lights** *($18)* gives you a slightly sticky, phosphorescent highlighter in the now-familiar click-pen with a brush-tip apparatus. The shiny effect is unusual (and not glittery), and this could be a fun change of pace if you don't mind a bit of stickiness. **Color Frequency Single** *($14)* and **Color Frequency Duo Eyeshadows** *($18)* have a far better gimmick than performance. Actually, the marketing copy for Frequency far surpasses any simple definition of the word "gimmick." The incredible concept for this product is that it contains chamomile and vitamins "for the physical," and color "for the metaphysical … [to] awaken your intuition with Color Frequency Eye Shadow. Clinically proven to aid in personal revelation." Eyeshadow can aid in personal revelation? Enlightenment via makeup—Can spirituality get any more superficial than this? The amount of chamomile and vitamins is at best negligible and these exceptionally basic, overpriced eyeshadows (I guess personal revelation doesn't come cheap) are sold alone or in a single-disc compact with two shades, available in either high shimmer, standard (which is slightly shimmery), or matte finishes. The texture of the shiny shades is powdery and sheer, while the matte shades are dry to chalky. When all is said and done, cosmic hype is all these eyeshadows have going for them.

☹ **Cosmic Lights** *($12)* uses "pure Crystalina" to create these eight shades of sparkly powder, similar to the Cosmetic above. The only difference is that these have a rough, grainy texture and do not adhere well to skin. That's not surprising, given that crystalina is made of iridescent translucent Mylar flakes (yes, like Mylar bags or balloons), which explains why it isn't so skin friendly, but it undeniably does shine. **Cosmic Liquid Lights** *($16)* continues "the sparkle revolution," but is a costly way to add lots of glitter to your makeup routine. This brush-on gel could work for smaller flashy accents, but not without looking childish.

<u>EYE AND BROW SHAPER:</u> ☺ $$$ **Herbal Eye Pencil** *($16)* and **Herbal Glitter Eye Pencil** *($18)* are standard, and I mean *standard*, pencils that have a creamy texture and glide on easily. These have a powdery finish, but are best used for a smoky look, as they smudge easily. These also promise to firm skin with cucumber, and fight eye irritation with chickweed, but, like the other claims here, they're just bogus.

☺ $$$ **Ultimate Brow Pencil** *($18)* is standard in every sense of the word, except for the misguided notion that this single gray color flatters all eyebrow shades. Talk about delusional!

☹ **Herbal Liquid Liner** *($18)* is below standard due to its odd distinction of applying too much product at once (and unevenly) while at the same time being sheer. The colors are trippy, but that's not enough to make up for the application drawbacks. **Herbal Char'Khol Eye Liner** *($18)* is a thick, wind-up, retractable pencil that is inordinately greasy and seems to smear by sheer will power. There is no reason to put up with this, and the fact that a product meant for use around the eye contains camphor is deplorable.

<u>LIPSTICK AND LIP PENCIL:</u> ☺ **Mood Balance Lipstick** *($15)* goes on and on about the lavender, rosemary, and St. John's wort it contains, but it's merely irritating window dressing for a rather standard, boring group of lipsticks. There are three finishes—creamy, semi-matte, and gloss—and all are barely distinguishable from each other.

They all have a creamy texture and slightly glossy finish, although some are more opaque than others. **Herbal Aromatherapy Lip Gloss** *($14)* is just standard, non-sticky lip gloss with some enticing, high-shine colors. Avoid the glitter-packed shades with a "Cosmic" prefix unless you like gritty-feeling lips.

☺ $$$ **Divine Lip Shine** *($16)* is, for all its New Age pretense, just a basic wand-type gloss that comes in sparkle-filled, sheer colors. This does contain tangerine oil for flavor and scent, which can be irritating to lips. **Herbal Lip Pencil** *($16)*. Once you get around all the hype about this pencil being "therapeutic," what you find is the same creamy lipliner that every other line has been selling for years, only the color range here is a bit strange.

☹ **Herbal Lip Glitter** *($18)* are chunky pencils infused with glitter. It gives this standard, creamy pencil an uninviting, grainy texture—but the shine is here for those who crave it.

<u>MASCARA:</u> ✔☺ $$$ **Herbal Eye Mascara** *($18)* is still a fantastic mascara that goes on beautifully and builds long, separated, lightly thickened lashes with minimal effort. It also holds up well and does not smear throughout the day. A Clear version and other colors are available, but the blue and purple shades are not recommended.

<u>BRUSHES:</u> ✔☺ $$$ Tony & Tina sought the assistance of Shu Uemura for their **Technology of Kindness Brushes** *($36–$98)*, and the benefit is apparent. These are wonderfully full, soft, 100% synthetic brushes with workable shapes. What a shame they are so exorbitantly priced! If you survive the sticker shock, you will find some exquisite, plush options, but you can absolutely ignore the ☺ $$$ **Lip Brush** *($48)*, as it's way too pricey for such a standard, very small brush.

☺ <u>SPECIALTY:</u> **Nail Paint** *($10)* is basic nail polish with some of the most imaginative colors and textures I've ever seen. For those of you wishing for shiny, polyester-infused blues, and fuchsias with enough glitter to blind oncoming traffic, welcome home! **Millennium Key** *($15)* is "the only nail polish packaging in the Museum of Modern Art" and it's not hard to see why. This clever, artful container allows you to paint your nails while resting the bottle between your fingers, and it does work well to keep things steady. Then again, so does setting the bottle on a flat surface as you manicure, but that would be far too logical for the mindset of Tony & Tina!

TRI-LUMA

If you have been struggling to lighten or remove the dark brown patches on your skin caused by sun damage, birth-control pills, or hormone problems, ☺ $$$ **Tri-Luma** *($90 for 30 grams/1.05 ounces)* may just become your best friend. This distinctive, pre-scription-only topical cream is a unique combination of fluocinolone acetonide 0.01% (a topical cortisone), hydroquinone 4%, and tretinoin 0.05% (the active ingredient in Renova). This triple-action cream has an interesting synergistic effect that can help reduce or eliminate brown skin discolorations. The 4% hydroquinone means this is a potent melanin-inhibiting product, and the tretinoin helps restore normal cell production. Together they can produce striking results, although both the hydroquinone and tretinoin have a strong potential for causing skin irritation. That's where the hydrocortisone comes in. Hydrocortisone is an effective topical agent that prevents irritation. Any negative effect of using hydrocortisone on the skin is mitigated by the tretinoin. In fact, Tri-Luma would have all of the positive aspects of using tretinoin on skin even without the other two ingredients.

Once the brown patching has dissipated, you would only use Tri-Luma as needed. Devoted, consistent use of a sunscreen with UVA-protecting ingredients can maintain the results. The only real drawbacks for this product are the price and the need for a prescription from your physician. That definitely adds up. Even so, considering that many high-priced products being sold to lighten skin at cosmetics counters and spas can cost nearly this much yet contain few to no ingredients that can have any impact on skin, Tri-Luma starts looking more and more like a bargain.

TRISH MCEVOY (MAKEUP ONLY)

Trish McEvoy remains a strong contender amongst the makeup artist–designed color lines. Her products excel when it comes to makeup brushes, eyeshadows, a few of the mascaras, a couple of good foundations, and the ingenious Face Planners. On the downside, a fair number of McEvoy selections lag behind some of the options her competitors, including Lauder-owned Bobbi Brown, M.A.C., and Stila have to offer.

As I visited McEvoy's counters, it was obvious that there were some transitions under way, with discontinued foundations waiting out their last days on the shelves before being replaced by their (ostensibly improved) successors. So bear in mind the best I can do is comment on any line's makeup products as I find them. It is entirely possible the next generation of McEvoy foundations will compete nicely with neighboring makeup artistry lines. For now, although there are some very satisfying choices, the scope and variety are limited, and that's not positive, especially when you consider the often higher than average prices.

One thing has been constant: Trish McEvoy makeup artists are typically well-trained, and are adept both at coordinating makeup wardrobes as well as using her multitude of brushes and passing that know-how on to you. More than many of her peers, McEvoy is fanatical about using the proper brush and teaching the best application techniques for achieving the look you want. That passion comes through in the brushes and organizational palettes she sells, and is a strength that needs to spill over into the ordinary and cool-concept, poor-execution products that keep Trish McEvoy makeup from where it ultimately could go. For more information about Trish McEvoy, call (800) 431-4306 or visit www.saksfifthavenue.com.

FOUNDATION: ☺ $$$ **Dual Powder** *($26)* works very well as a silky, talc-based powder foundation. This can go on a bit powdery (it's pressed quite softly), but it does blend well without looking cakey or opaque. The eight shades include some real winners, though Tan 7 can be too peach for most skin tones. **Cream Powder Makeup** *($35)* is substantially more creamy than powdery. In fact, the powder finish is minimal and will be brief when used over oilier areas. This formula is best for normal to dry skin that wants adjustable coverage. Blending this is a smooth proposition, and the result is a rather natural-looking finish. Of the nine shades, the following are too peach or pink: Cool 3, Shell, N5, and Warm 4 Honey. **All Over Face Color** *($26)* are pressed-powder tablets that come in a small range of neutral to brown-toned blush/contour colors, all with a soft shine. The silken texture applies and blends great, and this is worth considering as a multipurpose product to define and add color.

☺ $$$ **Natural Tint Foundation Oil-Free** *($38)* is becoming surprisingly dated, at least in terms of lacking the same silicone smoothness seen in foundations from Bobbi Brown, M.A.C., and Stila, though this is just fine for a standard liquid foundation. It offers sheer coverage, a moist feel, and a natural, almost matte finish. The 12 shades demonstrate McEvoy's keen eye for neutral tones, but there are a few missteps to watch out for, such as Warm Honey and Sun Bronze. **Face Shine** *($32)* is nothing more than creamy shine with a sheer powder finish. The color is very faint, so using this is primarily for those who want shine more than anything else—and haven't noticed that countless lines sell similar products for a lot less money.

☺ $$$ <u>CONCEALER:</u> **Protective Shield Concealer** *($21)*. I still don't understand why some makeup artist lines sell really creamy concealers that crease endlessly, and here's one more to add to the list. This castor oil–based concealer blends well and provides great coverage and a natural finish—it isn't nearly as thick as Bobbi Brown's Creamy Concealer is—but unless it's set with lots of powder, it will migrate into lines or creases. By and large, the colors are workable, but watch out for Honey, Tan, and Deep Tan—all are strikingly orange.

<u>POWDER:</u> ☺ $$$ **Loose Powder** *($20)* is talc-based, with a very silky, soft texture but the three color choices are appropriate only for light to medium skin tones. The number of McEvoy's darker foundation shades has been reduced, so it's no longer much of an issue that there are no darker powder colors. Avoid Nude Shimmer, which is extraordinarily shiny.

☺ $$$ **All Over Face Powder** *($28)* is a group of rather ordinary talc-based powders. The colors are fine, but I wouldn't choose these over pressed powders from L'Oreal or, in the same price range, Lancome—unless you're using it from one of McEvoy's makeup planners.

<u>BLUSH:</u> ☺ $$$ **Radiant Blush** *($19)* is very smooth, and each color applies well. Many of the latest colors have an intensity that was absent in the past, which may or may not be to your liking (I liked it). The only downside is that after searching high and low for a few matte options, I found none. If you don't want shiny cheeks, you'll need to look elsewhere. **Lip & Cheek Tint** *($18)* is another water-based cheek and lip stain à la BeneFit's

BeneTint and all the rest. This version offers very sheer colors, which may be preferred by some, as you can layer this to build intensity instead of living with too much color from the get-go. Considering its fluidity, this blends well without looking spotty, and it stays on well, too.

☺ $$$ **Cream Blush** *($32)* delivers a very creamy, almost greasy, blush. It blends out to just a hint of color, but doesn't measure up to the superior cream blush options from Laura Mercier or Bobbi Brown.

EYESHADOW: Four types of powder ☺ Eye Shadows *($15 each)* might sound like overkill, but in this case you can ignore the categories and just shop for the colors you like, because they are all fairly similar. The **Glazes** have some amount of shine; the **Shapers** are supposed to be softer colors (and most are); the **Definers** are intense, deep colors for liner; and the **Enhancers** are medium shades for the crease. All of the colors are interchangeable and the few matte ones are, of course, the best. However, even the shiniest shades blend and cling surprisingly well. The deepest colors are easy to overdo, and have a mild tendency to crease if you don't go easy with them.

☺ $$$ **Face Essentials** *($45)* is a compact quintet of colors with two squares of eyeshadow, a strip of eyeliner and one of lip gloss, and a rectangular blush. The colors are arranged so that it is easier to not intermix them, but they're still close enough that you wouldn't want to casually sweep your brush over them without watching where it's going! I am not a fan of buying sets, but most of these are fail-safe, especially if your makeup wish list includes shine. If you find a selection that meets all your needs, this can be an essential kit for you.

☺ $$$ **Nude Touch-Up Kit** *($24)* gives you all the basics to refresh your makeup on the fly (foundation, concealer, lip color, blush), but the amount of most of the colors is very small, and the large powder blush/face color is very shiny, which may work if you're heading out for cocktails rather than rushing to the boardroom or a business meeting. **The Card** *($24)* is a thin, credit card–sized compact filled with four shiny eyeshadows and four lip glosses. It's OK as a discreet addition to your evening bag, but you'd still have to pack application tools.

☹ **Water Stix Eye Shadow** *($20)* seems like an innocuous cream-to-powder, twist-up stick eyeshadow, available in an array of iridescent pastel and nude tones. However, things get ugly when you try to blend—this sticks to the skin, is incredibly stubborn, and stays sticky. Using more than one color (if you can stand that) results in a muddy-looking mess.

EYE AND BROW SHAPER: The ☺ Eye Pencils *($15)*, in a very typical assortment of colors, are incredibly standard. **Finish Line** *($15)* is a variation on using plain water to dampen an eyeshadow in order to get a more dramatic line. This is essentially a water-based gel that contains some slip agents and sheer thickeners, but lacks any film-forming agents. This works, but has little advantage over using tap water when you want to use a powder eyeshadow wet.

☺ **$$$ Brow Pencils** *($18)* are very stiff and difficult to apply, plus these dry-finish pencils need routine sharpening.

☺ **$$$ Brow Gel** *($18)* is as predictable as rain is wet. It functions perfectly well as a clear brow groomer, but so does Cover Girl's version, for one-third the price.

LIPSTICK AND LIP PENCIL: ☺ **$$$ Lip Colors** *($18)* come in a delectable range of full-coverage shades, but this traditionally creamy lipstick can be too greasy for anyone prone to lipstick bleeding. To remedy that, McEvoy came up with **Flawless Lip** *($20),* which is a clear, silicone-based pre-lipstick base designed to keep lipstick anchored firmly on the lips. It works marginally well, but still can't keep McEvoy's lipsticks from their forward march into lines around the mouth.

☺ **$$$ Sheers** *($16)* are like a gloss, and with the same staying power. **Sheers with SPF 15** *($16)* are identical to the Sheers except that they contain sunscreen, but not adequate UVA protection. **Moisture Stick SPF 15** *($18)* lacks effective UVA protection and is otherwise an extremely greasy, lanolin oil–based clear lipstick. **Highlights Lip Gloss** *($19)* offers an interesting array of colors, including reds, a shiny lavender, and a shiny gold, as well as soft, pale shades of pink, mauve, and peach. These glosses go on thinner than most yet still look rich and wet. However, the price is out of line, especially if you don't care for fairly sticky gloss. **Lip Liner** *($16)* comes in a nice assortment of colors, and one end of the pencil has a lip brush. It's a nice touch, but this is too creamy if you're concerned with keeping lipstick in place. Those who don't share that concern will find some versatile colors available. **Essential Pencil** *($20)* appears to be the darling of this line's lip color collection, as the number of shades available is hard to ignore. The fuss will be all for naught, though, as these are completely standard thick pencils that impart light to medium color saturation and are fairly greasy. **Maxed Out Kit** *($19)* is for serious McEvoy lip gloss fans, as this flat compact holds ten different colors and wisely includes a good lip brush. If the gloss had a better feel, this would be rated better; test it yourself and see what you think.

MASCARA: The original ✓☺ **$$$ Mascara** *($18)* is fantastic on all counts, building credible length, some thickness, and beautifully separated lashes. It's easy to get overzealous with this one, and that can cause some smearing, so try to contain yourself! ✓☺ **$$$ Lash Building Mascara** *($18)* takes its sweet time to get going, but with patience, this turns out to be an excellent thickening mascara that doesn't clump.

☺ **$$$ Lash Curling Mascara** *($25)* doesn't curl lashes any more than a lot of other mascaras, and the price of this one straddles the border between acceptable and obnoxious. This excels at lengthening, but it does take some time to "set," and keeping lashes wet too long increases the chance of smearing.

☺ **$$$ Waterproof Mascara** *($18)* smears a bit too easily during application, but it passes with flying colors as a waterproof mascara. This goes on much easier if the wand is wiped down first, but even so there are better and less expensive choices for waterproof mascara.

The Reviews T

☹ **Lash Builder** *($18)* is a basic primer that makes little difference in the fullness or appearances of your lashes, except for some clumping when a regular mascara is used over it. McEvoy's mascaras don't need this hinders-more-than-helps product.

BRUSHES: Trish McEvoy has a well-earned reputation for producing some of the softest, most exquisitely shaped ✔☺ $$$ **Brushes** *($14–$58)* anywhere, and, aside from the steep price tag that accompanies many of them, you won't be disappointed with their performance and longevity. There are some unconventional options whose purpose was explained to me, but I still wouldn't choose those over something more versatile. There's no doubt that makeup brush enthusiasts will have a field day among the 35 options here. The non-essential brushes include the awkwardly cut ☺ $$$ **Brush 42** *($25)* and **Eyeshadow Brush 10** *($26);* the **Crease Brush #35** *($30),* which is too soft and hard to control; and the **Groomer** *($14),* which works well (just like a cleaned-up mascara wand).

The ☺ $$$ **Foundation Brush** *($25),* for those so inclined, is softer and more flexible than many others, and that can indeed make application easier, because the brush comfortably flexes to fit the contours and hard-to-reach areas of the face. Also of note and highly recommended (price notwithstanding) are **Brush #5** *($48),* **Blush Brush #2B** *($40),* **Eyeshadow Brush #45** *($26),* **Eye Lining Brush #11** *($20),* **Lining Brush #9** *($18),* and **Lip Brush #7** *($18).* Among the pre-selected **Brush Sets** *($55–$95),* the ones to pay attention to are the **On the Go** *($55)* and **Lucite** *($95)* sets.

The ☺ $$$ **Makeup Brush Cleaner** *($14)* is a spray-on solution that primarily consists of water, mild detergent cleansing agents, and a tiny bit of witch hazel and preservatives. This will cleanse brushes, but it's rather pricey for what amounts to watered-down shampoo.

SPECIALTY: ✔☺ $$$ **Face Planners** *($48–$58 for the case, $12–$14 for the pages)* are a very clever way to assemble a makeup bag that resembles a day planner. A two-ring binder inside a zippered pouch holds covered plastic "pages" that can be filled (and refilled) with the colors of your choice. It's pricey, but the bags are handsomely made and exceedingly convenient, especially if you're loyal to Trish McEvoy's color line. You can assemble all the products you need for a complete makeup application, from foundation to lip color, and there are interior pockets that can hold several brushes or miscellaneous items that won't fit on the pages.

☺ $$$ **Luxury Compact** *($35)* is luxuriously sleek, and for the indulgent, an ultramodern way to powder one's nose in public. The refillable compact can hold your choice of pressed powder, concealer, blush, or one of McEvoy's solid fragrances.

TRUCCO (MAKEUP ONLY)

Trucco is a small line of makeup products developed by the hair-care company Sebastian International. The products have hardly changed at all since the previous edition of this book, though some have been discontinued. The tag line for Trucco is "Addicted to Colour," but although there are a few products worth checking out if you come across a salon or boutique that carries this line, nothing merits even a mild case of addiction. What you may want to investigate are the foundations and powders, which offer some good neutral colors, and the decent selection of matte eyeshadows and blushes. The rest of the lineup is a mixture of standard fare, ranging from problematic mascaras to terrible concealers. The cost of Trucco products varies from location to location, as salons that sell the line set their own retail price. Therefore, consider the prices listed here to be an average and decide from there whether or not Sebastian's Trucco makeup is as appealing to you as its enormous selection of hair-care products. If you are a licensed cosmetologist or hairdresser, you can purchase these products at the wholesale price, which is typically half of the suggested retail price. And a note to Sebastian: It wouldn't hurt to train the staff at your salons how to sell and use the makeup. In the salons I visited, they were often ignorant about the prices and apathetic about the products. For more information about Trucco, call (800) 829-7322 or visit www.sebastian-intl.com.

FOUNDATION: ☺ $$$ **Pro Coverage Foundation SPF 8** *($27.75)* is a slightly thick, but smooth-textured foundation that does contain a UVA-protecting ingredient (titanium dioxide), although it has a disappointingly low SPF (SPF 15 is the benchmark). The foundation blends on well and provides light to medium coverage and a satiny-soft finish. It would be suitable for normal to dry skin, and of the seven shades (with nothing for very light or very dark skin tones), only Bisque, Tan, and Sand are too peach for most skin tones. Olive, Beige, and Ivory are lovely neutral colors. **Prepair Duo Powder Foundation** *($28.75)* is a standard, talc-based powder foundation with a smooth, soft texture and medium coverage that blends very nicely. There are six colors, with no options for darker skin. Mood is the only one to steer clear of as it's too orange for most skin tones.

☺ $$$ **Studio Creme Foundation SPF 12** *($28.75)* is a creamy makeup that comes in a compact and almost dries to a powder finish. The SPF ingredient is not listed in the active ingredient list, which makes this misleading and definitely unreliable for sun protection. There are only three shades, which is shortsighted, and one (Compromise) is too peach for most skin tones. **Tinted Moisturizer SPF 8** *($17)* does not contain any UVA-protecting ingredients and is just a basic, very sheer (but emollient) tint for the face. The two available shades are fine.

☹ **CONCEALER:** Trucco's **Concealer** *($14.45)* comes in a pot and has a creamy, almost greasy texture that is only capable of light coverage and can easily crease into any lines around the eyes. The colors are right-on, but the negatives offset that. **All Purpose Color Corrector** *($13)* is similar to the Concealer above, but the instructions are to use this very peach-toned cream to neutralize unwanted skin tones, and the end result is exactly what you might expect: peach-tinted-looking skin.

☺ $$$ **POWDER:** **Touch Up Pressed Powder** *($20.50)* is talc-based, with a dry, soft texture and sheer application. Of the three colors, Shell and Ecru are very light and Bronze is best used as a matte bronzing powder instead of an all-over face powder. **Final**

Touch Loose Powder *($16.50)* is talc-based and has a smooth, even texture and three very good colors suited to lighter skin tones.

BLUSH: ☺ **One Blush** and **Trio Blush** *($13.75 singles, $24.25 trios)* have soft and sheer, slightly dry textures that blend decently, just not as easily as many other powder blushes. One Blush is a small but good group of matte shades, and the Trio Blush presents blush, contour, and highlighter colors in one compact. These can be a convenient option, but there are no dividers between the colors, so once you've used them they tend to spill over onto each other. The colors are well coordinated, which is always a plus.

☹ **Face Cremes** *($25)* are overpriced creamy, glittery colors for eyes, lips, and cheeks. Due to the glitter particles, the texture is somewhat rough. If you're interested in this type of product, a better place to start would be M.A.C.'s Creme Colour Base ($14).

☺ **EYESHADOW: Eye Colours** *($12.20)* are single eyeshadows with a smooth texture that is a bit stubborn when it comes to blending evenly. The shiny colors are labeled as Reflectives, while the Mattes are called just that. The Mattes are not entirely matte, but the shine is very soft.

EYE AND BROW SHAPER: ☺ **Pro Eye Pencil** *($11)* is a very standard pencil that glides on well and has a soft, dry finish. **Graphic Liquid Eyeliner** *($11.65)* has a great, quick-drying formula that goes on solid and heavy. Be careful when applying it, as the brush is too stiff and scratchy. If you can handle the discomfort of the applicator, which does make getting an even line tricky, it does wear well!

☺ **$$$ Hi-Brow Trio** *($25.50)* is virtually identical to Hard Candy's Training Brow Compact ($28). Trucco offers three matte colors, Light, Medium, and Dark, that have a dry finish and apply well, but most women would do just fine with one matte color for the brows, and these are too dry to double as eyeshadow. This may be worth it to makeup artists without any budget constraints, but others will get limited use from two of the three shades. **Brow Shaper** *($9)* is your basic, everyday clear brow gel that works as well as any.

☺ **LIPSTICK AND LIP PENCIL: Identity Lipsticks** *($13.50)* are marketed with a transcendent flair, but in reality they are just ordinary lipsticks. The **Cremes** are very creamy and rich with a glossy finish and mostly iridescent colors. The **Mattes** are not matte in the least but are nicely creamy and opaque. The texture is somewhat sticky, and feels that way on the lips. The **Sheers** have an SPF 12 sans UVA-protecting ingredients, but can be relied on for an emollient, very glossy lip tint (which is not all that sheer), and there are lots of colors. **Divinyls Lip Gloss** *($9.50)* is for serious gloss fans. This is a rich, thick, slightly sticky gloss that comes in a tube and leaves an extremely wet-looking finish. The colors go from bold to subtle, and many have iridescence. **Pro Lip Pencil** *($11)* is as standard as it gets. This pencil needs sharpening and has a creamy, but relatively solid, finish.

☹ **MASCARA: In Focus Mascara** *($12.50)* still goes on a little too wet and can make lashes look heavy and limp. It builds some length, but the side effects are not fun to live with. **In Focus Waterproof Mascara** *($14)* is barely passable for just average length and no thickness. Don't get caught in the rain with this one; it breaks down readily on contact with water.

☺ <u>BRUSHES:</u> Trucco has a handsome, well-crafted collection of six **Brushes** *($12–$26)*, but few salons stock them, so if you decide to pursue these, be prepared to hunt. You may want to visit Sebastian's Web site to locate a salon in your area that sells Trucco products and may also have their brushes. The prices are more than reasonable, and the only one to take lightly (or not at all) is the **Blending Brush** *($12)*.

ULTIMA II

Ultima II's counter displays and image need some serious renovation and restructuring. What's most disappointing is that Revlon, which owns Ultima II, seems to have taken an indifferent attitude toward this line and its products. Several calls to Revlon's customer service number made me feel as if I were running in circles, as I was consistently told to phone J.C. Penney (the department store that carries the line), and then when I did, the salespeople at J.C. Penney told me to call Revlon. When it comes to the hodge-podge of skin-care products here, you'll find some good stragglers left to consider, especially in the category of moisturizers. However, come prepared, as this is not an easy line to navigate and you'll more than likely need some assistance, if you can find anyone who knows something about the line, because Revlon is seemingly not offering any educational help to Ultima II's counter people. For more information about Ultima II, you can attempt to contact them at (800) 4-REVLON. There is no Web site for this line. **Note:** The "CHR" acronym stands for Collagen Hydrating Response. All of the CHR products do contain tiny amounts of collagen, but collagen is merely a good water-binding agent. It can't affect the collagen in your skin, much less alter the appearance of wrinkles (or what causes them) in any way. Also, all Ultima II products contain fragrance.

ULTIMA II SKIN CARE

☺ **CHR Cream Cleanser** *($18.50 for 4 ounces)* is a standard, mineral oil–based cleanser that must be wiped off and that can leave a greasy film on the skin, though it may be an option for someone with dry skin.

☹ **CHR Double Action Gentle Cleanser for Dry Skin** *($17.50 for 4.8 ounces)* is a standard, detergent-based, water-soluble cleanser that contains some fairly drying cleansing agents that are not the best for most skin types.

☹ **Vital Radiance Foaming Face Wash for Normal to Dry Skin** *($17.50 for 5 ounces)* is almost identical to the CHR Double Action Gentle Cleanser above, and the same comments apply.

☺ **Vital Radiance Foaming Face Wash for Normal to Oily Skin** *($17.50 for 5 ounces)* is a standard, detergent-based cleanser that can work well for normal to oily skin. It does contain sodium lauryl sulfate as one of the cleansing agents, and that can be a problem for causing irritation and sensitizing skin reactions.

☺ **Eye Makeup Remover for Sensitive Eyes** (*$12.50 for 3.6 ounces*) is a standard, detergent-based eye-makeup remover similar to almost every one of this kind in the industry.

☺ **Going Going Gone Makeup Remover** (*$13.50 for 4 ounces*) is just a mineral oil–based cold cream that can leave a greasy film on the skin, though it can be a makeup-removing option for dry skin.

☹ **Vital Radiance Skin Renewing Exfoliator for All Skin Types** (*$17.50 for 4.7 ounces*) lists sodium lauryl sulfate as the third ingredient, which makes this too potentially irritating and drying for all skin types.

☹ **CHR Double Action Gentle Toner for Dry Skin** (*$17.50 for 8 ounces*) contains menthol, which makes it anything but gentle for any skin type, much less for dry skin.

✔☺ **Vital Radiance Skin Renewing Toner Normal to Dry Skin** (*$17.50 for 8 ounces*) is a very good toner with about 2% salicylic acid (BHA). The pH of this product is about 4, which makes it fairly effective as an exfoliant. In addition to that it contains some very good water-binding agents and vitamins.

☹ **Vital Radiance Skin Renewing Toner Normal to Oily Skin** (*$17.50 for 8 ounces*) is similar to the Normal to Dry Skin version above except that this one contains witch hazel distillate as the second ingredient. Since that is composed mostly of alcohol, it makes this potentially too irritating and drying for all skin types.

☺ **CHR Lotion Concentrate** (*$32.50 for 3 ounces*) is about as basic a moisturizer as it gets. The teeny amount of collagen and vitamin E are inconsequential for skin.

☺ **CHR Cream Concentrate** (*$32.50 for 2 ounces*) is a very standard, ordinary moisturizer for someone with dry skin. It is exceptionally emollient, with several plant oils, mineral oil, and lanolin oil high on the ingredient list. But the small amount of collagen is just a good water-binding agent, it definitely isn't a concentrated amount.

✔☺ **CHR Double Action Night Cream** (*$45 for 2 ounces*) is a very emollient moisturizer for normal to dry skin that is loaded with water-binding agents and a small amount of antioxidants.

✔☺ **CHR Double Action Eye Cream** (*$22.50 for 0.5 ounce*) is similar to the CHR Double Action Night Cream above, and the same comments apply.

✔☺ **Light Captor-C Skin Reviving Day Lotion** (*$40 for 0.75 ounce*) is similar to the CHR Double Action Night Cream above, and the same comments apply.

✔☺ **Light Captor-C Skin Reviving Emulsion** (*$30 for 0.5 ounce*) is similar to the CHR Double Action Night Cream above, and the same comments apply.

☹ **ProCollagen Eyes with Sunscreen** (*$27.50 for 0.8 ounce*) doesn't contain the UVA-protecting ingredients of avobenzone, zinc oxide, or titanium dioxide, and for some strange reason no SPF is indicated. Without any way to know the amount of protection you're getting, you'd do well to avoid this product, especially as it has no UVA protection; it is not recommended.

☹ **ProCollagen Face and Throat with Sunscreen** (*$42.50 for 2 ounces*) is similar to the ProCollagen Eyes above, and the same comments apply.

☺ **Under-It-All Makeup Perfector SPF 25** *($13.50 for 1.25 ounces)* is a very good, titanium dioxide– and zinc oxide–based sunscreen in a very good moisturizing base with interesting water-binding agents and vitamins for someone with normal to dry skin.

☹ **Under Makeup Moisture Cream** *($22 for 2 ounces)* is a very ordinary emollient, though matte-finish moisturizer for dry skin. It is a completely unnecessary extra layer of product to apply.

☹ **Under Makeup Moisture Lotion** *($27.50 for 4 ounces)* is identical to the Under Makeup Moisture Cream above except that it is slightly less emollient, but the same basic comments apply.

☹ **Vital Radiance Skin Perfecting Lotion SPF 15** *($22.50 for 1.5 ounces)* and **Vital Radiance Skin Perfecting Cream SPF 15** *($22.50 for 1.5 ounces)* are supposed to be beta hydroxy acid (BHA—salicylic acid) formulations with SPF added. Even if they had a pH low enough to make the BHA effective as an exfoliant (which they don't), the sunscreen agents don't include the UVA-protecting ingredients of titanium dioxide, zinc oxide, or avobenzone to ensure protection against sun damage. Without those ingredients, these two products aren't vital in any way—at best they're trivial and unimportant.

☹ **Vital Radiance Skin Renewing Eye Reviver SPF 6** *($22.50 for 0.4 ounce)* has a dismal SPF number and doesn't contain the UVA-protecting ingredients of titanium dioxide, zinc oxide, or avobenzone; it is not recommended.

☺ **Vital Radiance Skin Renewing Night Serum** *($25 for 0.95 ounce)* is a very good, lightweight moisturizing lotion that contains several good water-binding agents and a small amount of antioxidants..

☹ **$$$ Brighten Up, Tighten Up Eye Cream** in **Amber**, **Rose**, and **Golden Tones** *($20 for 0.5 ounce)* is a very good moisturizer/concealer for dry skin. The ingredient list is immense; if you want to try almost every water-binding agent and antioxidant in the book (which isn't a bad idea), this is the product to buy. Unfortunately, the colors associated with this formulation are unrelated to skin tone, and despite the ingredient positives this won't be worth the tradeoff for most women.

ULTIMA II MAKEUP

Something has gone awry in the land of Ultima II makeup. The tester units have been compacted to include products from several different categories as well as haphazard new products. A formerly wonderful group of foundation colors has been whittled down to what amounts to an insignificant handful of options. Even more disappointing are the Glowtion products. What began as one innocuous, sheer, and shiny face tint has multiplied into an ever-expanding range of shiny companion products. For women who loved the luminescent shine they got from the original Glowtion, this is good news— they can now get more of that from companion products, including compact foundations, powders, lip glosses, and lipsticks. That much shine could serve as a beacon for passing ships! I mentioned in the previous edition that there would probably even be Glowtion

The Reviews U

mascara available so that the lashes won't feel all alone and boringly matte, but that day hasn't come … yet.

Perhaps most distressing is that this Revlon-owned line was once a pioneer when it came to offering women completely neutral foundations, powders, blushes, eyeshadows, and concealers. Few people know that the late Kevyn Aucoin helped create the refreshingly neutral, classic colors for Ultima II's crowning achievement, The Nakeds. What's left of today's Nakeds is barely worth mentioning, and it's almost embarrassing given what's taken their place. It's sad, but true—the Ultima II makeup you'll find nowadays is merely a shadow of its former self.

FOUNDATION: ☺ **Beautiful Nutrient Nourishing Makeup SPF 15** *($21.50)* has a great, in-part titanium dioxide–based sunscreen. This foundation has sheer coverage and a soft, lightweight texture that can feel a bit slippery while you're blending it, but dry skin will like this. There are now seven shades, with no options for darker skin tones. Note that Alabaster, Dawn, Almond, and Aurora Beige are too peach, rose, or orange for most skin tones. **Glowtion Skin Brightening Makeup SPF 15** *($17.50)* has ten wonderful colors with a smooth texture, but they are waylaid by this foundation's iridescent finish! Perhaps I can concede to a touch of shine for a special occasion, but for business day wear it's just too much. The sunscreen is in-part titanium dioxide, which is great. Note: This has a very strong fragrance.

☹ $$$ **Beautiful Nutrient Nourishing Compact Makeup SPF 12** *($23.50)* is a cream-to-powder foundation that is more cream than powder. It applies thick but blends well, and though the SPF is titanium dioxide, SPF 15 would have been better. There are seven mostly uninspired shades, with the only three to consider being Linen, Sand, and Natural. **Glowtion SPF 25** *($21)* is a tinted moisturizer with an in-part titanium dioxide–based sunscreen and a great SPF number. Almost all of the four shades for both the cream and lotion are iridescent and peach- to orange-toned. Fair is the only shade that looks like skin. The shine is on the subtle side, but it's still obvious. Glowtion is also available in a No Color version with an in-part avobenzone-based sunscreen with an SPF 15. The level of shine remains the same. **Glowtion Skin Brightening Moisture Cream for Dry Skin SPF 15** *($21.50)* has a creamy, whipped texture and feels moist while imparting a sheer iridescent glow to the skin along with in-part avobenzone UVA protection. Unfortunately, the colors are just as poor as for the Glowtion SPF 25 above, except for Fair. **Wonderwear Foundation SPF 6** *($21.50)* is one of the original ultra-matte foundations, and is essentially Ultima II's version of Revlon's ColorStay Makeup, and the same comments apply. The SPF is far too low to rely on for protection. Of the 12 shades, most are neutral, though Alabaster, Honey, Fawn, Almond, and Mocha (which is *very* orange) are too peach or rose for most skin tones. The long-wear technology is impressive (and this does wear on and on), but the tradeoff is a heavy look and dry finish that only those with very oily skin will love.

☹ **Wonderwear Cream Makeup SPF 6** *($21.50)* contains titanium dioxide as its sunscreen for UVA protection, but the SPF number is too low to offer adequate protec-

tion. This is a creamy foundation that provides full, opaque coverage; it's not for foundation beginners—and even pros may shy away from such a thick, hard-to-blend texture
that looks unavoidably obvious. If you decide to take on this foundation, Ginger and
Natural are best avoided. **Glowtion to Go Compact Tinted Moisturizer SPF 15** *($21.50)*
has a very good, part zinc oxide and part titanium dioxide sunscreen, but this is otherwise
an awful pink-copper iridescent cream-to-powder makeup that lays on enough shine to be
noticeable across a crowded concert hall. **Ultimate Coverage** *($18.50)* comes in a jar and
is a thick, full-coverage foundation that blends on quite well for such a heavy-duty product. This has been pared down to four shades, all with a rosy or peachy cast, which makes
this almost impossible to recommend. **Under-It-All Makeup Perfector SPF 25** *($13.50)*
gets high marks for its titanium dioxide and zinc oxide sunscreen, but otherwise it's just a
pale pink moisturizer sold as a makeup primer. The silicone-based lotion dries to a soft
matte finish, but the pink tint can mix with your foundation shade and create a third,
unexpected color. **The Nakeds Line Smoothing Makeup SPF 10** *($20)* won't smooth
lines, and, despite the claim to the contrary, it can settle into fine lines, like almost any
creamy foundation. The SPF is in-part titanium dioxide, but the three colors are too peach
or ash to recommend. This is all that's left of the once brilliant Nakeds foundation line!

CONCEALER: ✔☺ **Wonderwear Concealer SPF 6** *($13.50)* has a smooth, even
application that is neither too dry nor greasy, and that makes it an excellent choice. There
is only a small chance this will slip into the lines around the eyes. This is identical to
Revlon's ColorStay Concealer ($9.69), and the two shades are great. Though the SPF
number is far too low, the sunscreen is titanium dioxide.

POWDER: ☹ $$$ **The Nakeds Loose Powder** *($21.50)* is a talc-based powder that
comes in a huge tub and has shine, which fundamentally defeats the purpose of a powder.
Beautiful Nutrient Pressed Powder *($18.50)* has the requisite talc-based soft texture and
smooth application and looks light on the skin. There are only three shades, and Deep is
too peach for most skin tones.

☹ **Glowtion Translucent Powder** *($16.50)* is a pressed powder that has an almost
creamy feel, yet because it isn't tightly pressed, powder tends to get everywhere. The two
shades are clearly about shine more than color, and neither is appealing.

BLUSH: ☺ $$$ **Nourishing Blush Stick** *($17)* is a twist-up, cream-to-powder blush
that has a soft, beautiful texture and a sheer, even application. This is one to try if you
prefer this type of blush, and the colors are plentiful. Only Coral Sun and Warm Shimmer are shiny.

✔☺ **Gotta Blush Cheek Color** *($15)* is an outstanding powder blush that applies
evenly and color-true. There are only a few shades, but they're all beautiful and matte.

☺ $$$ **Wonderwear Cheek Color** *($16.50)* is smooth, but powdery, and all of the
shades have noticeable shine. Once on, it wears well, but there are more elegant blushes
to consider.

EYESHADOW: ☺ $$$ **Wonderwear Eye Color** *($15.50)* has some workable duos,
and they go on softly and evenly. The best duos are Wonder Taupe/Wonder Sand and

Wonder Mocha/Wonder Blush. The rest are too shiny or blue. It's sad that there are so few matte options when they were once so plentiful, but there's no doubt that shine sells.

☺ **Fade Not, Crease Not Eyeshadow Base** *($13.50)* is a silicone-based, pink-toned primer for the eyes. It does have a silky texture that dries to a soft powder finish almost immediately, but with mineral oil as the second ingredient the fading and creasing you were hoping to eliminate will only increase. **Re-Flektive Powder Eyeshadow** *($15)* are shiny eyeshadow duos that include a regular and a for-looks-only "speckled" color. These are acceptable as far as application goes, and most of the pairings work well together.

☹ **Peepers Wet/Dry Shadow** *($11)* are Ultima II's latest eyeshadow singles, and although there are some matte options and a smooth texture, this goes on a bit too powdery and tends to flake easily. **Swirlsational Cream Eyeshadow** *($15)* has very sheer, shiny colors sold as duos. The formula goes on well but stays slightly creamy, so creasing will eventually occur. These poorly formulated shadows make me long for Ultima's once wonderful eyeshadows.

☺ <u>EYE AND BROW SHAPER:</u> **Wonderwear Longwear Eyeliner** *($12)* is an extremely standard pencil that doesn't need sharpening; it's about as long wearing as most other pencils.

<u>LIPSTICK AND LIP PENCIL:</u> ☺ **Glowtion Luminous Lipcolor SPF 15** *($11.50)* does not have UVA-protecting ingredients and is quite greasy and sheer, with loads of iridescence.

☺ **Ultimate Edition Lipstick SPF 15** *($15)* is supposedly the ultimate due to its lipophilic spheres that continually release moisture as you wear one of these creamy, slightly greasy colors. Spheres or not, the best part of this lipstick is the avobenzone-based sunscreen. This is similar to (but not as nice as) Revlon's Absolutely Fabulous LipCream SPF 15 ($6.99). **Pucker & Pout Flowing Lipstick SPF 15** *($12.50)* contains avobenzone as one of the active sunscreen agents! That, combined with the traditional UVB-blocking sunscreens in this one, makes it a winner for those who want color *and* sun protection in one. I wish I liked the texture and application of this product as much as the sunscreen, but they both fall short. The thick, sticky texture can be likened to standard lip gloss, though you do get medium to opaque coverage along with a glossy finish. The lip color is fed from the base into a synthetic brush tip when you rotate the bottom of the container. It's a clever idea, but it is all too easy to click up more color than you need, and that makes application messy and uneven. However, if what is most important to you are more options for lipstick with adequate sunscreen these drawbacks are minor. **Beautiful Nutrient Nourishing Lipstick** *($13.50)* is another nice, but ordinary, creamy lipstick. Nothing to write home about, but not bad either. **Full Moisture Lipcolor SPF 25** *($13.50)* does not contain UVA-protecting ingredients, which is a shame, because the SPF rating is great. This is just a slick, slightly greasy lipstick that has a glossy finish and some amount of stain. **Glowtion Lip Brightener SPF 15** *($13.50)* has inadequate UVA protection, but is a nice sheer, lightly tinted iridescent lip gloss. **Lipsexxxy**

Lipliner *($12.50)* is a standard, twist-up, nonretractable lip pencil with only a handful of shades left.

☺ MASCARA: **Wonderwear Mascara** *($13)* builds relatively long lashes with no clumping or smearing, but it doesn't have any more staying power than other mascaras. The claim of keeping mascara smudge-free for 18 hours sounds impressive, but many mascaras can do that. **Lashfinder Mascara** *($11)* sounds like a detective for lashes, but it's just another good lengthening mascara that provides some thickness, albeit with effort. The dual-sided brush gives way to slight clumping, but it's manageable. The tube has a mirror on the side, so you can pretty much apply this anywhere.

UNIVERSITY MEDICAL SKIN CARE

What was true for this line in previous years is still the case today. And that means University Medical Skin Care just about wins the prize for the most ignominious claims and assertions about its products. First, there is no university associated with University Medical Skin Care (in earlier editions of this book, this line even quoted a physician in its ads, and when I interviewed the doctor who was supposedly quoted, he said he had never heard of these products—and this misinformation has since been deleted from the marketing materials I've seen for University Medical Skin Care). However, even if there were a host of doctors backing up the name University Medical Skin Care, they would all have to have their licenses revoked for endorsing such a distorted, overhyped line of products with dubious advertising practices. If you find the claims enticing and the prices seemingly benign, just keep in mind that almost all of these products contain nothing that can live up to even a small fraction of the claims being made for them, though several of them can be good moisturizers. After all, how many products in the same line can promise to erase wrinkles before we catch on that *none* of them are telling the truth? (Because if even a single one could erase wrinkles, why would you need more than that?) For more information about University Medical Skin Care, call (800) 535-0000 or visit www.universitymedical.com.

☹ **Face Lift Prima Hydroxy Daily Cleanser** *($19.99 for 4.1 ounces)* is just a detergent-based cleanser, though the third ingredient is alcohol, which makes this too potentially irritating and drying for all skin types. Plus, there are no AHA ingredients in this product to affect the skin (sugarcane and sugar maple are not alpha hydroxy acids).

☺ **Face Lift Collagen 5 C5 Serum** *($14.97 for 1 ounce)* contains a very good mix of antioxidants and water-binding agents, but it won't lift skin or collagen anywhere. It is an option for normal to slightly dry skin.

✓☺ **Face Lift Collagen 5 Cell Regeneration Cream** *($14.97 for 1.5 ounces)* is a very good emollient moisturizer for normal to dry skin that contains an impressive mix of water-binding agents and antioxidants.

✓☺ **Face Lift Collagen 5 Intensive Lifting Complex** *($12.97 for 1.5 ounces)* is similar to the Face Lift Collagen 5 Cell Regeneration Cream above only in lotion form, and the same basic comments apply.

☺ **Face Lift Collagen 5 Intensive Lifting Complex** *($12.97 for 1.5 ounces)* is an emollient moisturizer for normal to dry skin with some good water-binding agents, but only a small amount of antioxidants. There are some interesting plant extracts, ranging from mushroom to saw palmetto and wild yam; however, there is no research showing any of those to have benefit when applied topically to skin.

☺ **Face Lift Collagen 5 Concentrated Treatment Patch** *($9.97 for 12 patches)*. Skin receives no special benefit when a product is applied via a cloth patch placed over the skin. However, this does contain vitamin C, a water-binding agent, and an antioxidant. It is an option, but it doesn't add anything over and above what a well-formulated moisturizer can do.

☺ **Face Lift Vitamin C Anti-Wrinkle Patch** *($10.97 for 8 patches)* is almost identical to the Concentrated Treatment Patch above, and the same comments apply.

☺ **Face Lift Advanced Under Eye Therapy** *($10.97 for 0.5 ounce)* is a good moisturizer for the eye area if you have somewhat dry skin. Nothing in it will lift skin, but this does contain some very good water-binding agents and a small amount of antioxidants.

☺ **Face Lift Overnight Moisturizer with Lavender Aromatherapy** *($10.97 for 2.5 ounces)* is an OK moisturizer for normal to dry skin, but this does contain a lot of wafting fragrance, and that can be a problem for skin.

☹ **Face Lift Anti-Oxidant Moisturizer SPF 15** *($10.95 for 2.5 ounces)* does not contain the UVA-protecting ingredients of avobenzone, zinc oxide, or titanium dioxide, and is not recommended.

☺ **Daytime Advanced Retinol-A** *($13.97 for 1 ounce)* does not contain the UVA-protecting ingredients of avobenzone, zinc oxide, or titanium dioxide, and is not recommended. Plus, this product actually doesn't contain retinol at all; rather, it contains another form of vitamin A, retinyl palmitate, which is several generations removed from retinol (itself already several generations removed from the active ingredient in Renova and Retin-A).

☺ **Nighttime Advanced Retinol-A** *($13.97 for 1 ounce)* is an emollient moisturizer for dry skin that contains some good antioxidants and water-binding agents. However, like the Daytime version above this does not contain retinol.

☹ **Ease** *($19.95 for 2 ounces)* is one of those products aimed at baby boomers who are worried about the effects of menopause on their skin, and is also one of a growing number of products being sold with plant extracts that supposedly contain estrogen or progesterone. It does contain wild yam extract, but there is no research showing that this provides any benefit for skin, or has any bioavailable plant hormones that can be delivered to the skin. (For more on wild yam, see Chapter Seven.) None of the other plant extracts have any research showing them to have benefit for menopausal symptoms when applied topically on skin.

☹ **Thigh Cream** *($10.97 for 4.1 ounces)* does contain aminophylline, which was the original ingredient in the first thigh-cream product to be sold claiming to have scientific proof that it could reduce cellulite. However, research has established that this ingredient is not effective for that purpose (Sources: *Plastic and Reconstructive Surgery,* September 1999, pages 1110–1117; and *Annals of Pharmacotherapy,* March 1996, pages 292–293). Further, if this product did work, who would have cellulite? And wouldn't there be a lot more products containing this nonexclusive ingredient, instead of almost none?

☹ **Tummy Cream** *($9.97 for 4.1 ounces).* Well, why not? If you believe a cream can magically eliminate fat on your thighs, there should be something you can buy to magically take care of your stomach. This contains not one single ingredient that can remotely have any effect on fat anywhere on your body.

URBAN DECAY

Urban Decay (what a name for a cosmetics line!) wants you to know that "You are no ordinary beauty." According to the company's information, "The beauty of Urban Decay is in expressing that extraordinary beauty of yours any way you damn well please, even if you change your look every single day." Well all right, then, damn the torpedoes and full speed ahead, no matter what gets in your way! Their philosophy has an undercurrent of empowerment that's refreshing, and their products definitely walk the eccentric and somewhat wild side of makeup when it comes to creating your own unique look. Self-expression is a highly personal thing, and if Urban Decay's philosophy of "no rules, no formulas, just a lot of pretty pots, tubes, and vials of shimmery, shiny stuff" really speaks to your beauty ideals, by all means dive right in and color and glitter yourself from head to toe.

Urban Decay's formulations have recently improved in some respects. Along with their revised packaging, you'll find some changes—some for the better, others not so good, and still others for the worse. What definitely has not changed is the lineup of unusual nail-polish shades and all manner of sparkle-filled makeup that encourages you to "go for broke, not for average." You can say that again—talk about in-your-face makeup! This line has its image down pat, and how that fits into the image *you* want to project is a decision that only you can make. One quick comment about their skin-care products: They are little more than an afterthought, with names that are far more catchy than the formulations are clever. For more information about Urban Decay, call (800) 784-8722 or visit www.urbandecay.com.

URBAN DECAY SKIN CARE

☺ **Zen Cleanse 2-in-1 Cleanser and Toner** *($16 for 5 ounces)* is an extremely standard, detergent-based cleanser that would work well for someone with normal to oily skin. It can't function as a toner in the least because in a cleanser the water-binding agents and antioxidants would just be washed away.

☺ **Clean Up Gentle Makeup Remover for Face and Eyes** *($14 for 4.25 ounces)* is a standard, detergent-based makeup remover that is the same as almost every one of its type reviewed in this book. The inclusion of seawater is a bit bizarre, because getting salt

The Reviews U

water in the eye would be extremely irritating. I suspect it doesn't really contain that ingredient or it has been processed to be just plain water.

☹ **Detox Cocktail** *($16 for 4.5 ounces)*. There is nothing in this product that could detoxify anything. It is just an extremely lightweight toner with small amounts of water-binding agents and antioxidants. It could have been an option for most skin types, but this also contains camphor and lemon, and that makes it too potentially irritating.

☺ **Guardian Angel Protective Oil-Free Moisturizer SPF 15** *($20 for 1.7 ounces)* is a good, in-part avobenzone-based sunscreen in an exceedingly standard matte-finish base that is an option for normal to oily skin. However, there is no advantage to using this product versus Cetaphil's or Ombrelle's SPF 15 products, which both include more avobenzone than this version.

☺ **Guardian Angel Protective Moisture SPF 15** *($20 for 1.7 ounces)* is similar to the Guardian Angel Oil-Free version above, and the same basic comments apply, though this one is more emollient, which makes it better for normal to dry skin.

☺ **Magic Mud Pore Clearing 2-in-1 Mask & Scrub** *($16 for 3.4 ounce)* is as standard a clay mask as it gets, but it also includes ground-up plastic (polyethylene) as the scrub particles. It is an option for normal to oily skin. The claim that this has some magical property for skin due to the "10,000-year old Russian silt" it contains is sheer farce. It only contains a minute amount of the stuff anyway, and there is no research showing that silt, young or old, is good for skin.

URBAN DECAY MAKEUP

FOUNDATION: ✓☺ **$$$ Liquid Surreal Skin Liquid Foundation SPF 15** *($24)* is a fluid, almost runny foundation that includes an in-part titanium dioxide sunscreen. It applies smoothly, but blending must be swift, as it quickly dries to a solid matte finish. Coverage is very good—this starts at medium and can be layered from there for areas that need full coverage. Eight shades are available, and the first six are expert examples of what I mean by truly neutral colors—they're that good! The darkest shades, Vision and Mirage, are OK, but can be too orange for some skin tones. This is one to check out if you have normal to slightly oily skin and prefer more substantial coverage.

You can mix any of the foundation shades with Urban Decay's ☺ **Special Sauce** *($12)*, a sort of foundation "accessory" that comes in Glisten, Glow, or Matte formulas. The Matte formula has a dry finish and can prolong the matteness of the Surreal Skin Foundation, but not to a noticeable extent. The other two Sauces just add glitter or pink shine to the mix, and can be an option for special effects if you don't mind compromised coverage.

☺ **$$$ Surreal Skin Makeup 4 in 1 Powder** *($25)*. It must be the name that's surreal, because it can't be the quality of this fairly standard, talc-based powder that has a slightly thicker consistency so it can cover more like a foundation. It does have subtle shine, so those with oily skin need to consider the downside of adding more shine. If you have dry skin, a pressed-powder foundation can make skin look and feel drier. That leaves only normal skin types to use this version. The six shades are remarkably neutral, but for the money this isn't in the same league as Estee Lauder's So Ingenious Multi-Dimension Powder Makeup ($32.50) or Stila's Illuminating Powder Foundation ($23, $20 for refillable compact).

☹ **CONCEALER:** **Urban Camouflage Concealer** *($14)* is a very emollient, slightly waxy concealer that features a split pan of flesh-toned color with a mint green color. The mint shade is useless, and while the flesh tones are just fine, this will assuredly crease and is absolutely not a good idea to use to "treat hardcore zits," as the label states.

POWDER: ☺ $$$ **Surreal Skin Compact Face Powder** *($18)* is a talc-based, semi-opaque pressed powder that applies smoothly, albeit a bit thickly, which can cause a chalky look on some skin tones. The five shades are all slightly yellow-toned, and only Nirvana is too yellow to work for most skin tones. Pressed powder always works best if applied with a powder brush, and that is especially true for this version.

☺ $$$ **Universal Micronized Loose Powder** *($20)* is a talc-based, lemony yellow powder that goes on sheer, but this is definitely not a one-shade-fits-all product. Most will find it lends too strong a yellow cast to the skin, and that's a shame, because the texture is superb.

☹ **Baked Bronzing Powder** *($19)* is packaged in an aluminum baking pan that resembles a miniature potpie. This is one shiny bronzer, and the texture lays down very soft color, so you're left looking more shiny than tan.

☺ $$$ **BLUSH:** **Afterglow Blush** *($16)* has a supremely smooth texture and three workable shades, but the overpowering shine makes me hesitant to give this an all-out recommendation. If sparkly cheeks motivate you, this is one to try. **Cool Shimmer Stick** *($16)* is a pint-sized water-to-powder blush stick that goes on slightly wet and dissipates to a soft powder (in feel only) finish. The shine is very strong, and the glitter particles tend to flake outside of the application area, so be prepared to deal with way-ward glitter particles.

EYESHADOW: ☺ **Eye Shadow** *($15)* has an undercoat of smoothness that is compromised by the heavy dose of shine that each and every color has. Although the intensity of shine and levels of pigmentation vary, none of these shades are for anyone who wants a subtle glow. As you may expect, the shiniest shades flake terribly. **Liquid Metal Eye Color** *($15)* includes sponge-tip eyeshadow liquids that, surprise, come in intensely shiny, metallic hues. These have a dry, talc-based finish, so they do wear better and longer than traditional liquid or cream shadows.

☺ $$$ **Shadow Box** *($34)* is a set of eight eyeshadows (all very shiny) along with a highlighting cream. If you're sold on Urban Decay's colors and live by the motto "you can never be too rich or too shiny," this is for you. **One Stick Wonder** *($18)* actually gets you two powdery eyeshadow sticks shaped to look like thick pieces of chalk. These do have a dry finish, but they can be tricky to apply, especially with the glitter separating from the formula. For the experimental, the sticks can be used anywhere.

☹ **FX Powder** *($18)* is a test-tube vial of loose powder that is supposed to have a holographic effect on the skin; all it does is add shine. The texture is grainy and does not adhere that well, so you're left with shine everywhere except where you wanted it to go. **Pocket Rocket** *($17)* is a chunky standard pencil that's creamy and infused with flecks of glitter. This is a messy proposition for eyelining, and the glitter can flake onto the skin or into your eyes, so you may want to blast off with a shiny pencil from another line.

<u>EYE AND BROW SHAPER:</u> ☺ **Eye Pencil** *($12)* is quite standard and has a creamy finish that smears easily. **Smoke Out Eye Pencil** *($14)* is a standard, slightly creamy pencil that applies well and has a built-in sponge to facilitate the smokiness.

☹ $$$ **Sparkler Pen** *($16)* is a click pen with a fine brush tip that allows you to paint liquid glitter wherever you please. I am sure this is appealing to lots of women, but it's not a look I would encourage anyone to adopt.

☺ **Liquid Liner** *($14)* has a good, firm brush that applies the color evenly. This formula stays on very well. Even though the product itself is nice, the colors are truly bizarre and are either metallic or shiny, though Soot is a basic black.

<u>LIPSTICK AND LIP PENCIL:</u> Urban Decay's ☺ **Lipstick** *($12)* heavily favors unimpressive colors, although there are some beguiling options mixed in, particularly amid the reds. The thick, reasonably creamy texture isn't as nice (or opaque) as the previous formula, but clearly the unique colors speak louder than the performance. **Pleather Pencil** *($14)* is one of the greasiest pencil lipsticks that you'll find. The colors are bold and go on opaque, but expect this to smear and hitch a free ride into any lines around the mouth. **Skitz-O-Styx** *($14)* are overpriced, two-toned lipsticks that are very shiny and greasy. **Lip Gunk** *($13)* is a clever name for a standard, food-flavored gloss with a uniquely odd range of colors. These do apply smoother and feel less sticky that the former version, which is a plus for fans of blue, green, and silver gloss. **Lip Palette** *($10)* serves up ten of Urban Decay's lip colors in a credit card–sized compact. The amount of each shade is small, but half of these shades are among the best of this line's mostly unconventional colors. **Lip Arsenal** *($34)* is feast rather than famine for anyone who can't get enough of Urban's Lip Gunk. Here you will find eight shades in a compact, along with a lip brush— a necessary tool for applying this thick gloss.

✓☺ $$$ **Ink Lip Stain** *($17)* looks like a Magic Marker and delivers rich, fluid color that stains the lips for days. The color does fade, but not by much—even expert efforts to remove this will only reduce the color intensity by half. The three shades favor reds, and this is a surefire winner for ultra long-lasting color without any moisture or glossiness. As a bonus, this is quite easy to apply (but it must be applied quickly because it dries fast).

☺ **Lip Pencils** *($13)* are extremely standard pencils that need sharpening, though the small color selection is more intensely pigmented than most.

☹ **XXX Shine Cooling Lip Gloss** *($15)* is a tube gloss that has the runny texture of corn syrup, is just as sticky, and smells terrible. I don't know what they were thinking with this one!

MASCARA: ✓☺ $$$ **Skyscraper Mascara** *($16.50)* is an incredible mascara, but before I get into that, I need to mention Urban Decay's claim that the shu extract in here (also known as Fo-Ti) is included for its positive effect on hair loss and pigmentation, because this claim is based on folklore, not fact. This mascara won't stop lashes from falling out, and it only affects lash pigmentation when you wear it. However, the rather strange brush reaches each lash and allows you to lengthen, thicken, and separate lashes in just a few sweeps. It's a really nice balance of what a good mascara should do.

BRUSHES: ✓☺ $$$ Urban Decay has a small range of synthetic **Brushes** *($15–$35)*. Most of them are excellent, and they're made with firm, soft Taklon (a synthetic hairlike fiber), with enough density to apply color efficiently. The only one to be wary of is the **Concealer Brush** *($15)*, which has a strange square tip and is too flimsy for much accuracy or for even blending.

SPECIALTY: ☺ **Nail Enamel** *($9.50)* features all the funky, crazy colors you could possibly ever want, in an improved formula that's not much of a departure from the norm, except for the colors. If these shades strike your fancy, that's what you're really paying for. **Body Paints to Go** *($12)* is body paint in extreme colors along with temporary tattoo stencils, for those so inclined. There's not much more to say about it!

☺ $$$ **Liquid FX Sheer Sparkler SPF 15** *($16)* is nothing more than an iridescent tint for the face and body. The effect is glow with glitter and the SPF is without UVA protection. For that matter, it's without active ingredients! **Face Case** *($34)* is a face palette that includes four eyeshadows, two Lip Gunks, one lip gloss (which is indistinguishable from the Gunk), one powder blush, and two substandard applicators. I'm getting tired of saying it, but the shine is so prevalent you couldn't possibly choose this for any reason other than a strong desire to glisten and glow from head to toe. And yes, I am aware that rhymes.

USANA (SEE SENSE USANA)

UVAVITA (SKIN CARE ONLY)

I'm always stunned to see what warrants attention or headlines in the cosmetics world. In this case, it was grape seed oil that did it. With this simple ingredient added, what would otherwise be a completely unimpressive, innocuous, do-nothing group of products somehow becomes a miracle treatment for skin. Grape seed oil is now the answer for wrinkles because it is supposed to be the final answer for fighting free-radical damage. Or anyway, that's Uvavita's hook. Its products do contain grape seed oil. It probably won't shock you to learn that grape seed oil won't change or prevent a wrinkle on anyone's face, but even if it could, the minimal amount of it used in these products means that it isn't even all that helpful as an antioxidant. And despite the "Uva" in the company name, this small group of products doesn't include a sunscreen. (For your information, "uva" is the Spanish word for grape.)

The Reviews U

A lot of the buzz about anything involving grape extracts is from a story in *Consumer Reports* (November 1999) that ranked grape juice just above green tea and blueberries as having strong antioxidant properties. However, the benefits reported in both *Consumer Reports* and a lead story in *USA Today* (February 2, 2000) had to do with drinking the stuff, not putting it on the skin. There are no published studies indicating that grapes in any form, applied topically, can affect the wrinkling process (and vineyard workers are hardly wrinkle-free). But when it comes to skin care, there are lots of unpublished studies that "prove" all kinds of things. Uvavita loves to point to a Dr. Stephen Herber of the St. Helena Institute for Plastic Surgery (not surprisingly, St. Helena is in the heart of California's wine country), who conducted a study on the benefits of grape seed. In this "study," and I use that word loosely, 16 volunteers used pure milled grape seed extract as a topical application to their facial skin twice each day for six weeks. The results? What a surprise! Herber found that 88% of the volunteers reported improved texture for their facial skin. Other reported effects included evening-out of complexion pigmentation and excessive oil, a decrease in breakouts, and a decrease in dryness. But it only takes a cursory look to notice that this study wasn't done double-blind, that a placebo wasn't used (so we don't know if the results would have been the same with a similar or dissimilar type of extract), and that we have no idea of the status of the participants' skin before they started, or what their relation to the product line or researcher was. Even if you buy the results of this study, the study itself used a pure concentration of the substance on the skin, and Uvavita products use minuscule amounts of grape extract or grape oil, and there is no information on whether this watered-down version has any benefit whatsoever.

Right now, it's too early to suggest that we know which of the many antioxidants are the best, how much of them is needed, or even if they can conclusively work on the surface of skin to affect wrinkling. So when it comes to products that say they know best, we also can't be sure about which are a waste of money and don't help your skin. For more information about Uvavita, call (707) 967-8482 or visit www.uvavita.com. **Note:** A few Uvavita products contain a tiny amount of phenol, an extremely irritating preservative that is rarely, if ever, used in cosmetics anymore. As a matter of fact, this is one of only a very small number of product lines in this entire book that uses phenol.

☺ $$$ **Day Antioxidant Moisturizer** (*$53 for 2 ounces*) is an exceptionally ordinary moisturizer for normal to dry skin, though without sunscreen this is not a moisturizer to use during the day.

☺ $$$ **Night Antioxidant Nourishing Cream** (*$56 for 2 ounces*) is similar to the Day Antioxidant above and the same basic comments apply. The teeny amount of collagen in this product has no impact on skin.

☺ $$$ **Exfoliating Body Scrub** (*$34 for 6 ounces*) is a fairly gentle, extremely standard, detergent-based, overpriced body scrub that uses crushed grape seeds as the abrasive. Using this is taking a leap of faith that the crushed grape seeds have special properties for skin, though even if they did, they would be rinsed down the drain before they could have any benefit.

☺ $$$ **Exfoliating Dead Sea Mask** *($40 for 8 ounces)* is a standard clay mask with the most minuscule amount of grape seed oil imaginable. Aside from the grape seed oil, this product contains Dead Sea mud. While Dead Sea mud may have some benefit for certain skin diseases and it can absorb oil (just like earth minerals from any other source can), there is no research anywhere indicating it has any other unique benefit for wrinkles or skin discolorations.

☺ **Hydrating Body Lotion** *($30 for 6 ounces)* is just a decent moisturizer with a minuscule amount of grape seed extract.

VANIQA

Manufactured by Bristol-Meyers Squibb, Vaniqa *($37.50 for 1.05 ounces)* is FDA-approved as a prescription-only topical cream for reducing and inhibiting the growth of unwanted facial hair. (It has not been studied for its effect on hair on other parts of the body.) On the surface, Vaniqa might sound like a depilatory, like those nonprescription, drugstore products that topically "eat" away hair. However, Vaniqa's effect on hair and skin is unrelated to the way a depilatory works.

The active drug in Vaniqa is eflornithine hydrochloride, which has been used as an oral medication for certain cancers and to treat African sleeping sickness. There are many disconcerting side effects associated with this drug, ranging from anemia to diarrhea, vomiting, and hair loss. The notion that topical application of eflornithine hydrochloride could also affect hair loss probably stems from its hair-loss side effect when it's taken orally. However, the product information insert for the medication states that, when applied topically, eflornithine hydrochloride "is not known to be metabolized and is primarily excreted unchanged in the urine with no adverse systemic side effects."

The information insert also explains that eflornithine hydrochloride affects the skin because it "interferes with an enzyme found in the hair follicle of the skin needed for hair growth. This results in slower hair growth.… [However] Vaniqa does not permanently remove hair or 'cure' unwanted facial hair.… Your treatment program should include continuation of any hair removal technique you are currently using.… [Further] Improvement in the condition occurs gradually. Don't be discouraged if you see no immediate improvement. Improvement may be seen as early as 4 to 8 weeks of treatment … [and] may take longer in some individuals. If no improvement is seen after 6 months of use, discontinue use. Clinical studies show that in about 8 weeks after stopping treatment with Vaniqa, the hair will return to the same condition as before beginning treatment."

There are warnings that accompany this cream and there is still research to be done. Note that the insert warns, "You should not use Vaniqa if you are less than 12 years of age.…" Plus, there are animal studies that showed definite fetal problems. That means pregnant women should not use this drug, and lactating women probably should not either, though there is no research about that risk. Also, "Vaniqa may cause temporary redness, stinging, burning, tingling or rash on areas of the skin where it is applied. Folliculitis (hair bumps) may also occur," as well as acne.

So, should you consider Vaniqa? Well, that depends on how you look at the statistics, because clearly for some women it may work well to reduce facial hair. In addition, you must consider how often you have to use other methods such as tweezing, shaving, or waxing. And it sure beats the expense of laser hair-removal treatments.

What about those statistics? Vaniqa does not work for everyone. "In two randomized double-blind studies involving 594 female patients, approximately 32% of patients showed marked improvement or greater after 24 weeks of treatment compared to 8% [with a placebo]." It is important to note that 42% to 66% of those women in the study showed no improvement or actually believed their condition got worse. If you think it's worth it to find out if you fall into the group of those who might have success with Vaniqa, it may be worth the risk. Just keep in mind that this isn't a slam dunk. More than half of those who use it won't be happy with the results.

VERSACE

The Versace name is one that is well known to upscale, Italian style–savvy consumers. Widely known as the fashion world's "most extravagantly exotic designer," no other fashion figurehead from the last century so successfully merged urban chic with a pop-art rock-and-roll sensibility and celebrity as the late Gianni Versace. His couture and ready-to-wear collections were the epitome of fashion as abstract art, often commingling elegance and jaw-dropping edginess. Some of his most daring (and revealing) creations have adorned the bodies of luminaries like Madonna, Elizabeth Hurley, and Cindy Crawford, just to name a few.

Since 1982, Gianni Versace had steadily built a fashion empire, one that included his brother, Santo, and eventually, his younger sister, Donatella. Since his untimely passing in 1997, Santo and Donatella have continued to expand and propel the House of Versace into the upper echelons of luxury goods, encompassing all manner of fashion, perfume, housewares, and now, cosmetics.

Never one for subtlety, Versace's makeup line is a sight to behold. Each item is exquisitely packaged bearing the signature Versace logo of the Medusa. The Italian influence also goes beyond the eye of the beholder, as most of the makeup products have incredibly smooth, silky textures, and attractive finishes.

The Versace line is made in Italy—home to some of the best private-label cosmetics companies in the world—and they have no doubt been behind the scenes on many (if not all) of these products. What's ironic is that these cosmetics manufacturers offer exquisite products at low (and I mean *low*) prices, yet Versace is seemingly not interested in passing this savings on to cosmetics consumers. But why would they be? As an established prestige brand, it would be almost blasphemous to offer skin care and makeup at reasonable prices. Once the price drops, the illusion of affluence and exclusivity vanishes, and the products must stand on their own. Here, in the case of the foundations, powders, concealers, eye pencils, brushes, and mascaras, the line competes with the best of the best in all price ranges. Where it goes astray is with its oddly paired eyeshadow duos, ordinary brow and lip pencils, and good but pricey lipsticks. Another issue is with sun protection—three of the foundations and all of the lipsticks claim an SPF rating, but the sunscreen agents are not listed as active ingredients (an FDA mandate). Even when sunscreen ingredients are present in a product's formula, as they are here, unless they're listed as active they cannot be relied on for sun protection. Nevertheless, there are some completely worthwhile products to consider, despite the incomplete sunscreen claims and high prices.

The skin-care products, on the other hand, can't hold a candle to the quality of the makeup. In fact, the handful of facial and body-care products is so banal as to be a bit of an embarrassment by comparison. You'd be better off skipping over those and proceeding to the really interesting stuff that follows. Versace is sold in select Barneys New York and Nordstrom stores, and is available online at www.beauty.com. For more information about Versace, call (212) 317-0224. **Note:** All Versace skin-care products contain fragrance unless noted otherwise.

VERSACE SKIN CARE

☹ **Foaming Cleanser** *($33 for 5 ounces)* is a standard, detergent-based cleanser that contains sodium lauryl sulfate as one of the cleansing agents, which makes it too potentially irritating and drying for all skin types. At this price, that's a major mistake.

☺ **$$$ Creamy Cleanser** *($33 for 5 ounces)* is a fairly ordinary, wipe-off cleanser that includes alcohol high up on the ingredient list, which isn't the best for dry or sensitive skin. There is nothing about this product that isn't easily replaced with Neutrogena's Extra Gentle Cleanser ($5.49 for 6.7 ounces).

☺ **$$$ Perfect Zone Eye Cleanser** *($33 for 4.2 ounces)* is an extremely standard, and extremely overpriced, silicone-based eye-makeup remover similar to almost every one of its kind reviewed in this book. There isn't a reason in the world to spend this kind of money on such an ordinary product. This is fragrance-free.

☺ **$$$ Gentle Tonic Lotion** *($33 for 6.76 ounces)*. This is indeed gentle, but it is also void of any water-binding agents or antioxidants. It is merely water, slip agents, detergent cleansing agents, preservatives, and fragrance. It doesn't get much more mundane and tedious than this.

☺ **$$$ Rich Tonic Lotion** *($33 for 6.76 ounces)* is similar to the Gentle Tonic above only it includes a tiny amount of water-binding agent. That doesn't change much about this rather boring toner. The claims for this product far exceed its formulation.

☺ **$$$ Hydra-Effective Gel** *($63 for 1.37 ounces)* is a lightweight moisturizer that contains some good water-binding agents and a tiny amount of anti-irritant. There is nothing in this product worth the cost.

☺ **$$$ Hydra Effective Cream** *($63 for 1.37 ounces)* is a rather shockingly ordinary moisturizer that lacks any significant water-binding agents and is void of antioxidants.

☺ $$$ **Active Skin-Time Treatment** *($85 for 1.36 ounces)* is one of the more over-priced, exceedingly ordinary moisturizers for normal to dry skin reviewed in this book. It contains a modicum of water-binding agents and antioxidants. The teeny amount of whey and vitamin E in it isn't going to stop or change one second of aging.

☺ $$$ **Firming Anti-Wrinkles Treatment** *($100 for 1.29 ounces)* is similar to the Active Skin-Time Treatment above and the same comments apply.

☺ $$$ **Repairing Eye Zone Treatment** *($65 for 0.64 ounce).* This simple moistur-izer is about as lackluster as it gets. The fractional amounts of algae and plant extracts won't repair or change anything under the eye area.

VERSACE MAKEUP

FOUNDATION: ✓☺ $$$ **Cream Compact Foundation** *($42)* has a soft, ultra-smooth texture and a sheer matte finish. This talc-based powder foundation is on a par with favorites like Laura Mercier Foundation Powder ($38) or Lancome Dual Finish ($31). There are eight shades, and all are decidedly warm-toned. V2003 is too yellow for most skin tones, and V2002 has a slight shimmer, but the remaining shades are beautiful.

☺ $$$ **Lasting Hydrating Foundation SPF 15** *($47)* does not list any active ingre-dients, so it cannot be relied on for sun protection. However, if you're willing to pair this with an effective sunscreen, you will find this has an extraordinarily smooth, light texture that offers a seamless natural finish and light to medium coverage. This silicone-based foundation is best for normal to dry (but not very dry) skin, and the nine shades are wonderful. Shade V2003 is an excellent option for very light skin, while V2007 and V2008 are great for darker skin—neither color is too red or ashy. **Lasting Oil-Free Foun-dation SPF 12** *($45)* has the same issues of non-listed active sunscreen ingredients as the one above, but also shares the positive traits, although this formula is best for normal to oily skin. The slightly thick texture blends on evenly and dries down to a lightweight matte finish. The seven shades are mostly excellent, with the only cause for concern being the medium shades, which have a subtle peach tint that can darken into orange over oily areas. Otherwise, this is simply beautiful on the skin. **Smoothing Skin Founda-tion SPF 12** *($55)* follows suit and advertises sunscreen without listing any active ingredients, so it is unreliable in that regard. This creamy makeup has a dewy, very smooth texture that blends down to a natural finish. Coverage goes from sheer to light, and the silicone-based formula is best for normal to dry skin. This features six very good shades, with most falling between pale neutral yellow and golden. Only V2104 may be too gold for most skin tones.

CONCEALER: ✓☺ $$$ **Long-Lasting Hydrating Cream Concealer** *($30)* has a velvety cream texture that blends evenly over the skin and leaves a natural matte finish. The chances of this creasing into lines under the eye are good unless it is set with powder, yet the five shades go on less peachy than they appear, making this an expensive, though worthy, contender.

<u>POWDER:</u> ✔☺ $$$ **Natural Finish Loose Powder** *($42)* is a lightweight, talc-based powder that has a very smooth texture and a soft, dry finish. The shade range is excellent for both lighter and darker skin.

☺ $$$ **Invisible Pressed Powder** *($38)* also has a light, smooth texture, but it is noticeably more powdery and slightly drier than the Loose Powder above. This formula is talc-free, and contains mica and cornstarch, which explains the drier feel. Shade 2005 is too yellow for most skin tones, but the seven other shades are fine, especially 2006 and 2007, which are great bronzing powder colors. **Bronzing Powder** *($38)* is a talc-free pressed-powder bronzer that offers three believable tan shades, each with a subtle shine. The texture isn't as dry as the Invisible Pressed Powder above, and application is sheer and even. **Extra Glow Soft Loose Powder** *($45)* is talc-free loose powder with a smooth texture and a sheer, softly shiny finish. This is more of an occasional-use product, and when it comes to shiny powders, there are considerably less expensive options to try before this one.

☺ $$$ <u>BLUSH:</u> **Compact Blush** *($37)* has a dry (but smooth) texture and a collection of shades that favors vibrant hues over neutrals. These blush tones are not for the timid, though there are some workable options. Each shade has shine, and that makes this one hard to recommend over the plethora of smoother and matte powder-blush options from many other lines. **Glam Touch Blush** *($37)* has a delicate, silky powder texture and a soft, sheer application that is downgraded by the inclusion of noticeable iridescence. For nighttime glamour, this is an option, and the three shades are pleasant.

☹ <u>EYESHADOW:</u> **Eye Shadow Duo** *($32)* has some highly contrasting, vibrant color combinations, most of which are very shiny. There are a few OK color pairings, but the texture and application don't warrant the steep price. **Eye Shadow Single** *($24)* certainly reaffirms Gianni Versace's love of bold splashes of color. These are pigment-rich and all of them are shiny with a grainy texture that doesn't cling to skin very well, so some flaking is inevitable.

<u>EYE AND BROW SHAPER:</u> ✔☺ $$$ **Comfort Eye Pencil** *($24)* is a standard pencil with an excellent texture that's not too creamy or too dry. This includes a sharpener, and your best bets within the small selection of colors are the brown and black shades.

☺ $$$ **Eyebrow Pencil** *($24)* is your average dry-textured brow pencil that features a brow brush on one end for softening the color. It works, but at this price you may want to pass.

<u>LIPSTICK AND LIP PENCIL:</u> ☺ $$$ **Hydrating Lipstick SPF 16** *($21)* does not list any active sunscreen ingredients, so you can ignore the SPF claim. This is a thick-feeling, creamy, opaque lipstick that has a light glossy finish and richly pigmented shades, so most of the colors will have some stamina on the lips. Shade V2029 is a great universal red color. **Versace's Lips SPF 8** *($23)* is also without designated active sunscreen ingredients, but works beautifully as an ultra-light creamy-smooth lipstick. The intense colors offer full coverage and should wear well without needing perpetual touch-ups.

✔☺ **$$$ Wet Cream Lipgloss SPF 8** *($20)* is a pricey, though supremely smooth, non-sticky wand-applicator gloss that is a must-try if "great gloss at any cost" is your motto. The range of sheer to semi-opaque colors is excellent. The similarly named **Wet Lipgloss SPF 12** *($20)* is without active sun protection ingredients and is simply a slick, lipstick-style gloss.

☺ **$$$ Comfort Lip Pencil** *($24)* is a standard lip pencil that includes a sharpener. This has a creamy, slightly matte texture that drags a bit, but it also tends to stay put. The color selection makes this worth a look if premium-priced pencils don't faze you.

MASCARA: ✔☺ **$$$ Luxury Volume Mascara** *($21)* lets you easily and quickly create long, thick, nicely separated lashes without clumps. If you crave dramatic mascara, try this one.

☺ **$$$ Fabulous Mascara** *($21)* isn't my definition of what a fabulous mascara should be, but this does produce decent length and thickness in equal measure. This doesn't clump, but smears a bit unless you're very careful. **Gorgeous Curling Mascara** *($21)* is the in-between version of the two mascaras above. This provides more oomph than the Fabulous Mascara but isn't as striking in the thickness department as Luxury Volume. The amount of curl you'll get is not noteworthy, especially compared to less expensive options in other lines.

BRUSHES: ✔☺ **$$$** You are not likely to be disappointed by the feel and performance of most of Versace's **Brushes** *($18–$63)*. They are well-shaped and nicely tapered to fit the areas they're designed for, not to mention the softness of the natural-hair bristles. The ☺ **$$$ Lip Brush** *($21)* is rather unremarkable at this price, because it should be retractable or come with a cap, and it doesn't. The **Powder Brush** *($63)* is feather-soft but too floppy for even, controlled application of powders. But the rest of the collection is recommended.

VICHY (SKIN CARE ONLY/CANADA ONLY)

The Vichy line of skin-care products is owned by L'Oreal, and, much like L'Oreal, Vichy retails at drugstores, the prices are relatively inexpensive, and there are some OK products. The areas where Vichy excels are its sunscreens, though it falls short in its acne and moisturizing products. Vichy has chosen to set itself apart from other lines on the basis of the special water they use that comes from a mineral spring in the town of Vichy, France. (Of course, if this water is so special and great for skin it could make you wonder why all the L'Oreal and Lancome products don't use it.) Is there actually something helpful in the use of Vichy spring water for skin care? According to articles in the *International Journal of Cosmetic Science* (1996, volume 18, pages 269–277) and *Nouvelles Dermatologiques* (1998, volume 17), it seems that Vichy water has been used for local application in the treatment of certain dermatitis. But rather than having some mysterious quality, the most likely reason Vichy water helps is its high fluoride content. Two journal articles, one published in the *American Journal of Kidney Disorders* (August 1987, volume 10, number 2, pages 136–139) and the other in *Pathologie et Biologie* (Paris) (January 1986, volume 34, number 1, pages 33–39), indicate that Vichy water is "a highly mineralized water containing 8.5 mg/L of fluoride." Fluoride is a potent antimicrobial agent, and dermatitis conditions such as rosacea and psoriasis can be helped by topical antimicrobial agents, so it isn't surprising that the fluoride in the Vichy water may provide some of that benefit to skin. However, whether or not any of that benefit is retained once the Vichy water is mixed into a skin-care product is unknown.

What is clearly misleading are the claims about these products being hypoallergenic, because the fragrance in almost all of these products negates any notion of them having a reduced potential for allergic reactions. The company also claims they are dermatologist tested, but if a dermatologist did test them, he or she didn't know much about skin care in regard to irritation, or how an effective AHA or BHA product is formulated, or what ingredients can be a problem for combination skin. For more information about Vichy, call (514) 335-8000 or (888) 45-VICHY or visit www.vichy.com. **Note:** All prices are in Canadian dollars. All Vichy products contain fragrance unless otherwise noted.

☺ **Purete Thermale Demaquillant Integral One-Step Cleanser for Face and Eyes 3-in-1** *($15.50 for 200 ml)* is mostly a wipe-off cleanser with a teeny amount of detergent cleansing agent. It is an option for normal to dry skin and presents minimal risk of leaving a greasy film on the skin.

☹ **Dermatological Cleansing Bar** *($7.95 for 100 g)* is a standard, detergent-based bar cleanser that can be drying for most skin types.

☺ **Normaderm Express Cleansing Gel for Acne Prone Skin** *($9.99 for 150 ml)* is a standard, detergent-based cleanser with a teeny amount of AHA and a small amount of triclosan, a topical disinfectant. The amount of AHA isn't enough to exfoliate the skin, and the disinfectant would be rinsed down the drain before it could have much of an effect. Triclosan is an effective disinfectant, but there is no research showing it to be effective against the bacteria that cause blemishes.

☹ **Normaderm Express 2-in-1 Lotion for Acne Prone Skin** *($12.95 for 150 ml)* is mostly alcohol, and that hurts all skin types.

☺ **Purete Thermale Detoxifying Cleansing Milk for Normal & Combination Skin** *($15.95 for 200 ml)* is a standard, mineral oil–based wipe-off cleanser with a small amount of detergent cleansing agent. It is a good option for someone with normal to dry skin, but would not be suitable for combination skin.

☺ **Purete Thermale Detoxifying Cleansing Milk for Dry & Sensitive Skin** *($15.95 for 200 ml)* is a simple emollient formulation that is more of a cold cream than anything else. It would work well for normal to dry skin, though it isn't the best at removing makeup without the aid of a washcloth. It doesn't contain fragrance, which is best for all skin types.

☹ **Purete Thermale Detoxifying Rinse-Off Gel-Mousse for Normal & Combination Skin** *($15.95 for 125 ml)* is a detergent-based cleanser that uses some fairly drying cleansing agents that can be too drying for all skin types.

☺ **Demaquillant Yeux Sensibles Eye Makeup Remover for Sensitive Eyes** *($15.95 for 150 ml)* is a standard, detergent-based cleanser that contains way too many cleansing agents, as well as fragrance, which does not make it better for sensitive eyes, though as a standard makeup remover it is an OK option.

☺ **Purete Thermale Gentle Exfoliating Gel** *($15.95 for 50 ml)* is a standard, detergent-based scrub that uses synthetic scrub particles (ground-up polyethylene) as the abrasive. This also contains salicylic acid, but the pH of this product is too high for the BHA to be effective as an exfoliant.

☺ **Purete Thermale Hydra Fresh Detoxifying Toner** *($15.95 for 200 ml)* is an OK toner for most skin types, but it can't detoxify anything. This contains mostly water, glycerin, and an insignificant amount of antioxidants.

☺ **Purete Thermale Nutri-Gel Detoxifying Toner** *($15.95 for 200 ml)* is similar to the Hydra Fresh version above, and the same comments apply.

☺ **Thermal Spa Water** *($4.95 for 50 ml)*. The fluoride content of the water may have some antimicrobial benefit if you have dermatitis, but for general skin care it is not of help.

☹ **Lift-Activ** *($34 for 50 ml)*. The cornstarch in this product may make the skin feel tighter, though it is also drying and potentially problematic for dry skin. This is just an ordinary moisturizer with tiny amounts of water-binding agents and antioxidants.

☹ **Lift-Activ Eyes** *($26 for 15 ml)* is similar to the Lift-Activ product above, and the same comments apply.

☹ **Lift-Activ Night Intensive Detoxifying Firming Care** *($37.50 for 50 ml)* is similar to the other Lift-Activ products above, and the same basic comments apply.

☹ **Lift-Activ Dry Skin** *($34 for 50 ml)* is similar to the other Lift-Activ products above, and the same comments apply.

☺ **$$$ Lift-Activ Profil, Profiling Tightening Concentrate** *($37.50 for 30 ml)* is an emollient, though ordinary, moisturizer for normal to dry skin.

☹ **Lumiactive Rejuvenating Daily Filter-Care SPF 8** *($28 for 50 ml)*. While this does contain both avobenzone and Mexoryl SX, which are very good UVA-protecting sunscreen ingredients, the SPF 8 is far below the standard SPF 15 recommended by almost every medical association in the world, and this is not recommended.

☺ **Lumineuse Sheer Radiance Tinted Moisturizer, Dry Skin** *($24.50 for 30 ml)* is only a very basic moisturizer for dry skin, with teeny amounts of water-binding agents and antioxidants, and the color isn't the best.

☺ **Lumineuse Sheer Radiance Tinted Moisturizer, Normal to Combination Skin** *($24.50 for 30 ml)* is similar to the Tinted Moisturizer, Dry Skin above, only this version does have a matte finish and can be an OK option for normal to slightly oily skin.

☺ **Nutrilogie 1, Intensive Care for Dry Skin** *($30 for 40 ml)* is an OK, basic moisturizer for dry skin. Such minuscule amounts of vitamins and water-binding agents make them inconsequential for skin.

☺ **Nutrilogie 2, Intensive Care for Very Dry Skin** *($30 for 40 ml)* is similar to the Nutrilogie 1 above and the same basic comments apply.

☺ **Optalia Restructuring Eye Gel** *($30 for 15 ml)* is a good lightweight moisturizer for normal to slightly dry skin. However, the really interesting ingredients are listed well after the preservative, making them almost inconsequential for skin.

☺ **Thermal S1: Long Lasting Hydration** *($26 for 50 ml)* is a very good moisturizer for normal to dry skin with a very good mix of water-binding agents and antioxidants.

☺ **Thermal S2: Long Lasting Hydration for Very Dehydrated Skin** *($26 for 50 ml)* is similar to the Thermal S1 above, and the same basic review applies.

☹ **Thermal S Mat** *($26 for 50 ml)* contains alcohol high up on the ingredient list, which makes this too irritating and drying for all skin types, and it lacks any of the beneficial ingredients that are present in the other Thermal products.

☺ **Thermal S UV SPF 20** *($26 for 50 ml)* is a very good sunscreen that contains both avobenzone and Mexoryl SX, which are very good UVA-protecting sunscreen ingredients. Yet this ordinary moisturizing base lists cornstarch as the second ingredient, and that makes this problematic for most skin types.

☺ **$$$ Novadiol Intensive Re-Densifying Care, for Face & Neck** *($39 for 50 ml)* is an extremely ordinary moisturizer for normal to slightly dry skin.

☺ **Capital Soleil Protective Gel-Cream SPF 15** *($19.50 for 120 ml)* is a very good sunscreen for normal to dry skin; it contains three of the four known UVA-protecting ingredients: titanium dioxide, avobenzone, and Mexoryl SX. However, it also contains a good deal of alcohol, and that can be a problem for causing dryness and irritation. Do not use this one on your face.

☺ **Capital Soleil Protective Lotion SPF 15** *($19.50 for 120 ml)* is a very good UVA-protecting sunscreen for normal to dry skin; it contains titanium dioxide, avobenzone, and Mexoryl SX in an ordinary moisturizing base.

☺ **Capital Soleil Total Sunblock Lotion SPF 30** *($21 for 120 ml)* is a very good sunscreen for normal to dry skin; it contains titanium dioxide, avobenzone, and Mexoryl SX in a standard moisturizing base.

☺ **Capital Soleil Total Sunblock Cream SPF 45** *($21 for 50 ml)* is a very good sunscreen for normal to dry skin; it contains titanium dioxide, avobenzone, and Mexoryl SX in a very standard moisturizing base.

☺ **Capital Soleil Total Sunblock Cream SPF 60** *($19.50 for 50 ml)* is a very good sunscreen for all the same reasons the other Vichy sunscreens are so great, but the SPF 60 just doesn't make sense. The SPF 60 tells the average fair-skinned individual that they can stay in the sun for 20 hours, but there are very few places in the world that have that amount of daylight. SPF 60 doesn't offer "better" or more intensive protection, just unnecessarily longer protection.

☺ **Capital Soleil Sunblock Lotion for Children SPF 35** *($19.50 for 120 ml)* is a very good sunscreen for normal to dry skin that contains titanium dioxide, avobenzone, and Mexoryl SX; however, there is nothing about this product that makes it more appropriate for children.

☺ $$$ **Capital Soleil Sunblock Stick SPF 25** *($9 for 3 ml tube)* does contain in-part titanium dioxide; however, given that all the other sunscreens from Vichy also contain avobenzone and Mexoryl SX (which really add to the UVA protection you get) and cost less than this version, this is not the one to pick over those reviewed above.

☹ **Capital Soleil Self-Tan Cream-Gel for Face SPF 7** *($18 for 50 ml)* does contain very good UVA protection, but the SPF number is not enough for daily protection. It does contain dihydroxyacetone, the same ingredient used in all self-tanners to affect the color of skin, but the sunscreen protection is just misleading.

☺ **Capital Soleil Self-Tan Body Milk** *($19.50 for 100 ml)* contains dihydroxyacetone, the same ingredient all self-tanners use to affect the color of skin. This one will work as well as any.

☺ **Capital Soleil Express Self-Tanning Spray for Body** *($19.50 for 125 ml)* contains dihydroxyacetone, the same ingredient all self-tanners use to affect the color of skin. This one will work as well as any.

☹ **Capital Soleil After Sun Calming Reparative Gel for Sunburn** *($18 for 100 ml)* is an OK moisturizer for normal to dry skin, but the claim that it "encourages repair of damage to DNA caused by the sun" is a stretch of the imagination. There is not one ingredient in here that can repair the damage to a single skin cell that sunlight causes.

☹ **Capital Soleil Soothing and Hydrating After-Sun Milk** *($15.50 for 150 ml)* would have been a great moisturizer, but this one contains menthol, a skin irritant.

☹ $$$ **RETI-C Intensive Care, Retinol, Anti-Wrinkle Vitamin C, Radiance** *($34 for 30 ml)* is produced for all those women who will think that they now have the best of both worlds, a product that contains both retinol and vitamin C. However, this also contains aluminum starch (octenylsuccinate), cornstarch, and magnesium sulfate, which are all absorbent and drying and not the best in a product meant to help make skin look less wrinkled.

☺ $$$ **RETI-C Concentrate Night** *($37.50 for 30 ml)* does contain vitamin C and retinol in an ordinary emollient base. For a retinol and vitamin C product, this is as good as any.

☺ $$$ **RETI-C Yeux Eyes** *($30 for 15 ml)* is similar to the RETI-C Concentrate above and the same basic comments apply.

☹ **Normaderm Express (Tinted and Non-Tinted) Treatment Cream, for Acne Prone Skin** *($12.95 for 30 ml)* includes a teeny amount of glycolic acid that is not enough to exfoliate skin. It also contains triclosan, a topical disinfectant, but there is no research showing that this is effective against the bacteria that cause blemishes. This is an ordinary moisturizer with no benefit for any skin type, and definitely not for acne-prone skin.

☹ **Normaderm Patch Express, for Acne Prone Skin** *($10.99 for 24 patches)* contains a tiny amount of disinfectant and some BHA. The disinfectant triclosan has no research showing it is effective against the bacteria that cause blemishes. Plus, the pH isn't low enough for the BHA to be effective as an exfoliant.

☹ **Normaderm Stick Express Treatment Stick for Imperfections, for Acne Prone Skin** *($9.99 for 0.28 g)* contains lots of ingredients that would be a problem for blemish-prone skin, including castor oil, titanium dioxide, and thick waxes. What were they thinking?

☺ $$$ **Purifying Thermal Mask** *($19.95 for 50 ml)* is a very standard clay mask that can be good for normal to oily skin.

☺ $$$ **Rehydrating Thermal Mask** *($19.95 for 50 ml)* is a fairly emollient moisturizer, with a small amount of water-binding agents and antioxidants, that is being used as a mask, which is just fine.

VICTORIA JACKSON COSMETICS

Victoria Jackson Cosmetics was one of the first makeup and skin-care lines whose products were sold via infomercial, and it remains one of the most successful to hit the airwaves. Armed with everything from celebrity endorsements to impressive before-and-after pictures of women, Jackson's presentation is impressive. You almost feel like you're sitting on that overstuffed sofa, right next to Ali McGraw, taking turns exclaiming about how much you love this makeup, as Ms. Jackson nods in agreement.

It's hard to not fall under the spell of Jackson's concept of what it takes to look beautiful, especially when it's commingled with commonsense "when you look good, you feel good" philosophies. Though how good are you going to feel when you realize that Jackson's line hasn't been updated in years and that it lacks the benefit of many new technologies that allow for improved textures and application of powders, blushes, foundations, and concealers? The skin care is sparse and offers little that you won't conveniently find elsewhere, not to mention that there still isn't a sunscreen and the products are aimed at only one skin type, normal to dry. But this line isn't about skin care, it's about makeup—the very same makeup that (according to the infomercial) made "such a difference" in the lives of so many "Where are they now?" celebrities.

Note: All Victoria Jackson Cosmetics products have two prices. The lower price is wholesale, the higher price is retail. After you order a certain dollar amount, you will be allowed to buy at the wholesale prices. It seems like a great deal, but bear in mind that the poorer products in this line are not a bargain at any price. For more information about Victoria Jackson Cosmetics, call (800) V-MAKEUP or visit www.vmakeup.com.

VICTORIA JACKSON SKIN CARE

☺ **Facial Cleanser and Eye Makeup Remover** *($9.25, $13.50 for 4 ounces)* is a standard, detergent-based, wipe-off cleanser. This one would work as well as any.

☺ **Toning Mist** *($9.75, $14.50 for 4 ounces)* is a very good, nonirritating toner for all skin types, with some very good water-binding agents.

☺ **Moisturizer** *($13.75, $20.50 for 2 ounces)* is an OK moisturizer for normal to dry skin with a small amount of water-binding agents and antioxidants. It is not as impressive as the Skin Renewal System reviewed below.

✓☺ **Skin Renewal System** *($20.95, $40.95 for 0.14 ounce of Extra-Intensive Eye Cream and 1.25 ounces of Extra-Intensive Night Cream)* is somewhat unusual. The Night Cream is in the bottom half of the jar, and the Eye Cream is in the top half. Very cute. However, the ingredients in the two are not all that different, so the division is unnecessary. Both creams are very good moisturizers for dry skin, with an impressive mix of water-binding agents and antioxidants.

☹ **Firming Gel Masque** *($11.95, $17.50 for 4 ounces)* won't firm anything, and the second ingredient is a potential skin irritant. If your skin looks tighter after you take this mask off, it's due to the irritation.

☹ **Moisturizing Lip Conditioner** SPF 15 *($9.95, $15.95)* doesn't contain the UVA-protecting ingredients of avobenzone, zinc oxide, or titanium dioxide, and is not recommended for sun protection.

VICTORIA JACKSON MAKEUP

FOUNDATION: Victoria Jackson sells only one ☺ $$$ **Foundation** *($14.95, $25.95)*; it comes in a single compact that holds two shades for each of three categories of skin tones: Light, Medium, and Tan. The colors are marginally good, with the medium shades being a tad ashy green and the Light shades being a bit pink. The sole option for dark skin tones is best for Mediterranean or light Native American skin, but it is too light for most African-American skin tones. To create the right color for your skin, you are supposed to mix the two shades together, which is fine if you know how to mix them in the right proportions. If you don't, you're likely to have trouble. What's strange is that this emollient, almost greasy foundation claims to give you "all of the coverage you need, without a texture." Please! This is as thick and moist as the day is long, and if that's not a texture, I don't know what is. This truly has more cons than pros, but may be worth considering by those with dry skin who prefer adjustable coverage.

☹ **CONCEALER:** There is no individually packaged concealer in the Victoria Jackson line. Instead, she suggests using the lighter of the two foundation shades for the under-eye area. That would be fine if the foundation weren't so greasy. It's actually shocking that after all these years this line still lacks at least one good concealer. This one easily slips into lines around the eyes, and any liner you use afterward will probably smear.

☺ **POWDER:** Pressed Powder *($11.95, $17.95)* comes in three shades and is talc-based. The colors are all fine and the texture is sheer and light.

☺ **BLUSH:** Most of the Victoria Jackson kits come with at least one dual color **Blush Compact** *($11.95, $20.95)*, where one shade is either a pale pastel or vivid shade and the other is either a vivid or an earthy brown tone. The textures and colors are very good, although some of the color combinations do not work well with the rest of the kit's shades, and that can make blending one color into the next a challenge. In particular, the Beautiful Naturals II and Night Color Kits have blush tones that clash with the lip or eyeshadow shades.

☺ <u>EYESHADOW:</u> The **$$$ Eyeshadow Compact** *($11.95, $20.95)* is a single compact holding four different colors. Most of the color combinations are excellent, but there are a few odd mixes that would look a little off if applied for the same eye design. What's most problematic is that almost every shade in these quads is shiny, which is limiting if you're going for a subtle design or don't want this much shine all the time.

☺ <u>EYE AND BROW SHAPER:</u> All of the **Eye Pencils** *($7, $10.95)* and the **Taupe Brow Pencil** *($7, $10.95)* are standard, with a dry but workable texture. In most of the kits, you'll receive two twist-up eye pencils in black and brown. The Taupe Brow Pencil (which is not going to work for everyone) is available in the Introductory Kit.

<u>LIPSTICK AND LIP PENCIL:</u> Each Victoria Jackson Cosmetics color kit includes a ☺ **Lip Compact** *($11.95, $18.95)* that contains four different colors. In the original Peach, Pink, and Red kits, you get three fairly greasy lip colors and a lipcolor powder. The lip powder is a problem because it tends to cake on the lips and dry them out when used alone or for an extended period of time. The rest of Jackson's color kits contain the Lip Compacts in varying color combinations, and all four colors are the standard, greasy lipstick formula, this time with no lipcolor powder. Each kit includes a matching **Lip Pencil** *($7, $10.95)* that is just a standard, creamy, twist-up pencil. **Tube Lipsticks** *($9.95, $15.95)* are simply a traditional tube version of Jackson's lip compact colors. These are sold as a different formula, but, much like Jackson's compact lip colors, they remain fairly standard, opaque, and greasy lipsticks that are not for those prone to lip colors bleeding.

☺ **At Long Last** *($9.95, $15.95)* is a very creamy, full-coverage tube lipstick whose colors are not about subtlety. The eight shades stay on reasonably well (definitely longer than Jackson's other lipsticks) and their opacity and richness make them good choices for darker skin tones. This is still creamy enough to bleed into lines around the mouth, but it's a very good product that is definitely an improvement on the line's other lipsticks.

<u>MASCARA:</u> The Introductory Kit comes with ☺ **Dual Mascara** *($8.50, $13.95)*; this has a clear lash conditioner on one end and a black mascara on the other. The mascara is good, but the conditioner part is just glycerin and film-forming agent. It won't do much for the lashes, and you won't notice any difference when you use it. The black **Traditional Mascara** *($14.95)* is great all by itself, providing nice length and some thickness.

☹ **Fabulous Waterproof Mascara** *($9.50, $14.95)* goes on sketchy, smoothing evenly over some lashes while caking on others. It can make lashes feel heavy, and isn't exactly waterproof, so it ends up being a waste on all fronts.

☹ <u>BRUSHES:</u> For a line created and endorsed by a professional makeup artist, the Victoria Jackson brushes are a resounding letdown. A **Retractable Brush Set** *($9.95,*

$40) that includes a retractable Blush and Lip Brush is very overpriced (on the retail side) for what you get, and the blush brush can feel rough on the skin. The **Professional Brush Set** *($4.95, $18.95)* is available separately or as part of the Introductory Kit. It includes a lip brush, an eyebrow brush/comb, a two-sided eyeshadow brush, and a blush brush. The bristles on all of these brushes are sparse and not firm enough to hold color well. Avoiding these brushes is a very good idea.

☹ $$$ <u>SPECIALTY</u>: Victoria Jackson began her line with the **Introductory Kit** *($89.95, $234.35)* and it's still the backbone of the color line. The Introductory Kit is available in three different colorations (Peach, Pink, or Red) and essentially includes everything you need for a full makeup. You also get a copy of *The Victoria Jackson Difference* videotape, basically an expanded version of the infomercial, that gets a bit more detailed about how to use the products in the kit. For further explanation of the individual products in the kit, please refer to the respective reviews above. The regular **Color Kits** *($69.95, $162.50)* are condensed versions of the Introductory Kit above that include all the basics (foundation, powder, blush, eyeshadow, pencils, lip colors, and mascara) minus the makeup video and so-called Professional Brush Set. These kits do have their appeal, but it's likely you won't enjoy or use all of the colors equally, and the eyeshadow colors in the Red Kit contain shades that went by the wayside years ago. **Morning**, **Noon**, and **Night Collection** *($7 $11.95, $18.95 $20.95 per item)* aren't kits but are themed eyeshadow, blush, eye pencil, lip pencil, and lip compacts that are sold separately. The key concept is that the intensity of your makeup colors should be adjusted based on the time of day. Given that notion, should we then purchase three different sets of makeup and reapply it as the sun rises and sets? Hardly. It's more or less a marketing tactic that is a twist on the more straightforward terms Light, Medium, and Dark—which is exactly how the color gradations go as you segue from Morning to Night. There is also a **Shimmer On** kit that is a set of eyeshadow, pencil, and lip color, all with a pronounced metallic shine instead of the standard iridescent finish of most the other shades. The **Fine Wines**, **Subtle Dramatics**, and **Beautiful Naturals Color Kits** *($41.95, $82.75)* are more preselected kits that include blush, eyeshadow, pencils, and lip colors. The best-coordinated of the three sets is Fine Wines; the other two have one too many out-of-place, hard-to-combine colors.

Jackson's **Vanity Kit** *($52.95)* is dubbed the Ultimate Space-Saving Makeup Kit. It does look great in the picture and it does end up occupying only a small amount of room on your vanity. Yet for all the convenience and orderliness this kit provides, its containers are not refillable, so once products start running out, replacing them becomes an expensive proposition you have to start all over again. The James Bond-ish **Survival Kit** *($42.95)* is "so small, it fits in your hand," but this kit expands in every direction to reveal 23 makeup items, from lip colors to mascara and brushes. Of course, the amount of each product and the size of the brushes are minuscule, but this set was cute enough to play a pivotal role as a makeup prop in the film *Zoolander*. Overall, the packaging is very clever, but what's inside is easy to forgo.

VICTORIA'S SECRET COSMETICS
(MAKEUP ONLY)

Victoria's Secret makeup clearly tries to play up the same sleek, coy sexuality the rest of the Victoria's Secret merchandise is known for. And what could be a better environment for offering makeup! Victoria's Secret stores are all about a woman feeling sexy and beautiful, head to toe. Donning a silky teddy or lacy corset almost begs for full, glossed, pouty lips and softly blushed cheeks. Since the previous edition of this book, the focus has been tipped heavily toward emphasizing Victoria's Secret fragrances, of which there are now several. Just trying to reach the cosmetics (and not all stores stock the makeup) can involve several run-ins with saleswomen eager to determine your fragrance personality or spritz your wrist with scents named Very Sexy or Heavenly Angels. Once I reached the makeup without succumbing to the fragrances and ancillary bath products crowding the shelves (no easy feat, even for an "unscented" woman like me), I discovered it had barely changed at all since my last visit two years ago. The polished silvery containers and delicate pink boxes are indeed beautiful and the names are still sweet and winsome. Draw Me a Line Lip Pencil and Keep Your Secret Cream Concealer are irresistibly cute. Nevertheless, as I stated before, cute doesn't always mean quality, and beyond the packaging, there needs to be good product quality that works. The large display is inviting, though not nearly as well-maintained as it was in the past (another sign that the makeup has been downplayed in favor of perfume). The stores I visited had rather sloppy tester units, with many missing products, which made re-reviewing this line trickier than usual. Still, product after product touched down with just about the same results as last time around. Be wary of getting waylaid by the impulse buying this line (or any line for that matter) can encourage. A few of the products are worth your attention, but, as always, I encourage you to choose wisely. What won't be a secret after you read my review are which products work and which ones don't. For more information about Victoria's Secret Cosmetics, call (800) 888-8200 or visit www.victoriassecret.com.

☺ <u>MAKEUP REMOVER:</u> **Take It All Off Makeup Remover** *($8.50 for 4 ounces)* is a very standard, but effective and gentle silicone-based makeup remover. This is fragrance and colorant-free.

<u>FOUNDATION:</u> ☹ **Seamless Cover Oil-Free Cream-to-Powder Makeup SPF 10** *($19.50)* has a creamy-slick texture that quickly dries to a nice matte finish, and although the SPF of 10 is too low, the UVA protection is pure titanium dioxide. The 12 colors for this haven't gotten much better than they were when I first reviewed this line, but their excessive shininess has been eliminated. The following shades are too peach, pink, or rose: 05, 06, 07, 08, 09, 10, and 12.

☹ **Seamless Cover Moisture Rich Cream-to-Powder Makeup SPF 10** *($17.50)* has colors that are almost all poor, but what's even more disappointing is the lack of any UVA-protecting ingredients. The texture is rather thick and creamy, which isn't bad, just heavy and hard to blend. If you're up for the challenge, shade 04 is the only skin-realistic option. **All an Illusion Skin Tone Primer** *($17.50)* is your standard group of green-, peach-, and lavender-toned color correctors. They don't change skin tone, they only add a strange cast to the skin and interact even more strangely with your foundation. **Liquid Lingerie Moisture Rich Makeup SPF 10** *($17.50)* has become heavier, offering almost opaque coverage and a slight chalky finish in a poor selection of colors. Of the ten shades, the only decent options are 02, 03, and 05. The sunscreen now contains titanium dioxide, which is good, but the SPF number is still disappointing.

☺ **Liquid Lingerie Oil-Free Makeup SPF 10** *($17.50)* has far better colors than the Moisture Rich version above (there are 14, including shades for very light and dark skin tones) and a far more elegant texture. The application isn't as sheer as the name implies, but you do get light to medium coverage with a dry, smooth matte finish! This one is worth checking out if you have normal to oily skin, but watch out for shades 01, 04, 06, 08, 12, and 13. The too low SPF 10 is at least backed by titanium dioxide as the sole active ingredient.

<u>CONCEALER</u>: ☺ **Keep Your Secret Cream Concealer** *($10)* comes in a squeeze tube and offers three borderline neutral shades. It has a smooth, even finish, but it can crease, so test this one before you buy it.

☹ **Trick Stick Corrector Crayon** *($10)* has the same color-correcting concept as the Skin Tone Primer above, only in pencil form, and for some reason comes in only two shades, yellow and green. **Trick Stick Concealer Crayon** *($10)* is a pencil concealer that comes in some OK colors, but it's difficult to use and blending is sketchy. There is no reason to consider this over a liquid or cream concealer—almost any of them can outperform a pencil like this.

<u>POWDER</u>: ☺ **Powdered Silk Finishing Powder** *($15)* is a standard, talc-based pressed powder with a smooth, silky texture. Of the eight shades #2, #5, and #6 can be too rose, peach, or pink. The other five shades are excellent.

☺ **$$$ Sunny Cheeks Mosaic Bronzing Powder** *($17.50)* is pretty to look at, and the compact features five artfully arranged colors in one powder cake, but they're all shiny and impart little color. This works for shine over shading, but more than anything else this is prettier to look at than to wear.

<u>BLUSH</u>: ✓☺ **Sudden Blush Sheer Blushing Powder** *($15)* has a gorgeous silky texture in a beautiful range of colors, most of which have a touch of shine. The noticeably shiny shades are Honey, Mauve, and Sunny. This applies and blends extraordinarily well.

☹ **Dream Dust Face & Body Shimmer Powder** *($17.50)* is actually not all that shimmery, and the floury texture is not as soft and even as that of the other powders in this line. Although I'm not a fan of shine, this product wouldn't please even if I were crazy about it.

☺ <u>EYESHADOW</u>: **Silk Wear Eye Color** *($11)* is a good-looking group of very workable eyeshadow colors. Unfortunately, most of the shades are iridescent, but don't tell that to the sales staff, who more often than not call most of them matte. The only true matte shades were In the Buff, Shell, and Love at First Sight. **Party of 4 Transforming Eye Colour Quad** *($15)* is a set of four shiny shades of very pale pastel blue, pink, yellow, and green. The sales staff fawns over this as if it's the be-all and end-all of makeup, exclaiming how you can apply one of the iridescent shades over a pencil liner to change the color. Guess what? You can do that with any shiny powder, and these are no exception. The real question is, with all this shine going on, how is anyone who gazes upon you going to know where to focus his or her attention?

EYE AND BROW SHAPER: ☹ **Pencil Me in Brow Pencil** *($10)* has an exceptionally dry finish. That can make brows look less "penciled," but this one is hard to get on in the first place. If you want to put up with the tough application, this does stay put. **Dash Me a Line Eye Pencil** *($10)* not only needs regular sharpening, but is also so creamy that even those who have never had their eye pencil smear will find their track record broken upon using this, especially on the lower lashline.

☺ **Unruffled** *($12.50)* is brow mascara that comes in a clear gel (like a gel hairspray) and two sheer colors—blonde and dark brown. The color choice is limited, but this one works well enough.

LIPSTICK AND LIP PENCIL: ☺ **Smooth Talk Creamy Lip Color** *($12.50)* has an application that is definitely creamy, so if you have any lines around your lips this one will bleed in an instant. If not, the opaque colors are a great option. **Gentle Kiss Lip Conditioner SPF 15** *($12.50)* lacks significant UVA protection, so it's out as a broad-spectrum sunscreen for lips. However, as an emollient, glossy lip balm it works well. **Draw Me a Line Lip Pencil** *($10)* is a large range of standard lip pencils that have a creamier application than most, and they go on with ease. **Suede Touch Modern Matte Lipstick** *($13.50)* is what passes for matte these days, so I suppose the "modern" name makes sense. This is really a silky, creamy lipstick that feels lighter and provides less color impact than the Smooth Talk Lip Colors above. **Liquid Gleam** *($11)* is smooth, light lip gloss that has a wand applicator for glossing up whenever the mood is right. The silky texture of this is not likely to be a turn-off when it's time to kiss that special someone. **Mirror Mirror Shiny Lipgloss** *($10)* is a very good pot lip gloss that is thicker and more imbued with iridescence than the Liquid Gleam above. This has only a slight stickiness, which is more than tolerable.

☺ **Pure Reflection Ultra Shine Lipstick** *($13)* has a slippery, greasy texture that will slide off with even the softest kiss. The colors are almost all iridescent and are an option if that's the look you are going for, but it isn't the best for wear or texture. **Glamour Defined Swivel-Up Lip Liner** *($11)* is an automatic, retractable lipliner that's creamy but not nearly as smooth as the Draw Me A Line Lip Pencil above. The inclusion of a few dark brown to near-black colors is odd—but the label confirms these are indeed for lips, not eyes.

☹ **Pleasingly Plump Lip Enhancer** *($12.50)* is supposed to be a type of "spackle" that fills in the lips, making them smooth and perfect. It doesn't work. It's just an aluminum starch– and wax-based matte-finish concealer that sits on the surface of the lips for several minutes until it settles into the lines. It doesn't fill in anything or change the appearance of lips.

☹ <u>MASCARA:</u> **Brush with Greatness Thickening Mascara** *($12)* and **Exaggeration Lengthening Mascara** *($12)* remain unimpressive and barely capable of meeting basic expectations for mascara, and that's being generous. The Thickening version isn't much for thickness, but does add some length, while the Lengthening formula is the textbook definition of underachiever. **Push Up Plumping Lash Primer** *($12)* has a name that conjures up countless double entendres, but is merely a useless, sticky lash primer that would be easy to overlook if Victoria's Secret could find some way to ask, say, Lancome for its "secret" to superior mascaras!

☺ <u>BRUSHES:</u> If there is one solid area of interest for this line, it is the handful of handsome, silver-handled brushes. The feel is soft and the density great for application, though these fall a bit short of the best brushes. The **Face Powder Brush** *($17.50),* **Blush Brush** *($14.50),* and **Retractable Blush Brush** *($14.50)* work well, as do the **Eye Colour** *($10.50),* **Eye Liner** *($8.50),* and **Retractable Lip Brush** *($8.50).* The only one I question is the **Eye/Lip Definer Brush** *($8.50)*; it is really too small for the mouth and too big to use for the eyes. But if you need this specific size of brush (say, to smudge eyeliner), it is an option. This lacks a protective cap, so forget about using it to touch up lipstick while on the go.

VINCENT LONGO (MAKEUP ONLY)

Vincent Longo is a fashion makeup artist with a long list of celebrity and supermodel clients. To give a little background, Australian-born Vincent Longo has been in the business for quite a while. Believing "all women are beautiful," he studied makeup artistry in Italy and eventually migrated to New York, where he was the featured makeup artist for one of Cindy Crawford's first professional photo shoots, circa 1981. He has now joined the ranks of Bobbi Brown, Stila, Lorac, Trish McEvoy, NARS, and all the others with his own line of makeup products, though his line is in far more Sephora boutiques than department stores.

From a comparative point of view, Longo's line has strength in its foundation textures and colors, as the rest of the line is fairly standard and in some cases (for example, blush shades) woefully lacking. The eyeshadows have many positive qualities; yet, in contrast to those available from his competitors, almost all of Longo's eyeshadows have obvious shine. And then, in an effort to stand out, Longo's eyeshadow trios are embossed with floral and pinwheel designs that are eye-catching but impractical to use. The brushes aren't of the quality you might expect from an artistry line, and the mascaras pale in comparison to what you'll find from Lorac, Bobbi Brown, and M.A.C., among others. Knowing Vincent Longo's background and talents, it's genuinely surprising that his namesake line is such a mishmash of good and bad. If you decide to give this line a go, it's quite likely your experiences will echo mine. The superior products deserve to take a bow, while the bad ones need to be whisked offstage before the inevitable boos they'll elicit begin. For more information about Vincent Longo, call (877) LONGO-99 or visit www.sephora.com.

FOUNDATION: ✓☺ $$$ **Water Canvas** *($45, $12 for optional compact)* is Longo's trademark product, and though it has an interesting texture, it is not exclusive to Longo's line. For example, Awake's Hydro Touch Foundation ($30) and Borghese's Molto Bella Makeup ($35), like Longo's Water Canvas, are foundations that feel like liquid powder, have a watery rather than creamy feel, and then dry to a satiny-smooth, matte, slightly powdery finish. These are great for someone with normal to oily or combination skin, or slightly dry skin looking for light to medium coverage, and they all have beautiful textures and aren't the least bit greasy. Be aware that Longo's version can roll and chip out of the container if you aren't meticulous about keeping the compact tightly closed or if you get too zealous with your makeup sponge. Nevertheless, for color choice and the most natural finish, Longo wins hands down, with 16 mostly ideal light to dark shades. The only ones to avoid are Cafe Soleil, Golden Beige, Sienna, and Honey Pecan, which are too peach or ash for most skin tones. ✓☺ $$$ **Liquid Canvas Healthy Fluid Foundation SPF 6** *($35)* is extraordinary. This home-run liquid foundation is perfect on almost all counts: It has a modern texture, blends impeccably, and looks incredible on normal to slightly dry or slightly oily skin. The eight shades are benchmark neutral tones, though there are no colors for dark skin. The only peculiarity is the fact that no active ingredients are listed for the low SPF sunscreen.

☺ $$$ **Water Canvas Base Primer** *($40)* is sold as "the secret to foolproof results with virtually any foundation." Sounds good, doesn't it? Yet this is just a water-based silicone gel that disappears into skin and leaves a silky-smooth finish. It's fine as an expensive lightweight moisturizer, but in terms of enhancing a foundation's look or wear it isn't the dream product it's made out to be. The good news is that this would be a safe bet for blemish-prone skin with dry areas because it doesn't contain thickening agents or oils that can clog pores.

☹ **CONCEALER: Cream Concealer** *($16)* is disappointing, especially when compared to Longo's foundations. It's very thick and creamy, and the colors, though mostly adequate, are nothing to get excited about. This castor oil–based concealer will crease and crease and crease if you have even a hint of lines around your eyes. The same comments apply to the lipstick-style **Cream Duo Concealer** *($18)*, where you get two colors in one stick, with half of each shade being too pink or peach. Both of these pose a challenge when it comes to blending and wearability.

☺ $$$ **POWDER: Loose Powder** *($30)* is supposed to contain "triple milled lux silken fibers," and as exceptional as that sounds, this is just a standard, talc-based powder with a fairly standard feel and finish. It is a fine choice for loose powder, but price-wise it isn't preferred to the options from L'Oreal, Sonia Kashuk, or Clinique. Of the five shades, only Golden Oriental should be avoided, though Golden Banana may be too yellow for fair skin tones. **Bronzer** *($16)* comes in two of the best bronze tones around and is reasonably priced, but you'll still have to put up with a shiny finish, and that doesn't translate into a naturally tan appearance. If that's not your goal, give this a whirl.

<u>BLUSH:</u> The ☺ $$$ **Powder Blush** *($16)* has a beautiful, smooth texture but only two colors, which is a shame.

✓☺ $$$ **Lip & Cheek Gel Stain** *($18)* is a sheer, long-lasting liquid stain that you dot on with a wand applicator and immediately blend. The colors are a step above those of similar products from BeneFit, NARS, and Lorac, and that's saying something. The real tiebreaker with this one is how well it blends without streaking. The ✓☺ $$$ **Creme Blush** *($16)* has a small but good collection of intensely pigmented shades that blend on surprisingly sheer, though slightly greasy, leaving a slight cream-to-powder texture. If you're adept at applying cream blush, give this one a try—but remember, a little goes a long way!

☺ $$$ **Duo Powder Blush** *($18)* is a two-sided blush, with a matte cheek color and a shiny highlighter. It is difficult to separate the two with a brush, so you will end up with intense, chunky shine even if you're careful, which leaves me unimpressed.

<u>EYESHADOW:</u> ☺ $$$ **The Powder Eyeshadow** *($16)* consists of Matte, Glimmer, or Frost finishes, with a preference toward the ultra-shiny. That's regrettable because these all have a remarkably smooth, easy-to-blend texture and are dense enough to show up well on darker skin tones. The token mattes in this collection are beautiful, and most are deeper colors suitable for contouring or lining. Despite my distaste for overtly shiny colors, I have changed the face rating for these due to how well they apply and blend, without flaking. **Creme Powder Eyeshadow** *($16)* must be misnamed, as these are identical to (and as shiny as) the Glimmer Powder Eyeshadow reviewed above.

☺ $$$ **Eyeshadow Trio** *($20)* now has improved color combinations, but still shares three shades (all in one compact) that tend to spill into each other, making application difficult. They all have a silky, slightly creamy texture and apply beautifully. Many of these color combinations are stark contrasts and should be avoided; the ones worth considering are Autumn Rhythm and Evolution, which are matte. A nice touch is that each powder is labeled by number based on the order in which Longo recommends they be applied, and comes complete with a little instruction pamphlet.

☹ **Creme Frost Eyeshadow** *($16)* offers almost no color choices and has a slick texture and grainy finish courtesy of too much shine and glitter. **Alfresco-Matic Highlight Eye Shadow** *($25)* is absurdly expensive for what amounts to pastel, iridescent, cream-to-powder eye colors. The push-button pen dispenses product onto the brush tip, but tends to squirt out way more than you'll need, and there's no putting it back.

<u>EYE AND BROW SHAPER:</u> ☺ **Eyeliner Pencil** *($15)* is a standard pencil with a creamy texture that applies nicely but stays creamy, so be wary of smudging. The colors are plentiful, but Olive and Navy are best avoided.

☺ $$$ **Brush-On Brow** *($16)* is a slightly shiny brow powder that comes in four very good colors, each with a soft shine. I don't understand why eyebrows need shine, but it shows up often enough to be almost commonplace. This is easy to work with and allows you to build well-defined brows.

LIPSTICK AND LIP PENCIL: Vincent Longo's lipstick selection is large and not organized in any easily recognizable way. There are five purported finishes, and they are strewn throughout the collection with no rhyme or reason, a maddening prospect to say the least. The ☺ $$$ **Lipsticks** *($18)* for the most part are fine, though very standard and assuredly overpriced given their straightforward formulations. **Stain** is misnamed because it leaves no stain at all, though it provides greater color than the **Sheer**, which is more light-coverage color than sheer and has a slightly greasy finish. **Cream** is nicely creamy and opaque with a slightly glossy finish; **Frost** is similar to the Creams, except that they are heavy on the iridescence; **Satin Matte** is my favorite and is accurately named, since these have a slick texture, are opaque, and have a nice stain. **5 Pan Sheer Lip Palette** *($35)* includes five sheer, glossy lip colors (along with a good brush) in one package. This can be a fun splurge if you like the preselected colors.

☺ **Lip Pencil** *($15)* is an extremely standard pencil that needs sharpening. It tends to be on the creamy side, making it more likely to bleed into the lines around the mouth, but it does apply easily and the colors are nice.

☺ $$$ **Gel Crayons** *($18)* are standard, thick pencils that impart sheer, glossy color that can feel greasy, especially if used (as recommended) on the cheeks. As a sheer lip gloss that needs sharpening, it's a less than desirable option. **Alfresco-Matic Lip Gloss** *($25)* shares the same packaging as the Alfresco Highlight Eye Shadow above, but this is easier to work with and produces a smooth, moderately sticky iridescent lip gloss. **Lip Lux** *($16)* is gloss in a compact, and although it feels sticky, it has a high shine that gives a heightened dimensional quality to the lips. **Sheer Lustrous Lipstick** *($20)* are dual-sided lipsticks that feature sheer color and heavy shine in one. They are lighter and more slippery than Longo's other lipsticks, and not for those who want longevity from their lipstick.

MASCARA: Longo's ☹ $$$ **Mascara** *($16)* is only an option if you want minimal length and no thickness; otherwise, it is no competition for many of the superior lengthening and thickening mascaras available at the drugstore.

☹ **Waterproof Mascara** *($16)* builds decent length, but barely holds up if lashes get wet. There's no reason to consider this one over countless other waterproof mascaras that easily outdo it.

☺ $$$ **BRUSHES:** I was a bit surprised at the mostly unexceptional **Brushes** *($10– $35)* available from Longo. While some may find these shapes and textures workable, I have found far better options from M.A.C. to Laura Mercier than the selection offered here. One plus is that most of the brushes are available in short- and long-handled versions. The short-handled brushes can work well for travel, and the prices aren't atrocious, but for far silkier, more lush-feeling brushes this isn't the line to choose. If you're smitten by Longo's products, the best brushes to consider are the **Sable Lip Brush** *($24)*, **Jumbo Foundation Brush** *($33)*, and **Concealer Brush** *($28)*.

☺ **$$$ <u>SPECIALTY</u>:** Longo has launched the cool-looking, very sturdy **Spectralite Palm Palettes** *($20 for empty palette, $14 per blush, lip gloss, or eyeshadow tablet)* that look like something the cast of *Sex & the City* would rave about. Sadly, all is not what it seems and this ends up being an incredibly expensive way to assemble a makeup wardrobe. What's worse, most of the colors are bizarre and laced with sparkles (though they do have smooth textures), and the individual tablets are exclusive to Longo, so you can't purchase the case and fill it with someone else's colors. The salesperson confided to me that these had been on the counters for months, and not a one had sold, which, given the limitations, is not surprising. If the color selection was expanded or if the case were more versatile, this would compete nicely with similar offerings from Stila and Trish McEvoy.

WET 'N' WILD (MAKEUP ONLY)

Wet 'n' Wild is one of the few cosmetics companies around that prides itself on being extraordinarily cheap. But don't let its hokey name and its "cheap"-looking packaging deter you, because there are some great options available. The best-performing products will seem like steals, while the less impressive to horrible products will quickly have you thinking, "you get what you pay for." It is not very often that a line offers such a procession of clear-cut winners and dismal losers (almost all with the annoying prefix "mega-"), but once you know what to focus on, you won't get soaked by Wet 'n' Wild. For more information about Wet 'n' Wild, call (800) 325-6133.

<u>**FOUNDATION:**</u> ☹ **Twisted Cream Foundation Stick** *($2.99)* is a standard, cream-to-powder foundation with a poor, choppy texture and a limited color selection. The coverage is very sheer with a dry finish. It tends to disappear into the skin as if you hadn't applied it at all.

☺ **Keep It Real Oil Free Foundation** *($2.99)* is a very basic makeup that has a smooth, satiny texture that goes on sheer and light. This tends to stay moist once it has set, making it appropriate for normal to dry skin only. Among the small selection of shades, the best options are Naked, Honey, and Earth. **MegaPump Bronzer Gel** *($1.69)* offers little in terms of color, but is high on shine. I suppose it's nice that this is non-sticky.

☹ <u>**CONCEALER:**</u> **Cover All Stick** *($1.64)* is very greasy, easily creases under the eye, and the shades look nothing like real skin. How's that for "three strikes, you're out"? **Blemish Block** *($1.99)* is meant to be a medicated concealer for blemishes, and in reality is a transparent, shiny tint that uses willow bark extract as the blemish-fighter. Willow bark is distantly related to salicylic acid, but there isn't enough of it in this product to exfoliate skin, nor is the pH of the product low enough to allow it to be effective even if the amount was right.

<u>**POWDER:**</u> ☺ **Pressed Powder** *($2.49)* is a standard, talc-based powder, but considering the smooth, silky feel and even application, the standard classification is not so bad! The shades are slightly shiny, making these best for those who aren't worried about applying shine to their skin. ✔☺ **Bronzer** *($2.79)* comes in two shades—one is matte (#701,

a very believable tan color) and the other is orange and shiny (#702). The matte shade has an exceptional texture and would work beautifully as a bronzer or blush/contour color for most skin tones.

BLUSH: ☺ **Twist-Up Blush Stick** *($1.99)* is a great option for those who prefer cream-to-powder blush. These apply and blend well (much better than the Twisted Cream Foundation Stick above) and the colors are sheer and bright. Comparatively, you could pick up four of these for the price of one department-store blush stick, and you won't see much difference. These do leave a slight sheen on the skin, and Flirt is an opalescent shimmer that's best used for evening makeup, if at all. **Silk Finish Blush** *($2.59)* offers some excellent colors, a few of which are matte. If you find a suitable shade, these will work about as well as any other powder blush you may have tried, but bear in mind they go on sheer and are best for light skin tones. The Shimmer shade would make a decent shiny highlighting powder.

☹ **MegaGlo Face Illuminator** *($2.99)* is a Wet 'n' Wild misstep and not worth considering. This very greasy cream blush/highlighter is far less elegant than the shine-infused options from any other drugstore line, from Bonne Bell to Revlon.

☺ EYESHADOW: **Silk Finish Creative Eye Shadow** *($2.99)* are quad eyeshadows whose (mostly shiny) colors have improved, and for the most part the combinations make sense. This has a silky, slightly dry texture that is mildly prone to flaking. The same comments apply for the **Silk Finish Eyeshadow Singles** *($1.69)*, which include a small but decent selection of softly shiny shades. **MegaEyes Hi-Lighter** *($1.99)* is fine for silicone-based cream eyeshadow. The pale iridescent colors dry to a smooth finish, but can look a bit patchy on the skin. A shiny powder eyeshadow is much easier to apply and blend.

EYE AND BROW SHAPER: ☺ **Kohl Kajal Eye Liner Pencils** *($0.99)* are strikingly similar (if not identical) to all of the other standard pencils in the cosmetics world and work just as well. Don't let the price fool you; if you are used to using an eye pencil, these definitely work for lining the eye or filling in brows! Sharpening them is a pain, but that's true for any non-twist-up pencil.

☺ **Super Jumbo Body Crayon** *($2.39)* is a thick, chunky crayon that comes in shiny silver and glittery pastel hues that add shine wherever you use them. As long as you don't expect this to stay in place or last for long, you should be pleased. **Eyebrow/Eyeliner Pencils** *($1.69)* are dual-sided pencils, both with a smooth application but a too creamy texture that will easily smudge or smear. For a sheer, smoky look, these are an option.

☹ **MegaLiner Liquid Liner** *($1.99)* starts out as a promising liquid liner, but once it dries it tends to flake or peel off and you can remove this completely with plain water (convenient, but not good if you want long wear). **Eyeshadow Chalk** *($2.99)* does look like a small piece of chalk, and you may as well use plain chalk because this isn't too far from it. The shiny shades apply unevenly, ball up and flake, and are an all-around mess.

LIPSTICK AND LIP PENCIL: ✓☺ **MegaSlicks Liquid Lipcolor** *($1.69)* is a find for gloss fans! This smooth, fluid gloss comes in a dazzling array of colors (mostly of the "anything goes" variety) and has a light, non-sticky finish and light coverage. ✓☺ **MegaPlump Lipstick** *($1.99)* is a *Paula's Pick* because it is the best least-expensive lipstick in this book. This won't plump anything, but it provides rich, semi-opaque color and has a slightly greasy texture that never feels heavy and affords a soft gloss finish. This is slick enough to creep into lines around the mouth, but if that's not a worry, you should definitely audition this lipstick.

☺ **MegaColors Lipstick** *($1.69)* is more of a gloss than a lipstick, but it would work just fine for a sheer, wet look. **Silk Finish Lipstick** *($.94)* is Wet 'n' Wild's standard lipstick; it's a sheer formula with a glossy finish and has plenty of shades—and at this price, you could buy a dozen and experiment for weeks! **Precious Metals Lipstick** *($1.69)* is identical to the Silk Finish Lipstick above, except that these all have a shiny, metallic finish and less conventional colors. **Glassy Gloss Lip Gloss** *($1.69)* and **Mega Flavors Gourmet Lip Gloss** *($1.69)* are both standard pot glosses with a slight sticky feel and a very shiny finish. Look no further if you've ever wondered what bananas flambé lip gloss tastes like. **MegaSlicks Crystal Clear Lip Gloss** *($1.69)* is a very emollient gloss that isn't as sticky as the ones above, and you get a more sanitary, convenient wand applicator. **Lip Patrol Moisturizer for Lips** *($1.79)* is a standard castor oil– and wax-based lipstick that is available colorless as well as in iridescent gold or silver. Only the colorless version is recommended— the others look awful on the lips. **Lip Liner** *($.99)* is similar to the Kohl Kajal Eye Liner Pencil above, and the same basic comments apply. A few of the colors are excellent versatile shades that you really should check out if you can tolerate the sharpening aspect.

☺ **Lip Tricks Color Changing Lipstick** *($1.59)* may take you back to a time when these "mood lipsticks" were all the rage. It is just a light gloss with a hint of color. **MegaBrilliance Lip Gloss** *($1.69)* is a very standard, but certainly inexpensive, wand-type lip gloss. This is quite sticky and each shade is infused with flecks of glitter.

☹ **Glossy Gloss Lip Gel** *($2.99)* is lip gloss in a squeeze tube, and this one has a thick texture that's exceptionally sticky and highly fragranced. This is bound to be one of the most unpleasant glosses you'll ever come across. **Mega Core Lipstick** *($1.79)* is a greasy lipstick with a moisture "core" that's no different from the total lipstick formula. The color range is sheer, but mostly unattractive and of limited appeal.

☹ **MASCARA:** **Protein Mascara** *($1.69)* is one of the worst smear-prone mascaras in any price range. **MegaLash Lengthening Mascara** *($1.69)* is a complete disappointment in all areas, including regular smearing. **MegaVolume Thickening Mascara** *($2.99)* is an all-talk, no-action mascara that doesn't just keep the volume low—this sets it on mute. **MegaWink Lash Curling Mascara** *($2.49)* has nothing mega about it other then consistent smearing.

☹ **BRUSHES:** The too tiny **Brush Kit** *($2.09)* gives new meaning to the phrase "Why bother?"

☹ **SPECIALTY:** **MegaGlitter Body Gel** *($2.99)* comes in a pump bottle and is nothing more than water and alcohol mixed with film-forming agent and many glitter particles. I would advise you to check out similar alcohol-free options from Jane or N.Y.C. Color before choosing this.

YON-KA PARIS (SKIN CARE ONLY)

Yon-Ka Paris is a French line of cosmetics with a decidedly French accent, but that is where the élan of this pricey skin-care line starts and stops. The ads for Yon-Ka Paris declare that the company has a passion for the "world of plants … that nourish and heal the body and soul and restore the beauty of skin and spirit." At these prices, that's the least you should expect. Adding to the allure is a description of the name Yon-Ka. "Yon is a river in China known as a place of eternal beauty and renewal, chosen to symbolize the purity of the products; Ka is Egyptian for vital energy, representing the life force that all botanicals possess." Wow! But that is incredibly overblown for some fairly standard products that contain some incredibly unnatural ingredients that range from propylene glycol to polyethylene glycol-33, Vaseline, mineral oil, methylparaben, polyquaternium-11, diazolidinyl urea, triethanolamine, and on and on. Don't misunderstand me, I don't think any of those ingredients are terrible or awful for skin, but Yon-Ka Paris maintains that they are bad for skin. It is just inexplicably ironic that Yon-Ka Paris makes it abundantly clear from its piles of marketing information and stacks of training manuals that many of the ingredients in the company's own products are offensive to them! Didn't anyone else notice this?

I would love to challenge each and every outlandish claim made for these exceedingly standard formulations, but there just isn't room—it would take volumes. Let me just say this: For a line boasting about passion and blending science with nature, there is very little science to be found. No sunscreens are part of the daily skin-care routine, the products for oily or combination skin are destined to make matters worse instead of better, there is no disinfectant or effective AHA or BHA exfoliant, and the products for sensitive skin all contain sensitizing ingredients.

What is most shocking is that the company sells products encouraging sun tanning. Yon-Ka Paris must be in the dark about the fact that any amount of tanning or unprotected sun exposure can cause skin cancer and is the primary source of wrinkles and skin damage. Why anyone would trust their skin to a company that would settle for this kind of pathetic, and dangerous, information is beyond me.

The moisturizers are good and the cleansers are fairly run-of-the-mill, but many of the products contain irritating or sensitizing ingredients and, in comparison to many other lines that use a variety of water-binding agents and antioxidants and have well-formulated AHA and BHA exfoliants, these products just aren't that interesting or state-of-the-art. For more information about Yon-Ka Paris, call (800) 533-6276 or visit www.yonka-paris.com. **Note:** All Yon-Ka Paris products contain fragrance.

☺ $$$ **Gel Nettoyant Cleansing Gel** (*$34 for 6.7 ounces*) is a very good, but very basic, water-soluble, detergent-based cleanser for normal to oily skin.

The Reviews Y

☺ **$$$ Lait Nettoyant Cleansing Milk** *($34 for 6.8 ounces)* is as standard a mineral oil–based, wipe-off cleanser as it gets. It is little more than expensive cold cream, but it is an option for someone with dry skin.

☺ **$$$ Nettoyant Creme, Wash Cream for Very Sensitive Skin** *($31 for 3.5 ounces)* is similar to the Cleansing Milk above and the same basic comments apply, though given the amount of fragrance in here, there is nothing about this cleanser that makes it preferred for sensitive skin.

☹ **Gommage 303, Soft Clarifying Gel Peel with Botanical Extracts for Normal to Oily Skin** *($34 for 1.7 ounces)* contains way too many irritating ingredients, including lemon (the second ingredient), along with the added irritants orange oil, lemon oil, and lime oil, to be good for any skin type.

☹ **Gommage 305, Soft & Clarifying Gel Peel with Botanical Extracts for Dry or Sensitive Skin** *($34 for 1.7 ounces)* is similar to the Gommage 303 above, except that they left out most of the irritating ingredients except the lime oil. Why the company didn't know that the lime oil is also a potential irritant is anyone's guess.

☺ **$$$ Lotion, Alcohol Free Toner with Botanical Essential Oils for Normal to Dry Skin** *($34 for 6.6 ounces)* includes fragrant oils that may smell nice, but they are all serious potential skin irritants, and it contains no ingredients that are beneficial for skin. This is more like putting eau de cologne on the skin than using a skin-care product.

☺ **$$$ Lotion, Alcohol Free Toner with Botanical Essential Oils for Normal to Oily Skin** *($34 for 6.6 ounces)* is almost identical to the Normal to Dry Skin version above and the same basic comments apply.

☺ **$$$ Alpha-Complex Deep Retexturing Night Gel** *($59 for 0.5 ounce)*. The plant extracts in this gel are not AHAs and they do not have exfoliating properties. It does contain some good water-binding agents, but lacks antioxidants.

☹ **Alpha-Contour, Anti-Wrinkles Eye and Lip Contour, Renewing Gel with Fruit Acids** *($39 for 0.88 ounce)*. The mint oil this contains is a problem for all skin types, plus the fruit extracts are not AHAs and do not have exfoliating properties.

☹ **Creme 11, Calming Treatment Cream for Visible Redness** *($43 for 1.4 ounces)* would have been an OK (though extremely standard) moisturizer for dry skin, but the arnica, yarrow, and fragrant oils can cause skin irritation, which would only add redness to skin.

☹ **Creme 15, Purifying Treatment Cream with Botanical Extracts for Problem Skin** *($40 for 1.7 ounces)* is similar to the Creme 11 above, which makes it a problem for problem skin. In addition, this version contains coltsfoot, sage, and birch, along with the fragrant oils, which can cause problems for any skin type.

☺ **Creme 28, Protective and Hydrating Cream with Botanical Essential Oils for Dehydrated Skin** *($43 for 1.7 ounces)* is an OK moisturizer for dry skin that contains some good water-binding agents but only a negligible amount of antioxidants. It does contain retinol, but only a very minute amount.

☺ $$$ Creme 83, Protective and Environmental Cream with Botanical Essential Oils *($43 for 1.7 ounces)* is an OK, though extremely standard, moisturizer for dry skin. There is nothing in this product that would protect the skin from the environment, and there are far better-formulated moisturizers than this mundane formulation, which is void of any water-binding agents or antioxidants.

☺ $$$ Creme 93, Protective and Balancing Cream with Botanical Essential Oils, for Combination Skin *($43 for 1.7 ounces)* is almost identical to the Creme 83 above and the same basic comments apply. The exception is that, contrary to what the label indicates, this would absolutely not be appropriate for combination skin.

☺ $$$ Creme PG for Oily Skin *($43 for 1.7 ounces)* is similar to the Creme 93 above and would be completely inappropriate for oily skin.

☺ $$$ Creme PS, Protective and Nourishing Cream for Dry Skin *($43 for 3.52 ounces)* is an ordinary, though emollient, moisturizer for normal to dry skin with a tiny amount of water-binding agent and an inconsequential amount of antioxidants. This does contain a minute amount of retinol.

☺ $$$ Elastine Jour, Protective Age-Free Hydrating Cream for All Skin Types *($53 for 1.7 ounces)* is hardly appropriate for all skin types, and it won't stop one second of age, though it is an OK, though very standard moisturizer for dry skin with a minute amount of water-binding agents. Of course, without sunscreen, this is inappropriate for daytime use.

☺ $$$ Elastine Nuit, Age-Free Hydrating Cream for All Skin Types *($54 for 1.7 ounces)* is a fairly standard moisturizer with a small amount of water-binding agents that would be OK for dry skin. The inclusion of amniotic fluid is supposed to make you feel like your skin stands a chance of returning to the womb, but it can't.

☹ Emulsion Pure, Purifying Emulsion with Botanical Essential Oils for Blemishes *($40 for 1.7 ounces)* contains only water, a form of castor oil, and fragrance (essential oils). The claim that the essential oils can help blemishes has no proof or substantiation. Your face may smell nice, but with this product you also run the risk of making it irritated.

☺ $$$ Fruitelia for Dry Sensitive Skin *($60 for 1.7 ounces)*. Even the brochure that accompanies this product states that it has a pH of 5.4, which isn't low enough for an exfoliant to be effective (that calls for a pH of 3 to 4). Besides, the supposedly AHA content isn't the real deal, since it's only extracts of bilberry and lemon, which aren't AHAs.

☺ $$$ Fruitelia for Normal to Oily Skin *($60 for 1.7 ounces)* is similar to the Dry Sensitive Skin version above, and the same comments apply.

☺ $$$ Galbol 90 Firming Concentrate *($45 for 0.5 ounce)* is more of a toner than anything else, and a poorly formulated one at that. The plant extracts are mostly skin irritants and it simply contains water, glycerin, water-binding agent, and alcohol. This is neither great skin care nor firming.

☹ Nutri Contour, Eye & Lip Nourishing Protection Cream with Botanicals *($39 for 0.5 ounce)* contains peppermint, which is a potent skin irritant, particularly for the eye area.

☺ **$$$ Optimizer Cream** *($59 for 1.4 ounces)* is an exceedingly ordinary moisturizer for normal to dry skin with a small amount of water-binding agents and no antioxidants. It does contain a tiny amount of lactic acid (less than 1%), which isn't even vaguely enough to be effective for exfoliation.

☺ **$$$ Optimizer Fluid** *($59 for 1 ounce)* is an OK, lightweight moisturizer for normal to slightly dry skin with some very good water-binding agents, though it lacks antioxidants.

☹ **Pamplemousse, Protective and Vitalizing Cream with Botanical Essential Oils for Normal to Dry Skin** *($43 for 1.7 ounces)* contains grapefruit (pamplemousse) extract and lime oil, and that makes it a problem for dry skin.

☹ **Pamplemousse, Protective and Vitalizing Cream with Botanical Essential Oils for Normal to Oily Skin** *($43 for 1.7 ounces)* is almost identical to the Normal to Dry Skin version above, and that means it can be irritating for all skin types. However, the plant oils make it an even bigger problem for oily skin types. Why does someone with oily skin need olive, pumpkin, or coconut oil?

☺ **$$$ Phyto 52, Firming Treatment Cream with Rosemary Extracts for All Skin Types** *($50 for 1.4 ounces)* is an ordinary, though emollient moisturizer for dry skin that won't firm anything. The trace amount of vitamin E has no benefit for skin.

☺ **$$$ Phyto 54, Blending Treatment Cream for Visible Redness** *($43 for 1.4 ounces)* is similar to the Phyto 52 above, only with a different claim, one that it can't deliver on.

☺ **$$$ Phyto 58, Rejuvenation Treatment Cream with Rosemary Extracts, for Normal to Dry Skin** *($50 for 1.4 ounces)* is an ordinary, though emollient moisturizer for dry skin that won't firm anything.

☺ **$$$ Phyto Contour, Eye Firming Cream with Rosemary Extracts, for Puffiness, Dark Circles** *($39 for 0.53 ounce)*. The rosemary extract can be a skin irritant, which isn't great for puffy eyes, and the other ingredients just add up to a boring moisturizer for dry skin.

☺ **$$$ Yon-Ka Serum** *($43 for 0.5 ounce)* contains merely plant oils (corn, sunflower seed, and soybean) along with fragrance, and teeny amounts of vitamins E and F. Skip the fragrance, which is a problem for the skin, and use some olive oil from your kitchen, which has a similar benefit but without the irritating fragrance and expense of this product.

☺ **$$$ Creme 40 Lightening Cream** *($53 for 1.4 ounces)* actually doesn't contain one ingredient capable of affecting the color of skin. This is merely water, thickeners, plant oil, slip agent, preservative, and fragrance. It is an exceptionally dated formulation with a claim that is completely unattainable.

☹ **Dermol 1** *($38 for 0.5 ounce)* is more of a toner than anything else, but the inclusion of alcohol high up on the ingredient list makes it a problem for all skin types.

☹ **Dermol 2** *($38 for 0.5 ounce)* is similar to the Dermol 1 above, and the same comments apply.

The Reviews Y

☹ **Dermol 3** *($38 for 0.5 ounce)* is similar to the Dermol 1 above, and the same comments apply.

☹ **3 Creme 410, Protective Sun Cream with Botanicals for Dark Skin** *($28 for 1.7 ounces)* doesn't have an active ingredient list, and the regular ingredient list doesn't include any UVA-protecting ingredients. Further, this doesn't have an SPF (which is required by the FDA for real sunscreens), so even if it did contain UVA-protecting ingredients it's absolutely not recommended for reliable protection from any kind of sun exposure. It is just a very ordinary, dated moisturizing formula for normal to dry skin.

☹ **6 Creme 410, Protective Sun Cream with Botanicals for Fair Skin** *($21 for 1.7 ounces)* is similar to the 3 Creme 410 above, and the same comments apply.

☹ **6 Creme 410 Teintee, Tinted Sun Cream with Botanicals for Fair Skin** *($21.75 for 1.7 ounces)* is similar to the 3 Creme 410 above, and the same comments apply.

☹ **6 Lait Solaire, Protective Sun Tan Milk with Botanicals for Fair Skin** *($21.75 for 5 ounces)* is similar to the 3 Creme 410 above, and the same comments apply.

☺ **$$$ Ultra Protection, Age-Free Solar Block with AHAs and Botanicals, Water Resistant, SPF 25, UVA-UVB-IR** *($48 for 1 ounce)* is an in-part titanium dioxide–based sunscreen that contains no AHAs (the sugarcane and other plant extracts in this product are not the same as AHAs). It is a standard moisturizing sunscreen for normal to dry skin. To suggest that there are far less expensive as well as far better-formulated sunscreens than this is an understatement.

☺ **Auto-Bronzant, Self-Tanning Lotion with AHAs and Botanicals, for Face and Body SPF 4** *($28.25 for 5 ounces)* contains dihydroxyacetone, the same ingredient all self-tanners use to affect the color of skin. This one would work as well as any. The claim about AHAs is strange, given that it doesn't contain any, while the SPF rating is so low that it would be useless for sun protection, and just misleading as far as having any benefit for skin.

☺ **Lait Apres Soleil, Soothing Hydrating After Sun Milk with Botanicals, for All Skin Types** *($33 for 5 ounces)*. I would imagine that after not using a sunscreen you would want something to help your skin, but this standard, ordinary moisturizer isn't the one to use. For after-sun exposure, you would be better off using pure aloe vera, but you would be far, far better off if you used appropriate sun protection and didn't need these products, at least if you are interested in preventing skin cancer and wrinkles.

☺ **$$$ Hydratant 60, Hydrating Botanical Gel Mask for All Skin Types** *($39 for 1.7)* is just water, glycerin, slip agent, thickeners, a form of castor oil, preservatives, and fragrance. It is a completely ordinary skin-care product that is not worth the money or time to buy or use it.

☺ **$$$ Masque 103, Purifying and Clarifying Clay Mask, for Normal to Oily Skin** *($39 for 3.52 ounces)* is an exceptionally standard clay mask that contains more fragrance than most bottles of cologne. It is an option for absorbing oil, but it can't purify anything.

☺ **$$$ Masque 105, for Dry and Sensitive Skin** *($39 for 3.52 ounces)* is almost identical to the Masque 103 above and the same basic review applies. This would be a problem for someone with dry or sensitive skin.

☹ **Halo 70, "Instant Glow" Vials with Natural Essential Oils, for All Skin Types** *($43 for 0.5 ounce).* Hold on to your halo, because this contains water, glycerin, castor oil, fragrance, sulfur, and coloring agents. That means it borders on being one of the most useless and worthless products reviewed in this book, and that is really saying something!

YOUNGBLOOD

Aside from the catchy name, this line's claim to fame is an assortment of loose powders that perpetuate the trend of mineral makeup. These supposedly revolutionary talc-free powders are promoted as an all-in-one product—foundation, concealer, and powder. The brochure states, "You'll be amazed at how lightweight and long lasting this powder is," plus it's "water resistant, [it] won't run, smear, or fade," it contains no "talc, fillers, perfumes, [or] dyes," and it isn't supposed to cause breakouts. The good news is that half of Youngblood's claims are valid: This is an amazingly versatile foundation that can double as concealer or loose powder. The bad news is that the other half of its claims are embellished and misleading, although that doesn't diminish the positives. When considering this type of makeup base, keep in mind that if your skin is even slightly dry, the powder will cause flaking, and if your skin is very oily, it can pool into the pores and look patchy.

The brochure describes one of the ingredients, bismuth oxychloride, as a natural antiseptic that can be healing for problem skin. It can't. This earth mineral does have antiseptic properties, but it can also be a skin irritant, which doesn't make it very healing. In addition, the powders are supposed to give the skin "a translucent glow." The powder imparts a glow because it contains shiny, sparkly ingredients, including mica and iron oxides. If you have oily skin, you will not be happy with this much shine. However, these powders really do provide surprisingly even, smooth coverage that's easy to blend. They also stay on incredibly well, and for most of the day give the face a nice glow that only starts to look *too* shiny at day's end. Like nearly identical loose mineral foundations from Jane Iredale or bare escentuals, Youngblood's version did feel quite light, but it still provided completely opaque coverage and evened out most imperfections, especially when applied with a sponge instead of a brush. For more information about Youngblood, call (800) 216-6133 or visit www.ybskin.com.

☹ **Lyphazome SPF 30** *($22 for 4 ounces)* doesn't contain the UVA-protecting ingredients of titanium dioxide, zinc oxide, or avobenzone, and is not recommended.

<u>**FOUNDATION AND POWDER:**</u> ☺ **$$$ Natural Mineral Foundation** *($31.95)* is described in detail in the introductory paragraph above. This has a dry texture that is composed of titanium dioxide, bismuth oxychloride, mica (for the "glow"), and iron oxides (pigment). When used by itself, it's best for normal skin. There are 16 colors, with options for very light and dark skin tones, and most are wonderfully neutral and easy to blend. Be careful with Warm Beige (too gold), Sunglow and Coffee (both too ash), and Pearl (very shiny). The packaging has been improved, and the powder now comes in a wider, flatter container with a larger sponge. A word of caution: This product contains a

fair amount of titanium dioxide, which explains why, as a loose powder, it can provide opaque coverage and stay in place so well. When I asked about the lack of an SPF rating, the salesperson explained that it wasn't rated ("It hasn't undergone the expensive testing required to give it an SPF number"), but she said, "It rates an SPF 15." If Youngblood doesn't want to spend the money necessary to rate this product, that's up to them, but making any unsupported statement about sun protection is disingenuous and irresponsible. If a product doesn't have an SPF rating, you just can't know how much protection you're really getting. **Mineral Rice Setting Powder** *($17.90)* is talc-free, opting to use rice and cornstarch as its base. That can be problematic for those prone to breakouts because the bacteria that contribute to breakouts feed on such food-based ingredients. However, this has a finely milled, light, but very dry texture that provides very sheer coverage and comes in three good colors, though Deep may be too golden peach for dark skin tones. **Lunar Dust** *($25)* is very shiny loose powder than can go on a bit intense, and that coupled with the mess inherent to using such products makes it tough to recommend.

☺ $$$ **Pressed Mineral Compact Foundation** *($35.50)* has been reformulated, and no longer contains talc, which is good in the sense that Youngblood made much ado about their other powders being talc-free, as if it were an ingredient to eschew (it's not). Regardless, the latest version, which is rice powder–based, is much drier than and not nearly as silky-smooth as the previous powder. It's an OK option for a sheer application and dry finish, but not for those with dry skin. All of the six shades are soft and neutral.

BLUSH: ☹ **Crushed Mineral Blush** *($16.25)* is a shiny loose-powder blush that is messy to use and easy to apply unevenly. There really is no reason to try this, given the innumerable pressed-powder blushes available from almost every other line that are far easier to apply, and that includes the ones with visible shine.

☹ $$$ **Pressed Mineral Blush** *($19.50)* is certainly easier to apply than the Crushed Mineral Blush above, and the three colors are suitably neutral, but you still have to put up with a fair amount of shine and these do not blend as smoothly as they should.

☹ **EYESHADOW: Crushed Mineral Eyeshadow** *($15.50)* is also in loose-powder form and has the same application issues as the Crushed Mineral Blush above. There are 13 mostly pastel, ultra-shiny shades and a few labeled as matte that still have discernible shine, especially in daylight.

EYE AND BROW SHAPER: ✔☺ **Eye Liner Pencil** *($10)* is a very standard pencil that glides on smoothly and has a soft, dry finish, which means you'll have significantly less smearing and smudging.

LIPSTICK AND LIP PENCIL: The Youngblood ☺ **Lipsticks** *($14)* are creamy with a slightly too thick, waxy texture. It's nice that they're not greasy or too glossy, but the application could certainly be smoother. By the way, Youngblood makes a big deal over the "natural minerals" used to create its lipstick colors, but you only have to take a cursory glance at the ingredient list to see they contain the same minerals and FD&C colorants found in thousands of other lipsticks.

☺ **Lip Liner Pencil** *($12)* is just fine in terms of standard pencils, but you can find the same texture and finish in countless other less expensive pencils.

☹ **MASCARA:** The **Mascara** *($14)* is not worth all the effort it takes to obtain the mediocre results, plus it smears perpetually throughout the day.

☺ **BRUSHES:** Youngblood offers a small collection of mostly good brushes *($12–$20)* that aren't the fullest or softest you may find, but are certainly affordable. The **Small** and **Large Kabuki Brushes** *($14 and $16.50)* are very full and are attached to a small base instead of a handle. This can be awkward to use and it is not preferred to a standard, soft and full powder brush. The remaining brushes are worth a look if you happen upon a Youngblood display.

YVES ST. LAURENT

While the Yves St. Laurent haute couture label is considered synonymous with international standards of beauty and glamour, the makeup and skin-care products set no such comparative standards. In many ways this is one of the least impressive of all the French lines I've reviewed. The skin-care products are just OK, but truly ordinary and lacking recent innovations in formulary standards. Do you really want to overspend on something so ordinary? For more information about Yves St. Laurent, call (800) 268-2499 or visit www.ysl.com. **Note:** All Yves St. Laurent products contain fragrance unless otherwise noted.

YVES ST. LAURENT SKIN CARE

☺ **$$$ Soothing Creme Cleanser** *($27.50 for 5 ounces)* is a standard, mineral oil–based cleanser that can leave a greasy film on the skin, though it can be an option for dry skin.

☹ **Foaming Cleansing Gel** *($27.50 for 5 ounces)*. The cleansing agent is sodium C14-16 olefin sulfate, which can be very drying and may cause skin irritation.

☹ **Pure Cleansing Mousse** *($30 for 5 ounces)* is similar to the Foaming Cleansing Gel above and the same comments apply.

☺ **$$$ Instant Cleansing Milk** *($27.50 for 6.6 ounces)* is similar to the Soothing Creme Cleanser only in lotion form, and the same basic comments apply.

☺ **$$$ Gentle Eye Makeup and Lipstick Remover** *($24 for 2.5 ounces)* is just a synthetic emollient, slip agent, and preservatives; it doesn't contain fragrance. It will remove makeup, but it's just not worth the money.

☹ **Extra-Gentle Tonic Alcohol-Free** *($27.50 for 6.6 ounces)* is mostly fragranced water, and several of the plant extracts it contains can be skin irritants. It's about as do-nothing a skin-care product as you can imagine.

☹ **Mild Clarifying Tonic** *($27.50 for 6.6 ounces)* is an alcohol-based toner that can be drying and irritating for all skin types.

☹ **Matifying Beauty Toner** *($30 for 6.7 ounces)* is an alcohol-based toner that can be drying and irritating for all skin types, and that isn't beautiful in the least.

☹ **Hydra Tech Optimum Hydration Creme SPF 8** *($58 for 1 ounce)*. Although this does contain avobenzone for UVA protection, the SPF 8 falls far below the standard SPF 15 recommended by almost every medical association in the world.

☹ **Hydra Tech Optimum Hydration Lotion SPF 8** *($58 for 1 ounce)* is similar to the Creme SPF 8 version above, and the same comments apply.

☺ **$$$ Instant Grand Jour Daylight Creme** *($53 for 1.7 ounces)* is an emollient moisturizer for normal to dry skin that has a good mix, though only an extremely tiny amount, of some very good water-binding agents and antioxidants. This does not have sunscreen and should not be worn during the day.

☺ **$$$ Visible Energie Complete Day Creme for Combination Skin** *($55 for 1.7 ounces)* is a very ordinary moisturizer for normal to dry skin. For this price you would expect a lot more.

☺ **$$$ Visible Energie Oil Free Lotion** *($50 for 1.6 ounces)* contains several ingredients that could be problematic for combination skin. Aside from that, this is just a rather average moisturizer for normal to dry skin that contains a tiny amount of water-binding agents and an antioxidant.

☺ **$$$ Anti Wrinkle Concentrate** *($85 for 1 ounce)* is an exceedingly overpriced moisturizer. It has what amounts to an exceedingly mundane formulation with trace amounts of water-binding agents and antioxidant, and is a complete waste of money as well as a waste of effort to apply.

☺ **$$$ Firm Effects Eye Complex** *($48 for 0.5 ounce)*. It's almost embarrassing how ordinary a moisturizing formula this is. The teeny amounts of yeast, soybean, and plankton extracts may have some minor anti-irritant benefit, but given this ordinary group of ingredients, why bother?

☺ **$$$ Firm Effects Creme** *($65 for 1 ounce)*. Much like the Eye Complex above, this product contains minuscule amounts of yeast, soybean, and plankton extracts and a trace amount of vitamin E, which all adds up to an ordinary, mundane, and incredibly overpriced moisturizer.

☺ **$$$ Firm Effects Lotion** *($57 for 1 ounce)* is almost identical to the Firm Effects Creme above only in lotion form, and the same basic comments apply.

☺ **$$$ Firming Eye and Lip Creme** *($60 for 0.5 ounce)* is almost identical to the Firm Effects Creme above, only in lotion form, and the same basic comments apply. The only difference is the addition of a minuscule amount of cytochrome. Cytochrome is a protein found in blood cells that, with the aid of enzymes, serves a vital function in the transfer of energy within cells. There are three types of cytochromes, indicated by A, B, or C, with cytochrome C being the most stable. However, in order to be effective in their function of cellular respiration, cytochromes require a complex process that is triggered by a sequence of other components, and thus they can serve no function alone by themselves on the skin.

☺ **$$$ Firm Effects Instant Lift Concentrate** *($70 for 1 ounce)* is almost identical to the Firm Effects Eye Complex above and the same basic comments apply. There is nothing in this that can lift skin even a fraction of a millimeter.

☹ **Firm Effects Neck Serum, Emulsion and Gel** *($85 for 1.6 ounces)*. Both the Emulsion and Gel list alcohol as the second ingredient, and that is too drying and irritating for all skin types.

☺ **$$$ Fruit Jeunesse/Firming Renewal Complex Glucohydroxy Acid** *($57 for 1.6 ounces)* is an OK 4% malic acid (AHA) product. However, malic acid is not considered the best AHA—glycolic and lactic acids are considered better for penetration and reliable exfoliation. This product is an option, but there are far better and less expensive AHA formulations than this one.

☹ **Hydro-Light Day Lotion, SPF 15** *($50 for 1.3 ounces)* doesn't contain the UVA-protecting ingredients of titanium dioxide, zinc oxide, or avobenzone, and is not recommended.

☺ **$$$ Instant Firming Gel** *($60 for 1 ounce)* is an OK gel moisturizer that contains some good water-binding agents and a tiny amount of antioxidants.

☺ **$$$ Smoothing Eye Contour Gel** *($52 for 0.5 ounce)* includes some interesting water-binding ingredients, but they are listed well after the preservatives, which makes them useless. Other than that, this is a good, though very ordinary, lightweight moisturizer for normal to slightly dry skin. The yeast and collagen are present in such teeny amounts as to have no benefit for skin.

☺ **$$$ Temps Majeur Intensive Skin Supplement** *($280 for 1.6 ounces)*. The only thing major about this product is the price. It is a silicone-based moisturizer with a small amount of water-binding agents and a negligible amount of antioxidant. This product's claim to fame is that it contains *Ganoderma lucidum* extract; that is, mushroom stem extract. There are several animal and in vitro studies showing that this extract, when taken orally, may have properties that make it effective as an antitumor, immune modulating, anticoagulant, antiviral, and antibacterial substance (Sources: *International Journal of Cancer,* November 2002, pages 250–253; *Immunology Letters,* October 2002, pages 163–169; *Life Sciences,* June 2002, pages 623–638; *Cancer Letters,* August 2002, pages 155–161; and *Bioorganic and Medicinal Chemistry,* April 2002, pages 1057–1062). However, there is no research showing it to be effective when used topically on skin (Source: *Natural Medicines Comprehensive Database,* www.naturaldatabase.com). It most likely does have antioxidant properties (Source: *Journal of Agricultural and Food Chemistry,* October 2002, pages 6072–6077), but that hardly makes it a must-have ingredient for skin.

☺ **$$$ Time Prevention Day Creme** *($72 for 1.7 ounces)* is an overpriced, extremely standard moisturizer for dry skin with the most mundane formulation. The tiny amounts of antioxidant and water-binding agents make it a waste of your time.

☺ **$$$ Absolute Purifying Masque** *($33 for 2.5 ounces)* is a standard clay mask that won't purify anything, though it can absorb some amount of oil.

☺ **$$$ Hydra Tech Optimum Hydration Mask** *($48 for 2 ounces)* is an ordinary, mundane group of thickening and slip agents with teeny amounts of water-binding agents.

☺ **$$$ Natural Action Exfoliator Granule-Free** *($40 for 2.5 ounces)*. Rubbing this waxy cream over the skin helps to rub off dead skin cells. It works, but it's pricey for such a basic formulation.

YVES ST. LAURENT MAKEUP

Even though revered fashion designer Yves St. Laurent retired in early 2002, his ready-to-wear clothing, fragrances, and cosmetics live on under the ownership of Gucci. Tom Ford, the man who single-handedly revitalized Gucci in the minds of the fashion-conscious, is now Creative Director of the Yves St. Laurent brand. Perhaps Mr. Ford is being stretched too thin, because the changes that were made in Laurent's makeup products were not in the realm of raising the level of performance, but rather in honing the image. Of course, couture cosmetics lines especially rely on image to sell their wares. When you're charging four to ten times what dozens of other lines do for comparable products, you must have image to spare in order to get the consumer's attention. Yves St. Laurent makeup does have an improved tester unit that makes almost everything readily accessible, and the former gold compacts and caps are transitioning to sleek, gunmetal gray components. Yet for all the aesthetic improvements, most of the products still fall short of what other department-store lines offer, whether the influence is French (Lancome or Chanel), Italian (Versace), or American (Estee Lauder). The YSL foundations are bedecked with promises they cannot possibly fulfill given the ingredient lists and the predominantly poor colors. Other categories contain one disappointment after another, from problematic concealers to overly shiny blushes and eyeshadows, and unreasonably priced lipsticks. The mascaras are great, but so are countless others that don't cost this much. It's all exquisitely wrapped, but what's inside doesn't begin to match the quality of the package itself. In fact, you might say Yves St. Laurent's makeup is all dressed up with no place to go.

FOUNDATION: ☺ **$$$ Energie Teint Oil-Free Liquid Foundation SPF 12** *($46)* has a very good, avobenzone-based sunscreen for UVA protection, but SPF 15 would have been better. This one's creamy texture blends well and stays very moist on the skin, providing light to medium coverage. The seven shades are impressive compared to Yves St. Laurent's other choices, but there is nothing for very dark skin. Only #3, #6, and #8 are too peach for most skin tones. By the way, this comes in a pump bottle, which isn't the most economical way to use foundation, especially at this price. **Teint Compact Matite** *($52, $34.50 for refill)* is a very thick cream-to-powder foundation that initially feels like spackle but blends quickly to a surprisingly light feel with a solid powder finish. This is not for anyone with even a speck of dryness, since the finish will magnify any flakes tenfold. Coverage can go from sheer to full, and the four predominantly neutral shades stick out like a sore thumb against Laurent's other mostly peach or pink shades.

☺ **$$$ Premier Teint Long Lasting Radiant Primer** *($35)* is nothing more than a sheer, silicone-based shiny liquid that offers some strange colors and no coverage. For an artificial, tinted glow, it's fine, but this holds no advantage over less expensive products in the Revlon Skinlights line. **Teint Singulier Sheer Powder Creme Veil Foundation** *($38)* has a slippery texture that dries to a satin-matte finish, providing sheer coverage that would work for someone with normal to dry skin. Most of the four shades are off-color and tend toward pinks and peaches, but this so sheer it doesn't really matter. Contrary to the vastly inflated claims, this does not "perfectly shape the face" in any way, nor is it capable of concealing blemishes. **Teint Sur Mesure SPF 8** *($52.50)* is a contradictory, two-part foundation. Before you smooth on this creamy foundation, you're directed to apply the accompanying Perfecting Base, which "acts in synergy" with the foundation to reduce sebum (oil) and provide a matte finish. The **Perfecting Base** *($46 for a full-size jar)* does have a matte finish and leaves a sheer, pale pink cast on the skin. However, applying this before the foundation is futile, because the foundation's creaminess completely negates the underlying matte finish of the Base. Odd-couple pairings aside, the foundation is fine by itself and provides a silky, satin-matte finish. The sunscreen is part titanium dioxide, but SPF 8 is an embarrassingly low number for this so-called "perfectionist" foundation. Of the six shades, three are very rose or peach; Avoid #5, #7, and #9. **Teint De Jour Tinted Matte Moisturizer** *($38)* starts creamy and then, before you know it, it dries to a light-coverage matte finish. Unfortunately, this can look a bit chalky on the skin (titanium dioxide is a prominent ingredient), but at least the five sheer shades go on less rose and peach than they look.

☹ **Teint de Soie Line Smoothing Foundation** *($46)* is a moist foundation suitable for normal to dry skin seeking light to medium coverage and a soft, natural finish. However, all five shades are too pink, rose, or peach to look natural, though #7 is an OK option for fair skin.

<u>CONCEALER:</u> ☺ $$$ **Radiant Touch** *($35)* is a slightly shiny concealer/highlighter that comes packaged in a pen with a brush tip. You click the bottom to "feed" concealer to the brush, which can make it hard to control how much product comes out. As a highlighter it can work well, and the texture is smooth, but this has limited use. Of the three shades, #2 is slightly rose while #3 is fairly peach. Revlon's Skinlights Illusion Wand SPF 12 ($7.89) takes this concept even further by offering sun protection and some real skin colors.

☹ **Multi-Action Concealer** *($26).* It takes a lot of chutzpah to charge so much for such a greasy, heavy-looking concealer that creases in no time. If for some reason you prefer this type of product, there are significantly less expensive versions available at the drugstore.

<u>POWDER:</u> ✓☺ $$$ **Poudre Compact Matte** *($50, $27.50 for refill)* is an amazingly smooth, talc-based pressed powder that melds with skin to create a very natural nonpowdery finish. There are three decent flesh-toned shades and one shiny pink powder, which is best used for evening highlights, if at all.

☺ $$$ **Semi-Loose Powder** *($55)* comes in a cake form, but the container shaves off the top layer when you twist it, creating a loose powder. It's less messy than conventional loose powder, but this extra convenience doesn't come cheap. The talc- and aluminum starch–based formula goes on sheer and has a dry finish, and all four of the colors have a bit of shine, so this is not for those who want to use powder to keep shine at bay.

☹ **Bronzing Powder** *($40)* has too many weak points to make it a contender among other high-end pressed bronzing powders, including those from Chanel, Givenchy, and Guerlain. Try as they might, none of the three colors is great for creating a tanned appearance, and the shine ranges from barely there to a veritable sparklefest.

☺ $$$ **BLUSH: Blush Variations** *($36)* comes quad-style, with two matte and two intensely shiny colors, all subtle variations of the same shade. These apply superbly, and although the colors look bold and are perhaps too bright, they all go on sheer, so you can build intensity if desired. If only these weren't so distractingly shiny, they would be wholeheartedly recommended (assuming you're OK with the exorbitant price).

☹ **EYESHADOW: Eye Shadow Quartet** *($42)* offers a new formulation that is silkier than before, but these are a bit too dry to apply evenly, and that's key if you're going to offer colors this shiny. The four colors will have you wondering how to coordinate a nuanced eye design with such opposing hues as purple, green, orange, and burgundy. **Eye Shadow Duo** *($36)* are too powdery and flaky for a smooth, even application, and all of the duos are ultra-shiny, with poor color combinations.

EYE AND BROW SHAPER: ☺ $$$ **Kohl Eyeliner Pencil** *($24.50)* is oh-so-standard and has a creamy application, but it sets to a soft powder finish that does help this last longer. **Eyeliner Moire** *($25)* is a liquid liner with a thin brush that applies evenly, allowing you to lay down a solid line with one swift stroke. All of the colors (except black) are shiny, but this is much less smudge-prone than previous versions, so those who want an expensive shiny liquid eyeliner are bound to love it.

☺ $$$ **Perfecting Eye Crayon** *($19.50)* is a dual-ended standard pencil with one end white and the other black. Both colors have a cream-to-powder texture that stays slick, which will result eventually in smudging. **Eyebrow Enhancer** *($38)* is a compact providing two different, smooth-powder brow colors (blonde and taupe) that can double as eyeshadow, along with a charcoal-brown brow wax. Apparently, these three different tones are supposed to work for everyone, as no other colors are offered. Someone with blonde brows will find this severely limiting, while someone with dark brows will only be able to use the wax, if they want matted eyebrows that is. How strange!

☹ **Eyebrow Pencil** *($20)* has a too dry texture that makes it difficult to apply because it balls up on the skin as you draw it over the brow. **Long Lasting Eye Pencil** *($20)* is not as creamy as the Perfecting Eye Crayon above, but the colors go on so softly that they fade in no time. This needs-sharpening pencil needs a new name!

LIPSTICK AND LIP PENCIL: ☺ $$$ **Rouge Pur Pure Lipstick** *($26)* offers dozens of shades (including lots of unusually bright pinks and purples) in a fairly greasy lipstick formula that has a strong opaque finish. These are richly pigmented, which is nice, but they can easily bleed and feather into lines around the mouth. **Rouge Pur Matte Lipstick** *($26)* goes on opaque and creamy, but isn't matte in the least. The few colors are vivid with a strong stain, which will aid in longer wear. **Smoothing Lip Gloss** *($25)* is your everyday wand gloss that features sheer, unquestionably glossy colors with a tacky feel. **Lip Liner Pencil** *($18)* is a very good standard pencil that feels slightly creamy going on but ends up having a drier than usual finish, which helps keep it in place. The color range is one to consider for hard-to-find vivid pinks and bold purples.

☺ $$$ **Rouge Pur Transparent Lipstick SPF 8** *($24.50)* is an overpriced, extra-glossy lipstick with a bevy of frosted shades and a too low SPF and insufficient UVA protection. **Rouge Vibrations Lipstick** *($28)* is an exceptionally slick and greasy lipstick. The metallic colors are designed for a "magnetic glow," but it's bound to be short-lived. This is Yves St. Laurent's weakest lipstick offering.

☺ $$$ <u>MASCARA:</u> **Mascara Volume Luxurious Mascara** *($22.50)* has a slightly heavy feel, but does build substantial thickness. This comes up short when it comes to length, but it doesn't clump and it wears well throughout the day. **Mascara Aquaresistant** *($22.50)* is expertly waterproof, even if lashes get completely soaked. This applies well, producing enough length and thickness to surpass many other waterproof formulas. Yes, there are less expensive options, but for those who insist on buying designer mascara, this won't disappoint.

☹ <u>BRUSHES:</u> This line's **Brushes** *($20–$30)* are still lacking in most respects. The counter makeup artists I encountered were consistently embarrassed about the brushes, and it's not hard to see why.

Z. BIGATTI (SKIN CARE ONLY)

The trend of cosmetics companies selling more and more expensive skin-care products has found more and more lines jumping on that overpriced bandwagon hoping to ride the fad of selling what appears to be high-end skin care. The idea is to convince consumers that high prices reflect quality and are the answer to the skin-care needs of women who can afford the products (and especially for those women who can't, but who will spend their money anyway hoping that the expense really means the products are better). Z. Bigatti produces the line of products called Re-Storation, formulated by dermatologist Dr. Jennifer A. Biglow. Regardless of Biglow's credentials, these products are not worth their $65 to $195 price tags. I am bewildered at the limitations of this line. There are no sunscreens, no products for oily skin or breakouts, no effective AHA or BHA products, and no effective skin-lightening products. What these products do have is a lot of bells and whistles when it comes to antioxidants (superoxide dismutase and alpha lipoic acid show up in most of them), as well as very good water-binding agents and anti-irritants. But none of that will change a wrinkle, and nothing else about these products warrants the price. Moreover, though I haven't generally commented on specific packaging issues throughout this edition, it is important to point out that almost every container for this line ensures that the antioxidants won't be stable once the product is opened. It is also surprising that irritating plant extracts and fragrance show up in several products, and this in a line supposedly developed by a dermatologist! Suffice it to say there is nothing in this line worth $100+ per ounce. For more information about Z. Bigatti call (888) 430-1529. These products are also available at www.ibeauty.com and www.sephora.com.

☺ $$$ Re-Storation Champagne Gel Cleanser ($65 for 4 ounces) is a very standard, water-soluble, detergent-based cleanser with some interesting water-binding agents and antioxidants, although in a cleanser their benefit would just be washed down the drain.

☹ Re-Storation Silk Toner ($60 for 4 ounces) contains mostly water, slip agents, glycerin, plant extracts, antioxidants, vitamin E, preservatives, and coloring agents. The plant extracts are not exfoliants, though the lemon and menthol can be skin irritants.

☺ $$$ Re-Storation Deep Repair Facial Serum ($195 for 1 ounce) includes many bells and whistles, from grape seed extract to alpha lipoic acid and superoxide dismutase, along with some good water-binding agents, all of which contribute to making it a very good lightweight moisturizer for normal to dry skin. But the price tag alone can make your skin wrinkle, and there are many other less expensive products out there offering similar benefits, and without the pointless inclusion of the eucalyptus oil and comfrey in here, which can be skin irritants.

☺ $$$ Re-Storation Eye Return ($115 for 0.5 ounce) is similar to the Facial Serum above and the same basic comments apply. The only addition here is vitamin K, but there is no independent research showing that to be helpful for dark circles.

☺ $$$ Re-Storation Delicate Intensive Moisturizing Facial Treatment ($150 for 2 ounces) is a good emollient moisturizer with a decent amount of water-binding agents and antioxidants. It isn't as intense as other moisturizers in this line when it comes to state-of-the-art ingredients, but at least it left out some of the irritating plant extracts that show up in some of the other products. It is an option for normal to dry skin if the price doesn't make you choke.

☺ $$$ Re-Storation Skin Treatment Facial Lotion ($150 for 2 ounces) is a very good emollient moisturizer replete with great water-binding agents and antioxidants. It also contains about 4% AHA and 1% BHA, but the pH of 5 makes them ineffective for exfoliation.

☺ $$$ Re-Storation Vitamin and Antioxidant Skin Treatment ($150 for 2 ounces or $500 for 8 ounces) contains mostly water, plant oils, thickeners, glycerin, silicone, Vaseline, mineral oil, film-forming agent, AHA, BHA, vitamins, antioxidants, water-binding agents, preservatives, and coloring agents. This is a very good moisturizer for dry skin that contains many of the same bells-and-whistles ingredients as the other Re-Storation products; however, the pH of this product is too high for it to be effective as an exfoliant.

☺ $$$ Re-Storation Swan Neck Firming Treatment ($128 for 1 ounce) is similar to the Skin Treatment above, and the same basic comments apply. There is nothing about this that makes it special for the neck, not to mention the face. It does contain eucalyptus, which can be a skin irritant.

☺ **$$$ Re-Storation Enlighten Skin Tone Provider** *($174 for 1 ounce)* contains everything but the kitchen sink when it comes to antioxidants and water-binding agents, yet nothing that would be very effective to help diminish skin discolorations. The pH of this product is too high for the AHA and BHA in it to be effective for exfoliation, and the kojic acid and other potentially arbutin-containing plant extracts (which have some evidence showing they may be able to reduce melanin production) are present in such minute amounts as to be useless for that purpose. This is a good moisturizer but that's about it.

☹ **$$$ Re-Storation Impact Fruit Enzyme Facial Mask** *($124 for 2 ounces)* is an exceptionally basic clay mask that adds a bit of BHA (salicylic acid) to the mix, but the pH of the product is too high for the BHA to be effective as an exfoliant. It also contains bromelain, a very standard enzyme that can have exfoliating properties, though the likelihood that it will remain stable in this product is iffy. It also contains several potentially irritating plant extracts, including arnica, eucalyptus, and grapefruit. Ouch!

☹ **$$$ Re-Storation Dew Hydrating Facial Mask** *($98 for 1 ounce)* could have been a good, though exceedingly overpriced, mask for someone with normal to dry skin, but the eucalyptus can be a skin irritant. It contains mostly water, aloe, water-binding agents, film-forming agent, antioxidants, vitamins, and preservatives.

☹ **$$$ Re-Storation Lip Pout** *($55 for 0.2 ounce)* is little more than overpriced Chap Stick. Now that can make anyone want to pout!

ZAPZYT

If the name of a product line was ever meant to tell a woman exactly what to expect, this one is it. Though the name is clear enough, don't expect much skin "clearing" from this assortment of products. The bar soap is too alkaline, which can be irritating and encourage the growth of bacteria, and the pH of the BHA products is generally too high, which makes them relatively poor as exfoliants. The benzoyl peroxide gel is actually quite good, but it only comes in one strength, and not all skin types can handle the potency. For more information about ZAPZYT, call (800) 648-0833 or visit www.zapzyt.com.

☹ **Cleansing Bar** *($2.99 for 3 ounces)* contains 3% sulfur, which is too irritating and problematic for most skin types. While sulfur can be a good disinfectant, there are far more effective and less irritating options for skin. There is also well-documented research that points to a high pH as causing an increase in the presence of bacteria. With a pH of 10, this standard bar cleanser would definitely negate any positive effect from the disinfecting action of the sulfur.

☹ **Acne Wash Treatment** *($4.99 for 6.25 ounces)* is a standard, detergent-based cleanser that uses an exceptionally drying and potentially irritating cleansing agent, sodium C14-16 olefin sulfonate. It also includes 2% salicylic acid (BHA), but the pH of 5 means the BHA isn't all that effective as an exfoliant, and even if it were, in a cleanser it would quickly be rinsed down the drain, wasting its minimal opportunity to get inside the pore where it needs to be to have the most impact.

✔☺ **10% Benzoyl Peroxide** *($4.99 for 1 ounce)* is a great option for treating acne. It contains no fragrance or any other irritating ingredient—well, except for the 10% benzoyl peroxide—but that is a good option for killing the bacteria that can cause blemishes. Keep in mind that 10% benzoyl peroxide is at the high end of the options available and is potentially quite drying and irritating. It should only be considered after trying lower concentrations of 2.5% and 5%.

☺ **Pore Treatment Gel** *($5.29 for 0.75 ounce)* is an option for a topical BHA (it contains 2% salicylic acid). This gel formula contains no other irritants, and while the pH of 4 is on the high side for being effective as an exfoliant, it can still be helpful for some skin types.

ZIA NATURAL SKIN CARE

Zia Wesley Hosford is the founder of Zia Natural Skin Care, but due to a falling-out with her partners, the Zia line is no longer owned by Zia herself. However, the product philosophy remains the same and the "natural" bent is as hyped as ever. While there are plenty of plant oils and extracts in these products, there are synthetic ingredients as well. Keep in mind that just because an ingredient has a natural source does not mean it's automatically better for the skin. Poison ivy is natural and you don't want that on your skin. And there are lots of plants, particularly those with fragrant, volatile oils, that can cause skin irritation, which is bad for skin. There are some very good products to consider in this line, but there are also definitely those to stay away from, so choose carefully. For more information about Zia Natural Skin Care, call (800) 334-7546 or visit www.ziacosmetics.com. **Note:** All Zia products contain fragrance unless otherwise noted.

☹ **Absolutely Pure Aloe & Citrus Wash for Normal to Oily Skin** *($18.95 for 6 ounces)* definitely does contain citrus (it's actually the first ingredient), but just as orange juice would be drying and irritating to skin, so will the citrus perform here. This one also doesn't clean skin all that well and isn't the best for removing makeup.

☺ **Fresh Cleansing Gel for All Skin Types** *($15.50 for 8 ounces)* is a mild, detergent-based cleanser that should work well for normal to dry skin.

☺ **Moisturizing Cleanser for Normal to Dry Skin** *($15.50 for 8 ounces)* is basically a wipe-off cleanser with thickening agents and plant oils. It can leave a greasy film on the skin, so it is an option only for someone with dry skin.

☹ **$$$ Balancing Elixir** *($16.95 for 4 ounces)* is supposed to be aromatherapy for the face. The plant extracts it contains are all potential irritants, including lemon, grapefruit, lavender, and clary, which is disappointing, because the other ingredients make for a decent toner. The teeny amount of tea tree extract is not enough to have any effect as a disinfectant.

☹ **$$$ Hydrating Elixir** *($16.95 for 4 ounces)* is almost identical to the Balancing version above only with different, but equally problematic, plant extracts. This is more like applying eau de cologne to skin than a skin-care product.

The Reviews Z

☺ **$$$ Replenishing Elixir** *($16.95 for 4 ounces)* is almost identical to the Balancing version above only with different, but equally problematic, plant extracts.

☺ **Sea Tonic Aloe Toner for Normal to Oily Skin** *($11.95 for 6 ounces)* is a simple toner with a small amount of water-binding agents. There is nothing in it that makes it appropriate for oily skin, though it is an OK option for most skin types.

☺ **Sea Tonic Rosewater & Aloe Toner for Normal to Dry Skin** *($11.95 for 6 ounces)* is similar to the Sea Tonic Aloe Toner above, and the same basic comments apply.

☺ **Citrus Night Time Reversal Alpha Hydroxy Acid Creme for All Skin Types** *($25.95 for 1.5 ounces)* contains sugarcane extract, which is not related to glycolic acid (AHA), and the same lack of relation is true for the red wine (tartaric acid) and milk solids (lactic acid). Putting milk, wine, or sugarcane on your skin will not have the same effect as applying AHAs. Besides, even if they were effective AHAs, the pH isn't low enough for them to be effective as exfoliants—so this is just an exceedingly ordinary moisturizer, nothing more.

☹ **Ultimate Exfoliator** *($29.95 for 2 ounces)* contains lemon, lime, and citrus, which are too irritating for all skin types. And there is no research showing papaya to be effective as an exfoliant.

☺ **$$$ Essential Eye Gel** *($19.95 for 0.5 ounce)* includes plant extracts that can be good anti-irritants, and there are some interesting water-binding agents, but there's only a tiny amount of antioxidants. This is a good lightweight moisturizer for normal to slightly dry skin.

☺ **Everyday Moisturizer, Fragrance Free for Sensitive Skin** *($18.95 for 2 ounces)* is an emollient, though ordinary, moisturizer for normal to dry skin. Fragrance-free is great, but why not make all the products in this line fragrance-free, given that it's very clear that this line recognizes fragrance as a problem for sensitive skin? Because this product doesn't contain sunscreen, it should not be worn by itself during the day.

☺ **Herbal Moisture Gel for Oily/Blemished Skin** *($22.95 for 1.5 ounces)* is a very lightweight gel that contains an anti-irritant, thickeners, water-binding agent, and preservatives. This won't do much for skin, but if you have a touch of dry skin it isn't bad.

☺ **Nourishing Creme Cellular Renewal for Severely Dry Skin** *($32.75 for 1 ounce)* is a very good emollient moisturizer for dry skin, but it won't help cell renewal any more than any other emollient moisturizer.

✓☺ **$$$ Ultimate "C" Serum** *($39.95 for 0.5 ounce)* is a very good, emollient moisturizer for normal to dry skin that contains some very good water-binding agents and antioxidants. However, the amount of vitamin C it contains is hardly the "ultimate."

☺ **$$$ Ultimate Eye Creme** *($29.95 for 0.5 ounce)* contains a good deal of fragrance (the first ingredient), not the best for skin anywhere on the face, which is a shame, because otherwise this contains very good water-binding agents and antioxidants.

✓☺ **Ultimate Moisture** *($34.95 for 1.5 ounces)* is a very good moisturizer for normal to dry skin, with an impressive mix of antioxidants and water-binding agents.

☺ $$$ **Deep Moisture Repair Serum** *($34.95 for 0.3 ounce)* can't repair anything. However, it is a good moisturizer for normal to slightly dry skin.

☹ $$$ **Seaweed Lift Serum** *($34.95 for 0.5 ounce)*. The fact that this contains apple juice is strange, but it shouldn't be a problem for skin. This is still a good lightweight moisturizer for normal to slightly dry skin that contains some very good water-binding agents, but only a tiny amount of antioxidants. The algae in it can't lift skin anywhere.

☹ **Daily Moisture Sunscreen SPF 15** *($19.95 for 1.5 ounces)* does not contain the UVA-protecting ingredients of titanium dioxide, zinc oxide, or avobenzone, and is not recommended.

☺ **Hands-On Protection SPF 15** *($17.95 for 2 ounces)* is a very good, in-part zinc oxide–based sunscreen in an emollient moisturizing base that contains some good water-binding agents and a small amount of antioxidants. The small amount of kojic acid may have some melanin-inhibiting properties.

☹ **Solar Intelligence SPF 15 or 30 Body Spray** *($12.95 for 4 ounces)* does not contain the UVA-protecting ingredients of titanium dioxide, zinc oxide, or avobenzone, which makes it a completely unintelligent option for sun protection. This is not recommended.

☹ **Sunscreen SPF 15 Gel for the Face** *($15.95 for 1.8 ounces)* does not contain the UVA-protecting ingredients of titanium dioxide, zinc oxide, or avobenzone, and it is not recommended.

☹ **Sunscreen SPF 30 Gel for the Face** *($16.95 for 1.8 ounces)* does not contain the UVA-protecting ingredients of titanium dioxide, zinc oxide, or avobenzone, and is not recommended.

☺ **Sans Sun Self Tanning Creme for All Skin Types** *($16.95 for 5 ounces)*, like all self-tanning products, uses dihydroxyacetone to turn the skin brown, and would work as well as any.

☹ **15 Minute Face Lift** *($19.95 for 1.4 ounces of Lift Powder, 4 ounces of Sea Tonic Rosewater & Aloe Toner, and Application Brush)*. The Sea Tonic is reviewed above, but the "lift" part of this mask is mostly cornstarch and egg white! If you want to believe that will lift your skin, whatever I have to say won't stop you.

☹ **Acne Treatment Mask** *($14.95 for 3 ounces)* contains mostly alcohol, sulfur, and camphor. Any one of these would be enough to hurt blemish-prone skin, but together they can make skin red and irritated, plus they have no benefit for skin. Sulfur can be a topical disinfectant, but it poses many problems for skin that negate its benefit as a disinfectant.

☺ **Super Moisturizing Mask** *($14.95 for 3 ounces)* is an OK emollient moisturizer with lots of plant oils, lanolin, and thickeners. It would feel soothing for dry skin.

☺ **Ultimate Hydrating Mask** *($24.95 for 3 ounces)* is similar to the Super Moisturizing Mask above, only with some very good water-binding agents and antioxidants.

☺ **Fresh Papaya Enzyme Peel Non-Abrasive Exfoliant for All Skin Types** *($20.95 for 1.5 ounces)*. Papaya contains papain, an enzyme reputed to exfoliate skin, but papaya extract contains only minimal papain, plus there is no research demonstrating papain's effectiveness as an exfoliant.

☺ **Pumpkin Exfoliating Mask** *($22.95 for 1.2 ounces)* contains some very good water-binding agents and some antioxidants, but the claim that the showcase ingredient, pumpkin puree, has some special properties for skin is something more for trick or treat than for skin care.

ZIA MAKEUP

☺ **Natural Foundation SPF 8** *($14.95)* contains an excellent titanium dioxide and zinc oxide sunscreen, but why they stopped at the SPF 8 is a mystery; an SPF 15 would've been much better for this smooth-textured foundation. This foundation offers light to medium coverage and a natural finish, but of the ten shades, only the following four are worth considering: Alabaster and Moonstone (great for very light skin tones) and Sandstone and Mica. This is the first time I've seen a cosmetics company ask "Which rock are you?" when it comes to choosing a foundation shade. It's unique, but utterly useless in helping you determine which color to use.

☺ **Face Powder** *($14.95, $10.95 for refill)* is a talc-free pressed powder that has a very soft, silky texture and a satiny finish. The cornstarch can be problematic for those with breakout tendencies. This features six colors, best for light to medium skin tones. Avoid Pink Tourmaline (too ashy pink) and Bronze (too orange).

CHAPTER FOUR

Baby's Skin-Care Products

BABY'S SKIN

Simply based on the fact that a baby's skin has unique physical and functional characteristics, it is accepted and relatively self-evident that their skin is more delicate than an adult's and, thus, more vulnerable to problems with irritants and allergens. Therefore, the ideal cleansers, moisturizers, powders, and sunscreens for babies should be very mild to avoid irritation, allergic, or sensitizing skin reactions (Source: *Journal of the European Academy of Dermatology and Venereology*, September 2001, Supplemental, pages 12–15). Despite this fairly intuitive, commonsense information, it turns out that most skin-care products aimed at children are formulated to be anything but gentle and soothing. Many are often an irritation waiting to happen.

For all the women who are trying to clean, soften, and soothe their baby's skin (or the skin of any child in their life), let me warn you about baby products. Be alert and keep an eye out for the alarming number of these products, both inexpensive and expensive, that are marketed as better for young, delicate skin, when, for the most part, they are not.

Products for babies and young children are usually highly fragranced. That delicious, recognizable aroma you could smell a mile away is nothing more than added fragrance, which we know can cause irritation. Moreover, baby products almost always have a pretty yellow or pink tint, which is contrived by coloring agents, another group of ingredients in skin-care products that are potentially problematic for sensitive skin. If baby products were really gentler than those that adults put on their skin, they would be fragrance-free. Sadly, few of those exist.

Cosmetics and hair-care companies know that mothers feel an impulsive emotional pull toward scents that trigger the image of their babies. That subconscious pull is difficult for a marketer to ignore, given the way women gravitate to the fragrance generated by other perfume-laden products. In other words, hair-care and skin-care companies don't have much motivation to leave these problematic ingredients out. That means that you, as an advocate for your child, must pay attention to this issue and choose fragrance-free and color-free products whenever you can!

Aside from the issues of fragrance and coloring agents, it is even more shocking that baby products contain such skin irritants as peppermint, menthol, and citrus. The very idea of their presence is disturbing because these ingredients are all problematic for an adult's skin, and, thus even more so for a child's skin. It is essential to avoid products, for the sake of your child's skin (and yours for that matter), that contain any unnecessary irritants. Just paying attention to the ingredient list will give you far better information than the product description or the claims on the package or in the ads. Ignore the picture on the label of the sweet innocent child, especially when it can disguise a formula that is anything but sweet and innocent.

WHAT TO USE?

The basics for any child's skin are a gentle cleanser, a gentle shampoo, fragrance-free baby wipes, diaper ointment, sunscreen, and a lightweight, soothing moisturizer. But when it comes to fragrance-free, most of the versions available at the drugstore are those packaged for adults, such as Cetaphil Moisturizer, Eucerin Daily Replenishing Lotion Fragrance-Free, and Lubriderm Seriously Sensitive Moisturizing Lotion. These are also excellent for children. Fragrance-free zinc oxide–based and petrolatum-based diaper rash ointments are the best ones because they don't contain fragrance, and it hurts to put fragrance on red, rashy skin.

It is best not to use talc on a baby's skin, so choose talc-free dusting powder. Plain cornstarch is an excellent alternative. It is the primary ingredient in most talc-free baby powders anyway, and plain cornstarch from your kitchen cupboard doesn't contain fragrance.

During the day, if the child's skin is going to be exposed to the sun, even through windows indoors, a sunscreen is an absolute must. Sunscreen with SPF 15 or greater that contains the UVA-protecting ingredients of titanium dioxide, zinc oxide, or avobenzone is the basic essential. Formulations with only titanium dioxide or zinc oxide as the active ingredient are best because of their reduced risk of irritation compared to other sunscreen ingredients. (Avobenzone does protect from UVA rays, but it can be a skin irritant and the goal is to eliminate all sources of irritation as much as possible.) Keep in mind that babies don't care about the white cast these kinds of sunscreens sometimes give to the skin.

Remember: It's important to be alert in the defense of a baby's sensitive skin. There is no reason for a baby to put up with fragrance just because a parent thinks it smells better.

BABY SHAMPOO AND CLEANSERS

I can't stress enough how important it is that cleansers and shampoos for babies and children need to be gentle (Sources: *Dermatology*, 1997, volume 195, number 3, pages 258–262; and *Pediatric Clinics of North America*, August 2000, pages 757–782; and 2001, Supplemental pages 12–15).

When you read the label, look for the following ingredients, which are considered the most gentle cleansing agents for any skin type: cocamidopropyl betaine, cocamphocarboxyglycinate-propionate, sodium lauraminodipropionate, disodium monoleamide MEA sulfosuccinate, disodium monococamido sulfosuccinate, disodium cocamphodipropionate, disodium capryloamhodiacetate, cocoyl sarcosine, and sodium lauryl sarcosinate. These are all extremely gentle, and now you'll be able to recognize them on an ingredient list! Although they don't have great cleansing ability, they don't need it to wash a baby's skin.

Along with insisting on the gentleness of the shampoo formula, make sure it's fragrance-free, irritant-free, and coloring agent–free; all primary concerns for the health of your child's skin.

CRADLE CAP

The crusty, yellowish, thick layer of built-up skin on your baby's scalp is commonly called cradle cap, yet it has nothing to do with the cradle, how your baby sleeps, or what kind of sheets you use. Cradle cap is really seborrheic dermatitis, a skin problem typical of infants that usually disappears by their first birthday. It is always important to discuss any of your child's skin problems with your pediatrician before using anything on your baby's skin. A simple home remedy for cradle cap that you can discuss with your doctor is to gently massage a small amount of olive oil or plain, fragrance-free mineral oil all over the scalp (baby oil is just mineral oil with fragrance and your baby's skin doesn't need the fragrance). Leave the oil on overnight and then wash it off the next day with a gentle, fragrance-free baby shampoo. If several applications of this don't help, you should talk to your doctor about using an over-the-counter shampoo containing ketoconazole (Nizoral) for infantile seborrheic dermatitis. There is research showing this to be an effective option for resolving cradle cap in children (Source: *Pediatric Dermatology,* September-October 1998, pages 406–407).

MOISTURIZER FOR CHILDREN

Over and above the issue of fragrance-free skin-care products for children, it's important to use a moisturizer to help soothe skin and to deal with any potential dry skin. Dry skin can be a precursor to or an early warning sign of skin rashes and general skin irritation. For the most part, it has been believed that an extremely emollient, creamy moisturizer is best for a child's skin regardless of the condition. However, there is now research showing that a lightweight lotion or gel formula might be preferred (Source: *American Journal of Contact Dermatitis,* December 2000, pages 222–225). It may be helpful to start with a lightweight lotion and see how your child's skin responds. If you find that their skin still looks or feels dry, you can try a more emollient version, which may be better for your child's specific skin-care needs.

Most of the same concerns that apply to the quality of moisturizers for adult skin are also true for those used on a child's skin. Children also need water-binding agents that help maintain the integrity of the skin's intercellular matrix (the skin's outer barrier) as well as antioxidants and anti-irritants to help reduce inflammation and assist in skin healing. I rated products that contained these ingredients highly, as being the better option for a child's skin.

SUNSCREEN

The issue of sunscreen protection should absolutely be of primary concern for babies and small children. Their delicate skin is even more sensitive than adults' skin to the sun's damaging energy. Whether or not you are diligent about staying out of the sun or using sunscreen for yourself, you must be diligent when it comes to the health of your children.

An article in the *Archives of Pediatrics & Adolescent Medicine* (August 2001, pages 891–896) stated that "the regular practice of sun protection for children rarely takes place and primarily consists of applying sunscreen rather than methods that reduce sun exposure. This flies in the face of definitive knowledge that skin cancer, both melanoma and nonmelanoma, has reached epidemic proportions, that excessive sun exposure is associated with the subsequent development of most types of skin cancer, and that as much as 80% of lifetime sun exposure takes place during childhood.... [S]un protection should take its place among topics like car seats, smoke alarms, safe water temperature, and bicycle helmets...."

When should you start using sunscreen for children? According to an August 1999 press release from the American Academy of Pediatrics (AAP), www.aap.org, "it may be safe to use sunscreen on infants younger than 6 months of age when adequate clothing and shade are not available. Previously, the use of sunscreen on infants younger than 6 months old was not advised by the AAP. However, there is no evidence that using sunscreen on small areas of a baby's skin causes harm. Avoiding sun exposure and dressing infants in lightweight long pants and long-sleeved shirts are still the top recommendations from the AAP to prevent sunburn. However when adequate clothing and shade are not available, parents can apply a minimal amount of sunscreen to small areas, such as the infant's face and the back of the hands. In addition to possible sunburn, infants and children may be at increased risk for eye injury from the sun."

The Australian Cancer Society, in a Position Paper entitled, "Sun Protection and Babies," dated August 2000, supported by the Australasian College of Dermatologists, concluded that "There is no evidence that using sunscreen on infants is harmful. Although premature babies may have increased skin permeability consistent with incomplete development of the skin, the structure of the stratum corneum (the skin layer principally determining permeability) in full term babies is indistinguishable from that of adults [thus] providing an effective barrier. If infants are kept out of the sun or well protected from UVR [ultra-violet radiation] by clothing, hats and shade, then sunscreen need only be used occasionally on very small areas of a baby's skin. When used according to these guidelines, it is unlikely that the small amount of organic sunscreen components absorbed would exceed the metabolic capacities of the liver. In this position statement, the term 'infant' refers to babies from birth to 12 months of age."

Before you make a decision about sunscreen for your child, check with your physician for his or her recommendation.

When choosing a sunscreen for your child, it's easy to be attracted to the sunscreen products with pictures of cute babies on the label. However, despite these marketing tactics, products aimed at children are formulated no differently from those made for adults. All sunscreen formulations that have an SPF are regulated closely by the FDA; the formulations do not differ in any way because of the age of the intended user. The only difference I've ever noted in baby products is the use of added fragrance. Certain fragrances may make you think of little babies and children, but fragrance can be irritating for all skin types, and baby formulations tend to contain more fragrance than many adult products do. Of greater concern is that many sunscreens claiming to be for children do not contain the essential UVA-protecting ingredients of titanium dioxide, zinc oxide, or avobenzone. If one of these ingredients is not present in the active ingredient list on the label, do not buy the product; or, if you already own one, now that you know better, throw it out immediately and do not use the product again. For more information on why UVA protection is needed, see Chapter Seven, *Cosmetics Dictionary*.

If you are looking for a less irritating sunscreen for your kids, choose one that contains only pure titanium dioxide or zinc oxide as the active ingredient, because these are definitely less irritating than products with other inorganic sunscreen agents.

DIAPER RASH

If you can be sure of anything with your baby, it's that there is a strong chance he or she will develop diaper rash at some point. In some ways this is a confounding problem, because the very nature of diapering your baby and hoping he or she sleeps through the night sets up the perfect environment for developing diaper irritation. Urine and feces trapped next to a baby's bottom for long periods of time are the problem, but are there really other practical options? "The primary goals of preventing and treating diaper dermatitis include keeping the skin dry, protected, and infection free. Frequent diaper changes with the super-absorbent disposable diapers may be the best tactic for infants' skin, if not the environment. Also, the more time that infants spend without diapers, the less dermatitis they experience, but a practical balance must be struck. Gentle cleansing and barrier creams are beneficial, and [fungus or yeast] infections must be treated" (Source: *Pediatric Clinics of North America*, August 2000, pages 909–919).

Frequent diaper changes, fragrance-free baby wipes (so you are not adding to the irritation), gentle cleansing, and allowing your baby to go diaper free whenever it is practical are essential for getting diaper rash under control. When a child is wearing a diaper it is also extremely helpful to use an occlusive diaper ointment that prevents skin contact with urine or feces. Some of the best options are a traditional zinc oxide–based ointment, a zinc oxide– and petrolatum-based formulation, or just plain Vaseline (Source: *Journal of the European Academy of Dermatology and Venereology*, September 2001, Supplemental, pages 5–11).

Even if you diligently follow all the options for treating diaper rash, you may find your child still suffers from the irritation, redness, and swelling the condition produces. Pediatricians can offer prescription options that may settle matters. These can include any of the following: Nystatin, a topical antifungal (trade name Mycostatin); clotrimazole, another topical antifungal ointment (trade name Lotrimin); a combination product of nystatin and triamcinolone that blends an antifungal agent with a topical hydrocortisone to reduce inflammation); or just plain hydrocortisone to reduce or eliminate the irritation (Source: *Archives of Pediatric and Adolescent Medicine*, September 2000, pages 943–946).

TALC-FREE?

One of the ways to help keep a baby dry is with a dusting powder. However, it should be a talc-free powder because it is best not to use talc all over a baby's body, and, preferably, it should also be fragrance-free.

Why is talc not preferred? Talc is not preferred because, in pure, large concentrations, such as in talcum powder, it may be a health risk. Studies published in the 1990s, for example, found a significant increase in the risk of ovarian cancer from vaginal (perineal) application of talcum powder (Sources: *American Journal of Epidemiology*, March 1997, pages 459–465; *International Journal of Cancer*, May 1999, pages 351–356; *Seminars in Oncology*, June 1998, pages 255–264; and *Cancer*, June 1997, pages 2396–2401). It should be pointed out that subsequent and concurrent studies have cast doubt on the way these studies were conducted as well as on their conclusions (Sources: *Journal of the National Cancer Institute*, February 2000, pages 249–252; *American Journal of Obstetrics and Gynecology*, March 2000, pages 720–724; and *Obstetrics and Gynecology*, March 1999, pages 372–376). However, there are also issues when talc is inhaled (Source: *Inhalation Toxicology*, January-February 2000, pages 97–119). Given the potential for problems, and because it is easy to avoid using talcum power, there are other options that should be considered. Plain cornstarch is an excellent option for a diaper powder; it is the primary ingredient in most talc-free baby powders anyway, and plain cornstarch doesn't contain fragrance. (Cornstarch can be problematic for some sensitive skin types or in a pressed powder for an adult or teen struggling with breakouts.)

BABY MASSAGE

Bathing, shampooing, moisturizing, sunscreen application, diapering, and preventing diaper rash are all standard parts of baby skin care. One option to consider adding to this basic daily regime is regular massage, with the significant health benefits it can have for both mother and child. Researchers have demonstrated that many medical and emotional conditions can improve after a baby receives regular massage therapy from the parent. Healthier growth and better weight gain, reduced physical discomfort, enhanced immune functioning, and improved sleep patterns are a few of the advantages massage imparts to the baby. Added to this are equally important emotional benefits for the parent, particularly for the mother. Reduced maternal depression and a notable improvement in the quality of mother–infant interaction and bonding can also be achieved (Sources: *Medicine Clinics of North America,* January 2002, pages 163–171; *Journal of Affective Disorders,* March 2001, pages 201–207; and *Pediatrics,* October 2001, page 1053). Adding a few minutes of massage to the time you spend with your baby can create some of the most rewarding moments both of you will experience.

There are many options and routines you can follow to create an enjoyable massage experience. I offer one suggestion here, but do check with your physician or health care provider for what they consider to be best for you and your baby.

Choose a moment when both you and your child are relaxed and calm. A half hour or more after the baby has eaten is best. Be sure that the room temperature is comfortably warm (at least 78 degrees Fahrenheit) and that there are no drafts emanating from windows or doorways. Undress the baby completely, and if the weather is cold or damp cover the areas of the baby's body that are not being massaged. You can also keep the baby's socks on, and a warm hat on the baby's head to prevent a chill. Put the baby on a soft surface to provide a comfortable and secure surrounding area. Keep little pillows handy to cushion and protect various parts of the body while the massage is taking place.

It is a good idea to put a small amount of moisturizer, nonfragranced mineral oil, or a plant oil such as safflower or sunflower on your hands to facilitate a gentle stroking motion and to reduce friction. Be sure your hands are warm to the touch before starting the massage. There are many ways to proceed with a massage, but generally the movements flow from the head to the toes. With soft gentle motions, pressing very lightly, you can begin to touch the head, then the face, and then work toward the shoulders, arms, chest, stomach, and legs. Remember that your touches should be serene, smooth, and consistent—do not make mechanical, hard, or abrupt motions. As best you can, attempt to read how your baby is doing. Don't be set on any specific routine. If your baby seems happy lying face down then there is no reason to change. Whenever the baby wants to change position, you can assist in allowing that to happen. During the massage, it is best to have a calm demeanor and to speak lovingly and freely to your baby.

For more specifics about baby massage, there are some great books out there that provide comprehensive descriptions and explanations that can help you create the best routine for your baby. Here are a few: *Infant Massage, A Handbook for Loving Parents,* by V.S. McClure, Bantam Books, 2000; *Baby Massage: The Calming Power of Touch,* by Heath, Bainbridge, and Fisher, DK Publishing, 2000; and *Loving Hands: The Traditional Art of Baby Massage,* by F. Leboyer, Newmarket Press, 1997.

THE SEARCH FOR FRAGRANCE-FREE

Whether it is synthetic or comes in the form of plant extracts or oils, fragrance can be a potent skin irritant, sensitizer, and allergen. I stress the need to use fragrance-free products on a baby's skin because of the potential for irritation, although I realize it is almost a futile recommendation because so few baby products meet that criterion. Providing products that please the sensory wishes of the parent is the focus of almost every baby skin-care line. Aside from the problem that poses for finding the best baby products, it makes reviewing and rating baby products a challenge. Do all products receive a neutral face because of the fragrance component (which would be the vast majority of all baby products)? Or do I concentrate on other aspects of a product's formulation, such as the use of gentle cleansing agents, the exclusion of serious skin irritants, and the inclusion of significant water-binding agents, antioxidants, and anti-irritants, as I did when reviewing products aimed at teens and adults? I finally decided that the need to use fragrance-free products was far more significant (and beneficial) for a child's skin, keeping in mind the incidence of diaper rash and the extraordinary vulnerability of a baby's skin. As a result, the ratings of the following products are less than stellar. Although it may surprise you, it turns out that many products labeled "for adults" and that are fragrance-free end up being far better for a child's skin than those packaged and marketed as being best for your baby, and there's no reason not to use them.

I made one exception to this fragrance-free rule, in the ratings for sunscreens. Because suncare is so vital, and because sunscreens that contain titanium dioxide and zinc oxide as the only active ingredients are far more gentle on skin than sunscreens that contain other active ingredients, these products received a good rating whether or not they included fragrance.

ARBONNE BABY CARE

☺ **Hair and Body Wash** *($10.50 for 8.5 ounces)* is a standard, detergent-based cleanser that contains plant oils and water-binding agents that can help prevent dryness.

☺ **Body Lotion** *($10.50 for 8.5 ounces)* is an emollient moisturizer with some very good water-binding agents, plant oils, and antioxidants. What a shame it contains fragrance.

☺ **Body Oil** *($9.50 for 4 ounces)* contains more thickening agents than plant oil. (The plant oil is primarily safflower oil.) Given that this contains fragrance, your baby would do just as well if you used plain safflower oil from your kitchen cupboard.

☺ **Herbal Diaper Rash Ointment** *($10.50 for 4 ounces)* is a standard, zinc oxide–based diaper ointment with small amounts of plant oil, water-binding agents, and antioxidants. The fragrance makes this product something to avoid putting on a baby's rash.

BABY MAGIC BABY CARE

What would really be magical about the following is if these products didn't have such a noticeable scent to them!

☺ **Baby Bath, Original** *($3.49 for 15 ounces)* is an exceptionally gentle cleanser with way too much fragrance.

☺ **Baby Bath with Aloe** *($3.49 for 15 ounces)* is similar to the Baby Bath, Original above, only this one has a teeny amount of aloe, though that doesn't do anything to affect the problems caused by the fragrance.

☺ **Baby Shampoo, Original** *($1.99 for 9 ounces)* is similar to the Baby Bath, Original above, and the same comments apply.

☺ **Baby Lotion, Original** *($3.49 for 15 ounces)* is an ordinary, dated formulation of water, thickening agents, mineral oil, fragrance, and preservatives.

☺ **Baby Lotion with Aloe** *($3.49 for 15 ounces)* is almost identical to the Baby Lotion, Original above, but with a tiny amount of aloe thrown in, and that doesn't improve this mediocre product in any way.

✓☺ **Baby Wipes Unscented** *($3.99 for 80 wipes)* are soft wipes that contain gentle cleansing agents and have no fragrance, and that makes these a good option for baby's skin.

☺ **Baby Wipes Scented** *($3.99 for 80 wipes)* are virtually identical in every way to the Unscented version above, but the addition of scent in this one is the problem.

☺ **Baby Magic Oil Creamy Aloe** *($3.99 for 15 ounces)* is mostly just fragrance and mineral oil with some thickening agents and a teeny amount of aloe. Almost any plant oil in your kitchen, or just plain, nonfragranced mineral oil would be preferable to this.

☺ **Lite Baby Oil and Aloe** *($3.49 for 15 ounces)* is just mineral oil, silicone, a trace amount of aloe, and fragrance. The same comments for the Baby Magic Oil above apply here as well.

☺ **Magic Foaming Shampoo Extra Gentle** *($3.99 for 7 ounces)* is a standard, detergent-based cleanser, similar to most other baby shampoos. The only thing that would make this gentle is if it had no fragrance.

☺ **Foaming Hair and Body Wash Extra Gentle** *($3.99 for 7 ounces)* definitely contains gentle cleansing agents, but the fragrance doesn't make this gentle, much less extra gentle.

☺ **Hair and Body Wash** *($3.99 for 15 ounces)* is almost identical to the Foaming Hair version above and the same comments apply.

BABY POWDERS

Please refer to the "Talc-Free?" section in the introductory paragraphs above for information about the recommendation to avoid talc-based baby powders. Additional baby powders are reviewed in some of the product lines below.

☹ **Caldesene Protecting Powder, Fresh Scent** (*$4.79 for 5 ounces*) is mostly talc and fragrance.

☹ **Columbia Antiseptic Powder, Fragrance Free** (*$4.99 for 6 ounces*) is a talc-based powder that includes a small amount of zinc oxide and a phenol-based disinfectant, carbolic acid. You would want to discuss the use of this kind of topical disinfectant with your pediatrician.

☺ **Desitin Baby Powder, Cornstarch** (*$2.99 for 14 ounces*) is cornstarch with fragrance.

☹ **Gold Bond Medicated Baby Powder** (*$4.59 for 4 ounces*) is a talc-based powder that contains a tiny amount of zinc oxide and a good deal of fragrance.

☹ **The Healing Garden zzztherapy Tender Touch Soothing Baby Powder with Chamomile** (*$6.49 for 4.2 ounces*) is a talc-based powder that includes fragrance, and neither of those ingredients are healing for a baby's skin.

BABY WIPE PRODUCTS

Additional baby wipe products are reviewed in some of the product lines below.

☺ **Chubs Baby Wipe with Aloe** (*$3.79 for 80 towelettes*) uses very gentle cleansing agents soaked onto soft towelettes. These do contain fragrance, so forget this one, and use the others that are fragrance-free.

☺ **Diaparene Wash Cloths Fragrance Free** (*$2.49 for 100 wipes*) is almost identical to the Chubs version above and the same comments apply. Despite the label, this product does contain a fragrant component.

☺ **Huggies Baby Wipes, Scented** (*$3.49 for 80 wipes*) is similar to the Chubs version above and the same comments apply.

☺ **Huggies Natural Care Baby Wipes, Scented** (*$3.49 for 80 wipes*) is similar to the Chubs version above and the same comments apply.

✓☺ **Huggies Natural Care Baby Wipes, Unscented** (*$3.49 for 80 wipes*) contain gentle cleansing agents and don't contain fragrance, making these a good option for a baby's skin.

✓☺ **Huggies Supreme Care Baby Wipes, Fragrance Free** (*$3.49 for 64 wipes*) are virtually identical to the Huggies Natural Care Unscented version above and the same comments apply.

☺ **Huggies Supreme Care Baby Wipes, Lightly Scented** (*$3.49 for 64 wipes*). The fragrance doesn't help a baby's skin, so the Fragrance Free version above is a far better choice.

☺ **Pampers Baby Fresh Baby Wipes, Original** (*$3.99 for 80 wipes*). Without the fragrance these would have been a gentle option for a baby's skin.

☺ **Pampers Premium Baby Wipes Big Wipes** (*$3.99 for 65 wipes*) is almost identical to the Pampers Baby above and the same comments apply.

☺ **Pampers One-Ups! Baby Wipes, Original Alcohol Free** (*$3.69 for 80 wipes*) is almost identical to the Pampers Baby above and the same comments apply. Alcohol-free is a strange claim, but fragrance-free would have made this one-up on most of the competition.

☺ **Pampers One-Ups! Baby Wipes, with Aloe Alcohol Free** *($3.69 for 80 wipes)* is virtually identical to the One-Ups Original above and the same basic comments apply. The tiny amount of aloe isn't much of a help in this formulation.

☹ **Seventh Generation Unscented Baby Wipes with Aloe Vera & Vitamin E** *($3.49 for 80 wipes)* contains the preservative Kathon CG, which is not recommended for use in leave-on skin-care products. Even though it is being wiped away, some of the cleanser does remain on the baby's skin, making this not acceptable.

☹ **Tushies Baby Wipes with Aloe Vera** *($3.39 for 80 wipes)* contains the preservative Kathon CG, which is not recommended for use in leave-on skin-care products. Even though it is being wiped away, some of the cleanser does remain on the baby's skin.

☺ **Kleenex Cottonelle Flushable Moist Wipes with Aloe** *($2.49 for 50 towelettes)*. The Kleenex brand name is recognizable and the gentle cleansing agent is good, but the fragrance is what it would have been best to flush away before they put these in the box.

☹ **Wet Ones Moist Towelettes with Vitamin E & Aloe** *($2.49 for 40 wipes)* lists alcohol as the second ingredient, and that is just a bizarre ingredient to have in a baby product!

BOBBI BROWN BABY ESSENTIALS

☺ **$$$ Gentle Body Wash and Shampoo** *($18 for 6.7 ounces)* is a fairly gentle (though extremely ordinary and overpriced) cleanser. It does contain fragrance; without that, this would really have been gentle.

☺ **$$$ Soothing Body Balm** *($22.50 for 8.5 ounces)* is an emollient balm of thickening agents, plant oils, and a trace amount of antioxidants and water-binding agents. It does contain fragrance. There is no extra benefit to be gained from spending this kind of money when plain almond oil, the main oil in this product, would work as well, and it doesn't contain fragrance.

✓☺ **$$$ Diaper Balm** *($14.50 for 2.5 ounces)* is nicely fragrance-free and is an interesting option for a diaper ointment. It contains mostly castor oil, plant oils, film-forming agent, thickening agents, and Vaseline. It's pricey, but it's still a good, emollient option for a baby's skin.

☺ **$$$ Massage Oil** *($16 for 4 ounces)* is just overpriced plant oils and fragrance. Skip the fragrance and consider using just one of the main plant oils in this product such as soybean oil or almond oil.

☺ **$$$ Silkening Powder** *($18 for 3.5 ounces)* contains mostly cornstarch, along with oat flour and rice starch, as well as fragrance. Plain cornstarch would serve your baby's skin far better than this overpriced, overly fragranced formulation.

BURT'S BEES BABY PRODUCTS

☹ **Baby Bee Buttermilk Soap** *($5 for 3.5 ounces)* is indeed soap, which gives it an incredibly high pH of over 10. That extremely alkaline base is very drying and irritating for all skin types. It also contains fragrance.

☺ **Baby Bee Shampoo Bar** *($5 for 3.5 ounces)* is definitely more gentle than the Soap version above, but the fragrance doesn't make this an exciting preference for a baby.

☺ **Baby Bee Buttermilk Bath** *($15 for 7.5 ounces)*. If there is a reason why a mother would want to soak her child in milk, I don't know what it is. OK, let's say there is a reason; in that case, this product is only nonfat dry milk, whole dry buttermilk, and fragrance. Forget the fragrance and just dump some nonfat dry milk in the bath. I'm not saying it's a good idea, but it's better than using this product.

☺ **Baby Bee Skin Creme** *($11 for 2 ounces)* is an emollient moisturizer similar to the Buttermilk Lotion below, and the same basic comments apply.

☺ **Baby Bee Buttermilk Lotion** *($9 for 8 ounces)* contains mostly water, plant oils, glycerin, thickeners, vitamin E, aloe, buttermilk powder, more thickeners, water-binding agents, and fragrance. Without the fragrance this would have been an OK, emollient moisturizer for dry skin, but it is not preferred for a baby's skin.

✔☺ **Baby Bee Apricot Baby Oil** *($8 for 4 ounces)* is, as the name implies, mostly apricot seed oil, along with a small amount of grape seed oil, wheat germ oil, and vitamin E, and it contains no fragrance. This is a very good option for a baby's skin.

☺ **Diaper Ointment** *($7 for 1.75 ounces)* is just zinc oxide and plant oils along with fragrance. That does not make this preferable over fragrance-free zinc oxide versions that are available for less money at the drugstore.

☺ **Dusting Powder** *($8 for 2.5 ounces)* is mostly cornstarch, baking soda, clay, and fragrant plant extracts. The baking soda and clay don't add much, if any, benefit and you would be fine just using plain cornstarch.

☹ **Solid Perfume** *($7 for 0.3 ounce)*. I know there must be a reason why a mother would want to apply perfume to her child; I just can't think what it might be.

CALIFORNIA BABY

If you appreciate environmental scare tactics as a way to sell products for skin (and many companies do just that), then you will be happy to learn about California Baby's company story. According to their Web site, "California Baby was developed to meet the standards of a very particular mother. Jessica's son, Ian, was just a few months old when she realized the products available for his skin and hair were loaded with potential toxins…." That essentially means everybody else's products are dangerous for your baby except, of course, those from California Baby. One of the many astounding claims this line makes is that they use "decyl polyglucose (and combine … it with soapbark and yucca in the bubble baths) to take the place of the more typical sodium lauryl sulfate and

DEA, which can be damaging to the skin, retinas and stripping of delicate membranes." Although there are issues with using DEA or sodium lauryl sulfate in a skin-care product, there is no research suggesting that either of these ingredients can strip membranes or damage eyes (much less the retina, which is located at the far back interior of the eyeball where the likelihood of being at risk is remote). Besides, I have found no baby products that contain either of these ingredients.

Along with many other so-called all-natural product lines, California Baby also identifies mineral oil and petrolatum as being closely associated with crude petroleum. Not only is there nothing toxic or irritating about mineral oil or petrolatum (and not a shred of evidence to prove otherwise), but there is also research showing both of these to be great for healing skin (they are both antioxidants), and they have no risk of causing irritation to the skin.

Aside from what these products don't include, the real feature touted by this line is the essential oils they do contain. But using essential oils is just a different way of listing fragrance on an ingredient label. Although fragrance is pleasant for your nose, it isn't helpful for skin, and particularly not for a baby's skin. Of course there is no information from California Baby about the potential risk of contact irritation or the photosensitizing properties of many fragrant oils.

California Baby explains that they "…use food grade (used in cough syrups) parabens…" in tiny amounts for their preservative system. Their Web site erroneously states that "at these very low concentrations, we are not required to list them, but we do!" According to the FDA, *all* ingredients (except for fragrance) must be listed on the ingredient label regardless of the amount. This is a basic FDA guideline, yet one of many that California Baby chose to misrepresent. To top it off, perhaps the most flagrant inaccuracy is the notion that willow bark, coffee extract, and pansy extract are natural sunscreen ingredients! This notion is completely untrue and without any supporting evidence, and if parents assume that those ingredients can protect their baby's skin it could be dangerous. For more information about California Baby, call (800) 576-2825 or visit www.californiababy.com.

☺ **Shampoo & Body Wash-Calming Blend** (*$8.95 for 8.5 ounces*) is a very gentle moisturizing shampoo, but the essential oils it contains are nothing more than cleverly disguised fragrance.

✓☺ **Super Sensitive Shampoo & Body Wash** (*$8.95 for 8.5 ounces*) is the most noteworthy, worthwhile product in the entire line, but not because of what's in it. What is impressive is what's *not* included in this exceptionally gentle cleanser, namely, any type of fragrance. But why not provide this for all children? If the owners of this line recognize that fragrance can be a problem for babies (and what baby doesn't have super-sensitive skin), why not just do the same for all the products?

✓☺ **Bubble Bath, No Fragrance Super Sensitive** (*$9.99 for 13 ounces*) is almost identical to the Super Sensitive Shampoo above, and the same comments apply.

☹ **Calming Bubble Bath with Aromatherapy** *($11.50 for 13 ounces)*, **I Love You Bubble Bath** *($12.50 for 13 ounces)*, **Overtired & Cranky Bubble Bath with Aromatherapy** *($11.50 for 13 ounces)*, **Herbal Chamomile Bubble Bath** *($10.95 for 13 ounces)*, **Colds & Flu Bubble Bath** *($10.95 for 13 ounces)*, and **Light & Happy Bubble Bath** *($10.95 for 13 ounces)* all come in the exact same gentle cleansing base. However, all of these contain potent skin irritants that should be kept far away from baby skin, such as eucalyptus, Douglas fir, lavender, citrus, geranium, ylang-ylang, and tangerine. These may smell heavenly, but that does not translate to gentle or healthy baby skin care.

☹ **Diaper Rash Cream** *($9 for 2 ounces)* is a standard, overpriced zinc oxide diaper rash salve. But the arnica and fragrant oils it contains have no business being in a cream meant for an already delicate, tender area of skin.

☺ **100% Aloe Vera After Sun Lotion, for Face & Body** *($11.49 for 2.9 ounces)* isn't 100% aloe vera because it contains other ingredients. This otherwise simple, emollient body lotion would be better off without the fragrance. Pure aloe vera is still a viable option for a baby's skin, but you would do better with a version you buy at a health food store that is fragrance-free and costs less, too.

☺ **SPF 30 Sunscreen: No Fragrance** *($15.99 for 2.9 ounces)* is a good sunscreen that contains only titanium dioxide as the active sunscreen agent. That does make it better for a baby's skin. However, this product absolutely contains fragrance ("essential oils" are nothing more than fragrant oils). By comparison, Neutrogena's Sensitive Skin UVA/UVB Block SPF 17 ($8.39 for 4 ounces) and Sensitive Skin UVA/UVB Block SPF 30 ($8.39 for 4 ounces), both titanium dioxide–based sunscreens, are not only truly fragrance-free, but also far less expensive.

☺ **Citronella Bug Blend Sunscreen, SPF 30+** *($15.99 for 2.9 ounces)* is similar to the SPF 30 sunscreen above, but with the addition of citronella, a potential irritant. It would be best to check with your doctor as well as testing this on a small portion of your child's skin before choosing it as an all-over sunscreen option. Citronella is minimally effective as a bug repellant.

☺ **$$$ SPF 30+ Sunblock Stick: Everyday/Year-Round** *($10.99 for 0.5 ounce)* is a stick form of sunscreen with pure titanium dioxide as the only active ingredient, and although that could have made it a convenient take-along sunscreen, the price makes this a costly venture. To use it appropriately (meaning liberally), you would go through this in less than a few days. See the comments above for the SPF 30: No Fragrance, which also apply here.

☺ **SPF 30+ Sunscreen: Everyday/Year-Round** *($15.99 for 2.9 ounces)* is similar to the other SPF 30 products above, and with all the excessive fragrance, too.

☺ **Water Resistant, Hypo-Allergenic Sunscreen, SPF 30+** *($11.99 for 2.9 ounces)* is similar to the other SPF 30 products above, and with all the excessive fragrance, too, which makes it far from being anything related to hypoallergenic. This one is water-resistant.

☺ **Hair Conditioner** (*$8.50 for 8.5 ounces*) is a fairly emollient blend of plant oils that may be an option for dry to very dry hair. This would easily weigh down baby-fine hair. Willow bark, coffee, and pansy extracts are not natural sunscreens, as the label indicates. Suggesting that they have any sun protection capability is deceptive and potentially harmful to the consumer.

☺ **Hair Detangler** (*$9.25 for 8.5 ounces*) is a decent, though fairly emollient, spray-on conditioner (it contains a good amount of silicone) that is best for normal to dry hair. It does contain fragrant oils and several plant extracts.

☺ **Moisturizing Cream** (*$13.50 for 4 ounces*) contains mostly water, aloe, plant extracts, plant oil, fragrant extracts, thickeners, more plant oils, vitamins, preservatives, and fragrance. As a standard, ordinary moisturizer this is fine, but the fragrance is a problem for a baby's skin.

☺ **Calendula Cream** (*$9 for 2 ounces*) is an ordinary moisturizer for dry skin; it also contains fragrance.

☺ **Vitamin E & Aloe Baby Lotion** (*$9 for 4.5 ounces*) would be a decent moisturizer for normal to dry skin, but it contains too much fragrance for a baby's skin.

☺ **Apricot & Sesame Baby Oil** (*$9 for 4.5 ounces*) is a blend of plant oils that would be just fine for your baby's skin. However, the belief that fragrance is essential for a baby's skin mars this otherwise simple oil blend. Save the money, mix your own, and leave out the fragrance—your baby will be much happier if you do. (The oils in this are sesame seed oil, almond oil, apricot oil, safflower oil, and hazelnut oil, all easy to find at the health-food store.)

☺ **Offspring Overtired & Cranky MOMMY & DADDY Massage Oil** (*$9 for 4.5 ounces*), despite the cute name, is almost identical to the Apricot & Sesame Baby Oil above, and the same comments apply.

☹ **Offspring Diaper Rash Cream** (*$9 for 2 ounces*) is a standard, zinc oxide–based diaper ointment that includes lanolin, thickeners, and plant oil. Unfortunately, it also includes arnica and comfrey, and both of those are problematic for abraded skin. It also contains fragrance.

☹ **Baby Powder** (*$9.00 for 2.5 ounces*) is just cornstarch and clay with fragrance and arnica, a potent irritant that should not be used on abraded skin. For the comfort and health of your baby's skin, plain cornstarch would be a much better option.

CRABTREE & EVELYN

☹ **Soap Collection** (*$8 for 3 ounces*) is an assortment of standard, tallow-based bar soaps that can be drying and irritating for a baby's skin. These do contain fragrance.

☹ **Peter Rabbit Soap** (*$5 for 3.3 ounces*) is, as the enticingly cute name plainly indicates, soap—and that makes it potentially too drying and irritating. It does contain fragrance.

☺ **Tom Kitten Body Wash and Shampoo** (*$13.50 for 8.5 ounces*) is as standard a cleanser for a baby as it gets, using gentle cleansing agents, but then adding fragrance.

☺ **Tom Kitten Baby Lotion** *($15 for 8.5 ounces)* is an exceedingly standard, mineral oil–based moisturizer with fragrance that can easily be replaced with Cetaphil or Eucerin moisturizers at the drugstore, which are both fragrance-free and less expensive.

☺ **Cream for Baby** *($15 for 5.1 ounces)* is similar to the Lotion version above and the same comments apply.

☺ **Baby Powder** *($12 for 2.4 ounces)* is mostly cornstarch, shine (mica), and fragrance. Cornstarch all by itself is less expensive and better for a baby and the shine is just strange for a baby product.

DIAPER RASH OINTMENTS

Diaper rash ointments share more qualities in common than they have differences. They almost all contain varying concentrations of zinc oxide, oils (plant and mineral oils), lanolin, and thickening agents. Regrettably, most also contain fragrance, which is a problem for a baby's sensitive bottom. The different concentrations of zinc oxide are what cause the varying textures; the products with the higher concentrations are more occlusive and, therefore, are better for stubborn cases of diaper rash.

☺ **A+D Original Diaper Rash Ointment** *($4.29 for 4 ounces)* is exceptionally emollient, containing mostly petrolatum, lanolin, cod liver oil, fragrance, mineral oil, and wax. It would be best if it didn't contain fragrance, but this product is exceptionally moisturizing.

☺ **A+D Diaper Rash Ointment with 10% Zinc Oxide** *($5.49 for 4 ounces)* isn't as emollient as the A&D Original above, though the zinc oxide this contains makes it a better barrier ointment.

☺ **A+D Zinc Oxide Diaper Rash Cream with Aloe** *($3.99 for 4 ounces)* contains 10% zinc oxide, silicone, cod liver oil, mineral oil, thickeners, and fragrance.

✔☺ **Aveeno Diaper Rash Cream** *($4.49 for 4 ounces)* is a standard, emollient, zinc oxide–based diaper rash ointment similar to almost every other one in this group, except that this is one of the only fragrance-free versions available.

☹ **Balmex Diaper Rash Ointment** *($5.75 for 4 ounces)* contains balsam as one of the main ingredients, and that can be a skin irritant.

☹ **Boudreaux's Butt Paste** *($7.49 for 4 ounces)* has a great name, but the second ingredient is balsam, and that can be a skin irritant.

☺ **Desitin Diaper Rash Ointment** *($4.49 for 4 ounces)* is a very thick, white, mostly zinc oxide (40%) ointment that also includes Vaseline, lanolin, and fragrance.

☺ **Desitin Diaper Rash Ointment, Creamy, Fresh Scent** *($4.49 for 4 ounces)* is only 10% zinc oxide, along with mineral oil, silicones, and fragrance. It is lighter in weight than the Desitin version above.

☺ **Desitin Diaper Rash Ointment, Hypoallergenic** *($4.49 for 4 ounces)* is almost identical to the Desitin Rash Ointment with 40% zinc oxide above. There is nothing about this version that is hypoallergenic because it, too, contains fragrance.

☺ **Dr. Smith Diaper Ointment** *($8.99 for 2 ounces)* is a 10% zinc oxide ointment with Vaseline, lanolin, mineral oil, thickeners, and happily, no fragrance. This is a great option for protecting a baby's skin from diaper rash.

☹ **Palmer's Diaper Rash Cream, Cocoa Butter Formula** *($3.99 for 4.4 ounces)* actually doesn't contain much cocoa butter. Rather, it is mostly Vaseline (30%), silicone, mineral oil, thickeners, and fragrance. The tiny amount of antioxidants it contains offers no real benefit for skin.

☹ **RashStick Creamy Diaper Rash Ointment** *($4.99 for 2 ounces)* contains about 12% zinc oxide along with thickeners. The balsam of Peru can be a skin irritant. It does contain fragrance.

GERBER BABY PRODUCTS

☺ **Baby Moose Foaming Wash for Hair & Body, Lavender** *($3.99 for 10 ounces)* is a gentle cleanser with fragrance and tiny amounts of water-binding agents and antioxidants.

☺ **Hair and Body Baby Wash** *($3.79 for 15 ounces)* is just gentle cleansing agents and fragrance.

☺ **Teeny Bodies Moisturizing Cream** *($3.79 for 8 ounces)* is an emollient, Vaseline-based moisturizer with a small amount of water-binding agents and antioxidants. It does contain fragrance.

☹ **Skin Nutrients Baby Lotion with Lavender and Chamomile** *($3.79 for 15 ounces)* is a very standard moisturizer for dry skin with a tiny amount of water-binding agents and a minute amount of antioxidants. It does contain fragrance.

☹ **Skin Nutrients Lotion with Oatmeal Moisturizer** *($3.79 for 15 ounces)* is a very standard moisturizer for dry skin with a tiny amount of water-binding agents and a minute amount of antioxidants. It does contain fragrance.

☹ **Teeny Faces Moisturizing Stick** *($3.79 for 0.6 ounces)* is just Vaseline with thickeners, a tiny amount of plant oil, some emollients, and a minuscule amount of antioxidants. It does contain a fragrant plant extract. There is little benefit to be gained by using this rather than plain Vaseline.

☺ **Skin Nutrients Baby Wash for Hair and Body, with Oatmeal Moisturizers** *($3.79 for 15 ounces)* is a standard gentle cleanser that has some water-binding agents that can be helpful, though leaving out the fragrance would have made this even better for skin.

☺ **Skin Nutrients Baby Wash for Hair and Body with Lavender and Chamomile** *($3.79 for 15 ounces)* is identical to the Skin Nutrients version above only minus some of the water-binding agents and a different fragrance. The same basic comments apply.

☹ **Vapor Bath with Menthol Vapors** *($3.79 for 15 ounces)*. The menthol and eucalyptus in this product may be nice to smell, but they make this a problem for skin irritation.

Johnson & Johnson Baby
AND Kids Products

☺ **Baby Bar** *($2.29 for 3-ounce bar)* is a standard bar cleanser with fragrance. It can be somewhat drying.

☺ **Baby Bath** *($3.69 for 16 ounces)* is a gentle cleanser with fragrance.

☺ **Baby Bath, Bedtime** *($4.79 for 15 ounces)* is similar to the Baby Bath above.

☺ **Baby Bath, Soothing for Dry Skin** *($4.39 for 15 ounces)* uses somewhat gentler cleansing agents than the two Baby Bath products above, but only slightly. This still contains fragrance.

☺ **Moisturizing Baby Bath with Aloe Vera and Vitamin E** *($3.79 for 9 ounces)*. There is nothing moisturizing about this cleanser, which is almost identical to the Baby Bath above. The minute amounts of aloe and vitamin E are insignificant for skin.

☺ **Head to Toe Baby Wash, Original** *($3.79 for 15 ounces)* is a gentle cleanser with fragrance.

☹ **Soothing Vapor Bath** *($3.69 for 9 ounces)* is a gentle cleanser that includes eucalyptus and menthol, and while that is nice to smell these are skin irritants and should be kept away from a baby's skin.

☺ **Gentle Cleansing Cloths, Head to Toe** *($4.39 for 28 cloths)* is a gentle cleanser soaked on soft wipes. These do contain fragrance.

☺ **Gentle Cleansing Cloths, Moisturizing** *($4.39 for 28 cloths)* is virtually identical to the Head to Toe version above. There is nothing moisturizing about this version.

☺ **Ultra Sensitive Baby Cleansing Bar** *($2.29 for 3-ounce bar)* is a bar cleanser that doesn't contain fragrance. It can still be somewhat drying for skin, but the lack of fragrance is a plus.

☺ **Baby Shampoo, Natural Lavender** *($3.79 for 15 ounces)* is a gentle cleanser with fragrance.

☺ **Baby Shampoo, Honey & Vitamin E** *($4.49 for 20 ounces)* is a gentle cleanser with fragrance. The minute amount of vitamin E adds no benefit for skin or hair.

☺ **Baby Shampoo, Original** *($4.49 for 20 ounces)* is a gentle cleanser with fragrance.

☺ **Baby Shampoo, 2 in 1 Detangler** *($4.49 for 20 ounces)* is a gentle cleanser with fragrance that adds a detangling agent, something that can be helpful for a baby's hair as it is gets longer.

☺ **Baby Cream, Soothes and Protects** *($3.73 for 4 ounces)* is a very basic, very emollient (and fragranced) moisturizer.

☺ **Baby Lotion** *($3.79 for 15 ounces)* is an ordinary moisturizing lotion for dry skin; it does contain fragrance.

☺ **Baby Lotion with Aloe Vera and Vitamin E, Soothes and Nourishes Dry Skin** *($3.79 for 15 ounces)* is almost identical to the Baby Lotion above. The minute amounts of vitamin E and aloe are barely detectable.

☺ **Baby Lotion, Soothing for Dry Skin** *($4.39 for 15 ounces)* is an ordinary emollient lotion for dry skin. It does contain fragrance.

☺ **Baby Lotion, Bedtime** *($4.49 for 15 ounces)* is an ordinary emollient lotion for dry skin. It does contain fragrance.

☹ **Baby Lotion with Daily UV Protection with SPF 15** *($3.59 for 4 ounces)* is a good, in-part titanium dioxide–based sunscreen. However, this product uses the preservative Kathon CG, which is not recommended for use in leave-on skin-care products.

☺ **Baby Oil, Creamy** *($3.79 for 15 ounces)* is just mineral oil, thickeners, and fragrance.

☺ **Baby Oil, Original** *($4.49 for 20 ounces)* is just mineral oil and fragrance. Plain mineral oil without the fragrance would be a better choice. Ask your pharmacist for plain mineral oil.

☺ **Baby Oil, Aloe Vera & Vitamin E** *($4.49 for 20 ounces)* is similar to the Baby Oil, Original above, only with the addition of a minute amount of vitamin E and aloe.

☺ **Baby Oil Gel, Aloe & Vitamin E** *($3.79 for 6.5 ounces)* is similar to the Baby Oil, Aloe Vera & Vitamin E above, only in gel form.

☺ **Baby Oil Gel, Chamomile & Multi Vitamin** *($3.79 for 6.5 ounces)* is similar to the Baby Oil Gel above, only with the addition of a minute amount of antioxidants. This contains more fragrance than it does multivitamins.

☺ **Baby Powder, Medicated** *($3.79 for 15 ounces)* is just cornstarch, zinc oxide, and fragrance. Plain cornstarch would work as well.

☺ **Baby Powder, Cornstarch with Aloe & Vitamin E** *($4.49 for 22 ounces)* is just cornstarch and baking soda with a teeny amount of vitamin E and aloe. That's nice, but in such minute amounts they are not beneficial for a baby's skin. This does contain fragrance.

☺ **Baby Powder, Lavender & Chamomile** *($4.49 for 22 ounces)* is just cornstarch, baking soda, and fragrance. Plain cornstarch would work as well.

☹ **Baby Powder, Original** *($4.49 for 22 ounces)* is traditional talcum powder and is not recommended.

✓☺ **Diaper Rash Cream with Zinc Oxide** *($3.29 for 3 ounces)* contains 13% zinc oxide along with mineral oil, silicones, lanolin, Vaseline, thickeners, and a teeny amount of vitamin E. Note that it does not contain fragrance, making this good news for a baby's skin.

KIEHL'S BABY CARE

☺ **Mild Gentle Shampoo for Babies** *($8.50 for 4 ounces)* is a standard gentle cleanser that contains a small amount of plant oil, which can be helpful for dry skin. This also contains fragrant plant oil.

☺ **Baby Body Lotion** *($12.50 for 4 ounces)* is an emollient lotion containing several plant oils and a small amount of antioxidants. It doesn't contain fragrance.

☺ $$$ **Nourishing, Soothing Diaper Area Ointment** *($25.50 for 3 ounces)* is an emollient mix of thickening agents and plant oils along with some antioxidants and a tiny amount of anti-irritants. It is an option for a diaper ointment and it doesn't contain fragrance.

☺ **Baby Lip Balm** *($5.50 for 0.17 ounce)*. Although this has no benefit over other emollient lip balms, this one does lack fragrance and that is helpful for a baby!

☺ **Body Wash** *($9.50 for 4 ounces)* is a gentle cleanser with fragrant plant oil.

LITTLE FOREST BABY CARE

☹ **Baby Soap** *($4 for 3.65 ounces)* is, as the name indicates, soap, and it also contains fragrance. This can be drying for skin.

☹ **Baby Shampoo** *($8 for 4 ounces)* is a standard cleanser, though this one also contains tea tree oil and eucalyptus oil, both unnecessary skin irritants. This is not recommended.

☹ **Baby Cream (for Diaper Rash)** *($10.59 for 2 ounces)* contains tea tree oil and eucalyptus oil, both unnecessary skin irritants. This is not recommended.

☺ **Daily Barrier Cream** *($8 for 2 ounces)* is an emollient moisturizer for dry skin that contains mostly water, plant oils, thickeners, silicone, tiny amounts of vitamins, preservatives, and fragrance.

☹ **Baby Bug Block** *($7.99 for 4 ounces)* contains both eucalyptus oil and tea tree oil, and is not recommended.

☺ **Baby Soothing Cooler** *($7.99 for 4 ounces)* is a lightweight gel with some good soothing agents and antioxidants. It does contain fragrance.

☺ **Baby Powder** *($6.50 for 3 ounces)* contains rice flour and clay as the powder. It does contain fragrance. The plant extracts are a mix of anti-irritants and irritants, though the amounts are so small as to be insignificant for skin.

MUSTELA BABY PRODUCTS

☺ **Cleansing Lotion** *($10 for 6.8 ounces)* is just plant oils, thickeners, a tiny amount of cleansing agents, and fragrance. It can leave a slight greasy film on skin but is an option for dry skin.

☹ **Skin Freshener for Babies** *($11 for 6.8 ounces)* is an ordinary toner with too much fragrance that contains not a single beneficial ingredient for a baby's skin.

☺ **PhysiObebe** *($13.50 for 10 ounces)* is a wipe-off cleanser that contains gentle cleansing agents. It does contain fragrance.

☺ **Refreshing Cleansing Cloths** *($6 for 40 cloths)* are not the best of the cleansing cloths, as these contain only a minute amount of cleansing agents. These do contain fragrance.

☺ **Mild and Rich Soap with Cold Cream** *($5.50 for 5 ounces)* is a bar soap with a lot of fragrance. The small amount of mineral oil and castor oil won't prevent this soap from being drying for skin.

☺ **Dermo Cleansing** *($16 for 16.9 ounces)* is a gentle cleanser with fragrance.

☻ **2 in 1 Hair & Body Wash** *($10 for 6.8 ounces)* is a gentle cleanser with fragrance.

☺ **Foam Shampoo** *($10 for 5.1 ounces)*. The ingredients that make this product foam are not helpful for a baby's skin because they can be irritating to skin, which is why most baby products don't use them. This does contain fragrance.

☺ **Baby Shampoo** *($10 for 6.8 ounces)* is almost identical to the Foam Shampoo above and the same comments apply.

☺ **Bath Oil** *($9 for 6.8 ounces)* is just corn oil, thickeners, plant oils, fragrance, and an insignificant amount of vitamins. You would do just a well using plain corn oil from your cupboard.

☺ **Hydra Bebe Facial Hydrating Cream** *($9 for 1.4 ounces)* is a Vaseline-based, standard emollient moisturizer for dry skin. It does contain fragrance.

☺ **Hydra Bebe Body Lotion** *($12.50 for 10.1 ounces)* is similar to the Hydrating Cream above only in lotion form.

☹ **Bubble Bath for Babies** *($9 for 6.8 ounces)* contains sodium lauryl sulfate as one of the main cleansing agents, which makes this too potentially irritating and drying for a baby's skin.

☺ **Cold Cream** *($11 for 1.4 ounces)* is a Vaseline-based moisturizer with thickeners and plant oil. It does contain fragrance.

☺ **Hydra Stick** *($8 for 0.33 ounce)* is primarily just castor oil, thickeners, mineral oil, and fragrance. It is emollient, but ordinary.

☺ **Massage Oil** *($11.50 for 3.4 ounces)* is just mineral oil and sunflower oil, along with some fragrance. The minute amount of vitamins barely matters. You can easily make this up yourself and leave out the fragrance, which can be a problem for skin.

☺ **Extra Thick Cleansing Cloths** *($11 for 70 cloths)* contains mostly mineral oil and almond oil on fairly soft wipes. These can leave a slight greasy film on skin, and they do contain fragrance.

☺ **Vitamin Barrier Cream** *($10 for 1.9 ounces)* is just water, zinc oxide, mineral oil, thickener, fragrance, and preservatives. The minuscule amount of vitamins is inconsequential for skin.

☹ **Natural Soothing Powder** *($9.50 for 3.5 ounces)* is a talc-based powder and is not recommended.

☺ **Maximum Sun Protection Lotion SPF 30+** *($14.50 for 1.6 ounces)*, **Total Sun Protection Lotion SPF 25** *($17 for 4.2 ounces)*, and **Sunblock Stick SPF 20** *($9 for 0.35 ounce)* are all very good, in-part titanium dioxide– and zinc oxide–based sunscreens, though they do contain fragrance. These are pricey but they would work well, though they offer no benefit over using Neutrogena's Sensitive Skin UVA/UVB Block SPF 17 ($8.39 for 4 ounces) and Sensitive Skin UVA/UVB Block SPF 30 ($8.39 for 4 ounces), both titanium dioxide–based sunscreens that are truly fragrance-free and far less expensive.

PEDIAM

Other than the impressive name, there is very little that is particularly clinical about these products for a baby's skin, though there are some good products. First, despite the claim that these products are fragrance-free, one does contain lavender oil. Some of the products also include some irritating plant extracts, such as arnica, which should not be used on rashes or raw skin. Given the buildup about these products, and the high prices, you would expect more, especially for your baby. For more information about PEDIAM, call (480) 991-2580 or visit www.pediaderm.com.

☺ **Milky Cleanser** *($15 for 8 ounces)* contains mostly water, aloe, thickeners, slip agent, detergent cleansing agents, and preservatives. This is a fine cleansing option for most skin types, including a baby's skin. It is fragrance-free.

☹ **Moisturizer** *($15 for 8 ounces)*. Given the inclusion of ivy, pellitory, and arnica, which are well-known skin irritants, this product should not be used on a regular basis on anyone's skin.

☺ **Irritation Ointment** *($15 for 4 ounces)* contains Vaseline (disguised under the trade name Protopet on the ingredient list), lanolin, zinc oxide, aloe, thickeners, plant oil, and preservatives. For the most part this adds nothing to the benefits that a baby's bottom can receive (for far less money) from just a fragrance-free zinc oxide cream with a little Vaseline over it. This product is fragrance-free.

☺ **Healing Gel** *($18 for 8 ounces)* contains mostly aloe gel (water and aloe), slip agent, thickener, soothing agents, water-binding agents, vitamins, and preservatives. While the allantoin, aloe, and oatmeal it contains are definitely soothing to a baby's skin, I would first try pure aloe vera, the kind you buy at the health food store, before this version; that way you skip the preservatives and slip agent, and just get the real thing right next to your baby's skin. If that doesn't work, this one is definitely an option for soothing. This is fragrance-free.

☺ **Hair & Body Wash** *($15 for 8 ounces)* is a good, though standard, cleanser that would be as gentle as any other baby wash. This does contain fragrance (lavender oil).

✔☺ **Sun Block SPF 30** *($18 for 8 ounces)* is a very good sunscreen that contains only titanium dioxide and zinc oxide as the active ingredients. That's great for a baby's skin, and this simple formula would pose little to no risk of irritation. This is fragrance-free.

CHAPTER FIVE

Men's Skin-Care Products

SKIN CARE FOR MEN

Men are about as comfortable discussing skin care or any subject related to beauty as they are holding a woman's purse while she shops. Their aversion to these topics determines in advance that most men aren't going to read, or even see, this chapter, even though they should. That means I have to rely on you, my female readers, to share this section with the men in your lives. Men have faces too, and they definitely have skin-care needs, but you could never convince the vast majority of men to put even a fraction of the attention and energy into the issue that women do. One positive result of this lack of interest is that men don't waste their time on wrinkle creams or unnecessary products for their skin. Even the products sold to men cost far less than those sold to women. While this monetary savings is significant, it also probably means that most men don't use sunscreen on a consistent basis, leaving their skin at risk for cancer, not to mention wrinkles. On a less serious note, it also means that most men don't understand about staying away from irritating skin-care ingredients in their shaving products, and as a result end up with red, rashlike bumps and razor burn (which is really, more often than not, product burn).

What gives? Men definitely wrinkle as much as women (any notion suggesting otherwise is myth, and a bias about how much better men look with wrinkles than women do, related to the social stigma women endure in regard to having any wrinkles). Men also get dry skin, oily skin, breakouts, blackheads, rosacea, acne, rashes, ingrown hairs, and red irritated spots from shaving. So why don't men seem to care as much as women do about taking care of their skin? I suspect that not paying attention to "beauty issues" is a vestige of machismo some men hold on to. In fact, the very marketing angles about gentleness, soothing, antiaging, rejuvenating, and antiwrinkling that are included on the labels and that sell billions of dollars of skin-care products to women are usually left off of men's products, although that is changing. More often than not, men's skin-care products are merely labeled with simple concepts (such as cleansing and moisturizing) or with pragmatic descriptions of shaving products (for pre-, during-, and after-shave), and that is about as elaborate as it gets for men, with just a few "good for sensitive skin" claims occasionally tossed into the mix. Yet *simple* doesn't necessarily translate into *good* skin care.

Almost all of the information in this book pertains to men as well as to women. Very little distinguishes the skin-care needs of men from those of women, except for shaving. Well, maybe taking off makeup is an area most men don't have to pay attention to! But other than that, just because most men ignore their skin-care issues doesn't mean the problems and the solutions aren't there for them, too. Other than shaving products, the truth is that there really is no need for a separate category of men's skin-care products. In fact, the only major difference between men's and women's skin-care products is that the men's products have masculine-identified packaging, which caters only to the superficial requirements of image rather than to unique or special formulations.

FOR MEN IT'S REALLY IRRITATING

Ironically, the product lines that are supposedly designed to meet a man's special skin-care needs are actually the worst ones for him. Many of these products seem to be designed with nothing but irritation in mind. This happens because, in the same way cosmetics companies believe women want wrinkle creams, they believe men need menthol, peppermint, eucalyptus, camphor, lemon, grapefruit, orange, or alcohol in their skin-care products to create the "strong smell—strong man—tingling is good and refreshing" concept the male consumer seems to want. Both notions may be what this consumer *wants*, but neither is what the skin actually *needs*. All of those ingredients, particularly the sensation of tingling, are nothing more than needless irritation, and that is a serious problem for the health of skin.

Irritation is problematic for many reasons, but primarily it causes skin to become inflamed, red, and sore, and that isn't pretty. The consequences of such topical irritation are that it inhibits the skin's immune response, reduces the skin's ability to heal, prevents cell growth, diminishes the skin's structure, and can in the long run break down collagen and elastin, the building blocks of skin. While inflamed, red, and sore skin is often the way irritation manifests itself, that isn't always the case. It is important to understand that skin will not always tell you when it is being irritated; the damage can be taking place within or underneath the skin and not be apparent on the surface. Yet problems are nonetheless taking place (Sources: *Skin Pharmacology and Applied Skin Physiology*, November-December 2000, pages 358–371; *Toxicology*, October 2000, pages 55–63; *Archives of Dermatologic Research*, November 1998, pages 615–620; and *Contact Dermatitis*, June 1998, pages 311–315). That means it is crucial that you pay attention to what you apply to your skin, so you can be informed about what is really going on, beyond what you can see or feel.

Aside from all the basic needs outlined in Chapter Two of this book, the fundamental concern when selecting men's skin-care products is to avoid products that are irritating. This advice should not be ignored, as the results of such products are often evident in the mirror every morning. Fortunately, there are a lot of good alternatives out there, too.

SHAVING: BRACE YOURSELF

The morning shaving ritual is the most typical start to a man's day. Yet, if I may be so bold, it is also the first area where men make mistakes. Most shaving creams and preshave products contain irritating ingredients such as alcohol, menthol, mint, high levels of potassium or sodium hydroxide, and camphor. These skin irritants cause the hair follicle and skin to swell, forcing the hair up and away from the skin. While this does make the hair stand up to some extent, supposedly allowing for a closer shave, the irritation and resulting swelling also cause some of the hair to be hidden by the swollen follicle and skin. So, what might get the hair to rise to the occasion really doesn't make for a better shave, because the swollen skin prevents the razor from getting closer to the base of the hair. Additionally, after you shave, because some of the facial hair is hidden beneath swollen skin (which temporarily gives the impression of a close shave) the stubble will have a harder time navigating its way back out. If the hair begins to grow (which it does almost immediately) before the swelling is reduced, it increases the likelihood of ingrown hairs.

Moreover, a razor gliding over the face abrades the skin—granted, not all that much, but enough to cause havoc when an innocent-looking aftershave lotion with irritating ingredients is splashed over that broken skin. Think of splashing an aftershave on a cut or scrape or on any other part of your body where you have an abrasion. Now, why would you want to do that to your face (other than the erroneous notion that this somehow protects the skin or is healing after shaving)? Basic skin-care rule number one, for both men and women: If the skin-care product you're using repeatedly burns, irritates, tingles, causes the skin to become inflamed, or hurts, don't use it.

SKIN CARE BASICS FOR MEN

What should men use to take care of their skin when they shave? The list isn't all that different from the one that applies for women, and so Chapter Two applies to men as well. In summary, all men's skin types need a gentle, water-soluble cleanser; a gentle shave product (foam, cream, or gel); followed by a gentle, nonirritating aftershave or shaving lotion (which for all intents and purposes is just a masculine name for a gentle toner). The same options follow for treating breakouts (BHA and disinfectant), sun care (SPF 15 with UVA protection), or dealing with dry skin (a good moisturizer). The one exception to selecting a parallel routine is that, for some skin types, it can prove to be too irritating for men to follow shaving with an AHA or BHA product, and those should only be used at night.

MEN AND WRINKLES

When it comes to sun exposure and genetic aging, men and women age in exactly the same way, determined primarily by how much time they have spent in the sun without adequate sun protection (and for most of us, given how little we've known about sun protection until recently, that's likely to have been a lot of time).

However, in terms of surface-cell turnover, men who shave do have an advantage, because shaving regularly removes the top layer of dead skin cells, improving cell turnover. That's good, but it only accounts for a certain amount of surface smoothness over the shaved areas (encouraging cell turnover doesn't alter the way wrinkles are formed or lessen their occurrence). And it doesn't help the areas of the face where men don't shave. It also means that men don't have to pass up the advantages of using a retinoid—like Retin-A or Renova—or that they should omit using a reliable sunscreen. Men who shave daily are probably best off not using AHAs on the bearded area of the face because shaving exfoliates the skin more than adequately there, and it isn't necessary to do more by using an AHA product. However, cell turnover is not stimulated in nonshaved areas, so using an AHA or BHA product over the nonshaved areas of the face, neck, or forehead could be a good addition to a man's skin-care routine. Using a good sunscreen is the best answer of all.

RATING MEN'S SKIN-CARE PRODUCTS

All of the standards for rating skin-care products discussed in the introductory sections of Chapter Three apply to men's products as well. The only additional criterion for men's products is the expectation that all shaving-related products, including preshaves, shaving gels, creams, and lotions, as well as aftershaves, contain no irritating ingredients whatsoever. It would be best for a man's skin (just as it is for a woman's) if the products they use are fragrance-free, although that is almost a nonexistent possibility. In fact, except for some rare exceptions, all of the products reviewed in this chapter contain fragrance unless otherwise noted.

ANTHONY LOGISTICS

☺ **Algae Facial Cleanser** (*$20 for 4 ounces*) is a standard, detergent-based cleanser with the teeniest amount of algae imaginable. There is no advantage to using this cleanser versus far less pricey alternatives available at the drugstore.

☹ **Glycolic Facial Cleanser** (*$18 for 8 ounces*) is a standard, detergent-based cleanser that contains about 7% AHA. However, the pH of this product is too high for it to be effective as an exfoliant.

☹ **Glycerin Cleansing Bar** (*$8 for 5.5 ounces*) contains peppermint, which makes it potentially irritating for all skin types.

☺ **$$$ Facial Scrub** (*$18 for 4 ounces*) is a standard, detergent-based cleanser that uses ground-up plastic (polyethylene) as the abrasive. It is an option for normal to oily skin.

☺ **Alcohol Free Toner** (*$16 for 8 ounces*) is alcohol-free, but it is also free of any beneficial skin-care ingredients. It does contain a minute amount of water-binding agent and anti-irritants, but in such a small quantity the content is undetectable for skin.

☺ **Oil Free Facial Lotion** (*$25 for 2.5 ounces*) is an OK, ordinary moisturizer for normal to dry skin that contains a modicum of water-binding agents.

☺ **All Purpose Facial Moisturizer** (*$25 for 2.5 ounces*) is an OK moisturizer for dry skin that contains several plant extracts that sound like they are related to AHAs; however, they have no exfoliating properties.

☺ **Facial Moisturizer SPF 15** *($30 for 2.5 ounces)* is a very good, in-part avobenzone-based sunscreen in an ordinary moisturizing base. It contains plant extracts that sound like they are related to AHAs, but they have no exfoliating properties.

☺ **$$$ Sport Stick SPF 15 Lip & Eye Treatment** *($15 for 0.5 ounce)* is a very good, in-part avobenzone-based sunscreen in an ordinary emollient base of Vaseline, plant oil, and thickeners.

☺ **$$$ Eye Cream** *($28 for 0.75 ounce)* contains no ingredients that make it unique for the eye area. It is just an ordinary emollient moisturizer for normal to dry skin.

☹ **Pre-Shave Oil** *($18 for 2.5 ounces)* contains eucalyptus and peppermint oils, which make it too potentially irritating for all skin types. This is not the way to start off shaving.

☹ **Razor Burn Repair** *($22 for 4 ounces)* contains eucalyptus and peppermint oils, which won't repair any part of skin.

☹ **Electric Pre-Shave Solution** *($12 for 4 ounces)* contains mostly alcohol, as well as peppermint and eucalyptus oils, which add up to a prelude for irritation.

☹ **Astringent After Shave** *($18 for 8 ounces)* contains mostly alcohol, as well as peppermint, eucalyptus, and camphor, which is painful for me to even list.

☹ **After Shave Lotion** *($18 for 2.5 ounces)* contains eucalyptus oil and peppermint oil, which makes it too potentially irritating for all skin types.

☹ **Shave Gel** *($14 for 6 ounces)* is a standard shave gel that also contains benzocaine, a topical anesthetic. Benzocaine numbs the skin, and is probably intended to reduce shaving discomfort. Yet that would have been better served by eliminating the irritating ingredients of eucalyptus and peppermint this product contains.

☹ **Shave Cream** *($14 for 6 ounces)* contains eucalyptus oil and peppermint oil, which make this too potentially irritating for all skin types.

☺ **$$$ Deep Pore Cleansing Clay** *($22 for 4 ounces)* is an exceptionally standard, though extremely fragrant, clay mask for normal to oily skin

AQUA VELVA

☹ **Classic Ice Blue Cooling After Shave** *($4.79 for 7 ounces)* lists alcohol as the first ingredient, and in addition it contains menthol! Ouch!

☹ **Ice Sport Cooling After Shave** *($4.29 for 3.5 ounces)* is almost identical to the Ice Blue above, and the same painful comments apply.

☺ **After Shave Cologne, Musk** *($2.99 for 3.5 ounces)* is a fragrance that contains mostly alcohol. This should not be used on the face.

ARAMIS LAB SERIES

☹ **Dual Action Face Soap** *($10 for 5.5 ounces)* is a standard bar soap that is too drying and irritating for all skin types. This one also contains camphor, which only adds to the potential for more irritation and dryness.

☹ **Lift Off! Power Wash** *($14 for 8.5 ounces)* lists the main detergent cleansing agent as sodium lauryl sulfate, which makes this too potentially irritating and drying for all skin types.

☹ **Active Treatment Scrub** *($12.50 for 3.4 ounces)* lists alcohol as the second ingredient, and it also contains menthol. Together, that makes this too potentially irritating and drying for all skin types.

☹ **Close Call Shave Solution** *($12 for 0.5 ounce)* contains menthol and is not recommended.

☹ **Electric Shave Solution** *($11 for 3.4 ounces)* lists alcohol as the first ingredient and that makes this too drying and irritating for all skin types.

☹ **Maximum Comfort Shave Cream** *($10.50 for 3.4 ounces)* is a standard shave cream except for the addition of benzocaine, a topical anesthetic. Benzocaine is an interesting ingredient to include because it is meant to numb the skin, reducing irritation and discomfort from shaving. That purpose would have been better served by eliminating the irritating ingredients of eucalyptus, lemon, and coriander this product contains.

☺ **Razor Burn Relief Plus** *($25 for 3.4 ounces)* is just a simple moisturizing product with some good water-binding agents and a tiny amount of antioxidant. There is nothing in it that can reduce the irritation caused from shaving itself, much less irritating shaving products.

☹ **Razor Bump Relief** *($25 for 1.7 ounces)* contains aspirin, which can be helpful to alleviate irritated skin, but it also contains alcohol (the second ingredient) as well as eucalyptus, both of which cause irritation. This is a very confused product.

☺ **Tri-Gel Extra Shave Formula** *($12 for 4.2 ounces)* does contain a few problematic plant extracts, but they are far enough down on the ingredient list to make this a potentially irritant-free shave gel. It is extremely standard and overpriced, but still a good option.

☺ **Age Rescue Lotion** *($28 for 1.4 ounces)* is a very good moisturizer for normal to dry skin that contains a nice blend of anti-irritants, water-binding agents, and antioxidants. This won't rescue your skin from one minute of "age," but it is a very good moisturizer for normal to dry skin.

☺ **Age Rescue Skin Care Therapy** *($30 for 1.4 ounces)* is similar to the Age Rescue Lotion above, and the same basic comments apply.

☺ **$$$ Eye Rescue Undereye Therapy** *($23.50 for 0.5 ounce)* is similar to the Age Rescue Lotion above, and the same basic comments apply.

☺ **Sharp Shooter Anti Oxidant Vitamin Lotion** *($22.50 for 2 ounces)* is a good moisturizer for normal to dry skin that contains a nice blend of anti-irritants and some water-binding agents, but only a tiny amount of antioxidants. It is an option for someone with normal to dry skin.

☺ **Trifecta Triple Effect Formula for Oily Skin** *($32.50 for 1.7 ounces)* is a silicone-based moisturizer with some very good antioxidants and water-binding agents. This does contain a tiny amount of peppermint, but most likely not enough to be a problem for skin.

☺ **Fast Absorbing Sunless Tanning Spray** (*$12 for 3.4 ounces*) contains dihydroxy-acetone, the same ingredient all self-tanners use to affect the color of skin; it would work as well as any.

☹ **Waterproof, Sweatproof Sun Protection Spray SPF 15** (*$18 for 3.4 ounces*) doesn't contain the UVA-protecting ingredients of titanium dioxide, zinc oxide, or avobenzone, and is not recommended.

☹ **Super Lift Off! AHA/BHA Formula SPF 15** (*$37.50 for 3.4 ounces*) doesn't contain the UVA-protecting ingredients of titanium dioxide, zinc oxide, or avobenzone, and is not recommended.

☺ **Frequent Flyer Daily Face Lotion SPF 15** (*$20 for 1.7 ounces*) is a mediocre sunscreen for dry skin that contains a tiny amount of titanium dioxide, enough to be borderline effective for protecting against UVA sun damage.

☺ **$$$ Lift Off Deep Cleansing Clay Mask** (*$17.50 for 3.4 ounces*) is a very simple clay mask that also contains some BHA (salicylic acid) and charcoal. Charcoal can absorb oil, but the pH of this mask is too high for the BHA to have exfoliating properties. It would work well as a mask to absorb oil.

☹ **Skin Clearing Lotion** (*$10 for 3.4 ounces*) lists alcohol as the first ingredient, and that makes it too drying and irritating for all skin types. Irritation won't clear up anything, but will add up to more skin-care problems.

☺ **Stop Shine Oil Control Formula** (*$24.50 for 1.7 ounces*) won't stop oil—it's mostly a lightweight, silicone-based moisturizer that contains some good water-binding agents and a tiny amount of BHA (salicylic acid), although the pH of the product is too high for it to be effective as an exfoliant. Besides, BHA doesn't absorb oil or affect oil production in any way. What an effective BHA product can do is help improve the shape and size of the pore, thus improving the "natural" flow of oil and helping to prevent clogging and breakouts.

ARBONNE SKIN FITNESS

☺ **$$$ Cleansing Scrub** (*$15 for 4 ounces*) is a standard, detergent-based cleanser that also contains some cornmeal as the abrasive. As an occasional exfoliant, it's an option for normal to oily skin. The tiny amount of balm mint is most likely too small to be a problem for skin.

☺ **Soothing Shave Gel** (*$11 for 6 ounces*) lists peanut oil as the third ingredient, and except for a small amount of lemon oil this is a fairly irritant-free shave gel that would be an option for normal to dry skin.

☹ **Balancer** (*$13.50 for 4 ounces*) contains some irritating plant extracts, including camphor and lemon oil, and that doesn't balance anything.

☺ **Moisture Plus AHAs** (*$17.50 for 2 ounces*) contains about 8% lactic acid in a decent moisturizing base that includes some antioxidants and anti-irritants. Unfortunately, it also contains some problematic plant extracts, which aren't the best for skin.

AVEDA MEN'S SKIN CARE

☺ **After Shave Balm** *($13.50 for 1.7 ounces)* is a rather fragrant, though ordinary, moisturizer for normal to dry skin.

☹ **Shave Cream** *($11 for 7.9 ounces)* contains peppermint extract, and that can be a problem for irritation.

AVEENO

✓☺ **Aveeno Therapeutic Shave Gel** *($3.79 for 7 ounces)* is a very good, fragrance-free shave gel that would work well for all skin types. It does contain a tiny amount of triclosan, a topical disinfectant, and while that may help reduce some risk of infection, infection is not the real cause of red, irritated bumps on the skin after shaving.

BIOTHERM MEN

☺ **Anti Shine Face Cleanser** *($14.50 for 5.2 ounces)* is a standard, detergent-based cleanser that also contains some clay, which can help absorb oil. This is an option for normal to oily skin.

☺ **Non Drying Facial Cleansing Gel** *($12.50 for 3.4 ounces)* is an extremely standard, detergent-based cleanser that would work well for most skin types.

☹ **Detoxifying Cleanser** *($15.50 for 5 ounces)* is a fairly drying, detergent-based cleanser that won't detoxify skin in any way, though it can cause dryness and irritation.

☺ $$$ **Facial Exfoliator** *($14.50 for 1.7 ounces)* is a standard, detergent-based cleanser that uses ground-up plastic as the abrasive. This is an option for normal to dry skin, though it is incredibly overpriced for what you get. A basic cleanser from Neutrogena to Cetaphil mixed with some baking soda would do the job far better for far less money.

☹ **Face Purifying Scrub** *($14.50 for 2.53 ounces)* contains a far more drying detergent cleansing agent than the Facial Exfoliator above and that is not purifying in the least.

☺ **Active Anti-Shine Moisturizer** *($20 for 1.7 ounces)* lists alcohol as the fourth ingredient. That is drying, but it doesn't eliminate shine, it just dries up skin cells. This does contain some absorbents, such as silica and clay, which is helpful, but the alcohol gets in the way.

☺ **Detoxifying Moisturizer** *($27 for 1.7 ounces)* lists alcohol as the third ingredient, and that doesn't detoxify anything, although it can cause irritation and dryness.

☺ $$$ **Hydra Detox Yeux** *($24 for 0.5 ounce)* is an OK, silicone-based moisturizer for normal to dry skin that contains some very good water-binding agents and emollients, but lacks any significant antioxidants.

☺ **Active Moisturizer SPF 15** *($20 for 1.7 ounces)* is a very good, in-part avobenzone-based sunscreen, though the third ingredient is alcohol, which can be a problem for causing dryness and irritation.

☹ **D Stress Energy Booster** *($27 for 1.7 ounces)* lists alcohol as the second ingredient, making this a potential problem for dryness and irritation, not energy.

☹ **AquaPower Ultra Moisturizing Oligo-Thermal Care** *($25 for 2.53 ounces)*. The second ingredient listed is alcohol, making this a problem for dryness and irritation.

☺ **Total Care Revitalizer Gel** *($29 for 1.7 ounces)* is an OK, lightweight moisturizer for normal to slightly dry skin that contains a small amount of water-binding agents, but it lacks any significant antioxidants.

☺ **Active Shave Repair** *($15 for 1.7 ounces)* won't repair anything on the face, but it is an OK, though extremely ordinary, lightweight moisturizer for normal to slightly dry skin.

☺ **Express Bronzer Tinted Self Tanning Gel for the Face** *($15 for 1.7 ounces)* contains dihydroxyacetone, the same ingredient all self-tanners use to affect the color of skin. This overpriced option would work as well as any.

☺ **$$$ Anti Shine Mask** *($14.50 for 2.64 ounces)* is an extremely simple and basic (though overpriced) clay mask that is an option for absorbing oil.

☺ **Sensitive Skin Close Shave** *($11 for 5.1 ounces)* is a standard shave cream that is indistinguishable from any of the Edge products reviewed below, which are available for far less money.

☹ **Purifying Close Shave** *($12 for 5.1 ounces)* contains menthol and is not recommended.

THE BODY SHOP SKIN MECHANICS FOR MEN

☺ **Shaving Cream** *($11.50 for 6 ounces)* is a standard shave cream indistinguishable from any of the Edge products reviewed below and available at one-third this price.

☹ **After Shave Balm Lotion** *($10.50 for 3.2 ounces)* would be a good emollient moisturizer for dry skin, but the menthol makes it a problem for irritation and redness.

☺ **After Shave Gel** *($10.50 for 3.4 ounces)* is more like putting aloe vera with fragrance and coloring agents on your skin, which isn't bad, but you could just skip the unnecessary fragrance and dyes and use plain aloe that's available at the health food store.

☺ **Face Protector** *($10.50 for 3.4 ounces)* does not have an SPF rating (though it does contain sunscreen), so it can't be relied on for sun protection. Other than that, it is just a very ordinary, though emollient, moisturizer for dry skin.

BURT'S BEES MEN

☹ **Bay Rum Aftershave Balm** *($12 for 4 ounces)* lists alcohol as the second ingredient, and it also contains menthol, making this too irritating and drying for all skin types.

☹ **Bay Rum Moisturizing Cream** *($7 for 1.5 ounces)*. The number of irritating and sensitizing plant extracts in this standard moisturizer makes it a serious problem for skin.

☹ **Bay Rum Exfoliating Soap** *($5 for 3.25 ounces)*. The number of irritating and sensitizing plant extracts in this standard soap add up to a problem for skin.

☹ **Bay Rum Shaving Soap** *($6 for 3 ounces)* is similar to the Exfoliating Soap above, and is not recommended.

CALIFORNIA NORTH MEN'S SKIN CARE

☺ **Gel Skin Wash for Face and Body** *($20 for 7.8 ounces)* is a standard, detergent-based cleanser that is an option for normal to oily skin. It also contains several plant extracts, which means it has the potential for skin irritation, but they would probably be rinsed away before they could have an affect on skin.

☹ **Gel Skin Scrub** *($20. for 7 ounces)* lists alcohol as the second ingredient, and it also contains menthol, and that makes this too drying and irritating for all skin types.

☹ **Action Moisturizer for Body and Face, Oil Free, SPF 4** *($15 for 7 ounces)*. The SPF 4 is offensively low (SPF 15 is the minimum acceptable), not to mention this doesn't contain the UVA-protecting ingredients of titanium dioxide, zinc oxide, or avobenzone. It is not recommended.

☹ **After Shave Care Triple Action, Oil Free, 2% BHA and SPF 4** *($15 for 4 ounces)* is similar to the Action Moisturizer above, and the same comments apply.

☺ **Titanium 15 Sunblock Waterproof/Sweatproof** *($20 for 7 ounces)* is a very good, in-part titanium dioxide–based sunscreen in an extremely standard moisturizing base that would be an option for someone with normal to dry skin.

☺ **Titanium 30 Sunblock Waterproof/Sweatproof** *($22 for 7 ounces)* is similar to the Titanium 15 version above except that this version has an SPF 30.

☺ **Titanium Self Tanner** *($24 for 7 ounces)* contains dihydroxyacetone, the same ingredient all self-tanners contain to affect the color of skin. This one would work as well as any.

☺ $$$ **Men's Razor Shave Cream, Foamless Protective Blade Shave** *($16 for 7 ounces)* is a fairly basic shave cream that contains a minimum of problematic plant extracts. However, there is no advantage to using this over the far less expensive versions available at the drugstore.

☹ **Electric Glide Formula** *($14 for 4 ounces)* lists alcohol as the first ingredient, which makes this too drying and irritating for all skin types.

☹ **Foaming Shave Gel** *($14 for 5 ounces)* is a fairly basic shave gel, but it contains several problematic plant extracts that are best not applied to abraded, shaved skin.

CLARINS MEN'S

☺ $$$ **Active Face Wash** *($16 for 4.4 ounces)* is an exceptionally standard, detergent-based cleanser that is an option for most skin types.

☺ $$$ **Undereye Serum** *($26 for 0.7 ounce)* is an OK, lightweight moisturizer for normal to slightly dry skin with a tiny amount of water-binding agents and antioxidants.

☺ **Fatigue Fighter** *($26 for 1.7 ounces)*. You'd be better off with a cup of coffee than this mediocre moisturizer. The third ingredient listed is alcohol, which can cause dryness and irritation, but it also contains rice starch, which absorbs moisture, and that negates the other moisturizing ingredients in this self-contradicting lotion.

☺ **Moisture Gel** *($24 for 1.7 ounces)* is a silicone-based, lightweight moisturizing gel that contains a tiny amount of antioxidants and an unimaginably small amount of water-binding agents.

☺ **Moisture Balm** *($24 for 1.7 ounces)* is a fairly basic moisturizer for dry skin that lacks any significant water-binding agents or antioxidants. There are far better moisturizers to consider than this.

☺ **Smooth Shave** *($14 for 5.25 ounces)* is an exceptionally standard shave cream that has no advantage over and is no different from less expensive versions found at the drugstore.

☹ **Shave Ease** *($22 for 1 ounce)* contains menthol and eucalyptus, and that makes this too drying and irritating for all skin types.

☺ **$$$ Total Shampoo** *($16 for 7 ounces)* is an exceptionally standard, detergent-based shampoo that is embarrassingly overpriced for what you get. There is no advantage to using this over any shampoo from L'Oreal to TRESemme, which are available at the drugstore for a fraction of the price.

CLINIQUE SKIN SUPPLIES FOR MEN

☹ **Face Soap Regular Strength** *($11 for 6-ounce bar)* is a standard bar soap, which makes it not all that different from Ivory, and worth neither the price nor the dryness it can cause.

☹ **Scruffing Lotion 1½ for Sensitive Skin** *($10.50 for 6.7 ounces)* contains mostly alcohol, witch hazel distillate, and menthol. There is no reason to use those ingredients on any skin type, but it is thoughtless to have them in a product for someone with sensitive skin.

☹ **Scruffing Lotion 2½ for Dry to Average Skin** *($10.50 for 6.7 ounces)* is similar to the Sensitive Skin version above, and the same comments apply.

☹ **Scruffing Lotion 3½ for Oily Skin** *($10.50 for 6.7 ounces)* has the same problems as the 2½ version above, and the same comments apply.

☹ **Scruffing Lotion 4½ for Very Oily Skin** *($10.50 for 6.7 ounces)* has the same problems as the 2½ version above, and the same comments apply.

☹ **Face Scrub** *($15 for 3.4 ounces)* is a standard, detergent-based scrub that uses ground-up plastic (polyethylene) as the abrasive. However, it contains menthol, which makes it too irritating, especially in a scrub.

✓☺ **$$$ Eye Treatment Formula** *($26 for 0.5 ounce)* is a very good, silicone-based moisturizer with some good water-binding agents and antioxidants.

✓☺ **Moisture Surge Extra Oil Free Gel** *($31 for 1.7 ounces)* is a very good, silicone-based moisturizer with some good water-binding agents and a decent amount of antioxidants.

☺ **M Lotion** *($17 for 3.4 ounces)* is the male version of Clinique's Dramatically Different Moisturizer, and the only difference is in the packaging. This exceptionally ordinary, mineral oil–based moisturizer is so out of date it makes the typewriter look like new technology.

☺ **Turnaround Lotion** *($26 for 1.7 ounces)* is an OK, basic moisturizer for normal to dry skin. It does contain BHA, but the product's pH is too high for it to be an effective exfoliant.

☺ **Non-Streak Bronzer** *(15.50 for 2 ounces)* is a very sheer, relatively tan-looking bronzer in a lightweight gel base. It can add a bit of color, but on very light skin it can have a slightly too peach look.

☹ **Creme Shave** *($8 for 4.2 ounces)* would be a good basic shave cream, but it contains menthol, and that can cause redness and irritation.

✔☺ **M Shave Aloe Gel** *($11.50 for 4.4 ounces)* is a good, nonirritating shave gel, but it is also virtually identical to excellent versions from Gillette and Edge that are available at the drugstore for far less money. A major plus is that this is fragrance-free.

☹ **Post Shave Healer** *($14.50 for 2.5 ounces)* lists alcohol as the second ingredient and that doesn't help heal skin, though it will add to irritation and dryness.

COLGATE SHAVING CARE

☺ **Shave Cream, Aloe** *($1.29 for 11 ounces)*; **Shave Cream, Regular** *($1.29 for 11 ounces)*; **Shave Cream, Arctic Cool** *($1.29 for 11 ounces)*; **Shave Cream, Sensitive Skin** *($1.29 for 11 ounces)*; and **Shave Cream, Irish Spring** *($1.29 for 11 ounces)* are virtually identical except for a change in fragrance. These are standard shave creams that have minimal risk of irritation. They do contain a small amount of sodium lauryl sulfate, but probably not enough to be a problem for most skin types.

CRABTREE & EVELYN FOR MEN

☹ **Nomad Soap** *($15 for 2 bars)* contains eucalyptus, which makes it too irritating for all skin types (not to mention that this standard soap formulation can be drying and irritating in and of itself).

☹ **Sandlewood Soap** *($15 for 10.5 ounces)* is a standard, very fragrant bar soap that can be drying and irritating for skin.

☹ **Sienna Soap** *($15 for 10.5 ounces)* is identical to the Sandlewood Soap above except for the fragrance. The same basic comments apply.

☺ **Sienna After Shave Balm** *($30 for 4.2 ounces)* is a very ordinary, though fragrant, moisturizer for normal to dry skin. There is nothing in it that makes it worth the price.

☺ **Sandalwood Shaving Bowl** *($15 for 3.2 ounces)* is just the Sandalwood Soap in an attractive bowl that you lather up with a traditional shave brush. This traditional way of shaving was replaced with shave gel and creams because they were less drying and rough on skin, and this product doesn't change that problem.

☺ **Nomad Shave Gel** *($10 for 4.2 ounces)* is a good basic shave gel that would work well for all skin types, with minimal to no risk of irritation.

☺ **Nomad Shave Cream** *($10 for 3.5 ounces)* is a good, basic shave cream, but despite the product's claim that it's good for sensitive skin, it isn't, at least not any more so than other shave creams.

☹ **Nomad After Shave Balm** *($24 for 3.4 ounces)* lists witch hazel distillate (which is primarily alcohol) as the second ingredient, and that isn't soothing or helpful to shaven skin.

☺ **Shaving Cream** (comes in **Sweet Almond Oil**, **Sandalwood**, and **Sienna**) *($18.50 for 5.8 ounces)* is a standard shave cream that is identical to those available at the drugstore for far less money.

EDGE PRO GEL

☺ **Pro Gel Extra Moisturizing Shave Gel** *($2.59 for 7 ounces)* is a standard, but good, shave gel for most skin types, with minimal to no risk of irritation or dryness.

☺ **Extra Protection from Nicks and Cuts** *($2.49 for 7 ounces)* is similar to the Extra Moisturizing version above, and the same comments apply. There is nothing in this product to prevent cuts or nicks from shaving.

☹ **Extra Refreshing with Lime Splash** *($2.49 for 7 ounces)*. The lime in this product just adds to the risk of irritation.

☹ **Extra Soothing with Cooling Menthol** *($2.49 for 7 ounces)*. Menthol is indeed cooling, but it is also irritating and can increase the risk of redness and breakouts from shaving.

✓☺ **Fragrance-Free for Irritated Skin and Razor Bumps** *($2.49 for 7 ounces)* is similar to the Extra Moisturizing version above, and it is indeed fragrance-free, making this a rarity in the world of men's skin-care products. This does contain triclosan, a topical disinfectant that can be helpful to prevent infection, but infection is rarely the reason the skin becomes irritated and bumpy after shaving.

☺ **Normal Skin Shave Gel** *($2.49 for 7 ounces)* is almost identical to the Extra Moisturizing version above, and the same comments apply.

☺ **Sensitive Skin with Aloe Shave Gel** *($2.49 for 7 ounces)* is almost identical to the Extra Moisturizing version above, and the same comments apply. There is nothing about this formulation that makes it preferred for sensitive skin.

✓☺ **Skin Conditioning Shave Gel** *($2.49 for 7 ounces)* is almost identical to the Extra Moisturizing version above, and the same comments apply, but this is an even better option because it is fragrance-free!

☺ **Shaving Gel Tough Beards with Beard Softeners Formula** *($2.49 for 7 ounces)* is almost identical to the Extra Moisturizing version above, and the same comments apply. There is nothing different about this product (other than the name) that makes it more suitable for those with heavy beards.

ESTEE LAUDER PLEASURES FOR MEN

In their brochure for Pleasures, Lauder announces that it's a "Fact: A man's skin is different. It's oilier and thicker. And because it's shaved on a regular basis, it's open to all kinds of problems—red bumps, ingrown hairs and dry irritated patches." Of course, Pleasures is supposed to address those unique problems. Yet, in tackling these male issues, in many ways these products come up short. As seductive as the name sounds, the products still leave men's skin in need of a good nonirritating pre-shave, a soothing aftershave, and a sunscreen. Lauder recommends that men use the Pleasures Oil-Free Moisturizer (which has no sunscreen) twice a day! That recommendation is way off the mark, especially considering that Lauder has plenty of good sunscreens that would work beautifully for men.

☺ **Comfort Shave Gel** (*$13.50 for 6.7 ounces*) is an exceptionally standard shave gel with a good deal of fragrance. The teeny amount of green tea isn't enough to counter either the irritation from shaving or from the fragrance the product contains. There are plenty of gentle, fragrance-free shave gels available at the drugstore.

☹ **After Shave** (*$30 for 3.4 ounces*) is just alcohol, water, and fragrance, which adds up to cologne, not skin care. Do not put this on your face.

☹ **Close-Shave Cream** (*$10 for 3.4 ounces*) is standard shave cream that contains menthol, and that is too potentially irritating for all skin types.

☺ **Oil-Free Moisturizer** (*$25 for 2 ounces*) has a formula that is strikingly similar to Lauder's Idealist—a moisturizer marketed to women that sells for $70 for 1.7 ounces. It contains acetyl glucosamine, which is supposed to be a new exfoliating agent that doesn't irritate the skin (although its ability to exfoliate is doubtful). Overall, this is a very good, light-feeling moisturizer for normal to dry skin with very good water-binding agents and a teeny amount of anti-irritants. Unfortunately, there aren't enough anti-irritants to keep up with the potential for irritation from the strong fragrance in this product.

☺ **Skin Comfort Lotion** (*$18.50 for 1.75 ounces*) is an OK moisturizer for normal to dry skin that contains a small amount of water-binding agents and antioxidants. It is also highly fragranced.

GILLETTE

☺ **Foamy Shaving Cream, Aloe and Allantoin** (*$1.99 for 11 ounces*) is an extremely standard, but good, shaving cream. It does contain a small amount of sodium lauryl sulfate, but probably not enough to be a problem for skin. The small amounts of aloe and allantoin have little benefit for skin, though they can be soothing agents.

☺ **Foamy Shaving Cream, Regular** (*$1.99 for 11 ounces*) is an extremely standard, but good, shaving cream. It does contain a small amount of sodium lauryl sulfate, but probably not enough to be a problem for skin.

☺ **Foamy, Shaving Cream, Lemon-Lime** *($1.99 for 11 ounces)* is similar to the Foamy Shaving Cream, Regular above, and the same comments apply. The lemon-lime just refers to a change in fragrance.

☺ **Shaving Foam, Moisturizing** *($2.79 for 9 ounces)* is similar to the Foamy Shaving Cream, Regular above, only this one also contains mineral oil, which can be better for dry skin.

☺ **Shaving Foam, Sensitive Skin** *($2.79 for 9 ounces)* includes no ingredients that make it more appropriate for sensitive skin. It is virtually identical to the Shaving Foam, Moisturizing above.

☺ **Shaving Gel, Conditioning** *($2.79 for 7 ounces)* is similar to the Foamy Shaving Cream, Regular above, and the same comments apply. The formula difference is merely in texture.

☺ **Shaving Gel, Moisturizing** *($2.79 for 7 ounces)* is similar to the Shaving Foam, Moisturizing above, and the same comments apply. The formula difference is merely in texture.

☺ **Shaving Gel, Protection** *($2.79 for 7 ounces)* is similar to the Foamy Shaving Cream, Regular above, and the same comments apply. The formula difference is merely in texture.

☺ **Shaving Gel, Sensitive Skin** *($2.79 for 7 ounces)* is similar to the Foamy Shaving Cream, Regular above, and the same comments apply. There is nothing about this product that makes it especially appropriate for sensitive skin; the formula difference is merely in texture.

☺ **Shaving Gel, Clean Skin** *($2.79 for 7 ounces)* is similar to the Foamy Shaving Cream, Regular above, and the same comments apply. The formula difference is merely in texture. This also contains a tiny amount of tea tree oil, but not enough to be effective as a topical disinfectant, so it won't help prevent breakouts.

☹ **After Shave Gel, Normal to Dry Skin** *($2.89 for 2.54 ounces)*; **After Shave Gel, Protection** *($2.89 for 2.54 ounces)*; **After Shave Gel, Sensitive Skin** *($2.89 for 2.54 ounces)*; and **After Shave Gel, Conditioning** *($2.89 for 2.54 ounces)* all list alcohol as the second ingredient, which makes these too drying and irritating for all skin types.

☺ **After Shave Lotion, Protection** *($2.89 for 2.54 ounces)* is not much of a moisturizer, and is actually a rather confused product. The second ingredient is aluminum starch octenylsuccinate, an absorbing and thickening agent, which is good for a matte finish and good for absorbing oil, but it has no place as a primary ingredient in a moisturizer. The third ingredient is fragrance. That means the remaining ingredients make up less than 0.1 percent of the content, and that adds up to as mediocre a formulation as you will find.

☺ **After Shave Lotion, Conditioning** *($2.89 for 2.54 ounces)* is almost identical to the After Shave Lotion, Protection above, and the same comments apply.

☺ **After Shave Lotion, Sensitive** *($2.89 for 2.54 ounces)* is almost identical to the After Shave Lotion, Protection above, and the same comments apply.

☹ **After Shave Splash, Pacific Light** *($4.99 for 3.5 ounces).* Although this doesn't contain alcohol, which is refreshing, it does contain menthol, which makes this too potentially irritating for all skin types.

☹ **After Shave Splash, Wild Rain** *($4.99 for 3.5 ounces)* and **After Shave Splash, Cool Wave** *($4.99 for 3.5 ounces)* are mostly alcohol and fragrance, which makes them nothing more than eau de cologne. These should not be applied to the face.

KIEHL'S FOR MEN

☺ **Soothing, Nourishing Face Cream for Men, for Dry to Normal Skin Types** *($19.50 for 8 ounces)* is an extremely ordinary, mundane moisturizer for normal to dry skin. It is not worth the effort of applying it.

✓☺ **Close Shavers Squadron Ultimate Brushless Shave Cream, It's a "Goggle-Fogger" Formula, Blue Eagle with Aloe for Sensitive Skin** *($13.50 for 5 ounces)* has an impressive name that is attached to a rather standard, non-aerosol shave cream. However, this is thankfully fragrance-free, and would work well for most skin types.

☹ **Close Shavers Squadron Ultimate Brushless Shave Cream, "Take Off" Formula, Green Eagle** *($10.50 for 4 ounces)* contains peppermint oil. Ouch!

☹ **Close Shavers Squadron Ultimate Brushless Shave Cream, It's a "Hair Raizer" Formula, White Eagle** *($10.50 for 4 ounces)* contains menthol and camphor, which are indeed hair-raising, but in a shocking way, not a good way.

☹ **Light Flite Shave Cream for the Brush** *($25.50 for 4.5 ounces)* is an extremely confused product. It contains benzocaine, a topical anesthetic that numbs skin to help reduce shaving discomfort. That purpose would have been better served by eliminating the irritating ingredients of menthol and camphor this product contains.

☹ **Men's Alcohol Free Herbal Toner** *($17.50 for 8 ounces)* is definitely alcohol free, which is nice, but it contains some problematic plant extracts that can be irritating for skin. It also lacks any significant water-binding agents or antioxidants, which makes it a rather useless product for skin.

☹ **Blue Astringent Herbal Lotion** *($9 for 4 ounces)* lists alcohol as the second ingredient, and it also contains camphor and menthol. Ouch!

☺ **The Ultimate Men's After Shave All Day Moisturizer** *($20.50 for 8 ounces)* is an ordinary moisturizer for normal to dry skin. However, without sunscreen, it is ultimately a serious problem for daytime use.

☹ **The Ultimate Men's After Shave All Day Moisturizer (Mentholated)** *($20.50 for 8 ounces)* contains menthol and camphor, which are too irritating for all skin types, but especially for newly shaved skin. This product does contain benzocaine, a very mild anesthetic, but that wouldn't be necessary if this didn't contain so many irritating ingredients. And without sunscreen, this is a risky product to wear during the day if you take even one step outside.

MARY KAY MEN'S SKIN CARE

☹ **Cleansing Bar for All Skin Types** *($8.50 for 5.5 ounces)* is a standard bar cleanser with all the drying, irritating problems that can accompany this kind of product.

☺ **Enriched Shave Cream for All Skin Types** *($5.50 for 6.75 ounces)* is a standard shave cream similar to most of those available at the drugstore. This would work well for most skin types.

☹ **Cooling Toner for All Skin Types** *($8.50 for 6 ounces)* contains alcohol, balm mint, and peppermint, making it an irritation waiting to happen.

☹ **Conditioner with Sunscreen SPF 8 for Dry and Normal Skin** *($13 for 3.5 ounces)* doesn't contain the UVA-protecting ingredients of titanium dioxide, zinc oxide, or avobenzone. Also, with an SPF of only 8, it falls far below the standard SPF 15 set by the American Academy of Dermatology and the Skin Cancer Foundation, and is not recommended.

☹ **Oil Controller with Sunscreen SPF 8 for Combination and Oily Skin** *($13 for 3.5 ounces)* is similar to the Conditioner above, and is absolutely not recommended.

NEUTROGENA MEN

Given the wide range of men's products available in the mass market, you would think Neutrogena would have taken a critical look at the many alcohol- and menthol-laden men's products and gone in a different direction by offering truly irritant-free products. After all, Neutrogena is owned by Johnson & Johnson, the company that also owns the Aveeno line of skin-care products, which are based on being good for sensitive skin and that typically do not contain irritating skin-care ingredients. Alas, Neutrogena decided to maintain the status quo for men's products, and they've rolled out a copycat line that is packed with skin irritants. Even more disappointing, given how many great sunscreens are marketed by Johnson & Johnson (and Neutrogena), is the rather shocking *lack* of sun protection in their men's skin-care line. This omission is regrettable, as Neutrogena could have set an important precedent by including an effective sunscreen.

Precious few of these aggressively marketed products perform as well as they promise, chiefly because the key active ingredients are only on the skin for brief periods, meaning that their effectiveness against breakouts or in preventing ingrown hairs is, at best, limited. In terms of stopping razor irritation before it starts, that takes more than a protective shaving cream or gel, and it doesn't help when you add menthol, alcohol, and fragrance to the mix, because they can create a good deal of irritation all by themselves. There are some OK options here, but this is not the essential one-stop skin-care solution for men.

☺ **Skin Clearing Face Bar** *($2.99 for 3.5 ounces)* is a standard bar cleanser that contains fairly mild detergent cleansing agents. Interestingly, Neutrogena maintains that their claim for breakout and blackhead reduction does not apply to this product, which is absolutely true and I am a bit surprised they were so forthright about the limitations of a bar cleanser. This is one of the gentler bar cleansers available.

☹ **Skin Clearing Face Wash** *($5.99 for 5.1 ounces)* would have been a fairly gentle water-soluble cleanser if they had left out the menthol. If you're applying it over abraded skin (particularly from shaving), you're almost guaranteed an irritating or sensitizing reaction. This also contains 1.5% salicylic acid, which can be extremely helpful for unclogging pores, but its inclusion in a cleanser is fruitless because it's rinsed away before it has a chance to work.

☺ **Skin Clearing Shave Cream** *($4.49 for 5.1 ounces)* is a standard emollient shave cream that uses 1% salicylic acid, supposedly to minimize two common skin complaints—breakouts and ingrown hairs. However, putting this ingredient in a shave cream is pretty much as pointless as adding it to a cleanser. That's because salicylic acid needs to be left on the skin to have a positive impact, and what man wants to leave shaving cream on his skin longer than he has to?

☹ **Skin Clearing Astringent After Shave** *($5.49 for 3.4 ounces)* is a poor choice to use on freshly shaved skin because it contains alcohol and menthol. Neutrogena's Alcohol-Free Toner ($5.40 for 8.5 ounces) is not only cheaper but also a much better option for soothing skin after shaving, and you'll get over twice as much product. The claim that this standard, irritating astringent can minimize breakouts and ingrown hairs doesn't hold water.

☺ **Skin Clearing Targeted Acne Treatment** *($5.99 for 0.67 ounce)* is a fairly standard 2.5% benzoyl peroxide product that can kill acne-causing bacteria. The claims that it is clinically proven to work as well as a conventional 10% benzoyl peroxide formula without excessive redness, dryness, or irritation have no published or peer-reviewed information to back them up, so you would just have to take Neutrogena's word for it. This remains a standard blemish cream that can indeed disinfect the skin, but it may still cause dryness because bentonite (clay) is one of the main ingredients.

☺ **Razor Defense Shave Gel** *($4.49 for 7 ounces)* is preferred to the Skin Clearing Shave Cream above because it has a lighter texture and it does not contain any irritants, though it does contain a small amount of fragrance. This formula is almost identical to Aveeno's Therapeutic Shave Gel ($3.69 for 7 ounces), but Aveeno omits the fragrance.

☺ **Razor Defense Daily Face Scrub** *($5.99 for 4.2 ounces)* is a standard face scrub that uses polyethylene (ground-up plastic) as the abrasive agent. This contains fewer scrub particles than many other scrubs, and, except for the inclusion of menthyl lactate (a form of menthol), it is a fairly gentle option. Since most men get plenty of exfoliation from shaving, it is not necessary to use a scrub over the beard area. Even for the most gentle of formulas, that can still be overdoing things.

☺ **Razor Defense Face Lotion** *($5.99 for 2.5 ounces)* is a rather ordinary, lightweight moisturizer that would be an OK option for normal to slightly dry skin. The tiny amount of menthyl lactate (a form of menthol) can be an irritant. However, Neutrogena has lots of other moisturizers that have far better and gentler formulations than this one. Any of the Healthy Defense sunscreens or moisturizers in Neutrogena's regular product lineup would be far better for skin than this ho-hum product. That's especially true because this doesn't contain what would be the real defense sunscreen, meaning it shouldn't be worn during the day.

NIVEA FOR MEN

There are fundamental concerns about Nivea's line of men's skin-care products, the main one being the lack of a reliable SPF for sun protection (an absence that's just bizarre). The other issue is that all of the products contain fragrance—most are redolent with scent—yet the labels claim the products are fragrance-neutral. That might lead men to believe they are reducing their chances of irritation, when in fact they aren't, because fragrant ingredients over freshly shaved skin can cause red bumps and inflammation.

☺ **Moisture Rich Moisturizing Lotion SPF 4** *($5.99 for 1.7 ounces)*. With an SPF of 4, the claim that this product "helps protect skin from aging environmental influences; [and] helps skin regenerate…" is nonsense. The American Academy of Dermatology, Skin Cancer Foundation, American Cancer Society, and on and on, call for a minimum of SPF 15. Other than that, this is a standard, rather boring moisturizer with a matte finish. There are far more elegant moisturizers at the drugstore to consider than this one.

☺ **Double Action Face Wash** *($5.99 for 5.1 ounces)* is a standard, but very good, detergent-based, water-soluble cleanser that would work well for most skin types.

☺ **Exfoliating Face Scrub** *($5.99 for 2.5 ounces)* is just fine as a mechanical exfoliant, but given that shaving is enough exfoliation for any one face this would be an option only for areas of the face that men don't shave. It uses soft, synthetic polyethylene particles as the abrasive.

☹ **After Shave Balm, Mild** *($5.99 for 3.4 ounces)* lists alcohol as the second ingredient, so this is neither mild nor soothing, and it definitely won't hydrate the skin. Alcohol is drying and irritating for skin.

☺ **After Shave Balm, Sensitive** *($5.99 for 3.4 ounces)*. At least this version eliminated the alcohol, which makes it far better for all skin types. However, the "fragrance-neutral" claim is misleading, because while the product doesn't reek, it still contains fragrance, and that can be a skin irritant, especially over freshly shaved skin.

☺ **Moisture Rich Shaving Gel, Sensitive** *($2.89 for 7 ounces)*. Despite the "fragrance-neutral" claim, this product has a wafting fragrance. It's a good basic shave gel without other irritating ingredients, and that makes it an option, but given that Edge and Aveeno both have fragrance-free, nonirritating shave gels, why bother with this one?

☺ **Moisture Rich Shaving Gel, Refreshing** *($2.89 for 7 ounces)* is almost identical to the Sensitive version above, and the same comments apply.

OLD SPICE

☹ **Cool Contact Refreshment Towels** *($3.99 for 20 towels)* lists alcohol as the second ingredient, and there isn't one beneficial skin-care ingredient in this product.

☹ After Shave Lotion, Original *($6.29 for 6.37 ounces)* is just alcohol and fragrance. That's not skin care, it's eau de cologne, and this should not be used on the face.

PHYTOMEN BY PHYTOMER

☺ Softening Shaving Gel for Sensitive Skin *($12 for 5 ounces)* is a good, extremely standard, shave gel for most skin types. It does contain a tiny amount of triclosan, a topical disinfectant, and while that may help reduce some risk of infection, infection is not the real cause of red, irritated bumps on the skin after shaving.

☺ Soothing After Shave Balm with Hypericum *($15 for 1.6 ounces)* is an OK, though extremely standard, moisturizer for dry skin, and the price is unwarranted for what you're getting. Hypericum is the herb St. John's wort, and it has no real benefit for skin. In fact, recent studies indicate that St. John's wort can be photosensitizing if taken orally or applied topically in quantity (though it does takes a lot to have that effect). Most likely, manufacturers are hoping that by including St. John's wort in their product they will convey to the consumer that they can have some kind of tranquilizing effect on skin. St. John's wort can't do that from the outside in.

☹ Invigorating Body Splash *($35 for 6.76 ounces)*. Alcohol and fragrance may be considered invigorating, but by most real standards, they are just irritating and drying. This is nothing more than eau de cologne, which should not be applied over the face or body.

RALPH LAUREN POLO SPORT

☹ Face and Body Soap *($15 for 5.3 ounces)* is a standard soap that can be drying and irritating for skin.

☹ Scrub Face Wash *($15 for 2.5 ounces)* is a standard, detergent-based, water-soluble scrub that uses ground-up plastic (polyethylene) as the abrasive. That would be OK, but this product also contains eucalyptus, peppermint, grapefruit, and menthol, and that makes this just too irritating for words.

☹ After Shave *($40 for 4.2 ounces)* contains mostly alcohol and fragrance, which is just eau de cologne, not a skin-care product. This should not be applied to the face.

☺ $$$ Eye Fitness Complete Eye Therapy *($16.50 for 0.5 ounce)* is a rather ordinary moisturizer for normal to dry skin with tiny amounts of antioxidants and water-binding agents, which makes it unfit and incomplete for the eye area or any part of the face.

☹ Face Fitness AHA Moisture Formula, SPF 8 *($25 for 4.2 ounces)* doesn't contain the UVA-protecting ingredients of titanium dioxide, zinc oxide, or avobenzone. Also, with an SPF of only 8, it falls far below the standard SPF 15 set by the American Academy of Dermatology and the Skin Cancer Foundation, and is not recommended.

☹ Medicated Acne Gel *($12.50 for 0.5 ounce)* lists alcohol as the second ingredient, and also contains eucalyptus and peppermint, and none of that means this is medicated or that it can have any effect on acne. If anything, this will add irritation, redness, and dryness to blemish-prone skin.

SHISEIDO BASALA FOR MEN

☺ **Facial Cleansing Foam** *($17 for 3.8 ounces)* is similar to almost every other Shiseido skin cleanser, which makes this potentially too drying for most skin types.

☺ **Advanced Performance Emulsion** *($40 for 3.3 ounces)* is an exceptionally ordinary, Vaseline-based moisturizer that contains a minute amount of antioxidants. There is no reason to waste money or effort on this mundane formulation.

☺ **$$$ Advanced Performance Cream** *($40 for 1.7 ounces)* is similar to the Emulsion above only in cream form. The same basic comments apply.

☹ **After Shave Splash** *($30 for 5 ounces)* is almost entirely alcohol and fragrance, though it also includes camphor and menthol, making it an irritation waiting to happen. This should never be applied to the face, and especially over freshly shaved skin.

SKIN BRACER BY MENNEN

☹ **Original After Shave** *($5.99 for 7 ounces)*; **Pre-Electric Shave Lotion** *($3.59 for 5 ounces)*; and **After Shave, Cooling Blue** *($2.99 for 3.5 ounces)* all contain mostly alcohol and a good amount of menthol, making them too drying and irritating for all skin types.

TEND SKIN

☺ **Air Shave Gel** *($16 for 8 ounces)* is a good lightweight shave gel, though the price is steep given the rather basic, ordinary formulation.

☹ **Tend Skin Lotion** *($20 for 4 ounces)* contains mostly alcohol (that's the first ingredient), plus some aspirin. Aspirin is definitely a good anti-inflammatory agent, but the alcohol negates that benefit by causing dryness and irritation.

ZIRH MEN'S SKIN CARE

☹ **Clean** *($12.50 for 8 ounces)* contains lemon oil, menthol, and peppermint oil, and that isn't clean, it's just irritating, and makes this a problem for all skin types.

☹ **Scrub** *($12.50 for 4 ounces)* contains sodium lauryl sulfate as the main cleansing agent, which is too drying and potentially irritating for all skin types.

☺ **Prepare** *($14.50 for 1 ounce)* is a simple formulation of sunscreen (don't ask me why it contains that when this doesn't have an SPF) along with plant oil and some plant extracts. Basically, this is a waste of time and won't prepare the skin for anything.

☺ **Soothe** *($28.50 for 4 ounces)* is an exceptionally ordinary moisturizer for dry skin that is easily replaced by a wide range of less expensive and far better-formulated moisturizers from Cetaphil to Neutrogena.

☺ **Restore** *($22.50 for 1 ounce)* won't restore anything. It is just an OK moisturizer with a tiny amount of water-binding agents and antioxidant.

☺ **Correct** *($22.50 for 2 ounces)* contains several potentially irritating plant extracts. That's disappointing, because this version does contain some very good antioxidants.

☹ **Protect SPF 8** *($22.50 for 4 ounces)* doesn't contain the essential UVA-protecting ingredients of titanium dioxide, zinc oxide, or avobenzone. Also, with an SPF of only 8, it falls far below the standard SPF 15 set by the American Academy of Dermatology and the Skin Cancer Foundation, and is not recommended.

☺ **Block SPF 25** *($22.50 for 4 ounces)* is a very good, in-part titanium dioxide–based sunscreen in a rather standard moisturizing base. Still, there is little reason to consider this version over similarly formulated sunscreens at the drugstore.

☹ **Shield SPF 14** *($22.50 for 4 ounces)* has an SPF 14, which is strange, because that falls just shy of the standard SPF 15. While this does contain avobenzone, the other main ingredient is alcohol, and that makes this otherwise fine sunscreen a problem for skin. Your skin would be far better off with an Ombrelle product, which also contains avobenzone, available for half the price at the drugstore.

☺ **$$$ Facestick, Water Resistant Sunscreen SPF 28** *($14.50 for 0.31 ounce)* is a very good, titanium dioxide–based sunscreen in a standard moisturizing base. This can leave a white film on the skin. However, given its expense and the overall need to apply sunscreen liberally in order to get the full benefit, this basic formulation is easily replaced with Neutrogena's Sensitive Skin SPF 30 ($8.39 for 4 ounces) found at the drugstore.

☺ **Lip Guard SPF 19** *($12.50 for 1 ounce)* is a very good, in-part, titanium dioxide–based sunscreen in a rather standard, though emollient, moisturizing base.

☺ **Bronze** *($22.50 for 4 ounces)* contains dihydroxyacetone, the same ingredient all self-tanners use to affect the color of skin. This would work as well as any.

☺ **Cool** *($22.50 for 4 ounces)* is mostly water, aloe, plant extracts, fragrance, and preservatives. The plant extracts are a mix of irritants and anti-irritants, which cancels any benefit. Your skin would be far better off if you applied plain aloe vera that you can buy at the health food store.

☺ **Shave Gel** *($18.50 for 8 ounces)* is a very good, thick but rinsable, shave gel that is somewhat compromised by its intense fragrance.

☹ **Shave Cream** *($18.50 for 8 ounces)* is a standard shave cream that contains menthol, which makes it too potentially irritating for all skin types.

☺ **Clay Mask** *($14.50 for 4 ounces)* is a very standard clay mask that can absorb excess oil.

CHAPTER SIX

The Best Products Summary

NAVIGATING THE LISTS

The product lists that follow are derived from the individual reviews presented in Chapter Three and include all the products that received a happy face rating regardless of price. But, be sure to read the more-detailed product reviews in Chapter Three before making any final decisions about the best products for your individual skin-care needs and budget.

Over the years, many readers have complained that my list of "best" products is just too long, and some have asked me to reduce the number of recommendations to only the absolute favorites, or to create a top-ten list. Believe me, I understand the frustration of trying to make a decision based on such a huge range of good choices. When so many products are worthwhile (and are presented without the misleading, overhyped marketing sales pitches and claims that usually sway decisions), how do you decide what to use? For this edition, as you may already have noticed, I use more stringent criteria to determine what comprises a great product, which narrows the options substantially. Yet, even using the new and more strict criteria to assess the quality and effectiveness of a product, the lists are still daunting. There are just so many lines with so many good products to consider.

While the lists of great products are still lengthy, there is a new checkmark/happy face rating (✔☺), which denotes a **Paula's Pick** product. These products receive this rating because in some way they stand out from the crowd by excelling in a particular category. However, the products in these lists that don't qualify as a Paula's Pick still have merit and are a still a consideration as worthwhile options.

Keep in mind that not all product categories have a gold standard for excellence and the products within these categories cannot be rated as being better than any others. For example, cleansers, eye-makeup removers, scrubs, and self-tanners are rarely, if ever, uniquely formulated. Despite a company's claim to the contrary, there is absolutely nothing about these formulations that differs from one to another. Due to the repetitive, ordinary, and straightforward ingredients these products contain, and the glaring lack of any distinctive formulary considerations, there is no way to distinguish one from the other, and therefore, none of those receive a Paula's Pick rating. As long as these products are well-formulated and contain no problematic ingredients they receive a happy face rating. I apologize that I can't make these lists any shorter, but there are a lot of standard, though great, products in these categories. This is not the case, however, for moisturizers, toners, and specialty products such as topical disinfectants, skin-lightening products, sunscreens, foundations, concealers, pressed powders, blushes, pencils, eyeshadows, lipsticks, and mascaras. All of these products are held to specific and scrupulous standards because there are so many things that can create significant differences in quality. In these categories, Paula's Picks are denoted in the lists by the checkmark and happy face (✔☺) that precede the specific product.

As comprehensive as this book is, as it goes to press, there are new products being created and launched all the time, and there is ongoing publication and release of new research unveiling the promise of ingredients that may have increased benefits or risks for skin. To keep you up to date on all the information you need to take beautiful care of your skin and to find the best makeup products available, I offer my newsletter, *Cosmetics Counter Update* ($18.75 per year for 6 issues in the United States) and my free online Beauty Bulletin (sign up at www.cosmeticscop.com); I also add regularly to my Web site (www.cosmeticscop.com) so that you can stay informed and current on what works and what doesn't. These resources also provide more extensive explanations and clarification about specific topics than I can provide in this book. In the "Dear Paula" section of my newsletter, readers write to me about their particular concerns and needs, and I address those matters and make specific recommendations depending on the individual's situation and history. My newsletter and Beauty Bulletin also allow me to provide far more detail about a product's claims and its ingredients. In this book, the goal is to bring more general information together all in one place, giving consumers enough comparative information to find what works best for them among all the products with great, reliable formulations.

IT CAN GET CONFUSING

Do not automatically buy a company's group of products just because it is recommended for your skin type. Most cosmetics companies recommend skin-care routines for specific skin types. As helpful as this may seem, it often ends up being a waste of money and problematic for your skin-care concerns. I strongly suggest that you ignore their categories and the corresponding product names. A person with dry skin who automatically follows a cosmetics company's recommendations could end up using too many products that are too emollient or too heavy, which can cause skin cell buildup and result in dull, rough-feeling skin. Loading up dry skin with too many heavy products can also cause breakouts (particularly whiteheads). Conversely, someone with oily skin may be sold products that contain strong irritants that can cause skin to become dry, irritated, red, and flaky, while still leaving you with oily skin. Someone with blemish-prone skin often ends up purchasing products that are ineffective for that problem. Please consider each product individually for its quality and value to your skin, instead of by its placement within a series of products, its promotional ads or brochures, or the sales pitches you are likely to hear.

Product names are meant to be seductive, not factual. Please keep in mind that a cosmetics company's name for a product does not always correspond with my recommendations. Just because a product label says it "gets rid of wrinkles" or is "good for sensitive skin" or "is a firming and nourishing serum" doesn't mean the formulation itself supports that label or claim. The same is true for eye, chest, or throat creams; despite what the cosmetics industry wants you to believe, these products can be used anywhere on the face, and what counts is what skin type they are good for. There is absolutely nothing about any eye cream reviewed in this book that is unique for use in that area. What is most shocking is that eye creams are often identical to the face product, only you get less product and are charged more under the guise that it is "specially formulated." Of even greater concern is that many specialty eye and face products don't contain sunscreen. So, if you were being diligent about using a sunscreen on your face, but were only applying a designated eye or throat product that didn't contain sunscreen, you would be causing harm to the skin in those areas.

Additionally, you will find many selections in the following list of recommended products with names that sound like they should be in the dry-skin group, but that I have included in the oily-skin group, and vice versa. That's because what counts is how the product is formulated, not what the companies want you to believe about their products.

Putting together the best routine for your skin type and makeup needs is the goal. The sequence of applying products for a particular skin-care regime for a wide range of skin types is described at length in my book *The Beauty Bible*. As a general rule, the following sequence is a safe guideline, depending on the products your skin needs: cleanser; scrub; eye-makeup remover (if needed); toner; AHA, BHA, topical disinfectant; topical retinoid (retinoids cannot be used with benzoyl peroxide), azelaic acid, Differin, MetroGel, or MetroCream; skin-lightening product; and during the day sunscreen and at night a moisturizer. Sunscreen is always the last item you apply during the day because you must never dilute a sunscreen.

BEST CLEANSERS

The standard of excellence for the cleanser category of products, for almost all skin types (except dry to very dry skin), is that the cleanser be water-soluble, gentle, and able to thoroughly clean skin without leaving it feeling dry or greasy. It also must be free of harsh, irritating, or sensitizing ingredients. I never recommend bar soap because the ingredients that keep bar soap in a bar form can clog pores, and the cleansing agents in them are almost always drying. Emollient wipe-off cleansers may be the only types of cleansers that don't cause dry, sensitive skin to become drier, and I therefore recommend them for that skin type.

I do not specify a group of "medicated" or "anti-acne" cleansers supposedly designed for very oily or blemish-prone skin, for two reasons. First, cleansers identified as being good for those skin types generally contain ingredients that are too harsh or irritating, and that is not helpful for any skin type. Cleansing needs to be gentle and thorough, not harsh and drying. Second, cleansers for blemish-prone skin often contain topical disinfectants such as benzoyl peroxide, but in a cleanser, the effective ingredient, in this case benzoyl peroxide, will be rinsed down the drain before it has much chance to affect skin.

You will also notice that there are no Paula's Picks in the cleanser category. Cleansers, regardless of their price tag or claims of natural, gentle, moisturizing, hydrating, or soothing action, have far more in common than they do differences. A well-formulated cleanser is noted more by what it doesn't contain (i.e., harsh cleansing agents and irritating ingredients) than by what it does contain. In fact, the formulations of cleansers, whether for normal to oily skin or for normal to dry skin, are virtually identical. So, spending a lot of money on cleansers does not in any way, shape, or form mean you are getting a better product.

BEST WATER-SOLUBLE CLEANSERS FOR NORMAL TO OILY/COMBINATION AND/OR BLEMISH-PRONE SKIN TYPES: **Aesop** Amazing Face Cleanser ($35 for 6.9 ounces) and Fabulous Face Cleanser ($35 for 6.9 ounces); **Ahava** Deep Cleanser for All Skin Types ($20 for 3.4 ounces); **Almay** Milk Plus Foaming Facial Gel 2-in-1 Cleanser and Toner Normal to Oily Skin ($6.93 for 6.7 ounces); **Almay** Kinetin Skin Optimizing Cleanser ($8.50 for 5 ounces); **Aloette** Foaming Citrus Cleanser ($13.50 for 6 ounces); **Aloette AloePure** Simply Clear Clarifying Face Wash ($13 for 4 ounces); **Alpha Hydrox** Facial Moisturizing Cleanser ($5.99 for 5 ounces) and Foaming Face Wash for All Skin Types ($5.57 for 6 ounces); **Arbonne** Bio-Matte Oil-Free Cleanser ($16.50 for 2 ounces); **Aveda** Purifying Gel Cleanser ($17 for 5.5 ounces); **Aveeno** Skin Clarifying Cleanser ($7.99 for 6.7 ounces); **Avon** Anew Perfect Cleanser ($11 for 5.1 ounces) and Pore-Fection Porefection Cleanser ($7 for 6.7 ounces); **Avon beComing** Cool Current Purifying Gel Cleanser ($12 for 6.8 ounces); **B. Kamins** Vegetable Skin Cleanser ($32 for 8 ounces); **Basis** Cleaner Clean Face Wash ($4.99 for 6 ounces) and Comfortably Clean Face Wash ($4.99 for 6 ounces); **Bath & Body Works** Completely Clean Foaming Face Wash ($8 for 6 ounces) and Oil-Control Cleanser ($8 for 5.25 ounces); **BeautiControl** All Clear Skin Wash ($12 for 6 ounces), Gentle Wash ($14 for 5.7 ounces) and Purifying Cleansing Gel ($12 for 8 ounces); **Beauty Without Cruelty** 3% Alpha Hydroxy Facial Cleanser Normal/Oily Skin Types ($7.49 for 8.5 ounces); **Bioelements** Decongestant Cleanser ($21.50 for 6 ounces); **BioMedic** Purifying Cleanser ($26.95 for 6 ounces); **Biore** Foaming Cleanser ($5.99 for 5 ounces); **BioTherm** Biopur Pure Cleansing Gel ($15.50 for 5 ounces), Biosensitive Self-Foaming Gentle Cleanser ($19 for 5 ounces), Biosource Foaming Cleansing Gel ($15.50 for 5 ounces), and Biosource Enriched Cleansing Foam, for Dry Skin ($15 for 5 ounces); **Black Opal** Oil Free Cleansing Gel ($5.95 for 6 ounces); **Bobbi Brown** Purifying Gel Cleanser ($22 for 4.2 ounces); **The Body Shop** Skin Defensives Cleansing Face Wash ($15 for 3.4 ounces), Tea Tree Oil Facial Wash ($10 for 8.4 ounces), and Seaweed Purifying Facial Wash for Normal to Oily Skin ($10 for 3.4 ounces); **CamoCare** Camomile Light Foaming Cleanser ($9.95 for 4 ounces); **Caudalie** Instant Foaming Cleanser ($25 for 5 ounces); **Cellex-C** Betaplex Gentle Foaming Cleanser ($29 for 6 ounces);

Cetaphil Cetaphil Daily Facial Cleanser for Normal to Oily Skin ($5.99 for 8 ounces); **Chanel** Gel Purete Foaming Gel Face Wash ($30 for 5 ounces); **Christian Dior** iOd Clear Aqua Foam ($20 for 5.1 ounces) and Purifying Wash-Off Cleansing Foam ($22.50 for 6.8 ounces); **Clarins** Gentle Foaming Cleanser for All Skin Types ($22 for 4.4 ounces); **Cle de Peau Beaute** Gentle Cleansing Foam (Mousse Nettoyante Tendre) ($50 for 3.3 ounces); **Clean & Clear by Johnson & Johnson** Foaming Facial Cleanser for Sensitive Skin ($3.79 for 8 ounces), Foaming Facial Cleanser ($3.49 for 8 ounces), and Oil Free Daily Pore Cleanser ($3.99 for 5.5 ounces); **Clientele** Face Wash ($25 for 8 ounces), Blemish Free Face Wash ($35 for 8 ounces), Time Therapy Alpha Hydroxy Face Wash for Normal/Dry, Sensitive Skin ($25 for 4 ounces), and Elastology Gentle Soy Antioxidant Wash ($35 for 8 ounces); **Darphin** Purifying Foam Gel ($40 for 4.2 ounces); **DHC** Facial Wash for Oilier Skin ($18 for 6.7 ounces; **Doctor's Dermatologic Formula** Earthy Herbal Foaming Cleanser ($20 for 6.7 ounces), Laid Back Lavender Foaming Cleanser ($20 for 6.7 ounces), Pick-Me-Up Pink Grapefruit Foaming Cleanser ($20 for 6.7 ounces), Non-Drying Gentle Cleanser ($25 for 8.45 ounces), Sensitive Skin Cleansing Gel ($27.50 for 8.45 ounces), and Wash off Cleanser ($24 for 8.45 ounces); **Dr. Dennis Gross, M.D. Skin Care** All-in-One Facial Cleanser with Toner ($25 for 8 ounces); **Dr. Mary Lupo Skin Care System** Gentle Purifying Cleanser ($22 for 7 ounces); **Elizabeth Grant** Hydrating Cleanser with Torricelumn ($15.99 for 4 ounces); **Epicuren** Herbal Cleanser ($48 for 4 ounces) and Gelle Cleanser ($17 for 4 ounces); **Estee Lauder** Perfectly Clean Foaming Lotion Cleanser, Normal/Dry and Dry Skin ($16.50 for 4.2 ounces), Perfectly Clean Foaming Gel Cleanser, Normal/Oily and Oily Skin ($16.50 for 4.2 ounces), and WhiteLight Brightening Cleansing Foam ($26 for 4.2 ounces); **Eucerin** Gentle Hydrating Cleanser ($7.99 for 8 ounces); **Exuviance** Purifying Cleansing Gel ($19 for 8 ounces); **FACE Stockholm** Foaming Facial Cleanser Normal to Oily Skin ($18 for 4 ounces); **Fashion Fair** Botanical Cleansing Gel ($12.50 for 6.7 ounces); **Flori Roberts** My Everything Treatment Foaming Gel Cleanser ($12 for 6 ounces); **Givenchy** Regulating Cleansing Gel, Purifying Care for Radiant Skin Combination and Oily Skin ($22 for 4.5 ounces); **Glymed Plus** Gentle Facial Wash ($29 for 8 ounces); **H2O+ Skin Care** Oil Control Cleansing Mousse ($17.50 for 7.5 ounces) and Waterwhite Brightening Cleansing Mousse ($25 for 7.5 ounces); **Helena Rubinstein** Fresh Foaming Gel Gentle Water Dissolve Cleanser ($21.50 for 6.7 ounces); **Hydron** Oil Control Facial Cleansing Gel ($15.75 for 4 ounces); **Iman** Liquid Assets Gentle Cleansing Lotion ($14.50 for 4 ounces); **Jafra** Cleansing Gel for Oily Skin ($14 for 4.2 ounces); **Jan Marini Skin Research** C-Esta Cleansing Gel ($25 for 6 ounces) and Bioglycolic BioClean Cleanser ($25 for 8 ounces); **Jason Natural** Super-C Cleanser Gentle Face Wash ($10 for 6 ounces); **Joey New York** Calm & Correct Gentle Soothing Cleanser ($24 for 8 ounces); **Jurlique International** Tea Tree and Lavender Foaming Facial Cleanser ($33 for 6.8 ounces); **Kiehl's** Gentle Foaming Facial Cleanser for Dry to Normal Skin Types ($14.50 for 8 ounces), Rare-Earth Oatmeal Milk Facial Cleanser #1 (Mild) ($18.50 for 8 ounces), and Rare-Earth

Oatmeal Milk Facial Cleanser #2 (Medium Strength) ($18.50 for 8 ounces); **L'Oreal** HydraFresh Deep Cleanser Foaming Gel for Normal to Oily Skin ($4.99 for 6.5 ounces), HydraFresh Cleanser Foaming Cream for Normal to Dry Skin ($4.99 for 6.5 ounces), Shine Control Foaming Face Wash with Pro-Vitamin B5 ($5 for 6 ounces), and RevitaClean Gentle Foaming Cleanser ($5 for 6 ounces); **La Mer** The Cleansing Gel ($65 for 6.7 ounces); **La Roche-Posay** Effaclar Purifying Foaming Gel ($14.95 for 5 ounces) and Toleriane Foaming Cleanser ($12.95 for 3.38 ounces); **Lancaster** Aquamilk Fresh Foaming Cleanser ($26 for 13.5 ounces) and Energizing Cleansing Foam ($22 for 6.7 ounces); **Lancome** Ablutia Fraicheur Purifying Foam Cleanser ($21.50 for 6.4 ounces), Clarifiance Oil-Free Gel Cleanser ($21.50 for 6.8 ounces), Gel Controle ($19.50 for 4.2 ounces), Mousse Controle ($19.50 for 4.2 ounces), Gel Clarte ($19.50 for 4.2 ounces), Mousse Clarte ($25 for 6.8 ounces), and Mousse Confort ($19.50 for 4.2 ounces); **Laura Mercier** One Step Cleanser ($35 for 8 ounces); **Lorac** Oil-Free Face Wash ($17 for 8 ounces); **Marcelle** Aquarelle Oil-Free Purifying Cleansing Gel for Oily Skin ($11.95 for 170 ml) and Gentle Foaming Wash All Skin Types ($10.95 for 170 ml); **Marilyn Miglin** Skin Vitality Cleanser ($24 for 7 ounces) and Estrosoy Foaming Facial Cleanser with Collagen ($20 for 6.75 ounces); **Merle Norman** Luxiva Foaming Cleanser for Dry Skin ($18 for 4 ounces); **Moisturel** Sensitive Skin Cleanser ($8.49 for 8.75 ounces); **Morgen Schick** Marine Wash ($19.95 for 4 ounces); **Murad** Moisture Rich Skin Cleanser ($22 for 6 ounces) and Refreshing Skin Cleanser ($22 for 6 ounces); **Natura Bisse** China Clay Cleanser Purifying and Cleansing Paste ($37 for 4.2 ounces), Facial Cleansing Gel Foaming Cleanser ($28 for 7 ounces), and Sensitive Cleansing Cream for All Skin Types ($34 for 6.5 ounces); **Neostrata** NeoCeuticals Clarifying Facial Cleanser ($19.50 for 6 ounces); **Neutrogena** Fresh Foaming Cleanser Soap-Free Cleanser for Combination Skin ($5.49 for 5.5 ounces); **Neways Skin Care** Extra Gentle Cleanser ($8.70 for 4 ounces); **Nivea Visage** Foaming Facial Cleanser Deep-Cleansing Formula ($5.49 for 6 ounces) and Refreshing Cleansing Gel, Normal & Combination Skin ($5.99 for 6.8 ounces); **Noevir** Clear Control Clean Wash ($14 for 2.6 ounces); **Obagi Nu-Derm** Foaming Gel Cleanser ($29 for 6.7 ounces) and Nu-Derm Gentle Cleanser ($29 for 6.7 ounces); **Olay** Foaming Face Wash ($3.99 for 6.78 ounces) and Sensitive Skin Foaming Face Wash ($3.99 for 6.78 ounces); **Ole Henriksen Skin Care** On the Go Exhilarating Cleanser ($28 for 12 ounces); **Orlane** B21 Purifying Balancing Gel ($45 for 6.8 ounces); **Osmotics** Calming Cleansing Milk for Sensitive Skin ($27 for 6 ounces) and Hydrating Cleanser for Normal to Dry Skin ($27 for 6 ounces); **Parthena** 2 in 1 Cucumber Cleanser ($12 for 4 ounces); **Paula's Choice** One Step Face Cleanser, Normal to Oily/Combination Skin ($11.95 for 8 ounces); **Peter Thomas Roth** Chamomile Cleansing Lotion ($30 for 8 ounces), Gentle Cleansing Lotion ($30 for 8 ounces), Foaming Face Wash ($30 for 8 ounces), Extra Strength Cleansing Gel Oil-Free for Oily, Combination or Problem Skin ($30 for 8 ounces), Sensitive Skin Cleansing Gel ($30 for 8 ounces), and Combination Skin Cleansing Gel ($30 for 8 ounces), and Anti Aging Cleansing Gel ($30 for 8 ounces);

Pevonia Botanica RS2 Gentle Cleanser ($26 for 6.8 ounces); **Pharmagel** Hydra Cleanse Foaming Gel ($14.95 for 8 ounces); **Physicians Formula** Deep Pore Cleansing Gel for Normal to Oily Skin ($6.95 for 8 ounces); **Phytomer** Purifying Cleansing Gel ($26 for 5 ounces); **Pond's** Foaming Cleanser & Toner in One Normal to Oily Skin ($4.69 for 4 ounces); **Prada Beauty** Purifying Gel/Face ($50 for 3.4 ounces); **Prescriptives** All Clean Fresh Foaming Cleanser ($21 for 6.7 ounces); **Principal Secret** Advanced Gentle 4-in-1 Cleanser ($19 for 6 ounces) and Gentle Deep Cleanser ($17.25 for 6 ounces); **Purpose** Gentle Cleansing Wash ($5.29 for 6 ounces) and Moisturizing Foaming Cleanser ($5.49 for 6 ounces); **Re Vive** Cleanser Agressif for Normal to Oily ($65 for 16 ounces) and Cleanser Gentil for Normal to Dry ($65 for 16 ounces); **Rejuvenique** Purifying Cleanser ($18.50 for 4 ounces); **Reversa** 3 in 1 Mild Gel Cleanser ($17.99 for 130 ml); **Revlon** Vitamin C Reviving Cleanser ($7.69 for 6.6 ounces); **RoC** Deep Action Facial Wash with Beta Hydroxy ($6.99 for 5.07 ounces) and Protient Lift Daily Firming Cleanser ($7.79 for 5 ounces); **Sea Breeze** Foaming Face Wash for Sensitive Skin ($3.99 for 6 ounces); **Sense Usana** Gentle Daily Cleanser ($20 for 6 ounces); **Sephora** Cleansing Gel for Face & Eyes ($6 for 3.3 ounces); **Serious Skin Care** C-Clean Vitamin C Cleanser ($19.95 for 4 ounces); **Shaklee** Purifying Cleansing Gel ($16.50 for 6 ounces); **Shiseido** Cleansing Water ($23 for 4.2 ounces); **Shu Uemura** Cleansing Water ($30 for 8.4 ounces); **SkinCeuticals** Simply Clean ($24 for 8 ounces); **Sothys Paris** Purifying Foaming Gel ($23 for 4.2 ounces); **St. Ives** Foaming Facial Apricot Cleanser ($3.99 for 10 ounces); **Suave** Balancing Facial Cleansing Gel ($2.75 for 8 ounces) and Foaming Face Wash ($2.75 for 8 ounces); **T. Le Clerc** Purifying Gel Cleanser ($25 for 4.16 ounces); **Thalgo** Silky Cleansing Cream ($30 for 5.07 ounces) and Thalgodermyl Cleansing Gel ($24 for 1.7 ounces); **Urban Decay** Zen Cleanse 2-in-1 Cleanser and Toner ($16 for 5 ounces); **Vichy** Normaderm Express Cleansing Gel for Acne Prone Skin ($9.99 for 150 ml); **Yon-Ka Paris** Gel Nettoyant Cleansing Gel ($34 for 6.7 ounces); **Z. Bigatti** Re-Storation Champagne Gel Cleanser ($65 for 4 ounces); **Zia** Fresh Cleansing Gel for All Skin Types ($15.50 for 8 ounces).

BEST CLEANSERS FOR NORMAL TO DRY OR VERY DRY SKIN: **Aesop** Purifying Facial Cream Cleanser ($35 for 6.9 ounces); **Ahava** Advanced Cleansing Milk for Normal to Dry Skin ($24 for 8.5 ounces); **Almay** Milk Plus Rinse-Off Facial Cream 2-in-1 Cleanser and Toner for Normal to Dry Skin ($6.93 for 6.7 ounces); **Aloette** Essential Cleansing Oil ($16 for 2 ounces); **Annemarie Borlind** LL Bi Aktiv Regeneration LL Cleansing Milk ($33.75 for 5.07 ounces), Rose Cleansing Milk ($24 for 5.07 ounces), Absolute Cleanser ($46.50 for 5.07 ounces), and Peach Skin Cleansing Cream ($16.75 for 3.4 ounces); **Arbonne** Cleansing Cream ($16 for 2 ounces) and Cleansing Lotion ($15 for 3.25 ounces); **Artistry by Amway** Moisture Rich Vitalizing Cleansing Creme for Normal to Dry Skin ($17.20 for 4.4 ounces) and Delicate Care Cleanser for Sensitive Skin Types ($17.20 for 4.2 ounces); **Aveda** Purifying Cream Cleanser ($17 for 5.5 ounces); **Aveeno** Skin Replenishing Cleansing Lotion ($7.99 for 6.7 ounces); **Avon** Anew Ultra Cream

Cleanser ($14 for 5.1 ounces); **Avon beComing** All Gone Cleansing Makeup Remover ($12 for 3.4 ounces); **B. Kamins** Vitamin Face Cleanser ($42 for 8 ounces); **Bath & Body Works** Hydrating Facial Cleanser ($8 for 6 ounces); **BeautiControl** Chamomile Balancing Cleansing Lotion for Combination Skin ($14 for 8 ounces) and Mild Rosemary Cleansing Fluide for Dry Skin ($14 for 8 ounces); **Beauty Without Cruelty** Extra Gentle Facial Cleansing Milk ($9.95 for 8.5 ounces); **BeneFit** All Types Skin Wash ($16 for 4 ounces); **Bioelements** Moisture Positive Cleanser ($21.50 for 6 ounces); **BioTherm** Biosensitive High Tolerance Fluid Cleansing Milk ($20 for 5 ounces), Biosource Normal to Combination Skin Biosource Invigorating Cleansing Milk ($15.50 for 8 ounces), and Biosource Dry Skin Biosource Softening Cleansing Milk ($15.50 for 5 ounces); **BlissLabs** Fully Loaded Cleansing Milk for Dry Skin ($23 for 8.5 ounces) and Quiet Type Cleansing Milk for Sensitive Skin ($23 for 8.5 ounces); **Bobbi Brown** One-Step Cleanser and Long-Wear Makeup Remover ($22 for 3.4 ounces), Rich Cream Cleanser ($22 for 4.2 ounces), and Extra Balm Rinse ($50 for 6.8 ounces); **The Body Shop** Soy & Calendula Gentle Cleanser, for Dry/Sensitive Skin ($10 for 6.7 ounces), Vitamin C Hydrating Cleanser ($14 for 8 ounces), and Vitamin E Cream Cleanser ($10 for 6.8 ounces); **Borghese** Fango Effetto Immediato Spa Comforting Cleanser ($29.50 for 8.4 ounces); **Calvin Klein** Balancing Milk Cleanser ($20 for 6 ounces); **CamoCare** Camomile Moisturizing Cleanser ($9.95 for 4 ounces); **Cellex-C** Betaplex Gentle Cleansing Milk ($29 for 6 ounces); **Cetaphil** Gentle Skin Cleanser ($8.99 for 16 ounces); **Chantecaille** Flower Infused Cleansing Milk ($43 for 3.4 ounces); **Christian Dior** Prestige Cleansing Cream ($55 for 6.9 ounces), Cleansing Milk for Face and Eyes ($22.50 for 6.8 ounces), and Softening Wash-Off Cleansing Creme ($22.50 for 6.8 ounces); **Clarins** One-Step Facial Cleanser with Orange Extract ($26 for 6.8 ounces); **Clinique** Comforting Cream Cleanser ($16.50 for 5 ounces); **Club Monaco** Face Lotion Wash ($14 for 6.8 ounces) and Face Soothing Wash ($17 for 6.8 ounces); **Decleor** Nutrivital Cleansing Cream ($29 for 8.4 ounces), Velvet Cleansing Milk, with Plant Extracts ($27.50 for 8.4 ounces), and Gentle Cleansing Wash with Plant Extracts ($33.50 for 8.4 ounces); **Dermalogica** Essential Cleansing Solution ($37.50 for 16 ounces); **Diane Young** Age Lift Hydrating Cleansing Milk ($28.50 for 2.5 ounces); **DHC** Deep Cleansing Oil ($22 for 6.7 ounces) and Mild Cleansing Cream for Drier Skin ($14 for 4.9 ounces); **Dr. Jeannette Graf, M.D.** Retinol Facial Cleanser ($17.50 for 4 ounces); **Ella Bache** Cleansing Milk, for Dry and Sensitive Skin ($26 for 6.7 ounces) and Rinse-Off Cleansing Cream for Sensitive Skin ($21 for 2.50 ounces); **Ellen Lange Skin Care** Daily Maintenance Cleanser ($24 for 6 ounces); **Elizabeth Arden** Millennium Hydrating Cleanser ($27 for 4.4 ounces), Ceramide Purifying Cream Cleanser ($21 for 4.2 ounces), and Hydra-Gentle Cream Cleanser ($15 for 5 ounces); **Elizabeth Grant** Gentle Cleansing Milk ($16.99 for 4 ounces) and Torricelumn Pur Cleanser ($34.99 for 4 ounces); **Epicuren** Apricot Cream Cleanser ($31 for 4 ounces); **Estee Lauder** Soft Clean Milky Lotion Cleanser ($16.50 for 6.7 ounces), Tender Creme Cleanser ($26 for 8 ounces), Re-Nutriv Intensive Hydrating Cream Cleanser ($35 for

4.2 ounces), and Verite Light Lotion Cleanser ($22.50 for 6.7 ounces); **Exuviance** Gentle Cleansing Creme, Sensitive Formula ($19 for 6.8 ounces); **FACE Stockholm** Aloe Vera Cleansing Cream ($18 for 4 ounces) and Aloe Vera Cleansing Lotion ($18 for 4 ounces); **Fashion Fair** Cleansing Creme with Aloe Vera ($14.25 for 4 ounces) and Deep Cleansing Lotion Balanced for All Skin Types ($15 for 8 ounces); **Gatineau** Soothing Cleanser ($28 for 13.5 ounces); **Glymed Plus** Cell Science High Purification Skin Cleanser ($29 for 8 ounces); **Guerlain** Issima Flower Cleansing Cream ($42 for 6.8 ounces); **Guinot** Moisture Rich Cleansing Milk ($25 for 6.7 ounces), Wash-Off Cleansing Cream ($28.50 for 5 ounces), and Refreshing Cleansing Milk ($25 for 6.7 ounces); **H2O+ Skin Care** Moisturizing Marine Cleansing Cream ($21 for 8 ounces) and Sea Mineral Cleanser ($14.50 for 5.7 ounces); **Helena Rubinstein** Fresh Cleansing Fluid Express Face and Eye Cleanser ($23.50 for 6.7 ounces); **Hydron** Best Defense Gentle Cleansing Creme ($16.50 for 6 ounces); **Jafra** Cleansing Lotion for Dry to Normal Skin ($12.50 for 8.4 ounces), Cleansing Lotion for Normal to Oily Skin ($4 for 8.4 ounces), and Cleansing Cream for Dry Skin ($14 for 4.2 ounces); **Jason Natural** Fresh Face Rehydrating Cleanser ($9 for 8 ounces); **Karin Herzog Skin Care** Cleansing Milk ($30 for 7.05 ounces); **Kiehl's** Ultra Moisturizing Cleansing Cream ($17.50 for 8 ounces) and Washable Cleansing Milk a Moisturizing Cleanser for Dry or Sensitive Skin ($14.50 for 8 ounces); **Kiss My Face** Gentle Face Cleanser for Normal to Dry ($10 for 4 ounces); **L'Occitane** Extra Gentle Cleansing Milk ($18 for 8.4 ounces); **L'Oreal** RevitaClean Cold Cream for Dry or Maturing Skin ($5.29 for 5 ounces); **La Mer** The Cleansing Lotion ($65 for 6.7 ounces); **La Prairie** Purifying Creme Cleanser ($60 for 6.8 ounces); **La Roche-Posay** Toleriane Dermo-Cleanser ($12.95 for 6.76 ounces); **Lancaster** Soft Milk Cleanser ($26 for 13.5 ounces) and Suractif Cleansing Treatment ($35 for 13.5 ounces); **Lancome** Galatee Comfort Milky Creme Cleanser ($37.50 for 13.5 ounces); **Linda Sy** Oil-Free Cleansing Lotion ($11 for 8 ounces); **M.A.C.** Cold Cream Cleanser ($15 for 4 ounces), Everyday Lotion Cleanser ($15 for 5 ounces), and Super Cleansing Oil ($15 for 5.1 ounces); **Marcelle** Cleansing Milk for Dry to Normal Skin ($11.25 for 240 ml) and Hydractive Water Rinseable Cleansing Lotion for Dehydrated/Normal to Dry Skin ($11.95 for 180 ml); **Mario Badescu** Seaweed Cleansing Soap ($12 for 8 ounces), Orange Cleansing Soap ($12 for 8 ounces), and Keratoplast Cream Soap ($10 for 8 ounces); **Mary Kay** Deep Cleanser Formula 3 ($10 for 6.5 ounces); **M.D. Formulations** Facial Cleanser Basic ($18 for 8 ounces); **Merle Norman** Cleansing Lotion ($16.50 for 14 ounces), Cleansing Cream ($12.50 for 7.5 ounces), and Luxiva Collagen Cleanser ($18.50 for 6 ounces); **Natura Bisse** Dry Skin Milk Cleanser ($24 for 6.5 ounces); **Neutrogena** Extra Gentle Cleanser ($5.49 for 6.7 ounces) and Non-Drying Cleanser Lotion ($6 for 5.5 ounces); **Neways Skin Care** TLC/Facial Cleansing Lotion ($6.95 for 4 ounces) and Milky Cleanser ($16.15 for 4.2 ounces); **Nu Skin** Creamy Cleansing Lotion for Normal to Dry Skin ($15 for 5 ounces); **Olay** Facial Cleansing Lotion ($3.99 for 6.78 ounces); **Orlane** B21 Vivifying Cleansing Care ($42.50 for 6.8 ounces), B21 Oligo Vit-A-Min, Vitalizing Cleanser for

Dry or Sensitive Skin Types ($35 for 8.4 ounces), and Claircilane Hydro Clarifying Cleanser ($35 for 6.8 ounces); **Paula's Choice** One Step Face Cleanser, Normal to Dry Skin ($11.95 for 8 ounces) and Skin Recovery Cleanser, Normal to Very Dry Skin ($11.95 for 8.5 ounces); **Peter Thomas Roth** Silky Cleansing Cream ($30 for 8 ounces); **Pevonia Botanica** Sensitive Skin Cleanser ($23 for 6.8 ounces); **pHisoDerm** Deep Cleaning Cleanser, Normal to Dry Skin ($3.99 for 8 ounces), Deep Cleaning Cleanser, Normal to Oily Skin ($3.99 for 8 ounces), and Deep Cleaning Cleanser, Sensitive Skin ($3.99 for 8 ounces); **Phytomer** Gentle Cleansing Milk ($25 for 6.8 ounces), Neutralizing Cleanser ($34 for 6.8 ounces), and Whitening Cleansing Milk ($24 for 6.8 ounces); **Pola Pelenna** Pure Skin Cleanser ($22 for 3.5 ounces); **Pond's** Cleansing Lotion & Moisturizer in One Normal to Dry Skin ($3.99 for 4 ounces); **RoC** Retinol Actif Pur Anti-Wrinkle Cleansing Lotion ($8.99 for 4.2 ounces), Endrial Dermo Calming Cleanser ($14.50 for 200 ml), and Cleansing Milk Dry Skin, Extra Gentle ($14.50 for 200 ml); **Shaklee** Hydrating Cleansing Lotion ($18.15 for 6 ounces); **Shiseido** Benefiance Creamy Cleansing Emulsion ($29.50 for 6.7 ounces), Make Up Cleansing Gel ($23 for 4.4 ounces), and Cleansing Foam ($23 for 4.9 ounces); **Sothys Paris** Lait Demaquillant Douceur Softening Beauty Milk for Dry Skin ($21 for 6.7 ounces); **St. Ives** Cream Cleanser with Soothing Chamomile ($2.79 for 6 ounces); **T. Le Clerc** Gentle Cleansing Milk ($27.50 for 6.7 ounces); **Ultima II** CHR Cream Cleanser ($18.50 for 4 ounces) and Ultima II Going Going Gone Makeup Remover ($13.50 for 4 ounces); **Vichy** Purete Thermale Demaquillant Integral One-Step Cleanser for Face and Eyes 3-in-1 ($15.50 for 200 ml), Purete Thermale Detoxifying Cleansing Milk for Normal & Combination Skin ($15.95 for 200 ml), and Purete Thermale Detoxifying Cleansing Milk for Dry & Sensitive Skin ($15.95 for 200 ml); **Yon-Ka Paris** Lait Nettoyant Cleansing Milk ($34 for 6.8 ounces); **Yves St. Laurent** Soothing Creme Cleanser ($27.50 for 5 ounces) and Instant Cleansing Milk ($27.50 for 6.6 ounces); **Zia** Moisturizing Cleanser for Normal to Dry Skin ($15.50 for 8 ounces).

BEST SCRUBS

Exfoliating the skin (getting rid of unwanted, dead, or built-up layers of sun-damaged skin cells and improving skin-cell turnover) can be beneficial for almost all skin types, and especially those with sun-damaged skin or a tendency toward breakouts or clogged pores, but even dry-skin types can benefit for many reasons. Despite the fact that most beauty experts, as well as dermatologists and plastic surgeons, agree that exfoliating the skin is a wonderful way to take care of both oily and dry skin, how to exfoliate remains a bone of contention.

During most of the '70s and '80s, the only choices for exfoliation were topical, mechanical scrubs with ingredients such as honey and almond pits, cleansers with scrub particles, facial masks, and irritating toners. Most of these options took a toll on the face, and irritation or dry patches of skin with redness were typical problems. That has definitely changed and there are far gentler scrubs and masks than ever before that still have effective exfoliating properties. AHAs and BHA (reviewed in the next section) add another level of improved exfoliation for skin.

For normal to oily skin, a scrub is rated by how gently and effectively it cleans and exfoliates the skin without being irritating or harsh. For normal to dry skin, a scrub is rated by how gentle and emollient it is, while maintaining exfoliating properties. While there are some very effective topical scrubs, there are none that rate a Paula's Pick. Scrub formulations are exceedingly mundane, with repetitive formulations that have no distinctive considerations setting one apart from another. Almond pits, ground-up rock, jojoba beads, and synthetic scrub particles do not function differently enough to recommend one over the other as being a better choice for skin. **Note:** What was true in the first edition of this book is still true today: I feel strongly that Cetaphil Gentle Skin Cleanser ($9 for 16 ounces) mixed with baking soda, or just plain baking soda by itself, is a great topical scrub for most skin types.

BEST SCRUBS FOR NORMAL TO OILY/COMBINATION AND/OR BLEMISH-PRONE SKIN: **Aloette** Gentle Citrus Scrub ($14 for 4 ounces); **Astara** Daily Refining Scrub ($28 for 4 ounces); **The Body Shop** Peachy Clean Exfoliating Wash ($10 for 3.4 ounces); **Aveeno** Skin Brightening Daily Scrub ($6.99 for 5 ounces); **bare escentuals Cush** Turning Tide Fresh Face Exfoliator ($36 for 2.3 ounces); **BeautiControl** Balancing Scrub for Combination Skin ($14.50 for 3 ounces) and Renewing Scrub/Masque ($14 for 3 ounces); **Biore** Mild Daily Cleansing Scrub ($5.99 for 5 ounces); **BioTherm** Biopur Double Purifying Exfoliator ($16.50 for 2.5 ounces) and Biosource Clarifying Exfoliating Gel ($14.50 for 2.5 ounces); **Club Monaco** Face Mild Exfoliant ($15 for 3.3 ounces); **Darphin** Oil Free Exfoliating Foam Gel ($40 for 4.2 ounces); **Doctor's Dermatologic Formula** Almond, Bergamot, Herbal, Strawberry; and Coconut Face & Body Polish ($23 for 8 ounces), Face & Body Scrub ($23 for 8 ounces), and Pumice Acne Scrub ($26 for 8 ounces); **Elizabeth Arden** Smooth the Way Cleansing Scrub for Face and Body ($16.50 for 6.8 ounces); **Gatineau** Oxygenating Exfoliating Treatment ($34 for 3.3 ounces); **H2O+ Skin Care** Oil-Controlling Exfoliator ($17.50 for 4 ounces) and Sea Mineral Scrub ($17.50 for 4 ounces); **Jason Natural** Original Apricot Scrub Facial Wash and Scrub ($4.50 for 4.5 ounces) and Citrus 6-in-1 Facial Wash & Scrub with Ester-C ($6 for 4.5 ounces); **Lancome** Exfoliance Delicate Exfoliating Gel ($21 for 3.5 ounces) and Exfoliance Clarte Clarifying Exfoliating Gel ($21 for 3.4 ounces); **Neutrogena** Deep Clean Gentle Scrub ($5.99 for 4.2 ounces); **Nivea Visage** Oil Control Cleansing Gel Oily Skin ($5.99 for 6.8 ounces); **Nu Skin** Exfoliant Scrub Extra Gentle ($11.95 for 2.5 ounces); **Osmotics** Balancing Cleanser for Normal to Oily Skin ($27 for 6 ounces); **Pond's** Clear Solutions Deep Pore Scrub ($5.69 for 3 ounces); **Principal Secret** Gentle Exfoliating Scrub ($16.75 for 4 ounces); **Sephora** Deep Cleansing Facial Scrub ($8 for 3.3 ounces); **Serious Skin Care** Daily Ritual Acne Medication Cleanser ($21 for 4 ounces).

BEST SCRUBS FOR NORMAL TO DRY SKIN: Ahava Advanced Gentle Mud Exfoliator for All Skin Types ($24 for 3.4 ounces); **Artistry by Amway** Exfoliating Scrub ($23.10

for 3.4 ounces); **BeneFit** Pineapple Facial Polish ($24 for 5.5 ounces); **BioTherm** Biosource Softening Exfoliating Cream ($14.50 for 2.5 ounces); **Chanel** Maximum Radiance Delicate Exfoliator ($30 for 2.6 ounces); **Clarins** Gentle Exfoliating Refiner for Face ($21 for 1.7 ounces); **Clinique** 7 Day Scrub Cream Rinse Off Formula ($15 for 3.4 ounces); **Dr. Hauschka** Cleansing Cream ($18 for 1.7 ounces); **Dr. LeWinn's Private Formula** Mega-C Facial Polishing Gel ($39.50 for 178 ml); **Ella Bache** Deep Cleansing Scrub, for Combination to Oily Skin ($21 for 6.17 ounces); **Givenchy** Gentle Exfoliating Massage ($45 for 1.7 ounces); **Guerlain** Issima Smoothing Gentle Exfoliator ($37 for 2.5 ounces); **Hydron** Best Defense Micro-Exfoliating Creme ($16.75 for 3.6 ounces); **Kiehl's** Ultra Moisturizing Buffing Cream with Scrub Particles ($11.50 for 4 ounces); **L'Oreal** Turning Point Instant Facial Scrub ($8.99 for 1.7 ounces); **La Prairie** Essential Exfoliator ($60 for 7 ounces); **Lancaster** Aquamilk Soft Touch Exfoliant ($28 for 3.4 ounces); **Lancome** Exfoliance Confort ($21 for 3.4 ounces); **Laura Mercier** Face Polish ($24 for 3.7 ounces) **Nu Skin** Facial Scrub ($11.45 for 2.5 ounces); **Ole Henriksen Skin Care** New Beginning Skin Smoothing Scrub ($22 for 2 ounces); **Pevonia Botanica** Gentle Exfoliating Cleanser ($25.50 for 5 ounces); **Physician's Choice** pHaze 4 Gentle Exfoliant ($14.95 for 6 ounces); **Prescriptives** Vibrant Scrub ($19 for 3.4 ounces); **RoC** Gentle Exfoliating Cream ($14 for 50 ml); **Serious Skin Care** Phyto-Pumpkin Scrub Acid-Free ($21 for 2 ounces); **Sothys Paris** Biological Skin Peeling ($23 for 1.7 ounces).

BEST MAKEUP REMOVERS AND CLEANSING WIPES

There are no makeup removers that receive a Paula's Pick rating. It's not that there aren't well-formulated makeup removers, because there are, it's just that there isn't a formulary value that distinguishes one from another. Makeup removers are shockingly similar. Those that are more emollient are almost always either silicone-based (and these are better for removing waterproof makeup or for those with dry skin) or contain gentle detergent cleansing agents (better for normal to oily or normal to slightly dry skin). From Chanel to Almay, Bobbi Brown, Clinique, or Lancome, the ingredient lists are endlessly monotonous and mundane. Aside from price or token plant extracts, there is absolutely no way to differentiate one from the other.

Using an eye-makeup remover is about preference and need. If you are using waterproof mascara, then silicone-based or more emollient versions are preferred. If you just want a way to remove eye makeup without leaving a residue on the skin (albeit a silky residue that silicone-based makeup removers provide), then those with gentle cleansing agents are preferred.

BEST MAKEUP REMOVERS THAT USE GENTLE CLEANSING AGENTS CONSIDERED BETTER FOR NORMAL TO OILY SKIN, BUT CAN WORK FOR ALL SKIN TYPES: **Ahava** Eye Makeup Remover ($18 for 6.8 ounces); **Alexandra de Markoff** Gentle Eye Makeup Remover ($18 for 4 ounces) and Professional Secrets Makeup Solvent ($42 for 2 ounces); **Almay** Non-Oily Eye Makeup Remover Gel ($4.49 for 1.5 ounces), Non-Oily Eye Makeup

Remover Lotion ($4.29 for 2 ounces), and Non-Oily Eye Makeup Remover Pads ($3.49 for 35 pads); **Aveda** Pure Gel Eye Makeup Remover ($15 for 3.7 ounces); **bare escentuals Cush** Eye Makeup Remover ($14 for 4.4 ounces); **Basis** So Refreshing Cleansing Towelettes ($4.99 for 30 cloths) and Facial Cleansing Cloths, Individually Wrapped ($4.99 for 20 cloths); **Bath & Body Works** Completely Clean Facial Cloths ($8 for 20 cloths) and Soothing Eye Makeup Remover ($7 for 4 ounces); **BeautiControl** Lash & Lid Bath ($9.50 for 4 ounces); **BeneFit** Clean Sweep ($14 for 4 ounces) and Make Up Remover and Brush Cleaner Baby! ($21 for 12 ounces); **BioTherm** Biocils Soothing Eye Make-up Remover ($14 for 4.2 ounces); **BlissLabs** Lid and Lash Wash ($22 for 8.5 ounces); **Bobbi Brown** Eye Makeup Remover ($18.50 for 3.4 ounces); **The Body Shop** Chamomile Eye Make-up Remover, for All Skin Types ($12 for 8.4 ounces) and Chamomile Makeup Wipes ($10 for 30 wipes); **Borghese** Gel Delicato Gentle Makeup Remover ($29.50 for 8.4 ounces); **Calvin Klein** Makeup Remover ($16 for 4 ounces); **Chanel** Gel Tendre Non-Foaming Makeup Remover Face and Eyes ($30 for 5 ounces); **Christian Dior** Instant Eye Makeup Remover ($18.50 for 3.4 ounces); **Clean & Clear by Johnson & Johnson** Daily Pore Cleansing Cloths ($4.99 for 25 cloths); **Clientele** Eye Makeup Remover ($14 for 2 ounces); **Clinique** Naturally Gentle Eye Makeup Remover ($14.50 for 2.5 ounces) and Rinse-Off Eye Makeup Solvent ($13.50 for 4.2 ounces); **Club Monaco** Eye Colour Remover ($12 for 3.4 ounces); **Decleor** Eye Make Up Remover with Plant Extracts ($21.50 for 4 ounces); **Dermalogica** Soothing Eye Makeup Remover ($21 for 4 ounces); **DHC** Make Off Sheet ($6 for 50 sheets) and Oil-Free Makeup Remover ($15 for 3.3 ounces); **Doctor's Dermatologic Formula** Eye Make-Up Remover Pads ($15 for 60 pads); **Dove** Daily Hydrating Cleansing Cloths, Sensitive Skin ($6.99 for 30 cloths) and Daily Hydrating Cleansing Cloths, Regular ($6.99 for 30 cloths); **Ellen Lange Skin Care** Daily Maintenance Eye Makeup Remover ($12 for 2.8 ounces) and Daily Maintenance Singles ($20 for 36 packets); **Erno Laszlo** pHelitone Gentle Eye Makeup Remover ($18 for 3 ounces); **Estee Lauder** Gentle Eye Makeup Remover ($13.50 for 3.4 ounces); **Gatineau** Gentle Eye Make-Up Remover ($15 for 1.6 ounces); **Guinot** Gentle Eye Cleansing Gel ($19.50 for 4.2 ounces); **H2O+ Skin Care** Water-Activated Eye Makeup Remover ($14.50 for 4 ounces); **Jason Natural** Quick Clean Eye Makeup Remover for All Skin Types, Oil Free ($7.49 for 75 pads); **Joey New York** Extra Gentle Eye Makeup Remover ($17 for 6 ounces) and Gentle Makeup Remover Pads ($12 for 50 pads); **La Roche-Posay** Toleriane Eye Make-Up Remover ($15.95 for 30 capsules); **Lancome** Effacile Gentle Eye Makeup Remover ($17.50 for 4 ounces); **Laura Mercier** Eye Make Up Remover ($18 for 4 ounces); **Lorac** Oil-Free Makeup Remover ($17 for 6.5 ounces); **M.A.C.** Pro Eye Makeup Remover ($15 for 5 ounces); **Marcelle** Eye Make-Up Remover Lotion Oil-Free ($8.50 for 120 ml); **Merle Norman** Instant Eye Makeup Remover ($8.50 for 3 ounces); **Morgen Schick** Perfectly Gentle Eye Makeup Remover ($10 for 2 ounces); **Nivea Visage** Eye Make-Up Remover ($4.99 for 2.5 ounces); **Ole Henriksen Skin Care** Purifying Eye Make-Up Remover ($18 for 75 pads); **Origins** Well-Off Fast and Gentle Eye

Makeup Remover ($11 for 3.4 ounces); **Physicians Formula** Eye Makeup Remover Lotion for Normal to Dry Skin ($4.75 for 2 ounces); **Pond's** Cleansing and Make-Up Remover Towelettes ($5.99 for 30 towelettes); **Prescriptives** Quick Remover for Face Makeup ($18.50 for 4.2 ounces); **Remede** Dissolve ($33 for 6.7 ounces); **RoC** Eye Makeup Remover Lotion ($14.50 for 125 ml); **Sephora** Soothing Eye Makeup Remover ($8 for 4.9 ounces); **Shaklee** Eye Makeup Remover ($9.15 for 2 ounces); **St. Ives** Apricot Exfoliating Cleansing Cloths ($5.99 for 30 cloths); **T. Le Clerc** Lip and Eye Make-Up Remover ($19 for 4.16 ounces); **Thalgo** Double Action Cleanser and Toner ($32 for 10.14 ounces) and Cleansing Lotion for Eyes and Lips ($18 for 4.2 ounces); **Ultima II** Eye Makeup Remover for Sensitive Eyes ($12.50 for 3.6 ounces); **Urban Decay** Clean Up Gentle Makeup Remover for Face and Eyes ($14 for 4.25 ounces); **Victoria Jackson Cosmetics** Facial Cleanser and Eye Makeup Remover ($13.50 for 4 ounces).

BEST MAKEUP REMOVERS THAT ARE SILICONE-BASED AND CONSIDERED BETTER FOR NORMAL TO DRY SKIN, BUT CAN WORK FOR ALL SKIN TYPES: **Almay** Dual Phase Eye Makeup Remover ($5.69 for 4 ounces); **Artistry by Amway** Eye & Lip Makeup Remover ($12.80 for 4 ounces); **Avon** Perfect Wear Makeup Remover ($4.50 for 2 ounces); **BioTherm** Biocils Waterproof Eye Make-up Remover ($14.50 for 4.2 ounces); **The Body Shop** Chamomile Gentle Eye Makeup Remover Gel ($10 for 3.4 ounces) and Soothing Eye Makeup Remover Gel ($10 for 3.38 ounces); **Calvin Klein** Oil Control Hydrator ($30 for 1.7 ounces); **Chanel** Demaquillant Yeux Intense Gentle Biphase Eye Makeup Remover ($23.50 for 3.4 ounces); **Christian Dior** iOd Mineral Aqua Gelee ($20 for 5.1 ounces), Purifying Cleansing Gelee for Face and Eyes ($22.50 for 6.8 ounces), and Duo-Phase Eye Makeup Remover ($20 for 3.4 ounces); **Cle de Peau Beaute** Absolute Eye Makeup Remover (Demaquillant Pour Les Yeux) ($35 for 2.5 ounces); **Clinique** Take the Day Off Makeup Remover, for Lids, Lashes and Lips ($15.50 for 4.2 ounces); **Epicuren** Crystal Clear Makeup Remover ($27 for 4 ounces); **Givenchy** Make-off Emulsion ($28 for 6.7 ounces); **Guerlain** Perfect Eye and Lip Makeup Remover ($28 for 3.3 ounces); **H2O+ Skin Care** Dual Action Eye Makeup Remover ($16 for 4.5 ounces); **Helena Rubinstein** All Mascaras! Complete Eye Make Up Remover ($22 for 4.2 ounces); **Hydron** Best Defense Gentle Eye Make Up Remover ($17 for 4 ounces); **Jafra** Dual-Action Eye Makeup Remover ($9 for 2 ounces); **La Prairie Cellular** Cellular Eye Make-Up Remover ($45 for 4.2 ounces); **Lancome** Bi-Facil Double-Action Eye Makeup Remover ($20 for 4 ounces); **M.A.C.** Wipes ($12.50 for 45 sheets); **Merle Norman** Luxiva Dual Action Eye Makeup Remover ($14.50 for 4 ounces); **Paula's Choice** Gentle Touch Makeup Remover ($12.95 for 4 ounces); **Shiseido** Eye & Lip Makeup Remover ($19 for 2.5 ounces); **Stila** H2Off ($18 for 40 cloths); **Versace** Perfect Zone Eye Cleanser ($33 for 4.2 ounces).

BEST MAKEUP REMOVERS THAT ARE MINERAL OIL– OR PLANT OIL–BASED AND WORK BEST FOR DRY TO VERY DRY SKIN: **Almay** Moisturizing Eye Makeup Remover Lotion ($4.29 for 2 ounces), Moisturizing Eye Makeup Remover Pads ($3.49 for 35 pads), and Moisturizing Gentle Gel Eye Makeup Remover ($4.49 for 1.5 ounces); **Aubrey Or-**

ganics Herbessence Makeup Remover ($6.95 for 2 ounces); **Chanel** Lait Tendre Gentle Makeup Remover Face and Eyes ($30 for 6.8 ounces); **Clientele** Time Therapy Eye Makeup Remover Oils ($15 for 2 ounces) and Elastology Makeup Remover ($25 for 2 ounces); **Decleor** Whitening Cleanser ($34 for 8.4 ounces) and Cleansing Oil for the Face and Eyes, with Sweet Almond Oil ($35 for 8.4 ounces); **Elizabeth Arden** All Gone Eye and Lip Make-up Remover ($16 for 3.4 ounces); **Kiehl's** Oil-Based Cleanser and Makeup Remover ($11.50 for 4 ounces); **Marcelle** Eye Make-Up Remover Pads ($8.50 for 60 pads) and Creamy Eye Make-Up Remover ($6.99 for 50 ml); **Mario Badescu** Cucumber Makeup Remover Cream ($10 for 4 ounces); **Merle Norman** Very Gentle Eye Makeup Remover ($8.50 for 2 ounces); **Parthena** Dissolve Eye Makeup Remover ($9.50 for 2 ounces).

BEST LOTION-STYLE MAKEUP REMOVERS THAT WORK BEST FOR DRY TO VERY DRY SKIN: Clinique Extremely Gentle Eye Makeup Remover ($10 for 2 ounces); **DHC** Deep Cleansing Oil ($22 for 6.7 ounces); **Estee Lauder** Take It Away Makeup Remover ($18 for 6.7 ounces); **Marcelle** 2 in 1 Face and Eye Cleanser ($11.25 for 170 ml); **Tony & Tina** Herbal Aromatherapy Make-Up Remover ($18 for 6 ounces); **Yves St. Laurent** Gentle Eye Makeup and Lipstick Remover ($24 for 2.5 ounces).

BEST TONERS

Regrettably, toners are the one product category that has seen the least improvement over the past several years. Although there are more and more alcohol-free toners being sold, many still contain other irritating ingredients or are extremely fragranced. In many instances, the toner contains so much fragrance that it's more like applying eau de toilette or cologne, and that isn't helpful or beneficial for skin. More often than not, toners are simplistic formulations (water and glycerin) with little to no interesting or state-of-the-art ingredients.

What do toners tone? The answer: not a thing. However, a well-formulated toner can provide some worthwhile advantages that can be helpful for most skin types. Toners and all the products that fall into this category (refining lotions, clarifying lotions, soothing tonics, stimulating lotions, fresheners, and astringents) are primarily an extra cleansing step. These products often contain gentle cleansing agents that can help remove the last traces of makeup that a cleanser can leave behind. The better formulated toners have water-binding, moisturizing, anti-irritant, and antioxidant properties. There is little difference between toners for normal to oily skin and toners for normal to dry skin because all should leave skin soft and clean, but not dry. For oily skin, a good toner can be the only moisturizer that is needed.

There are OK to good toners in all price ranges, but overall the formulations are amazingly redundant, with the primary components being water, glycerin, anti-irritants, water-binding agents, and fragrance. As a result of my being more critical of formulations in this edition, the list of good toners is far shorter than in earlier editions of this book, and there are very few Paula's Picks in this category as well.

BEST TONERS FOR ALL SKIN TYPES: Aesop Oil Free Hydrating Mist ($37.50 for 3.35 ounces); **Alexandra de Markoff** Luxury Skin Toner ($28 for 6 ounces); **Aloette** Nutrition Vitamin Complex ($17 for 8 ounces) and Sensitive Skin Toner ($14 for 8 ounces); **Arbonne** Awaken Rejuvenating Mist ($14 for 4 ounces); **Avon beComing** Get Supple Hydrating Mist ($12 for 5 ounces) and Get Vital Rejuvenating Mist ($12 for 5 ounces); **BeautiControl** ✓☺ Calming Rinse ($15.50 for 5.7 ounces) and Moisturizing Toner ($14.50 for 8 ounces); **Beauty Without Cruelty** Balancing Facial Toner for All Skin Types ($7.95 for 8.5 ounces); **BioTherm** ✓☺ Biosource Softening Toner ($14.50 for 8 ounces); **Bobbi Brown** Soothing Face Tonic ($22 for 6.7 ounces); **Clarins** Extra-Comfort Toning Lotion Very Dry or Sensitized Skin ($23 for 6.8 ounces); **Doctor's Dermatologic Formula** ✓☺ Aloe Toning Complex ($22 for 8 ounces); **H2O+ Skin Care** Oasis Mist ($15 for 6 ounces); **Hydron** ✓☺ Best Defense Botanical Toner ($14.50 for 6.5 ounces); **Jafra** Soothing Results Calming Toner for Sensitive Skin ($15 for 8.4 ounces); **L'Occitane** Essential Water for the Face ($20 for 6.7 ounces); **La Prairie Cellular** ✓☺ Cellular Refining Lotion ($65 for 8.2 ounces); **La Prairie** Age Management Balancer ($70 for 8.4 ounces); **Marcelle** Hydractive Reviving Toner, Dehydrated and Normal to Dry Skin ($11.25 for 180 ml); **Marilyn Miglin** Perfect C Skin Toner ($20 for 6 ounces); **M.D. Formulations** ✓☺ Moisture Defense Antioxidant Spray ($28 for 6 ounces); **Nu Skin** ✓☺ NaPCA Moisture Mist ($10 for 8.4 ounces); **Osmotics** Firming Tonic Facial Mist ($35 for 6.8 ounces); **Paula's Choice** ✓☺ Final Touch Toner, Normal to Oily/Combination Skin ($9.95 for 8 ounces) and ✓☺ Final Touch Toner, Normal to Dry Skin ($9.95 for 8 ounces); **Serious Skin Care** Super Hydrate Oil Free Mist ($19.95 for 4 ounces); **Shiseido** Whitening Softener I ($43 for 5 ounces); **Shu Uemura** Moisture Lotion ($35 for 8.4 ounces), Refreshing Lotion ($35 for 8.4 ounces), and Whitening Lotion ($33 for 5 ounces); **Victoria Jackson Cosmetics** Toning Mist ($14.50 for 4 ounces).

BEST TOPICAL DISINFECTANTS

For someone who struggles with blemishes, a topical disinfectant is a fundamental way to start effectively treating this condition. One of the primary causes of blemishes is the presence of a bacterium, and killing this bacterium can be of great help to many of those suffering with varying degrees of acne. Benzoyl peroxide is considered the most effective topical disinfectant for the treatment of blemishes. Generally, benzoyl peroxide products come in concentrations of 2.5%, 5%, and 10%, and as a rule, it's best to start with a lower concentration to see if that will work for you. If not, you can then try the next higher concentration. If the higher concentrations don't work, then it would be essential for you to consult a dermatologist or health care provider for a prescription topical disinfectant and/or for other topical acne treatments such as Retin-A, Avita, Tazorac, or generic versions of these (active ingredient tretinoin).

Alternative sources of topical disinfectants such as tea tree oil are an option, but there are only two products that meet the criterion for the appropriate concentration (at least

5%) to have an impact on disinfecting blemishes. **Note:** Almost all of the following benzoyl peroxide products are Paula's Picks because they include appropriate concentrations with no other irritating or harsh ingredients.

BEST TOPICAL DISINFECTANTS FOR BLEMISH-PRONE SKIN: BeautiControl ✓☺ All Clear Outta Sight Nighttime Clearing Complex ($14 for 1 ounce); **Bioelements** ✓☺ Breakout Control ($35 for 1 ounce); **BioMedic** ✓☺ Antibac Spot Treatment ($16.95 for 0.5 ounce); **Clean & Clear by Johnson & Johnson** ✓☺ Persa-Gel 10, Maximum Strength ($3.49 for 1 ounce); **Clinique** ✓☺ Acne Solutions Emergency Gel Lotion ($13.50 for 0.5 ounce); **Dermalogica** ✓☺ Special Clearing Booster ($37 for 1 ounce); **Doctor's Dermatologic Formula** ✓☺ 5% Benzoyl Peroxide Gel with Tea Tree Oil ($18 for 2 ounces); **Glymed Plus** ✓☺ Serious Action Skin Medication No. 5 ($26.95 for 4 ounces) and ✓☺ Serious Skin Medication No. 10 ($26.40 for 4 ounces); **Jan Marini Skin Research** ✓☺ Benzoyl Peroxide 2.5% ($25 for 4 ounces), ✓☺ Benzoyl Peroxide 5% ($25 for 4 ounces), and ✓☺ Benzoyl Peroxide 10% ($25 for 4 ounces); **Mary Kay** ✓☺ Acne Treatment Gel ($7 for 1.25 ounces); **M.D. Formulations** ✓☺ Benzoyl Peroxide 5% ($20 for 4 ounces) and ✓☺ Benzoyl Peroxide 10% ($20 for 4 ounces); **Neutrogena** On-the-Spot Acne Treatment Tinted Formula 2.5% Benzoyl Peroxide ($5.49 for 0.75 ounce) and ✓☺ On-the-Spot Acne Treatment Vanishing Formula 2.5% Benzoyl Peroxide ($6.75 for 0.75 ounce); **Oxy Balance** ✓☺ Sensitive Skin Acne Treatment, Vanishing Formula ($5.52 for 1 ounce), ✓☺ Maximum Acne Treatment, Tinted ($5.25 for 1 ounce), and ✓☺ Maximum Acne Treatment, Vanishing ($5.25 for 1 ounce); **PanOxyl** ✓☺ Aqua Gel Treatment ($9.99 for 1.5 ounces); **Paula's Choice** ✓☺ Blemish Fighting Solution, All Skin Types ($13.95 for 4 ounces) and Extra Strength Blemish Fighting Solution ($13.95 for 4 ounces); **Peter Thomas Roth** ✓☺ BPO Gel 2.5% ($20 for 3 ounces), ✓☺ BPO Gel 5% ($22 for 3 ounces), and ✓☺ BPO Gel 10% ($24 for 3 ounces); **ProActiv** ✓☺ Repairing Lotion ($21.75 for 2 ounces); **Serious Skin Care** ✓☺ Clearz-it Daytime Blemish Preventor ($17.50 for 2 ounces); **ZAPZYT** ✓☺ 10% Benzoyl Peroxide ($4.99 for 1 ounce).

BEST AHA AND BHA

Alpha hydroxy acids (AHAs, such as glycolic acid and lactic acid) and beta hydroxy acid (BHA, which is salicylic acid) work by exfoliating the skin chemically instead of mechanically via abrasion. For many reasons, these can be less irritating and can create more even and smoother results than scrubs, which is why facial scrubs have become less and less a part of most daily skin-care routines. There is also research showing that AHAs and BHA can improve skin thickness and cell turnover, increase collagen content, and improve pore function (reducing the amount of clogged pores and breakouts).

The goal is to use one effective AHA (between 5% and 10% concentration) or one BHA (1% to 2% concentration) product, and only as needed—which may be twice a day, once a day, or once every other day, depending on your skin type and its response.

The AHA and BHA products recommended below not only have formulations with the appropriate concentrations but also have a pH between 3 and 4, which is critical if those ingredients are to be effective as exfoliants.

AHAs are best for someone with normal to dry skin and BHAs for those with normal to oily or blemish-prone skin. AHAs cannot penetrate oil and, therefore, cannot get into the pore. BHA can penetrate oil and, therefore, can be absorbed into the pore where it can improve and repair pore function.

All of the products listed below are effectively formulated AHA and BHA products. Those that receive a Paula's Pick rating have a few more bells and whistles, such as anti-oxidants, water-binding agents, or anti-irritants, which are worthwhile additions to almost any product because they contribute to the overall health of skin.

If you decide to use an AHA or BHA product, particularly one from my list of recommendations, the question is, do you still need to use a mechanical scrub? The answer isn't all that easy, and you will have to judge that for yourself. Most women with normal to dry and/or sensitive skin should probably use only the AHA product and no other exfoliant (except maybe once in awhile). Someone with normal to oily skin should use a good BHA product, but may also find benefit from using a mechanical scrub once a day or once every other day. Whatever you choose, always listen carefully to your skin and remember that irritation is never the goal.

BEST ALPHA HYDROXY ACID PRODUCTS FOR NORMAL TO OILY OR COMBINATION SKIN: Alpha Hydrox Extra Strength AHA Oil-Free Formula, 10% AHA Facial Treatment ($9.29 for 1.7 ounces); **Artistry by Amway** Alpha Hydroxy Serum Plus ($43.15 for 1 ounce); **BioMedic** Phospholipid Gel ($20.95 for 2 ounces) and Phospholipid Lotion ($20.95 for 2 ounces); **Clientele** Roll-On Alpha Hydroxy Wrinkle Treatment ($25 for 0.35 ounce); **Doctor's Dermatologic Formula** Glycolic Moisturizer 10% ($32.50 for 2 ounces); **Dr. Mary Lupo Skin Care System** AHA Renewal Gel I ($25 for 3.5 ounces) and AHA Renewal Gel II ($25 for 3.5 ounces); **Exuviance** ✔☺ Vespera Bionic Serum ($55 for 1 ounce); **Glymed Plus** AHA Accelerator ($59.95 for 4 ounces) and Treatment Cream ($69.55 for 2 ounces); **Jan Marini Skin Research** Bioglycolic Cream ($60 for 2 ounces) and Bioglycolic Facial Lotion ($45 for 2 ounces); **Lac-Hydrin** Five Lotion ($10.99 for 8 ounces) and 12 Lotion ($34.98 for 7.6 ounces); **Neostrata** ✔☺ Bionic Face Serum PHA 10 ($45 for 1 ounce); **Paula's Choice** ✔☺ 8% Alpha Hydroxy Acid Solution ($13.95 for 4 ounces); **Peter Thomas Roth** Glycolic Acid 5% Moisturizer ($40 for 2 ounces) and Glycolic Acid 10% Moisturizer ($40 for 2 ounces); **Principal Secret** AHA Booster Complex ($45 for 1 ounce); **ProActiv** Revitalizing Toner ($16 for 4 ounces); **Serious Skin Care** Home Spa Facial Peel Six Week Facial Peel Program ($19 for 6 towelettes).

BEST ALPHA HYDROXY ACID PRODUCTS FOR NORMAL TO DRY SKIN: Alpha Hydrox AHA Creme 8% AHA Facial Treatment for Normal Skin ($9.29 for 2 ounces), AHA Enhanced Creme 10% AHA Facial Treatment, for Dry to Normal Skin ($8.41 for 2 ounces), and AHA Lotion 10% AHA Facial Treatment, for Dry Skin ($9.29 for 6 ounces);

BeautiControl **Regeneration** Regeneration Face and Neck Creme ($32 for 2 ounces), Regeneration 2 Face and Neck Creme ($32 for 2 ounces), Regeneration Face and Neck Cream, Oily Skin ($32 for 2 ounces), Regeneration 2 for Oily Skin ($32 for 2 ounces), and Regeneration Gold ($56 for 1.8 ounces); **BioMedic** Conditioning Cream ($24.95 for 2 ounces); **Dr. Mary Lupo Skin Care System** AHA Renewal Lotion I ($25 for 3.5 ounces) and AHA Renewal Lotion II ($25 for 3.5 ounces); **M.D. Formulations** Smoothing Complex with 10% Glycolic Compound ($35 for 0.5 ounce); **M.D. Forte** ✓☺ Skin Rejuvenation Lotion I, 5% Glycolic Compound ($34 for 1 ounce); **Murad** Night Reform ($52.50 for 1.4 ounces) and ✓☺ Advanced Sensitive Skin Smoothing Cream ($48 for 3.3 ounces); **Neostrata** Skin Smoothing Cream AHA 8 ($18.75 for 1.75 ounces), Skin Smoothing Lotion AHA 10 ($20 for 6.8 ounces), Eye Cream PHA 4 ($28 for 0.5 ounce), and Ultra Moisturizing Face Cream PHA 10 ($27 for 1.75 ounces); **Neutrogena** ✓☺ Healthy Skin Face Lotion ($9.99 for 2.5 ounces) and ✓☺ Healthy Skin Face Lotion Delicate Skin ($9.99 for 2.5 ounces); **N.V. Perricone, M.D.** Alpha Lipoic Acid Face Firming Activator with NTP Complex ($85 for 2 ounces); **Obagi Nu-Derm** Nu-Derm Exfoderm Forte ($48 for 2 ounces); **Osmotics** Facial Renewal ($75 for 1.7 ounces); **Peter Thomas Roth** Glycolic Acid 10% Hydrating Gel ($45 for 2 ounces) and AHA 12% Hydrating Ceramide Repair Gel ($45 for 2 ounces); **Pevonia Botanica** Glycocides Cream ($46 for 1.7 ounces); **Pond's** Age Defying Complex Cream ($10.99 for 2 ounces), Age Defying Lotion ($10.99 for 3 ounces), Dramatic Results Advanced Anti-Aging Care Active Face & Neck Moisturizer ($13.24 for 1.7 ounces), and Dramatic Results Anti-Wrinkle Cream ($14.99 for 1.25 ounces); **Reversa** Eye Contour Cream ($23.99 for 15 ml), Skin Smoothing Cream 5% ($26.99 for 60 ml), Skin Smoothing Cream 8% ($26.99 for 60 ml), and Corrective Night Cream ($26.99 for 50 ml); **SkinCeuticals** C + AHA ($115 for 1 ounce).

BEST BETA HYDROXY ACID PRODUCTS FOR NORMAL TO OILY OR COMBINATION SKIN: BeautiControl All Clear Skin Moisture ($14 for 4 ounces); **Clinique** Mild Clarifying Lotion ($10.50 for 6.7 ounces); **M.A.C.** Oil Control Lotion ($22 for 1.7 ounces); **Neutrogena** Deep Pore Treatment ($6.29 for 2 ounces) and Clear Pore Treatment Nighttime Pore Clarifying Gel Salicylic Acid Acne Treatment ($6.75 for 2 ounces); **Paula's Choice** ✓☺ 2% Beta Hydroxy Acid Liquid Solution, Normal to Oily Skin ($13.95 for 4 ounces) and ✓☺ 2% Beta Hydroxy Acid Lotion, All Skin Types ($13.95 for 4 ounces); **philosophy** hope in a bottle, oil-free moisturizer normal to oily skin ($32.50 for 2 ounces); **Serious Skin Care** Clarify Clarifying Treatment ($17.50 for 2 ounces); **Ultima II** ✓☺ Vital Radiance Skin Renewing Toner Normal to Dry Skin ($17.50 for 8 ounces); **ZAPZYT** Pore Treatment Gel ($5.29 for 0.75 ounce).

BEST BETA HYDROXY ACID PRODUCTS FOR NORMAL TO DRY SKIN: Estee Lauder ✓☺ Fruition Extra Multi-Action Complex ($70 for 1.7 ounces) and Clear Difference Oil-Control Hydrator for Oily Normal/Oily and Blemish-Prone Skin ($27 for 1.7 ounces); **Origins** Clearance Time ($22.50 for 1 ounce); **Paula's Choice** ✓☺ 1% Beta Hydroxy Acid Solution, All Skin Types ($13.95 for 4 ounces).

BEST BETA HYDROXY ACID AND ALPHA HYDROXY ACID COMBINATION PRODUCTS FOR NORMAL TO DRY OR COMBINATION SKIN: **Clientele Elastology** Lotus Vitamin C Serum ($65 for 1 ounce); **Jan Marini Skin Research** Bioglycolic BioClear ($50 for 1 ounce); **La Prairie** Cellular Purifying Systeme Hydro Repair ($125 for 1 ounce); **M.D. Formulations** Vit-A-Plus Night Recovery Complex ($50 for 1 ounce); **Neutrogena** Multi-Vitamin Acne Treatment ($5.99 for 2.5 ounces); **Olay** Age Defying Series Daily Renewal Cream ($9.29 for 2 ounces); **Pond's** Clear Solutions Combination Skin Moisturizer ($6.99 for 4 ounces); **Serious Skin Care** Renewal Gel Glycolic Skin Perfector ($20 for 4 ounces).

BEST MOISTURIZERS

Regardless of what they are called on the label—wrinkle creams, day creams, firming creams, eye creams, throat creams, lotions, serums, replenishing gels, and nourishing creams—all these concoctions and combinations do the same thing—moisturize the skin—and, for the most part, they do an excellent job. What is offensive is that many of the moisturizer formulations don't warrant the outlandish claims, ridiculous prices, or your belief that you've finally found the fountain of youth.

Moisturizers for oily skin are difficult to evaluate. As a rule, if oily skin is not being irritated or assaulted with harsh skin-care products, it does not need a moisturizer. Lotions and creams in general can be problematic for oily skin. Even gels and serum-type moisturizers can feel heavy on oily skin. For this reason I rate moisturizers, regardless of their designation as serums, gels, lotions, antiwrinkle, antiaging, or otherwise, on the basis of their value for normal to dry or dry to slightly dry skin. As a result, there is no group for oily skin moisturizers. Even when a product is labeled as being for someone with oily or combination skin, it is meant to be used only over dry areas and not over oily areas.

If you are not using harsh or irritating skin-care products, but still have dry, red patches of skin in areas that are oily, it can be indicative of a skin disorder such as rosacea, dermatitis, psoriasis, or seborrhea. That doesn't require a moisturizer, but rather a change in how you are taking care of your skin or an appointment with a dermatologist.

If you have oily skin but also have dry areas (and you are certain you have no skin disorders and are not using irritating skin-care products), consider using the moisturizers in the slightly dry or dry skin group below, but use them only over dry areas, not all over.

Because many of you are curious about products containing retinol (vitamin A), and because there is new research indicating that it can have benefits on skin similar to the benefits of the active ingredient tretinoin in the prescription drugs Renova and Retin-A, I list the products that contain relatively reliable concentrations (though exactly what amount to rely on is unknown) and that are packaged in a way that will keep the product stable.

I did not create a list of vitamin C products. It is an understatement to say that there is no consensus on which is the best form of vitamin C, or much less how much of it to use. There isn't even a consensus among companies selling vitamin C products. Even the physician lines declaring antiwrinkle properties for their vitamin C products also sell other products making equally amazing claims for other ingredients. Like all antioxidants, there can be impressive benefit for skin, but vitamin C is not a standout over other forms such as superoxide dismutase, grape extract, green tea, vitamin E, and on and on.

The moisturizer you use on your face will also work around your eyes and throat, on your chest, or wherever. Try to disregard the scare tactics at the cosmetics counters and the brochures that carry on about special formulations designed exclusively for the eye, throat, or chest areas. These claims are not substantiated by the ingredients in the products, which are identical to products supposedly designed just for the face.

Please keep in mind that products claiming that they are antiaging, antiwrinkling, lifting, firming, repairing, or rejuvenating; can give the skin oxygen; or contain any number of miracle ingredients are spinning fairy tales (except for well-formulated sunscreens). What isn't a fantasy is the fact that there are a lot of great moisturizers that can help soothe the skin and eliminate dryness (at least while you wear them—the effect is gone once you wash you face), and help make wrinkles look less pronounced—but when you stop using the product, whatever the exotic name, promise, or claim, the wrinkles are back in short order. The most frustrating aspect of the moisturizer craze is the belief that using moisturizers can somehow slow down or stop the wrinkling process, so a lot of women end up searching for the best moisturizer, when in fact the search for the best sunscreen would be a much more productive task.

Paula's Picks are assigned to the moisturizer products that are loaded with antioxidants, water-binding agents, and anti-irritants. A staggering amount of research has proven that these ingredients are extremely beneficial for skin. (I explain why these types of ingredients are so important for skin in the beginning of Chapter Three, and provide details in Chapter Seven, *Cosmetics Dictionary*.) But it is shocking how many products include only trace amounts of these ingredients (just so they can make a claim that the products contain them), which makes them useless and ineffectual.

Note: There are no products that can change dark circles under the eye (unless the dark circling is caused by sun damage, which requires a well-formulated skin-lightening product).

Important reminder: Because none of the moisturizers in this section contain sunscreen, they are absolutely not to be used for daytime unless another effective sunscreen is worn over it. The only real difference between daytime moisturizers and nighttime moisturizers should be whether or not the one for daytime contains a sunscreen.

BEST LIGHTWEIGHT MOISTURIZERS FOR NORMAL TO SLIGHTLY DRY OR COMBINATION SKIN: Aloette ✓☺ Line Control Eye Gel ($12.50 for 0.5 ounce), Time Restore Firming Serum ($45 for 1 ounce), and Simply Clear Clarifying Moisture Balance ($13.50 for 2 ounces); **Arbonne** NutriMin C with Bio-Hydria NutriMin C Lift with Bio-Hydria ($36 for 3.3 ounces); **Artistry by Amway** Time Defiance Nighttime Renewal Lotion ($63.05 for 1.7 ounces); **Astara** Botanical Eye Treatment ($48 for 1 ounce); **Aveda** Firming Fluid ($32 for 1 ounce); **Avon Anew** Anew Force Extra Triple Lifting Eye Cream

($18 for 0.5 ounce), ✔☺ Anew Retroactive Eye Age Reversal Serum ($18 for 0.4 ounce) and Anew Skintrition Multi-Vitamin Skin Primer ($16 for 1.7 ounces); **Avon beComing** Soothing Booster ($20 for 0.5 ounce), Detoxifying Booster ($20 for 0.5 ounce), Pack Your Bags De-Puffing Eye Gel ($24 for 0.5 ounce), and Off Line Anti-Wrinkle Quick Click ($24 for 0.5 ounce); **Awake** Hydro-Force Oil-Free Treatment ($45 for 1.7 ounces) and Serum Up-Sign Face Essence ($70 for 1.4 ounces); **Bath & Body Works** Illuminating Face Lotion ($20 for 1 ounce); **Beauty Without Cruelty** ✔☺ Green Tea Nourishing Eye Gel ($14.49 for 1 ounce), Vitamin C Vitality Serum ($24.95 for 1 ounce), and ✔☺ Vitamin C Revitalizing Eye Cream ($24.95 for 1 ounce); **BeneFit** Eye Lift ($25 for 1 ounce); **BioMedic** Hydro Active Emulsion ($22.95 for 2 ounces), Hydrating Serum ($56.25 for 3 ounces) and ✔☺ High Density Gel ($23.95 for 0.5 ounce); **Bobbi Brown** Shine Control Hydrating Face Gel ($38 for 1.7 ounces); **Borghese** ✔☺ Advanced Spa Lift for Eyes ($45 for 1 ounce), ✔☺ Cura Notte Night Therapy, for Normal to Oily Skin ($43.50 for 1.7 ounces), ✔☺ Equilibrio Equalizing Restorative ($42.50 for 1.7 ounces), and Hydra-Puro Moisture Renewing Oil Free Fluid ($35 for 1.7 ounces); **Cellex-C** ✔☺ Advanced-C Eye Toning Gel ($70 for 0.5 ounce), ✔☺ Advanced-C Serum ($115 for 1 ounce), Advanced-C Skin Hydration Complex ($79 for 1 ounce), ✔☺ Eye Contour Gel ($51 for 0.5 ounce), and Fade-Away Gel ($55 for 0.84 ounce); **Chanel** ✔☺ Age Delay Eye Rejuvenation Eye Gel ($50 for 0.5 ounce), ✔☺ Age Delay Rejuvenation Serum ($60 for 1 ounce), ✔☺ HydraMax Balanced Hydrating Gel ($40 for 1.7 ounces), and HydraMax Oil-Free Hydrating Gel ($40 for 1.7 ounces); **Clarins** Multi-Active Day Cream-Gel ($55 for 1.7 ounces); **Clientele** ✔☺ Night Serum, for Normal/Oily Skin ($49 for 1 ounce); **Clinique** Anti-Gravity Firming Lift Lotion ($35 for 1.7 ounces), ✔☺ Moisture in Control ($31 for 1.7 ounces), ✔☺ Moisture Surge Eye Gel ($26 for 0.5 ounce), and ✔☺ Moisture Surge Extra Thirsty Skin Relief ($31 for 1.7 ounces); **DHC** AntioxC ($32 for 1.4 ounces), Hydrating Nighttime Moisture ($28 for 1 ounce), Oil-Free Hydrator for Oilier Skin ($22 for 3.3 ounces), and Water Base Moisture ($12 for 2 ounces); **Diane Young** Years Younger Serum ($45.50 for 1 ounce) and Years Younger Soothing Serum ($50 for 1 ounce); **Doctor's Dermatologic Formula** ✔☺ EPF Eye Serum C3 ($39 for 0.5 ounce), ✔☺ EPF Serum C3 Environmental Protection ($60 for 1 ounce), ✔☺ Ultra Lite Oil Free Moisturizing Dew ($28 for 1.67 ounces), ✔☺ Bio-Molecular Firming Eye Serum ($75 for 0.5 ounce), and ✔☺ Soothing Eye Gel ($37 for 1 ounce); **Dr. Jeannette Graf, M.D.** ✔☺ Skin Energizing Booster AM/PM ($24.50 for 1 ounce); **Dr. LeWinn's Private Formula** Mega-C Bio-Deliverant Serum ($95 for 30 ml); **Ella Bache** Eye Lift Gel ($45 for 0.53 ounce) and Intensive Anti-Wrinkle Serum ($90 for 1.07 ounces); **Ellen Lange Skin Care** Velvet Vinyl ($45); **Epicuren** Enzyme Concentrate ($56 for 1 ounce) and Live Enzyme Gel Plus ($68 for 2 ounces); **Glymed Plus** Eye and Lip Renewal Complex ($36.75 for 0.75 ounce); **G.M. Collin** ✔☺ Ultraderm Native Collagene Gel ($49.90 for 1.7 ounces), ✔☺ Ultraderm Hydro Nutritive Cream ($52.50 for 1.7 ounces), ✔☺ Ultraderm Hydro Restorative Cream ($69 for 1.7 ounces), and

✓☺ Time Corrector Eyelid Gel-Cream ($43 for 0.8 ounce); **H2O+ Skin Care** Marine Enzyme Serum ($22.50 for 1 ounce) and ✓☺ Waterwhite Brightening Essence ($45 for 0.85 ounce); **Hydron** Oil Balancing Serum ($19.75 for 0.45 ounce); **Jafra** ✓☺ Optimeyes Eye Treatment ($21 for 0.5 ounce); **Jan Marini Skin Research** Antioxidant Group Recover-E ($40 for 1 ounce), ✓☺ C-Esta Eye Repair Concentrate ($55 for 0.5 ounce), and ✓☺ C-Esta Serum ($75 for 1 ounce); **Jason Natural** Natural NaPCA Moisturizing Creme ($7 for 4 ounces); **Joey New York** Lift Up Eye Gel ($20 for 0.5 ounce); **Jurlique International** Eye Gel ($65 for 0.53 ounce) and Herbal Extract Recovery Gel ($61 for 1 ounce); **La Prairie** ✓☺ Cellular Lipo-Sculpting Systeme Face Serum ($125 for 1 ounce) and ✓☺ Cellular Desensitizing Serum ($150 for 1 ounce); **La Roche-Posay** Active C Facial Skincare ($34.95 for 1 ounce) and Active C Light Facial Skincare ($34.95 for 1 ounce); **Lancome** Oligo Mineral Lotion ($95 for 1.7 ounces); **Mario Badescu** Cellufirm Drops ($25 for 1 ounce); **Merle Norman** Luxiva Energizing Concentrate ($37.50 for 1 ounce), ✓☺ Luxiva Fine Line Minimizer ($44.50 for 1 ounce), and Luxiva Triple Action Eye Gel ($18.50 for 0.5 ounce); **Murad** Cellular Serum ($42 for 1.4 ounces), Energizing Pomegranate Treatment ($30 for 0.5 ounce), and ✓☺ Perfecting Serum ($52 for 1 ounce); **Neutrogena** Pore Refining Mattifier ($11.99 for 0.5 ounce); **Neways Skin Care** Circles & Lines ($21 for 1 ounce); **Nivea Visage** Soothing Eye Gel ($8.99 for 0.5 ounce); **Noevir** ✓☺ Eye Treatment Gel ($65 for 0.52 ounce); **Nu Skin** ✓☺ Celltrex Skin Hydrating Fluid ($29 for 0.5 ounce), Enhancer Skin Conditioning Gel ($29 for 2.5 ounces), HPX Hydrating Gel ($49 for 1.5 ounces), and NaPCA Moisturizer ($21 for 2.5 ounces); **Nutrifirm Isomers** Absolute A + C Serum ($49.99 for 1 ounce), Absolute A + E Serum ($59.99 for 1 ounce), and Vitamin C Serum ($39.99 for 1 ounce); **Obagi Nu-Derm** Cffectives Eye Contour Serum 5% ($32.95 for 0.5 ounce) and Cffectives High Potency Serum 10% ($57.95 for 1 ounce); **Origins** ✓☺ Line Chaser, Stop Sign for Lines ($25 for 0.5 ounce); **Parthena** Daily Support Gel ($9.95 for 2 ounces), Daisy Gel ($14.50 for 1 ounce), Eye Wonder Serum ($21.50 for 0.5 ounce), and Blanc de Blanc Cream ($16 for 0.5 ounce); **Paula's Choice** ✓☺ Completely Non-Greasy Moisturizing Lotion, Normal to Oily Skin ($13.95 for 4 ounces) and ✓☺ Skin Balancing Moisture Gel, Normal to Oily Skin ($14.95 for 2 ounces); **Peter Thomas Roth** Environmental Repair Hydrating Gel ($35 for 2 ounces), Power C 10 Serum Liquid ($75 for 1 ounce), Power C 10 Anti-Oxidant Serum Gel ($80 for 1 ounce), and Power C 20 Anti-Oxidant Serum Gel ($80 for 1 ounce); **Pharmagel** Complexe Eye Firme Firming Eye Gel ($18.95 for 1 ounce) and Pharma C Serum Vitamin C Facial Treatment ($29.95 for 1 ounce); **Pond's** Revitalizing Eye Capsules for Delicate Eye Area ($10.99 for 20 capsules totaling 0.26 ounce), Skin Smoothing Capsules ($10.99 for 26 capsules totaling 0.33 ounce), and Soothing Cucumber Eye Treatments ($8.99 for 24 pads); **Prescriptives** Px Uplift Active Firming Cream ($45 for 1 ounce) and Super Line Preventor ($45 for 1 ounce); **Serious Skin Care** C-Eye Vitamin C Eye Beauty Treatment ($19.50 for 0.5 ounce), C-Serum Vitamin C Skin Conditioner ($26.50 for 1 ounce), ✓☺ Acid-Free Skin Resurfacing Serum ($26.50

for 1 ounce), ✔☺ Eye Firming Gel Acid-Free ($19.50 for 0.5 ounce), Haven Stabilizing Serum for All Skin Types ($26.50 for 2 ounces), and Megamins Multi Vitamin Beauty Serum ($28 for 1 ounce); **SkinCeuticals** ✔☺ SkinC Serum 10 ($60 for 1 ounce), ✔☺ SkinC Serum 15 ($75 for 1 ounce), ✔☺ Eye Gel ($42 for 0.5 ounce), Hydrating B5 Gel ($55 for 1 ounce), Intense Line Defense ($50 for 1 ounce), Phyto Corrective Gel ($45 for 1 ounce), and Serum 20 ($95 for 1 ounce); **St. Ives** Cucumber & Elastin Eye & Face Stress Gel ($2.79 for 4 ounces); **Ultima II** Vital Radiance Skin Renewing Night Serum ($25 for 0.95 ounce); **University Medical Skin Care** Face Lift Collagen 5 C5 Serum ($14.97 for 1 ounce), Face Lift Collagen 5 Concentrated Treatment Patch ($9.97 for 12 patches), and Face Lift Vitamin C Anti-Wrinkle Patch ($10.97 for 8 patches); **Vichy** Optalia Restructuring Eye Gel ($30 for 15 ml); **Zia** Essential Eye Gel ($19.95 for 0.5 ounce) and Deep Moisture Repair Serum ($34.95 for 0.3 ounce).

BEST MOISTURIZERS FOR NORMAL TO DRY SKIN: **Adrien Arpel's Signature Club A** Anti-Sag Extra-Firming Cream Duo with Caviar ($28.50 for 2 ounces of Eye Gel and 2 ounces of Eye Creme), Flower Acid Wrinkle Remedy Night Face Creme ($23.50 for 2 ounces), and Flower Acid Wrinkle Remedy Day Eye Creme ($15.50 for 1 ounce); **Ahava** Advanced Night Replenisher ($48 for 1.7 ounces); **Alexandra de Markoff** Advanced Daily Nourisher ($75 for 2 ounces) and Compensation Skin Serum ($68.50 for 2 ounces); **Almay** Milk Plus Illuminating Eye Cream ($10.93 for 0.5 ounce); **Almay** Kinetin Repair & Rejuvenate Night Concentrate ($18 for 1.7 ounces), Anti-Wrinkle Booster Serum ($18 for 0.3 ounce), Rejuvenating Eye Treatment ($18 for 0.5 ounce), and De-Aging Neck & Chest Treatment ($18 for 3.75 ounces); **Aloette** Nutri-C Moisture Cream ($15.50 for 3 ounces); **Annemarie Borlind** LL Bi Aktiv Regeneration LL Day Cream ($49 for 1.7 ounces), LL Regeneration Ampoules ($49 for 7 vials), Rose Day Cream ($36.50 for 1.7 ounces), Rose Night Cream ($37.75 for 1.7 ounces), Absolute Day Cream ($98 for 1.7 ounces), Absolute Firming Fluid ($50 for 0.5 ounces), Absolute Night Cream ($98 for 1.7 ounces), and Peach Skin Facial Cream ($16.75 for 1.7 ounces); **Arbonne** Rejuvenating Cream for All Skin Types ($31 for 2 ounces) and NutriMin C with Bio-Hydria NutriMin C Night Cream with Bio-Hydria ($62.50 for 2 ounces); **Artistry by Amway** ✔☺ Delicate Care Calming Moisturizer for Sensitive Skin Types ($24.45 for 2.5 ounces), Advanced Daily Eye Creme ($20.25 for 0.5 ounce), and Time Defiance Nighttime Renewal Creme ($63.05 for 1.7 ounces); **Astara** Anti-Oxidant Light Moisturizer ($42 for 2.2 ounces), Microcluster Anti-Oxidant Infusion ($72 for 2.2 ounces), and Anti-Oxidant Rich Moisturizer ($52 for 2.2 ounces); **Aubrey Organics** Sea Buckthorn Rejuvenating Serum with Ester-C ($15.75 for 0.36 ounce) and Rosa Mosqueta Rose Hip Seed Oil ($12.50 for 0.36 ounce); **Aveda** ✔☺ Night Nutrients ($38 for 1 ounce), Tourmaline Charged Eye Creme ($30 for 0.5 ounce), Balancing Infusion for Dry Skin ($18 for 0.33 ounce), and Balancing Infusion for Sensitive Skin ($18 for 0.33 ounce); **Aveeno** Radiant Skin Daily Moisturizer ($13.99 for 4 ounces); **Avon** Anew Positivity Recharging P.M. Replenisher ($25 for 1 ounce), Botanisource Comforting Moisture Cream ($9.50 for 1.7

ounces), ✔☺ Hydrofirming Night Cream ($11.50 for 1.7 ounces), ✔☺ Hydrofirming Eye Cream ($9.50 for 0.5 ounce), Lighten Up Plus Undereye Treatment ($15 for 0.5 ounce), and ✔☺ Moisture 24 Long-Lasting Hydrating Cream ($11 for 1.7 ounces); **Avon beComing** ✔☺ Hydrating Booster ($20 for 0.5 ounce), Luminous Transfirm Contouring Treatment ($35 for 1.7 ounces), and Evening Retreat Moisture Cream ($20 for 1.7 ounces); **B. Kamins** Cellular Renewal Serum ($59 for 1.7 ounces), Eye Cream ($52 for 0.6 ounce), and Night Cream for All Skin Types ($78 for 2.2 ounces); **Bath & Body Works** Hydrating Night Cream ($12 for 2 ounces), ✔☺ Nourishing Eye Cream ($12 for 0.5 ounce), and Skin Renewal Serum ($20 for 1 ounce); **BeautiControl** ✔☺ Cell Block-C PM Cell Protection ($30 for 0.95 ounce), ✔☺ Microderm Eye-X-Cel Daily Therapy Creme ($19 for 0.5 ounce), Platinum Regeneration Eye ($30 for 0.6 ounce), ✔☺ Relaxing Moisture ($16 for 4 ounces), and Balancing Moisturizer ($16 for 4.5 ounces); **Beauty Without Cruelty** ✔☺ Vitamin C Renewal Cream ($18.95 for 2 ounces); **BeneFit** Daily Hyaluronic Creme for Seriously Sensitive Skin ($22 for 2 ounces); **Bioelements** Recovery Serum ($52 for 1 ounce) and ✔☺ Urban Detox ($35 for 1 ounce); **BioMedic** Conditioning Eye Cream ($23.95 for 0.5 ounce) and ✔☺ Extra Rich Moisturizer ($31 for 1 ounce); **BioTherm** D-Stress Yeux Anti-Fatigue Eye Care ($26 for 0.5 ounces); **BlissLabs** Fully Loaded Moisture Lotion for Dry Skin ($36 for 1.7 ounces), Quiet Type Moisture Lotion for Sensitive Skin ($36 for 1.7 ounces), and All Around Eye Cream ($26 for 0.5 ounce); **Bobbi Brown** Hydrating Eye Cream ($32.50 for 0.5 ounce), Hydrating Face Cream ($38 for 1.7 ounces), and Intensive Skin Supplement ($50 for 1 ounce); **The Body Shop** ✔☺ Grapeseed Daily Hydrating Moisture Cream, for Normal to Dry Skin ($12 for 1.7 ounces), ✔☺ Grapeseed Extra Rich Night Cream, for Normal to Dry Skin ($15 for 1.7 ounces), ✔☺ Vitamin C Super Charged Serum ($20 for 1 ounce), Vitamin E Under Eye Cream ($12.50 for 0.5 ounce), and Hydrating Moisture Lotion, for Normal to Dry Skin ($16 for 3.38 ounces); **Borghese** ✔☺ Cura Notte Night Therapy, for Normal to Dry Skin ($43.50 for 1.7 ounces), ✔☺ Dolce Notte ReEnergizing Night Creme ($50 for 1.85 ounces), Energia Skin Recovery Creme ($49.50 for 1.7 ounces), and Fluido Protettivo Advanced Spa Lift for Eyes ($45 for 1 ounce); **Burt's Bees** Marshmallow Vanishing Creme ($9.99 for 1.5 ounces); **CamoCare** ✔☺ Intense Facial Therapy ($20.69 for 1 ounce); **Caudalie** Vinolift ($75 for 1 ounce); **Cellex-C** ✔☺ Advanced-C Eye Firming Cream ($90 for 1 ounce), Advanced-C Neck Firming Cream ($115 for 2 ounces), ✔☺ Advanced-C Skin Tightening Cream ($135 for 2 ounces), ✔☺ Eye Contour Cream ($64 for 1 ounce), ✔☺ High Potency Serum ($90 for 1 ounce), ✔☺ Serum for Sensitive Skin ($90 for 1 ounce), ✔☺ Skin Firming Cream ($105 for 2 ounces), ✔☺ Skin Firming Cream Plus ($114 for 2 ounces), G.L.A. Dry Skin Cream ($58 for 2 ounces), and G.L.A. Eye Balm ($54 for 1 ounce); **Chanel** ✔☺ HydraMax Balanced Hydrating Cream ($40 for 1.7 ounces), ✔☺ Rectifiance Nuit Night Lift Restoring Cream ($50 for 1.7 ounces), and Skin Recovery Eye Cream ($95 for 0.5 ounce); **Chantecaille** ✔☺ Vital Essence ($78 for 1.7 ounces); **Christian Dior** ✔☺ Capture Rides Wrinkle Creme for

Eyes ($45 for 0.5 ounce) and Vitalmine Radiance Activator ($45 for 1 ounce); **Clarins** Total Double Serum Age-Control Extra-Firming Serum ($75 for two 0.5-ounce bottles), Extra-Firming Day Cream for Dry Skin ($63 for 1.7 ounces), Eye Contour Balm "Special" ($38.50 for 0.7 ounce), and Energizing Morning Cream ($52.50 for 1.7 ounces); **Clientele Time Therapy** Nourishing Night Oils ($100 for 10 vials), Time Therapy ($75 for 1.1 ounces), ✔☺ Night Serum, for Normal/Dry, Sensitive Skin ($49 for 1 ounce), and ✔☺ Sacred Lotus Seed Wrinkle Serum ($49 for 1 ounce); **Clientele Elastology** ✔☺ Anti-Aging Activator Plus ($50 for 1.3 ounces), ✔☺ Firming Eye Cream ($45 for 0.5 ounce), ✔☺ Firming Night Cream ($75 for 1.1 ounce or kit 3 for $84), and ✔☺ Lotus Firming Serum ($65 for 1 ounce); **Clinique** ✔☺ Advanced Stop Signs Visible Anti-aging Serum ($35 for 1.7 ounces), ✔☺ All About Eyes ($26 for 0.5 ounce), Anti-Gravity Firming Lift Cream ($35 for 1.7 ounces), Anti-Gravity Firming Eye Lift Cream ($28.50 for 0.5 ounce), ✔☺ Moisture On-Call ($31 for 1.6 ounces), ✔☺ Moisture On Line ($31 for 1.7 ounces), Skin Texture Lotion Oil-Free Formula ($21 for 1.25 ounces), Total Turnaround Visible Skin Renewer ($30 for 1.7 ounces), and Turnaround Lotion Oil Free ($26 for 1.7 ounces); **Darphin** Soleil Douceur ($48 for 5 ounces); **Decleor** Vitalite Nourishing and Firming Face Cream, with Plant Extracts and Essential Oils ($62 for 1.69 ounces); **Dermablend** Advanced Enzyme Moisturizer with Ultrasomes ($35 for 1 ounce), Eye Revitalizing Complex ($20 for 0.5 ounce), and Hydrating Complex Cream ($30 for 3.75 ounces); **Dermalogica** Intensive Eye Repair ($37 for 0.5 ounce), Multivitamin Power Firm for Eye and Lip Area ($42 for 0.5 ounce), Intensive Moisture Balance ($37 for 1.75 ounces), and Skin Smoothing Cream ($46 for 3.5 ounces); **DHC** Emollient Balm ($30 for 3.3 ounces), Rich Moisture for Normal to Drier Skin ($24 for 3.3 ounces), Moisturizer ($28 for 3.3 ounces), Pure Squalane ($25 for 1 ounce), Retino A Essence ($36 for 0.17 ounce), Tocophero E Cream ($26 for 1.2 ounces), and Wrinkle Relief ($28 for 0.7 ounce); **Doctor's Dermatologic Formula** ✔☺ Cellular Revitalization Age Renewal ($125 for 1.7 ounces), Dramatic Radiance TRF Cream ($95 for 1.7 ounces), ✔☺ Nourishing Eye Cream ($37 for 1 ounce), and After Sun Security ($22 for 8 ounces); **Dr. Jeannette Graf, M.D.** ✔☺ Overnight Recovery Treatment ($24.50 for 2 ounces); **Dr. LeWinn's Private Formula** ✔☺ Advanced Night Cream ($54.50 for 56 grams); **Dr. Mary Lupo Skin Care System** Intensive Target Moisturizer ($39.70 for 1 ounce) and Vivifying Serum C ($39.95 for 1 ounce); **Ellen Lange Skin Care** ✔☺ MicroThera Eye Care ($32 for 0.5 ounce), MacroThera P.M. ($42 for 1.4 ounces), MacroThera Eye Care ($34 for 0.35 ounce), and ✔☺ MultiDose Serum Therapy ($36 for 1 ounce); **Elizabeth Arden** Ceramide Advanced Time Complex Capsules ($59 for 60 capsules), Ceramide Defining Eye Brightener ($42.50 for 0.5 ounce), ✔☺ Ceramide Defining Skin Brightener ($49.50 for 1.7 ounces), ✔☺ Ceramide Firm Lift, Intensive Lotion for Face and Throat ($46 for 1 ounce), ✔☺ Ceramide Night Intensive Repair Cream ($46 for 1 ounce), ✔☺ Ceramide Time Complex Moisture Cream ($46 for 1.7 ounces), ✔☺ Millennium Energist Revitalizing Emulsion ($60 for 1.7 ounces), and Visible Difference

Perpetual Moisture ($30 for 1.7 ounces); **Elizabeth Grant** Intensive Eye Cream ($29.99 for 0.5 ounce); **Epicuren** Botanical Elixir ($48 for 1 ounce), CXc Stabilized Vitamin C Topical ($172 for 2 ounces), Eye Cream ($56 for 0.5 ounce), Pro-Collagen III ($30 for 0.33 ounce), and Ultra Rose Treat Emulsion ($71 for 4 ounces); **Erno Laszlo** ✔☺ Antioxidant Concentrate for Eyes, Intensive Therapy for the Eye Area ($48 for 0.5 ounce), ✔☺ Antioxidant Moisture Complex Cream for Extremely Dry to Normal Skin ($67 for 2 ounces), ✔☺ Retexturizing SAP Complex ($67 for 1 ounce), HydrapHel Emulsion AM Moisturizer for Extremely Dry and Dry Skin ($50 for 2 ounces), and ✔☺ C10 Radiance Cream ($62 for 1.05 ounces); **Estee Lauder** Re-Nutriv Creme ($78 for 1.75 ounces), Re-Nutriv Firming Throat Creme ($55 for 1.7 ounces), Re-Nutriv Intensive Lifting Creme ($150 for 1.7 ounces), Estee Lauder Re-Nutriv Intensive Lifting Series ($250 for 14 vials, total 0.95 ounce), ✔☺ Re-Nutriv Ultimate Lifting Cream ($250 for 1.7 ounces), Resilience Lift Overnight ($70 for 1.7 ounces), ✔☺ Verite Calming Fluid ($60 for 1.7 ounces), ✔☺ Verite Special Eye Care ($50 for 1.7 ounces), ✔☺ Advanced Night Repair Protective Recovery Complex ($70 for 1.7 ounces), ✔☺ Advanced Night Repair Eye Recovery Complex ($45 for 0.5 ounce), ✔☺ Estoderme Emulsion ($27.50 for 4 ounces), ✔☺ Future Perfect Micro-Targeted Skin Gel ($45 for 1.75 ounces), ✔☺ Idealist ($42.50 for 1 ounce), Skin Perfecting Creme Firming Nourisher ($35 for 1.75 ounces), and ✔☺ Nutritious Bio Protein ($45 for 1.7 ounces); **Exuviance** Evening Restorative Complex ($27.50 for 1.75 ounces) and Hydrating Lift Eye Complex ($24.50 for 0.5 ounce); **Gatineau** Melatogenine Eye-Care Cream ($45 for 0.5 ounce), Laser Radiance Contour Serum ($45 for 0.5 ounce), Laser Radiance Day Moisturizer ($55 for 0.8 ounce), and Laser Radiance Night Moisturizer ($65 for 1.6 ounces); **Glymed Plus** ✔☺ Cell Science Daily Skin Repair Cream ($68.25 for 2 ounces), ✔☺ Cell Science Daily Cell Repair Serum ($68.25 for 0.5 ounce), ✔☺ Vitamin C Cream ($82.95 for 2 ounces), and Vitamin C Serum ($67.95 for 0.5 ounce); **G.M. Collin** ✔☺ Sensiderm Cream ($34 for 1.7 ounces), Hydramucine Cream ($30 for 1.7 ounces), ✔☺ Nutrivital Cream ($33.50 for 1.7 ounces), and ✔☺ Phyto-Lipidic Complex ($35 for 0.8 ounce); **H2O+ Skin Care** ✔☺ Eye Mender Restorative Firming Treatment ($25 for 0.5 ounce), ✔☺ Eye Oasis Moisture Replenishing Treatment ($22.50 for 0.5 ounce), ✔☺ Face Oasis Hydrating Treatment ($32 for 1.7 ounces), ✔☺ Green Tea Antioxidant Face Complex ($32 for 1.7 ounces), ✔☺ Instant Lift Eye Serum ($28 for 0.95 ounce), ✔☺ Intensive Night Recovery Complex ($30 for 1.7 ounces), Intensive Night Repair Supplement ($24 for 1 ounce), and Waterwhite Brightening Night Cream ($40 for 1.7 ounces); **Helena Rubinstein** Face Sculptor Line Lift Cream ($75 for 1.7 ounces), Throat Sculptor Lift Up Cream ($65 for 1.7 ounces), Eye Sculptor with Pro Phosphor ($52 for 0.5 ounce), Face Sculptor Concentrated Line Lift Serum ($78 for 1 ounce), Force C Premium Super Anti Fatigue Eye Care ($42 for 0.5 ounce), and Force C Premium Super Energizing Cream ($56 for 1.7 ounces); **Hydron** Best Defense Fragile Eye Moisturizer ($22.50 for 0.5 ounce), ✔☺ Best Defense Moisture Balance Restorative Overnight Liposome Complex ($29.75 for 2 ounces), and ✔☺ Hydronamins Moisturizing Vitamin Therapy Night Creme ($36.75 for 2 ounces); **Iman** Time Control Renewal Complex ($29.50 for 1 ounce); **Jafra** ✔☺ Time Corrector Firming Moisture Cream ($38 for 1.7 ounces), Time Protector Eye Cream ($21 for 0.5 ounce), Night Cream Moisturizer for Dry to Normal Skin ($17.50 for 1.7 ounces), and ✔☺ Elasticity Recovery Hydrogel ($35 for 1 ounce); **Jan Marini Skin Research** Age Intervention Face Cream ($75 for 1 ounce), Age Intervention Face Serum ($75 for 1 ounce), ✔☺ C-Esta Cream ($75 for 1 ounce), and ✔☺ C-Esta Eye Contour Cream ($40 for 0.5 ounce); **Jason Natural** Hemp Plus Oil Enriched with Natural EFA's Moisturizing Creme ($9 for 1 ounce), Hemp Plus Oil Enriched with EFA's ($9.50 for 4 ounces), Perfect Solutions Ester-C Moisture Creme, Daily Age Defense ($16.50 for 2 ounces), Suma Moist Active Creme Concentrate with Live Yeast Cell Extracts ($9 for 2 ounces), Super E Creme, Super Moisture Creme, 25,000 I.U. ($11 for 4 ounces), Vitamin E All Purpose Moisturizing Creme, 5,000 I.U. ($6 for 4 ounces), Pure Vitamin E Oil 14,000 I.U. ($6 for 1 ounce), Vitamin E Oil 5,000 I.U. ($6 for 4 ounces), Vitamin E Oil Blend 45,000 I.U. ($10.50 for 2 ounces), Vitamin K Creme with Bioflavonoids and Calendula ($20 for 2 ounces), ✔☺ Hyper-C Serum Anti-Aging Therapy ($50 for 1 ounce), ✔☺ Ultra-C Eye Lift Treatment ($20 for 0.5 ounce), New Cell Therapy 3-1/2 Plus Gentle Eye Gel with Alpha Hydroxy Acids ($12.99 for 1 ounce), Skin-amins Topical Vitamin Therapy Hi-Vitamin A Complex with MSM, 10,000 I.U. ($10 for 2 ounces), Skin-amins Topical Vitamin Therapy Hi-Vitamin B Complex with MSM, 3,000 milligrams ($10 for 2 ounces), Skin-amins Topical Vitamin Therapy Hi-Vitamin C Complex with MSM, 3,000 milligrams ($10 for 2 ounces), Skin-amins Topical Vitamin Therapy Hi-Vitamin D Complex with MSM, 12,000 I.U. ($7.99 for 2 ounces), Skin-amins Topical Vitamin Therapy Hi-Vitamin E Complex with MSM, 10,000 I.U. ($7.99 for 2 ounces), and Skin-amins Topical Vitamin Therapy Hi-Vitamin H,F,K, Complex with MSM, 6,000 mg ($11.99 for 2 ounces); **Jurlique International** Day Care Face Cream ($30.50 for 1.4 ounces), Day Care Face Lotion ($33 for 1 ounce), Wrinkle Softener Beauty Cream ($24 for 0.3 ounce), and Skin Bronzer ($34 for 1 ounce); **Kiehl's** Panthenol Protein Moisturizing Face Cream ($23.50 for 4 ounces) and All Night Olive & Aloe Moisture Creme ($10 for 3.75 ounces); **Kiss My Face** Vitamin C & A Ultra Rich Moisturizer ($15 for 1 ounce), A, C, & E Eye Opener ($15 for 0.5 ounce), and Organic Botanical Lifting Serum ($12 for 1 ounce); **L'Oreal** ✔☺ Age Perfect Anti-Sagging and Ultra-Hydrating Cream Eye ($13.99 for 0.5 ounces); **La Mer** Serum de la Mer ($175 for 1 ounce); **La Prairie** ✔☺ Cellular Hydrating Serum ($150 for 1 ounce), ✔☺ Age Management Eye Repair ($100 for 0.5 ounce), Age Management Night Cream ($125 for 1 ounce), and Extrait of Skin Caviar Firming Complex ($100 for 1 ounce); **Lancome** Impactive Multi Performance Silkening Moisturizer ($38 for 1.7 ounces); **Laura Mercier** ✔☺ Eyedration Firming Eye Cream ($35 for 0.5 ounce); **Liz Earle Naturally Active Skin Care** Daily Eye Repair ($21.68 for 0.5 ounce); **M.A.C.** Moisture Feed Eye ($25 for 0.5 ounce), ✔☺ Fast Response Eye Cream ($25 for 0.5 ounce), Studio Moisture Fix ($22 for 1.7 ounces), and

✔☺ Strobe Cream ($25 for 1.7 ounces); **Marcelle** Anti-Wrinkle Cream with Collagen & Elastin ($15.75 for 40 ml); **Marilyn Miglin** Estrosoy Concentrate with Collagen ($35 for 0.5 ounce); **Mario Badescu** Ceramide Complex with NMF and AHA ($35 for 1 ounce), Dermonectin Eye Cream ($18 for 0.5 ounce), Vitacel Moist Cream ($18 for 1 ounce), and Revitalizing Night Cream ($40 for 1 ounce); **Mary Kay** Instant Action Eye Cream ($15 for 0.65 ounce); **M.D. Formulations** ✔☺ Moisture Defense Antioxidant Creme ($55 for 1 ounce), ✔☺ Moisture Defense Antioxidant Hydrating Serum ($42 for 1 ounce), Moisture Defense Antioxidant Treatment Masque ($26 for 2.5 ounces); **M.D. Forte** ✔☺ Replenish Hydrating Cream ($39 for 2 ounces); **Merle Norman** Luxiva Delicate Balance Moisturizer, for Sensitive Skin ($38 for 1.7 ounces), Luxiva Firming Neck and Chest Creme ($34.50 for 2 ounces), Luxiva Moisture Rich Facial Treatment ($20 for 3 ounces), and Luxiva Nighttime Recovery Creme ($38 for 2 ounces); **Murad** ✔☺ Environmental Shield Essential Night Moisture ($48 for 1.4 ounces), Environmental Shield Daily Renewal Complex ($80 for 1.4 ounces), and ✔☺ Perfecting Night Cream ($34 for 2.25 ounces); **Natura Bisse** Essential Shock Night Cream for Dry Skin ($95 for 2.5 ounces), ✔☺ Diamond Bio-Lift Eye Contour Cream ($130 for 0.8 ounce), and ✔☺ Diamond Anti-Aging Bio-Regenerative Cream for Dry Skin ($235 for 1.7 ounces); **Neutrogena** Eye Cream ($11.99 for 0.5 ounce); **Neways Skin Care** Retention Plus ($34.60 for 1 ounce), Skin Brightener ($31.50 for 4.2 ounces), Skin Enhancer Beauty Lotion ($31.50 for 4 ounces), Wrinkle Drops ($85 for 0.5 ounce), Wrinkle Gard ($37.90 for 1 ounce), and Rebound After Sun Lotion ($29.40 for 4.2 ounces); **Noevir** ✔☺ Intensive Anti-Wrinkle Treatment ($35 for 0.6 ounce); **Nu Skin** Intensive Eye Complex Moisturizing Cream ($36 for 0.75 ounce), Moisture Restore Intense Moisturizer ($28 for 2.5 ounces), Night Supply Nourishing Cream ($35 for 1.7 ounces), Night Supply Nourishing Lotion ($35 for 1.7 ounces), and Night Complex ($64 for 1 ounce); **Nutrifirm Isomers** Absolute Wrinkle Defense Cream ($39.99 for 3 ounces), Enzyme Therapy Treatment Cream ($39.99 for 2 ounces), Gemmotherapy Cream ($39.99 for 3 ounces), and Resurgence Gemmotherapy Nucleus Cream ($39.95 for 2 ounces); **N.V. Perricone, M.D.** Vitamin C Ester Amine Complex Face Lift with NTP Complex ($75 for 2 ounces), Vitamin C Ester 15% Concentrated Restorative Cream with NTP Complex ($90 for 1.86 ounces), Vitamin C Ester Eye Area Therapy ($45 for 1 ounce), Alpha Lipoic Acid Anti Spider-Vein Face Treatment with Tocotrienols ($80 for 1 ounce), Phosphatidyl-E Lipid Bi-Layer Repair Face Treatment with Tocotrienols ($120 for 2 ounces), Olive Oil Polyphenols Day Face Treatment ($85 for 2 ounces), Olive Oil Polyphenols Night Face Treatment ($85 for 2 ounces), Olive Oil Polyphenols Face Hydrator ($65 for 1.7 ounces), and Pore Refining Moisturizer ($55 for 2 ounces); **Olay** Total Effects Intensive Restoration Treatment ($19.99 for 1.01 ounces) and Total Effects Night Firming Creme for Face and Neck ($19.99 for 1.7 ounces); **Ole Henriksen Skin Care** ✔☺ Fresh Start Eye Cream ($35 for 1 ounce); **Origins** ✔☺ Calm Balm Sensitive Skin Eye Creme ($25 for 0.5 ounce), Look Alive Vitality Moisture Cream ($18.50 for 1.7 ounces), Night-A-Mins

Cream ($27.50 for 1.7 ounces), Night-A-Mins Lotion (28.50 for 1.7 ounces), Steady Drencher, If Your Young Skin Acts Dry ($22.50 for 1.7 ounces), and Time Mender, If Your Skin Acts Older Than You'd Like ($22 for 1.7 ounces); **Orlane** B21 Purete Hydro Matifying Care ($100 for 1.7 ounces), B21 Bio-Energic Absolute Youth Concentrate Age Defense Protective Oxytoning System for All Skin Types ($300 for 0.7 ounce), B21 Oligo Gentle Soothing Cream for Sensitive Fragile & Allergic Skin Types ($65 for 1.7 ounces), and B21 Oligo Light Smoothing Cream ($65 for 1.7 ounces); **Osmotics** ✓☺ Blue Copper Firming Elasticity Repair ($98 for 2 ounces), ✓☺ Triceram ($30 for 3.4 ounces), Kinetin Cellular Renewal Serum ($78 for 1.7 ounces), Kinetin Intensive Eye Repair ($75 for 0.5 ounce), and Intensive Moisture Therapy ($65 for 2 ounces); **Parthena** ✓☺ Longevity Daily Line Smoothing Fluid ($5.95 for 1 ounce) and ✓☺ Longevity Wonder Serum ($32.50 for 1 ounce); **Paula's Choice** ✓☺ Completely Emollient Moisturizer, Normal to Dry Skin ($13.95 for 4 ounces), ✓☺ Hydrating Treatment Cream, Normal to Dry Skin ($12.95 for 2 ounces), and ✓☺ Super Antioxidant Concentrate, Normal to Dry Skin ($17.95 for 1 ounce); **Peter Thomas Roth** Ceramide Moisture Renewal ($45 for 2 ounces), Power C Eye Complex ($48 for 0.75 ounce), Power C Souffle ($85 for 1.5 ounces), Power K Eye Rescue ($100 for 0.5 ounce), and Power K Skin Brightener ($110 for 1 ounce); **Pevonia Botanica** Evolutive Eye Cream ($36 for 0.7 ounce), Combination Skin Care Cream ($49 for 1.7 ounces), O2ptimale Dry Skin Care Cream ($56 for 1.7 ounces), ✓☺ Collastin Eye Fluid ($52 for 1 ounce), Marine Elastin Cream ($51 for 1.7 ounces), and Marine DNA Cream ($53 for 1.7 ounces); **philosophy** eye believe, eye cream ($27.50 for 0.5 ounce), hope in a jar for dry, sensitive skin ($35 for 2 ounces), and dark shadows, eye balm ($27.50 for 0.5 ounce); **Physician's Choice** pHaze 12 Eye Wrinkle Cream ($25 for 0.5 ounce); **Prescriptives** ✓☺ Px Comfort Lotion ($35 for 1.7 ounces), Px Comfort Cream 24 Hour Care for Sensitive Skin ($37.50 for 1.7 ounces), and Vibrant Vitamin Infuser for Dull, Stressed Skin, Lotion or Cream ($45 for 1.7 ounces); **Principal Secret** ✓☺ Advanced Continuous Lift Serum ($40 for 0.5 ounce), Advanced Eye Conditioner ($34.50 for 0.5 ounce), Advanced EyeSaver Gel ($27 for 0.5 ounce), and ✓☺ Advanced Nighttime Treatment ($35 for 1 ounce); **Rachel Perry** Immediately Visible Eye Renewal Gel-Cream with Liposomes ($27 for 0.5 ounce); **Remede** Alchemy ($72 for 1.7 ounces), Night Eye Contour Barrier Balm Intensive Treatment Creme with SR-38 ($80 for 0.5 ounce), Sensitive Intensive Cream Soothing Skin Formula with SR-38 Night ($135 for 1.7 ounces), and Soothing Treatment Creme Complex Sensitive Delicate Skin Day ($125 for 1.7 ounces); **Revlon** ✓☺ Vitamin C Absolutes Overnight Renewal Cream ($14.89 for 1.6 ounces) and ✓☺ Eye Contour Radiance Cream ($14.89 for 0.45 ounce); **RoC** Revitalizing Night Cream ($30 for 40 ml); **Sense Usana** ✓☺ Night Renewal ($36 for 1.7 ounces), Eye Nourisher ($16.50 for 0.5 ounce), and ✓☺ Perfecting Essence ($45 for 1 ounce); **Serious Skin Care** ✓☺ C-Repair Vitamin C Moisturizing Night Cream ($22.50 for 2 ounces) and ✓☺ Acid-Free Skin Resurfacing Moisturizer ($22 for 4 ounces); **Shaklee** ✓☺ Balancing Moisturizer

($22 for 2 ounces), ✔☺ Eye Treatment ($22 for 0.5 ounce), ✔☺ Hydrating Moisturizer ($22 for 1.7 ounces), and C+E Repair P.M. ($45 for 1 ounce); **Shu Uemura** Regenerate Accelerator ($60 for 0.6 ounce); **SkinCeuticals** ✔☺ Eye Cream ($53 for 0.67 ounce), Skin Firming Cream ($85 for 1.67 ounces), Primacy Eye Balm with Triple Age Defense Technology ($68 for 0.5 ounce), and ✔☺ Primacy Face Cream with Triple Age Defense Technology ($128 for 1.67 ounces); **Sothys Paris** ✔☺ Immuniscience Cream for Sensitive Skin ($32 for 1.7 ounces), ✔☺ Immuniscience Fluid for Ultra-Sensitive Skin ($32 for 1.7 ounces), and Moisturizing Intensive Care Liposomes Hydrogel ($62 for 1.7 ounces); **St. Ives** Hypo-Allergenic Oil-Free Moisturizer ($2.99 for 4 ounces); **Thalgo** Marine Replenishing Serum with BHA ($120 for 1 ounce) and La Creme Day Moisturizer ($70 for 1.7 ounces); **Ultima II** ✔☺ CHR Double Action Night Cream ($45 for 2 ounces), ✔☺ CHR Double Action Eye Cream ($22.50 for 0.5 ounce), ✔☺ Light Captor-C Skin Reviving Day Lotion ($40 for 0.75 ounce), and ✔☺ Light Captor-C Skin Reviving Emulsion ($30 for 0.5 ounce); **University Medical Skin Care** ✔☺ Face Lift Collagen 5 Cell Regeneration Cream ($14.97 for 1.5 ounces), ✔☺ Face Lift Collagen 5 Intensive Lifting Complex ($12.97 for 1.5 ounces), and Face Lift Advanced Under Eye Therapy ($10.97 for 0.5 ounce); **Vichy** Thermal S1: Long Lasting Hydration ($26 for 50 ml) and Thermal S2: Long Lasting Hydration for Very Dehydrated Skin ($26 for 50 ml); **Victoria Jackson Cosmetics** ✔☺ Skin Renewal System ($40.95 for 0.14 ounce of Extra-Intensive Eye Cream and 1.25 ounces of Extra-Intensive Night Cream); **Z. Bigatti** Re-Storation Deep Repair Facial Serum ($195 for 1 ounce), Re-Storation Eye Return ($115 for 0.5 ounce), Re-Storation Delicate Intensive Moisturizing Facial Treatment ($150 for 2 ounces), Re-Storation Skin Treatment Facial Lotion ($150 for 2 ounces), Re-Storation Vitamin and Antioxidant Skin Treatment ($150 for 2 ounces or $500 for 8 ounces), and Re-Storation Swan Neck Firming Treatment ($128 for 1 ounce); **Zia** Nourishing Creme Cellular Renewal for Severely Dry Skin ($32.75 for 1 ounce), ✔☺ Ultimate "C" Serum ($39.95 for 0.5 ounce), and ✔☺ Ultimate Moisture ($34.95 for 1.5 ounces).

BEST MOISTURIZERS FOR DRY TO VERY DRY SKIN: **Alexandra de Markoff** Skin Tight Firming Eye Cream ($52.50 for 0.35 ounce); **Annemarie Börlind** LL Bi Aktiv Regeneration, LL Wrinkle Cream ($41.75 for 1 ounce); **Arbonne** Skin Conditioning Oil ($16.50 for 1 ounce); **Avon beComing** Evening Retreat Intensive Moisture Cream ($20 for 1.7 ounces); **Beauty Without Cruelty** ✔☺ Maximum Moisture Cream Benefits Dry/Mature Skin ($14.49 for 2 ounces); **BioTherm** D-Stress Fortifying Anti-Fatigue Radiance Cream Dry Skin ($28.50 for 1.7 ounces) and D-Stress Relaxing Night Care Anti-Fatigue Radiance Cream Dry Skin ($35 for 1.7 ounces); **Caudalie** Facial Treatment Oil for Dry Dehydrated Skin ($51 for 1 ounce); **Dr. Jeannette Graf, M.D.** Moisturizing Face Cream ($22.50 for 2.25 ounces); **Ellen Lange Skin Care** MicroThera P.M. ($40 for 1.5 ounces); **Estee Lauder** ✔☺ Swiss Performing Extract Moisturizer ($25 for 1.7 ounces); **Paula's Choice** ✔☺ Extra Emollient Moisturizer, Normal to Extra Dry Skin ($13.95 for 4 ounces), ✔☺ Skin Recovery Moisturizer, Dry to Extra Dry Skin ($13.95 for 4 ounces),

Peter Thomas Roth Ceramide Ultra-Rich Night Renewal ($55 for 2 ounces) and Ceramide Eye Complex ($48 for 0.75 ounce).

BEST MOISTURIZERS CONTAINING RETINOL: **Alpha Hydrox** Retinol Night ResQ Anti-Wrinkle Firming Complex ($11.99 for 1.05 ounces); **Aveeno** ✔☺ Skin Brightening Daily Moisturizer SPF 15 ($14.99 for 1 ounce) and Skin Brightening Daily Moisturizer ($14.99 for 1 ounce); **Avon** Anew Line Eliminator Dual Retinol Treatment ($16 for 1 ounce); **Avon beComing** ✔☺ Skinfusion Renewal Complex Night ($40 for 1.7 ounces); **BeautiControl** Regeneration Time to Go with Retinol ($35 for 1 ounce); **BioMedic** Retinol Creme 15 ($30.95 for 1 ounce), Retinol Creme 30 ($30.95 for 1 ounce), and Retinol Creme 60 ($30.95 for 1 ounce); **BioTherm** Retinol Smoothing Anti-Wrinkle Care ($35.50 for 1 ounce) and Retinol Eye & Lip ($35 for 0.5 ounces); **Cetaphil** ✔☺ Nighttime Facial Moisturizer with Retinol ($12.95 for 1.05 ounces); **Doctor's Dermatologic Formula** Retinol Energizing Moisturizer ($85 for 2 ounces); ✔☺ Retinol Energizing Serum with Protein Complex ($70 for 1 ounce), ✔☺ Retinol Eye Renewal ($49 for 0.5 ounce), and ✔☺ Silky-C Serum ($65 for 1 ounce); **Erno Laszlo** Retinol Reparative Therapy ($87 for 1 ounce) and Retinol Reparative Therapy for Eyes ($69 for 0.5 ounce); **Estee Lauder** ✔☺ Re-Nutriv Intensive Lifting Serum ($170 for 1 ounce) and ✔☺ Diminish Retinol Treatment ($70 for 1.7 ounces); **G.M. Collin** ✔☺ Retinol Action + Q10 Vitamin A Skin Care ($56 for 1.7 ounces); **H2O+ Skin Care** Line Defense Retinol Complex ($38 for 1 ounce); **Helena Rubinstein** Power A for Eyes Pure Retinol Repair System ($55 for 0.5 ounce); **Jafra** Intensive Retinol Treatment ($40 for 30 capsules); **Jan Marini Skin Research** Factor-A Cream ($45 for 1 ounce) and Factor-A Lotion ($40 for 1 ounce); **Karin Herzog Skin Care** Additional Night Cream ($32 for 1.76 ounces); **L'Oreal** Line Eraser Pure Retinol Concentrate ($14.99 for 1 ounce); **La Prairie** Cellular Retinol Complex PM ($150 for 1 ounce) and Age Management Stimulus Complex for the Eyes ($125 for 0.5 ounce); **Lancome** ReSurface ($52.50 for 1 ounce) and ReSurface Eye ($44 for 0.5 ounce); **Mary Kay** Lumineyes Dark Circle Diminisher ($28 for 0.5 ounce); **M.D. Forte** Rejuvenating Eye Cream ($46 for 0.5 ounce); **Neutrogena** Healthy Skin Anti-Wrinkle Cream with Retinol ($10.99 for 1.4 ounces); **Neways Skin Care** Night Science ($29.95 for 2 ounces); **Nu Skin** ✔☺ Ideal Eyes Vitamins C & A Eye Refining Creme ($40 for 0.5 ounce); **N.V. Perricone, M.D.** ✔☺ Alpha Lipoic Acid Evening Facial Emollient with NTP Complex and Retinol ($80 for 2 ounces); **Parthena** Cream International AM ($16.50 for 2 ounces); **Pevonia Botanica** ✔☺ Youthful Lip Cream ($40 for 0.7 ounce) and ✔☺ Youthful Lip Serum ($36 for 0.5 ounce); **philosophy** help me, retinol night cream ($45 for 1.05 ounces); **Prescriptives** Px Retinol LSW ($50 for 1 ounce); **RoC** ✔☺ Retinol Actif Pur Anti-Wrinkle Treatment, Day, SPF 15 ($16.99 for 1.01 ounces), Retinol A+C+E Triple Action Day/Night ($38 for 30 ml), Retinol Actif Pur Skin Refining Treatment ($17.99 for 1.35 ounces), and Retinol Actif Pur, Eye Contour Cream ($16.99 for 0.51 ounce); **Serious Skin Care** A-Eye Vitamin A Eye Cream with Retinol ($21 for 0.5 ounce); **Sothys Paris** Retinol 15 ($48 for 1.05 ounces); **St. Ives**

Multi-Vitamin Retinol Anti-Wrinkle Cream ($8.99 for 1.05 ounces), Vitamin A Anti-Wrinkle Serum ($6.99 for 14 0.16-ounce capsules), and Vitamin K Dark Circle Diminisher Under Eye Treatment ($8.99 for 0.5 ounce); **University Medical Skin Care** Nighttime Advanced Retinol-A ($13.97 for 1 ounce); **Vichy** RETI-C Concentrate Night ($37.50 for 30 ml) and RETI-C Yeux Eyes ($30 for 15 ml).

BEST SUNSCREENS

Many, if not most, of the changes that take place on our skin over the years, such as wrinkles, skin discolorations, loss of elasticity, texture problems, and dryness, are the result of sun damage from exposure to the sun without appropriate or adequate sun protection. Sunscreens are essential for skin care day in and day out, 365 days a year. If applied correctly (meaning liberally and frequently reapplied), they are the only true antiwrinkle product. They can also potentially help prevent some forms of skin cancer. If you are not using a sunscreen of some kind (lotion, cream, gel, serum, or foundation with sunscreen) with SPF 15 or greater and that contains the UVA-protecting ingredients of either avobenzone, zinc oxide, or titanium dioxide (or Mexoryl SX outside of the United States), then you are doing nothing of value for the long-term health of your skin. All of the antiwrinkle, firming, antiaging, or rejuvenating products in the world are completely and totally useless if you are not protecting your skin from the sun. It is of vital importance to the health of your skin to include a well-formulated sunscreen in your daily skin-care regime. Arguably, the most unethical thing the cosmetics industry does is sell women a plethora of skin-care products that more often than not do not include reliable sun protection.

As you look over the lists for this category, you will notice there are many more sunscreens for normal to dry skin than for normal to oily skin. The reason for this, which is not reassuring for those with oily skin or skin prone to breakouts, is that sunscreen agents work better in an emollient emulsion than in a matte base or liquid. When a lightweight liquid is available, the base often includes alcohol, and that is hard on skin due to the irritation it can cause. Plus, on oily skin, the non-sensitizing UVA-protecting ingredients of zinc oxide and titanium dioxide can clog pores or feel heavy.

For the face, someone with oily skin may prefer to use a foundation with a good SPF, and from the neck down a well-formulated sunscreen. This is one area of skin care that is difficult for someone with oily skin, and it takes experimentation to find what works well for you.

All of the following sunscreens are awarded happy faces because they have an SPF of 15 or greater and they contain either avobenzone, titanium dioxide, or zinc oxide (or Mexoryl SX outside of the United States) as one or more of the active ingredients (if these are listed someplace else on the ingredient list, it does not count toward reliable sun protection). Avobenzone may be listed on an ingredient label as Parsol 1789 or butyl methoxydibenzoylmethane. The difference in the costs of the different sunscreen products are strictly the result of the caprice of cosmetics companies, and are not indicative of any special qualities whatsoever. However, products rated as Paula's Picks contain decent to impressive amounts of water-binding agents, antioxidants, or anti-irritants because there is research indicating that using antioxidants during the day helps reduce the amount of free-radical damage resulting from the sun, oxygen, and pollution.

BEST SUNSCREENS FOR NORMAL TO SLIGHTLY DRY OR COMBINATION SKIN: **Adrien Arpel's Signature Club A** Flower Acid Wrinkle Remedy Day Face Creme with Sunscreen SPF 20 ($15.50 for 2 ounces); **Almay** Kinetin Age Decelerating Daily Lotion SPF 15 ($18 for 4 ounces) and Age Decelerating Daily Cream SPF 15 ($18 for 1.6 ounces); **Artistry by Amway** ✓☺ Clarifying Balancing Moisturizer for Normal to Oily Skin SPF 15 ($24.45 for 2.5 ounces); **Bain de Soleil** Oil-Free Protecteur Sunscreen Spray, SPF 25 ($8.99 for 4 ounces), VitaSkin Lotion Facial Care SPF 30 ($9.99 for 5.7 ounces), VitaSkin Lotion SPF 15 ($9.99 for 6 ounces), and VitaSkin Lotion SPF 30 ($9.99 for 6 ounces); **Banana Boat** Ultra Sunblock Quick Dry Spray SPF 30 ($8.99 for 6 ounces) and Active Sport Sunblock Gel SPF 30 ($8.99 for 6 ounces); **BioMedic** Facial Shield SPF 20 ($19.95 for 2 ounces); **BioTherm** Age Fitness Active Revitalizing Age Treatment SPF 15, for Normal to Combination Skin ($35 for 1.7 ounces) and Special Wrinkle Sun Block SPF 15 ($15 for 1.7 ounces); **The Body Shop** Aloe & Chamomile Oil Free Face Lotion SPF 25 ($12 for 2.5 ounces); **Calvin Klein** Protective Moisture Lotion SPF 15 ($30 for 1.7 ounces); **Chanel** Fluide Multi-Protection Daily Protection Lotion SPF 25 ($26 for 1 ounce), Skin Conscience Total Health Oil-Free Moisture Fluid SPF 15 ($45 for 1.7 ounces), and Skin Conscience Total Health Moisture Cream SPF 15 ($45 for 1.7 ounces); **Clarins** Moisture Quenching Hydra-Balance Lotion SPF 15 ($48.50 for 1.7 ounces); **Club Monaco** Face Day Protection Fluid SPF 15 ($19 for 1.7 ounces); **Coppertone** Sunblock Lotion SPF 30 ($6.99 for 4 ounces), Sunblock Lotion Spray SPF 30 ($8.99 for 7 ounces), Shade Sunblock Lotion, SPF 45, UVA/UVB Protection ($7.99 for 4 ounces), and Oil Free Sunblock Lotion for Faces SPF 30 ($7.99 for 3 ounces); **Dr. Mary Lupo Skin Care System** Full Spectrum Sunscreen UVA/UVB SPF 27 ($17.50 for 3 ounces); **Elizabeth Arden** Triple Protection Oil Free Sunblock SPF 15 ($18.50 for 4.2 ounces), ✓☺ Triple Protection Face Block SPF 30 ($19.50 for 4.2 ounces), and Triple Protection Sunblock Spray SPF 15 ($18.50 for 4.2 ounces); **Epicuren** ✓☺ YouthTeen SPF 30 Sun Protection ($34 for 4 ounces); **G.M. Collin** SPF 30 Total Sunblock ($27 for 5 ounces), SPF 15 Sun Protection ($25 for 5 ounces), and SPF 14 Spray Lotion ($25 for 5 ounces); **Helena Rubinstein** Force C Premium Super Energizing Fluid Vitamin C Time Release SPF 15 ($56 for 4.2 ounces) and Golden Defense SPF 15 Moisturizing Sun Lotion ($26.50 for 5.07 ounces); **Hydron** Best Defense Daily Facial Moisturizer Oil-Free with SPF 15 ($26 for 2 ounces) and Sunblock Cream SPF 15 ($12.50 for 4.2 ounces); **Jafra** Sunblock Cream SPF 30 ($12 for 4.2 ounces); **Jan Marini Skin Research** Bioglycolic Facial Lotion SPF 15 ($45 for 2 ounces); **Jason Natural** Moisture Plus SPF 15 ($9 for 4 ounces); **Kiehl's** Klaus Heidegger's All-Sport Water-Resistant Skin Protector with SPF 25 ($19 for 4 ounces); **L'Occitane** Protective Lotion SPF 15 ($34 for 1 ounce); **Lancome** SPF 15

Face and Body Lotion with Pure Vitamin E ($25 for 5 ounces), UV Expert SPF 15 Water Light Fluid ($31 for 1 ounce), and SPF 25 Face and Body Lotion with Pure Vitamin E ($25 for 5 ounces); **Neostrata** ✓☺ Oil Free Lotion SPF 15 PHA 4 ($28 for 1.75 ounces); **Nu Skin** Sunright Body Block SPF 30 ($13 for 3.4 ounces) and Sunright Body Block SPF 15 ($13 for 3.4 ounces); **Olay** ProVital Protective Moisture Lotion SPF 15 ($8.99 for 4 ounces); **Parthena** Intercept SPF 30 Spray ($6.95 for 2 ounces); ✓☺ **Paula's Choice** Essential Non-Greasy Sunscreen SPF 15, Normal to Oily Skin ($12.95 for 6 ounces) and ✓☺ Extra Care Non-Greasy Sunscreen SPF 30+ with Antioxidants Water-Resistant, Normal to Oily Skin ($12.95 for 6 ounces); **philosophy** shelter, moisturizing SPF 15 facial sunblock ($16 for 2 ounces); **Pola** 1/f Sunscreen Face SPF 30 ($24 for 1 ounce); **ProActiv** Oil Free Moisture with SPF 15 ($25 for 1.7 ounces); **Purpose** Intensive Daily Moisturizer SPF 15 Protection ($8.49 for 4 ounces); **Shiseido** Ultra Light Sun Block Lotion SPF 30 ($27 for 3.3 ounces); **Urban Decay** Guardian Angel Protective Oil-Free Moisturizer SPF 15 ($20 for 1.7 ounces).

BEST SUNSCREENS FOR NORMAL TO DRY AND EXTRA DRY SKIN: **Almay** Milk Plus Nourishing Facial Lotion SPF 15 Normal to Oily Skin ($10.93 for 4.2 ounces) and Nourishing Facial Cream SPF 15 Normal to Dry Skin ($10.93 for 2 ounces); **Arbonne** ✓☺ Take Cover for Face and Body SPF30+ (18.50 for 4 ounces); **Artistry by Amway** ✓☺ Moisture Rich Moisturizer for Normal to Dry Skin SPF 15 ($24.45 for 2.5 ounces); **Aubrey Organics** Sun Shade Ultra 15 Tanning Cream SPF 15 ($7.25 for 4 ounces), Green Tea Sunblock for Children SPF 25 ($8.50 for 4 ounces), and Titania Full Spectrum Sunblock SPF 25 ($8 for 4 ounces); **Aveda** ✓☺ Daily Light Guard SPF 15 ($16.50 for 5 ounces); **Aveeno** ✓☺ Radiant Skin Daily Moisturizer SPF 15 ($13.99 for 4 ounces); **Avon** ✓☺ Anew Force Extra Triple Lifting Day Cream SPF 15 ($22 for 1.7 ounces), ✓☺ Anew Force Extra Triple Lifting Day Lotion SPF 15 ($22 for 1.7 ounces), Anew Luminosity Skin Brightener SPF 15 ($20 for 1.7 ounces), ✓☺ Anew Positivity Empowering A.M. Fortifier, SPF 15 ($20 for 1 ounce), Anew Instant Eye Smoother, SPF 15 ($16.50 for 0.5 ounces), ✓☺ Anew Perfect Eye Care Cream SPF 15 ($13.50 for 0.53 ounce), ✓☺ Age Block Environmental Protection Cream SPF 15 ($12.50 for 1.7 ounces), ✓☺ Sun-So-Soft SPF 25 Sunscreen Stick ($7.50 for 0.42 ounce), Sun-So-Soft SPF 40 Sunscreen Lotion for Kids ($9 for 4.2 ounces), Sun-So-Soft Sunscreen Lotion SPF 15 ($8.50 for 4.2 ounces), and Sun-So-Soft Sunscreen Lotion SPF 30 ($8.50 for 4.2 ounces); **Avon beComing** ✓☺ Skinfusion Revitalizing Complex SPF 15 ($40 for 1.7 ounces), Resist the Elements SPF 15 Sunscreen Body ($13.50 for 2 ounces), and ✓☺ Resist the Elements SPF 30 Sunscreen Face ($13.50 for 2 ounces); **B. Kamins** Maple Treatment Cream SPF 15 ($88 for 2 ounces) and Sunbar Sunscreen SPF 30, Fragrance and Fragrance-Free versions ($29 for 4 ounces); **Banana Boat** VitaSkin Lotion SPF 50 ($9.99 for 6 ounces), Sunblock Spray Lotion SPF 48 ($8.99 for 6 ounces), Baby Block Sunblock Lotion SPF 50 ($8.99 for 4 ounces), and Kids Sunblock Spray Lotion SPF 48 ($8.99 for 6 ounces); **Bath & Body Works** Hydrating Day Creme with SPF 15 ($12 for 2 ounces);

BeautiControl Cell Block-C New Cell Protection SPF 20 ($30 for 0.95 ounce) and Sunlogics Waterproof Sunblock SPF 30 ($15 for 4.5 ounces); **Beauty Without Cruelty** ✔☺ SPF 15 Daily Facial Lotion, Benefits All Skin Types ($9.49 for 4 ounces); **Bioelements** ✔☺ Year-Round Protector SPF 30+ Moisturizer ($45 for 2.5 ounces); **BioMedic** Gentle Moisturizing Emulsion SPF 20 ($17.95 for 2 ounces); **BioTherm** Age Fitness Age Fitness Active Revitalizing Age Treatment SPF 15, for Dry Skin ($35 for 1.7 ounces), Aquasource UV SPF 15 ($25 for 1.7 ounces), UV Protect SPF 25 ($14.50 for 1 ounce), High Protection Sun Block SPF 30 ($15 for 1.7 ounces), High Protection Sun Block SPF 25 ($15 for 1.7 ounces), Sun Block Lotion High Protection SPF 25 ($15 for 5 ounces), and Protective Lotion SPF 15 ($15 for 5 ounces); **Bobbi Brown** Hydrating Face Lotion SPF 15 ($38 for 1.7 ounces) and Extra Moisturizing Balm SPF 25 ($75 for 1.7 ounces); **The Body Shop** ✔☺ Vitamin C Protective Daywear Moisturizer with SPF 15 ($12 for 2.5 ounces), Vitamin E Facial Day Lotion SPF 15 ($12 for 2.5 ounces), Aloe & Chamomile Sun Protection Body Lotion SPF 25 ($15 for 5.7 ounces), and Shea Self-Tanning Lotion SPF 15 ($15 for 6 ounces); **Calvin Klein** Protective Moisture Cream SPF 15 ($30 for 1.7 ounces); **Cellex-C** Sun Care SPF 30 ($35 for 4 ounces), Sun Care SPF 30+ ($25 for 3.3 ounces), and Sun Care SPF 15 ($33 for 4 ounces); **CamoCare** EPF Daily Facial Moisturizer SPF 15 ($19.95 for 1 ounce); **Cetaphil** Daily Facial Moisturizer SPF 15 ($7.99 for 4 ounces); **Chanel** ✔☺ Rectifiance Day Lift Refining Cream SPF 15 ($60 for 1.7 ounces) and ✔☺ Rectifiance Day Lift Refining Lotion SPF 15 ($50 for 1.7 ounces); **Christian Dior Snow** Ultra Protection UV 30 Face Coat ($31 for 1 ounce) and Snow UV SPF 35 ($60 for 1.9 ounces); **Clarins** Extra-Firming Day Lotion SPF 15 ($57.50 for 1.7 ounces), ✔☺ Hydration-Plus Moisture Lotion SPF 15 for All Skin Types ($38.50 for 1.7 ounces), Sun Care Cream SPF 20 ($30 for 7 ounces), Sun Wrinkle Control Cream SPF 15 ($24 for 2.7 ounces), and Sun Wrinkle Control Cream SPF 30 ($24 for 2.7 ounces); **Clientele Time Therapy** ✔☺ Day Serum SPF 25 for Normal/Dry, Sensitive Skin ($49 for 1 ounce) and Day Serum SPF 25 for Normal/Oily Skin ($49 for 1 ounce); **Clientele Elastology** ✔☺ Age Blocker with SPF 25 ($75 for 1.1 ounces) and ✔☺ Saving Face Oil Free SPF 30 ($65 for 1 ounce); **Clinique** ✔☺ Weather Everything Environmental Cream SPF 15 ($18.50 for 1 ounce), Sun Care Body SPF 15 Sun Block ($15.50 for 3.4 ounces), ✔☺ Sun-Care Body SPF 25 Sun Block ($15.50 for 3.4 ounces), ✔☺ Body SPF 30 Sun Block ($16.50 for 5 ounces), and ✔☺ Face SPF 30 Sun Block ($16.50 for 2.5 ounces); **Darphin** Ecran Soleil SPF 30 ($50 for 1.7 ounces), Soleil Filtrant SPF 25 ($48 for 5 ounces), and Vital Protection Day Fluid SPF 15 ($75 for 1 ounce); **Dermablend** Advanced Enzyme Moisturizer with Photosomes, SPF 15 ($35 for 1.7 ounces); **Dermalogica** Total Eye Care SPF 15 ($33 for 0.75 ounce); **DHC** Dual Defense SPF 25 ($24 for 3.5 ounces); **Diane Young** De-Aging Sunscreen Oil Free Firming Moisturizer SPF 15 ($38.50 for 1.5 ounces); **Doctor's Dermatologic Formula** ✔☺ Moisturizing Photo-Age Protection SPF 15 ($22 for 4 ounces), Moisturizing Photo-Age Sunscreen SPF 30 ($22 for 4 ounces), and ✔☺ Sport Proof SPF 30 ($22 for 4 ounces); **Dr. Dennis Gross, M.D. Skin**

Care Waterproof Sunscreen SPF 15 ($28 for 7 ounces) and Waterproof Sunscreen SPF 30 ($28 for 7 ounces); **Dr. Mary Lupo Skin Care System** Daily Age Management Oil Free Moisturizer SPF 15 ($23 for 2 ounces); **Elizabeth Arden** Extreme Conditioning Cream SPF 15 ($35 for 1.7 ounces) and Let There Be Light Lotion SPF 15 ($25 for 1.7 ounces); **Erno Laszlo** R.E.M. SPF 30 ($68 for 2.5 ounces); **Estee Lauder** ✔☺ Resilience Lift Face and Throat Cream SPF 15 ($65 for 1.7 ounce), ✔☺ Resilience Lift Face and Throat Lotion SPF 15 ($45 for 1 ounce), LightSource Transforming Moisture Creme SPF 15 ($45 for 1.7 ounces), LightSource Transforming Lotion SPF 15 ($45 for 1.7 ounces), ✔☺ Day Wear Super Anti-Oxidant Complex SPF 15 ($37.50 for 1.7 ounces), ✔☺ Sunblock for Body SPF 25 ($18.50 for 5 ounces), ✔☺ Sun Block for Face SPF 15 ($18.50 for 1.7 ounces), ✔☺ Sun Block for Face SPF 30 ($18.50 for 1.7 ounces); **Eucerin** Daily Sun Defense Sensitive Skin Lotion SPF 15 ($7.99 for 6 ounces) and Facial Moisturizing Lotion, SPF 25 ($8 for 4 ounces); **Exuviance** Essential Multi-Defense Day Creme SPF 15 ($25 for 1.75 ounces), Essential Multi-Defense Day Fluid SPF 15 ($23 for 2 ounces), Fundamental Multi-Protective Day Creme SPF 15 Sensitive Formula ($25 for 1.75 ounces), and Fundamental Multi-Protective Day Fluid SPF 15 Sensitive Formula ($23 for 2 ounces); **Glymed Plus** ✔☺ Cell Science Photo-Sunscreen SPF 35 ($40.95 for 2 ounces); **Guinot** ✔☺ Pigmentation Mark Prevention SPF 15 ($25 for 1.7 ounces), ✔☺ Skin Defense SPF 15 ($48 for 1.6 ounces), Sun Screen SPF 30 ($27 for 2.6 ounces), and Moisturizing Sun Spray SPF 15 ($27.50 for 5.4 ounces); **H2O+ Skin Care** ✔☺ Solar Block SPF 30 ($15 for 1.7 ounces); **Helena Rubinstein** Urban Active Age Defense System Fluid SPF 15 ($50 for 1.76 ounces) and Urban Active Age Defense System Cream SPF 15 ($50 for 1 ounce); **Hydron** ✔☺ Hydronamins Moisturizing Vitamin Therapy Day Creme SPF 15 ($29.75 for 1.9 ounces); **Jafra** ✔☺ Time Protector Daily Defense Cream, SPF 15 ($38 for 1.7 ounces) and Ecko the Gecko Kids Sunblock SPF 35 ($10 for 3.5 ounces); **Jason Natural** SPF 16 Sun Block ($8 for 4 ounces), SPF 26 Sun Block Sport Stick ($9 for 4 ounces), SPF 26 Total Sun Block ($8 for 4 ounces), SPF 36 Family Sun Block ($10.50 for 4 ounces), SPF 40 Active Sun Block ($10.75 for 4 ounces), and SPF 46 Kids Sun Block ($11 for 4 ounces); **Joey New York** Double Stuff Day and Night Moisturizer ($40 for 1 ounce of Green Tea with Multivitamins SPF 30 and 1 ounce of Red Marine Algae Vitamin Enriched Moisturizer) and Outdoor Activities SPF 20 ($22 for 4 ounces); **Jurlique International** Sun Cream, SPF 30+ ($36 for 3.5 ounces); **Kiehl's** All-Sport "Non-Freeze" Face Protector SPF 30 ($15 for 1.4 ounces); **Kiss My Face** Hot Spots Certified Organic Formula Sunscreen, SPF 30 ($9 for 0.5 ounce) and Oat Protein Sunblock SPF 30 ($10 for 4 ounces); **L'Occitane** Sun Block Cream SPF 30 ($21 for 2.6 ounces) and High Protection Sun Lotion SPF 20 ($27 for 8.4 ounces); **L'Oreal** Visible Results Skin Renewing Moisture Treatment SPF 15 Fragrance Free ($18.96 for 1.6 ounces); **La Mer** The SPF 18 Fluid ($50 for 1 ounce); **La Prairie** ✔☺ Cellular Brightening System Day Emulsion with SPF 15 ($125 for 1 ounce), ✔☺ Cellular Moisturizer SPF 15 The Smart Cream ($140 for 1 ounce), ✔☺ Cellular Eye Moisturizer SPF

15 The Smart Eye Cream ($125 for 0.5 ounce), Cellular Purifying Systeme Hydrating Fluid SPF 15 ($100 for 1.7 ounces), ✔☺ Cellular Time Release Moisture Lotion SPF 15 ($125 for 1.7 ounces), and ✔☺ Age Management Stimulus Complex SPF 25 ($150 for 1 ounce); **Lancome** Bienfait Total UV Eye SPF 15 ($28.50 for 0.5 ounce), Vinefit Complete Energizing Lotion SPF 15 ($37.50 for 1 ounce), Vinefit Cream SPF 15 ($37.50 for 1.7 ounces); Water-Light Spray SPF 15 with Pure Vitamin E ($25 for 5 ounces), High Protection SPF 30 Face Creme with Pure Vitamin E ($24 for 1.7 ounces), Soleil Expert Sun Care SPF 30 High Protection Sun Stick ($19.50 for 0.26 ounce), Soleil Ultra Eye Protection SPF 40 ($25 for 1.2 ounces), and Soleil Ultra Face and Body Lotion SPF 40 ($25 for 1.2 ounces); **Laura Mercier** Mega Moisturizer Cream with SPF 15 ($38 for 2 ounces) and Moisturizer Cream with SPF 15 ($38 for 2 ounces); **M.A.C.** ✔☺ Day SPF 15 Light Moisture ($22 for 1.7 ounces); **Mary Kay** Day Solutions SPF 15 ($30 for 1 ounce); **M.D. Formulations** Total Daily Protector SPF 15 ($20 for 2.5 ounces) and Total Protector 30 ($22 for 2.5 ounces); **M.D. Forte** Total Daily Protector SPF 15 ($13 for 2.5 ounces) and Environmental Protector SPF 30 ($18 for 2.5 ounces); **Merle Norman** Luxiva Changing Skin Treatment SPF 15 ($42 for 1 ounce), ✔☺ Luxiva Preventage Firming Defense Creme for Dry Skin SPF 15 ($38 for 2 ounces), ✔☺ Luxiva Preventage Firming Eye Creme SPF 15 ($21.50 for 0.5 ounce), and ✔☺ Luxiva Preventage Firming Defense Creme for Oily and Normal/Combination Skin Types SPF 15 ($38 for 2 ounces); **Murad** Energizing Pomegranate Moisturizer SPF 15 ($25 for 2 ounces), ✔☺ Environmental Shield Oil Free Sunblock SPF 15 ($20 for 2 ounces), ✔☺ Environmental Shield Hydrating Sunscreen SPF 15 ($23 for 4.2 ounces), and ✔☺ Environmental Shield Waterproof Sunblock SPF 30 ($25 for 4.2 ounces); **Natura Bisse** Sensitive Sun Fluid SPF 25 ($45 for 4.2 ounces), Extreme Sun Protector SPF 35 ($40 for 4.2 ounces), and Sun Protector SPF 30 Hydrating Sun Block for All Skin Types ($60 for 4.2 ounces); **Neostrata** ✔☺ Daytime Protection Cream SPF 15 PHA 4 ($27 for 1.75 ounces), ✔☺ Daytime Skin Smoothing Cream SPF 15 ($25 for 1.75 ounces), and Daily Protection Sunscreen SPF 29 ($30 for 3.4 ounces); **Neutrogena** Healthy Defense Daily Moisturizer SPF 30 ($11.49 for 1.7 ounces), Pore Refining Cream SPF 15 ($13.99 for 1 ounce), ✔☺ Visibly Even Moisturizer SPF 15 ($12.49 for 1 ounce), Visibly Firm Face Lotion SPF 20 ($19.99 for 1.7 ounces), Healthy Defense Oil-Free Sunblock Stick SPF 30 ($6.99 for 0.47 ounce), Healthy Defense Oil-Free Sunblock SPF 45 ($8.39 for 4 ounces), and Sunblock Lotion with SPF 45 ($8.39 for 4 ounces); **Neways Skin Care** Sunbrero SPF 30 ($11 for 4.2 ounces); **Nu Skin** ✔☺ Moisture Restore Day Protective Lotion SPF 15 for Normal to Oily Skin ($30 for 1.7 ounces) and ✔☺ Moisture Restore Day Protective Lotion SPF 15 for Normal to Dry Skin ($30 for 1.7 ounces); **Olay** Complete UV Protective Moisture Lotion SPF 15 (Fragrance and Fragrance Free) ($7.99 for 4 ounces), Complete UV Protective Moisture Cream SPF 15 (Fragrance and Fragrance Free) ($6.99 for 2 ounces), Total Effects Moisturizing Vitamin Complex SPF 15 Fragrance Free ($8.99 for 1.7 ounces), Age Defying Series Protective Renewal Lotion Beta Hydroxy Complex, SPF 15 ($8.91

for 4 ounces), and ProVital Protective Moisture Cream SPF 15 ($8.99 for 1.7 ounces); **Ombrelle** Sunscreen Lotion SPF 15 ($7.95 for 4 ounces), Sunscreen Lotion SPF 30 ($7.95 for 4 ounces), Sunscreen Lotion Extreme SPF 40 ($7.95 for 4 ounces), Sunscreen Lotion for Kids SPF 44 ($7.95 for 4 ounces), and Sunscreen Spray for Kids SPF 28 ($8.69 for 4 ounces); **Orlane** Anti-Wrinkle Sun Cream for the Face and Sensitive Areas SPF 30 ($75 for 1 ounce); **Osmotics** ✔☺ Balancing Complex SPF 15 ($55 for 3.4 ounces), ✔☺ Illuminating Hydrating Complex SPF 15 ($60 for 3.4 ounces), Protection Extreme Total Body SPF 15 ($32 for 4.25 ounces), and Protection Extreme Total Body SPF 25 ($35 for 4.25 ounces); **Paula's Choice** ✔☺ Essential Moisturizing Sunscreen SPF 15, Normal to Dry Skin ($12.95 for 6 ounces) and ✔☺ Extra Care Moisturizing Sunscreen SPF 30+ with Antioxidants Water-Resistant, Normal to Dry Skin ($12.95 for 6 ounces); **Peter Thomas Roth** All Day Moisture Defense Cream SPF 20 ($30 for 1.7 ounces), Max All Daily Moisture Defense Moisture Cream SPF 30 ($37 for 1.7 ounces), Oil-Free Sunblock SPF 20 ($25 for 4 ounces), Oil-Free Sunblock SPF 30 ($25 for 4 ounces), Water Resistant Sunblock SPF 20 ($25 for 4 ounces), Water Resistant Sunblock SPF 30 ($25 for 4 ounces), Max Sheer All-Day Moisture Defense Lotion SPF 30 ($37 for 1.7 ounces), and Ultra Lite Oil-Free Sunblock SPF 30 ($25 for 4 ounces); **Physician's Choice** pHaze 6+ Hydrator Plus SPF 15 ($26.95 for 2 ounces), pHaze 7 Protecting Hydrator SPF 15 ($25 for 2 ounces), and ✔☺ pHaze 8 Face & Body Hydrator SPF 15 ($12.95 for 12 ounces); **Pola** 1/f Suncut Milk SPF 30 ($24 for 1 ounce); **Pond's** Nourishing Moisture Lotion with SPF 15 ($5.99 for 2.5 ounces); **Prescriptives** ✔☺ All You Need Broad Spectrum Moisture Lotion SPF 15 ($40 for 1.7 ounces), ✔☺ All You Need Broad Spectrum Moisture Cream SPF 15 ($40 for 1.7 ounces), and ✔☺ Px Insulation Anti-Oxidant Vitamin Cream with SPF 15 ($40 for 1.7 ounces); **Rachel Perry** ✔☺ Environmental Skin Protector SPF 18 ($27 for 4 ounces); **Reversa** UV Ultra Vigilance Restorative Skin Tone Cream SPF 15 ($25.99 for 50 ml), UV Ultra Vigilance Anti-Wrinkle Cream SPF 15 ($25.99 for 60 ml), UV Anti-Wrinkle Fluid SPF 15 ($25.99 for 50 ml), and UV Anti Wrinkle Eye Contour Cream SPF 15 ($25.99 for 15 ml); **Revlon** Age Defying Performance Skin Care Face Cream, SPF 15 ($12.61 for 1.75 ounces), Age Defying Performance Skin Care Oil-Free Face Lotion, SPF 15 ($12.61 for 1.7 ounces), ✔☺ Daily Radiance Cream SPF 15 ($12.99 for 1.6 ounces), and ✔☺ Oil-Free Radiance Lotion SPF 15 ($14.89 for 1.6 ounces); **RoC** ChronoBlock Daily Moisturizing Care SPF 15 ($32 for 40 ml), ChronoBlock Yeux (for Eyes) SPF 15 ($25 for 15 ml), Hydra + Effet Reservoir for Normal Skin SPF 15 ($13.99 for 1.35 ounces), and Hydra + Effet Reservoir for Dry Skin SPF 15 ($13.99 for 1.35 ounces); **Sense Usana** ✔☺ Daytime Protective Emulsion SPF 15 ($28.45 for 1.7 ounces), Body Sunblock Lotion SPF 15 ($12.95 for 4 ounces), and Body Sunblock Lotion SPF 30 ($16.50 for 4 ounces); **Shiseido** Luminizing Day Essence SPF 24 ($50 for 1.4 ounces), Ultimate Sun Block Lotion SPF 50 ($35 for 3.3 ounces), Sun Block Compact SPF 32 ($25 for 0.42 ounce), Sun Block Face Cream SPF 35 ($24 for 1.7 ounces), Sun Block Stick SPF 35 ($21 for 0.31

ounce), Translucent Sun Block Stick SPF 30 ($21 for 0.31 ounce), and Day Protective
Moisturizer SPF 15 ($30 for 1.4 ounces); **Sisley** Botanical Facial Sun Cream SPF 15 ($100
for 1.4 ounces), Broad Spectrum Sun Protection SPF 25 ($100 for 2.1 ounces), and Bo-
tanical Sun Block SPF 20 ($100 for 1.5 ounces); **SkinCeuticals** Daily Sun Defense SPF 20
($28 for 3 ounces), Ultimate UV Defense SPF 30 ($34 for 3 ounces), and Ultimate UV
Defense SPF 45 ($34 for 3 ounces); **Sothys Paris** High Protection Cream SPF 15 ($21 for
2.5 ounces), Sunblock for Exposed Areas SPF 30 ($16.50 for 0.8 ounce), and SPF 25
Sunblock ($23 for 2.5 ounces); **Stila** Skin Visor SPF 30 ($22 for 2.5 ounces); **Thalgo**
Hydra Protective Emulsion SPF 15 ($28 for 4.2 ounces), Sun Shield Cream SPF 30 ($30
for 1.7 ounces), Sun Shield Emulsion SPF 25 ($30 for 3.4 ounces), and Unizone Protec-
tive Day Cream SPF 15 ($58 for 1 ounce); **Urban Decay** Guardian Angel Protective Moisture
SPF 15 ($20 for 1.7 ounces); **Vichy** Capital Soleil Protective Lotion SPF 15 ($19.50 for
120 ml), Capital Soleil Total Sunblock Lotion SPF 30 ($21 for 120 ml), Capital Soleil
Total Sunblock Cream SPF 45 ($21 for 50 ml), Capital Soleil Total Sunblock Cream SPF
60 ($19.50 for 50 ml), Capital Soleil Sunblock Lotion for Children SPF 35 ($19.50 for
120 ml), and Capital Soleil Sunblock Stick SPF 25 ($9 for 3 ml tube); **Yon-Ka Paris** Ultra
Protection, Age-Free Solar Block with AHAs and Botanicals, Water Resistant, SPF 25,
UVA-UVB-IR ($48 for 1 ounce).

BEST SUNSCREENS WITH ONLY TITANIUM DIOXIDE AND/OR ZINC OXIDE AS THE
ACTIVE INGREDIENTS, WHICH WOULD BE BEST FOR NORMAL TO DRY OR SENSITIVE
SKIN: **BioMedic** Pigment Shield SPF 18 ($19.95 for 2 ounces); **Clinique** ✔☺ City Block
Sheer SPF 15 ($15.50 for 1.4 ounces), ✔☺ Super City Block SPF 25 Oil-Free Daily Face
Protector ($15.50 for 1.4 ounces), and City Block Oil-Free Daily Face Protector SPF 15
($14.50 for 1.4 ounces); **Doctor's Dermatologic Formula** ✔☺ Organic Sunblock SPF
30 ($22 for 4 ounces); **Dr. Hauschka** Sunscreen Lotion SPF 15 ($18.50 for 3.4 ounces),
Sunscreen Lotion SPF 20 ($21 for 3.4 ounces), and Sunscreen Cream for Children SPF
22 ($21.95 for 3.4 ounces); **Epicuren** ✔☺ Zinc Oxide Sunblock Sunscreen SPF 20 ($28
for 2 ounces); **Glymed Plus** Photo-Age Environmental Protection Gel SPF 20 ($47.25
for 7 ounces); **Kiss My Face** Oat Protein Sunblock SPF 18 ($9 for 4 ounces); **La Prairie**
Suisse De-Sensitizing Systeme Barrier Shield SPF 15 ($100 for 1 ounce), Soleil Suisse
Cellular Anti-Wrinkle Sun Cream SPF 30 ($100 for 1.7 ounces), and Soleil Suisse Cellu-
lar Anti Wrinkle Sun Block SPF 50 ($125 for 1.7 ounces); **Linda Sy** ✔☺ ZincO Cream
SPF 20 Regular or Tinted ($28 for 3 ounces); **Marcelle** Moisture Cream Eye with Gingko
Biloba SPF 15 ($12.50 for 15 ml), Protective Block No Chemical Sunscreen Cream SPF
25 ($12.95 for 50 ml), Protective Block No Chemical Sunscreen Lotion SPF 25 ($12.95
for 120 ml), and Protective Block No Chemical Sunscreen Spray SPF 15 ($12.95 for 120
ml); **Neutrogena** Sensitive Skin UVA/UVB Block SPF 17 (8.39 for 4 ounces); **Noevir**
✔☺ Sun Defense Face SPF 15 ($30 for 1.6 ounces) and ✔☺ Sun Defense Body SPF
30+ ($30 for 4.2 ounces); **Obagi Nu-Derm** Sunblock SPF 25 ($38 for 2 ounces);
Origins Silent Treatment Instant UV Face Protector SPF 15 ($15 for 1.7 ounces);

Paula's Choice ✔☺ Pure Mineral Sunscreen SPF 15, Normal to Dry or Sensitive Skin ($12.95 for 6 ounces); **Peter Thomas Roth** Max Tinted Protective Day Cream SPF 30 ($40 for 2.3 ounces), Titanium Dioxide Sunblock SPF 15 ($25 for 4 ounces), and Titanium Dioxide Sunblock SPF 30 ($25 for 4 ounces); **Pevonia Botanica** ✔☺ Sunblock Dry to Sensitive Skin SPF 15 ($31 for 2.5 ounces), ✔☺ Sunblock Combination to Oily Skin SPF 15 ($31 for 2.5 ounces), and ✔☺ Sunblock Body Milk SPF 15 ($29.25 for 5 ounces); **RoC Canada** Minesol High Protection Sun Cream SPF 25 ($16 for 118 ml) and Minesol Mineral Sunblock Cream Very High Protection SPF 40 ($16 for 50 ml); **Shiseido** Gentle Sun Block Cream SPF 22 ($20 for 3.8 ounces); **Ultima II** Under-It-All Makeup Perfector SPF 25 ($13.50 for 1.25 ounces).

BEST FOUNDATIONS WITH SUNSCREEN FOR NORMAL TO DRY SKIN: See the section below for Best Foundations. An asterisk denotes those products that have adequate UVA protection and an SPF 15.

BEST FOUNDATIONS WITH SUNSCREEN FOR OILY/COMBINATION AND/OR BLEMISH-PRONE SKIN: See the section below for Best Foundations. An asterisk denotes those products that have adequate UVA protection and an SPF 15.

BEST LIP BALMS WITH SUNSCREEN: **Clientele Elastology** ✔☺ Sun Kiss Lip Conditioner SPF 15 ($15 for 0.24 ounce); **The Body Shop** Shea Sun Protection Facial Stick, SPF 30 ($6.50 for 0.6 ounce); **Clinique** Lip/Eye SPF 30 Sun Block ($15.50 for 0.21 ounce); **Epicuren** YouthTeen SPF 20 Lip Balm ($8 for 0.33 ounce); **Exuviance** Essential Multi-Protective Lip Balm, SPF 15 ($8.50 for 0.14 ounce); **Jason Natural** SPF 20 Natural Lip Protection on a String ($5 for 0.16 ounce); **Kiss My Face** Certified Organic Lip Balm, SPF 15 ($3.50 for 0.15 ounce); **Neostrata** Lip Conditioner SPF 15 ($6 for 0.14 ounce); **Nu Skin** Sunright Lip Balm 15 ($5.65 for 0.25 ounce); **Paula's Choice** ✔☺ Protective Lip Balm SPF 15 ($7.95 for 0.5 ounce) and Moisturizing Lipscreen SPF 15 ($6.95); **Physicians Formula** Sun Shield Lip Care SPF 15 ($2.50 for 0.15 ounce); **Prada Beauty** Shielding Balm SPF 15 ($60 for 30 packets each containing 0.05 ounce, for a total of 1.5 ounces) and Shielding Balm SPF 15/Lip Tint ($38 for 10 packets each containing 0.05 ounce, for a total of 0.5 ounce); **Reversa** UV Moisturizing Lip Balm SPF 15 ($5.99 for 15 ml); **RoC** Minesol High Protection Lipstick SPF 20 ($10 for 3 grams).

BEST SELF-TANNERS

Almost all self-tanners use the exact same ingredient, dihydroxyacetone, to turn the skin brown, and there is no way to differentiate one from another: they all perform essentially the same. Where self-tanners do differ is in the amount of dihydroxyacetone they contain; however, there is no way for the consumer to determine how much is actually in each product. The concentration determines how deep a color the skin will turn, but exactly what that color will be on your skin cannot be predicted by the formulation or by the company making the product. The way skin cells interact with the active ingredient varies so widely that there isn't any reliable way to tell what amount is too much or too little, and whether that's either a positive or a negative thing. It all depends on your skin and, even more primarily, on your application technique. For evaluations that are more subjective, please visit the Web site www.sunless.com; it is both an entertaining and informative look at dozens upon dozens of self-tanners.

The only exceptions to dihydroxyacetone-based self-tanners are those that contain erythrulose. Erythrulose is chemically similar to dihydroxyacetone, but the color change that results from erythrulose is neither as reliable nor as consistent as the color change that results from dihydroxyacetone. Further, while dihydroxyacetone completely changes the color of skin within two to six hours, erythrulose takes about two to three days for the skin to show a color change. For those who have not been successful using typical self-tanners (those that contain dihydroxyacetone), those that contain erythrulose are an option and are listed in this summary.

BEST SELF-TANNERS FOR ALL SKIN TYPES: **Aloette** Self Tanning Lotion ($18 for 4.5 ounces); **Arbonne** Self Tanner for Face and Body ($16.50 for 4 ounces); **Artistry by Amway** Self Tanning Lotion ($18.20 for 4.23 ounces); **Aveda** Sun Source ($16.50 for 5 ounces); **Avon** Sun-So-Soft Self-Tanning Lotion ($7.99 for 4.2 ounces); **BeneFit** Aruba in a Tuba Ultra Sunless Tan ($22 for 5 ounces); **Bain de Soleil** Auto-Bronzant Self Tanning Creme, Dark ($8.99 for 3.12 ounces), Auto-Bronzant Self Tanning Spray, Dark ($8.99 for 3.5 ounces), Auto-Bronzant Self Tanning Spray, Deep Dark ($8.99 for 3.5 ounces), Faces, Tinted Self-Tanning Creme for All Skin Tones ($8.99 for 2 ounces), Radiance Eternelle Self Tanning Creme, Dark ($13.99 for 3.2 ounces), Radiance Eternelle Self Tanning Creme, Medium Dark ($13.99 for 3.2 ounces), Streakguarde Self Tanning Creme, Dark ($8.99 for 3.12 ounces), Streakguarde Self Tanning Creme, Dark, Dark ($8.99 for 3.12 ounces), and Streakguarde Self Tanning Creme, Deep Dark ($8.99 for 3.12 ounces); **Banana Boat** Sunless Tanning Creme, Soft Medium ($7.99 for 3.75 ounces), Sunless Tanning Creme, Deep Dark ($7.99 for 3.5 ounces), and Sunless Tanning Spray Soft Medium and Deep Dark ($5.99 for 3.75 ounces); **Bioelements** Serious Self Tanner for Face and Body ($31 for 6 ounces); **BioMedic** Self Tan ($22.95 for 4 ounces); **Bobbi Brown** Sunless Tanning Gel for Face and Body ($27.50 for 4.2 ounces); **Christian Dior** Auto-Bronzant Face Self Tanner SPF 10 ($22.50 for 1.7 ounces), Auto-Bronzant Golden Self Tanner for Body ($25 for 1.7 ounces), and Auto-Bronzant Instant Glow Tinted Body Self-Tanner ($25 for 4.2 ounces); **Clarins** Self Tanning Gel without Sunscreen ($21 for 4.4 ounces) and Radiance Plus Self Tanning Cream Gel ($45 for 1.7 ounces); **Clinique** Face Quick Bronze Tinted Self Tanner ($15.50 for 1.7 ounces) and Self Tanning Lotion ($15.50 for 4.2 ounces); **Coppertone** Endless Summer Sunless Tanning Lotion, Light/Medium or Dark ($10.99 for 3.7 ounces) and Oil-Free Sunless Tanner ($7.99 for 4 ounces); **Darphin** Self Tanning Face and Body Cream ($45 for 4.2 ounces); **Doctor's Dermatologic Formula** Sun Free Self Tanner ($22 for 4 ounces); **Dr. LeWinn's Private Formula** Sunless Tanning Lotion ($34.50 for 227 ml); **Elizabeth Arden** Daily Bronzer Self Tanning Boost for the Face ($18.50 for 1.7 ounces), Modern Skin Care Oil

Free Self Tanning Lotion for Face & Body ($21 for 4.2 ounces) and Quick Spray Oil-Free Spray Self Tanner ($21 for 4.2 ounces); **Estee Lauder** Go Bronze Tinted Self Tanner for Face ($18.50 for 1.7 ounces), Go Bronze Tinted Self Tanner for Body ($25 for 5 ounces), and Stay Bronze Moisturizing Tan Extender for Face ($19.50 for 1.7 ounces); **Glymed Plus** Tan-In Self-Activating Tanning Cream ($21 for 7 ounces); **Guinot** Self Tanning Cream ($25 for 5.5 ounces); **H2O+ Skin Care** Express Bronzer Medium Tan or Deep Tan ($16.50 for 4 ounces); **Helena Rubinstein** Golden Beauty Sun Tan Express Crystal Self Tanning Gel ($25 for 1.7 ounces); **Jafra** Sunless Tanner for Body ($11.50 for 4.2 ounces) and Sunless Tanner for Face ($10.50 for 1.7 ounces); **Jan Marini Skin Research** Bioglycolic Sunless Self Tanner ($25 for 4 ounces); **Kiss My Face** Instant Sunless Tanner ($10 for 4 ounces); **Lancome** Flash Bronzer Self Tanning Face Gel with Pure Vitamin E, available in Medium, Deep, and Extra Deep ($24 for 1.7 ounces), Flash Bronzer Oil Free Tinted Self Tanning Face Lotion for the Face with Vitamin E available in Medium or Dark ($24 for 1.7 ounces), and Flash Bronzer Tinted Self Tanning Mousse ($27 for 5 ounces); **Marcelle** Self-Tanning Lotion with Alpha-Hydroxy Acid Moisturizing Formula for Face ($11.25 for 50 ml); **Mary Kay** Sunless Tanning Lotion ($10 for 4.5 ounces); **Merle Norman** Sun Free Self Tanning Creme Light ($12.50 for 4 ounces); **Murad** Environmental Shield Age Proof Self Tanner SPF 15 ($25 for 4.2 ounces); **Neutrogena** Instant Bronze, Sunless Tanner and Bronzer for the Face ($8.99 for 2 ounces), Instant Bronze, Sunless Tanner and Bronzer in One (Medium and Deep) ($8.99 for 4 ounces), Sunless Tanning Foam, Deep ($8.99 for 4 ounces), Sunless Tanning Spray ($8.99 for 3.5 ounces), and Sunless Tanning Lotion (Light and Medium) ($8.99 for 4 ounces); **Neways Skin Care** Body Bronzer ($16.70 for 4.2 ounces); **Ocean Potion** Sunless Potion Streak Free Sunless Tanner ($6.49 for 6 ounces); **Ombrelle** Sunless Tanning Cream SPF 15 ($7.95 for 2 ounces); **Origins** Summer Vacation, The Natural-Looking Self Tanner ($17.50 for 5 ounces); **Osmotics** Extremely Natural Self Bronzer ($28 for 3.7 ounces); **Parthena** Spray On Sun Sunless Tanning Spray ($6.50 for 2 ounces); **Paula's Choice** Almost the Real Thing Self-Tanning Gel ($12.95 for 6 ounces); **Pevonia Botanica** Self-Tanning Emulsion Spray ($33 for 5 ounces); **philosophy** the healthy tan, self tanning gel ($16 for 3.3 ounces); **Phytomer** Intensive Self-Tanning Spray ($33.50 for 4.23 ounces) and Rapid Self-Tanning Gel ($31 for 1.7 ounces); **Reversa** Self Tanning Spray ($13.49 for 125 ml); **RoC** Auto Bronzant Self-Tanner ($18 for 100 ml); **Serious Skin Care** Instant Bronze Sunless Tanning Lotion ($16.50 for 4 ounces); **SkinCeuticals** Sans Soleil ($28 for 4 ounces); **Sothys Paris** Illuminating Express Self-Tanner ($21 for 4.2 ounces); **Thalgo** Scintillating Gel ($28 for 1.7 ounces) and Sublime Self Tanning Spray ($28 for 4.2 ounces); **Vichy** Capital Soleil Self-Tan Body Milk ($19.50 for 100 ml) and Capital Soleil Express Self-Tanning Spray for Body ($19.50 for 125 ml); **Zia** Sans Sun Self Tanning Creme for All Skin Types ($16.95 for 5 ounces).

SELF-TANNERS WITH ERYTHRULOSE: Marcelle Self-Tanning Spray with Erythrulose ($13.95 for 120 ml); **Principal Secret** Sun Secret Tan Sustainer SPF 15 ($18.25 for 4 ounces).

BEST FACIAL MASKS

Although I am rarely a woman of few words, I'm not one to get too excited about facial masks. First, I feel quite comfortable stating that there are not many exciting, interesting, or particularly helpful facial masks. Many facial masks use clay as their main ingredient, with some thickening agents, and although that can be beneficial for absorbing oil, the improvement is short-lived, not long-term. Other masks use clay as well, but also include water-binding agents and plant oils, and that can be better for normal to combination or slightly dry skin. Masks for normal to dry skin are often just moisturizers and nothing more and don't necessarily warrant the extra time it takes to apply them. They aren't bad for skin, they just aren't a necessary step.

There are also masks that use a plasticizing agent that is then pulled or peeled off the skin. These do impart a temporary soft feeling to the skin because they pull off a layer of skin, but that is hardly beneficial or lasting.

Facial masks can be a pampering, relaxing interval for women, but for good skin care, what you do daily is vastly more important than what you do once a week or once a month. The lack of Paula's Picks in this category reflects the repetitive nature of these products; there isn't a stand-out formulation among them. Even when a mask contains impressive water-binding agents, antioxidants, and anti-irritants, because the products are left on the face only briefly, there is doubt whether you would receive any benefit from those ingredients anyway.

BEST MASKS FOR NORMAL TO OILY/COMBINATION AND/OR BLEMISH-PRONE SKIN:
Aloette Skin Renewal Mud Masque ($14 for 4 ounces); **Arbonne** Mild Masque ($17.50 for 5 ounces); **Beauty Without Cruelty** Purifying Facial Mask ($8.95 for 4 ounces); **Borghese** Fango Active Mud for Face and Body ($30 for 7 ounces); **CamoCare** Revitalizing Mask ($13.39 for 2 ounces); **Chanel** Masque Purete ($28.50 for 2.6 ounces); **Clarins** Normalizing Facial Mask ($22.50 for 1.7 ounces); **Darphin** Fibrogene Mask ($75 for 1.7 ounces); **DHC** Hydrating Facial Mask ($16 for 3.5 ounces) and Mineral Mask ($31 for 3.5 ounces); **Doctor's Dermatologic Formula** Detoxification Mud Mask ($23 for 2 ounces); **Estee Lauder** So Clean Deep Pore Mask ($19.50 for 3.4 ounces); **FACE Stockholm** Detoxifying Green Clay Masque ($32 for 2.6 ounces); **Gatineau** Laser Radiance Energizing Mask ($35 for 2.5 ounces); **G.M. Collin** Exfozyme Exfoliant ($27.90 for 2.7 ounces) and Vitalift Mask-Gel ($25 for 1.7 ounces); **H2O+ Skin Care** Purifying Exfoliation Mask ($18 for 3 ounces) and Sea Mineral Mud Mask ($24 for 4 ounces); **Jurlique International** Deep Penetrating Cream Mask ($36 for 1.7 ounces) and Moor Purifying Mask ($35 for 1.7 ounces); **La Mer** Refining Facial ($75 for 3.4 ounces); **Lancaster** Aquamilk Clear-It-All Mask ($26 for 2.5 ounces); **Mary Kay** Clarifying Mask Formula 3 ($12 for 4 ounces); **Murad** Purifying Clay Masque ($22.50 for 2.25 ounces); **Nu Skin** Clay Pack ($13 for 2.5 ounces); **Ole Henriksen Skin Care** Firm Action Pore Refining Mask ($25 for 2 ounces) and Repair Formula Mask ($25 for 2 ounces); **Origins**

Clear Improvement Active Charcoal Mask to Clear Pores ($18.50 for 3.4 ounces); **Paula's Choice** Oil-Absorbing Facial Mask, Oily/Combination Skin ($10.95 for 6 ounces); **Peter Thomas Roth** Hydrating Nutrient Masque ($40 for 5 ounces); **Phytomer** Gentle Mask for Sensitive Skin ($28 for 1.7 ounces) and Hydrating Seaweed Facial Mask ($26 for 1.7 ounces); **Serious Skin Care** C-Mask Vitamin C Conditioning Mask ($21 for 3 ounces); **Thalgo** Nourishing Cream Mask with Marine Nutrients ($30 for 1.7 ounces); **Urban Decay** Magic Mud Pore Clearing 2-in-1 Mask & Scrub ($16 for 3.4 ounce); **Vichy** Purifying Thermal Mask ($19.95 for 50 ml); **Yves St. Laurent** Absolute Purifying Masque ($33 for 2.5 ounces).

BEST MASKS FOR NORMAL TO DRY SKIN: **Ahava** Advanced Mud Masque for Normal to Oily Skin ($28 for 4.2 ounces); **Astara** Golden Flame Hydration Mask ($39 for 1.9 ounces); **Aveda** Deep Cleansing Herbal Clay Masque ($19 for 4.5 ounces); **Awake** Skin Renovation Mask ($80 for 2.2 ounces; 8 single-use containers) and Vital Express Mask ($50 for 4 ounces; 12 sheets); **Bioelements** Restorative Clay Active Treatment Mask ($23.50 for 2.5 ounces); **Dermalogica** MultiVitamin Power Recovery Masque ($36 for 2.5 ounces); **Diane Young** Dry Parts Moisture Mask Salon Treatment ($56.50 for 1.5 ounces); **Doctor's Dermatologic Formula** Collagen Dry Skin Mask ($18 for 2 ounces); **Estee Lauder** Re-Nutriv Intensive Lifting Mask ($70 for 1.7 ounces), So Moist Hydrating Mask ($19.50 for 3.4 ounces), Stress Relief Eye Mask ($27.50 for ten 0.4-ounce packets), and Triple Creme Hydrating Mask ($27.50 for 2.5 ounces); **FACE Stockholm** Hydrating Rose Petal Antioxidant Face Masque ($32 for 2 ounces); **H2O+ Skin Care** Hydrating Marine Moisture Mask ($24 for 4 ounces); **Jafra** Soothing Results Cooling Yogurt and Honey Mask, for Sensitive Skin ($12.50 for 2.6 ounces); **Jan Marini Skin Research** C-Esta Facial Mask ($50 for 2 ounces); **Jason Natural** Vita-C Max One Minute Facial ($30 for 4 ounces); **Jurlique International** OPC Beauty Face Mask ($68 for 4.2 ounces); **Kiehl's** Algae Masque ($24 for 2 ounces) and Moisturizing Masque ($37 for 2 ounces); **L'Occitane** Moisturizing Mask ($25 for 2.6 ounces) and Soothing Exfoliating Face Mask ($26 for 2.6 ounces); **Lancaster** Aquamilk Absolute Moisture Mask ($26 for 2.5 ounces); **Marcelle** Gentle Purifying Mask ($10.95 for 50 ml); **Mary Kay** Indulging Soothing Eye Mask ($15 for 4 ounces); **Origins** Drink Up 10 Minute Moisture Mask ($18.50 for 3.4 ounces); **Parthena** Live Cell Derivative Soothing Eye Area Mask ($9.95 for 0.5 ounce) and Eyelasticity Line Smoothing Mask ($16.50 for 1 ounce); **Pevonia Botanica** Sensitive Skin Mask ($35 for 1.7 ounces); **Prada Beauty** Soothing Mask/Face ($85 for 15 packets each containing 0.01 ounce, for a total of 1.5 ounces); **Sense Usana** Nutritious Creme Masque ($16.95 for 3.7 ounces); **Zia** Ultimate Hydrating Mask ($24.95 for 3 ounces) and Super Moisturizing Mask ($14.95 for 3 ounces).

BEST SKIN-LIGHTENING PRODUCTS

This category includes only a small group of products that are effective as skin-lightening treatments. The preponderance of evidence indicates that the best ingredient for effectively inhibiting melanin production is hydroquinone. Over-the-counter hydro-quinone products are available in strengths of 1% to 2%, and higher concentrations are available from dermatologists and plastic surgeons. Some formulations include kojic acid, magnesium ascorbyl palmitate, mulberry extract, bilberry extract, or arbutin as alterna-tives. While all of those have been shown to inhibit melanin production to one degree or another (mostly in animal or in vitro studies), very few products contain enough of them to have an effect. Keep in mind that no skin-lightening product will work if an effective sunscreen is not used on a daily basis. For a prescription skin-lightening option, please see the review for Tri-Luma in Chapter Three.

BEST SKIN-LIGHTENING PRODUCTS THAT CONTAIN HYDROQUINONE FOR ALL SKIN TYPES: Avon ✓☺ Banishing Cream Skin Lightening Treatment ($8.50 for 2.5 ounces); BeautiControl ✓☺ Skin Lightening Complex ($25 for 1 ounce); Bioelements Pigment Discourager ($21 for 0.5 ounce); Black Opal ✓☺ Advanced Dual Complex Fade Gel ($11.95 for 0.75 ounce); Fashion Fair Vantex Skin Bleaching Creme with Sunscreens ($17.50 for 2 ounces); Flori Roberts My Everything Treatment Chromatone Plus Fade Creme ($15 for 3.75); Glymed Plus ✓☺ Derma Pigment Bleaching Fluid ($33.60 for 2 ounces); Iman Perfect Response Even-Tone Fade Gel with AHA ($20 for 1.7 ounces); Neostrata ✓☺ NeoCeuticals Skin Lightening Cream SPF 15 ($24 for 1.4 ounces); Obagi Nu-Derm Nu-Derm Blender ($54 for 2 ounces); Paula's Choice ✓☺ Remarkable Skin Lightening Lotion, All Skin Types ($13.95 for 4 ounces); Peter Thomas Roth ✓☺ Po-tent Botanical Skin Brightening Gel Complex ($45 for 2 ounces); Physician's Choice ✓☺ pHaze 13 Light Block Pigment Cream SPF 25 ($33.95 for 1 ounce); ProActiv ✓☺ Skin Lightening Lotion ($22 for 1 ounce); Serious Skin Care Fading Cream Skin Lightening Formula ($24.50 for 2 ounces), Fading Mask Skin Lightening Formula with 2% Hydroquinone ($22.50 for 2 ounces), and Fading Pads Skin Lightening Formula with 2% Hydroquinone ($24.50 for 30 pads); St. Ives ✓☺ Dark Spot Fade Cream with Vitamins E & A ($8.99 for 1 ounce).

BEST SKIN-LIGHTENING PRODUCTS THAT CONTAIN INGREDIENTS OTHER THAN HYDROQUINONE FOR ALL SKIN TYPES: Doctor's Dermatologic Formula ✓☺ Inten-sive Holistic Lightener ($45 for 1 ounce), ✓☺ Vitamin K Cream ($47 for 1 ounce), and ✓☺ Erase Eye Gel ($39 for 0.5 ounce); Christian Dior Anti-Spot Whitening Night Essence ($57 for 1 ounce); DHC White Cream ($34 for 1.4 ounces); Ella Bache Intensive Clearing Serum Special for Brown Spots ($63 for 1.05 ounces); Elizabeth Arden ✓☺ Visible Whitening Block SPF 20 ($42.50 for 1.7 ounces); Erno Laszlo ✓☺ Antioxidant Complex for Eyes, Lightening, Firming, Protective Eye Treatment for All Skin Types ($42 for 0.5 ounce); Estee Lauder Spotlight Skin Tone Perfector ($30 for 1.7 ounces), WhiteLight Brightening Treatment Lotion ($30 for 4.2 ounces), WhiteLight Brightening Moisture Creme ($37.50 for 1 ounce), WhiteLight Brighten-ing Protective Base, SPF 30 ($30 for 1.7 ounces), and WhiteLight Concentrated Brightening Serum ($65 for 1.3 ounces); Glymed Plus Derma Pigment Skin Brightener ($33.60 for 2 ounces) and ✔☺ Living Cell Clarifier ($33.60 for 2 ounces); **Guinot** ✔☺ Newlight Deep Action Lightening Serum ($64 for 1.07 ounces); **H2O+ Skin Care** ✔☺ Waterwhite Brightening Lotion SPF 15 ($35 for 1.5 ounces) and ✔☺ Waterwhite Brightening Tonic ($22.50 for 6 ounces); **Helena Rubinstein** Future White Whitening Fluid SPF 40 ($60 for 1.11 ounces) and Future White High Precision Whitening Essence ($90 for 1.01 ounces); **Jason Natural** C-Light Skin Tone Balancer ($19.99 for 1 ounce); **M.D. Formulations** Vit-A-Plus Illuminating Serum ($65 for 1 ounce); **Peter Thomas Roth** Ultra Gentle Botanical Skin Lightening Gel Complex ($45 for 2 ounces) and Potent Botanical Skin Brightening Lotion Complex ($45 for 2 ounces); **Pevonia Botanica** ✔☺ Lightening Gel ($38 for 1 ounce); **Pola** Milky White Night ($72 for 2 ounces), Cream White ($132 for 1 ounce), and Essence White ($132 for 0.8 ounce); **Sothys Paris** Blanc Perfect Serum ($52 for 4 vials, each containing 0.17 ounce); **Shu Uemura** ✔☺ Whitening Lipo ($67 for 0.11 ounce); **Z. Bigatti** Re-Storation Enlighten Skin Tone Provider ($174 for 1 ounce); **Zia** Hands-On Protection SPF 15 ($17.95 for 2 ounces).

SPECIALTY SKIN-CARE PRODUCTS

BEST OIL ABSORBING PAPERS: Bath & Body Works Oil Absorbing Tissues ($3 for 75 tissues); **The Body Shop** Facial Blotting Tissues ($10 for 2 packs, 65 sheets each); **Burt's Bees** Wings of Love Powdered Facial Tissue ($3 for 65 sheets); **Clean & Clear by Johnson & Johnson** Clear Touch Oil Absorbing Sheets ($4.95 for 50 sheets); **Paula's Select** Oil Blotting Papers; **Shiseido** Pureness Oil-Blotting Paper ($13.50 for 100 sheets).

BEST LIP BALMS WITHOUT SUNSCREEN: Avon On Everyone's Lips Daily Lip Refiner ($8.50 for 0.5 ounce); **bare escentuals Cush** Buzz Latte Lip Balm ($8 for 0.25 ounce); **BeneFit** Smoooch ($18 for 0.25 ounce); **The Body Shop** Cocoa Butter Lip Care Stick ($4.50 for 0.15 ounce) and Hemp Lip Protector ($6.50 for 0.30 ounce); **Caudalie** Grape Seed Lip Conditioner ($15 for 0.14 ounce); **Clinique** Moisture Stick ($13.50 for 0.14 ounce); **Dr. Hauschka** Lip Balm ($10 for 0.15 ounce) and Dr. Hauschka Lip Care Stick ($7.50 for 0.16 ounce); **Erno Laszlo** Lip Therapy ($42 for 0.5 ounce); **Gatineau** Lip Care Balm ($26 for 0.5 ounce); **Kiehl's** Lip Balm #1 ($4.95 for 0.7 ounce); **M.A.C.** Lip Conditioner ($8 for 0.5 ounce); **Noevir** Lip Conditioner ($9 for 0.12 ounce); **Origins** Mind Your Mouth ($6.50 for 0.15 ounce); **philosophy** kiss me lip balm ($10 for 0.5 ounce) and kiss me red lip balm ($10 for 0.5 ounce); **Rachel Perry** Lip Lover ($3.50 for 0.2 ounce); **Serious Skin Care** Vitamin A Moisture Stick ($15.75 for 0.17 ounce); **SkinCeuticals** Antioxidant Lip Repair ($30 for 0.3 ounce).

BEST MANUAL LIP EXFOLIATORS: Diane Young Coneflower Lipline Firmer ($41 for 0.5 ounce); **G.M. Collin** Kerato-Peel Gommage ($27.90 for 2.7 ounces); **Paula's Choice** Exfoliating Treatment ($7.95 for 0.5 ounce); **Yves St. Laurent** Natural Action Exfoliator Granule-Free ($40 for 2.5 ounces).

BEST FOUNDATIONS

Choosing the right foundation color is not only time-consuming, but also exceedingly frustrating. The only way to discover your ideal match is to apply the foundation on your facial skin, perhaps two different colors on either side of your face, and then to check it in the daylight. If the color isn't an exact match, you have to go back in and try again. Another hurdle is to find a foundation with a pleasing texture, one that feels soft and silky, but doesn't streak, cake, or look thick, and that takes experimentation, too. Determining how much coverage you want is another factor, and then there's what type of foundation (liquids or creams or stick formulas). Now tell me that isn't a challenge!

If you can splurge on only one cosmetic product, foundation is it. This is the one area where spending a little bit more is the best option, not because expensive means better, but because it's just way too risky to buy a foundation you can't try on first. Still, many mass market outlets and drugstores have very good hassle-free return policies for used makeup, and it's wise to inquire about that before purchasing makeup in these environments. Do not keep a foundation that ends up being the wrong color—return it and keep trying until you get it right.

Many women love the convenience and hands-free application of pressed powder–style foundations. Yet these have limitations that make them best for normal to slightly dry or slightly oily skin. These are a unique group of products to use as foundation, and the decision to use them is based more on personal preference than on actual skin type. I've included them in a separate category. Remember that most stick or cream-to-powder foundations are best for those with normal to slightly dry or slightly oily skin, because the ingredients that keep these types of foundations in their cream or stick form can be problematic for oily or blemish-prone skin, and the often powdery finish can be too drying for dry skin.

The number of excellent foundation formulas has increased noticeably. Improvements in silicone and pigment technology have led to more silky-smooth, neutral-toned foundations than ever before. These are truly good days to shop for foundation! And if you have stayed away from foundation because of a previous misstep or negative experience, there has never been a safer time to try it again. All of the selections listed below have wonderful textures, even coverage, smooth application, good wearability, and suit the needs and general preferences of the recommended skin type.

Very Important Note: The foundations with SPF listed below do not necessarily have UVA-protecting ingredients. The foundations with effective sun protection (meaning that they do contain UVA-protecting ingredients and have an SPF 15 or greater) have an asterisk before the product name.

BEST FOUNDATIONS FOR VERY OILY SKIN: **Almay** Amazing Lasting Sheer Makeup SPF 12 ($10.38); **BeautiControl** Color Freeze Liquid Makeup SPF 12 ($20); **Black Opal** True Color Liquid Foundation Oil Free ($7.99); **Clinique** ✔☺ SuperFit Makeup ($19.50); **DHC** Liquid Makeup ($27) and Water Base Face Color ($19); **Exuviance** *Skin Caring

Foundation SPF 15 ($26); **Guerlain** *Divinora Ultra-Fluid Foundation SPF 15 ($36); **Helena Rubinstein** Double Agent Skin Adjusting Makeup ($38.50); **Illuminare** ✓☺ *Ultimate All Day Foundation/Concealer Matte Finish Makeup SPF 21 ($20); **Lancome** ✓☺ Maquicontrole Oil-Free Liquid Makeup ($32.50) and ✓☺ Teint Idole Enduringly Divine Makeup ($32.50); **Make Up For Ever** Mat Velvet Oil-Free Foundation SPF 20 ($36); **Maybelline** EverFresh Makeup SPF 14 ($7.49); **Prescriptives** 100% Oil Free Matte Finish SPF 15 ($32.50); **Revlon** ✓☺ *ColorStay Lite Makeup SPF 15 ($11.29).

BEST FOUNDATIONS FOR NORMAL TO OILY/COMBINATION SKIN: Aloette Oil-Free Liquid Makeup ($12.50); **Anna Sui** Fluid Foundation ($35); **Artistry by Amway** *Absolute Oil Control Foundation SPF 15 ($24.25) and Self-Defining Sheer Foundation SPF 15 ($22.45); **Avon** Incredible Finish Foundation SPF 8 ($7); **Avon beComing** Pure Brilliance Perfect Balance Foundation SPF 8 ($15) and ✓☺ Redefine Airbrush Foundation SPF 10 ($19.50); **Awake** Oil Free Foundation ($32); **Bobbi Brown** Oil-Free Even Finish Makeup SPF 15 ($35); **CARGO** Liquid Foundation ($24); **Chanel** Teint Lift Eclat SPF 8 ($52) and ✓☺ *Double Perfection Fluide Matte Reflecting Makeup SPF 15 ($40); **Christian Dior** ✓☺ Teint Diorlight SPF 10 ($34.50); **Clarins** Multi-Matte Foundation ($32.50); **Cle de Peau Beaute** Teint Naturel Crème Foundation ($100) and Color Control Foundation ($85); **Clinique** ✓☺ Stay-True Makeup Oil-Free Formula ($16.50); **Cover Girl** CG Smoothers All Day Hydrating Makeup ($7.59) and ✓☺ *Fresh Look Makeup Oil-Free for Combination to Oily Skin SPF 15 ($7.59); **Elizabeth Arden** Flawless Finish Skin Balancing Makeup ($25) and Flawless Finish Mousse Makeup ($28); **Estee Lauder** Double Wear Stay-in-Place Makeup SPF 10 ($29.50), Enlighten Skin-Enhancing Makeup SPF 10 ($29.50), Re-Nutriv Intensive Lifting Makeup ($65), and ✓☺ Equalizer Smart Makeup SPF 10 ($32.50); **FACE Stockholm** Matte Foundation ($24); **Fashion Fair** Oil-Free Perfect Finish Souffle ($20); **Giorgio Armani** ✓☺ Luminous Silk Foundation ($42); **Guerlain** Divinora Silky Smooth Foundation SPF 12 ($37); **Helena Rubinstein** Illumination Natural Radiance Reviving Makeup SPF 15 ($40); **Jane** Oil Free Foundation ($3.47) and Stay Calm Face Makeup SPF 8 ($4.99); **L'Oreal** Ideal Balance Balancing Foundation for Combination Skin ($11.99), AirWear Breathable Long-Wearing Foundation SPF 14 ($11.99), and Visible Lift Line Minimizing Makeup SPF 12 ($10.29); **La Mer** The Foundation SPF 15 ($65); **La Prairie** Skin Caviar Concealer/Foundation SPF 15 ($150); **Lancaster** ✓☺ Light Enhancing Matte Finish Foundation ($28); **Lancome** Photogenic Skin-Illuminating Makeup SPF 15 ($32.50); **Laura Mercier** ✓☺ Oil-Free Foundation ($38); **Lorac** Oil-Free Makeup ($30); **Marcelle** True Radiance SPF 15 Oil-Free Liquid Makeup ($10.25); **Mary Kay** Day Radiance Oil-Free Foundation ($14); **Maybelline** Shine Free Oil Control Makeup ($6.49); **Neutrogena** ✓☺ *Visibly Firm Moisture Makeup SPF 20 ($14.99) and *Healthy Skin Liquid Makeup SPF 20 ($9.99); **N.Y.C.** Smooth Skin Liquid Makeup ($2.99); **Origins** Stay Tuned Balancing Face Makeup ($15); **Paula Dorf Cosmetics** Moisture Foundation Oil-Free ($34); **Paula's Select** ✓☺ *Best Face Forward Foundation SPF 15, Normal to Oily Skin ($12.95); **Prescriptives** Traceless Skin Responsive Tint SPF 8

($32.50) and ✔☺ Virtual Skin Super Natural Finish SPF 10 ($32.50); **Principal Secret** Liquid Foundation SPF 15 ($30); **Shiseido** *Benefiance Enriched Revitalizing Foundation SPF 15 ($42); **Shiseido** <u>The</u> **Makeup** *Cream Foundation SPF 16 ($32); **Shu Uemura** *UV Liquid Foundation SPF 21 ($32.50); **Stila** ✔☺ Liquid Makeup ($30); **Stila Sport** ✔☺ Pivotal Skin Foundation SPF 8 ($25); **Sue Devitt Studio Makeup** 70% Triple Seaweed Gel Foundation ($36); **Urban Decay** ✔☺ *Liquid Surreal Skin Liquid Foundation SPF 15 ($24); **Versace** Lasting Oil-Free Foundation SPF 12 ($45); **Victoria's Secret Cosmetics** Liquid Lingerie Oil-Free Makeup SPF 10 ($17.50); **Vincent Longo** ✔☺ Liquid Canvas Healthy Fluid Foundation SPF 6 ($35).

BEST FOUNDATIONS FOR NORMAL TO DRY SKIN: **Alexandra de Markoff** Sheer Illusion Lightweight Foundation ($37); **Almay** ✔☺ *Skin Smoothing Foundation with Kinetin SPF 15 ($11.99); **Arbonne** About Face Line Defiance Makeup SPF 8 ($26) and About Face Luminous Color Wand SPF 8 ($24); **Aveda** Base Plus Balance ($18); **Awake** Skin Renovation Fluid Makeup ($55); **Bobbi Brown** Moisture-Rich Foundation SPF 15 ($38) and Fresh Glow Cream Foundation ($35); **Body & Soul** ✔☺ Beauty Make-Up ($35); **The Body Shop** Oil-Free Face Base SPF 8 ($15.50) and *Moisture Face Base SPF 15 ($15.50); **Borghese** Hydro-Minerali Crème Makeup ($32.50) and Hydro-Minerali Natural Makeup ($31.50); **Chanel** Vitalumiere Satin Smoothing Fluid Makeup SPF 15 ($50); **Christian Dior** Teint Diorlift SPF 10 ($34.50); **Clarins** Hydrating Liquid Foundation ($32.50) and Extra Firming Foundation ($36); **Clinique** Balanced Makeup Base ($15.50), Soft Finish Makeup ($19.50), and ✔☺ *Dewy Smooth Anti-Aging Makeup SPF 15 ($19.50); **Club Monaco** Oil-Free Foundation ($19) and Liquid Foundation ($19); **Cover Girl** Continuous Wear Makeup ($7.79); **Elizabeth Arden** Flawless Finish Radiant Moisture Makeup SPF 8 ($25) and Flawless Finish Bare Perfection Makeup SPF 8 ($25); **Estee Lauder** ✔☺ So Ingenious Multi-Dimension Makeup SPF 8, Futurist Age-Resisting Makeup SPF 15 ($32.50) and Lucidity Light-Diffusing Makeup SPF 8 ($29.50); **FACE Stockholm** Liquid Foundation ($24); **Fashion Fair** Perfect Finish Creme Makeup ($18.50); **Helena Rubinstein** Face Sculptor Makeup Rich Lifting Foundation ($44); **Illuminare** Fantastic Finish Moisturizing Sunscreen Makeup SPF 21 ($20); **I-Iman** Liquid Foundation ($27); **La Prairie** *Cellular Treatment Foundation Satin SPF 15 ($60); **Lancaster** Light Enhancing Adaptive Foundation SPF 6 ($30); **Lancome** Photogenic Ultra-Comfort Skin Illuminating Makeup SPF 15 ($32.50), Maqui-Libre Skin-Liberating Makeup SPF 15 ($32.50), Teint Optim'age Minimizing Makeup SPF 15 ($32.50), and Maquivelours Hydrating Foundation ($32.50); **Laura Mercier** ✔☺ Moisturizing Foundation ($38); **Lorac** Translucent Cream Makeup ($35) and ✔☺ Satin Makeup ($35); **M.A.C.** Studio Finish Satin Foundation SPF 8 ($19.50) and Studio Finish Matte Foundation SPF 8 ($19.50); **Make Up For Ever** ✔☺ Face and Body Liquid Makeup ($37); **Mary Kay** Day Radiance Liquid Foundation with Sunscreen SPF 8 Normal/Combination Skin ($14); **Maybelline** True Illusion Makeup SPF 10 ($8.49); **NARS** Balanced Foundation ($38); **Neutrogena** Skin Clearing Makeup Flawless Finish Blemish Treatment ($11.39); **Orlane** Ultra Naturel Revealing Ultra-Fluid Foundation ($40); **Paula's Select** ✔☺ *All Bases Covered Foundation SPF 15, Normal to Dry Skin ($12.95); **Prescriptives** Custom Blend Foundation Oil Free ($55) and Custom Blend Foundation Moisturizing Formula ($55); **Revlon** Age Defying Makeup with SPF 10 ($11.49), ✔☺ *Age Defying Makeup and Concealer Compact SPF 20 ($13.89), and ✔☺ *Age Defying All Day Lifting Foundation SPF 20 ($12.49); **Rimmel** Natural Sensation All Day Natural Smooth Finish Makeup ($4.97); **Shiseido** <u>The</u> **Makeup** *Fluid Foundation SPF 15 ($32); **Shu Uemura** Fluid S Foundation SPF 8 ($30) and Fluid N Foundation SPF 8 ($30); **Sisley** Transmat Cucumber Makeup Cream ($66); **smashbox** Studio Seamless Liquid Foundation ($28); **Sonia Kashuk** Perfecting Liquid Foundation ($9.99); **Stila** ✔☺ Complete Coverage ($40) and ✔☺ Illuminating Liquid Foundation ($35); **Sue Devitt Studio Makeup** Balanced Foundation SPF 10 ($36); **Trucco** Pro Coverage Foundation SPF 8 ($27.75); **Ultima II** *Beautiful Nutrient Nourishing Makeup SPF 15 ($21.50); **Versace** Lasting Hydrating Foundation SPF 15 ($47) and Smoothing Skin Foundation SPF 12 ($55); **Yves St. Laurent** Energie Teint Oil-Free Liquid Foundation SPF 12 ($46); **Zia** Natural Foundation SPF 8 ($14.95).

BEST SHEER FOUNDATIONS/TINTED MOISTURIZERS FOR ANY SKIN TYPE (EXCEPT VERY OILY): **M.D. Formulations** *Total Protector Color Tint SPF 30 ($22); **Aveda** ✔☺ *Moisture Plus Tint SPF 15 ($25); **BeneFit** *I Am Rebel SPF 15 ($26); **Bobbi Brown** ✔☺ *SPF 15 Tinted Moisturizer ($35); **The Body Shop** Skin Re-Leaf Kinetin Tinted Moisturizer ($18); **Burt's Bees** Tinted Facial Moisturizer ($11); **Calvin Klein** ✔☺ *Sheer Coverage Foundation SPF 20 ($29); **Clinique** ✔☺ *Almost Makeup SPF 15 ($17.50); **Cover Girl** ✔☺ *CG Smoothers SPF 15 Tinted Moisture ($7.59); **Dermalogica** Treatment Foundation ($30); **Dr. Dennis Gross, M.D. Skin Care** *All-in-One Tinted Moisturizer SPF 15 ($32); **Hard Candy** *Hint Tint SPF 15 ($29.50); **Helena Rubinstein** Color Fitness Energizing Tinted Moisturizer SPF 12 ($30); **Lancome** ✔☺ *Bienfait Total UV Tinted SPF 15 ($36); **NARS** Gel Fraicheur ($30); **Neutrogena** ✔☺ *Healthy Defense Sheer Makeup SPF 30 ($10.99); **Origins** *Nude and Improved Bare-Face Makeup SPF 15 ($15); **Remede** *Translucent UV Coat Tinted SPF 30 ($36); **Revlon Skinlights** *Diffusing Tint SPF 15 ($12.29); **Shiseido** *Essential Tinted Moisturizer SPF 15 ($30 for 1.4 ounces); **Shu Uemura** *UV Underbase SPF 17 ($30).

BEST FOUNDATIONS FOR EXTRA DRY SKIN: **Alexandra de Markoff** Countess Isserlyn Creme Makeup ($47.50); **Avon** Face Lifting Moisture Firm Foundation Cream Souffle ($9); **Chanel** Vitalumiere Satin Smoothing Crème Makeup SPF 15 ($55); **Guerlain** Issima Foundation ($55); **M.A.C.** *Sheer Coverage Foundation SPF 15 ($22); **Origins** Dew Gooder Moisturizing Face Makeup ($15); **Paula Dorf Cosmetics** ✔☺ Perfect Glo Foundation ($42); **Rimmel** Hydrasense Flawless Hydrating Makeup ($4.97); **Sue Devitt Studio Makeup** ✔☺ Triple C-Weed Whipped Foundation ($39).

BEST FOUNDATIONS FOR MAXIMUM COVERAGE REGARDLESS OF SKIN TYPE: **Black Opal** True Color Maximum Coverage Foundation ($7.99); **Exuviance** ✔☺ *CoverBlend

Concealing Treatment Makeup SPF 20 ($22); **Illuminare** *Extra Coverage Foundation/Concealer Semi-Matte Finish Sunscreen Makeup SPF 21 ($20).

BEST PRESSED-POWDER FOUNDATIONS (GENERALLY BEST FOR NORMAL TO SLIGHTLY DRY OR SLIGHTLY OILY SKIN AND BEST USED AS POWDER, NOT FOUNDATION) AND LOOSE-POWDER FOUNDATIONS (BEST USED AS FOUNDATION): **Anna Sui** Compact Powdery Foundation ($25 for powder cake; $8.50 for compact); **Artistry by Amway** Versatile Matte Pressed Powder Foundation ($18.20); **Aveda** ✔☺ Dual Base Minus Oil ($19.50 without compact, $30 with); **Awake** Fine Finish Foundation ($38 with compact, $28 refill, $4 for sponge) and ✔☺ Skin Renovation Powder Makeup ($48); **BeautiControl** Perfecting Wet/Dry Finish Foundation ($20.50); **Body & Soul** Two-in-One Face Powder ($35); **The Body Shop** All in One Face Base ($15.50); **CARGO** Wet/Dry Powder Foundation ($24); **Chanel** Double Perfection Matte Reflecting Powder Makeup SPF 10 ($45); **Chantecaille** Compact Makeup ($47); **Christian Dior** Teint Dior Poudre Foundation ($42.50, $29.50 for refills); **Clarins** Matte Powder Compact Foundation SPF 15 ($32.50); **Cle de Peau Beaute** Creamy Powder Foundation ($110; $95 for refills); **Corn Silk** Zero Shine Powder Makeup ($6.99) and Shine Control Mattifying Loose Powder Makeup ($5.96); **Cover Girl** Fresh Complexion Oil Control Makeup ($6.49); **Elizabeth Arden** Flawless Finish Dual Perfection Makeup SPF 8 ($28); **English Ideas** *Perfect Powder SPF 15 Pressed Powder Foundation ($28); **Estee Lauder** ✔☺ So Ingenious Multi-Dimension Powder Makeup ($32.50); **FACE Stockholm** Powder Foundation ($27); **Giorgio Armani** ✔☺ Silk Foundation Powder ($40); **Jane Iredale** *Amazing Base Loose Mineral Powder Base SPF 20 ($42) and *PurePressed Base SPF 17 ($48); **L'Oreal** AirWear Breathable Long-Wearing Powder Foundation SPF 17 ($11.69); **La Prairie** Cellular Treatment Powder Finish SPF 10 ($60); **Lancome** ✔☺ Dual Finish Versatile Powder Makeup ($31); **Laura Mercier** ✔☺ Foundation Powder ($38); **Lorac** ✔☺ Oil-Free Wet/Dry Makeup ($35); **M.A.C.** ✔☺ StudioFix Powder Plus Foundation ($22.50); **Make Up For Ever** Powder Foundation ($40); **Maybelline** PureStay Powder Plus Foundation SPF 15 ($7.19); **Origins** Original Skin Pressed Makeup ($22.50); **Orlane** Dual Compact Cake Foundation ($42.50); **Quo Cosmetics** ✔☺ Wet and Dry Foundation ($21); **Shiseido** The Makeup *Powdery Foundation SPF 15 ($26 for powder cake, $6 for compact); **Shu Uemura** *UV Powder Foundation SPF 26 ($32.50); **smashbox** Wet/Dry Foundation ($32); **Sonia Kashuk** ✔☺ Dual Coverage Powder Foundation ($9.99); **Stila** ✔☺ Illuminating Powder Foundation SPF 12 ($23 for powder; $20 for compact); **T. Le Clerc** Powder Compact Foundation ($45); **Trish McEvoy** Dual Powder ($26); **Trucco** Prepair Duo Powder Foundation ($28.75); **Versace** ✔☺ Cream Compact Foundation ($42); **Youngblood** Pressed Mineral Compact Foundation ($35.50).

BEST CREAM-TO-POWDER AND LIQUID-(WATER)-TO-POWDER FOUNDATIONS (GENERALLY BEST FOR NORMAL TO SLIGHTLY DRY OR SLIGHTLY OILY SKIN): **Aloette** Creme-to-Powder Foundation ($14); **Aveda** Cooling Calming Cover Sheer Face Tint

($18); **Avon** Hydra Finish Stick Foundation SPF 8 ($9); **Avon beComing** ✓☺ *Bases Covered Cream to Powder Compact SPF 15 ($15); **Awake** ✓☺ *Hydro-Touch Foundation SPF 18 ($40 with compact, $30 for refills); **Black Opal** Perfecting Powder Makeup SPF 8 ($7.99); **Bobbi Brown** Oil-Free Even Finish Compact Foundation ($38); **Borghese** Molto Bella Makeup SPF 8 ($35); **Chantecaille** *Real Skin Foundation SPF 15 ($49 with compact; $31 for refill) and *Real Skin Foundation SPF 30 ($53 with compact; $31 for refill); **Christian Dior** Teint Diorlift Compact SPF 10 ($34.50); **Clinique** ✓☺ *City Base Compact Foundation SPF 15 ($21); **Cover Girl** ✓☺ *AquaSmooth Makeup SPF 15 ($8.50); **Fashion Fair** Oil-Free Perfect Finish Creme to Powder Makeup ($21); **Guerlain** ✓☺ *Terracotta Ultimate Bronze Compact Foundation SPF 15 ($32.50); **Iman** Second to None Cream to Powder Foundation ($18.50); **L'Oreal** Feel Naturale Compact Light Softening One-Step Makeup SPF 15 ($11.29); **Lancaster** Light Enhancing Cream Compact Foundation ($30); **M.A.C.** Studio Tech Foundation ($26); **Marcelle** Dual Cream Powder Makeup ($12.25); **Mary Kay** Creme-to-Powder Foundation ($14 for foundation, $9 for refillable compact); **Prescriptives** ✓☺ *Photochrome Light Adjusting Compact Makeup SPF 15 ($37); **Revlon** ✓☺ *New Complexion One Step Compact Makeup SPF 15 ($12.79); **Shu Uemura** *UV Cream Foundation SPF 31 ($32.50); **Trish McEvoy** Cream Powder Makeup ($35); **Vincent Longo** ✓☺ Water Canvas ($45, $12 for optional compact); **Yves St. Laurent** Teint Compact Matite ($52; $34.50 for refill).

BEST STICK FOUNDATIONS (GENERALLY BEST FOR NORMAL TO SLIGHTLY DRY OR SLIGHTLY OILY SKIN): **Almay** *One Coat Light and Easy Liquid Stick Makeup SPF 15 ($12.49); **BeneFit** PlaySticks ($30); **Chanel** ✓☺ Teint Cristallin Waterlights Sheer Makeup Stick ($37.50); **Chantecaille** New Stick Concealer & Foundation SPF 8 ($40); **Clarins** ✓☺ Smart Stick Foundation ($32.50); **Clinique** ✓☺ *City Stick SPF 15 ($21); **Elizabeth Arden** ✓☺ Flawless Finish Makeup Stick SPF 15 ($18); **Estee Lauder** *Minute Makeup Creme Stick Foundation SPF 15 ($29.50); **I-Iman** Stick Foundation ($30); **Jafra** *Stick Makeup SPF 15 ($15); **L'Oreal** *Quick Stick Long Wearing Foundation SPF 14 ($10.99); **Laura Mercier** ✓☺ Foundation Stick to Go ($35); **Maybelline** *3 in 1 Express Makeup SPF 15 ($8.39) and *Express Makeup Shine Control SPF 15 ($8.39); **Prescriptives** ✓☺ *Exact Matchstick Foundation SPF 15 ($37); **Revlon** ✓☺ *ColorStay Stick Makeup SPF 15 ($11.29); **Shiseido** The Makeup ✓☺ *Stick Foundation SPF 15 ($32); **smashbox** Foundation Stick ($28).

BEST SHINY/SHIMMERY FOUNDATIONS OR HIGHLIGHTERS (GENERALLY BEST FOR EVENING MAKEUP): **Avon** Illuminating Stick ($7.50); **Chanel** ✓☺ Sheer Brilliance ($36.50); **Giorgio Armani** ✓☺ Fluid Sheer ($42); **Jafra** White Souffle Highlighter ($9.50); **Make Up For Ever** Metalizer ($19); **Prescriptives** ✓☺ Magic lluminating Liquid Potion ($30); **Revlon** Skinlights *Face Illuminator SPF 15 ($10.99); **Sonia Kashuk** ✓☺ Illuminating Color Stick ($7.99); **Ultima II** *Glowtion Skin Brightening Makeup SPF 15 ($17.50).

BEST CONCEALERS

Finding a good under-eye concealer is an easier task than ever before, regardless of where you shop for makeup. Well-formulated concealers abound that aren't too drying, too greasy, don't fill in lines around the eye, apply effortlessly, and offer beautiful colors that blend easily onto skin. Paula's Pick concealers excel in all these criteria and are outstanding in this category. I do not recommend color-correcting concealers, as they rarely (if ever) look convincing in natural light, and often substitute one visible discoloration for another. Concealers in the list below that are marked with an asterisk provide effective sun protection with an SPF 15 or higher that includes UVA-protecting ingredients.

BEST MATTE-FINISH CONCEALERS: Almay ✓☺ Amazing Lasting Concealer SPF 6 ($5.97); **Avon** Incredible Finish Concealer ($4.50); **Calvin Klein** ✓☺ Concealer ($17); **Chanel** ✓☺ Quick Cover ($32.50); **Christian Dior** ✓☺ Teint Diorlift Smoothing Anti-Fatigue Concealer ($22.50); **Clinique** Soft Conceal Corrector ($12.50); **Club Monaco** ✓☺ Concealer ($11); **Corn Silk** Liquid Powder Concealer ($3.76); **Cover Girl** ✓☺ Invisible Concealer ($4.69); **Elizabeth Arden** ✓☺ Flawless Finish Concealer ($14); **Estee Lauder** Double Wear Stay in Place Concealer SPF 10 ($17) and Lucidity Light-Diffusing Concealer SPF 8 ($18); **L'Oreal** ✓☺ AirWear Long-Wearing Concealer ($9.89), ✓☺ Visible Lift Line Minimizing Concealer ($9.99), and Feel Naturale Concealer ($7.69); **La Mer** The Concealer ($50); **Lancome** ✓☺ *Photogenic Skin- Illuminating Concealer SPF 15 ($21); **M.A.C.** ✓☺ Select Cover-Up ($12.50); **Mary Kay** ✓☺ MK Signature Concealer ($9.50); **Maybelline** ✓☺ Great Wear Concealer ($5.19); **Neutrogena** Skin Clearing Oil-Free Concealer ($7.99) and ✓☺ Visibly Firm Eye Treatment Concealer ($9.99); **Origins** Quick, Hide! Easy Blend Concealer ($11); **Paula's Select** ✓☺ No Slip Concealer ($7.95); **Revlon** ✓☺ ColorStay Concealer SPF 6 ($9.69); **Revlon Skinlights** Illusion Wand SPF 12 ($7.89); **Rimmel** Hydrasense Flawless Concealer ($3.97); **Shiseido** The Makeup Concealer ($17); **Ultima II** ✓☺ Wonderwear Concealer SPF 6 ($13.50); **Versace** ✓☺ Long-Lasting Hydrating Cream Concealer ($30).

BEST CREAMY CONCEALERS: Almay *Wake-Up Call! Energizing Concealer SPF 15 ($6.89); **Aloette** Concealer ($10); **Aveda** Conceal Plus Protect ($13.50); **Avon beComing** Hide the Evidence Concealing Quick Stick ($14), ✓☺ *Beyond Color Line Diminishing Concealer SPF 15 ($6); **Black Opal** Flawless Perfecting Concealer ($3.79); **Cover Girl** ✓☺ Fresh Complexion Undereye Concealer ($4.99); **Estee Lauder** Smoothing Creme Concealer ($17); **Exuviance** *CoverBlend Multi-Function Concealer SPF 15 ($16); **I-Iman** Concealer ($18); **L'Oreal** Cover Expert Exact Match Concealer ($8.99); **Lancaster** Light Enhancing Cream Concealer ($14.50); **Lancome** ✓☺ Effacernes Waterproof Protective Undereye Concealer ($21); **M.A.C.** *Concealer SPF 15 ($12.50); **Prescriptives** ✓☺ Camouflage Cream ($16.50); **Principal Secret** Perfect Concealer SPF 8 ($14); **Quo Cosmetics** Concealer ($12); **Revlon** *Age Defying All Day Lifting Concealer SPF 20 ($8.89); **Shiseido UV White** *Whitening Pre-Makeup Stick SPF 25 ($30); **Three Custom Color** Creme Concealer ($19.50, $15 for refill) and Professional Concealer Palette ($58).

BEST CREAM-TO-POWDER OR STICK CONCEALERS: Avon ✓☺ Perfect Wear Total Coverage Concealer ($5.50) and ✓☺ Precise Coverage Concealing Stick ($5); **Bobbi Brown** Blemish Cover Stick ($20); **Bonne Bell** 2X Stick No Shame Concealer ($3.49); **Cle de Peau Beaute** ✓☺ Concealer ($65); **N.Y.C.** Cover Stick ($1.99); **Stila** Cover-Up Stick ($17).

BEST POWDERS

Pressed- and loose-powder options have improved greatly. New processing technology and ingredient combinations have created the most amazing silky-feeling powders imaginable, and that is true in all price ranges. Expense does not distinguish powders one from the other; there are equally beautiful options at the drugstore as there are at the department store. Pressed and loose powders are rated on their silky texture, even application, and skin tone color options. You will also find a plethora of loose and pressed shiny powders, and there are some that are distinctly preferred over others due to their attractive finish, ability to cling to the skin, and ease of application.

A separate category of pressed powders are those that contain sunscreen with an SPF 15 and the mineral-based UVA-protecting ingredients of titanium dioxide or zinc oxide. These are excellent options as a way to touch up makeup and add sunscreen protection over your foundation to be sure you have all-day coverage. Because of their thicker texture, these can also double as powder foundation, though they are best used over a regular sunscreen or a foundation with sunscreen to ensure excellent sun protection.

Note: The recommendations for skin type that follow are more interchangeable than you might think. Choosing a powder truly has more to do with your preference (what kind of finish you like), how much of the product you use, and what kind of foundation you wear. However, powders listed as best for dry skin typically have a satiny (as opposed to dry matte) finish, which is a more attractive choice for women with dry skin who use powder.

BEST FINISHING POWDERS (BOTH LOOSE AND PRESSED) FOR ALL SKIN TYPES (EXCEPT VERY DRY SKIN): Alexandra de Markoff Countess Isserlyn Loose Powdermist ($40) and Countess Isserlyn Pressed Powdermist ($35); **Almay** Skin Stays Clean Pore Minimizing Pressed Powder ($10.89) and Luxury Finish Loose Powder ($9.19); **Arbonne** Translucent Pressed Powder ($16.50); **Artistry by Amway** Loose Powder ($17.50); **Aveda** Pressed Powder Plus Antioxidants ($17.50 without compact, $28.50 with) and Loose Powder Plus Replenish ($17 in tub with puff); **Avon** Incredible Finish Loose Powder ($7.50), Clear Finish Great Complexion Pressed Powder ($8.50), and ✓☺ Incredible Finish Pressed Powder ($7.50); **Avon beComing** ✓☺ Smooth Finish Pressed Powder ($14); **Awake** Loose Powder ($28); **bare escentuals** bareMinerals mineral veil ($19); **BeautiControl** Secret Agent Private Detective Pressed Powder ($15); **Black Opal** Color Fusion Pressed Powder ($7.99) and ✓☺ Oil Absorbing Pressed Powder ($7.99); **BlissLabs**

Skin Twin Pressed Powder ($25); **Body & Soul** Loose Face Powder ($30) and Perfect Face Powder ($32); **Bonne Bell** No Shine Pressed Powder with Tea Tree Oil ($3.89); **Calvin Klein** Pressed Powder ($26) and Loose Powder ($32); **CARGO** Pressed Powder ($24) and ✔☺ Loose Powder ($24); **Chanel** Natural Finish Pressed Powder ($40) and ✔☺ Natural Finish Loose Powder ($45); **Christian Dior** Diorlight Pressed Powder ($35); **Cle de Peau Beaute** Perfect Enhancing Powder ($56); **Clinique** ✔☺ Blended Face Powder & Brush ($16.50), Stay Matte Sheer Pressed Powder Oil-Free ($16.50), and Superpowder Double Face Powder ($16.50); **Club Monaco** Pressed Powder ($20) and ✔☺ Loose Powder ($19); **Cover Girl** CG Smoothers Fresh Look Pressed Powder Combination to Oily Skin ($5.79), CG Smoothers Fresh Look Pressed Powder Normal to Dry Skin ($5.79), and Clean Pressed Powder Fragrance-Free Normal Skin ($5.49); **Elizabeth Arden** Flawless Finish Loose Powder ($20); **Erno Laszlo** Duo-pHase Face Powder ($30) and Duo-pHase Pressed Powder ($27); **Estee Lauder** Lucidity Translucent Loose Powder ($27), Lucidity Translucent Pressed Powder ($22), Enlighten Skin-Enhancing Powder ($22), Double-Matte Oil-Control Loose Powder ($22), and Double-Matte Oil-Control Pressed Powder ($22); **Exuviance** CoverBlend Anti-Aging Finishing Powder ($18); **FACE Stockholm** Loose Powder ($21); **Giorgio Armani** ✔☺ Sheer Powder ($38) and ✔☺ Micro-fil Loose Powder ($42); **Helena Rubinstein** Softwear Loose Powder with Micro Fibres ($35) and Double Agent Mattifying Pressed Powder ($30); **Iman** ✔☺ Luxury Loose Powder ($17.50) and ✔☺ Luxury Pressed Powder ($18); **I-Iman** Pressed Powder ($25); **L'Oreal** Visible Lift Line Minimizing Powder ($11.99), Feel Naturale Ultrafine Light Softening Powder SPF 15 ($11.59), and ✔☺ Translucide Naturally Luminous Powder ($9.89); **Lancaster** Light Enhancing Loose Powder ($26) and Light Enhancing Pressed Powder ($24); **Lancome** ✔☺ Photogenic Sheer Pressed Powder ($25) and ✔☺ Matte Finish Shine Control Sheer Pressed Powder ($22); **Laura Mercier** ✔☺ Loose Powder ($30) and Pressed Powder ($28); **Linda Sy** Translucent Loose Powder ($18); **Lorac** Face Powder ($28) and ✔☺ Translucent Touch Up Powder ($32); **M.A.C.** Studio Finish Face Powder ($18.50), Studio Finish Pressed Powder ($18.50), and Blot Powder ($15); **Make Up For Ever** Compact Powder ($28) and ✔☺ Super Matte Loose Powder ($28); **Marcelle** Face Powder Loose ($10.50); **Mary Kay** MK Signature Loose Powder ($12.50); **Maybelline** True Illusion Pressed Powder SPF 10 ($6.99) and Shine Free Translucent Pressed Powder ($5.19); **NARS** Loose Powder ($30); **N.Y.C.** Loose Face Powder ($2.99) and Pressed Face Powder ($1.99); **Origins** Silk Screen Refining Face Powder ($22.50); **Orlane** Transparent Loose Powder ($35) and Velvet Pressed Powder ($35); **Paula Dorf Cosmetics** Loose Powder ($30) and ✔☺ Pressed Powder ($25); **Paula's Select** ✔☺ Soft Pressed Powder ($10.95); **Posner** Finishing Touch Pressed Powder for All Skin Types ($4.39); **Prescriptives** Powderful Adjustable Coverage Pressed Powder ($28) and ✔☺ Virtual Skin Pressed Powder ($25); **Quo Cosmetics** Mosaic Perfecting Powder ($18) and Mosaic Highlighter ($18); **Revlon** New Complexion Powder Normal to Oily Skin ($11.69); **Shu Uemura** Face Powder ($30); **smashbox** Flash Powder ($28) and Pressed

Powder ($26); **Sonia Kashuk** ✓☺ Bare Minimum Pressed Powder ($7.99) and ✓☺ Barely There Loose Powder ($7.99); **Stila** Loose Powder ($27) and Pressed Powder ($17 for powder cake, $15 for refillable compact); **Sue Devitt Studio Makeup** ✓☺ Triple C-Weed Loose Powder ($29) and Silky Pressed Powder ($26); **Tony & Tina** Herbal Environmental Protector Pressed Powder ($28); **Trish McEvoy** Loose Powder ($20); **Trucco** Touch Up Pressed Powder ($20.50) and Final Touch Loose Powder ($16.50); **Urban Decay** Surreal Skin Compact Face Powder ($18); **Versace** ✓☺ Natural Finish Loose Powder ($42) and Invisible Pressed Powder ($38); **Victoria Jackson Cosmetics** Pressed Powder ($17.95); **Victoria's Secret Cosmetics** Powdered Silk Finishing Powder ($15); **Vincent Longo** Loose Powder ($30); **Wet 'n' Wild** Pressed Powder ($2.49).

BEST FINISHING POWDERS (BOTH LOOSE AND PRESSED) FOR DRY SKIN: Aloette Fresh Finish Loose Powder ($15); **Christian Dior** Diorlight Loose Powder ($42.50) and Teint Poudre ($35); **Clarins** ✓☺ Face Powder ($33); **Clinique** Soft Finish Pressed Powder ($16.50); **DHC** Face Powder ($12); **Erno Laszlo** Controlling Face Powder ($30) and Controlling Pressed Powder ($27); **Estee Lauder** Equalizer Smart Loose Powder ($28) and So Ingenious Multi-Dimension Loose Powder ($30); **Hard Candy** Peace Powder ($26); **Jafra** Translucent Face Powder ($14) and Pressed Powder ($14); **Joey New York** Finishing Powder ($26); **La Mer** The Powder ($60) and The Pressed Powder ($55); **Lancome** ✓☺ Photogenic Sheer Loose Powder ($30); **Maybelline** Finish Matte Pressed Powder ($5.89); **Prescriptives** Magic Liquid Powder ($32.50); **Principal Secret** Loose Face Powder ($23); **Rimmel** Stay Matte Pressed Powder ($2.97); **Shiseido** <u>The</u> Makeup Pressed Powder ($20 for powder cake, $6 for compact); **Shu Uemura** Compact Powder M ($30); **Yves St. Laurent** ✓☺ Poudre Compact Matte ($50, $27.50 for refill).

BEST BRONZING PRODUCTS (POWDER, GEL, CREAM, OR LIQUID): BeautiControl Sun Faux You Bronzing Powder ($15); **BeneFit** Hoola ($26) and ✓☺ Glamazon ($26); **Black Opal** Color Fusion Bronzer ($8.99); **Bobbi Brown** Bronzing Stick ($28) and Bronzing Powder ($26); **Bonne Bell** Gel Bronze Face and Body Bronzer ($3.69) and Powder Bronze ($3.89); **Calvin Klein** Bronzing ($24); **Chanel** ✓☺ Bronze Universal de Chanel ($40) and Sunlit Powder ($45); **Clarins** Bronzing Powder Duo ($29); **Club Monaco** Bronzer ($22); **Estee Lauder** Bronze Goddess Soft Matte Bronzer ($27); **FACE Stockholm** Bronzer ($20); **Giorgio Armani** ✓☺ Sheer Bronzer ($33); **Helena Rubinstein** Compact Bronzer SPF 30 ($30); **I-Iman** Bronzer ($27); **Laura Mercier** ✓☺ Bronzing Stick ($30); **Make Up For Ever** Sun Tan Bronzing Powder SPF 8 ($30); **NARS** Bronzing Powder ($24); **Origins** Sunny Disposition Liquid Bronzer ($15); **Paula's Select** ✓☺ Soft Matte Bronzing Powder ($10.95); **Quo Cosmetics** Mosaic Bronzer ($18) and Bronzing Powder ($19); **Revlon** New Complexion Bronzing Powder ($11.99); **Stila** Sun ($36); **Stila Sport** Pivotal Sun Bronzing Tint ($25); **Sue Devitt Studio Makeup** Gold Coast Bronzing Powder ($28); **Versace** Bronzing Powder ($38); **Vincent Longo** Bronzer ($16); **Wet 'n' Wild** ✓☺ Bronzer ($2.79).

BEST PRESSED POWDERS WITH SPF 15 OR HIGHER AND UVA-PROTECTING IN-GREDIENTS FOR ALL SKIN TYPES: **Neutrogena** ✓☺ Healthy Defense Protective Powder

SPF 30 ($9.99); **Paula's Select** ✓☺ Healthy Finish Pressed Powder SPF 15 ($11.95); **Pola** SunPowder SPF 15 ($40).

BEST SHINY LOOSE AND PRESSED POWDERS: Aveda Color Plus Definition ($15); **Giorgio Armani** Sheer Shimmer ($33); **L'Oreal** On the Loose Shimmering Powder ($5.99); **Lancome** Poudre Blanc Neige Light-Reflecting Compact Powder ($30); **Laura Mercier** Shimmer Pressed Powder ($32) and ✓☺ Loose Powder [Star Dust or Sun Dust] ($30); **Make Up For Ever** Shine-On Powder ($25); **Prescriptives** Magic Soft Powder ($28); **Stila** Illuminating Pressed Powder ($35); **Tony & Tina** Universal Color Dust ($15); **Versace** Extra Glow Soft Loose Powder ($45).

BEST BLUSHES

Today's powder blushes have predominantly silky-smooth textures, apply evenly, don't fade, and come in a range of pigment density (so you can create either a dramatic or soft appearance with little effort). For the most part, blush is probably one of the easiest cosmetics to get right because it is hard to buy a bad blush. Not that there aren't some real losers out there, but there are far more winners. The problem with blush is usually with application, and that is where good brushes come into play. Using the proper brushes is essential for getting blushes to go on correctly. With very few exceptions, the mini-brushes that come packaged with a blush should be discarded in favor of an elegant, professional-sized blush brush.

Sensing that women wanted something new when it came to blush options, many cosmetics companies launched cream-to-powder stick blushes, liquid cheek tints, and gel-based blushes. Of course, to seasoned cosmetics veterans this onslaught was merely the same old song with a different, contemporary-sounding title. Yet, among the copycat formulas, there are a few winners that emerged as viable alternatives for those looking for a change of pace from traditional powder blush. As for true cream blush, there are fewer of these available today than there were just two years ago. This class of blush is OK for very dry skin, but not much different from dabbing a bit of lipstick on your cheeks and blending. If anything, the interminable color range for lipsticks that can double as cream blush is staggering compared to the color range of actual cream blushes.

Blushes (both powder and cream) receive high marks if most of the colors are matte; have a soft, non-grainy texture; blend on smoothly; do not fade or dissipate with time; and come in a good selection of colors. Paula's Pick options excel in all these areas. There are plenty that qualify, so don't spend a lot of money on blush unless you need to test the color first. Many inexpensive blushes from the drugstore are of superior quality and provide the same results as those from the department store.

BEST POWDER BLUSHES: Almay Beyond Powder Blush ($7.47); **Aloette** ✓☺ Cheek Color Powder ($12.50); **Anna Sui** Blush Face Colors ($22); **Aveda** Blush Minus Mineral Oil ($13 for blush tablet; compacts sold separately), Cooling Calming Color ($18); **Avon** True Color Powder Blush ($7.50); **Awake** Blush ($18); **Bath & Body Works** First Blush

Cheek Color ($10); **BeautiControl** Unbelievable Blush ($13.50); **Bobbi Brown** Blush ($19); **Calvin Klein** Blush ($24); **CARGO** ✔☺ Blush ($20); **Chanel** Powder Blush ($37.50); **Chantecaille** Cheek Color Powder ($21); **Christian Dior** ✔☺ Diorlight Blush Final ($32) and Effets Blush Powder Blush Trio ($35); **Clarins** ✔☺ Powder Blush ($25); **Cle de Peau Beaute** Cheek Color ($40 for powder cake; $30 for compact; $15 for brush); **Clientele** Contour Blush ($25); **Clinique** Sheer Powder Blusher ($16.50) and Soft Pressed Powder Blusher ($16.50); **Club Monaco** ✔☺ Blush ($16); **Dr. Hauschka** Rouge Powder ($23.50); **Elizabeth Arden** Cheekcolor ($20); **Estee Lauder** Blush All Day Natural CheekColor ($21.50); **FACE Stockholm** Blush ($15) and Blush Shimmer ($15); **Guerlain** Divinora Radiant Blush ($34); **Jafra** Powder Blush ($12); **Jane** Blushing Cheeks ($3.22); **Jane Iredale** PurePressed Blush ($26); **L'Oreal** ✔☺ Feel Naturale Light Softening Blush ($10.99); **Lancome** ✔☺ Blush Subtil Delicate Oil-Free Powder Blush ($25.50); **Laura Mercier** Face Tint ($20); **Lorac** ✔☺ Blush ($16); **M.A.C.** Blush ($16); **Make Up For Ever** Powder Blush ($15); **Mary Kay** MK Signature Cheek Color ($9 for blush tablet, $8 for refillable compact); **Maybelline** Brush/Blush ($5.19); **Merle Norman** Luxiva Lasting Cheekcolor ($14.50); **NARS** ✔☺ Blush ($20); **Neutrogena** Soft Color Blush ($9.49); **Paula Dorf Cosmetics** ✔☺ Cheek Color ($18); **Paula's Select** ✔☺ Soft Matte Blush ($7.95); **Posner** Natural Blush ($4.95); **Prescriptives** Powder Cheekcolor ($16.50 for blush tablet; $6 for refillable compact); **Quo Cosmetics** ✔☺ Blush ($16); **Revlon** Smooth-On Blush ($8.89); **Rimmel** Blush ($2.97); **Shu Uemura** ✔☺ Glow On Blush ($22); **Sisley** Double Blush ($56); **Sonia Kashuk** Beautifying Blush ($7.99); ✔☺ **Sue Devitt Studio Makeup** Silky Blush ($20); **Trish McEvoy** All Over Face Color ($26) and Radiant Blush ($19); **Ultima II** ✔☺ Gotta Blush Cheek Color ($15); **Victoria Jackson Cosmetics** Blush Compact ($20.95); **Victoria's Secret Cosmetics** ✔☺ Sudden Blush Sheer Blushing Powder ($15); **Vincent Longo** Powder Blush ($16); **Wet 'n' Wild** Silk Finish Blush ($2.59).

BEST CREAM-TO-POWDER OR STICK BLUSHES: Avon ✔☺ Split Second Blush Stick ($7.50); **Avon beComing** Light De-Light ($13); **BlissLabs** blissglows ($15); **Christian Dior** Multi-Touch ($27.50); **Clarins** ✔☺ Multi Blush ($22); **Estee Lauder** Minute Blush Creme Stick for Cheeks ($26) and BlushLights Creamy CheekColor ($25); **Lancome** Couleur Flash Blush Stick ($28.50); **Laura Mercier** ✔☺ Cheek Colour Stick to Go ($26); **M.A.C.** Cheekhue ($17.50); **Make Up For Ever** ✔☺ Blush Pencil Mat ($14); **Maybelline** Express Blush ($7.29); **Parthena** Play on Lights Light Diffusing Face Color ($12.50); **Paula Dorf Cosmetics** ✔☺ Cheek Color Cream ($18); **Prescriptives** Mystick Swivel Cheekcolor ($25); **Revlon** Sleek Cheeks Creme Blush Duo ($9.49); **Three Custom Color** Creme to Powder Blush ($20.50); **Ultima II** Nourishing Blush Stick ($17); **Wet 'n' Wild** Twist-Up Blush Stick ($1.99).

BEST LIQUID OR GEL BLUSHES: BeneFit ✔☺ BeneTint ($26); **CARGO** ColorTube ($24); **Clinique** Gel Blush ($10.50); **Hard Candy** ✔☺ Stain for Lip & Cheek ($18); **Illuminare** *Perfect Color Blush SPF 21 ($20) and *Perfect Color Blush Ultimate SPF 21

($20); **L'Oreal** Translucide Luminous Gel Blush ($9.49); **Lorac** Sheer Wash ($24); **Morgen Schick** Schick Stick ($15) and High Roller ($15); **NARS** ✓☺ Color Wash ($24); **Origins** Pinch Your Cheeks ($10); **philosophy** the supernatural lip & cheek tint ($15); **Sephora** ✓☺ Aqua Tints ($14); **Tony & Tina** ✓☺ Herbal Cheek Gel ($15); **Trish McEvoy** Lip & Cheek Tint ($18); **Vincent Longo** ✓☺ Lip & Cheek Gel Stain ($18).

BEST TRADITIONAL CREAM BLUSHES: **Alexandrea de Markoff** Outlasting Cream Blush ($31.50); **BeneFit** ✓☺ Cheekies ($20); **Bobbi Brown** Cream Blush Stick ($25); **Giorgio Armani** ✓☺ Color Retouch ($35); **I-Iman** Stick Blush ($20); **Make Up For Ever** Blush Cream ($18); **Merle Norman** Luxiva Creme Blush ($14.50); **Sonia Kashuk** Luminous Creme Blush ($7.99); **Stila** Convertible Color Dual Lip and Cheek Cream ($28); **Stila Sport** Color Push-Ups All Over Color ($20); **Vincent Longo** ✓☺ Creme Blush ($16).

BEST EYESHADOWS

By now many of you know my opinions about shiny, as well as blue, green, or any brightly colored eyeshadow. It still is my goal to find the best matte shades available, and I am thrilled to say that the cosmetics industry does deliver (though the never-ending parade of shine has made finding these somewhat more difficult). There are plenty of matte shades available in all price ranges. You can shop the cosmetics counters in both drugstores and department stores and find wonderful textures and colors, though when it comes to variety of matte shades, the scales are tipped in favor of the department stores. Those of you who love eyeshadow with some shine will find these options almost limitless, regardless of where you shop.

BEST POWDER EYESHADOWS: **Avon** True Color Powder Eyeshadows ($3.50 singles; $4.25 duos; $6 quads); **BlissLabs** blisslids ($17); **Bobbi Brown** Eye Shadow ($18); **Bonne Bell** Powder Pak ($2.39 for two shadows, $2.39 for compact); **Calvin Klein** Eye Shadow ($15) and Eye Shadow Palette ($25); **CARGO** Eyeshadow ($15); **Chanel** Quadra Eyeshadow ($52.50) and Shadowlights ($27); **Club Monaco** Eyeshadow ($12); **Elizabeth Arden** Eyeshadow Singles ($10 for eyeshadow pan, $3 for duo compact); **Estee Lauder** ✓☺ Color Intensity Microfine Powder Eyeshadow ($13.50), ✓☺ Color Intensity Duos ($25), ✓☺ Color Intensity Quads ($35), and ✓☺ Pure Color Eyeshadow ($20); **FACE Stockholm** ✓☺ Pearl Shadow and ✓☺ Matte Shadow ($15); **Giorgio Armani** Eyeshadow ($22); **Guerlain** Divinora Radiant Color Single Eyeshadow ($22); **Helena Rubinstein** Color Statement for Eyes Radiant Eyeshadow ($18.50); **Jane Iredale** PurePressed Eyeshadows ($17.50) and Duo Eye Shadows ($27); **Lancome** Colour Focus Exceptional Wear EyeColour ($16.50); **Laura Mercier** Eye Colour ($18) and Eye Paints ($50); **Laura Mercier** Eye Shadows ($16) and Jewel Eye Shadow Box ($37.50); **M.A.C.** Eye Shadows ($12.50 small, $14 large) and Colour Theory No. 9 ($15); **Make Up For Ever** Eyeshadow ($15); **Marcelle** Eyeshadow Singles ($6.25); **Origins** Eyeshadow ($12.50); **Paula Dorf Cosmetics** Eye Color Glimmers ($17) and ✓☺ Eye Color ($17); **Paula's**

Select ✔☺ Soft Matte Eyeshadow ($7.95); **Physicians Formula** ✔☺ Quad Eye Shadow ($6.49); **Prescriptives** Pick 2 Eyeshadow ($13 each, $3 for refillable duo compact) and Eyepaints Wet/Dry Eyeshadow ($20); **Prestige Cosmetics** Shadow ($3.89) and Shadow Quads ($5.99); **Principal Secret** Eye Shadow Quad ($25); **Quo Cosmetics** ✔☺ Eye Shadow ($12) and ✔☺ Eyeshadow Quads ($20); **Rimmel** Special Eyes Eyeshadow ($1.97); **Shu Uemura** ✔☺ Pressed Eyeshadows ($18); **Sonia Kashuk** Enhance Eye Color ($4.99) and Eyeshadow Palette ($12.99); ✔☺ **Stila** Eyeshadow ($16); **Sue Devitt Studio Makeup** ✔☺ Silky Matte Eyeshadow ($18) and Silky Sheen Eyeshadow ($18); **Three Custom Color** Eyeshadow Singles ($17, $12.50 for refill); **Trish McEvoy** Eye Shadow ($15) and Face Essentials ($45); **Ultima II** Wonderwear Eye Color ($15.50); **Vincent Longo** Powder Eyeshadow ($16).

BEST CREAM-TO-POWDER, GEL, LIQUID, AND CREAM EYESHADOWS: **Bobbi Brown** Shimmer Eye Shadow ($18); **Cover Girl** CG Smoothers Gel Eye Color ($5.79); **Illuminare** ✔☺ *All Day Eye Colors SPF 15 ($15); **Laura Mercier** Eye Basics ($22); **M.A.C.** Paints ($15) and Sheer Colour Extract ($12.50); **Mary Kay** MK Signature Eyesicles Eye Color ($10); **Revlon** ✔☺ Illuminance Creme Eyeshadown($6.29); **Revlon Skinlights** Color Lighting for Eyes/Cheeks ($7.89).

BEST EYE AND BROW SHAPERS

Some cosmetics companies sell two different eye pencils, one for the brow and the other for lining the eye. Other cosmetics companies are more straightforward and sell only one that does both jobs. The latter is the practical and honest approach. There is often little to no difference between eye and brow pencils; the contrasts mainly involve color choice. When there is a difference, it's usually that the brow pencil has a drier, harder consistency, which can make drawing on a brow difficult, though it does tend to look less greasy. So, what you choose is a matter of personal preference and experimentation. (As an option, I strongly recommend that you fill in the brow with a powder, either an eyeshadow or a specific eyebrow powder.)

An eye pencil with a dry texture makes it difficult to line the eyelid after you've applied your eyeshadows; if the pencil is on the greasy side, it will line the lid more easily, but it is also more likely to smear under the lower lashes in a very short time.

For pencils, you can shop the more expensive lines, but it is a waste of money because, regardless of the price, almost all the pencils I tested in all price ranges had more similarities than differences. The few pencils awarded a Paula's Pick designation are about as groundbreaking as it gets in the world of standard pencils, but definitely a step above the norm.

Several companies sell colored eyebrow gels as a way to fill, lift, and define the brow. There are also a few companies that make a clear brow gel that isn't much different from using hairspray on a toothbrush and brushing it through the brow. For the most part, the natural-colored brow gels are great. I strongly recommend them as another way to make eyebrows look fuller but not artificial. If you can learn how to use the eyebrow "mascaras," they can be a great alternative to pencils.

The only pencils on the following "Best" list are the ones that have a Paula's Pick rating. This is because almost every line has its share of extremely standard, but overall good and mostly reliable, pencils. On the other hand, the liquid liners, brow powders, and brow gels do differ, and often vary widely, and this group includes products that are rated with just a happy face and others that are rated as a Paula's Pick, with the Paula's Pick products being the creme de la creme.

BEST LIQUID OR CAKE EYELINERS: **Alexandra de Markoff** Professional Secrets Liquid Eyeliner ($19); **Almay** ✓☺ Amazing I-Liner Liquid Liner ($5.79); **Aloette** ✓☺ Liquid Eyeliner ($12.50); **Anna Sui** Liquid Eye Liner ($19); **Avon beComing** Defining Moment Liquid Liner ($12); **Awake** Liquid Eye Liner ($20); **Bobbi Brown** ✓☺ Long Wear Gel Eyeliner ($18); **Chanel** Liquid Eyelines ($28.50); **Christian Dior** Diorliner ($30); **Clarins** Liquid Eye Liner ($18); **Clinique** Eye Defining Liquid Liner ($13.50); **Cover Girl** ✓☺ Liquid Pencil Felt Tip Eyeliner ($5.69); **FACE Stockholm** Cake Eyeliner ($12); **Guerlain** ✓☺ Eye-Liner ($26); **L'Oreal** ✓☺ Line Intensifique Extreme Wear Liquid Liner ($7.89) and Super Liner Perfect Tip Eyelining Pen ($7.19); **La Prairie** Cellular Treatment Wet/Dry Eyeliner ($32); **Lancome** ✓☺ Artliner Precision Point EyeLiner ($25); **M.A.C.** Creme Liner ($11.50) and Liquid Liner ($15); **Make Up For Ever** Color Liner ($19); **N.Y.C.** Liquid Eyeliner ($1.99); **Prestige** Cosmetics ✓☺ Liquid Eyeliner ($4.89); **Urban Decay** Liquid Liner ($14); **Yves St. Laurent** Eyeliner Moire ($25).

BEST EYEBROW POWDERS: **Awake** Stardom Eye Brow ($26); **BeautiControl** Brow Powder ($15); **Body & Soul** Brow Powder ($16.50); **FACE Stockholm** Brow Shadow ($18); **Lancome** Brow Artiste ($28); **Merle Norman** Only Natural Brow Powder ($12); **Paula Dorf Cosmetics** Brow Duet ($18); **Three Custom Color** Brow Powder ($17.50, $12.50 for refill); **Trucco** Hi-Brow Trio ($25.50); **Vincent Longo** Brush-On Brow ($16).

BEST EYEBROW PENCILS: **Awake** ✓☺ Brow Pencil ($16); **BlissLabs** ✓☺ Powder Brows ($16); **Chanel** ✓☺ Sculpting Brow Pencil ($26) and ✓☺ Precision Brow Definer ($26); **Christian Dior** ✓☺ Powder Eyebrow Pencil ($21); **Hard Candy** ✓☺ Training Brow Pencil ($16); **Lancome** ✓☺ Le Crayon Poudre for the Brows ($19.50); **M.A.C.** ✓☺ Eye Brow Pencil ($12.50); **Marcelle** ✓☺ Accent Eyebrow Crayon ($7.50).

BEST EYE PENCILS: **BlissLabs** ✓☺ Lidstick ($15); **Bonne Bell** ✓☺ Eye Definer ($2.39); **Cover Girl** ✓☺ Perfect Blend Eye Pencil ($4.69) and ✓☺ Perfect Point Plus ($5.39); **Giorgio Armani** ✓☺ Smooth Silk Eye Pencil ($22); **Marcelle** ✓☺ Kohl Eye Liner ($7.50); **Maybelline** ✓☺ Expert Eyes Defining Liner ($5.09); **Paula Dorf Cosmetics** ✓☺ Eye Pencil ($15); **Prestige Cosmetics** ✓☺ Eye Liner ($3.29); **Revlon** ✓☺ Softstroke Powderliner ($6.79); **Rimmel** ✓☺ Exaggerate Full Colour Eye Definer ($1.97); **Versace** ✓☺ Comfort Eye Pencil ($24); **Youngblood** ✓☺ Eye Liner Pencil ($10).

BEST BROW GELS AND TINTS (CAN ALSO BE USED FOR HAIR AS WELL): **bare escentuals** Brow Finishing Gel ($12); **Bobbi Brown** ✓☺ Natural Brow Shaper ($16.50); **The Body**

Shop Brow & Lash Tint ($10.50); **Bonne Bell** Lash Gloss Clear Mascara ($3.49); **Borghese** ✓☺ Brow Milano ($20); **Calvin Klein** Brow Groomer ($16); **Christian Dior** Brow Gel ($16); **Estee Lauder** Brow Gel ($15); **FACE Stockholm** Brow Fix ($13); **Jane** Fan Club Lash & Brow Mascara ($3.22); **Jane Iredale** ✓☺ PureBrow Colour ($20) and PureBrow Fix ($20); **L'Oreal** Brow Stylist Sculpting Brow Mascara ($7.49); **Laura Mercier** Eye Brow Gel ($18); **Lip Ink** Miracle Brow Liner ($15) and Miracle Brow Tint ($15); **M.A.C.** Brow Set ($12) and Colored Brow Set ($12); **Merle Norman** Tinted Brow Sealer ($12.95); **Origins** Just Browsing ($12) and **Brow Fix** ($12); **Paula Dorf Cosmetics** Perfect Brow ($14) and Brow Tint ($15); **Paula's Select** ✓☺ Brow/Hair Tint ($8.95); **Revlon** ColorStay Brow Color ($8.19); **Sonia Kashuk** Brow Gel ($5.99); **Trish McEvoy** Brow Gel ($18); **Trucco** Brow Shaper ($9); **Victoria's Secret Cosmetics** Unruffled ($12.50).

BEST LIPSTICKS AND LIP PENCILS

There are no truly bad lipsticks. If anything, most lipsticks are worthwhile—it just depends on your color and texture preferences. There are a handful of products with decent to very good stains that have surprising staying power (lasting for almost the whole day), but those still do not look or feel like traditional lipstick. Almost without exception, the greasier or glossier the lipstick, the less likely it is to last, and the more matte the lipstick, the longer it is likely to stick around, although if it is too matte it may be too drying. If you don't have a problem with dry lips and you want to try a matte look, mattes and ultra-mattes are certainly preferred for their longevity.

It is very difficult to make lipstick suggestions, because this is one area where preference plays a bigger role than any other issue (and women change their impressions and selections all the time). Still, after reviewing hundreds of lipsticks for this edition, I did come across a select few that deserve the elevated status of Paula's Pick. This is primarily due to their sublime textures, long wear, near-perfect color selection, and/or the inclusion of an effective broad-spectrum sunscreen of at least SPF 15.

For the most part, almost every cosmetics company's lipsticks, and especially lip pencils, work very well, with differences reflected only in terms of your personal preference (opaque rather than sheer coverage, creamy or glossy finish) rather than in performance. Instead of listing every product or product line that receive happy faces— which is virtually every company—I include only a list of Paula's Picks and specialty lipstick products that are relatively unique. Just keep in mind that price has nothing to do with how well a lipstick performs.

BEST MATTE LIPSTICKS: FACE Stockholm ✓☺ Matte Lipstick ($17); **Lancaster** ✓☺ Velvet Matte Comfort Lipstick ($14.50); **M.A.C.** ✓☺ Retro Matte Lipstick ($14) and ✓☺ Matte Lipstick ($14); **Make Up For Ever** ✓☺ Rouge Pinceau Mat Lipstick and Brush ($19); **Paula's Select** ✓☺ Soft Matte Lipstick ($7.95).

BEST CREAM LIPSTICKS: Aloette ✓☺ Lip Color ($9.50); **Awake** ✓☺ True-Rich Lipstick ($22); **Calvin Klein** ✓☺ Lip Color ($16); **Clarins** ✓☺ Le Rouge Lipstick

($21.50); **Clinique** ✓☺ Long Last Soft Shine Lipstick ($12.50) and ✓☺ Long Last Soft Matte Lipstick ($12.50); **Club Monaco** ✓☺ Matte Lipstick ($14); **Giorgio Armani** ✓☺ Smooth Lipstick ($21); **L'Oreal** ✓☺ Colour Riche Rich Creamy LipColour ($7.19) and ✓☺ Colour Riche Crystal Shine LipColour ($7.19); **Lorac** ✓☺ Cream Lipstick ($17.50) and ✓☺ Matte Lips ($17.50); **M.A.C.** ✓☺ Satin Lipstick ($14); **NARS** ✓☺ Semi-Matte Lipstick ($21); **Paula's Select** ✓☺ Soft Cream Lipstick ($7.95); **Prescriptives** ✓☺ Soft Suede Lipstick ($17.50) and ✓☺ Paints Liquid Lipcolor ($20); **Prestige Cosmetics** ✓☺ Moisture Intense Lipcolor ($3.99); **Quo Cosmetics** ✓☺ Lipstick ($14.50); **Rimmel** ✓☺ Lasting Finish Lipstick ($3.97), ✓☺ Rich Moisture Lipstick ($3.97), and ✓☺ Exaggerate HydraColor Lipstick ($3.97); **Three Custom Color** ✓☺ Lipstick ($15, $18.50 for Special Shades); **Wet 'n' Wild** ✓☺ MegaPlump Lipstick ($1.99).

    Best lipsticks with effective UVA/UVB sunscreen: **Almay** ✓☺ PureTints Protective Lip Care SPF 25 ($4.89) and ✓☺ Lip Vitality Smoothing Lipcolor with Kinetin SPF 15 ($8.69); **Borghese** ✓☺ Lip Treatment Moisturizer with SPF 15 ($18.50); **Cover Girl** Triple Lipstick SPF 15 ($5.89); **Revlon** ✓☺ Absolutely Fabulous Lip Cream SPF 15 ($6.99); **Ultima II** Ultimate Edition Lipstick SPF 15 ($15) and Pucker & Pout Flowing Lipstick SPF 15 ($12.50).

    Best lip glosses: **Aveda** ✓☺ Brilliant Lip Shine ($11.50); **Christian Dior** ✓☺ Diorific Plastic Shine Lip Gloss ($22); **L'Oreal** ✓☺ Glass Shine High Shine Lip Gloss ($7.99); **Make Up For Ever** ✓☺ Super Lip Gloss ($16) and ✓☺ Liquid Lip Color ($18); **Mary Kay** ✓☺ MK Signature Lip Gloss ($12); **N.Y.C.** ✓☺ Brush-On Lip Color ($2.99); **Paula's Select** ✓☺ Soft Shine Moisturizing Lip Gloss ($7.95); **Revlon** ✓☺ LipGlide Color Gloss ($9.49); **Shiseido** <u>The</u> **Makeup** ✓☺ Lip Gloss ($19); ✓☺ **Three Custom Color** Lip Gloss ($15) and Lip Gloss Palette ($53); **Versace** ✓☺ Wet Cream Lipgloss SPF 8 ($20); ✓☺ **Wet 'n' Wild** MegaSlicks Liquid Lipcolor ($1.69).

    Best lip pencils: **Aloette** ✓☺ Waterproof Lipliner ($10); **English Ideas** ✓☺ Kolour Crayon ($13.50); **L'Oreal** ✓☺ Rouge Pulp Anti-Feathering Lip Liner ($8.49); **Merle Norman** ✓☺ Definitive Lip Liner ($12); **N.Y.C.** ✓☺ Lip Liner Pencil (99 cents); **Paula Dorf Cosmetics** ✓☺ Lip Pencil ($15); **Paula's Select** ✓☺ Long-Lasting Anti-Feather Lipliner ($6.95); **Prescriptives** ✓☺ Deluxe Lip Pencil ($17.50).

    Best ultra-matte lipsticks: **Jafra** Always Color Stay-On Lipstick ($10); **L'Oreal** Colour Endure Stay On LipColour ($9.39).

    Best lipstains: **Cover Girl** ✓☺ Outlast All Day Lipcolor ($10.99); **Lip Ink** Starter Kit ($45), Aliens Color ($15), and Ultra ($15); **Max Factor** ✓☺ Lipfinity ($8.99); **Urban Decay** ✓☺ Ink Lip Stain ($17).

Best Mascaras

    I must hand it to the cosmetic chemists involved in formulating mascaras, because the wealth of superior choices is expanding almost monthly! I should also mention the wide variety of mascara brushes available, from a thin rod to a tightly packed full row of bristles. Performance of any mascara comes down to the perfect marriage of brush and formula, with packaging components coming in a close second. The rest is preference-related depending on the lash look you want. I am ecstatic to report there are excellent mascaras in all price ranges. Obviously, it is not logical to buy the most expensive mascara when reasonably priced ones are equally good. Given that this is one product you can't readily test at the counters, try a few of the inexpensive ones I suggest and see if that isn't the most sensible and beautiful decision. **Note:** Paula's Pick mascaras are those that have an almost instant "wow factor"; that is, those that offer impressive results quickly and go the distance when it comes to superior application and wear.

BEST MASCARAS: Almay ✓☺ One Coat Mascara Lengthening ($6.19), One Coat Mascara Thickening ($6.19), and Longest Lashes Mascara ($6.19); **Anna Sui** Mascara ($19); **Artistry by Amway** Smudgeproof Mascara 200 ($14.50); **Avon** Incredible Lengths Long and Strong Mascara ($6) and ✓☺ Curl-Ascious Maximum Curling Mascara ($6); **Avon beComing** On the Fringe All Purpose Mascara ($11); **Awake** ✓☺ Volumizing Mascara ($17); **Bobbi Brown** Defining Mascara ($16), Thickening Mascara ($16), and Lash Glamour Lengthening Mascara ($19); **CARGO** Mascara ($16); **Chanel** ✓☺ Instant Lash Mascara ($21.50), Sculpting Mascara Extreme Length ($21.50), ✓☺ Extreme Length Fine Lashes ($21.50), and ✓☺ Extreme Cils Drama Lash Mascara ($21.50); **Christian Dior** Mascara Parfait ($20) and ✓☺ Mascara Fascination ($20); **Clarins** Lengthening Mascara ($19.50), ✓☺ Pure Volume Mascara ($19.50), and ✓☺ Pure Curl Mascara ($19.50); **Clientele** Mascara ($15); **Clinique** Naturally Glossy Mascara ($12), Full Potential Mascara ($12), Long Pretty Lashes Mascara ($12.50), and ✓☺ Lash Doubling Mascara ($12.50); **Cover Girl** Super Thick Lash ($5.49) and Triple Mascara ($6.29); **Darphin** Mascara ($20); **Erno Laszlo** Multi-pHase Mascara ($19); **Estee Lauder** Futurist Lash-Extending Mascara ($18); **Giorgio Armani** ✓☺ Soft Lash Mascara ($20); **Givenchy** Thickening Lash by Lash Mascara ($19) and Lengthening and Curling Lashes Mascara ($19); **Helena Rubinstein** Generous Mascara ($22), Long Lash Mascara ($22), ✓☺ Spectacular Mascara ($22), ✓☺ Crescendo Mascara ($22), and ✓☺ Extravagant Mascara ($22); **Jane** ✓☺ Fan Club Curling Mascara ($3.22); **L'Oreal** Superior Longitude Extreme Lengthening Mascara ($9.29), Lash Out Curved Brush ($5.99), Voluminous Volume Building Mascara ($6.69, straight or curved brush), ✓☺ Lash Intensifique Lash by Lash Body Building Mascara ($6.69), ✓☺ Lash Intensifique Curved Brush Mascara ($6.69), ✓☺ Lash Architect 3-D Dramatic Mascara ($7.49, straight or curved brush), and ✓☺ Le Grand Curl ($7.39); **Lancome** Flextencils Full Extension Curving Mascara ($20), Amplicils Panoramic Volume Mascara ($20), ✓☺ Definicils High Definition Mascara ($20), ✓☺ Intencils Full Intensity Mascara ($20), and ✓☺ Magnificils Full Lash Precision Mascara ($20); **Laura Mercier** ✓☺ Thickening and Building Mascara ($19); **Lorac** Lorac Lashes ($17.50); **M.A.C.** ✓☺ Pro Lash Mascara ($9.50); **Make Up For Ever** Mascara ($16); **Mary Kay** Endless Performance Mascara ($8.50); **Max Factor** S-T-R-E-T-C-H Mascara ($3.97) and ✓☺ 2000 Calorie Mascara ($3.97); **Maybelline**

Lash Expansion Mascara ($5.59), Illegal Lengths Mascara ($5.09), ✔☺ Full N' Soft Mascara ($6.39 regular or curved brush), ✔☺ Lash Discovery Mascara ($5.99 regular or curved brush), and ✔☺ Volum' Express Mascara ($4.69; regular or curved brush); **Nu Skin** Water Resistant Mascara ($15); **Origins** Fringe Benefits Mascara ($12); **Paula Dorf Cosmetics** Mascara ($15); **Paula's Select** ✔☺ Lush Mascara ($7.95) and ✔☺ Epic Lengths Mascara ($7.95); **Physicians Formula** To Any Lengths Lash Extending Mascara ($4.89); **Quo Cosmetics** ✔☺ Lush Mascara ($12); **Revlon** ColorStay Lash Color ($6.49) and ColorStay Extra Thick Lashes Mascara ($6.49); **Rimmel** Extra Super Lash Mascara ($3.97), ✔☺ Exaggerate Extra Volume Mascara ($3.97), and ✔☺ Curly Mascara ($3.97); **Shiseido The Makeup** Volume Mascara ($18) and Distinguish Mascara ($19); **Shu Uemura** Mascara Basic ($27); **Sonia Kashuk** ✔☺ Lashify Mascara ($5.99); **T. Le Clerc** ✔☺ Mascara ($19); **Tony & Tina** ✔☺ Herbal Eye Mascara ($18); **Trish McEvoy** Lash Curling Mascara ($25), ✔☺ Mascara ($18), and ✔☺ Lash Building Mascara ($18); **Ultima II** Wonderwear Mascara ($13) and Lashfinder Mascara ($11); **Urban Decay** ✔☺ Skyscraper Mascara ($16.50); **Versace** Fabulous Mascara ($21), Gorgeous Curling Mascara ($21), and ✔☺ Luxury Volume Mascara ($21); **Victoria Jackson Cosmetics** Dual Mascara ($13.95) and Traditional Mascara ($14.95); **Yves St. Laurent** Mascara Volume Luxurious Mascara ($22.50).

BEST WATERPROOF MASCARAS: Avon beComing ✔☺ Swim Wear Waterproof Mascara ($11); **Bobbi Brown** Lash Lustre Waterproof Mascara ($16); **Clinique** Gentle Waterproof Mascara ($12.50); **Club Monaco** Waterproof Mascara ($12); **Cover Girl** ✔☺ Professional Waterproof Mascara ($5.49); **Guerlain** Super-Cils Mascara Waterproof ($22); **Jane** ✔☺ Fan Club Waterproof Mascara ($3.22); **L'Oreal** ✔☺ Lash Intensifique Waterproof Mascara ($6.69) and ✔☺ Le Grand Curl Waterproof Mascara ($5.99); **Lancome** Eternicils Enduring Mascara Waterproof ($20) and Aquacils Waterproof Mascara with Keratine ($20); **Max Factor** 2000 Calorie Aqualash Mascara ($3.97) and Lashfinity Mascara ($5.99); **Maybelline** Illegal Lengths Waterproof Mascara ($5.09), ✔☺ Wonder Curl Waterproof Mascara ($5.09 regular or curved brush), and ✔☺ Volum' Express Waterproof Mascara ($4.69); **Merle Norman** Waterproof Mascara ($13.50); **Revlon** ColorStay Extra Thick Lashes Mascara Waterproof ($6.49); **smashbox** Mascara ($16); **Stila Sport** ✔☺ Lash Visor Waterproof Mascara ($16); **Yves St. Laurent** Mascara Aquaresistant ($22.50).

BEST BRUSHES

More than ever before, professional-sized brushes are available in all price ranges. Keep in mind that the texture of the brush is more important than the source of the bristles. While many cosmetics companies love to brag about the type and grade of animal hair used, you are not buying a mink coat. What counts is softness, shape, and firmness, no matter the source. There are a few companies offering synthetic brushes that are often exquisite replications of natural-hair brushes that must be felt to be believed.

These synthetic brushes are perfectly worthwhile options, and an easy solution for anyone conflicted about using animal-hair brushes for applying makeup. Companies that offer a good selection of excellent synthetic brushes are indicated with an asterisk. Please note that not every single brush in the lines below is rated with a happy face. For comments on individual brushes and individual Paula's Pick brushes, please refer to the reviews in Chapter Three. A brush collection that rates a Paula's Pick represents a superior combination of performance, craftsmanship, and value.

BEST MAKEUP BRUSHES AND BRUSH SETS: Aloette ✓☺ Professional 7-Piece Brush Set ($66.50); Anna Sui Brushes ($12–$50); Arbonne ✓☺ 9-Piece Precision Brush Set ($35); Aveda ✓☺ Brushes ($8–$27.50); bare escentuals Brushes ($12–$24); Bath & Body Works Brushes ($7–$13); BeneFit ✓☺ Brushes ($11–$27); Bobbi Brown Brushes ($18.50–$62.50); Body & Soul Brushes ($20–$55); The Body Shop ✓☺ Brushes ($8.50–$24.50); CARGO ✓☺ Brushes ($12–$68); Chanel Brushes ($22.50–$45); Chantecaille Brushes ($20–$70); Clarins Brushes ($16–$28); Club Monaco Brushes ($6–$38); Darphin Brushes ($30 or $50); Dr. Hauschka Face Powder Brush ($56.50) and Blush Brush ($38.95); Elizabeth Arden Brushes ($20–$40); FACE Stockholm Brushes ($6–$30); Giorgio Armani Brushes ($20-$54); Guerlain Terracotta Brush ($28.50) and Meteorites Brush ($28.50); Jane Iredale Brushes ($9–$39); La Prairie Brushes ($28–$65, $125–$250 for collections); Lancaster Brush Set ($40); Laura Mercier Brushes ($20–$52; $100–$250 for sets); Lorac Brushes ($9–$35); M.A.C. Brushes ($8.50–$62.50); *Make Up For Ever ✓☺ Brushes ($13–$54); Maybelline Brushes ($3.89–$4.99); Merle Norman Eyeshadow Brushes ($5.50–$6.50) and Concealing Brush ($6.50); Morgen Schick Brushes ($13–$42.50); NARS Brushes ($18–$50); Nu Skin Nu Colour Brush Collection ($115); *Origins Brushes ($15–$50); *Paula Dorf Cosmetics Brushes ($6–$60); Paula's Select ✓☺ Brushes ($7.95–$16.95); Prescriptives Brushes ($16–$50); Prestige Cosmetics Makeup Brushes ($2.49–$12.99); Quo Cosmetics ✓☺ Brushes ($12–$20); Revlon Beauty Shapers Brushes ($5.99–$7.99); Sephora ✓☺ Brushes ($4–$42); ✓☺ *Shu Uemura Brushes ($5–$260); Sisley Brushes ($30–$44); smashbox #13 Foundation Brush ($32); Sonia Kashuk Brushes ($1.99–$9.99); Stila ✓☺ Brushes ($15–$58); Sue Devitt Studio Makeup Brushes ($15–$70); Three Custom Color ✓☺ Brushes ($3.50–$55); *Tony & Tina ✓☺ Technology of Kindness Brushes ($36–$98); Trish McEvoy ✓☺ Brushes ($14–$58); Trucco Brushes ($12–$26); *Urban Decay ✓☺ Brushes ($15–$35); Versace ✓☺ Brushes ($18–$63); Victoria's Secret Cosmetics Brushes ($8.50–$17.50); Youngblood Brushes ($12–$20).

BEST SPECIALTY PRODUCTS

The following is a list of miscellaneous products that have interesting effects or an intriguing premise that just doesn't fit squarely into the above categories. For more details please refer to the reviews for these products in Chapter Three.

Aloette Makeup Planner ($66.50); **BeautiControl** ✔☺ Lip Control Creme ($7); **The Body Shop** Matt It Face and Lips ($12.50) and Facial Blotting Tissues ($10 for 130 sheets); **I-Iman** Matte Spray ($27); **M.A.C.** Matte Creme Matifiance ($16.50); **Paula Dorf Cosmetics** Brush Out Brush ($12); **smashbox** Anti-Shine Foundation ($26); **philosophy** ✔☺ the little black book ($37.50); **Prescriptives Magic** Invisible Line Smoother ($35 for 0.5 ounce); **Sephora** ✔☺ Makeup Bags ($4–$38) and Train Cases ($65–$98); **Shiseido** <u>The</u> **Makeup** Eraser Pencil ($15); **Sonia Kashuk** ✔☺ Face Palette ($19.99); **Stila** ✔☺ 4-Pan Compact ($12); **Urban Decay** Special Sauce ($12).

CHAPTER SEVEN

Cosmetics Dictionary

Over the past several years, the amount of research that has taken place on cosmetic ingredients of all kinds, and especially on plants and their components, is nothing less than astounding. In recognition of that, this chapter is the most completely overhauled, reworked, and updated part of this book. You'll find that almost every ingredient has new data, studies, and research into its use and efficacy.

All of my comments regarding the efficacy of the plant extracts used in products throughout this edition and in the following list are based on published research as indicated by the sources cited in the entries for specific extracts.

Please keep some basic things in mind. First, and frequently stated in the literature describing research or studies for plant extracts, their efficacy depends on the part of the plant being used (stems, for example, may have very different contents and benefits than the leaves or roots), the time of year plants are collected, the type of extraction or preservation methods used, and the amount of the extract contained in the product. Second, because the cosmetics industry has no standards for any of these issues, even a general comment about the effectiveness of an extract cannot be translated with any certainty into how effective that extract will be when it is included as an ingredient in a cosmetic product. So, what the research provides is basically a collective or overall approach to understanding something about the benefit you may be gaining from an ingredient.

When valid studies and research do exist for various plant extracts, it is important to realize that most of the comments regarding efficacy are the result of research that examined a pure concentrate or a pure tincture (a plant substance in a simple solution). There are very few studies for any plant extract with respect to its use and efficacy when mixed into a cosmetic at fractional amounts or in combination with a host of other ingredients.

All of the following comments relate primarily to external (topical) application only. Benefits listed as obtainable when the plant extracts or vitamins are taken into the system orally as supplements do not necessarily relate to and/or can be very different from those obtainable from topical application. For oral and systemic benefits, please refer to www.drweil.com.

I strongly suggest you use this dictionary to help gain an understanding of the significance of an ingredient in terms of its claims and its potential for irritation, and then to help you make comparisons between products.

For a specific condition, like clogged pores, determining whether it is best to avoid a particular formulation because it might cause breakouts is very hard to do just by interpreting of the formulation. In this case, your best approach for determining a product's chance of causing breakouts is how thick it is and how emollient (rich) it feels. The thicker a product, the more likely that the thickening/emollient ingredients it contains could find their way into a pore and cause problems. The lighter in weight a product is (as long as it doesn't contain irritating ingredients), the far less likely it is to cause problems.

The following is a list of all the major ingredients found in cosmetic products.

2-bromo-2-nitropropane-1,3-diol. Trade name bronopol, a formaldehyde-releasing preservative (Source: *Contact Dermatitis,* December 2000, pages 339–343). *See* formaldehyde-releasing preservative.

***Acacia dealbata* leaf wax.** *See* gums.

***Acacia farnesiana* extract.** Fragrant extract from a type of acacia tree. There is no research showing it to have any benefit for skin (Source: *Natural Medicines Comprehensive Database,* http://www.naturaldatabase.com). *See* gums.

***Acacia senegal*.** Herb that can have anti-inflammatory properties, but that is used primarily as a thickening agent. *See* gums.

Accutane. Generic name: isotretinoin. A prescription-only drug derived from vitamin A, and which is taken orally. It essentially stops the oil production in sebaceous glands (the oil-producing structures of the skin) and literally shrinks these glands to the size of a baby's. This prevents sebum (oil) from clogging the hair follicle, mixing with dead skin cells, and rupturing the follicle wall to create an environment where a bacterium *(Propionibacterium acnes)* can thrive, which can result in pimples or cysts. Normal oil production resumes when treatment is completed, and the sebaceous glands slowly begin to grow larger again, but rarely as large as they were before treatment. "Because of its relatively rapid onset of action and its high efficacy with reducing more than 90% of the most severe [acne] inflammatory lesions, Accutane has a role as an effective treatment in patients with severe acne that is recalcitrant to other therapies" (Source: *Journal of the American Academy of Dermatology,* November 2001, Supplemental pages 188–194). However, Accutane is controversial for many reasons, principally because of its most insidious side effect: It has been proven to cause severe birth defects in nearly 90% of the babies born to women who were pregnant while taking it. Other commonly reported, although temporary, side effects of Accutane include dry skin and lips, mild nosebleeds (your nose can get really dry for the first few days), hair loss, aches and pains, itching, rash, fragile skin, increased sensitivity to the sun, headaches, and peeling palms and hands. More serious, although much less common, side effects include severe headaches, nausea, vomiting, blurred vision, changes in mood, depression, severe stomach pain, diarrhea, decreased night vision, bowel problems, persistent dryness of eyes, calcium deposits in tendons, an increase in cholesterol levels, and yellowing of the skin.

acerola fruit extract. Acerola contains vitamin C (*See* vitamin C). However, the dry acerola fruit and powder are unlikely to be a good source of vitamin C because much of the vitamin C is destroyed during the drying and processing (Source: *Natural Medicines Comprehensive Database,* http://www.naturaldatabase.com).

acetic acid. Acid found in vinegar, some fruits, and human sweat. It can be a skin irritant and drying to skin, though it also has disinfecting properties.

acetone. Strong solvent. Used to remove nail polish.

acetyl carnitine HCL. *See* L-carnitine.

acetyl glucosamine. Amino acid sugar and primary constituent of mucopolysaccharides and hyaluronic acid. It is an agent that has good water-binding properties for skin. In large concentrations it can be effective for wound healing. There is research showing that chitosan (which is composed of acetyl glucosamine) can help wound healing in a complex process (Sources: *Cellular-Molecular-Life-Science,* February 1997, pages 131–140; and *Biomaterials,* June 2001, pages 1667–1673). However, that is a few generations removed from the tiny amount of acetyl glucosamine used in cosmetics. Further, there is no research demonstrating that wrinkles are related to wounds.

acetyl glyceryl ricinoleate. Used as an emollient and thickening agent in cosmetics. *See* glyceryl ester.

acetyl hexapeptide-3. Synthetically derived peptide. The company selling acetyl hexapeptide-3 (trade name Argireline), Centerchem (www.centerchem.com), is based in Spain and, according to their Web site, "Argireline works through a unique mechanism which relaxes facial tension leading to a reduction in superficial facial lines and wrinkles with regular use. Argireline has been shown to moderate excessive catecholamines release." I strongly doubt that any of that is true because there isn't a shred of research substantiating any part of it. However, even if it were vaguely true, that would not be good news for your body because you wouldn't want a cosmetic without any safety data, efficacy documentation, or independent research messing around with your catecholamines. Catecholamines are compounds in the body such as epinephrine, adrenaline, and dopamine that serve as neurotransmitters. Epinephrine is a substance that prepares the body to handle emergencies such as cold, fatigue, and shock. A deficiency of dopamine in the brain is responsible for the symptoms of Parkinson's disease. None of that sounds like something you want a cosmetic to inhibit or reduce. What if you accidentally overuse the product or apply too much? It isn't known what excessive catecholamine release would mean for your body.

acetylated castor oil. Used as an emollient and thickening agent. *See* glyceryl ester.

acetylated hydrogenated cottonseed glyceride. Used as an emollient and thickening agent. *See* glyceryl ester.

acetylated lanolin. Emollient derived from lanolin. *See* lanolin.

acetylated palm kernel glycerides. Used as an emollient and thickening agent. *See* glyceryl ester.

Achillea millefolium. *See* yarrow extract.

acid. Anything with a pH lower than 7 is acid—above 7 is alkaline. Water has a pH of 7. Skin has an average pH of 5.5.

acne soap. Soaps that often contain very irritating ingredients in addition to harsh cleansers that, especially when combined with other acne treatments, can super-irritate the skin. There is no reason to overclean the skin, because breakouts have nothing to do with how clean your skin is! A study reported in *Infection* (March-April 1995, pages 89–93) demonstrated that "in the group using soap the mean number of inflammatory [acne] lesions increased…. Symptoms or signs of irritation were seen in 40.4% of individuals…." Furthermore, if the acne cleanser does contain antibacterial agents, the benefit would be washed down the drain.

acrylate. *See* film-forming agent.

acrylates/C10-30 alkyl acrylate crosspolymer. *See* film-forming agent.

Actaea racemosa. *See* black cohosh.

active ingredient. The active ingredients list is the part of an ingredient label that must adhere to specific regulations mandated by the FDA. Active ingredients must be listed first on an ingredient label. The amount and exact function of each active ingredient is controlled and must be approved by the FDA. Active ingredients are considered to have a pharmacological altering effect on skin, and these effects must be documented by scientific evaluation and approved by the FDA. Active ingredients include such substances as sunscreen ingredients, skin-lightening agents, and benzoyl peroxide. *See* inactive ingredient.

adenine. Component of DNA that carries genetic information to the cell. *See* DNA.

adenosine triphosphate. All living things need a continual supply of energy in order to function. Animals obtain their energy by oxidizing foods, plants obtain energy by using chlorophyll to trap sunlight. However, before the energy can be used, it must first be changed into a form that the organism can readily use. This special form, or carrier of energy, is the molecule adenosine triphosphate (ATP). In humans, ATP serves as the major energy source within the cell to drive a number of biological processes such as protein synthesis. However, for the cell to use ATP it must be broken down by hydrolysis to yield adenosine diphosphate (ADP), which is then further broken down to yield adenosine monophosphate (AMP). Whether or not ATP applied topically on skin can affect cellular energy has not been shown. It is unlikely that this complicated chemical molecular process can be generated from the outside in.

advanced glycation endproduct. Advanced glycation endproducts, also known as AGEs, are caused by the body's major fuel source, namely glucose. This simple sugar is essential for energy, yet it also can bind strongly to proteins (the body's fundamental building blocks) and form abnormal structures (AGEs) that progressively damage tissue elasticity. Once AGEs are generated, they begin a process that prevents many systems from behaving normally by literally causing tissue to cross-link and become hardened (Source:

Proceedings of the National Academy of Sciences, USA, March 14, 2000, pages 2809–2813). The theory is that by breaking these AGE bonds you can undo or stop the damage they cause. There are studies showing aminoguanidine and carnosine to be AGE inhibitors that can prevent glucose cross-linking of proteins and the loss of elasticity associated with aging and diabetes, but many other substances are potential candidates as AGE inhibitors as well. One study examined over 92 substances and 29 of them showed some degree of inhibitory activity, with 9 compounds proving to be 30 to 40 times stronger than aminoguanidine (Source: *Molecular Cell Biology Research Communications,* June 2000, pages 360–366). AGE and free-radical damage may be inextricably linked (Sources: *European Journal of Neuroscience,* December 2001, page 1961; and *Neuroscience Letters,* October 2001, pages 29–32), this has not been shown to be relevant to topical application of cosmetics that include these substances.

Aerocarpus santalinus. *See* red sandalwood.

Aesculus hippocastanum. *See* horse chestnut.

agar. *See* algae.

age spot. There is no such thing as an "age spot." The skin can develop brown patches for many reasons, but the characteristic small ones on the hands, arms, and face are caused by sun damage. These are possibly indications of precancerous conditions and should be watched carefully for changes. *See* melasma.

AGE. *See* advanced glycation endproduct.

AHA. Acronym for alpha hydroxy acid. AHAs are derived from various plant sources or from milk. However, 99% of the AHAs used in cosmetics are synthetically derived. In low concentrations (less than 3%) AHAs work as water-binding agents. At concentrations over 4% and in a base with an acid pH of 3 to 4, these can exfoliate skin cells by breaking down the substance in skin that holds skin cells together. The most effective and well-researched AHAs are glycolic acid and lactic acid. Malic acid, citric acid, and tartaric acid may also be effective but are considered less stable and less skin-friendly; there is little research showing them to have benefit for skin.

AHAs may irritate mucous membranes and cause irritation. However, AHAs have been widely used for therapy of photodamaged skin, and also have been reported to normalize hyperkeratinization (over-thickened skin) and to increase viable epidermal thickness and dermal glycosaminoglycans content. A vast amount of research has substantially described how the aging process affects the skin and has demonstrated that many of the unwanted changes can be improved by topical application of AHAs, including glycolic and lactic acid (Sources: *Cutis,* August 2001, pages 135–142; *Journal of the European Academy of Dermatology and Venereology,* July 2000, pages 280–284; *American Journal of Clinical Dermatology,* March-April 2000, pages 81–88; *Skin Pharmacology and Applied Skin Physiology,* May-June 1999, pages 111–119; *Dermatologic Surgery,* August 1997, pages 689–694 and May 2001 pages 1–5; *Journal of Cell Physiology,* October 1999, pages 14–23; and *British Journal of Dermatology,* December 1996, pages 867–875).

Ahnfeltia concinna **extract.** *See* algae.

ahnfeltia extract. *See* algae.

Ajuga turkestanica **extract.** The only research about this plant indicates that it may have anabolic steroid properties (Source: *Eksperimental'naya i Klinicheskaya Farmakologiya* [Russian scientific journal], May 1997, pages 41–44). There is no other research showing this to be of benefit for skin.

alanine. *See* amino acid.

Alaria esculenta. *See* algae.

albumin. Found in egg white, and can leave a film over skin. It can constrict skin temporarily, which can make it look smoother temporarily, but it can also cause irritation and is not helpful for skin.

Alchemilla vulgaris. Plant with antimicrobial properties. Its high tannin content can cause skin irritation (Source: *Journal of Ethnopharmacology,* July 2000, pages 307–313).

alcloxa. Technically known as aluminum chlorhydroxy allantoinate, alcloxa has constricting properties that can be irritating for skin.

alcohol. Group of organic compounds that have a vast range of forms and uses in cosmetics. In some benign forms they are glycols used as humectants that help deliver ingredients into skin. When fats and oils (*See* fatty acid) are chemically reduced, they become a group of less-dense alcohols called fatty alcohols that can have emollient properties or can become detergent cleansing agents. When alcohols have low molecular weights they can be drying and irritating. The alcohols to be concerned about in skin-care products are ethanol, denatured alcohol, ethyl alcohol, methanol, benzyl alcohol, isopropyl alcohol, and SD alcohol, which can be extremely drying and irritating to skin (Sources: "Skin Care—From the Inside Out and Outside In," *Tufts Daily,* April 1, 2002; *eMedicine Journal,* May 8, 2002, volume 3, number 5, http://www.emedicine.com; *Cutis,* February 2001, pages 25–27; and *Contact Dermatitis,* January 1996, pages 12–16).

Aleurites fordii **oil.** Oil from the Polynesian tung tree. May have antimicrobial properties for skin (Source: *Journal of Ethnopharmacology,* November 1995, pages 23–32).

alfalfa extract. Can be an antioxidant in skin-care products (Source: *Journal of Agricultural Food Chemistry,* January 2001, pages 308–314).

algae. Very simple, chlorophyll-containing organisms, in a family that includes more than 20,000 different known species. A number of these have been used for drugs, where they work as anticoagulants, antibiotics, antihypertensive agents, blood cholesterol reducers, dilatory agents, insecticides, and anti-tumorigenic agents. In cosmetics, algae are used as thickening agents, water-binding agents, and antioxidants. Some algae are also potential skin irritants. For example, the phycocyanin found in blue-green algae has been suspected of allergenicity and of causing dermatitis on the basis of patch tests (Source: *Current Issues in Molecular Biology,* January 2002, pages 1–11). Other forms of algae, such as Irish moss and carrageenan, contain proteins, vitamin A, sugar, starch, vitamin B1, iron, sodium, phosphorus, magnesium, copper, and calcium. These are all useful as sources for skin care, either as emollients or antioxidants (Source: *Journal of Agricultural Food Chemistry,* February 2002, pages 840–845). However, the claims that algae can stop or eliminate wrinkling, heal skin, or provide other elaborate benefits are completely unsubstantiated.

algin. Brown algae. *See* brown algae and algae.

alginic acid. Obtained by treating dry seaweed with acid to create a very thick, gelatin-like substance. Used as a thickening agent in cosmetics. *See* algae.

aliphatic hydrocarbon. Hydrocarbon contained in natural gas and mineral oils. It is a synthetic fluid with varying properties that range from solvent to slip agent. *See* slip agent, and solvent.

alkaline. Anything with a pH higher than 7 is alkaline (below 7 is acid). Water has a pH of 7; skin has an average pH of 5.5. Skin irritation can be caused by products with a pH of 8 or over (Sources: *eMedicine Journal,* January 7, 2002, volume 3, number 1, http://www.emedicine.com; *Cutis,* December 2001, Supplemental pages 12–19; and *Contact Dermatitis,* April 1996, pages 237–242). Also, research indicates that the bacterium that causes acne, *Proprionibacterium acnes,* proliferates when the skin is more alkaline (Sources: *Infection,* March-April 1995, pages 89–93; and *Journal of Antimicrobial Chemotherapy,* September 1994, pages 321–330).

alkanet extract. *See Alkanna tinctoria* extract.

***Alkanna tinctoria* extract.** There is research showing this extract to have antiviral and antibacterial properties (Sources: *Planta Medica,* August 1997, page 384, and January 1979, pages 56–60). However, information on some Web sites about hepatitis C has shown that this extract is toxic to the liver when consumed (Sources: HCV Advocate, http://www.hcvadvocate.org/HERBS.pdf; and Hepatotoxic Herbs, http://home.caregroup .org/clinical/altmed/interactions/Herb_Groups/Hepatotoxic.htm).

alkyloamides. Identified on skin-care product labels as DEA (*See* diethanolamine), TEA (triethanolamine), and MEA (monoethanolamine), these are used primarily for their foaming ability in shampoos, but can also be used as thickening or binding agents. They can be skin irritants. In addition, alkyloamides contain a free amine that can combine with formaldehyde-releasing preservatives in cosmetics, and there is concern that they may form carcinogens.

allantoin. By-product of uric acid extracted from urea and considered an effective anti-irritant.

all-trans retinoic acid. Active ingredient in Retin-A and Renova. *See also* tretinoin.

almond oil PEG-6 esters. Used as emollient and thickening agents in cosmetics. *See* glyceryl ester.

almond oil. Oil extracted from the seeds of almonds and used as an emollient. *See* natural moisturizing factors.

Aloe barbadenis. *See* aloe vera.

aloe extract. *See* aloe vera.

aloe juice. *See* aloe vera.

aloe vera. There is no real evidence that aloe vera (*Aloe barbadenis*) helps the skin in any significant way. An article in the *British Journal of General Practice* (October 1999, pages 823–828) stated that "Topical application of aloe vera is not an effective preventative for radiation-induced injuries…. Whether it promotes wound healing is unclear…. Even though there are some promising results, clinical effectiveness of oral or topical aloe vera is not sufficiently defined at present." There is research indicating that isolated components of aloe vera, such as glycoprotein, can have some effectiveness for wound healing and as an anti-irritant (Sources: *Journal of Ethnopharmacology*, December 1999, pages 3–37; *Free-Radical Biology and Medicine*, January 2000, pages 261–265; and *British Journal of Dermatology*, October 2001, pages 535–545). In pure form, aloe vera's benefits on skin are probably its lack of occlusion and the refreshing sensation it provides.

alpha bisabolol. *See* bisabolol.

alpha glucan oligosaccharide. Used as an emollient and has water-binding properties. *See* mucopolysaccharide.

alpha hydroxy acid. *See* AHA.

alpha lipoic acid. Enzyme that, when applied topically on skin, can be a very good antioxidant. While studies of alpha lipoic acid do exist, none of them have been carried out on people, and none have been double-blind or placebo-controlled to evaluate its effect on wrinkling (Source: *Clinical & Experimental Dermatology*, October 2001, pages 578–582). Most of the research has been done on human dermal fibroblasts in vitro (test tube) in cell-culture systems. In vitro results are interesting, but it's not known if the results translate to human skin. These models do mimic human skin, but something that mimics human skin is still not the same as living skin. There is research showing that alpha lipoic acid, when taken orally, can have benefit in preventing cellular damage via its antioxidant properties (Source: *Annals of the New York Academy of Sciences*, April 2002, pages 133–166). Again, whether all that translates to the effect on skin is unclear. It is clear from the research that alpha lipoic acid is a potent antioxidant, but this isn't the only one, and to date, there is no one that is best. *See* antioxidant.

alpha-tocopherol. *See* vitamin E.

***Alpinia officinarum* root extract.** May have antioxidant properties (Source: *Mutation Research*, May 2001, pages 135–150).

***Alteromonas* ferment extract.** *Alteromonas* is a gram-negative bacteria found in seawater. It may have water-binding properties for skin, but there is scant research supporting this.

Althaea rosea. *See* mallow.

Althea officinalis. Latin name for marshmallow plant. *See* mallow.

alumina. Aluminum oxide, used as an abrasive, thickening agent, and absorbent.

aluminum chlorohydrate. Chemically a salt, and used in antiperspirant preparations. It can be extremely irritating on abraded skin.

aluminum magnesium silicate. Salt that has absorbent properties.

aluminum silicate. Salt that has absorbent and abrasive properties.

aluminum starch octenylsuccinate. Powdery thickening agent, absorbent, and anticaking agent used in cosmetics.

aluminum sulfate. Topical disinfectant and typical ingredient in deodorants. It can be a skin irritant.

amino acid. Fundamental constituents of all proteins found in the body, such as: alanine, arginine, asparagine, aspartic acid, cysteine, cystine, glutamic acid, glutamine, glycine, histidine, isoleucine, leucine, lysine, methionine, phenylalanine, proline, serine, threonine, tryptophan, tyrosine, and valine. Some of these amino acids can be synthesized by the body; others, the essential amino acids, must be obtained from protein in the diet. In skin-care products, these types of ingredients work primarily as water-binding agents, and some have antioxidant properties and wound-healing abilities as well. However, these substances cannot affect, change, or rebuild wrinkles. Whether the protein in a skin-care product is derived from an animal or a plant, the skin can't tell the difference. *See also* protein, and natural moisturizing factors.

aminobutyric acid. Amino acid that has water-binding properties for skin and may be an anti-inflammatory. It supposedly also increases growth hormone when taken orally, but the only support for this is a single obscure study that was conducted more than two decades ago in fewer than 20 subjects, and the results have yet to be replicated by other scientists.

aminomethyl propanediol. Used to adjust pH in cosmetics.

ammonium chloride. Alkaline salt used as a pH balancer in skin-care products; it is not used in concentrations that would be problematic for skin.

ammonium laureth sulfate. Can be derived from coconut; used primarily as a detergent cleansing agent and is considered gentle and effective. *See* surfactant.

ammonium lauryl sulfate. Can be derived from coconut; used primarily as a detergent cleansing agent and is considered gentle and effective. *See* surfactant.

amniotic extract or fluid. There is some research showing pure concentrations of amniotic fluid (human) have some benefit for wound healing (Sources: *Journal of Hand Surgery*, March 2001, pages 332–339; and *Cornea*, September 1996, pages 517-524). However, there is no research showing amniotic fluid to be effective for wrinkles or other skin-care needs or when diluted in cosmetic formulations.

amodimethicone. *See* silicone.

amyl cinnamate. Fragrant component.

amyl salicylate. Fragrant component.

amyris oil. Fragrant oil. It has no known benefit for skin.

Ananas sativus **fruit extract.** *See* pineapple extract.

Anacyclus pyrethrum. *See* pellitory.

Anacystis nidulans **extract.** *See* algae.

andiroba oil. Extracted from the Brazilian mahogany tree; it has anti-inflammatory properties (Source: http://www.rain-tree.com/andiroba.htm).

andrographolide. Component of *Andrographis paniculata,* an herb common to India and China. It has anti-inflammatory and antioxidant properties (Source: *British Journal of Pharmacology,* January 2002, pages 399–406).

Angelica polymorpha sinensis **root extract.** *See* dong quai.

anisaldehyde. Synthetic fragrance used in cosmetics.

anise. Also known as aniseed; it can have potent antioxidant and antibacterial properties (Source: *Phytotherapy Research,* February 2002, pages 94–95), but its fragrant component makes this a potential skin irritant and it can cause photosensitivity (Source: *Natural Medicines Comprehensive Database,* http://www.naturaldatabase.com).

annato extract. Natural plant colorant derived from the flesh surrounding the seed of *Bixa orellana,* a shrub native to South America. Used as a coloring agent, it produces a deep yellow-orange to red color.

Anthemis nobilis **flower extract.** *See* chamomile.

Anthyllis vulnera. There is no research showing this plant to have any benefit for skin.

antibacterial. Any ingredient that destroys or inhibits the growth of bacteria. In the case of cosmetics, it destroys or inhibits the bacteria that cause blemishes.

anti-inflammatory. Any ingredient that reduces certain signs of inflammation, such as swelling, tenderness, pain, irritation, or redness.

anti-irritant. Any ingredient that reduces certain signs of inflammation, such as swelling, tenderness, pain, itching, or redness.

antioxidant. Describes the function a specific ingredient can have on skin to reduce the effects of free-radical damage. Free-radical damage can be caused by the presence of oxygen or any compound that contains an oxygen molecule (such as carbon monoxide, hydrogen peroxide, and superoxide), sunlight, and pollution. Any substance that impedes or slows free-radical damage by preventing the oxidative action of molecules is referred to as an "antioxidant." Many vitamins have antioxidant properties, including vitamins A, C, and E, as do amino acids such as methionine, L-cysteine, and L-carnitine; enzymes such as superoxide dismutase and ecatalase; and coenzymes such as alpha lipoic acid and coenzyme Q10. Other antioxidant compounds include glutathione and methylsufonylsulfate.

No one is exactly sure what free-radical damage and antioxidants have to do with wrinkles or skin damage, but, theoretically, when free-radical damage originates from natural environmental factors and fails to be cancelled out by antioxidant protection, then wrinkles appear. If people don't get enough antioxidant protection, either from the body's production, from dietary sources, or from other sources (including antioxidants put on skin), free-radical damage continues unrestrained, causing cells to break down and impairing or destroying their ability to function normally. Free-radical damage destroys collagen and other skin components. There are problems, however, with the hope that stopping free-radical damage with antioxidants can protect your skin, and these problems are that free-radical damage is constant and extensive. How could you ever use enough antioxidants to stop it? How much is needed? How much oxygen, sunlight, or pollution can you really keep away from all skin cells, or even some skin cells? How fast do the antioxidants you apply to your skin get used up? Do they last 20 minutes, one hour, two hours, or more on the skin? At this time, no one knows the answers to any of these questions for sure. Major investigations are currently under way in this fascinating area of human aging (intrinsic aging) and sun damage (extrinsic aging), factors that most unquestionably influence wrinkling. However, even though many respected researchers are working on this issue, the research is still in its infancy, and suggesting anything beyond that is sheer fantasy. *See* free-radical damage.

aorta extract. Obtained from hearts of animals. It is supposed to have rejuvenating properties for skin, but this has never been proven in research of any kind. Much like any part of a human or animal body, the heart tissue is a source of proteins, amino acids, and other water-binding agents for skin. Because of the concerns regarding Mad Cow Disease, ingredients like these are best avoided in skin-care products.

apple cider vinegar. *See* vinegar.

apricot kernel. Seed that, especially when finely ground, is a natural exfoliant.

apricot kernel oil. Emollient plant oil pressed from the seeds of apricots. Similar to other nonfragrant plant oils. *See* natural moisturizing factors.

arachidic acid. Derived from peanut oil and used as an emollient and thickening agent.

arachidonic acid. Produced from phospholipids and fatty acids. There is research showing that this is potentially unsafe and mutagenic when used topically, though more study is needed to decide this conclusively (Sources: *Journal of Cellular and Molecular Life Sciences,* May 2002, pages 799–807; and *Journal of Environmental Pathology, Toxicology, and Oncology,* 2002, volume 21, number 2, pages 183–191).

arachidyl alcohol. Waxy substance used as a thickening agent and emollient.

arachidyl propionate. Waxy substance used as a thickening agent and emollient.

***Arachis hypogaea* extract.** Extract of the plant commonly known as the peanut. It can have emollient and anti-inflammatory properties for skin, though peanut allergy is one of the five most frequent food allergies in children and in adults (Source: *Allergy,* 2002, volume 57, supplemental number 72, pages 88–93).

arbutin. Hydroquinone derivative isolated from the leaves of the bearberry shrub, cranberry, blueberry, and most types of pears. Because of arbutin's hydroquinone content, it can have melanin-inhibiting properties (Sources: *Analytical Biochemistry,* June 2002, pages 260–268, and June 1999, pages 207–219; *Pigment Cell Research,* August 1998, pages 206–212; and *Journal of Pharmacology and Experimental Therapeutics,* February 1996, pages 765–769). Although the research describing arbutin's effectiveness is persuasive (even if almost all of the research has been done on animals or in vitro), concentration protocols have not been established. That means we just don't know how much arbutin it takes to have an effect in lightening the skin. Moreover, most cosmetics companies don't use arbutin in their products because there are Shiseido-owned patents controlling its use in skin-care products for skin lightening. To get around this problem, many cosmetics companies use plant extracts that contain arbutin, such as bearberry. There is limited research, mostly animal studies or in vitro, showing that the plant extracts that contain arbutin have any impact on skin. Whether or not these extracts are effective in the small amounts present in cosmetics has not been established. *See* hydroquinone.

Arctium lappa. *See* burdock root.

Arctostaphylos uva ursi leaf. *See* bearberry.

argan oil. Derived from the nuts of the argania tree; it is an emollient oil (similar to peanut oil) that may have anti-inflammatory properties, but there is no research supporting that claim.

Argania spinosa kernel oil. *See* argan oil.

Argania spinosa oil. *See* argan oil.

arginine. Amino acid that has antioxidant properties and can be helpful for wound healing (Sources: *Journal of Surgical Research*, June 2002, pages 35–42; *Nitric Oxide*, May 2002, pages 313–318; and *European Surgical Research*, January-April 2002, pages 53–60). *See* amino acid.

Argireline. Trade name for acetyl hexapeptide-3. *See* acetyl hexapeptide-3.

arnica extract. Extract from the plant *Arnica montana*. It is repeatedly stated in all herbal journals used for the compilation of this dictionary that arnica should not be applied to abraded skin because it is a significant skin irritant. *The PDR Family Guide to Natural Medicines & Healing Therapies* says: "Repeated contact with cosmetics containing arnica can cause itching, blisters, ulcers, and dead skin." (Other Sources: IFA—International Federation of Aromatherapists; and http://www.int-fed-aromatherapy.co.uk). It is also associated with a high incidence of skin sensitization (Source: *American Journal of Contact Dermatitis*, June 1996, pages 94–99).

arrowroot. Thickening agent; it has no known benefit for skin.

Artemisia absinthium extract. *See* mugwort extract.

Artemisia annua. *See* wormwood.

Artemisia vulgaris. *See* mugwort extract.

artemia extract. *See* algae.

artichoke extract. May have antioxidant benefits for skin (Sources: *Journal of Agricultural Food Chemistry*, June 2002, pages 3458–3464; and *Free Radical Research*, August 2001, pages 195–202).

Ascophyllum nodosum. Form of seaweed. *See* algae.

ascorbic acid. Form of vitamin C that has antioxidant properties (Sources: *Advances in Experimental Medicine and Biology*, 2002, number 505, pages 113–122; and *Journal of Investigative Dermatology*, February 2002, pages 372–379) and anticancer properties when taken orally (Source: *Cancer Detection and Prevention*, 2000, volume 24, number 6, pages 508–523). It can be difficult to stabilize in formulations (Source: *International Journal of Pharmaceutics*, October 1999, pages 233–241). Its acid component is considered a skin irritant.

ascorbyl glucosamine. Form of vitamin C that has little research showing it to have the antioxidant or skin-lightening properties of other forms of vitamin C. The only study that does exist showed it to be ineffective for skin lightening (Source: *Dermatology*, 2002, volume 204, number 4, pages 281–286).

ascorbyl glucoside. Form of vitamin C combined with glucose. It can function as an antioxidant, though only minimal research substantiates this.

ascorbyl palmitate. Stable and nonacidic form of vitamin C that is effective as an antioxidant (Source: *Biochemical and Biophysical Research Communications*, September 1999, pages 661–665).

asiatic acid. *See Centella asiatica.*

asparagine. *See* amino acid.

***Asparagopsis armata* extract.** Derived from seaweed. *See* algae.

***Asparagus officinalis* stem extract.** There is no research showing asparagus extract to have any benefit for skin.

aspartic acid. *See* amino acid.

***Aspergillus/Aspidosperma quebracho* ferment.** Fungus compound that is considered problematic for health (Sources: *Current Opinion in Microbiology*, August 2002, page 386; and *Annual Review of Microbiology*, July 2002, http://micro.annualreviews.org/cgi/content/abstract/012302.160625v4). *Aspidosperma quebracho* is the bark of a tree that has no known benefit for skin (Source: *Natural Medicines Comprehensive Database*, http://www.naturaldatabase.com). There is no research showing that the combination of *Aspergillus* and *Aspidosperma quebracho* have any benefit for skin.

Astragalus membranaceus. Scientific name for the Chinese herb Huang qi, also known as milk vetch. *See* milk vetch root.

Astragalus sinicus. *See* milk vetch root.

ATP. *See* adenosine triphosphate.

Avena sativa. Oat plant. Oat extract can have anti-irritant and anti-inflammatory properties (Source: *Skin Pharmacology and Applied Skin Physiology*, March-April 2002, pages 120–124).

Avens extract. Derived from the geum plant family; can be a skin irritant due to its tannin and eugenol content.

avobenzone. Synthetic sunscreen ingredient (also known as Parsol 1789 and butyl methoxydibenzoylmethane) that can protect against the entire range of the sun's UVA rays (Sources: *Photodermatology, Photoimmunology, Photomedicine*, August 2000, pages 147–155; and *International Journal of Pharmaceutics*, June 2002, pages 85–94). *See* UVA.

avocado oil. Emollient oil similar to other nonfragrant plant oils. *See* natural moisturizing factors.

awapuhi. English name for wild ginger. *See* ginger.

Ayurveda. Alternative health practice historically developed in India. The term "Ayurveda" is based on two Sanskrit words: *ayu,* meaning life, and *veda,* meaning science. According to an article in the *Indian Journal of Experimental Biology* (May 2000, pages 409–414), the Ayurvedic system of treatments believes that the "living system is made of panch-mahabuta, in the form of vata, pitta and kapha at the physical level and satwa, raja and tama at the mental level. This covers the psychosomatic constitution and [is] commonly known as the Tridosh theory. The imbalance in these body humours [mechanisms] is the basic cause of any type of disease manifestation." Another interpretation of Ayurvedic theory, in *Alternative Therapies Health Medicine* (March 7, 2001), noted that "The body is composed of 3 body doshas, 3 mental doshas, 7 dhatus, and malas. The harmony among the body doshas of vata (nervous system), pitta (enzymes), and kapha (mucus) and the gunas, or mental doshas (which are human attributes: satogun [godly], rajas [kingly], and tamas [evil]), constitutes health, and their disharmony constitutes disease. The management of illness requires balancing the doshas back into a harmonious state through lifestyle interventions, spiritual nurturing, and treatment with herbo-mineral formulas based on one's mental and bodily constitution." There is no research showing how or if Ayurvedic principles of any kind can affect skin (though they do not prevent sun damage—that, at least, is certain).

Azadirachta indica. See neem extract.

azelaic acid. Trade name Azelex; a component of grains such as wheat, rye, and barley. It is effective for a number of skin conditions when applied topically in a cream formulation at a 20% concentration. For the most part, azelaic acid is recommended as an option for acne treatment, but there is also some research showing it to be effective for the treatment of skin discolorations. For example, "The efficacy of 20% azelaic acid cream and 4% hydroquinone cream, both used in conjunction with a broad-spectrum sunscreen, against melasma was investigated in a 24-week, double-blind study with 329 women. Over the treatment period the azelaic acid cream yielded 65% good or excellent results; no significant treatment differences were observed with regard to overall rating, reduction in lesion size, and pigmentary intensity. Severe side effects such as allergic sensitization or exogenous ochronosis were not observed with azelaic acid" (Source: *International Journal of Dermatology,* December 1991, pages 893–895). However, other research suggests that azelaic acid is more irritating than hydroquinone mixed with glycolic acid or kojic acid (Source: *eMedicine Journal,* http://www.emedicine.com, November 5, 2001, volume 2, number 11). Azelaic acid is a consideration for skin lightening if you have had problems using hydroquinone along with tretinoin. *See* hydroquinone, and tretinoin.

Azelex. *See* azelaic acid.

azuki beans. Legumes ground and used as abrasives in scrub products.

azulene. Chamomile extract used primarily as a coloring agent in cosmetics. It can have antioxidant and anti-inflammatory properties (Sources: *Journal of the European Academy of Dermatology and Venereology,* September 2001, pages 486–487; and *Biochemical and Biophysical Research Communications,* 1996 volume 92, number 3, pages 361–364). *See* chamomile.

babassu oil. Plant oil that can have emollient properties for skin. There is no research showing it to have special properties for skin.

Bacillus subtilis. Naturally occurring widespread bacterium that can be used to control plant diseases, fungal plant infestation, and several types of mildew. Based on available information, the bacterium appears to have no adverse effects on humans or the environment (Source: Environmental Protection Agency, http://www.epa.gov/pesticides/biopesticides/factsheets/fs006479e.htm). There is no known benefit when applied to skin.

balm mint extract. Derived from a fragrant plant; it poses some risk of skin irritation. It also has some reported antiviral properties (Source: *Phytomedicine,* 1999, volume 6, pages 225–230). Claims that it can help heal wounds are not substantiated.

balsam peru. Also balsam of Peru, a fatty resin that topically can cause allergic skin reactions and contact dermatitis. It also has the potential to cause photodermatitis and phototoxicity. Balsam peru is a standard used in patch tests for skin sensitivity due to its high incidence of causing reactions (Sources: *Natural Medicines Comprehensive Database,* http://www.naturaldatabase.com; and *Journal of the American Academy of Dermatology,* December 2001, pages 836–839).

banana extract. Has weak antioxidant properties (Source: *Free Radical Research,* February 2002, pages 217–233).

bar cleanser. Although these are often advertised as being gentle or specially formulated, they are no better than or different from what you can buy at the drugstore. The irritating and pore-clogging ingredients are still included regardless of the price or claim.

barberry. Plant whose primary component, berberine, is an alkaloid that can have antibacterial properties and some cellular anti-inflammatory response. However, it can also be a skin irritant because of its effect on cells (Sources: *Alternative Medicine Review,* April 2000, pages 175–177; and *Healthnotes Review of Complementary and Integrative Medicine,* http://www.healthwell.com/healthnotes/herb).

barium sulfate. Earth mineral used as a whitening agent. It can be a skin irritant.

barley extract. From barley plants. Can have antioxidant properties when ingested, but there is no research showing this to be the case when applied topically (Source: *Journal of Agricultural Food and Chemistry,* March 2001, pages 1455–1463).

bay leaf oil. Can be a potent antioxidant (Source: *Biological and Pharmaceutical Bulletin,* January 2002, pages 102–108). However, it can also be a potent skin irritant due to its fragrant component.

bearberry extract. Contains arbutin (Sources: *Phytochemical Analysis,* September-October 2001, pages 336–339; and *Phytochemical Analysis,* September 2001, pages 336–339).

Arbutin can inhibit melanin production, though this has only been shown in vitro and in pure form, not in a cosmetic formulation. The fractional amounts of bearberry extract used in cosmetics and the small amount of arbutin the extract contains mean this is unlikely to affect skin or melanin. *See* arbutin.

bee pollen. Can have antioxidant properties (Source: *Journal of Agricultural Food Chemistry,* April 2001, pages 1848–1853), but there is no research showing this to be true when applied topically. Bee pollen can also be a skin irritant and allergen (Source: *International Archives of Allergy and Immunology,* June 2001, pages 96–111).

beeswax. Substance made by bees to build the walls of their honeycomb. It is a thickening agent and has some emollient properties.

behenic acid. Fatty acid used as a thickening agent and surfactant. *See* fatty acid.

behenyl alcohol. Thickening agent. It is not related to irritating forms of alcohol.

Bellis perennis. See daisy flower extract.

bentonite. Claylike material used as an absorbent in cosmetics. It can be drying for skin.

benzalkonium chloride. Antimicrobial agent used as a preservative in skin-care products. There is no research showing it to have any effect against the acne bacterium *Propionibacterium acnes.*

benzephenone-3. Also called oxybenzone. Sunscreen agent that protects primarily from the sun's UVB rays and some, but not all, UVA rays (Sources: http://www.photoderma tology.com/sunprotection.htm; and *Skin Therapy Letter,* Volume 2, Number 5, 1997). *See* UVA.

benzocaine. Topical anesthetic (Source: *Dermatologic Surgery,* December 2001, pages 1010–8; and *Pediatric Dentistry,* January-February 2001, pages 19–23).

benzoic acid. Preservative used in skin-care products; considered less irritating than other forms of preservatives.

benzoin extract. Balsam resin that has some disinfecting and fragrant properties; may also be a skin irritant (Source: *Natural Medicines Comprehensive Database,* http://www.naturaldatabase.com).

benzoin siam. *See* benzoin extract.

benzophenones. Sunscreen agents used to protect mostly from UVB radiation and from some, but not all, UVA radiation (Sources: http://www.photodermatology.com/sunprotection.htm; and *Skin Therapy Letter,* Volume 2, Number 5, 1997). *See* UVA.

benzothonium chloride. Used as a preservative in cosmetics. It is generally considered less irritating than other forms of preservatives.

benzoyl peroxide. Considered the most effective over-the-counter choice for a topical antibacterial agent in the treatment of blemishes (Source: *Skin Pharmacology and Applied Skin Physiology,* September-October 2000, pages 292–296). The amount of research demonstrating the effectiveness of benzoyl peroxide is exhaustive and conclusive (Source: *Journal of the American Academy of Dermatology,* November 1999, pages 710–716). Among benzoyl peroxide's attributes is its ability to penetrate into the hair follicle to reach the bacteria that are causing the problem, and then kill them—with a low risk of irritation. It also doesn't pose the problem of bacterial resistance that some prescription topical antibacterials (antibiotics) do (Source: *Dermatology*, 1998, volume 196, issue 1, pages 119–125). Benzoyl peroxide solutions range in strength from 2.5% to 10%. It is best to start with less potent concentrations, because a 2.5% benzoyl peroxide product is much less irritating than a 5% or 10% concentration, and it can be just as effective. The necessary concentration completely depends on how stubborn the strain of bacteria in your pores happens to be.

benzyl alcohol. *See* alcohol.

Berberis aristata. *See* barberry.

bergamot oil. When used topically, it is a photosensitizer and has photomutagenic properties, meaning it can induce malignant changes to cells (Sources: *Natural Medicines Comprehensive Database*, http://www.naturaldatabase.com; *Journal of the American Academy of Dermatology*, September 2001, pages 458–461; and *Journal of Dermatology*, May 1994, pages 319–322).

Bertholletia excelsa **extract.** *See* Brazil nut extract.

beta hydroxy acid. *See* salicylic acid.

beta sitosterol. Plant extract, similar to cholesterol, that can have antimicrobial properties (Source: *Journal of Ethnopharmacology*, January 2002, pages 129–132) and, therefore, may be a problem for healthy skin cells. There is a small amount of research showing it to have anti-inflammatory properties (Source: *Biological & Pharmaceutical Bulletin*, May 2001, pages 470–473).

beta-carotene. Member of the carotenoid family. There are hundreds of carotenoids including lycopene and lutein. Beta-carotene is a precursor that helps form retinol (vitamin A). It is converted to vitamin A in the liver as needed. Topically, beta-carotene is a potentially good antioxidant and can reduce the effects of sun damage, though this benefit is dose dependent. There is research showing that too much beta-carotene can generate oxidative damage (Sources: *Photochemistry and Photobiology*, May 2002, pages 503–506; *Federation of American Societies for Experimental Biology Journal*, August 2002, pages 1289–1291; and *Berkeley Wellness Newsletter*, http://www.berkeleywellness.com/html/ds/dsBetaCarotene.php).

beta-glucan. Polysaccharide, meaning it is a sugar (such as starch and cellulose) that can be derived from yeast. It has some antioxidant properties and is a strong anti-inflammatory agent (Source: *Free Radical Biology and Medicine*, February 2001, pages 393–402). *See* mucopolysaccharide.

Betula alba. *See* birch bark.

BHA. Abbreviation for **b**utylated **h**ydroxy**a**nisole, a synthetic, potent antioxidant (Sources: *Journal of Agricultural Food Chemistry*, May 2002, pages 3322–3327; and *Free Radical Biology and Medicine*, 1996, volume 20, number 2, pages 225–236), but also a suspected carcinogen (Source: *Mutation Research and Genetic Toxicology and Environmental*

Mutagenesis, July 2002, pages 123–133). The abbreviation BHA should not be confused with beta hydroxy acid (salicylic acid), which is an exfoliant. Salicylic acid is abbreviated in discussions as BHA, but it would never be shown that way on a cosmetic ingredient list.

BHA. *See* salicylic acid.

BHT. Butylated hydroxytoluene, a synthetic, potent antioxidant that also has carcinogenic properties (Sources: *Mechanisms of Ageing and Development,* May 2002, pages 1203–1210; and *Free Radical Biology and Medicine*, February 2000, pages 330–336). *See* BHA.

bifida ferment lysate. Type of bacteria found in the digestive system. It has no known effect on skin.

bifidus extract. Carbohydrate in human milk that stimulates the growth of *Lactobacillus bifidus* in the intestine. In turn, the *Lactobacillus bifidus* lowers the pH of intestinal contents and suppresses the growth of *Escherischia coli* and other pathogenic bacteria. Whether or not bifidus extract can have benefit for skin is unknown.

bilberry extract. Some research shows bilberry to be effective as an antioxidant, but this effect has not been demonstrated on skin (Source: *Journal of Agricultural Food Chemistry,* September 2001, pages 4183–4187).

bioflavonoid. Diverse range of substances that are components of many fruits and vegetables. Many of these have been shown to have potent antioxidant and gene-regulatory activity (Sources: *Annals of the New York Academy of Science,* May 2002, pages 70–77; *Planta Medica,* August 2001, pages 515–519; and *Free Radical Biology and Medicine*, June 1998, pages 1355–1363).

biotin. Also known as vitamin H, a water-soluble vitamin produced in the body by certain types of intestinal bacteria and obtained from food. Considered part of the B complex group of vitamins, biotin is necessary for the metabolism of carbohydrates, fats, and amino acids (the building blocks of protein). However, it has no reported benefit for skin when applied topically.

birch bark. Derived from the plant *Betula alba* (commonly called white birch). It can have potent antioxidant properties (Source: *Journal of Agricultural Food Chemistry,* October 1999, pages 3954–3962), but it can also have astringent properties, which makes it a potential irritant for skin.

birch leaf extract. *See* birch bark.

bisabolol. Can be extracted from chamomile or derived synthetically. It is an anti-irritant.

bis-diglyceryl polyacyladipate. Used as an emollient and thickening agent in cosmetics. *See* glyceryl ester.

bitter orange flower. *See* orange blossom.

black cohosh. Perennial herb of eastern United States. There is research showing that black cohosh when taken orally can have some effect on menopausal and pre-menopausal symptoms (Source: *Journal of the American Pharmaceutical Association,*

March-April 2000, pages 327–329). However, there is no research showing that black cohosh can have this or any effect when applied topically on skin (Source: http://www.herbmed.org).

black currant oil. *See* gamma linolenic acid.

black elderberry. Has potent antioxidant properties (Source: *Journal of Agricultural Food Chemistry,* May 2000, pages 1588–1592).

black locust extract. Plant extract that can have antioxidant properties, though it may have toxic components as well (Source: FDA, Center for Food Safety & Applied Nutrition, "Poisonous Plant Bibliography," http://www.fda.gov).

black mulberry. There is no research showing this to have any benefit when applied topically to skin.

black pepper extract and oil. Used topically as a counter-irritant, but that means it can cause significant skin irritation (Source: *Natural Medicines Comprehensive Database,* http://www.naturaldatabase.com). *See* counter-irritant.

black raspberry. Fruit that has potent antioxidant properties (Source: *Journal of Agricultural Food Chemistry,* June 5, 2002, pages 3495–3500).

black tea. *See* green tea.

black walnut shell extract. There is a small amount of research showing this has antioxidant properties (Source: *Phytotherapy Research,* June 2002, pages 364–367).

blackberry. Berries that have potent antioxidant properties (Source: *Journal of Agricultural Food Chemistry,* June 5, 2002, pages 3495–3500).

bladderwrack extract. Derived from a seaweed; it can be an effective antioxidant and has water-binding properties for skin (Sources: *Journal of Cosmetic Science,* January-February 2002, pages 1–9; and *Journal of Agricultural Food Chemistry,* February 2002, pages 840–845).

***Bletilla striata* extract.** Some research (Chinese and German) shows this to be effective for preventing blood clots and stemming bleeding, when taken orally, and it may stem bleeding when applied topically. There is extremely limited information about this plant extract in regard to skin.

bloodroot. Potent skin irritant (Source: *Cornell University Poisonous Plants Informational Database,* http://www.ansci.cornell.edu/plants/alphalist.html).

bloodwort. Also known as yarrow. *See* yarrow extract.

bluet extract. *See* cornflower.

bois oil. Fragrant oil that has no research showing it to have benefit for skin (Source: *Natural Medicines Comprehensive Database,* http://www.naturaldatabase.com).

Bora cocos. *See Poria cocos.*

borage seed extract. From the plant *Borago officinalis.* Can have anti-irritant and anti-inflammatory properties (Source: *Biofactors,* 2000, volume 13, pages 179–185).

borage seed oil. Contains gamma linolenic acid (Source: *Natural Medicines Comprehensive Database,* http://www.naturaldatabase.com). *See* gamma linolenic acid.

borates. Used in cosmetics in small quantities primarily as pH adjusters (they have a pH of 9 to 11) or as antimicrobial agents (Source: *Biological Trace Element Research*, Winter 1998, pages 343–357). In larger amounts, due to the high pH, they can be significant skin irritants.

borax. Also known as sodium borate decahydrate, a mineral composed of sodium, boron, oxygen, and water. It has fungicide, preservative, insecticide, herbicide, and disinfectant properties. Borax functions as a bleaching agent by converting some water molecules to hydrogen peroxide (H_2O_2), which generates free-radical damage and is a problem for skin. The pH of borax is about 9 to 11 and it can therefore be a significant skin irritant when used in cosmetics.

boric acid. May have wound-healing benefits (Source: *Journal of Trace Elements in Medicine and Biology*, October 14, 2000, pages 168–173), but in cosmetics is used primarily as an antimicrobial agent.

boron nitride. Synthetic, inorganic powder. It has absorbent properties in cosmetics similar to organic powders such as talc.

Boswellia carterii. *See* frankincense extract.

Botox. Brand name of the nontoxic form of botulinum toxin type A. When injected into specific areas of the face (or body), particularly the forehead, it prevents movement by partially and almost completely paralyzing the muscles of that area. The resulting inability to use particular facial muscles causes certain wrinkles to disappear completely. This helps eliminate almost all of the wrinkles of the forehead, in the crow's-feet area (by the eyes), and the lines that run from the nose to the mouth (the naso-labial folds). Over 800,000 Botox treatments were administered in 2001. Since 1973, Botox has been used by ophthalmologists to treat patients with disabling eye ticks, and crossed eyes. It is also used by other medical specialists to treat spasmodic neck muscles, spasmodic laryngeal muscles, multiple sclerosis, cerebral palsy, some post-stroke states, spinal cord injuries, nerve palsies, Parkinson's disease, facial spasms, and, most recently, migraine headaches. This extensive use (and the corresponding research) has shown that Botox has a great success rate, with minimal risk of detrimental side effects. In rare cases, depending on what parts of the face are injected, the patient may experience temporary facial or eye-area drooping, bruising, or jaw and neck weakness, but it lasts only for the duration of the Botox effect, so it goes away in three to six months (Sources: FDA *Consumer* magazine, July-August 2002, http://www.fda.gov; *Plastic and Reconstructive Surgery*, August 2002, pages 601–611; *The Medical Letter*, May 2002, pages 47–48; *Clinical and Experimental Dermatology*, October 2001, pages 619–630; and *Journal of the American Academy of Dermatology*, June 2002, pages 840–849.)

bovine spongiform encephalopathy. *See* Mad Cow Disease.

boxwood extract. Can have constricting properties, which makes it a skin irritant.

boysenberry. Berry that can have potent antioxidant properties (Source: *Journal of Agricultural Food Chemistry*, June 5, 2002, pages 3495–3500).

Brassica campestris. See rapeseed oil.

Brazil nut extract. There is a small amount of research showing it can have antioxidant properties (Source: *Chemosphere,* February 1995, pages 801–802).

Brewer's yeast. *See* yeast.

broad spectrum. Meant to refer to a sunscreen's ability to protect the skin from both UVA and UVB rays from the sun. This term is not regulated by the FDA, so a cosmetic can make this claim even when the product does not actually provide adequate broad-spectrum protection. *See* UVA.

bromelain. Enzyme found in pineapple. Theoretically bromelain breaks down the connecting structure that holds surface skin cells together, which causes exfoliation, but it can also cause irritation. However, exactly how much bromelain is needed, whether it is stable, and in what bases and pH it works best have not been established. There is little to no research demonstrating how bromelain reacts on skin.

bronopol. Technical name 2-bromo-2-nitropropane-1,3-diol, a formaldehyde-releasing preservative (Source: *Contact Dermatitis,* December 2000, pages 339–343). *See* formaldehyde-releasing preservative.

brown algae. There is no research showing this to be beneficial for skin (Source: *Natural Medicines Comprehensive Database,* http://www.naturaldatabase.com). *See* algae.

bumetrizole. Sunscreen ingredient that absorbs primarily UVB light.

Bupleurum falcatum **extract.** There is no research showing extracts of this plant to have any benefit for skin, though it may have some wound-healing properties for peptic ulcers. It does contain glucoside and polysaccharide, but whether these can affect skin following topical application of the extract is unknown (Source: *Phytotherapy Research,* February 2002, pages 91–93). *See* mucopolysaccharide.

burdock root. A small amount of research shows this plant to be an effective anti-inflammatory agent and antioxidant (Source: http://www.herbmed.org).

butcher's broom extract. There is evidence showing that it can reduce edema and venous problems when taken orally (Source: *Journal of Alternative Complementary Medicine,* December 2000, pages 539–549). It may also have anti-inflammatory properties for skin, but there is little evidence of this.

butyl acetate. Solvent used in nail polish and many other products.

butyl methoxydibenzoylmethane. *See* avobenzone.

butylene glycol. *See* propylene glycol.

butylparaben. *See* parabens.

Butyrospermum **fruit.** Fruit from the karite tree, scientific name *Butyrospermum parkii,* used to obtain the fat that makes shea butter. *See* shea butter.

Buxus chinensis. See jojoba oil.

Buxus sempervirens. See boxwood extract.

C10-18 triglycerides. Used as an emollient and thickening agent in cosmetics. *See* glyceryl ester.

C12-15 alkyl benzoate. Used as an emollient and thickening agent. *See* glyceryl ester.

C12-18 acid triglyceride. Used as an emollient and thickening agent. *See* glyceryl ester.

C18-36 acid triglyceride. Used as an emollient and thickening agent. *See* glyceryl ester.

cabbage rose extract. Highly fragrant substance that can be a skin irritant.

cactus flower extract. There is little information about this plant extract when applied topically, but it may be a skin irritant that causes itching and skin pustules (Sources: *Botanical Dermatology Database,* http://bodd.cf.ac.uk/BotDermFolder/BotDermC/CACT.html; and *Natural Medicines Comprehensive Database,* http://www.naturaldatabase.com).

caffeic acid. Potent antioxidant that may have some anticarcinogenic properties (Sources: *Bioorganic & Medicinal Chemistry Letters, June 2002, pages 1567–1570;* and *Nutrition and Cancer,* 1998, volume 32, number 2, pages 81–85).

caffeine. One of a group of alkaloids called methylxanthines; a substance with a high tannin content, which constricts skin and can cause irritation. When consumed in coffee, caffeine can be a strong diuretic, but there is no evidence that this occurs when caffeine is applied to skin (so it would not have the effect of "flushing away" fluid in tissues around the eyes that can accumulate as you sleep). However, there is research that caffeine can have anticancer benefits when consumed along with green or black tea (adding caffeine to the decaffeinated versions of the teas did not work as well as using the caffeinated versions of the teas) (Source: *Cancer Research,* July 1997, pages 2623–2629). Whether there is any correlation between the effects of consuming caffeine and its effects when applied topically is unknown.

cajeputi oil. *See Melaleuca cajeputi* oil.

calamine. Preparation of zinc carbonate, colored with ferric oxide (a form of rust). Zinc carbonate is considered a counter-irritant and is used to reduce itching. *See* counter-irritant.

calcium ascorbate. Form of vitamin C; others include ascorbic acid, L-ascorbic acid, ascorbyl palmitate, and magnesium ascorbyl phosphate. There is very little research concerning its health benefits, either topically or orally, in regard to its antioxidant benefits. *See* Ester-C.

calcium carbonate. Chalk; used as an absorbent in cosmetics.

calcium d-pantetheine-s-sulfonate. *See* calcium pantetheine sulfonate.

calcium gluconate. Calcium is an essential mineral for the body. A small amount of research shows it to be a good anti-inflammatory and healing agent when applied topically (Source: *Annals of Emergency Medicine,* July 1994, pages 9–13).

calcium pantetheine sulfonate. A small amount of in vitro research shows this to have melanin-inhibiting properties (Source: *Pigment Cell Research,* June 2000, pages 165–171).

calcium pantothenate. Also known as pantothenic acid. *See* pantothenic acid.

calcium silicate. *See* silicate.

calendula extract. Derived from the plant commonly known as pot marigold; there is little research showing it to have any effect on skin, though it may have antibacterial and antioxidant properties for skin.

Calophyllum inophyllum **seed oil.** *See* tamanu oil.

Calophyllum tacamahaca. Source of a plant oil that has emollient and antimutagenic properties (Source: *Phytochemistry,* October 2001, pages 571–575).

Camellia kissi **oil.** *See Camellia sasanqua* oil.

Camellia oleifera. *See* green tea.

Camellia sasanqua **oil.** Plant extract that has emollient properties for skin. There is a small amount of research showing it to have anti-inflammatory properties as well (Source: *Phytochemistry,* May 1998, pages 301–305).

Camellia sinensis. *See* green tea.

camphor. Aromatic substance obtained from the wood of a southeast Asian tree, *Cinnamomum camphora,* or manufactured synthetically. When applied to the skin it produces a cooling effect and dilates blood vessels, which can cause skin irritation and dermatitis with repeated use (Sources: *British Journal of Dermatology,* November 2000, pages 923–929; and *Clinical Toxicology,* December 1981, pages 1485–1498). *See* counter-irritant.

cananga extract. Fragrance that can be a skin irritant, much like ylang-ylang.

Cananga odorata. *See* ylang-ylang.

candelilla wax. Derived from candelilla plants; used as a thickening agent and emollient to give products such as lipsticks or stick foundations their form.

Cannabis sativa **L. oil.** *See* hemp seed oil.

canola oil. Plant lipid that has barrier-repair and anti-inflammatory properties (Source: *British Journal of Dermatology,* February 1996, pages 215–220). *See* natural moisturizing factors.

caprylic/capric triglyceride. Derived from coconut, and considered to be a good emollient and thickening agent in cosmetics.

capsaicin. Component of capsicum. When used topically, capsaicin can prevent the transmission of pain. It is also a potent topical irritant and can trigger dermatitis. *See* capsicum.

capsicum. Large group of plants consisting primarily of the pepper family, including chili peppers and paprika. These are used as counter-irritants to relieve muscle aches. Capsicum and substances derived from it can cause allergic reactions or skin irritation and should never be applied to abraded skin (Source: *Natural Medicines Comprehensive Database,* http://www.naturaldatabase.com). *See* counter-irritant.

capsicum oleoresin. Fatty resin derived from capsicum plants. It can be a skin irritant and should not be applied to abraded skin. *See* capsicum.

caramel. Natural coloring agent.

carbomers. Thickening agents used primarily to create gel-like formulations.

carbopol. *See* carbomers.

cardamom. Plant of the ginger family, used as fragrance in cosmetics. Terpene is one of its major constituents, which can be a skin irritant and sensitizer.

carmine. Natural red color that comes from the dried female cochineal beetle. It is sometimes used to color lip gloss, lipsticks, and other cosmetics.

carnauba wax. Vegetable wax that has a hard, firm texture; it is used in cosmetics as a substantial thickening agent.

carnitine. *See* L-carnitine.

carnosic acid. Component of rosemary that is considered a potent antioxidant (Sources: *Free Radical Biology and Medicine,* June 2002, pages 1293–1303; and *Journal of Agricultural Food Chemistry,* March 2002, pages 1845–1851).

carnosine. Composed of amino acids, it has anti-inflammatory and antioxidant properties. There is some research showing it to have antiglycation properties (Source: *Life Sciences,* March 2002, pages 1789–1799).

carnosol acid. *See* carnosic acid.

carob fruit extract. May have antioxidant properties (Source: *Journal of Agricultural and Food Chemistry,* January 2002, pages 373–377).

carrageenan. Seaweed gum used in cosmetics as a thickening agent with water-binding properties.

carrot extract. Can have antioxidant properties (Source: *International Journal of Food Sciences and Nutrition,* November 2001, pages 501–508), but whether it can have that effect when applied topically on skin is not known.

***Carthamus tinctorius* oil.** *See* safflower oil.

carrot oil. Emollient plant oil similar to other nonfragrant plant oils. *See* natural moisturizing factors.

carvone. Essential oil used as a flavoring agent and fragrance component in cosmetics. It can be a significant skin sensitizer or allergen (Sources: *Planta Medica,* August 2001, pages 564–566; and *Contact Dermatitis,* June 2001, pages 347–356).

***Carya illinoensis* oil.** *See* pecan oil.

casein. Substance derived from milk protein that may have some antioxidant properties when applied topically, although the research for this is limited (Source: *International Journal of Food Science and Nutrition,* July 1999, pages 291–296).

***Cassia angustifolia* seed.** May have anti-inflammatory properties (Source: *Fitoterapia,* March 2001, pages 221–229).

castile soap. Contains olive oil instead of animal fat, but can still be drying to skin.

castor oil. Vegetable oil derived from the castor bean. It is used in cosmetics as an emollient, though its unique property is that when dry it forms a solid film that can have water-binding properties. It is rarely associated with skin irritation or allergic reactions but it can have a slightly sticky feel on skin.

catalase. Enzyme that decomposes hydrogen peroxide into water and oxygen and that has significant antioxidant properties (Source: *Journal of Investigative Dermatology,* April 2002, pages 618–625).

Catharanthus roseus. See Madagascar periwinkle.

Caulerpa taxifolia **extract.** *See* algae.

cedarwood. Fragrant plant extract. There is evidence that cedarwood oil is allergenic and can cause skin irritation. There is also a small amount of research showing it produces tumors on mouse skin (Sources: *Natural Medicines Comprehensive Database,* http://www.naturaldatabase.com).

Cedrus atlantica **bark extract.** Fragrant oil that can be a skin irritant.

celandine. Extract from the plant *Chelidonium majus* that has some amount of research showing it to have antiviral properties. There is no research showing it to have benefit when applied topically.

Celastrus paniculatus. Shrub native to India. May have antioxidant properties, although the research for this has been on animal models or in vitro (Source: *Phytomedicine,* May 2002, pages 302–311).

cellulose. Primary fiber component of plants. Used in cosmetics as a thickening agent and to bind other ingredients together.

Centaurea cyanus. See cornflower.

Centella asiatica. Herb that may appear on labels as asiatic acid, hydrocotyl, or gotu kola. It has antibacterial, anti-psoriatic, and wound-healing properties (Sources: *Aesthetic Plastic Surgery,* May-June 2000, pages 227–234; *Phytomedicine,* May 2001, pages 230–235; and *Contact Dermatitis,* October 1993, pages 175–179).

Centipeda cunninghami **extract.** Derived from an Australian plant commonly known as sneezeweed or old man's weed. It has been used by aborigines to treat burns, wounds, and skin infections. The only research confirming the effectiveness of this plant extract as an anti-inflammatory is from the company that owns the patent for its use.

cephalin. Phospholipid. *See* fatty acid, and natural moisturizing factors.

cera alba. Beeswax; used as a thickening agent in cosmetics.

cera microcristallina. See petrolatum.

ceramides. Naturally occurring skin lipids (fats) that are major structural components of the skin's outer structure (Source: *Journal of Investigative Dermatology,* November 2001, pages 1126–1136). Ceramides are necessary for the skin's water-retention capacity as well as cell regulation (Source: *Skin Pharmacology and Applied Skin Physiology,* September-October 2001, pages 261–271).

Ceratonia siliqua **gum.** *See* carob fruit extract.

ceresin. Waxy ingredient used as a thickening agent in cosmetics; derived from clay. It can be sensitizing for some skin types.

Cereus grandiflorus **extract.** *See* cactus flower extract.

ceteareth-20. Fatty alcohol that is used to thicken cosmetics and keep ingredients mixed together and stable.

cetearyl alcohol. Fatty alcohol used as an emollient, emulsifier, thickener, and carrying agent for other ingredients. Can be derived naturally, as in coconut fatty alcohol, or synthetically.

cetyl alcohol. Fatty alcohol used as an emollient, emulsifier, thickener, and carrying agent for other ingredients. Can be derived naturally, as in coconut fatty alcohol, or synthetically. It is not an irritant and is not related to SD alcohol or ethyl alcohol.

chamomile. Herb that has research showing it to have anti-irritant, soothing, and anti-oxidant properties (Sources: http://www.herbmed.org; *European Journal of Drug Metabolism and Pharmacokinetics,* October-December 1999, pages 303–308; and *Planta Medica,* October 1994, pages 410–413).

chaparral extract. There is conflicting research about its efficacy as an anticancer agent, though it does contain a component that has antioxidant properties (Source: *Society for Experimental Biology and Medicine,* January 1995, pages 6–12; and http://www.healthwell. com/healthnotes/). When ingested, it may cause liver toxicity (Sources: *Molecular and Cellular Biochemistry,* June 1999, pages 157–161; *Archives of Internal Medicine,* April 1997, pages 913–919; and http://www.quackwatch.com/01QuackeryRelatedTopics/OTA/ota04.html). Topically it can have antimicrobial properties (Source: *Journal of Ethnopharmacology,* June 1996, pages 175–177).

charcoal. Baked wood that is mainly carbon. One teaspoonful of Activated Charcoal USP has a surface area of more than 10,000 square feet, which gives charcoal unique absorption properties. It also can disinfect wounds.

chaste tree fruit extract. One research report says, "In a randomized, double-blind, placebo-controlled trial reported in the *British Medical Journal* (January 20, 2001), German researchers assigned 170 women diagnosed with PMS to a daily [oral] dose of *Vitex agnus-castus* (chaste tree) extract or to placebo for three menstrual cycles. The women assessed themselves before and after treatment on measures of irritability, mood, anger, headache, bloating, and breast fullness. Clinicians evaluated symptom severity and treatment effects. More than half of the women taking chaste tree fruit extract (popularly known as chasteberry)—compared to slightly less than one-quarter of those on placebo—had a 50% or greater improvement in PMS symptoms (with the exception of bloating)" (Source: *Harvard Women's Health Watch* newsletter, May 2001). There is no evidence that it can have any effect on skin.

chaulmoogra oil. Once the treatment for leprosy worldwide due to its antimicrobial properties (Source: *Proceedings of the National Academy of Sciences, USA,* February 2000, pages 1433–1437). It can be a skin irritant.

chayote extract. *See Sechium edule* extract.

chicory extract. Has antioxidant properties and may also have anti-inflammatory properties (Sources: *Archives of Pharmacal Research,* October 2001, pages 431–436; and *Natural Medicines Comprehensive Database,* http://www.naturaldatabase.com).

China clay. *See* kaolin.

chitosan. Derived from chitin, a polysaccharide found in the exoskeleton of shellfish such as shrimp, lobster, and crabs. It is used widely in pharmaceuticals as a base in formulations. There is also extensive research showing it can be effective in wound healing, as well as having antibacterial and anti-inflammatory properties (Sources: *Biomaterials,* November 2001, pages 2959–2966; *International Journal of Food Microbiology,* March 2002, pages 65–72; and *Journal of Pharmacy and Pharmacology,* August 2001, pages 1047–1067). *See* mucopolysaccharide.

chloasma. *See* melasma.

chlorella. *See* algae.

chlorhexidine. Topical antiseptic, it can cause irritation (Source: *Toxicology in Vitro,* August-October 2001, pages 271–276).

chlorophene. Used as a preservative in cosmetics.

chlorphenesin. An alcohol used as a preservative in cosmetics.

chocolate. *See* cocoa extract.

cholesterol. Phospholipid (a type of human or animal fat) used in cosmetics as a stabilizer, an emollient, and a water-binding agent. *See* natural moisturizing factors.

choline. Part of the vitamin B complex and a constituent of many other biologically important molecules, such as acetylcholine (a neurotransmitter) and lecithin.

chondroitin sulfate. *See* glycosaminoglycans.

Chondrus crispus. Form of red seaweed. *See* algae, and carrageenan.

chrysanthemum extract. Can have anti-inflammatory benefit for skin.

Chrysanthemum parthenium extract. *See* feverfew extract.

Cichorium intybus. Source of a plant extract with antioxidant properties (Source: *Archives of Pharmaceutical Research,* October 2001, pages 431–436).

Cichorium intybus. *See* chicory extract.

Cimicifuga racemosa root extract. *See* black cohosh.

Cinchona succirubra bark extract. In folk medicine, it is used topically as an astringent, bactericidal, and anesthetic. There is no research supporting any of its uses for skin (Source: *Natural Medicines Comprehensive Database,* http://www.naturaldatabase.com).

Cinnamomum camphora. *See* camphor.

Cinnamomum. *See* cinnamon.

cinnamon. Can have antimicrobial properties (Source: *Letters in Applied Microbiology,* January 2002, pages 27–31) and can also be a skin irritant.

Cistus ladaniferus oil. *See* labdanum.

citric acid. Derived from citrus and used primarily to adjust the pH of products to prevent them from being too alkaline.

citrulline. Amino acid involved in the formation of the amino acid, arginine. Citrulline has been identified in the surface layers of human skin (Source: *Journal of Investigative Dermatology,* April 2000, pages 701–705). There is no research showing it to have benefit when applied topically. However, like all amino acids, it most likely has water-binding properties. *See* amino acid, and natural moisturizing factors.

Citrullus colocynthis. Bitter apple; considered a skin irritant.

Citrus amara. See orange blossom.

Citrus aurantifolia. See lime.

Citrus aurantium extract. Bitter orange extract. It can have antioxidant properties when ingested (Source: *Journal of Agricultural Food Chemistry,* December 1999, pages 5239–5244); however, used topically its methanol content makes it potentially irritating for skin.

Citrus aurantium. See orange blossom.

Citrus medica limonium. See lemon.

clary oil. Used as fragrance, and can be a skin irritant or sensitizer.

clay. *See* bentonite, and kaolin.

Clematis vitalba. Plant that may have antifungal properties (Source: *Journal of Ethnopharmacology,* February 2002, pages 155–163) and may also be a skin sensitizer.

Clintonia borealis extract. There is no research showing this to have any benefit for skin (Source: *Phytotherapy Research,* February 2002, pages 63–65).

clove leaf. *See* clove oil.

clove oil. Potent skin irritant and inflammatory when used repeatedly (Sources: IFA— International Federation of Aromatherapists, www.int-fed-aromatherapy.co.uk; *Natural Medicines Comprehensive Database,* www.naturaldatabase.com; and *Contact Dermatitis,* March 2002, pages 141–144).

clover blossom. Contains eugenol, which can be a skin sensitizer and cause photosensitivity.

clover leaf oil. *See* clover blossom.

cobalt gluconate. Element found in trace amounts in tissues of the body. While cobalt plays a vital role in the formation of some body systems, there is no evidence it serves any purpose topically on skin, though it may act as an antioxidant.

cocamide DEA and MEA. *See* alkyloamides, and diethanolamine.

cocamidopropyl betaine. Considered one of the more gentle surfactants used in skin-care products. *See* surfactant.

cocamidopropyl hydroxysultaine. Mild surfactant. *See* surfactant.

cocoa butter. Oil extracted from cocoa beans, used as an emollient and with properties similar to those of all nonfragrant plant oils. *See* natural moisturizing factors.

cocoa extract. Can have potent antioxidant properties (Sources: *Experimental Biology and Medicine,* May 2002, pages 321–329; and *Journal of Agricultural Food Chemistry,* July 2001, pages 3438–3442).

cocoglycerides. Used as an emollient and thickening agent in cosmetics. *See* glyceryl ester.

coconut oil. Non-volatile plant kernel oil that has emollient properties for skin.

coconut. Has degreasing and cleansing properties, which is why detergent cleansing agents are frequently derived from coconut oil. *See* surfactant.

Cocus nucifera. See coconut oil.

Codium tomentosum **extract.** *See* algae.

coenzyme Q10. Only a handful of studies have shown coenzyme Q10 (CoQ10) to have any effect on wrinkles (Sources: *Biofactors,* September 1999, pages 371–378; and *Zeitschrift für Gerontologie und Geriatrie,* April 1999, pages 83–88). However, neither of these studies was double-blind or placebo-controlled, so there is no way to tell whether other formulations could net the same results. There is also research showing that sun exposure depletes the presence of CoQ10 in the skin (Source: *Journal of Dermatological Science Supplement,* August 2001, pages 1–4). This isn't surprising, because many of the skin's components become diminished upon exposure to the sun. But whether or not taking CoQ10 supplements or applying them to skin stops or alters sun damage is not known.

Coffea arabica **extract.** *Coffea arabica* is the coffee plant, and there is research showing coffee extract to have antioxidant properties (Source: *Journal of Agricultural and Food Chemistry,* June 2002, pages 3751–3756).

Cola acuminata **seed extract.** *See* kola nut.

Coleus barbatus. Member of the mint family; can be a skin irritant. *See* counter-irritant.

collagen. Major component of skin that gives it structure. Sun damage causes collagen in skin to deteriorate. Collagen can be derived from both plant and animal sources and is used in cosmetics as a good water-binding agent. Collagen in cosmetics, regardless of the source, has never been shown to have an effect on the collagen in skin.

collagen amino acid. Amino acids hydrolyzed from collagen. These have good water-binding properties for skin. *See* amino acid, and natural moisturizing factors.

colloidal oatmeal. *See* oatmeal.

colloidal silver. Refers to ground-up silver suspended in solution. *See* silver.

colostrum. Clear/cloudy "pre-milk" that female mammals secrete prior to producing milk. Colostrum contains immunoglobulins (disease resistance factors). While there is a small body of evidence indicating that adult consumption of colostrum may have disease-fighting potential, this is hardly substantiated, and there is no known benefit when colostrum is applied topically. The only study that does exist showed colostrum to have no wound-healing function on skin (Source: *Journal of Dermatologic Surgery and Oncology,* June 1985, pages 617–622).

coltsfoot. According to *The PDR Family Guide to Natural Medicines & Healing Therapies* and a German Commission E Monograph, coltsfoot is potentially carcinogenic due to its pyrrolizidine alkaloid content and is not recommended for repeated use on skin.

comfrey extract. Several studies have shown that comfrey extract can have carcinogenic or toxic properties when taken orally. Whether those properties translate to topical application of the extract is unknown, but its alkaloid content makes it a potential skin irritant (Sources: *Chemical Research in Toxicology,* November 2001, pages 1546–1551; and *Public Health Nutrition,* December 2000, pages 501–508).

Commiphora myrrha **extract.** *See* myrrh.

***Commiphora wightii* extract.** Has been shown to have cytotoxic components that may have a toxic effect on skin cells (Source: *Phytochemistry*, April 2001, pages 723–727).

coneflower. *See* echinacea.

***Conium maculatum*.** Also known as poison hemlock. When taken orally all parts of hemlock, including seeds, flowers, and fruits, are considered toxic and poisonous. Death has resulted after ingestion of hemlock. Prompt medical attention is advised after ingestion of hemlock. There is no research showing it to have any effect when applied topically on skin (Source: *Natural Medicines Comprehensive Database*, http://www.naturaldatabase.com).

***Copaifera officinalis*.** *See* balsam.

copper gluconate. Copper is an important trace element for human nutrition. The body needs copper to absorb and utilize iron, and copper is also a component of the powerful antioxidant enzyme superoxide dismutase. Copper supplements have been shown to increase superoxide dismutase levels in humans (Source: *Healthnotes Review of Complementary and Integrative Medicine*, http://www.healthnotes.com). The synthesis of collagen and elastin is in part related to the presence of copper in the body, and copper is also important for many other processes. For example, there is research showing that copper is effective for wound healing (Sources: *Journal of Clinical Investigation*, November 1993, pages 2368–2376; and *Federation of European Biochemical Sciences Letter*, October 1988, pages 343–346). However, wound healing is the result of many biophysical processes that have nothing to do with wrinkling. *See* superoxide dismutase.

copper peptides. *See* copper gluconate.

copper sulfate. Chemical effective for topical wound healing (Source: *American Journal of Physiology Heart Circulation and Physiology*, May 2002, pages 1821–1827). However, wound healing is the result of many biophysical processes that have nothing to do with wrinkling.

***Corallina officinalis* extract.** *See* algae.

coriander. Herb and spice plant, the source of a fragrant component; it can be a potential skin irritant (Source: *Natural Medicines Comprehensive Database*, http://www.naturaldatabase.com). It may also have some antibacterial and antifungal properties, but these properties have not been established for topical use on skin (Source: *Journal of Food Protection*, July 2001, pages 1019–1024).

corn glycerides. Used as an emollient and thickening agent in cosmetics. *See* glyceryl ester.

cornmint. Also known as wild mint; it can be a skin irritant. *See* counter-irritant.

corn oil. Emollient oil with properties similar to those of other nonfragrant plant oils (Source: *British Journal of Dermatology*, June 1994, pages 757–764).

cornstarch. Starch obtained from corn and sometimes used as an absorbent in cosmetics instead of talc. However, when cornstarch becomes moist, it can promote fungal and bacterial growth (Source: http://www.radiation-oncology.com/homecare/html/skin_13.htm).

cornflower. Can have anti-inflammatory properties (Source: *Journal of Ethnopharmacology*, December 1999, pages 235–241).

Cornus **extract.** *See* dogwood.

corticosteroids. *See* hydrocortisone.

Corylus americana. *See* hazelnut oil.

Corylus avellana. *See* hazelnut oil.

costus root. Has anti-inflammatory properties (Source: *European Journal of Pharmacology*, June 2000, pages 399–407), but there is research showing that it can also inhibit the immune response (Source: *Phytochemistry*, January 2002, pages 85–90).

coumarin. Organic compound found in plants and derived from the amino acid phenylalanine. It creates the fragrance found in fresh-mowed hay. More than 300 coumarins have been identified from natural sources, especially green plants. These varying substances have disparate pharmacological, biochemical, and therapeutic applications. However, simple coumarins are potent antioxidants (Sources: *Journal of Natural Products*, September 2001, pages 1238–1240; *Chemistry and Physics of Lipids*, December 1999, pages 125–135; and *General Pharmacology*, June 1996, pages 713–722).

counter-irritant. Ingredients such as menthol, peppermint, camphor, and mint are considered counter-irritants (Sources: *Archives of Dermatologic Research*, May 1996, pages 245–248; and *Code of Federal Regulations* Title 21—Food and Drugs, Revised as of April 1, 2001, CITE: 21CFR310.545, http://www.fda.gov). Counter-irritants are used to induce local inflammation for the purpose of relieving inflammation in deeper or adjacent tissues. In other words, they substitute one kind of inflammation for another, which is never good for skin. Irritation or inflammation, no matter what causes it or how it happens, impairs the skin's immune and healing response (Source: *Skin Pharmacology and Applied Skin Physiology*, November-December 2000, pages 358–371). And although your skin may not show it, or doesn't react in an irritated fashion, if you apply irritants to your skin the damage is still taking place and is ongoing, so it adds up over time (Source: *Skin Research and Technology*, November 2001, pages 227–237).

Crataegus monogina **extract.** *See* hawthorn extract.

Crithmum maritimum. Extract of algae that has weak antioxidant properties (Source: *Planta Medica*, December 2000, pages 687–693).

cucumber extract. Claims of cucumber having anti-inflammatory or soothing properties are anecdotal, as there is no research supporting this contention.

Cucumis sativus **extract.** *See* cucumber extract.

Curcuma longa **root.** *See* turmeric.

curcumin. Potent antioxidant that can be effective in wound healing (Source: *Journal of Trauma*, November 2001, pages 927–931). *See* turmeric.

Cyamopsis tetragonoloba. *See* guar.

cyanocobalamin. *See* vitamin B12.

Cyanopsis tetragonalba. Form of guar gum. *See* guar.

Cyanotis arachnoidea **extract.** There is no research showing this to have any benefit for skin.

Cyatheaceae **extract.** Derived from a neotropic plant; an extract that has no research showing it to have benefit for skin.

cyclamen aldehyde. Synthetic fragrant component; it can be a skin irritant.

cyclohexasiloxane. *See* silicone.

cyclomethicone. Silicone with a drier finish than dimethicone. *See* silicone.

cylopentasiloxane. *See* silicone.

Cymbopogon citrates. See lemongrass.

Cymbopogon martini. See geranium.

Cynara scolymus. See artichoke extract.

Cyperus rotundus **extract.** From the plant also known as nut grass and *xiang fu.* There is no research establishing this plant to have any benefit for skin. In a small number of animal experiments it has been shown, when administered orally, to have anti-inflammatory properties.

cysteine. *See* amino acid.

cystine. *See* amino acid.

cystosine. Component of DNA that carries genetic information to the cell. *See* DNA.

cytochrome. Protein found in blood cells that, with the aid of enzymes, serves a vital function in the transfer of energy within cells. There are three types of cytochromes, indicated by A, B, or C, with cytochrome C being the most stable. However, because cytochromes require a complex process that is triggered by a sequence of other components in order to be effective in their function of cellular respiration, they serve no function alone on skin.

cytokines. Diverse, potent, and extremely complex chemical messengers secreted by immune system cells. They stimulate the production of other substances to help protect the body. Cytokines encourage cell growth, promote cell activation, direct cellular traffic, and destroy target cells—including cancer cells. Interleukins, transforming growth factor, and interferon are types of cytokines. It is also important to note that cytokines can also cause unwanted, potentially serious side effects (Sources: http://www.medlineplus.com; and the National Cancer Institute, http://www.nci.nih.gov or http://www.cancer.gov). Even the notion that skin-care products can directly affect cytokine production in some way to change the appearance of skin is a scary thought, since cosmetic ingredients are not tested for safety the way pharmaceuticals or drugs are.

D&C. According to the FDA, D&C is an identification that indicates a coloring agent that has been approved as safe in **d**rug **a**nd **c**osmetics products, but not in food.

daisy flower extract. There is no research showing this to be beneficial for skin (Source: *Natural Medicines Comprehensive Database,* http://www.naturaldatabase.com).

dandelion extract. Can be a potent allergen (Source: *Archives of Dermatology,* January 1999, pages 67–70).

Daucus carota. Also known as wild carrot. It can have antioxidant properties, but topically it can cause dermatitis (Source: *Natural Medicines Comprehensive Database,* http://www.naturaldatabase.com).

DEA. *See* diethanolamine.

dead nettle extract. *See* white nettle.

Dead Sea minerals. Several studies demonstrate that Dead Sea minerals can have a positive effect on psoriatic skin (Sources: *Israel Journal of Medical Sciences,* November 2001, pages 828–832; *British Journal of Dermatology,* June 2001, pages 1154–1160; *International Journal of Dermatology,* February 2001, pages 158–159; and *Journal of the American Academy of Dermatology,* August 2000, pages 325–326). Psoriasis is a skin condition characterized by rapidly dividing, overactive skin cells. No one is quite sure how the Dead Sea minerals and salts affect psoriasis. One of the more popular theories is that the water's mineral content slows down the out-of-control cell division. Some research indicates that the benefit is cumulative and that the results can last for up to five months. However there is no research showing that these minerals have any effect on wrinkles, dry skin, or acne.

decyl glucoside. Used as a gentle detergent cleansing agent. *See* surfactant.

deer antler velvet. Soft epidermis that covers the hard inner structure of the growing bone and cartilage that will become deer antlers. Deer antler velvet is marketed as a remedy for a wide range of disorders and health benefits. However, there is a lack of information in the scientific literature to support these claims, and there is also a lack of information on potential toxicity. Areas of potential concern include drug residues, possible deleterious androgenic effects on fetuses and neonates, and allergic reactions (Source: *Veterinary and Human Toxicology,* February 1999, pages 39–41). Further, there is concern about the humane treatment of the animals when the substance is collected.

dehydroepiandrosterone (DHEA). Male hormone produced in the adrenal glands that contributes to bone density, muscle mass, and skin tone. DHEA production peaks when we are in our 20s and, like all male and female hormones, declines shortly thereafter. Its popularity as an oral supplement comes from its reputation for increasing strength, boosting the immune system, enhancing memory and concentration, reducing depression, preventing weight gain, and heightening libido function. The research on DHEA is interesting, albeit controversial. Libido function improvement was shown in research published in the *New England Journal of Medicine* (September 30, 1999) and brain function improvement was discussed in *Brain Research Reviews* (November 2001, pages 287–293). However, Dr. Andrew Weil (http://www.drweil.com) warns that DHEA "can increase the risk of breast and prostate cancer, and may elevate the risk of a heart attack." What does any of this have to do with skin? Aside from the suggested association between DHEA and male hormone levels, and hormone levels having an effect on skin, there is no research showing DHEA has any impact on skin in regard to wrinkling or aging (Source: *Clinics in Geriatric Medicine,* November 2001, pages 661–672). Besides, it isn't the male hormones that improve the texture and appearance of female skin; the feel and suppleness of a woman's skin are affected by the levels of her estrogen and progesterone production.

deionized/demineralized water. Filtered water used in cosmetics. All water used in cosmetic formulations goes through this deionization/demineralization process to remove components that could interfere with a product's stability and performance.

***Delesseria sanguinea* extract.** *See* algae.

denatured alcohol. *See* alcohol.

deodorant soap. Soap that contains ingredients to reduce the bacteria that cause body odor. The ingredients are too harsh for the delicate skin of the face and they don't stay on the skin long enough to have any real disinfecting effect.

deoxyribonucleic acid. *See* DNA.

detergent cleansing agent. *See* surfactant.

deuterium oxide. *See* heavy water.

dextran. Polysaccharide that has water-binding properties for skin. *See also* mucopolysaccharide.

dextrin. Carbohydrate that is classified as a polysaccharide. It is used as an adhesive when mixed with water. For skin it can have water-binding properties.

DHA. *See* dihydroxyacetone.

DHEA. *See* dehydroepiandrosterone.

diatomaceous earth. Light-colored porous rock composed of skeletons of minute sea creatures called diatoms, used typically as an abrasive material in scrub products.

diazolidinyl urea. Formaldehyde-releasing preservative (Source: *Contact Dermatitis*, December 2000, pages 339–343). *See* formaldehyde-releasing preservative.

dibutyl phthalate. Very common ingredient in almost every nail polish and synthetic fragrance sold. It is used as a plasticizer and is a key component in giving nail polish its unique properties. The Centers for Disease Control and Prevention (CDC, published the *National Report on Human Exposure to Environmental Chemicals—Results for Monobutyl phthalate* [which is] *(metabolized from Dibutyl phthalate)*. The report noted measurable levels of phthalate were found in the urine of the participants in the study. However, the CDC also stated that "Finding a measurable amount of one or more phthalate metabolites in urine does not mean that the level of one or more phthalates causes an adverse health effect. Whether phthalates at the levels of metabolites reported here are a cause for health concern is not yet known; more research is needed" (Sources: CDC, http://www.cdc.gov/nceh/dls/report/results/Mono-butylPhthalate.htm; and *Environmental Health Perspectives,* December 2000, volume 108, issue 12). In animal tests, dibutyl phthalate has been shown to produce detrimental effects. The Environmental Working Group (EWG, http://www.ewg.org), a nonprofit environmental research organization, found that "DBP is a developmental and reproductive toxin that in lab animals causes a broad range of birth defects and lifelong reproductive impairment in males [when] exposed in utero and shortly after birth. DBP damages the testes, prostate gland, epididymus, penis, and seminal vesicles. These effects persist throughout the animal's life." At this time, there is no conclusive or agreed-upon research pointing to phthalates as being a problem for humans.

diethanolamine (DEA). In 1999 the National Toxicology Program (NTP) completed a study that found an association between cancer in laboratory animals and the application of DEA and certain DEA-related ingredients to their skin (Source: Study #TR-478, Toxicology and Carcinogenesis Studies of Diethanolamine (CAS No. 111-42-2) in F344/N Rats and B6C3F1 Mice (Dermal Studies), July 1999—http://ntp-server.niehs.nih.gov/). For the DEA-related ingredients, the NTP study suggested that the carcinogenic response is linked to possible residual levels of DEA. However, the NTP study did not establish a link between DEA and the risk of cancer in humans. According to the FDA (Source: *Office of Cosmetics and Colors Fact Sheet,* December 9, 1999), "Although DEA itself is used in very few cosmetics, DEA-related ingredients (e.g., oleamide DEA, lauramide DEA, cocamide DEA) are widely used in a variety of cosmetic products. These ingredients function as emulsifiers or foaming agents and are generally used at levels of 1% to 5%. The FDA takes these NTP findings very seriously and is in the process of carefully evaluating the studies and test data to determine the real risk, if any, to consumers. The Agency believes that at the present time there is no reason for consumers to be alarmed based on the usage of these ingredients in cosmetics. Consumers wishing to avoid cosmetics containing DEA or its conjugates may do so by reviewing the ingredient statement required to appear on the outer container label of cosmetics offered for retail sale to consumers."

***Digenea simplex* extract.** *See* algae.

dihydroxyacetone. Ingredient in all self-tanners that affects the color of skin. It reacts with amino acids in the top layers of skin to create a shade of brown; the effect takes place within two to six hours and it can build color depth with every reapplication.

dimethicone copolyol. *See* silicone.

dimethicone. *See* silicone.

dimethyl sulfoxide. *See* DMSO.

dimethylaminoethanol (DMAE). What little research there is about DMAE relates to its effect as an oral supplement, and the findings are mixed. DMAE, known chemically as 2-dimethyl-amino-ethanol, has been available in Europe under the product name Deanol for over 30 years. As an oral supplement it is popularly believed to improve mental alertness, much like *Ginkgo biloba* and coenzyme Q10. However, the research about DMAE does not show the same positive results found with the other two supplements. Because DMAE is chemically similar to choline, DMAE is thought to stimulate production of acetylcholine. And because acetylcholine is a brain neurotransmitter, it's easy to see how it could be associated with brain function. However, only a handful of studies have looked at DMAE for that purpose and they have not been conclusive in the least, while some have shown that DMAE may be problematic or not very effective (Sources: *Mechanisms of Aging and Development,* February 1988, pages 129–138; *Neuropharmacology,* June 1989, pages 557–561; and *European Neurology,* 1991, pages 423–425). Despite the lack of evidence supporting DMAE as having any effect on skin, there are hundreds of Web sites claiming that it does. It is possible that DMAE can help protect the cell membrane, and keeping cells intact can have benefit, but so far that appears to be only conjecture and not fact.

***Dioscorea villosa* extract.** *See* wild yam extract.

***Dipsacus sylvestris* extract.** There is no research showing this to have benefit for skin (Source: *Natural Medicines Comprehensive Database,* http://www.naturaldatabase.com).

Dipotassium glycyrrhizinate. *See* anti-irritant, and licorice extract.

dismutin. Trade name for superoxide dismutase. *See* superoxide dismutase.

disodium ascorbyl sulfate. Form of vitamin C. There is no research showing it to have any benefit on skin.

disodium diglyceryl phosphate. Emollient and thickening agent. *See* glyceryl ester.

disodium EDTA. *See* EDTA.

disodium glyceryl phosphate. Emollient and thickening agent. *See* glyceryl ester.

disodium lauraminopropionate. Mild surfactant. *See* surfactant.

disodium laureth sulfosuccinate. Mild surfactant. *See* surfactant.

DMAE. *See* dimethylaminoethanol.

DMDM hydantoin. Formaldehyde-releasing preservative (Source: *Household and Personal Products Industry,* May 2001, "Preserving Personal Care and Household Products"). *See* formaldehyde-releasing preservative.

DMSO. Dimethyl sulfoxide; an intriguing substance because of its contradictory benefits and problems. Topically, it is a potent skin irritant and sensitizer and it can cause burning, blistering, drying, and scaling skin. Yet it easily penetrates the skin and facilitates topical penetration of other ingredients. DMSO also has some evidence of having antioxidant properties and can prevent skin from freezing. Given these divergent properties and the well-established risk of skin irritation, it is not recommended to have this as a primary ingredient in skin-care products (Sources: *Natural Medicines Comprehensive Database,* http://www.naturaldatabase.com; *Skin Research and Technology,* May 2001, pages 73–77; and *Contact Dermatitis,* February 1998, pages 90–95, and April 2000, pages 216–221).

DNA. Abbreviation for **d**eoxyribo**n**ucleic **a**cid. DNA is found in all cells, and is the primary component of genes—and genes are the way cells transmit hereditary characteristics. DNA is the basis for all genetic structure; its components include adenine (A), guanine (G), thymine (T), and cytosine (C). It is the mapping of these substances that makes up the genetic code of all human traits and cellular functions. DNA is the genetic material that is required for all cellular division and growth. DNA in a skin-care product is useless, as it cannot in and of itself affect a cell's genetic elements. The production of DNA is a complex system within the cell that requires a multitude of proteins and enzymes in order to have an effect on the body's genetic material. It is also doubtful you would want to ever put anything on your skin that could impact genetic material, particularly not via a cosmetic that has no safety or efficacy regulations. Beyond that, any successful attempt to affect what DNA does would potentially create a significant risk of cancer.

docosahexaenoic acid. Fatty acid. *See* fatty acid.

dog rose. *See* rose hip.

dogwood. There is a small amount of research showing dogwood to have antioxidant and anti-inflammatory properties (Source: *Journal of Agricultural Food Chemistry*, April 2002, pages 2519–2523).

dong quai. Herb that has been shown in some studies to have estrogenic activity and a positive effect in mitigating menopausal and pre-menopausal symptoms (Source: *Journal of Agricultural Food Chemistry*, May 2001, pages 2472–2479), although several other studies disprove this (Sources: *Journal of the American Pharmaceutical Association*, March-April 2000, pages 327–329; and *Fertility and Sterility*, December 1997, pages 981–986). There is also research showing that it can stimulate the growth of breast cancer cells (Source: *Menopause*, March-April 2002, pages 145–150). There are no studies showing dong quai to have any effect topically on skin.

***Duboisia leichardtii* leaf extract.** Can be a potent skin irritant due to its alkaloid content (Source: *Phytochemistry*, April 2002, pages 697–702).

***Dulcamara* extract.** Can have anti-inflammatory properties for skin (Source: *The Complete German Commission E Monographs: Therapeutic Guide to Herbal Medicines*, American Botanical Council, 1998, Integrative Medicine Communications).

dulse. *See* algae.

***Durvillaea antarctica* extract.** Derived from a form of algae. *See* algae.

echinacea. There are several types of echinacea plants, but only *Echinacea purpurea* and *E. pallida* have been shown to be effective. These may have antibacterial and anti-inflammatory properties on skin (Source: *Phytomedicine*, April 2002, pages 249–253).

***Echium lycopsis* extract.** Small amount of research shows it to have antibacterial properties (Source: *Planta Medica*, April 1982, pages 234–236).

***Echium lycopsis* oil.** Emollient oil that also has potent antioxidant properties (Source: *Phytochemistry*, February 2000, pages 451–456).

EDTA. Abbreviation for ethylenediaminetetraacetic acid. Stabilizer used in cosmetics to prevent ingredients in a given formula from binding with trace elements (particularly minerals) that can exist in water and other ingredients to cause unwanted product changes such as texture, odor, and consistency problems. The technical term for a compound with this function is a chelating agent.

egg yolk. Consists mostly of water and lipids (fats), especially cholesterol, which makes it a good emollient and water-binding agent for skin.

eicosapentaenioc acid. Fatty acid derived from salmon oil; it is a good emollient for skin. *See* fatty acid.

Elaeis guineensis. See palm oil.

elastin. Major component of skin that gives it flexibility. Sun damage causes elastin in skin to deteriorate. Elastin can be derived from both plant and animal sources and is used in cosmetics as a good water-binding agent. Elastin in cosmetics has never been shown to affect the elastin in skin or have any other benefit, though it most likely functions as a water-binding agent.

elderberry. Has potent antioxidant properties (Source: *Free Radical Biology and Medicine,* July 2000, pages 51–60).

elecampane. Can be very irritating to the skin and can trigger allergic reactions (Source: *Contact Dermatitis,* October 2001, pages 197–204).

Emblica officinalis. See Indian gooseberry.

emollient. Group of supple, waxlike, lubricating, thickening agents that prevent water loss and have a softening and soothing effect on the skin. They can be natural, like plant oils; manufactured, like silicones; or processed from a natural substance, like mineral oil. The assortment of technical-sounding names for all these ingredients is nothing less than astounding; there are more of them than you can imagine. They range from cetearyl alcohol to isopropyl myristate, triglycerides, myristic acid, palmitic acid, PEG-60 hydrogenated castor oil, glyceryl linoleate, cyclomethicone, dimethicone, hexyl laurate, isohexadecane, methyl glucose sesquioleate, decyl oleate, stearic acid, octyldodecanol, and thousands more. There are also more understandable, or at least more familiar, "natural" versions of emollients, such as lanolin, hydrogenated plant oils, shea butter, and cocoa butter.

emu oil. The emu is a large, flightless bird indigenous to Australia, and emu oil has become an important component of the Australian economy. As a result there is research from that part of the world showing it to be a good emollient that can help heal skin. But there is no research showing it to have antiaging or antiwrinkling effects. A study published in the *Australasian Journal of Dermatology* (August 1996, pages 159–161) looked at the "Cosmetic and moisturizing properties of Emu oil … assessed in a double-blind clinical study. Emu oil in comparison to mineral oil was found overall to be more cosmetically acceptable and had better skin penetration/permeability. Furthermore it appears that Emu oil in comparison to mineral oil has better moisturizing properties, superior texture, and lower incidence of comedogenicity, but probably because of the small sample size [number of people tested] these differences were not found to be statistically significant. Neither of the oils were found to be irritating to the skin." That's good, but it's hardly a reason to run out and by a product containing emu oil. Further, another study published in *Plastic and Reconstructive Surgery* (December 1998, pages 2404–2407) concluded that applying emu oil on a fresh wound actually delayed wound healing. Emu oil's reputation is driven mostly by cosmetics company claims and not by any real proof that emu oil is an essential requirement for skin.

English ivy extract. Can be a skin irritant due to its stimulant and astringent (skin-constricting) properties (Source: *Natural Medicines Comprehensive Database,* http://www.naturaldatabase.com).

Enteromorpha compressa **extract.** Extract from a form of green algae. *See* algae.

enzymes. Whether in the form of papaya fruit or in a substance such as papain (a proteinase derived from unripe papaya) or bromelain (derived from pineapple), enzymes (proteases) have long been used in their pure form as exfoliants (Source: *Burns,* November 1999, pages 636–639). However, there is limited (if any) research showing that enzymes perform as well or are as stable as alpha hydroxy acids or beta hydroxy acid. There is one study showing forms of enzymes such as papain or bromelain to be effective in pure form for exfoliation (Source: *Archives of Dermatological Research,* November 2001, pages 500–507). New enzymes are now being put in skin-care products that are claimed to stimulate your skin's own biological processes that have slowed down because of age or sun damage. However, all enzymes are proteins that function as biological catalysts. They accelerate chemical reactions in a cell, reactions that would proceed minimally or not at all if enzymes weren't there. Most enzymes—and a lot of different enzymes affect skin cells—are finicky about how they interact. Sometimes it takes several enzymes to produce one chemical reaction. Some enzymes depend on the presence of smaller enzymes, called coenzymes, in order to function. It would take an exceptionally complicated process to stimulate enzyme activity in the skin, and one tiny amount of an enzyme in a skin-care product won't turn on your skin's ability to make collagen or elastin. *See* AHA, and salicylic acid.

Ephedra sinica **extract.** Extract from a Chinese herb also known as Ma huang; it has a high tannin and volatile oil content and toxic properties (Source: *Toxicological Sciences,* August 2000, pages 424–430).

epidermal growth factor (EGF). Compound that stimulates cell division of many different cell types. There is research showing it to be helpful for wound and burn healing (Sources: *Journal of Burn Care and Rehabilitation,* March-April 2002, pages 116–125; and *Journal of Dermatologic Surgery and Oncology,* July 1992, pages 604–606), but there is also research showing that its effect is no different from that of a placebo and that it may not be effective (Sources: *Wounds,* 2001, volume 13, number 2, pages 53–58; and *Plastic and Reconstructive Surgery,* August 1995, pages 251–254). It can have anti-inflammatory properties when applied to skin (Source: *Skin Pharmacology and Applied Skin Physiology,* January-April 1999, pages 79-84), though it can also promote tumor growth (Source: *Journal of Surgical Research,* April 2002, pages 175–182). *See* human growth factor.

Epilobium angustifolium **extract.** Derived from a plant commonly known as fireweed or willow herb. Can have antimicrobial (Source: *Il Farmaco,* May-July 2001, pages 345–348) and anti-irritant properties for skin (Source: *Journal of Agricultural Food Chemistry,* October 1999, pages 3954–3962).

Equisetum arvense. See horsetail extract.

Equisetum hiemale **extract.** *See* horsetail extract.

ergocalciferol. Technical name for vitamin D. *See* vitamin D.

ergothioneine. Component of animal tissue that has potent antioxidant properties (Source: *Food and Chemical Toxicology,* November 1999, pages 1043–1053).

Eriobotrya japonica. See loquat extract.

erucic acid. Fatty acid. *See* fatty acid.

erythritol. Naturally occurring sugar found in plants and animals. Like all sugars, it has water-binding properties.

erythropoietin (Epo). Compound that stimulates the growth of cells that carry oxygen throughout the body. *See* human growth factor.

erythrulose. Substance chemically similar to the self-tanning agent dihydroxyacetone. Depending on your skin color, there can be a difference in the color effect with erythrulose. Erythrulose needs about two to three days for the skin to show a color change, while dihydroxyacetone completely changes the color of skin within two to six hours.

escin. Component of horse chestnut. It is considered therapeutically useful in the treatment of leg veins by protecting the elastic tissue of the vein (Sources: *Lancet,* 1996, volume 347, pages 292–294; and *Archives of Dermatology,* 1998, volume 134, pages 1356–1360). However, the amount needed for this potential benefit is far greater than what is used in cosmetic formulations.

esculin. Component of horse chestnut, it is considered a toxin and not recommended for skin (Source: *Clinical Pharmacology,* 2002, http://cponline.hitchcock.org/).

essential oil. *See* volatile oil.

Ester-C. Trade name for a combination form of vitamin C that contains mainly calcium ascorbate, but in addition contains small amounts of the vitamin C metabolites dehydroascorbic acid (oxidized ascorbic acid), calcium threonate, and trace levels of xylonate and lyxonate. In their literature, the manufacturers state that the metabolites, especially threonate, increase the bioavailability of the vitamin C in this product, and that they have performed a study in humans demonstrating the increased bioavailability of vitamin C in Ester-C. This study has not been published in a peer-reviewed journal. A small published study of vitamin C bioavailability in eight women and one man found no difference between Ester-C and commercially available ascorbic acid tablets with respect to the absorption and excretion of vitamin C (Source: *The Bioavailability of Different Forms of Vitamin C,* The Linus Pauling Institute, Oregon State University, http://www.orst.edu/dept/lpi/ss01/bioavailability.html). There are studies showing Ester-C to have no differences when compared to ascorbic acid (*Biochemical Pharmacology,* June 1996, pages 1719–1725).

estradiol. One of the three main forms of estrogen produced by the body; the other two are estrone and estriol. Estradiol is the most physiologically active form of estrogen. Many hormone replacement therapy (HRT) and birth control prescription drugs contain estradiol. Decreased production of estrogen by the ovaries can lead to symptoms such as hot flashes, night sweats, vaginal dryness, urinary tract infections, depression, and irritability. Physicians may prescribe a combination of natural estrogens. Whether or not natural estrogens are safe has not been well-researched.

Even though HRT can prevent problems associated with loss of estrogen in perimenopausal and menopausal women, it is now prescribed only with caution because of studies showing there to be an increased risk of breast cancer, heart attacks, strokes, gallbladder disease, and blood clots (Source: *Annals of Internal Medicine*, http://www.acponline.org/journals /annals/hrt.htm).

Topically, according to the FDA (http://www.fda.gov), "The estrogen content of an OTC product, be it a drug or a drug as well as cosmetic, may not exceed 10,000 IU per ounce, and users must be directed to limit the amount of product applied daily so that no more than 20,000 IU of estrogen or equivalent be used per month. Some estrogen-containing products have been claiming to prevent or reduce wrinkles, treat seborrhea, or stimulate hair growth. The Advisory Review Panel on OTC Miscellaneous External Drug Products has concluded that there are inadequate data to establish the safety of these products and that they are ineffective and may therefore be misbranded, even if marketed as cosmetics without making medicinal claims.... In a Final Rule, published in the Federal Register of September 9, 1993, 58 FR 47608, the FDA accepted this panel's recommendation and determined that all topically-applied hormone containing drug products for OTC human use are not generally recognized as safe and effective and are misbranded."

ethanol. *See* alcohol.

ethyl acetate. Compound made from acetic acid and ethyl alcohol, used as a solvent in nail polish and nail-polish removers. May irritate skin.

ethyl alcohol. *See* alcohol.

ethylene glycol. *See* propylene glycol.

ethylparaben. *See* parabens.

etidronic acid. *See* alcohol.

eucalyptus extract. Can have antibacterial, antifungal, and antiviral properties on the skin (Source: *Skin Pharmacology and Applied Skin Physiology*, January-February 2000, pages 60–64). It can also be a skin irritant, particularly on abraded skin (Sources: *Clinical Experimental Dermatology*, March 1995, pages 143–145; and http://www.alternativedr.com/conditions/ConsHerbs/Eucalyptusch.html). *See* counterirritant.

eucalyptus oil. *See* eucalyptus extract.

Eugenia aromatica. *See* clove oil.

Eugenia caryophyllus. *See* clove oil.

eugenol. *See* clove oil, and methyleugenol.

Euglena gracilis. *See* algae.

Eupatorium ayapana **extract.** May have antibacterial and antifungal properties (Source: *Fitoterapia,* April 2002, pages 168–170).

Euphrasia officinalis. See eyebright.

evening primrose oil. Can have anti-inflammatory and emollient benefits for skin (Sources: *Skin Pharmacology and Applied Skin Physiology,* January-February 2002, pages 20–25; and *Journal of Agricultural Food Chemistry,* September 2001, pages 4502–4507). However, whether or not evening primrose oil can mitigate certain symptoms of premenstrual syndrome (PMS) is unknown. "Trials of evening primrose oil have also had conflicting results; the two most rigorous studies showed no evidence of benefit" (Source: *Journal of the American College of Nutrition,* February 2000, pages 3–12). *See* gamma linolenic acid.

ex vivo. Describes a biological process or reaction taking place outside of a person or animal; it involves the extraction of cells from an animal or person and then testing these in a laboratory setting.

Ext. D&C. Type of coloring agent. According to the FDA (http://www.fda.gov), when Ext. D&C is followed by a color, it means the color is certified as safe for use only in drugs **and** cosmetics to be used **ext**ernally, but not around the eyes or mouth. It is not safe for foods.

eyebright. Herb of the genus *Euphrasia*. While the name sounds like it is beneficial for the eye area, there are no studies demonstrating it to have any benefit for the eye area or skin. The information about this plant's effect on the skin or eyes is strictly anecdotal.

faex. *See* yeast.

Fagus sylvatica **extract.** Beech tree extract; there is no research showing it to be beneficial for skin.

farnesol. Extract of plants that in cosmetics is used primarily for fragrance. A few animal studies and some in vitro research have investigated farnesol's antibacterial properties (Source: *Chemotherapy,* July 2002, pages 122–128), and it may also have some antioxidant properties (Source: *Journal of Bacteriology,* September 1998, pages 4460–4465), but there is no research showing it to have benefit on skin.

farnesyl acetate. *See* farnesol.

fatty acid. Substances typically found in plant and animal lipids (fat). Fatty acids include compounds such as glycerides, sterols, and phospholipids. They are used in cosmetics as emollients, thickening agents, and, when mixed with glycerin, cleansing agents. Fatty acids are natural components of skin and are components of a complex mixture that makes up the outermost layer protecting the body against oxidative damage (Sources: *Free Radical Research,* April 2002, pages 471–477; and *Journal of Lipid Research,* May 2002, pages, 794–804). Fatty acids can help supplement the skin's intercellular matrix. *See* natural moisturizing factors.

fatty alcohols. Made from fatty acids; in cosmetics these are used as thickening agents and emollients. *See* fatty acid.

FD&C. Type of coloring agent. According to the FDA, when FD&C is followed by a color, the color is certified as safe for use in **f**ood, **d**rugs, **and c**osmetics.

fennel extract. Derived from the fennel plant; it can be a skin irritant (Source: *Allergy and Immunology,* April 2002, pages 135–140).

fennel oil. Volatile, fragrant oil that can cause skin irritation and sensitivity. *See* fennel extract.

fennel seed extract. Can have antioxidant properties, but on skin it can be a skin irritant and photosensitizer (Source: *Natural Medicines Comprehensive Database,* http://www.naturaldatabase.com).

fenugreek. Spice plant; some research shows it to have antioxidant properties when taken orally. Whether it has similar properties when applied topically is unknown.

Ferula galbaniflua. See galbanum.

feverfew extract. Can be very irritating to the skin and can trigger allergic reactions (Source: *Contact Dermatitis,* October 2001, pages 197–204). When taken orally it has been shown to relieve migraines and have anti-inflammatory properties (Source: *Natural Medicines Comprehensive Database,* http://www.naturaldatabase.com).

fibroblast growth factor (FGF). Within the body, stimulates growth of the nervous system and bone formation. *See* human growth factor.

fibronectin. Type of protein found in the skin's intercellular matrix similar to collagen and elastin. Fibronectin's deterioration from sun damage and other factors is an element in skin aging and wrinkling. As is true for all proteins, regardless of their origin, it is probably a good water-binding agent for skin. However, applying fibronectin topically on skin doesn't help reinforce or rebuild the fibronectin in your skin.

Filipendula rubra. See meadowsweet.

film-forming agent. Large group of ingredients that are typically found in hair-care products but are also widely used in skin-care products, particularly moisturizers. These range from PVP to acrylates, acrylamides, and copolymers. When applied they leave a pliable, cohesive, and continuous covering over the hair or skin. This film has excellent water-binding properties and leaves a smooth feel on skin. Film-forming agents can be skin sensitizers for some individuals.

fir needle oil. Volatile, fragrant oil that can cause skin irritation and sensitivity.

fireweed. From the *Epilobium angustifolium* plant; also known as willow herb. *See Epilobium angustifolium.*

fish cartilage extract. May have water-binding properties, but there is no research showing this to have any benefit for skin.

flavonoid. *See* bioflavonoid.

flax. Plant source of linen and edible seeds. Seeds and seed oil have antioxidant properties (Source: *Biofactors,* 2000; volume 13, pages 179–185). Seeds are also a source of linolenic acid. *See* linolenic acid.

flaxseed oil. From seeds of the flax plant; a source of fatty acids. *See* flax.

floralozone. One of a number of synthetic fragrant components.

Foeniculum vulgare **extract.** *See* fennel seed extract.

folic acid. Part of the B-vitamin complex; when taken orally, it is considered a good antioxidant. That benefit has not been demonstrated when it is applied topically on skin.

Fomes officinalis. The scientific name for a fungus (mushroom) commonly called brown trunk rot. There is no research showing this to have benefit for skin.

formaldehyde-releasing preservative. Common type of preservative found in cosmetics (Source: *Contact Dermatitis,* December 2000, pages 339–343). There is no higher level of skin reaction to formaldehyde-releasing preservatives than to other preservatives (Source: *British Journal of Dermatology,* March 1998, pages 467–476). In fact, there is a far greater risk to skin from a product without preservatives, owing to the contamination and unchecked growth of bacteria, fungus, and mold that can result. However, there is concern that when formaldehyde-releasing preservatives are present in a formulation with amines, such as triethanolamine (TEA), diethanolamine (DEA), or monoethanolamine (MEA), that nitrosamines can then be formed, because nitrosamines are carcinogenic substances that can potentially penetrate skin (Source: *Fundamental and Applied Toxicology,* August 1993, pages 213–221). Whether or not that poses a health risk of any kind has not been established. *See* preservatives.

fragrance. One or a blend of either volatile and/or fragrant plant oils (or synthetically derived oils) that impart aroma and odor to products. These are often skin irritants (Sources: *Dermatology,* 2002, volume 205, number 1, pages 98–102; *Contact Dermatitis,* December 2001, pages 333–340; and *Toxicology and Applied Pharmacology,* May 2001, pages 172–178). *See* volatile oil.

frangipani. *See Plumeria alba* flower extract.

Frangula alnus **extract.** Extract from the Alder Buckthorn or Dogweed tree. Used orally as a laxative. There is no research showing this extract to have any benefit for skin (Source: *Natural Medicines Comprehensive Database,* http://www.naturaldatabase.com).

frankincense extract. Fragrant component used in skin-care products; it can be a skin irritant. There is no research showing frankincense to have any benefit for skin (Sources: http://www.herbmed.com; and *Natural Medicines Comprehensive Database,* http://www.naturaldatabase.com).

free-radical damage. It is now medically recognized that degenerative skin conditions, such as wrinkles and skin discolorations, are caused primarily by free-radical damage (Source: *Bioelectrochemistry and Bioenergetics,* May 1999, pages 453–461). The primary causes of free-radical damage are air and sunlight, but it can also be triggered by cigarette smoke, herbicides, pesticides, pollution, and solvents. Antioxidants are a way to reduce and potentially neutralize the rampage of free-radical damage (Sources: *Journal of Clinical Pathology,* March 2001, pages 176–186; and *Drugs and Aging,* 2001, volume 18, number 9, pages 685–716).

Free-radical damage takes place on an atomic level. Molecules are made of atoms, and a single atom is made up of protons, neutrons, and electrons. Electrons are always found in pairs. However, when oxygen molecules are involved in a chemical reaction, they can lose one of their electrons, and an oxygen molecule that has only one electron is called a free radical. With only one electron the oxygen molecule must quickly find another electron, and it does this by taking the electron from another molecule. When that molecule in turn loses one of its electrons, it too must seek out another, in a continuing reaction. Molecules attempting to repair themselves in this way trigger a cascading event called "free-radical damage." The action of free-radical damage takes place in a fraction of a second. Antioxidants are substances that prevent oxidative damage from being triggered. *See* antioxidant.

fructose. Often called fruit sugar; a type of sugar composed of glucose. It has water-binding properties for skin. *See* water-binding agent.

fruit acid. *See* sugarcane extract.

Fu ling. *See Poria cocos* extract.

***Fucus serratus* extract.** *See* algae.

***Fucus vesiculosus* extract.** *See* bladderwrack.

fuller's earth. Mineral substance that is similar to kaolin (a clay). Composed mainly of alumina, silica, iron oxides, lime, magnesia, and water, it is used as an absorbent and thickening agent in cosmetics.

***Fumaria officinalis* extract.** May have antibacterial properties (Source: *Natural Medicines Comprehensive Database,* http://www.naturaldatabase.com).

fumaric acid. Naturally occurring acid that has been proven effective for systemic and topical treatment of severe psoriasis vulgaris (Source: *Journal of Investigative Dermatology,* February 2001, pages 203–208); however, it can also cause serious skin irritation (Source: *Dermatology,* 1994, volume 188, number 2, pages 126–130). In small amounts it can be used as a pH adjuster in cosmetics.

galactoarabinan. Polysaccharide extracted from the western larch tree. *See* mucopolysaccharide.

galbanum. Fragrant substance that, because of its resin and volatile oil content, can be extremely irritating and sensitizing on abraded skin. There is no research showing it to have any benefit on skin.

gamma linolenic acid (GLA). Fatty acid used in cosmetics as an emollient, antioxidant, and cell regulator. GLA is believed to promote healthy skin growth and is an anti-inflammatory agent. GLA is found in black currant oil or seeds, evening primrose oil, and borage oil (Source: *Biochemical and Biophysical Research Communications,* March 17, 1998, pages 414–420). However, there is no research showing GLA to be effective in the treatment of wrinkles (Sources: *British Journal of Dermatology,* April 1999, pages 685–688; and *Dermatology,* 2000, volume 201, number 3, pages 191–195). When taken orally, GLA has been shown to have some anticancer properties, but there is no research showing that effect translates to skin. *See* fatty acid.

Gan jiang. See ginger.

Ganoderma lucidum **extract.** Mushroom stem extract. There are many animal and in vitro studies showing that this extract, when taken orally, has potentially effective antitumor, immune modulating, anticoagulant, cholesterol lowering, antiviral, and antibacterial properties (Sources: *International Journal of Cancer,* November 2002, pages 250–253; *Immunology Letters,* October 2002, pages 163–169; *Life Sciences,* June 2002, pages 623–638; *Cancer Letters,* August 2002, pages 155–161; and *Bioorganic and Medicinal Chemistry,* April 2002, pages 1057–1062). However, there is no research showing it to be effective when used topically on skin (Source: *Natural Medicines Comprehensive Database,* http://www.naturaldatabase.com), though it does have antioxidant properties (Source: *Journal of Agricultural and Food Chemistry,* October 2002, pages 6072–6077).

Gaultheria shallon. May have antioxidant activity for skin (Source: *Phytotherapy Research,* February 2002, pages 63–65).

gelatin. Protein obtained from plants or animals and used in cosmetics as a thickening agent.

Gellidiela acerosa **extract.** Derived from a type of algae. *See* algae.

gentian violet extract. Has anti-irritant and antibacterial properties (Sources: *Dermatology,* 2001, volume 203, number 4, pages 325–328; *International Journal of Dermatology,* December 2000, pages 942–944; and *Journal of Hospital Infection,* November 1995, pages 225–228).

geranium extract. Can have potent antioxidant properties (Source: *Phytomedicine,* June 2000, pages 221–229).

geranium oil. Fragrant oil that has antimicrobial properties but can also be a skin sensitizer or irritant (Sources: *Contact Dermatitis,* June 2001, pages 344–346; and *Journal of Applied Microbiology,* February 2000, pages 308–316).

Geranium pretense. Geranium plant. *See* geranium extract, and geranium oil.

Germaben II. Trade name for diazolidinyl urea. *See* diazolidinyl urea.

germanium. According to the FDA there is an import ban aimed at germanium, a trace element used in the production of computer chips, which sometimes is identified as vitamin O. The FDA noted that consumption of germanium has caused kidney injury and death when used chronically by humans, even at dosages suggested on product labels. It has banned germanium imports intended for human consumption on the grounds that these products are either poisonous and deleterious to health or are unapproved new drugs (Source: http://www.fda.gov). However, there is research showing it to have anti-inflammatory properties when taken as a drug (Source: *Journal of Interferon and Cytokine Research,* June 2001, pages 389–398). There is no research showing it to have any benefit topically on skin.

Gigartina stellata **extract.** Extracted from algae. There is no research showing this to have special properties for skin, though it may have water-binding benefits. *See* algae.

ginger oil. *See* ginger.

ginger. From a plant in the zingiber family that has research showing it to have anti-inflammatory and anti-carcinogenic activity when taken orally (Sources: *Carcinogenesis*, May 2002, pages 795–802; and *Food and Chemical Toxicology*, August 2002, pages 1091–1097). However, topically it can be a skin irritant (Source: IFA—International Federation of Aromatherapists, http://www.int-fed-aromatherapy.co.uk).

Ginkgo biloba. Tree with leaves having components that are effective as an anti-inflammatory and an aid in collagen production; ginkgo also has antioxidant properties (Sources: *Planta Medica*, April 2002, pages 316–321; *Skin Pharmacology and Applied Skin Physiology*, July-August 1997, pages 200–205; *Journal of Pharmacy and Pharmacology*, December 1999, pages 1435–1440; and *Methods in Enzymology*, 1994, volume 234, pages 462–475).

ginseng. From a family of herbs (Araliaceae) native to Asia. A small number of studies carried out on animals have shown that ginseng may have antitumor and anticancer properties (Sources: *Journal of Korean Medical Science*, December 2001, Supplemental, pages 38–41; and *Cancer Letter*, March 2000, pages 41–48), though there is also research showing that it can stimulate the growth of breast cancer cells (Source: *Menopause*, March-April 2002, pages 145–150). There is no evidence showing any benefit or risk when applied topically.

GLA. *See* gamma linolenic acid.

glabridin. Main ingredient in licorice extract. It has anti-inflammatory properties and there is research showing it to be effective in reducing skin discolorations (Source: *Pigment Cell Research*, December 1998, pages 355–361).

gluconolactone. *See* polyhydroxy acid.

glucosamine hydrochloride. When taken orally, it can have anti-inflammatory properties, but there is no research showing the same effect for skin when it is applied topically.

glucosamine sulfate. Needed by the body to form glycosaminoglycans such as hyaluronic acid, which is a major constituent of skin tissue as well as joint cartilage. There is no research demonstrating this to be effective topically on skin in generating hyaluronic acid; most likely it functions as a water-binding agent.

glucose oxidase. Enzyme that has antibacterial and water-binding properties when used on skin.

glucose tyrosinate. *See* tyrosine.

glucose. Monosaccharide that has water-binding properties for skin. *See* water-binding agent, and mucopolysaccharide.

glutamic acid. Amino acid derived from wheat gluten. It can have water-binding properties for skin. There is no research showing glutamic acid to have special properties when used in topical cosmetic formulations. *See* amino acid.

glutamine. Can help improve the barrier function of skin (Source: *Journal of Biological Chemistry*, July 1998, pages 1763–1770). *See* amino acid.

glutathione. Potent antioxidant (Source: *Free Radical Research,* March 2002, pages 329–340). *See* antioxidant.

glycereth-17 cocoate. Used as an emollient and thickening agent. *See* glyceryl ester.

glycereth-20 stearate. Used as an emollient and thickening agent. *See* glyceryl ester.

glycereth-26 phosphate. Used as an emollient and thickening agent. *See* glyceryl ester.

glycereth-6 laurate. Used as an emollient and thickening agent. *See* glyceryl ester.

glycerin. Also called glycerol; it is present in all natural lipids (fats), whether animal or vegetable. It is produced naturally by the hydrolysis of fats and by the fermentation of sugars, and can also be synthetically manufactured. For some time it was thought that too much glycerin in a moisturizer could pull water out of the skin instead of drawing it into the skin; that theory now seems to be completely unfounded. What appears to be true is that glycerin shores up the skin's natural protection by filling in the area known as the intercellular matrix and by attracting just the right amount of water to maintain the skin's homeostasis. There is also research indicating that the presence of glycerin in the intercellular layer helps other skin lipids do their jobs better (Sources: *American Journal of Contact Dermatitis,* September 2000, pages 165–169; and *Acta Dermato-Venereologica,* November 1999, pages 418–421). *See* intercellular matrix, and natural moisturizing factors.

glycerine. *See* glycerin.

glycerol monostearate. Used as an emollient and thickening agent. *See* glyceryl ester.

glycerol triacetate. Used as an emollient and thickening agent. *See* glyceryl ester.

glycerol trioleate. Used as an emollient and thickening agent. *See* glyceryl ester.

glycerol. *See* glycerin.

glyceryl cocoate. Used as an emollient and thickening agent. *See* glyceryl ester.

glyceryl dipalmitate. Used as an emollient and thickening agent. *See* glyceryl ester.

glyceryl distearate. Used as an emollient and thickening agent. *See* glyceryl ester.

glyceryl ester. Large group of ingredients that are composed of fats and oils. At room temperature, the fats are usually solid and the oils are generally liquid. Some tropical oils are liquids in their sites of origin and become solids in cooler climates or different applications. These multitudinous fats and oils are used in cosmetics as emollients and lubricants as well as water-binding and thickening agents.

glyceryl glycyrrhetinate. Used as an emollient and thickening agent. *See* glyceryl ester, and glycyrrhetinate.

glyceryl hydroxystearate. Used as an emollient and thickening agent. *See* glyceryl ester.

glyceryl isopalmitate. Used as an emollient and thickening agent. *See* glyceryl ester.

glyceryl isostearate. Used as an emollient and thickening agent. *See* glyceryl ester.

glyceryl myristate. Used as an emollient and thickening agent. *See* glyceryl ester.

glyceryl oleate. Used as an emollient and thickening agent. *See* glyceryl ester.

glyceryl palmitate. Used as an emollient and thickening agent. *See* glyceryl ester.

glyceryl ricinoleate. Used as an emollient and thickening agent. *See* glyceryl ester.

glyceryl stearate. Used as an emollient and thickening agent. *See* glyceryl ester.

glyceryl tricapryl-caprate. Used as an emollient and thickening agent. *See* glyceryl ester.

glycine. *See* amino acid.

Glycine soja **oil.** Oil derived from wild soybeans; it has emollient properties. *See* natural moisturizing factors.

glycogen. Polysaccharide that has water-binding properties for skin. *See* polysaccharide.

glycolic acid. *See* AHA.

glycolipid. Type of lipid composed of sugar (monosaccharide) and fat (lipid) that forms an important component of cell membranes and ceramides. Glycolipids coat cell walls, forming a barrier that holds skin and water content in place. *See* ceramide, lipid, and mucopolysaccharide.

glycoproteins. When combined with saccharides, these form the skin's intercellular matrix, holding skin cells and the skin's structure intact. They are used as water-binding agents. *See* natural moisturizing factors, protein, and mucopolysaccharide.

glycosaminoglycans. Also known as mucopolysaccharides; these are a fundamental component of skin tissue, and are essentially a group of complex proteins. Chondroitin sulfate and hyaluronic acid are part of this ingredient group. *See* chondroitin sulfate, hyaluronic acid, and natural moisturizing factors.

glycosphingolipid. *See* glycolipid, and natural moisturizing factors.

glycyrrhetic acid. Extract from licorice that has anti-inflammatory properties (Sources: *American Journal of Respiratory and Cellular Molecular Biology,* November 1998, pages 836–841; and *Planta Medica,* August 1996, pages 326–328). *See* licorice extract.

Glycyrrhiza glabra. Licorice plant. *See* glycyrrhetic acid, and licorice extract.

Gnaphalium leontopodium **flower extract.** Fragrant plant extract; it has no known benefit for skin.

gold. Relatively common allergen that can induce dermatitis about the face and eyelids (Source: *Cutis,* May 2000, pages 323–326). There is no research showing it to have benefit when applied topically to skin.

goldenseal. Perennial herb that may have antibacterial or antiviral properties when taken orally. There is no evidence that such an effect occurs when applied topically on skin. It can be a skin irritant.

gotu kola. *See Centella asiatica.*

grape seed extract. There are no published studies indicating that grapes in any form, applied topically, can affect the wrinkling process. However, grape seed extract contains proanthocyanidins, which are considered very potent antioxidants, helpful for diminishing the sun's damaging effects and lessening free-radical damage (Sources: *Current Pharmaceutical Biotechnology,* June 2001, pages 187–200; and *Toxicology,* August 2000, pages 187–197). It has also been shown to have wound-healing properties (Source: *Free Radical Biology and Medicine,* July 2001, pages 38–42). There is no difference in the antioxidant potential between different types of grapes (Source: *Journal of Agricultural Food Chemistry,* April 2000, pages 1076–1080).

grape seed oil. Emollient oil that also has good antioxidant properties. *See also* grape seed extract, and linoleic acid.

grapefruit oil. Can have antibacterial properties (Source: *Journal of Agricultural Food Chemistry,* July 2001, pages 3316–3320), but can also be a potent skin irritant, especially on abraded skin.

green tea. Significant amounts of research have established that teas, including black, green, and white, deliver many intriguing health benefits. Dozens of studies point to tea's potent antioxidant as well as anticarcinogenic properties. However, a good deal of this research was conducted on animal models that do not directly relate to human skin (Source: *Skin Pharmacology and Applied Skin Physiology,* 2001, pages 69–76). There is only limited information about its effect on human skin. The *Journal of Photochemistry and Photobiology* (December 31, 2001) stated that the polyphenols "are the active ingredients in green tea and possess antioxidant, anti-inflammatory and anticarcinogenic properties. Studies conducted by our group on human skin have demonstrated that green tea polyphenols (GTP) prevent ultraviolet (UV)-B…-induced immune suppression and skin cancer induction." Thus, green tea and other teas show a good deal of promise for skin, but they are not quite the miracle that cosmetics and health food companies make them out to be. As the *Annual Review of Pharmacology and Toxicology* (January 2002, pages 25–54) put it, "Tea has received a great deal of attention because tea polyphenols are strong antioxidants, and tea preparations have inhibitory activity against tumorigenesis. The bioavailability and biotransformation of tea polyphenols, however, are key factors limiting these activities in vivo [in humans]. Epidemiological studies … have not yielded clear conclusions concerning the protective effects of tea consumption against cancer formation in humans." What is not disputed are the anti-inflammatory properties of tea (black, green, and white). These are also definitely potent antioxidants. All of that is very good for skin, but whether it has any effect on wrinkles or scars is speculation, not fact.

***Grindelia Robusta* extract.** Also known as tar weed or gum weed. This extract can be a potential skin irritant (Source: *Natural Medicines Comprehensive Database,* http://www.naturaldatabase.com).

gromwell extract. *See Lithospermum officinale.*

guaiac wood. Used as a fragrant extract in cosmetics; it is a potent skin irritant.

***Guaiacum officinale*.** *See* guaiac wood.

guanine. Component of DNA that carries genetic information to the cell. *See* DNA.

guanosine. Ribonucleoside component of ribonucleic acid (RNA). RNA holds part of the body's genetic material. Guanosine is needed in a vital, complicated chemical process that creates DNA and RNA. However, guanosine topically on skin cannot affect the function of DNA or RNA. The production of DNA and RNA occurs in a complex process that requires a multitude of proteins and enzymes to have an effect on the body's genetic material. It is doubtful you would ever want to put anything on your skin that could impact genetic material, and particularly not via a cosmetic that has no safety or efficacy regulations. From any viewpoint, trying to impact DNA and RNA randomly would create a significant risk of cancer. *See* DNA, and RNA.

guar gum. Plant-derived thickening agent.

guarana. Herb that contains two and a half times more caffeine than coffee. It can have constricting properties on skin and can therefore be a skin irritant. *See* caffeine.

guava extract. Fruit extract that can have constricting properties on skin, which makes it a potential skin irritant when used regularly. When part of the diet, it has been found to have antioxidant properties (Source: *Journal of Agricultural Food Chemistry,* November 2001, pages 5489–5493), but there is no research demonstrating it has such an effect topically on skin.

gums. Substances that have water-binding properties but that are primarily used as thickening agents in cosmetics. Some gums have a sticky feel and are used as film-forming agents in hairsprays, while others can constrict skin and have irritancy potential. Natural thickeners such as acacia, tragacanth, and locust bean are types of gums.

Hamamelis virginiana. *See* witch hazel.

hamamelitannin. Tannin that is found in witch hazel. It can be a skin irritant but it also has potent antioxidant properties. *See* tannin.

Haslea ostrearia **extract.** Derived from a water plant also known as blue algae. In pure concentrations this extract can have antiviral properties on skin. *See* also algae.

hawthorn extract. When taken orally hawthorn may improve circulation (Source: *Phytomedicine,* 1994, volume 1, pages 17–24). The bioflavonoids in hawthorn are potent antioxidants (*Planta Medica,* 1994, volume 60, pages 323–328). But there is no research showing that this extract has any benefit for skin.

hayflower extract. Plant extract that, due to its constricting effect on skin, can be an irritant. There is no research supporting the claim that it can have any effect on skin.

hazelnut oil. Oil extracted from the hazelnut; used as an emollient. *See* natural moisturizing factors.

heavy water. Water in which hydrogen atoms have been replaced by deuterium; it is used chiefly as a coolant in nuclear reactors. It has no known benefit for skin or use in skincare products.

Hedera helix. *See* English ivy.

hedione. Synthetic fragrant component in products; can also be a skin irritant.

helianthus oil. *See* sunflower oil.

Helichrysum italicum. One species of a plant family that includes strawflower. Extracts of these plants can have potent antioxidant and anti-inflammatory properties for skin (Sources: *Journal of Pharmacy and Pharmacology,* March 2002, pages 365–371; and *Life Sciences,* January 2002, pages 1023–1033).

hematin. Iron-containing portion of blood. It has no known benefit for skin.

hemolymph extract. Extract of crustacean blood. It can be a source of proteins or other water-binding agents, but there is no research showing it to have special benefit when applied topically on skin.

hemp seed oil. From the hemp plant, *Cannabis sativa*. Because both hemp and marijuana are from the genus *Cannabis,* they are often thought (erroneously) to have similar properties. Yet because hemp contains virtually no THC (delta-9-tetrahydrocannabinol), which is the active ingredient in marijuana, it is not used as a drug of any kind. In cosmetics, hemp seed oil is used as an emollient. Other claims about its effect on skin are not substantiated. *See* fatty acid.

hepatocyte growth factor. Stimulates division in cells lining the liver, skin cells, and cells that produce skin color. *See* human growth factor.

heptamethylnonane. *See* isohexadecane.

hesperidin. Bioflavinoid that has antioxidant and water-binding properties for skin. Also called "vitamin P." *See* bioflavonoid.

hexylene glycol. *See* propylene glycol.

Hibiscus sabdariffa **flower extract.** There is some research showing extracted components of the plant have antioxidant, antitumor, and anti-inflammatory properties (Sources: *Food and Chemical Toxicology,* May 2000, pages 411–416, and June 1999, pages 591–601). Whether these potential benefits are from the flower extract itself or from its components has not been evaluated.

Hierochloe odorata **extract.** Commonly known as sweet grass, it may have antioxidant properties (Source: *Journal of Agricultural and Food Chemistry,* May 2002, pages 2914–2919).

Himanthalia elongate **extract.** Component of algae. *See* algae.

histidine. *See* amino acid.

Hoelen. *See Poria cocos* extract.

honey. Has antibacterial, preservative, wound-healing, and water-binding properties when applied topically (Sources: *BioMed Central [BMC] Complementary and Alternative Medicine,* 2001, volume 1, issue 1, page 2; and *Burns,* March 1998, pages 157–161).

honeysuckle extract. Fragrant plant extract that can be a skin irritant, but may also have anti-irritant properties (Source: *International Journal of Molecular Medicine,* January 2001, pages 79–83).

hops. There is no research showing that hops have any benefit for skin. However, components in hops may have antioxidant and antibacterial properties. The plant may also have estrogenic properties, though not when applied to skin.

Hordeum vulgare **extract.** *See* barley extract.

horse chestnut extract. May have anti-inflammatory properties for skin. When taken orally it has been shown to reduce edema in the lower leg by improving the elastic tissue surrounding the vein (Sources: *Pharmacological Research,* September 2001, pages 183–193; *Phytotherapy Research,* March 2002, number S1, pages 1–5; and *American Journal of Clinical Dermatology,* 2002, volume 3, number 5, pages 341–348). *See* escin.

horse elder. *See* elecampane.

horseradish. Can irritate skin and should never be applied to abraded skin.

horsetail extract. Derived from flowerless plants of genus *Equisetum*. Has a high tannin, alkaloid, and nicotine content, which can have skin-constricting properties and be irritating to skin (Source: http://www.herbmed.org). It also has antioxidant properties, but there are many other potent antioxidants that don't cause any skin irritation.

Huang qi. *See* milk vetch root.

human growth factor. It is important to make it clear that the topic of human growth factors (HGFs) is exceedingly complicated. The physiological intricacies of the varying HGFs and their actions challenge any layperson's comprehension. Nonetheless, because the use of HGFs seems to be the direction some skin-care companies are taking, and because there is a large body of research showing its efficacy for wound healing (but not for wrinkles), it does deserve comment.

HGFs make up a complex family of hormones that are produced by the body to control cell growth and cell division in skin, blood, bone, and nerve tissue. Most significantly, HGFs regulate the division and reproduction of cells, and they also can influence the growth rate of some cancers. HGFs occur naturally in the body but they are also synthesized and used in medicine for a range of applications, including wound healing and immune system stimulation. HGFs are chemical messages that bind to receptor sites on cell surfaces (receptor sites are places where cells communicate with a substance to let them know what or what not to do). HGFs must communicate with cells to instruct them to activate the production of new cells, or to instruct a cell to create new cells that have different functions. Another way to think of HGFs is that they are messengers designed to be received or "heard" by specific receptor sites or "ears" on the cell. HGFs, such as transforming growth factor (TGF, stimulates collagen production) and epidermal growth factor (EGF, stimulates skin cell production) play significant roles in healing surgical wounds. The main task of HGFs is to cause cell division, which is helpful; however, at certain concentrations and lengths of application they can cause cells to over-proliferate, which can cause cancer or other health problems.

But what happens when you put HGFs on skin, particularly TGF and EGF, which some companies claim their products contain? The risk is that they could accelerate the growth of skin cancer by stimulating the overproduction of skin cells. In the case of TGF, which stimulates collagen production, it can encourage scarring. This is because scars are the result of excessive collagen production, and if you make too much collagen you get a scar or a knot on the skin such as a keloidal scar. Most of the research on the issue of HGFs for skin has looked primarily at the issue of wound healing, and at short-term use of HGFs. In skin-care products, they would be used repeatedly, possibly over long periods of time. A shortcoming of HGFs, according to an article by Dr. Donald R. Owen in the March 1999 issue of *Global Cosmetic Industry*, is that "The body produces these [HGFs] in exquisitely small concentrations at just the right location and time.... Actual growth factors such as [EGF and TGF-B] are [large] configurations, which do not penetrate the skin.... They [also] lose their activity within days in water or even as solids at normal temperatures.... [Yet], even after all these complications, the siren's song is too strong. We [the cosmetics chemists] will use them." The research into HGFs is without question intriguing, but there is much that's not known, especially in terms of long-term risk or stability when they're used in cosmetics and applied to skin. In this arena, if cosmetics companies continue to use HGFs, it is the consumer who will be the guinea pig.

humectant. *See* water-binding agent.

***Humulus lupulus* extract.** *See* hops.

hyaluronic acid. Component of skin tissue that is used in skin-care products as a good water-binding agent. *See* natural moisturizing factors.

***Hydnocarpus anthelmintica*.** *See* chaulmoogra oil.

***Hydrastis canadenis*.** *See* goldenseal.

hydrocortisone. Hormone from the adrenal gland that can also be created synthetically. It has potent anti-inflammatory properties for skin, but prolonged use can destroy collagen in the skin and cause skin fragility (Sources: American Academy of Dermatology *Guidelines of Care for the Use of Topical Glucocorticosteroids*, http://www.aadassociation.org/Guidelines/topicalglu.html; *Journal of the American Academy of Dermatology*, 1996, volume 35, pages 615–619; and *Cosmetic Dermatology*, July 2002, pages 59–62).

hydrocotyl extract. *See Centella asiatica*.

hydrogen peroxide. There is a great deal of current research showing that hydrogen peroxide is problematic as a topical disinfectant because it can greatly reduce the production of healthy new skin cells (Source: *Plastic and Reconstructive Surgery*, September 2001, pages 675–687). Hydrogen peroxide is also a significant oxidizing agent, meaning that it generates free-radical damage. While it can function as a disinfectant, the cumulative problems that can stem from impacting the skin with a substance that is known to generate free-radical damage, impair the skin's healing process, cause cellular destruction, and reduce optimal cell functioning are serious enough that it is better to avoid its use (Sources: *Carcinogenesis*, March 2002, pages 469–475; and *Anticancer Research*, July-August 2001, pages 2719–2724). *See* free-radical damage.

hydrogenated castor oil hydroxystearate. Used as an emollient and thickening agent. *See* glyceryl ester.

hydrogenated coco-glycerides. Used as an emollient and thickening agent. *See* glyceryl ester.

hydrogenated lecithin. *See* lecithin.

hydrogenated palm glyceride. Used as an emollient and thickening agent. *See* glyceryl ester.

hydrolyzed actin. Form of protein that has water-binding properties for skin. *See* water-binding agent.

hydrolyzed conchiolin protein. Component of oyster shell. It can have water-binding properties for skin. *See* protein.

hydrolyzed reticulin. Reticulins are a type of fibers found in skin and thought to be part of a systematic network that surrounds collagen fibers and helps hold them together. There is no evidence that applying reticulin externally to skin can have any effect on collagen whatsoever. Moreover, the hydrolyzing process needed to mix reticulin into a skin-care product also alters its form, which may change or stop anything it might do.

hydrolyzed silk. *See* silk.

hydroquinone. Substance that is known to successfully reduce the intensity of freckles, melasma, and general brown patching by inhibiting melanin production. For continued and increased effectiveness it must be used long term. Unprotected sun exposure should be avoided, because it reverses the effect of hydroquinone by increasing melanin production. Occasionally, at higher concentrations, persons with darker skin will experience increased pigmentation, but this is rare. It can cause mild skin irritation and there is the possibility of an allergic reaction. Hydroquinone in 1% to 2% concentrations is available in over-the-counter products; 4% and greater concentrations are available by prescription only (Source: *American Journal of Clinical Dermatology*, September-October 2000, pages 261–268).

There is concern that hydroquinone is a potentially carcinogenic substance. In vitro, hydroquinone has a toxic effect on cells containing melanin (Source: *Biochemical Pharmacology*, March 1999, pages 663–672). Aside from what was shown by in vitro studies (done in test tubes), the only other harmful effects are reported in animal studies where hydroquinone is fed to animals. In these studies, tumor creation or DNA damage was noted. However, this is not the case in epidemiological studies in which production workers (meaning those workers involved in the manufacture of hydroquinone) have been shown to have lower death rates and reduced cancer rates when compared with the population as a whole. Adverse effects associated with skin-lightening products that contain hydroquinone in FDA-regulated products have been limited to a small number of cases of hyperpigmentation (Sources: *Critical Reviews in Toxicology*, May 1999, pages 283–330; and *Food and Chemical Toxicology*, November 1999, pages 1105–1111).

hydroxylated lecithin. *See* lecithin.

hydroxypalmitoyl sphinganine. Sphinganine is a sphingoid base found concentrated in mammalian epidermis, and that may serve as a natural antifungal barrier preventing infection by pathogenic fungi. However, it may also inhibit ceramide production (Source: *Food Chemistry and Toxicology*, January 2002, pages 25–31).

hydroxyproline. Derived from the amino acid proline, it is a fundamental component of collagen and other structural proteins. The skin's ability to heal is partly determined by the presence of hydroxyproline within it. Whether topical application of hydroxyproline on the skin can help with wound healing has not been substantiated. However, it does have water-binding properties similar to those of collagen.

hypericum **extract.** *See* St. John's wort.

Hypnea musciformis **extract.** *See* algae.

hypoallergenic. Term used by the cosmetics industry to lead consumers to believe they are using a product that will not cause them to have an allergic or sensitizing skin reaction to a product. However, the word "hypoallergenic" is not regulated in any manner by the FDA and it is therefore used indiscriminately by cosmetics companies without any substantiation or requirement to show proof of the claim.

hyssop. Fragrant plant extract that may have some antibacterial properties (Source: *International Journal of Food Microbiology*, August 2001, pages 187–195). It may also be a skin irritant.

Ilex paraguariensis. *See* yerba mate extract.

Illicium vernum. *See* anise.

imidazolidinyl urea. Formaldehyde-releasing preservative (Source: *Contact Dermatitis*, December 2000, pages 339–343). *See* formaldehyde-releasing preservative.

Imperata cylindrica **root extract.** There is no research to support the claims that this extract has any benefit for skin (Source: U.S. Food and Drug Administration Center for Food Safety and Applied Nutrition, Office of Nutritional Products, Labeling, and Dietary Supplements September 10, 2001, http://vm.cfsan.fda.gov/~dms/ds-ingrd.html).

in vitro. Literally means "in glass." It refers to a biochemical process or reaction tested in a petri dish or test tube, rather than one taking place in a living cell, organism, animal, or person.

in vivo. Refers to a biological or chemical process or reaction taking place in a living cell, organism, animal, or person.

inactive ingredient. The inactive ingredients list is the part of an ingredient label that is not regulated by the FDA, although the FDA does require that all ingredients be listed. These are listed in descending order of concentration; that is, the ingredient with the highest concentration is listed first, then the next largest, and so forth. Thousands and thousands of inactive ingredients are used in cosmetics, and there is controversy as to how truly inactive some of these substances are in regard to safety as well as about their long-term or short-term effects on skin or the human body.

Indian gooseberry. Can have anti-inflammatory, antioxidant, and anti-mutagenic properties (Sources: *International Journal of Oncology*, July 2002, pages 187–192; and *Planta Medica*, 1997, volume 63, number 6, pages 518–524).

inositol. Major component of lecithin that may have water-binding properties for skin. It is not a vitamin, though it is sometimes mistakenly thought of as a B vitamin.

insulinlike growth factor (IGF). Stimulates fat cells and connective tissue cells. *See* human growth factor.

intercellular matrix. "Mortar" that holds layers of skin cells together, creating a firm natural barrier. Preserving the intercellular layer intact keeps bacteria out, moisture in, and the skin's surface smooth. *See* natural moisturizing factors.

interleukins (IL). Stimulate growth of white blood cells. *See* human growth factor.

International Units. Often abbreviated as IU; a system used to measure vitamin dosage. However, there is no fixed definition for IU, as there is for grams, milligrams, or ounces. The actual amount in a particular international unit depends on the specific substance being measured. For example, 1000 IU of vitamin A (retinol) has a different weight than 1000 IU of natural vitamin E, and natural vitamin E has a different weight than synthetic vitamin E. For example, 1 IU of vitamin A (retinol) weighs 0.3 micrograms or 0.0003 milligrams; 1 IU of vitamin C weighs 25 nanograms or 0.000025 milligrams; and 1 IU of natural vitamin E weighs 0.67 milligrams (Sources: National Institutes of Health, http://www.nih.gov; and Center for Food Safety and Applied Nutrition, http://vm.cfsan.fda.gov/).

Inula helenium. *See* elecampane.

inulin. Natural plant carbohydrate. It is used in foods due to its fatlike feel and texture yet low caloric content. Inulin yields about 1.5 calories per gram, compared to 4 calories per gram for carbohydrates like sugar and 9 calories per gram for fat. In cosmetics it is used as a thickening agent.

iodopropynyl butylcarbamate. Used as a preservative in cosmetics. *See* preservatives.

Iris florentina **extract.** *See* orris root.

Irish moss extract. Type of red algae. *See* algae.

iron oxides. Compounds of iron that are used for coloring in some cosmetics. They are used as a metal polish called jewelers' rouge, and are well-known in their crude form as rust.

Irvingia gabonensis **kernel extract.** Used medicinally in West Africa to relieve pain. It has been shown to have narcotic analgesic properties. There is no research showing the extract to be of benefit for skin (Source: *Journal of Ethnopharmacology*, February 1995, pages 125–129).

isocetyl salicylate. *See* sodium salicylate.

Isodonis japonicus **extract.** Fragrant plant extract that contains terpenes. It can be a skin irritant. *See* volatile oil.

Isodonis trichocarpus **extract.** Fragrant plant extract that contains terpenes. It can be a skin irritant. *See* volatile oil.

isoflavone. Plant estrogen with potent antioxidant properties (Source: *Free Radical Biology and Medicine*, December 2001, pages 1570–1581).

isohexadecane. Used as a detergent cleansing agent, emulsifier, and thickening agent.

isoleucine. *See* amino acid.

isoparaffin. *See* paraffin.

isopropyl alcohol. *See* alcohol.

isopropyl lanolate. Derived from lanolin, it is used as a thickening agent and emollient.

isopropyl myristate. Used in cosmetics as a thickening agent and emollient. Historically, animal testing has shown it to be a cause of clogged pores (Source: *Archives of Dermatology*, June 1986, pages 660–665). That type of testing was eventually considered unreliable and there is no subsequent research showing this ingredient to be any more of a problem for skin than other emollient, waxy ingredients used in cosmetics.

isopropyl palmitate. Used in cosmetics as a thickening agent and emollient. As is true for any emollient or thickening agent, it can potentially clog pores, depending on the amount used in the product.

isotretinoin. *See* Accutane.

IU. *See* International Units.

ivy extract. *See* English ivy.

Japan wax. Vegetable wax obtained from sumac berries. It is used as a thickening agent and emollient in cosmetics.

Japanese dandelion. There is a small amount of research showing it to have anti-tumor properties on mouse skin (Source: *Biological and Pharmaceutical Bulletin,* June 1999, pages 606–610). But it can also be a skin irritant. *See* dandelion.

jasmine oil. Fragrant oil, often used as a source of perfume, that can be a skin irritant or a skin sensitizer (Sources: *Natural Medicines Comprehensive Database,* http://www.naturaldatabase.com; *Contact Dermatitis,* June 2001, pages 344–346; and *Cutis,* January 2000, pages 39–41). It may have antifungal properties (Source: *Mycoses,* April 2002, pages 88–90).

Jasminium grandiflorum. See jasmine oil.

jewelweed. Has antifungal properties (Sources: *Natural Medicines Comprehensive Database,* http://www.naturaldatabase.com; and *Plant Physiology,* April 2002, pages 1346–1358). There is one animal study showing that, when taken orally, it can stop itching associated with dermatitis (Source: *Phytotherapy Research,* September 2001, pages 506–510), however, when applied topically there is no benefit when compared to a placebo in cases using jewelweed to reduce itching related to dermatitis or poison ivy (Source: *American Journal of Contact Dermatitis,* September 1997, pages 150–153).

jojoba oil. Emollient oil similar to other nonfragrant plant oils. *See* natural moisturizing factors.

jojoba wax. The semi-solid portion of jojoba oil. *See* natural moisturizing factors.

jonquil extract. Fragrant plant extract that poses a strong risk of skin irritation.

Ju hua. See chrysanthemum extract.

juniper berry. Can have anti-inflammatory properties for skin (Source: *Pharmacology and Toxicology,* February 1998, pages 108–112), though the methanol content, with repeated application, can cause skin irritation.

Juniperus communis. See juniper berry.

kaolin. Natural clay mineral (silicate of aluminum) that is used in cosmetics for its absorbent properties.

Kathon CG. Trade name of preservative that is a combination of methylchloroisothiazolinone and methylisothiazolinone. Introduced in the mid-1970s, it was found to be very irritating when left on skin, and elicited a great number of sensitizations in consumers. Subsequently it was withdrawn from use in cosmetics except for in rinse-off products (Sources: *Contact Dermatitis*, November 2001, pages 257–264 and *European Journal of Dermatology*, March 1999, pages 144–160). When included in a cosmetic product, it is usually listed as methylchloroisothiazolinone or methylisothiazolinone. *See* preservatives.

katrafay oil. Emollient plant oil that may have anti-inflammatory properties; however there is no research supporting this use.

kava-kava extract. Extract of the *Piper methysticum* plant that has analgesic (anti-inflammatory) properties, but can also cause skin irritation and dermatitis (Sources: *Alternative Medicine Review*, December 1998, pages 458–460; and *Clinical Experimental Pharmacology and Physiology*, July 1990, pages 495–507).

kawa extract. *See* kava-kava extract.

kelp extract. *See* algae.

kelpadelie extract. Common name for an extract from *Macrocystis pyrifera*. *See* algae.

Khaya senegalensis **extract.** May have some antimicrobial properties (Sources: *Phytochemistry*, November 20, 1998, pages 1769–1772; and *Phytomedicine*, July 1999, pages 187–195).

Khus khus **extract.** *See* vetiver oil or extract.

Kigelia africana **extract.** Extract of an African plant commonly known as the sausage tree. African lore about this extract is that it can firm breast tissue, but there is no supporting research for this myth or that indicates this plant has any other benefit for skin.

kinetin. The trade name for kinetin is N6-furfuryladenine. It is a plant hormone responsible for cell division. As a "natural" skin-care ingredient it is primarily being promoted as having been clinically proven to reduce the signs of aging, improve sun damage, reduce surfaced capillaries, and offer many other skin benefits of particular interest to aging baby boomers. There is a good deal of research on kinetin when it comes to plants or in test tubes (in vitro), with cells, or even on flies, but there is no published research on kinetin's topical effect, either on animal or human skin (Source: *Dermatologic Clinics*, October 2000, pages 609–615).

However, there are two unpublished clinical studies responsible for much of the attention kinetin is getting. Both were sponsored by Senetek, the company licensing the use of kinetin. On a closer look, according to MedFaq.com (an Internet source evaluating the legitimacy of medical research), the data are far less convincing than Senetek would want you to know. The two studies, paid for by Senetek, were both done by Dr. Jerry L. McCullough, professor of dermatology, University of California, Irvine. According to MedFaq, "The first study was well-designed—there was a control group and [it was done] double-blind…. After 24 weeks, a good response was noted in 30% of the subjects treated with kinetin … [but] there was no statistically significant difference between the people taking kinetin and the people just getting the placebo." Another study was then performed that did not use a placebo control group, but in which everyone was using a product that contained some amount of kinetin. Not surprisingly, in this protocol the results for skin were much better. "Essentially all of the subjects reported improvement after 24 weeks …" regardless of how much kinetin the product contained. As MedFaq states, "This outcome could also have a variety of causes unrelated to kinetin: It could reflect an improvement over time, a change across seasons, the subjects' enthusiasm, or it could have been caused by the cream or lotion the kinetin is in. In the first study, all of the subjects followed 'a standard skin care regimen consisting of a gentle-skin cleanser and daily use of sunscreen.' If that regimen was followed in the second experiment, it too might explain the improvement."

Despite the overly indulgent interpretation of these two studies by Senetek and by those companies that buy kinetin from Senetek, there is intriguing fruit-fly and in vitro research concerning kinetin in regard to its cellular antiaging affects (Sources: *Biochemical and Biophysical Research Communications,* June 1994, pages 665–672, and November 1999, pages 499–502). Almost all of this published research was conducted by Dr. Suresh I.S. Rattan, PhD, DSc. In my interview with Dr. Rattan, associate professor of biogerontology at the University of Aarhus, Denmark, he stated that "Topically no one knows how or if N6-furfuryladenine is being taken up or used by the cell … [but] We are curious about negative effects.… In cell cultures when a concentration of, say, 250 micromolars of N6-furfuryladenine was used, we got good results, but when we used 500 micromolars of N6-furfuryladenine, the cells started dying." In other studies Rattan conducted, flies that were fed kinetin sometimes lived, but they died if the dose was varied just slightly. The possibility that kinetin may cause cell death has been investigated in other research as well (Source: *Cell Growth and Differentiation,* January 2002, pages 19–26). That may not be good news. I suspect that when applied topically kinetin can't exert any effect on the life span of the cell, which *is* good news. Even if it could somehow be utilized, there probably isn't enough kinetin in any product to have a negative or positive impact, but that is only a guess, no one knows for sure.

One recent study showed kinetin to have no antioxidant properties (Source: *Bioorganic and Medicinal Chemistry,* May 2002, pages 1581–1586), though there is other research suggesting it does (Source: *Biochemical and Biophysical Research Communications,* October 2000, pages 1265–1270).

kiwi fruit extract. As a food, kiwi has significant antioxidant properties that may even be greater than those of vitamin C (Source: *Nutrition and Cancer,* 2001, volume 39, number 1, pages 148–153). Whether that benefit translates to its use on skin has not been demonstrated. The acid component of the kiwi can be a skin irritant.

Kniphofia uvaria **nectar.** Derived from the plant also known as red hot poker or torch lily. There is no research showing this to have any benefit for skin.

Ko ken. See kudzu root.

kojic acid. By-product of the fermentation process of malting rice for use in the manufacture of sake, the Japanese rice wine. There is definitely convincing research, both in vitro and in vivo, and also in animal studies, showing that kojic acid is effective for inhibiting melanin production (Sources: *Biological and Pharmaceutical Bulletin*, August 2002, pages 1045–1048; *Analytical Biochemistry*, June 2002, pages 260–268; *Cellular Signaling*, September 2002, pages 779–785; *American Journal of Clinical Dermatology*, September-October 2000, pages 261–268; and *Archives of Pharmacal Research*, August 2001, pages 307–311). Both glycolic acid and kojic acid, as well as glycolic acid with hydroquinone are highly effective in reducing the pigment in melasma patients (Source: *Dermatological Surgery*, May 1996, pages 443–447). So why aren't there more products available containing kojic acid? Kojic acid is an extremely unstable ingredient in cosmetic formulations. Upon exposure to air or sunlight it turns a strange shade of brown and loses its efficacy. Many cosmetics companies use kojic dipalmitate as an alternative because it is far more stable in formulations. However, there is no research showing that kojic dipalmitate is as effective as kojic acid, though it is a good antioxidant. There is a small amount of research showing kojic acid to be a skin irritant (Source: http://www.emedicine.com, "Skin Lightening/Depigmenting Agents," November 5, 2001).

kola nut. One of the major components of the kola nut is caffeine, which can be a skin irritant. However, kola nut also has a primary amine content that can form nitrosamines, which are potential carcinogens (Source: *Food and Chemical Toxicology*, August 1995, pages 625–630). *See also* caffeine.

konjac powder. Dietary fiber that is highly absorbent, but no more so than other food substances (cornstarch for example) or nonfood substances (like talc, magnesium, or other minerals). If you have problems with breakouts, any oil-absorbing substance can be helpful for skin; however, adding absorbents in the form of food ingredients can increase the bacteria content in skin.

Krameria triandra **extract.** Derived from the plant commonly known as rhatany, it has a high tannin content and skin-constricting properties, making it a potential skin irritant. However, it also has antioxidant properties (Source: *Planta Medica*, March 2002, pages 193–197).

kudzu root. Source of isoflavone, genistein, and daidzein, all plant estrogens (Sources: *Phytochemistry*, June 2002, pages 205–211; and *Journal of Alternative Complementary Medicine*, Spring 1997, pages 7–12). It can be a potent antioxidant.

kukui nut oil. Non-volatile oil from a plant native to Hawaii; it has emollient properties for skin (Source: *Journal of the Society of Cosmetic Chemists*, September-October 1993).

L-ascorbic acid. Common form of vitamin C. It is considered a potent antioxidant and anti-inflammatory (Sources: *Bioelectrochemistry and Bioenergetics*, May 1999, pages 453–461; and *International Journal of Radiation Biology*, June 1999, pages 747–755), but claims that it can eliminate or prevent wrinkles when applied topically are not substantiated in any published studies. In addition, it is stable only in a formulation with a low pH, and that is potentially irritating for skin (Source: *Dermatologic Surgery,* February 2001, pages 137–142).

L-carnitine. Carboxylic acid that may be erroneously labeled an amino acid (which it is not). It has been claimed to have miraculous properties (unsubstantiated) for enhancing the metabolization of fat when taken orally. There is also research in animal studies showing it to have antiaging benefits when taken orally (*Annals of the New York Academy of Sciences,* April 2002, pages 133–166). However, there is no known benefit for skin when it is applied topically, though it may have antioxidant properties. *See* antioxidant.

L-cysteine. *See* antioxidant.

***Labdanum* oil.** Also known as rockrose oil. It is used as a fragrance and film-forming agent in cosmetics. This highly fragrant resin hardens to create a solid film. It may have antibacterial and antifungal properties (Source: *Natural Medicines Comprehensive Database,* http://www.naturaldatabase.com).

lactic acid. Alpha hydroxy acid extracted from milk, though most forms used in cosmetics are synthetic. It exfoliates cells on the surface of skin by breaking down the material that holds skin cells together. It may irritate mucous membranes and cause irritation. *See* AHA.

Lactobacillus bifidus. *See* bifidus extract.

lactobionate. Polysaccharide that has water-binding properties for skin.

lactobionic acid. *See* polyhydroxy acid.

lactoferrin. Protein usually derived from milk (particularly breast milk); also found in saliva. It can have antiviral, antibacterial, and anti-inflammatory effects on skin (Sources: *Biochemistry and Cell Biology,* 2002, volume 80, number 1, pages 103–107; and *British Journal of Dermatology,* April 2001, pages 715–725).

lactoperoxidase. Enzyme derived from milk; it has antibacterial properties for skin.

lady's mantle extract. *See Alchemilla vulgaris.*

lady's thistle extract. There is a great deal of research showing extracts of lady's thistle to have many medical health applications when taken orally. There is no research showing it to be beneficial for skin, though it may cause allergic reactions (Source: *Natural Medicines Comprehensive Database,* http://www.naturaldatabase.com).

Laminaria digitata. *See* algae.

Laminaria japonica. *See* algae.

Laminaria longicruris. *See* algae.

Laminaria saccharine. *See* algae.

Lamium album. Sometimes called dead nettle. *See* white nettle.

lanolin. Derived from the sebaceous glands of sheep. Lanolin has long been burdened with the reputation of being an allergen or sensitizing agent. That has always been a disappointment to formulators because lanolin is such an effective moisturizing agent for skin. A recent study in the *British Journal of Dermatology* (July 2001, pages 28–31) may change all that. The study concluded "that lanolin sensitization has remained at a relatively low and constant rate even in a high-risk population (i.e., patients with recent or active eczema)." Based on a review of 24,449 patients who were tested with varying forms of lanolin, it turned out that "The mean annual rate of sensitivity to this allergen was 1.7%" and it was lower than that for a 50% concentration of lanolin. It looks like it's time to restore lanolin's good reputation. That's a very good thing for someone with dry skin, though it can be a problem for someone with oily skin, because lanolin closely resembles the oil from human oil glands. However, in Europe, due to Mad Cow Disease, animal-derived ingredients are banned from cosmetics and lanolin is no longer used.

lanolin alcohol. Emollient derived from lanolin. *See* lanolin.

lappa extract. *See* burdock root.

Larrea divaricata **extract.** *See* chaparral extract.

Larrea tridentata. *See* chaparral extract.

lauramphocarboxyglycinate. Mild detergent cleansing agent. *See* surfactant.

laureths. Substances that in various combinations create a wide range of mild detergent cleansing agents called surfactants. *See* surfactant.

Laurus nobilis. *See* bay leaf oil.

lauryl alcohol. *See* surfactant.

Lavandula angustifolia. *See* lavender extract and oil.

Lavandula officinalis. *See* lavender extract and oil.

lavender extract and oil. Primarily a fragrance, though it may have antibacterial properties. There is no research showing it to have any benefit for skin (Sources: *Phytotherapy Research,* June 2002, pages 301–308; and *Healthnotes Review of Complementary and Integrative Medicine,* http://www.healthwell.com/healthnotes/Herb/). It can be a skin irritant (Source: *Contact Dermatitis,* August 1999, page 111) and a photosensitizer (Source: Family Practice Notebook, http://www.fpnotebook.com/DER188.htm).

lecithin. Phospholipid found in egg yolks and the membranes of plant and animal cells. It is widely used in cosmetics as an emollient and water-binding agent. *See also* natural moisturizing factors.

lemon balm. *See* balm mint.

lemon oil. Can be a skin irritant, especially on abraded skin.

lemon. Potent skin sensitizer and irritant. Though it can have antibacterial properties, the irritation can hurt the skin's immune response.

lemongrass extract. Can have antibacterial properties (Source: *Journal of Applied Microbiology,* 2000, volume 88, pages 308–316), but it may also be a skin irritant.

lemongrass oil. Can be effective as a mosquito repellant (Source: *Phytomedicine,* April 2002, pages 259–262).

lempuyang extract. Form of ginger. There is no research showing it to be effective or to have benefit for skin.

***Lentinus edodes* extract.** Extract from the shiitake mushroom that may have antimicrobial and antibacterial properties, although it could be a potential skin irritant (Source: *International Journal of Antimicrobial Agents,* February 1999, pages 151–157). There is research showing it also has antitumor activity when taken orally (Source: *Mutation Research,* September 2001, pages 23–32).

***Leptospermum scoparium* oil.** *See* manuka oil.

lettuce extract. Has weak antioxidant and anti-inflammatory properties (Source: *Free Radical Research,* February 2002, pages 217–233).

leucine. Amino acid. *See* amino acid, and natural moisturizing factors.

leukocytes. White blood cells. These defend the body against infecting organisms and foreign agents, both in skin and other tissue and via the bloodstream. An abnormal increase in the production of leukocytes is known as leukemia. Conversely, a sharp decrease in the number of leukocytes (leukopenia) prevents the body from fighting infection. There is no research showing that topical application of leukocytes is helpful for skin in any way.

***Levisticum officinale* root extract.** *See* lovage root extract.

licorice extract. Has anti-inflammatory properties (Source: *Healthnotes Review of Complementary and Integrative Medicine,* http://www.healthwell.com/healthnotes/Herb/). *See* glycyrrhetic acid.

licorice root. *See* licorice extract.

lignoceryl erucate. Form of erucic acid. *See* erucic acid, and fatty acid.

***Lilium candidum* bulb extract.** Derived from the white lily bulb. There is no research showing this to have benefit for skin.

lime oil or extract. Can be a skin irritant and a photosensitizer (Source: *Natural Medicines Comprehensive Database,* http://www.naturaldatabase.com).

Limnanthes alba. *See* meadowfoam.

linalool. Fragrant component of lavender that can be a potent skin irritant, allergen, or sensitizer (Source: *Contact Dermatitis,* May 2002, pages 267–272).

linden extract. The major active constituents in linden are flavonoids and glycosides. Flavonoids are potent antioxidants; glycosides are monosaccharides and have water-binding properties (Source: *Healthnotes Review of Complementary and Integrative Medicine,* http://www.healthwell.com/healthnotes/Herb/).

linoleic acid. Unsaturated fatty acid used as an emollient and thickening agent in cosmetics. There is some research showing it to be effective in cell regulation and skin-barrier repair, as well as an antioxidant and anti-inflammatory (Sources: *Archives of Dermatological Research,* July 1998, pages 375–381; *Clinical and Experimental Dermatology,* March 1998, pages 56–58; *Journal of Investigative Dermatology,* May 1996, pages 1096–1101; and *Seminars in Dermatology,* June 1992, pages 169–175). *See* fatty acid, and natural moisturizing factors.

linseed oil. Linoleic acid is a component of linseed oil. *See* linoleic acid.

Linum usitatissimum **extract.** *See* linseed oil.

lipid. Wide range of ingredients found in plants, animals, and human skin. Lipids include fatty acids, sebum, and fats. In skin-care products, these are emollients and thickening agents. *See* fatty acid, and natural moisturizing factors.

liposomes. Delivery system (not an ingredient) capable of holding other ingredients and releasing them after the liposome is absorbed into the skin. Liposomes are microscopic lipid (fat) sacs that are widely used to deliver other ingredients into skin (Source: *Journal of Pharmaceutical Sciences,* March 2002, pages 615–622).

Lithocarpus densiflorus **extract.** Evergreen bark. There is no research showing this to have any benefit for skin.

Lithotamnium calcarum **extract.** Extract of red algae. *See* algae.

Lithospermum officinale. Plant that can cause cell damage when applied topically (Source: American Herbal Products Association (AHPA), http://www.ahpa.org).

Lithospermum erythrorhizon **extract.** *See* shikonin.

Litsea cubeba. *See* lemongrass.

lysine. *See* amino acid.

locust bean. *See* gums.

Long xu cai. *See* algae.

longifolene. Component of plants that has some antifungal and antimicrobial properties (Sources: *Natural Toxins,* 1999, volume 7, number 6, pages 305–309; and *Bulletin of Environmental Contamination and Toxicology,* February 1997, pages 268–274).

Lonicera japonica. *See* honeysuckle.

loquat extract. Derived from a subtropical flower that has antioxidant and antitumor properties similar to those of green tea (Sources: *Journal of Agricultural Food Chemistry,* April 2002, pages 2400–2403; and *Phytochemistry,* February 2002, pages 315–323). *See also* green tea.

lotus seed extract. Can have anti-inflammatory and antioxidant properties (Sources: *Planta Medica,* August 1997, pages 367–369; and *Journal of Plant Physiology,* May 2001, pages 39–46).

lovage root extract. Orally it is used as a diuretic. In cosmetics, it is used as a fragrance. Theoretically, it can cause phototoxic reactions including photosensitivity dermatitis (Source: *Natural Medicines Comprehensive Database,* http://www.naturaldatabase.com).

Lu rong **extract.** *See* deer antler velvet.

Luffa cylindrica **seed oil or extract.** Components of this plant have antifungal properties (Source: *Peptides,* June 2002, pages 1019–1024) and antitumor properties, by preventing synthesis of certain proteins (Source: *Life Sciences,* January 2002, pages 899–906). It can also have anti-inflammatory properties (Source: *Natural Medicines Comprehensive Database,* http://www.naturaldatabase.com). It may also be toxic to skin cancer cells (Source: *Melanoma Research*, October 1998, pages 465–467). When the fruit of the luffa plant is dried it is used as an abrasive sponge.

lupine. Legume that is a source of isoflavones, a form of plant estrogen that has antioxidant properties (Sources: *Phytochemistry,* January 2001, pages 77–85; and *Bioscience, Biotechnology, and Biochemistry,* June 2000, pages 1118–1125). *See* isoflavone, and plant estrogen.

lupine oil. Extract of *Lupinus albus,* a legume; it has emollient and antioxidant properties, though it may also have significant allergen or skin-sensitizing potential. *See* lupine.

Lupinus albus **extract.** *See* lupine, and lupine oil.

Lupinus luteus **seed extract.** There is no research showing this plant extract to have any benefit for skin (Source: *Natural Medicines Comprehensive Database,* http://www.naturaldatabase.com).

lutein. Carotenoid that has antioxidant properties (Source: *Photochemistry and Photobiology,* May 2002, pages 503–596).

lycopene. Carotenoid that has antioxidant properties (Source: *Photochemistry and Photobiology,* May 2002, pages 503–596).

lye. *See* sodium hydroxide and/or potassium hydroxide.

lysine. Amino acid. *See* amino acid.

Ma huang. *See Ephedra sinica* extract.

macadamia nut oil. Used in cosmetics as an emollient for dry skin.

Macrocystis pyrifera. See algae.

Mad Cow Disease. Mad Cow Disease (technically known as **b**ovine **s**pongiform **e**ncephalopathy, or BSE) is a chronic degenerative disease affecting the central nervous system of cattle. The concern for humans is the risk of eating meat or meat products that contain the BSE pathogen. Whether bovine-derived ingredients used in cosmetics can harbor the disease and cause health risks is unknown, but theoretically a remote possible risk does exist. Some researchers believe that there is no evidence BSE can be contracted through the skin (Source: *Cosmetic Dermatology,* December 2001, pages 43–47); however, neither cooking, preserving, nor any of the other processing that most cosmetics go through can eliminate BSE pathogens. That means if animal by-products are used in cosmetics (in particular placenta and spleen bovine extracts), they can pose a risk, albeit remote, to the user. The British BSE Committee (http://www.bse.org.uk), in varying reports, has mentioned a concern that people could become infected if the creams were used on broken skin. It is important to realize that very few products use these kinds of ingredients. If you are thinking of buying cosmetics that contain animal organ extracts of any kind, you may want to reconsider, or discard them if you have already made a purchase.

Madagascar periwinkle. Plant that has anti-tumor properties (Sources: *Oncologist,* 2000, volume 5, number 3, pages 185–198; and *Journal of Agricultural Food Chemistry,* November 2001, pages 5165–5170). However, Madagascar periwinkle is considered toxic and has limited use for cancer treatment (Sources: *Natural Medicines Comprehensive Database,* http://www.naturaldatabase.com; and *FDA Poisonous Plant Database,* http://www.fda.gov).

magnesium. Element commonly found in earth minerals that has strong absorbent properties and some disinfecting properties.

magnesium aluminum silicate. Powdery, dry-feeling, white solid that can be used as a thickening agent and powder in cosmetics.

magnesium ascorbyl palmitate. Stable derivative of vitamin C that can be an effective antioxidant. *See* vitamin C.

magnesium ascorbyl phosphate. Form of vitamin C that is considered stable and an effective antioxidant for skin (Sources: *Photochemistry and Photobiology,* June 1998, pages 669–675; and *Journal of Pharmaceutical and Biomedical Analysis,* March 1997, pages 795–801). For skin lightening, there is only a single study showing it to be effective for inhibiting melanin production (Source: *Journal of the American Academy of Dermatology,* January 1996, pages 29–33). The study concluded that a moisturizer with a 10% concentration of magnesium ascorbyl phosphate "suppressed melanin formation…. The lightening effect was significant in 19 of 34 patients with chloasma or senile freckles and in 3 of 25 patients with normal skin." One study is not exactly anything to write home about, not to mention that at present there are no products on the market that contain 10% magnesium ascorbyl phosphate.

magnesium gluconate. Magnesium is an essential mineral the body uses to maintain circulatory and nervous system function. There is a small amount of research showing that it has antibacterial properties (Sources: *Bulletin of Experimental Biology and Medicine,* February 2001, pages 132–135; and *Journal of Pharmacy and Pharmacology,* May 1998, pages 445–452). There is also research showing it may be helpful for healing burns.

magnesium hydroxide. Active ingredient in milk of magnesia. It is an absorbent and has antibacterial properties for skin.

magnesium laureth sulfate. Mild detergent cleansing agent. *See* surfactant.

magnesium oleth sulfate. Mild detergent cleansing agent. *See* surfactant.

magnesium stearate. Used as a thickening agent in cosmetics.

mahanimba. *See* neem extract.

malic acid. *See* AHA.

malkagni. *See Celastrus paniculatus.*

mallow. Can be used as a thickening agent in cosmetics and may have anti-inflammatory and soothing properties for skin due to its content of mucilage, flavonoids, and anthocyanidins (Source: *Healthnotes Review of Complementary and Integrative Medicine,* http://www.healthwell.com/healthnotes/Herb/Mallow.cfm).

Malvaceae extract. From a plant family, Malvaceae, that includes over 1,000 species, found in tropical and temperate regions the world over. Their varying benefits and problems are diverse. Consequently, if this name alone appears on a cosmetic ingredient label it is misleading, given that each of the 1,000 species has its own pros and cons.

mandarin orange oil or extract. Primarily used as a fragrance; it can be a skin irritant. There is no research showing it to have benefit when applied topically.

manganese gluconate. Mineral found in trace amounts in tissues of the body. While manganese plays a vital role in the processes of many body systems, there is no evidence it serves any purpose topically on skin, though it may be an antioxidant.

Mangifera indica **root.** Derived from the mango tree; it can have antioxidant properties (Source: *Journal of Agricultural Food Chemistry,* February 2002, pages 762–766).

mannan. Any of a group of polysaccharides that have good water-binding, antioxidant, and anticancer properties (Source: *Mutation Research/Genetic Toxicology and Environmental Mutagenesis,* October 2001, pages 213–222). *See* mucopolysaccharide, and natural moisturizing factors.

mannitol. Component of plants that has potent antioxidant properties (Source: *Photochemistry and Photobiology,* August 1999, pages 191–198).

manuka oil. Derived from the New Zealand tea tree; the oil is similar to that of the Australian tea tree, *Melaleuca alternifolia.* Manuka oil has antifungal and antibacterial properties (Sources: *Phytotherapy Research,* December 2000, pages 623–629; and *Pharmazie International Journal of Pharmaceutical Sciences,* June 1999, pages 460–463). *See also* tea tree oil.

mare milk palmitate. Protein derivative from female horses that can have water-binding properties for skin. *See* natural moisturizing factors.

marigold. *See* calendula extract.

marionberry. Fruit that has potent antioxidant properties (Source: *Journal of Agricultural Food Chemistry,* June 5, 2002, pages 3495–3500).

marjoram. Herb with a fragrant component used in cosmetics; can be a skin irritant.

marshmallow. *See* mallow.

Mastocarpus stellatus. *See* algae.

mate extract. *See* yerba mate extract.

Matricaria **oil.** *See* chamomile extract.

Matrixyl. *See* palmitoyl pentapeptide 3.

MEA. *See* alkyloamides and triethanolamine.

Meadowsweet extract. Can have anti-inflammatory properties (Source: *Journal of Agricultural Food Chemistry,* October 1999, pages 3954–3962).

Medicago sativa. *See* alfalfa extract.

Melaleuca alternifolia. *See* tea tree oil.

Melaleuca cajeputi **oil.** There is no research showing this oil, derived from the same plant family as tea tree oil, to have antibacterial properties. It may cause skin irritation (Source: *The Illustrated Encyclopedia of Essential Oils,* Rockport, MA, Element Books, 1995, page 170).

melamine. Derived from urea, it is used as a film-forming agent. *See* film-forming agent.

melanin. Pigment in cells that creates the color in skin and hair.

melasma. Melasma or chloasma are brownish discolorations of the face, hands, chest, and neck. Pregnancy is a common cause of melasma, as well as taking oral contraceptives. However, unprotected exposure to sunlight is also a major cause.

Melia azadirachta. *See* neem extract.

melibiose. Saccharide that can have good water-binding properties. *See* mucopolysaccharide, and natural moisturizing factors.

Melissa officinalis. *See* balm mint, and counter-irritant.

Mentha arvensis. *See* cornmint.

Mentha piperita. *See* counter-irritant, and peppermint.

Mentha spicata. *See* counter-irritant, and spearmint oil.

Mentha viridis. *See* counter-irritant, and spearmint oil.

menthol. Derived from peppermint; it can have the same irritating effect as peppermint on skin (Source: *Archives of Dermatologic Research,* May 1996, pages 245–248). *See* counter-irritant, and peppermint.

menthone. Major constituent of peppermint. *See* peppermint.

menthyl lactate. Used as a cooling agent and fragrance in cosmetics. It is a derivative of menthol thought it is supposed to be less irritating. *See* counter-irritant, and menthol.

methanol. *See* alcohol.

methionine. *See* amino acid, and antioxidant.

methoxypropylgluconamide. Alpha hydroxy acid that may be less irritating than glycolic acid and lactic acid. However, there is almost no research about this ingredient and very little is known about its benefit or function (Source: *Dermatologic Surgery,* May 1996, pages 469–473). It most likely functions more as a water-binding agent than anything else. This ingredient was originally patented by Revlon and the study cited above was carried out by Revlon.

methylchloroisothiazolinone. *See* Kathon CG.

methyldibromo glutaronitrile. Formaldehyde-releasing preservative (Source: *Contact Dermatitis,* December 2000, pages 339–343). *See* formaldehyde-releasing preservative.

methyldihydrojasmonate. Synthetic fragrant components.

methyleugenol. Natural constituent of such plant oils as rose, basil, blackberry, cinnamon, and anise. According to the November 9, 1998, issue of *The Rose Sheet* (an insider cosmetics industry newsletter), the National Toxicology Program Board of Scientific Counselors concluded that "methyleugenol, a component of a number of essential oils, has shown clear evidence of carcinogenic activity in male and female rats and mice." The study is an animal model and so the results may or may not be applicable to humans.

methylisothiazolinone. *See* Kathon CG.

methylparaben. *See* parabens, and preservatives.

methylrosaniline chloride. *See* gentian violet.

methylsilanol mannuronate. *See* silicone.

methylsilanol PEG-7 glyceryl cocoate. Used as an emollient and thickening agent in cosmetics. *See* glyceryl ester, and silicone.

methylsulfonylmethane (MSM). There is no published research to back up claims made regarding any benefit this sulfur compound may have for arthritis or other physical ailments; nor is there research about its effect when applied topically. Sulfur is stored in every cell of the body, particularly in the hair, nails, and connective tissue of joints and skin, where it is an important structural protein component. An MSM manufacturer has sponsored two very small trials, but the results have not been published. Until additional research is published, MSM enthusiasm should be tempered. MSM is available in capsules and powder for oral intake or in creams for topical use. So far, there have been no reports of toxicity (Sources: *Harvard Health Letter,* August 2000, http://www.health.harvard.edu; *Healthnotes Review of Complementary and Integrative Medicine,* http://www.healthwell.com/healthnotes/herb; and http://www.drweil.com).

methylsufonylsulfate. *See* antioxidant.

mica. Earth mineral used to give products sparkle and shine.

micrococcus lysate. Enzyme derived from bacteria. It can break down foods and is present in the human body. It has no known benefit in skin care.

Microcystis aeruginosa. Latin name for spirulina. *See* algae.

milk protein. *See* protein.

milk vetch root. There is a good deal of research showing that the root of this plant has antioxidant properties (Source: *Natural Medicines Comprehensive Database,* http://www.naturaldatabase.com), but there is little evidence it has that function when applied topically.

mimosa oil or extract. Used as a fragrance in cosmetics.

Mimosa tenuiflora **extract.** Called Tepescohuite in Mexico, where it is used traditionally to treat wounds and burns. (Source: *Revista de Biologia Tropical,* December 2000, pages 939–954; and *Journal of Ethnopharmacology,* March 1993, pages 153–157). But there is conflicting evidence whether or not this extract is really effective and potentially toxic to skin (Source: *Revista de Investigacion Clinica,* July-September 1991, pages 205–210).

mineral oil. Clear, odorless oil derived from petroleum that is widely used in cosmetics because it rarely causes allergic reactions and can't become a solid and clog pores. Despite mineral oil's association with petroleum and the hype that it is bad for skin, keep in mind that petroleum is a natural ingredient derived from the earth and that once it becomes mineral oil, it has no resemblance to the original petroleum. Cosmetics-grade mineral oil and petrolatum are considered the safest, most nonirritating, and effective moisturizing ingredients ever found (Sources: *Cosmetics & Toiletries,* February 1998, pages 33–40, and January 2001, page 79; and *Cosmetic Dermatology,* September 2000, pages 44–46). Yes, they can keep air off the skin to some extent, but that's what a good antioxidant is supposed to do; they don't suffocate skin! Moreover, mineral oil and petrolatum are known to be efficacious in wound healing (Source: *Cosmetics & Toiletries,* February 1998, pages 33–40).

mink oil. Considered similar to human sebum and, therefore, an effective emollient. The miraculous claims made for this ingredient are not proven, and in moisturizers it is neither preferable to, nor more effective than, plant oils.

mint. Can be a skin irritant and cause contact dermatitis. *See* counter-irritant.

Mitracarpe scaber **extract.** Extract from a plant native to West Africa; it has been shown to have some antimicrobial properties (Source: *Letters in Applied Microbiology,* February 2000, pages 105–108).

mixed fruit extracts. *See* sugarcane extract.

montmorillonite. *See* bentonite.

Moor extract. Trade name for silt extract, a type of mud or clay that has absorbent properties. There is no research showing it to have special benefit for skin.

Moringa pterygosperma **extract.** Extract from the horseradish tree. It can have antioxidant and anti-inflammatory properties when taken orally (Source: *Nigerian Journal of Natural Products and Medicine,* November 2001, volume 5, http://www.inasp.org.uk/ajol/journals/njnpm/vol5abs.html), but there is no research showing it has those benefits when applied topically.

Morus bombycis **root extract.** *See* mulberry extract.

Morus nigra **root extract.** *See* black mulberry.

Mourera fluvitalis extract. There is no research showing this to have any benefit for skin.

mucopolysaccharide. Also known as glycosaminoglycans, this is a large class of ingredients that includes hyaluronic acid, which is found universally in skin tissue. These substances, in association with protein, bind water and other cellular elements so they remain intact, forming a matrix that holds skin cells together. *See* natural moisturizing factors.

mugwort extract. There is no research showing this extract to be beneficial for skin (Sources: *Natural Medicines Comprehensive Database,* http://www.naturaldatabase.com; and http://www.pubmed.com).

mulberry extract. Due to its arbutin content, this extract can have some value in preventing melanin production. Although there is limited research showing this to be the case, the research has been done only in vitro (Sources: *eMedicine Journal,* November 5, 2001, volume 2, number 11, http://www.emedicine.com; and *Biophysical Research Communications,* volume 243, number 3, pages 801–803). *See* arbutin.

Musa paradisica. *See* banana extract.

Myobloc. Aalternative to Botox. Myobloc is the botulinum toxin type B. *See* Botox.

myristates. Generally these are forms of fatty acids used in cosmetics as thickening agents and emollients. As is true for any emollient, they can potentially clog pores, depending on the amount used in the product. *See* fatty acid.

myristic acid. Detergent cleansing agent that also creates foam and can be drying. *See* surfactant.

myristyl myristate. Used in cosmetics as a thickening agent and emollient.

myrrh. Fragrant gum resin that can be a skin irritant. There is little research showing it to have any benefit for skin (Source: *Healthnotes Review of Complementary and Integrative Medicine,* http://www.healthwell.com/healthnotes/), though there is a small amount of research showing it may have antifungal and antibacterial properties (Source: *Planta Medica,* May 2000, pages 356–358).

myrtle extract. Contains volatile oil and tannins. It can have fungicidal, disinfectant, and antibacterial properties. It contains 1,8-cineole, a constituent responsible for toxicity. It is recommended that this extract should not come in contact with skin (Sources: *Journal of Natural Products,* March 2002, pages 334–338; and *Natural Medicines Comprehensive Database,* http://www.naturaldatabase.com).

***Myrtus communis* extract.** *See* myrtle extract.

***Mytilus edulis byssus* extract.** Extract of the blue mussel. There is no research showing it to have benefit for skin.

N6-furfuryladenine. Technical name for kinetin. *See* kinetin.

N-acetyl-L tyrosine. *See* tyrosine.

NaPCA. *See* natural moisturizing factors, and sodium PCA.

***Narcissus poeticus* wax.** Fragrant flower extract that can cause irritation and dermatitis (Source: *Natural Medicines Comprehensive Database,* http://www.naturaldatabase.com).

Nardost achys jatamaus. *See* spikenard.

natto gum. Fermentation product of soy protein. It may be a potent antioxidant (Source: *Journal of Agricultural Food Chemistry,* June 2002, pages 3592–3596).

natural ingredients. The FDA has tried to establish official definitions and guidelines for the use of certain terms such as "natural" and "hypoallergenic," but its regulations were overturned in court. That means that cosmetics companies can use these terms on ingredient labels to mean anything they want, and the result is that almost always they mean nothing at all. The term "all-natural" has considerable market value in promoting cosmetic products to consumers, but a close look at an ingredient label reveals that the plant extracts make up only a small percentage of the product. Plus, when a plant is added to a cosmetic, preserved, and stabilized with other ingredients, it loses its natural qualities (Source: FDA *Consumer* magazine, May-June 1998, revised May 1998 and August 2000).

natural moisturizing factors. One of the primary elements in keeping skin healthy is making sure the structure of the epidermis (outer layer of skin) is intact. That structure is defined and created by skin cells that are held together by the intercellular matrix. The intercellular matrix is the "glue" within the skin that keeps skin cells together, helps prevent individual skin cells from losing water, and creates the smooth, non-flaky appearance of skin. The components that do this are called natural moisturizing factors (NMFs). Lipids are the oil and fat components of skin that prevent evaporation and provide lubrication to the surface of skin. It is actually the intercellular matrix along with the skin's lipid content that gives skin a good deal of its surface texture and feel. When the lipid and NMF content of skin is reduced, we experience surface roughness, flaking, fine lines, and a tight, uncomfortable feeling (Source: *Skin Research and Technology*, August 2000, pages 128–134); moreover, the skin's healing process is impaired. NMFs and lipids make up an expansive group of ingredients that include ceramide, hyaluronic acid, cholesterol, fatty acids, triglycerides, phospholipids, glycosphingolipids, amino acids, linoleic acid, glycosaminoglycans, glycerin, mucopolysaccharide, and sodium PCA (pyrrolidone carboxylic acid). Mimicking the lipid content of skin ingredients are apricot oil, canola oil, coconut oil, corn oil, jojoba oil, jojoba wax, lanolin, lecithin, olive oil, safflower oil, sesame oil, shea butter, soybean oil, squalane, and sweet almond oil, which can all be extremely helpful for skin.

All of the skin's supporting NMFs and lipids are present in the intercellular structure of the epidermis, both between skin cells and in the lipid content on the surface of skin. When any of these ingredients are used in skin-care products, they appear to help stabilize and maintain this complex intercellular-skin matrix. Although none of these very good NMFs and lipids can permanently affect or change skin, they are great at temporarily keeping depleted skin from feeling dry and uncomfortable. More important, all of these ingredients, and many more, can help support the intercellular area of the skin by keeping it intact. This support helps prevent surface irritation from penetrating deeper into the skin, works to keep bacteria out, and aids the skin's immune/healing system.

neem extract or oil. From leaves of the neem tree; it has potential toxic effects, although it has also been shown to have antimicrobial properties (Sources: *Life Sciences*, January 2001, pages 1153–1160; *Journal of Ethnopharmacology*, August 2000, pages 377–382; *Phytotherapy Research*, February 1999, pages 81–83; and *Mutation Research*, June 1998, pages 247–258).

Nelumbo nucifera. *See* lotus seed extract.

neopentanate. Used in cosmetics as a thickening agent and emollient.

neopentyl glycol dicaprylate/dicaprate. Used as an emollient and thickening agent.

neptune kelp extract. *See* algae.

neroli. *See* orange blossom.

neroli oil. Fragrant plant oil; it can be a skin irritant and sensitizer.

nettle extract. May have anti-inflammatory properties (Source: *Healthnotes Review of Complementary and Integrative Medicine*, http://www.healthwell.com/healthnotes/Herb/Nettle.cfm).

niacin. *See* niacinamide.

niacinamide. Also called vitamin B3, niacin, and nicotinic acid. There are a handful of studies demonstrating that a 4% concentration of niacinamide applied topically in gel form can have effects similar to those of clindamycin, a prescription-only topical antibiotic. However, most of the research was performed by the company that makes this product (Papulex, 4% Niacinamide), and it can cause dryness and inflammation. Some animal and in vitro studies on human fibroblasts (cells that produce connective tissue such as collagen) have demonstrated that niacinamide may have a mitigating effect on skin tumors (Source: *Nutrition and Cancer,* 1997, volume 29, number 2, pages 157–162). Topical application of niacinamide has been shown to increase ceramide and free fatty acid levels in skin and to prevent skin from losing water content (Source: *British Journal of Dermatology,* September 2000, pages 524–531).

niaouli oil. Extracted from a plant related to melaleuca. It has properties similar to those of tea tree oil, making it a possible topical disinfectant. It is a weak antibacterial agent (Source: *Pharmazie,* June 1999, pages 460–463), but it can also be a potent skin irritant (Source: *Natural Medicines Comprehensive Database,* http://www.naturaldatabase.com). *See also* tea tree oil.

nicotinamide. *See* niacinamide.

nicotinic acid. *See* niacinamide.

***Nigella sativa seed* extract.** May have anti-inflammatory and immune-enhancing properties (Source: *Journal of Ethnopharmacology,* June 2001, pages 45–48). It can also be a skin sensitizer and there is little research showing it to have benefit for skin (Source: *Natural Medicines Comprehensive Database,* http://www.naturaldatabase.com).

nitrogen. Used as a propellant for products by the cosmetics industry; it can generate free-radical damage and cause cell death (Source: *Mechanisms of Ageing and Development,* April 2002, pages 1007–1019).

nitrosamines. Can be formed in cosmetics when amines (such as DEA, MEA, or TEA) are combined with a formaldehyde-releasing preservative (bronopol or quaternium-15, among others). Nitrosamines are known for their carcinogenic properties. There is controversy as to whether or not this poses a real problem for skin given the small concentrations that are used in cosmetics and the question of whether nitrosamines can even penetrate skin. *See* formaldehyde-releasing preservative.

nonacnegenic. Term used by the cosmetics industry to lead consumers to believe they are using a product that will not cause their skin to break out. However, "nonacnegenic" is not regulated in any manner by the FDA and, therefore, is used indiscriminately by cosmetics companies without any substantiation or proof of claim (Source: http://www.fda.gov).

noncomedogenic. Term meant to indicate that a product will not clog pores. This term is not regulated by the FDA or any other organization, so a cosmetics company can make this claim without proof or substantiation of any kind (Source: http://www.fda.gov).

nonoxynols. Used as mild surfactants. *See* surfactant.

nordihydroguaiaretic acid. Component of some plants that has been shown to have anticancer properties for skin and may also protect the skin from sun damage (Sources: *British Journal of Cancer,* April 2002, pages 1188–1196; *Molecular Carcinogenesis,* June 2002, pages 102–111; and *Biochemical Pharmacology,* March 2002, pages 1165–1176).

nylon-12. Powder substance that is used as an absorbent and thickening agent.

oak root extract. May have antibacterial properties on skin but can also be a skin irritant.

oatmeal. Can have anti-irritant and anti-inflammatory properties (Source: *Skin Pharmacology and Applied Skin Physiology,* March-April 2002, pages 120–124).

oatmeal soap. Soap containing oatmeal and supposed to be better at absorbing oil and soothing sensitive skin than other soaps or bar cleansers. There are studies demonstrating that oatmeal can have anti-irritant properties. How that translates into a bar cleanser is unknown, but the benefits are probably nonexistent given the brief amount of time the oatmeal is actually on the skin and the presence of other irritating ingredients. Plus, when rubbed over the skin the pieces of oat particles can be scratchy and irritate some skin types. *See* oatmeal.

octinoxate. *See* octyl methoxycinnamate.

octocrylene. Sunscreen agent that protects skin from the UVB range of sunlight (Sources: http://www.photodermatology.com/sunprotection.htm; and *Skin Therapy Letter,* 1997, volume 2, number 5, http://www.dermatology.org/skintherapy).

octyl methoxycinnamate. Sunscreen agent used to protect skin primarily from the sun's UVB rays (Sources: http://www.photodermatology.com/sunprotection.htm; and *Skin Therapy Letter,* 1997, volume 2, number 5, http://www.dermatology.org/skintherapy).

octyl palmitate. Used in cosmetics as a thickening agent and emollient.

octyl salicylate. Sunscreen agent used to protect skin primarily from the sun's UVB rays (Sources: http://www.photodermatology.com/sunprotection.htm; and *Skin Therapy Letter,* 1997, volume 2, number 5, volume 2, number 5, http://www.dermatology.org/skintherapy).

octyl stearate. Used in cosmetics as a thickening agent and emollient.

o-cymen-5-ol. Preservative used in cosmetics. *See* preservatives.

oleic acid. Mild surfactant. *See* surfactant.

oleic/linoleic triglyceride. Used as an emollient and thickening agent. *See* glyceryl ester.

oleths. Mild surfactants. *See* surfactant.

olibanum extract. *See* frankincense extract.

olive oil. Emollient plant oil similar to all nonfragrant plant oils. The concept of olive oil having antiaging properties stems from some evidence that diets high in olive oil may help prevent heart disease (Sources: *European Journal of Clinical Nutrition,* January 2002, pages 72–81; and *Lipids,* November 2001, pages 1195–1202, and Supplemental pages S49–S52). There are also a small number of animal tests showing that topically applied olive oil can protect against UVB damage (Sources: *Carcinogenesis,* November 2000, pages 2085–2090; *Journal of Dermatological Science,* March 2000, Supplemental pages S45–S50). It does seem that olive oil is a good antioxidant and assuredly it's a good moisturizing ingredient, but research shows similar results for other oils as well. *See* natural moisturizing factors.

olive oil PEG-6 esters. Used as an emollient and thickening agent. *See* glyceryl ester, and olive oil.

opium poppy seed. Potent analgesic (Source: *Phytotherapy Research,* September 2000, pages 401–418), though there is no research showing this to be effective when applied topically.

ornithine. Primary component of arginine (an amino acid) that shares many of the biopharmacologic effects of arginine, which include enhanced wound healing, particularly with regard to collagen synthesis, when taken orally (Sources: *Journal of Surgical Research,* June 2002, pages 35–42; *Nitric Oxide,* May 2002, pages 313–318; and *European Surgical Research,* January-April 2002, pages 53–60). Whether ornithine has that effect when applied topically is not known.

***Opuntia ficus-indica* extract.** Extract from the Indian fig or prickly pear cactus that has a small amount of research showing it to have wound-healing properties (Source: *Fitoterapia,* February 2001, pages 165–167) and anti-inflammatory properties (Source: *Archives of Pharmacal Research,* February 1998, pages 30–34).

orange blossom. Fragrant extract that can also be a skin irritant.

Orbignya martiana. *See* babassu oil.

Orbignya oleifera. *See* babassu oil.

orchid. Fragrant extract that can be a skin irritant.

oregano. Has potent antibacterial and antifungal properties, but can also be a skin irritant (Source: *Journal of Food Protection,* July 2001, pages 1019–1024).

Origanum majorana. *See* marjoram.

***Origanum vulgare* flower extract.** *See* oregano.

***Orobanche cernua* extract.** May have antibacterial properties (Source: *Journal of Basic Microbiology,* volume 39, number 5-6, pages 377–380).

***Orobanche rapum* extract.** May have antioxidant properties (Source: *Phytochemistry,* June 2000, pages 295–300).

orris root. Used primarily as a fragrant component due to its violet-like scent (Source: http://www.botanical.com/botanical/mgmh/i/irises08.html). It can cause allergic or sensitizing skin reactions and there is no research showing it to be beneficial for skin (Source: *Botanical Dermatology Database,* http://bodd.cf.ac.uk/BotDermFolder/BotDermC/CACT.html).

Ortho Tri-Cyclen. Low-dosage type of birth-control pills (generic norgestimate/ethinyl estradiol) approved for use in the United States for the treatment of acne. In Canada, Diane-35, a combination of cyproterone acetate and ethinyl estradiol, is approved for the treatment of acne (Source: *Skin Therapy Letter,* 1999, volume 4, number 4, http://www.dermatology.org/skintherapy). According to a double-blind, placebo-controlled study published in *Fertility and Sterility* (September 2001, pages 461–468), other "low-dose birth-control pills can be an effective and safe treatment for moderate acne." The double-blind, placebo-controlled, randomized clinical trial found that the birth-control pill containing levonorgestrel (Alesse) reduced the appearance of acne.

***Oryza sativa* oil.** *See* rice oil.

oryzanol. Component of plants and their products, such as rice bran, that has potent antioxidant properties.

osmanthus. Fragrant plant; used in perfumes, it can also be a skin irritant.

oxybenzone. Sunscreen agent that protects primarily from the sun's UVB rays, and some, but not all, UVA rays (Sources: http://www.photodermatology.com/sunprotection.htm; and *Skin Therapy Letter,* 1997, volume 2, number 5, http://www.dermatology.org/skintherapy). *See* UVA.

oxygen. Many cosmetic products contain *anti*oxidants, ingredients that reduce the negative effect of oxygen or oxidative substances on skin. At the same time, the cosmetics industry also sells products that contain hydrogen peroxide (H_2O_2) or other oxygen-releasing ingredients, which supposedly deliver an oxygen molecule when they come into contact with skin, although that generates free-radical damage (Source: *Human and Experimental Toxicology,* February 2002, pages 61–62). Why the concern about supplying oxygen to the skin? Oxygen depletion is one of the things that happens to older skin, regardless of whether it's been affected by sun damage or any other health-related factors. Why or how that happens is completely unknown, though it is thought to have something to do with blood flow and a reduction in lung capacity as we age. It is also believed that, with age, the issue isn't so much the amount of oxygen but rather a change in the blood's ability to use the oxygen it has.

However, when wound healing is a problem, regenerating the tissue often demands, in addition to other factors, increased topical oxygen, because wound repair can be facilitated by oxygen therapy. Yet this method of wound care lacks research showing it to be effective or to be the best option for skin (Source: *Annals of the New York Academy of Sciences,* May 2002, pages 239–249).

Oxidative stress is an unavoidable consequence of life in an oxygen-rich atmosphere. The "Oxygen Paradox" is that oxygen is dangerous to the very life forms for which it has become an essential component of energy production. The first defense against oxygen toxicity is the sharp reduction in the amount of oxygen present in cells, from the level present in air of 20% to a tissue concentration of only 3% to 4% oxygen. These relatively low tissue levels of oxygen prevent most oxidative damage from ever occurring. Cells, tissues, organs, and organisms have multiple layers of anti-oxidant defenses, plus damage replacement and repair systems to cope with the stress and damage that oxygen engenders (Source: *Journal of the International Union of Biochemistry and Molecular Biology,* October-November 2000, pages 279–289). *See* free-radical damage.

oxygenated water. Claims regarding the benefit of enhanced oxygenated water are unsubstantiated, and have been debunked by medical, sports, and physiology experts. All water that has been exposed to the air is "oxygenated" to a small extent. This can be increased a small amount by pressurizing the water with oxygen gas, but it adds less oxygen than what is contained in a single breath. Further, once the oxygenated water is exposed to air the oxygen goes back into the atmosphere (Source: *Penn State Sports Medicine Newsletter,* http://www.psu.edu/ur/NEWS/news/april98sportsmed2.html).

ozokerite. Mineral that is used as a thickening agent in cosmetics, especially for lipsticks and stick foundations.

P. elisabethae. The "*P.*" is short for *Pseudopterogorgia. See* sea whip extract.

PABA. *See* para-aminobenzoic acid.

padimate O. Sunscreen agent that protects skin primarily from the sun's UVB rays (Sources: http://www.photodermatology.com/sunprotection.htm; and *Skin Therapy Letter,* 1997, volume 2, number 5, http://www.dermatology.org/skintherapy).

Padina pavonica **extract.** *See* algae.

Paeonia albiflora **extract.** *See* peony flower.

Paeonia suffruticosa **extract.** *See* peony root extract.

palm glyceride. Used as an emollient and thickening agent. *See* glyceryl ester, and palm oil.

palm oil. Has emollient and antioxidant properties for skin (Source: *Free Radical Biology and Medicine,* 1997, volume 22, number 5, pages 761–769). *See* antioxidant, and natural moisturizing factors.

Palmaria palmata **extract.** Extract from sea plant, common name is dulse. *See* algae.

palmarosa oil. *See* geranium.

palmitates. Generally these are forms of fatty acids used in cosmetics as thickening agents and emollients. As is true for any emollient, they can potentially clog pores, depending on the amount used in the product. *See* fatty acid.

palmitic acid. Detergent cleansing agent that also creates foam and can be drying. *See* surfactant.

palmitoyl pentapeptide 3. Trade name Matrixyl, it is a fatty acid mixed with amino acids. The only research showing this to have significance for skin was carried out by the ingredient manufacturer, Sederma. In their research, three different "half-face" studies with a total of about 45 participants showed it to be better than a retinol or vitamin C product (Source: *Journal of Cosmetic Science,* January-February 2001, pages 77–78). Without independent substantiation, however, there is no way to know how accurate this company-funded research is. Further, according to Sederma's research, the recommended concentration for this ingredient is 3% to 5% and there are few, if any, products using more than just a trace amount in their products. *See* amino acid, and fatty acid.

Panax schinseng. See ginseng.

pansy extract. There is a small amount of research showing it to have anti-inflammatory and antioxidant properties (Source: *Natural Medicines Comprehensive Database,* http://www.naturaldatabase.com).

pantethine. Also known as pantothenic acid. *See* pantothenic acid.

panthenol. Alcohol form of vitamin B. *See* pantothenic acid.

pantothenic acid. Also called vitamin B5, and often touted as being effective for acne. However, there is only one study supporting this notion and it dates from the early 1980s (Source: *International Journal of Dermatology*, 1981, volume 20, pages 278–285). There is no current research showing this to be an effective treatment for acne, but there is a small amount of research showing that it can be effective for hydration and wound healing (Source: *American Journal of Clinical Dermatology*, 2002, volume 3, number 6, pages 427–433).

papain. Enzyme extracted from papaya. Applied topically, papain can cause severe irritation, itching, and allergic reactions (Source: *Natural Medicines Comprehensive Database*, http://www.naturaldatabase.com). There is one study showing it to be effective for exfoliation, but only in pure concentration (Source: *Archives of Dermatological Research*, November 2001, pages 500–507). *See* enzymes.

Papaver somniferum **seed.** Latin name for the opium poppy seed. *See* opium poppy seed.

papaya extract. Source of papain that theoretically can have exfoliating properties on skin, though almost none of the research has been performed on skin. Papaya can be a skin irritant. *See* enzymes.

para-aminobenzoic acid (PABA). Sunscreen ingredient rarely used since the 1990s because of strong potential for allergic reactions.

parabens. Group of preservatives used in cosmetics to prevent bacterial and fungal growth in products. While these are considered to cause less irritation than some preservatives, there is research showing that in animal models (and in vitro) parabens can have weak estrogenic activity. Whether that poses any health risk is unknown (Source: *Journal of Steroid Biochemistry and Molecular Biology*, January 2002, pages 49–60). *See* preservatives.

paraffin. Waxy, petroleum-based substance. Used as a thickener for cosmetics.

Paraffinum liquidum. *See* mineral oil.

Parietaria officinalis **extract.** Extract from a plant also known as pellitory. It can have antibacterial properties for skin, but also has strong allergic and irritant potential when applied topically (Sources: *European Journal of Clinical Chemistry and Clinical Biochemistry*, July 1996, pages 579–584; and *Natural Medicines Comprehensive Database*, http://www.naturaldatabase.com).

parsley extract. Can have antioxidant properties (Sources: *Phytotherapy Research*, August 2000, pages 362–365; and *British Journal of Nutrition*, June 1999, pages 425–426), but whether it has that effect when applied topically is not known.

Parsol 1789. *See* avobenzone.

Passiflora edulis **extract.** *See* passion fruit extract.

passion fruit extract. There is no research showing this to have benefit for skin.

patchouli. Fragrant oil derived from mint. It contains eugenol and can be a skin sensitizer and irritant. *See* counter-irritant.

Paullinia cupana. *See* guarana.

pawpaw extract. *See* papaya.

Pea extract. May have antioxidant properties (Source: *Plant Physiology*, June 2002, pages 251-257 and May 1997, pages 275-284)

peanut oil. Emollient plant oil.

pecan oil. Emollient plant oil.

pectin. Natural substance found in plants, especially apples, and used in cosmetics as an emulsifier and thickening agent.

PEG compound. PEG stands for polyethylene glycol. Various forms of PEG compounds are mixed with fatty acids and fatty alcohols to create a variety of substances that have diverse functions in cosmetics, including surfactants, binding agents (to keep ingredients blended), stabilizers, and emollients. *See* polyethylene glycol.

PEG-80 sorbitan laurate. Mild surfactant. *See* surfactant.

***Pelargonium graveolens* oil.** *See* geranium oil.

pellitory. *See Parietaria officinalis* extract.

pentadecalactone. Synthetic fragrance used in cosmetics.

pentasodium penetate. Used as a chelating agent in cosmetics to prevent varying mineral components from binding together and negatively affecting the formulation.

peony root extract. There is research showing that the root of the peony plant can have anticancer properties as well as antioxidant properties (Sources: *Cancer Letters,* December 2001, pages 17–24; *Archives of Pharmaceutical Research,* April 2001, pages 105–108; and *Chemical and Pharmaceutical Bulletin,* January 2001, pages 69–72). However, there is no research showing it to have that benefit for skin (Source: *Natural Medicines Comprehensive Database,* http://www.naturaldatabase.com).

peppermint. Both the oil and the extract can have antimicrobial properties (Source: *Journal of Agricultural and Food Chemistry,* July 2002, pages 3943–3946), but they can also have an irritating, sensitizing effect on skin (Source: *Natural Medicines Comprehensive Database,* http://www.naturaldatabase.com). *See* counter-irritant.

peptide. Short chain of amino acids. This is in contrast to proteins, which are long chains of amino acids. In the body, peptides regulate the activity of other molecules, such as proteins, by interacting with the target molecule. Peptides have many functions, as some can have hormonal activity and others antibiotic activity. Whether peptides can have benefit when applied topically to skin for wound healing, skin barrier repair, or as disinfectants is difficult to ascertain, as they generally cannot penetrate skin and remain stable (Source: *Biotechniques,* July 2002, pages 190–192).

perfluoropolymethylisopropyl ether. Film-forming agent. *See* film-forming agent.

***Perilla ocymoides* oil.** Derived from the seeds of the *Perilla ocymoides* plant. Perilla contains multiple flavones and the oil is high in alpha-linolenic acid. It has antioxidant and anti-cancer properties; however it may also be a significant skin irritant (Source: *Natural Medicines Comprehensive Database,* http://www.naturaldatabase.com).

periwinkle extract. There is no research showing this extract to have benefit for skin. It is not to be confused with Madagascar periwinkle, *Catharanthus roseus*, that has anti-tumor properties (Sources: *Oncologist*, 2000, volume 5, number 3, pages 185–198; and *Journal of Agricultural Food Chemistry*, November 2001, pages 5165–5170). However, Madagascar periwinkle is considered toxic and has limited use for cancer treatment (Sources: *Natural Medicines Comprehensive Database*, http://www.naturaldatabase.com; and FDA Poisonous Plant Database, http://www.fda.gov).

Persea gratissima **oil.** *See* avocado oil.

petitgrain mandarin. *See* mandarin orange.

petrolatum. Vaseline is pure petrolatum. For some unknown and unsubstantiated reason, petrolatum has attained a negative image in regard to skin care, despite good research to the contrary. Topical application of petrolatum can help the skin's outer layer recover from damage, reduce inflammation, and generally heal the skin (Source: *Acta Dermato-Venereologica*, November-December 2000, pages 412–415). *See also* mineral oil.

Pfaffia paniculata **extract.** Also known as suma extract and Brazilian ginseng. There is a small amount of research showing it to have anti-inflammatory properties (Source: *Natural Medicines Comprehensive Database*, http://www.naturaldatabase.com).

PHA. *See* polyhydroxy acid.

Phellodendron amurense **extract.** Extract of the Amur corktree; it can have anti-inflammatory and antifungal benefits (Sources: *Journal of Antimicrobial Chemotherapy*, May 1999, pages 667–674; and *Fitoterapia*, March 2001, pages 221–229).

phenoxyethanol. Common cosmetic preservative that is considered one of the less irritating ones to use in formulations. It does not release formaldehyde. *See* preservatives.

phenyl trimethicone. Silicone with a drier finish than dimethicone. *See* silicone.

phenylalanine. *See* amino acid.

phosphatidylcholine (PC). Active ingredient found in lecithin. Every cell membrane in the body requires PC. It is also a major source of the neurotransmitter acetylcholine. Acetylcholine is used by the brain in areas that are involved in long-term planning, concentration, and focus. PC is considered a very good water-binding agent and aids in the penetration of other ingredients into the skin. It absorbs well without feeling greasy or heavy (though other ingredients can perform similarly, including glycerin, ceramides, and hyaluronic acid) (Sources: *Skin Pharmacology and Applied Skin Physiology*, September-October 1999, pages 235–246; and *Journal of Controlled Release*, March 29, 1999, pages 207–214.) *See* lecithin, and water-binding agent.

phosphatidylethanolamine. *See* cephalin.

phospholipid. Type of lipid (fat) composed of glycerol, fatty acids, and phosphate. Phospholipids are essential to the function of cell membranes because they provide a stable surrounding structure. Lecithin and cholesterol are phosopholipids. *See* glyceryl ester, and natural moisturizing factors.

phosphoric acid. Used as a pH adjuster in cosmetic and skin-care products.

photosensitizer. Ingredients that can cause the skin to have an irritated or inflamed reaction when exposed to sunlight.

Phyllanthus emblica **fruit extract.** Has antioxidant and anti-inflammatory properties (Sources: *Journal of Ethnopharmacology,* May 2000, pages 171–176; and *Planta Medica,* December 1997, pages 518–524).

phytic acid. A component of plants that has antioxidant properties.

phytoalexins. Antimicrobial substances that are produced by a plant in response to infection by fungi or bacteria and that help to defend the plant by inhibiting the growth of invading microbes. Phytoalexins can also be potent antioxidants, and the combination of those two properties is thought to have benefit for skin, particularly for wound healing (Sources: *Free Radical Research,* June 2002, pages 621–631; and *Biochemical Pharmacology,* January 2002, pages 99–104). How that relates to daily skin care or wrinkles is unknown, but it is probably a good antioxidant.

phytoestrogen. *See* plant estrogen.

phytol. Subcomponent of vitamin E and also a component of chlorophyll. It has antioxidant properties, but there is limited research about phytol having any effect on skin.

phytonadione. *See* vitamin K.

Phytoplenolin. Trade name for plant extract of *Centipeda cunninghami.* See *Centipeda cunninghami* extract.

phytosterol. Cholesterol-like molecules found in all plant foods, with the highest concentrations occurring in vegetable oils. Phytosterols in the natural diet may lower cholesterol (Sources: *Annual Reviews of Nutrition,* 2002, volume 22, pages 533–549; and *Metabolism,* May 2002, pages 652–656). However, regarding topical application, there is research showing that the high lipid content of phytosterols can make the skin extremely sensitive to light (Source: *Photochemistry and Photobiology,* September 1997, pages 316–325).

pilewort extract. *See Ranunculus ficaria* extract.

Pimpinella anisum. *See* anise.

pine cone extract. Components of this extract, specifically linolenic and linoleic acid, can have antioxidant properties (Source: *Tree Physiology,* June 2002, pages 661–666) and antibacterial properties for skin (Source: *International Journal of Food Microbiology,* May 2000, pages 3–12).

pine needle extract. *See* pine oil.

pine oil. Can have disinfectant properties (Source: *Antimicrobial Agents and Chemotherapy,* December 1997, pages 2770–2772), but it can also be a potent skin irritant and should never be used on abraded or chafed skin.

pineapple extract. Contains the enzyme bromelain, which can break down the connecting layers between skin cells to exfoliate skin. However, bromelain used alone is a more effective source of exfoliation, without the other irritating properties of the pineapple. *See* bromelain.

***Pinus lambertiana* wood extract.** Pine extract that may have skin-sensitizing properties (Source: *Botanical Dermatology Database,* http://bodd.cf.ac.uk/index.html).

***Pinus sylvestris* extract.** *See* pine cone extract.

Piper nigrum. *See* black pepper.

***Pistacia vera* seed oil.** *See* pistachio seed oil.

pistachio seed oil. Emollient plant oil.

***Pisum sativum* extract.** *See* pea extract.

placenta extract. Obtained from the afterbirth of animals, it is supposed to have rejuvenating properties for skin, but this claim has never been proven in research of any kind. Much like any part of a human or animal body, the placenta is a source of proteins and amino acids that have water-binding and antioxidant properties (Sources: *Placenta,* July 2002, pages 497–502; and *Bioscience, Biotechnology, and Biochemistry,* November 2000, pages 2478–2481). These are helpful for skin, but no more so than hundreds of other ingredients with similar or superior attributes. Due to the concern about Mad Cow Disease, ingredients of this nature are best avoided.

placental enzymes. Obtained from either human or animal placentas. *See* placenta extract, and placental protein.

placental lipid. Lipid obtained from either human or animal placentas. *See* placenta extract, and placental protein.

placental protein. Obtained from either human or animal placentas, and used in cosmetics with varying, though completely unsubstantiated, claims about miraculous effects on skin. Use of animal- and human-derived ingredients are prohibited under the provisions of the European Union Cosmetics Directive (www.colipa.com/publication_17.html). For animal-derived ingredients, this directive is based on concerns about transmission of bovine spongiform encephalopathy (Mad Cow Disease); for human-derived ingredients the concern is viral diseases such as human immuno-deficiency virus (HIV) (Source: *International Journal of Toxicology,* 2002, volume 21, Supplement 1, pages 81–91). There is no way to know from a cosmetic ingredient label what the source of the extract is. *See* placenta extract.

plant estrogen. Current understanding regarding oral supplements of plant estrogens is that they may work by interfering with the body's own estrogen, thus preventing it from being out of balance. Plant estrogens may fool the body into thinking it has the right amount of this hormone by filling the receptor areas on cells sensitive to human estrogen. If the body has too much estrogen, the plant estrogen may prevent the body from using it (thereby preventing estrogen-related cancers); if the body has too little estrogen (as during the stages of menopause), plant estrogen might make the body think it has more, thus reducing some of the more uncomfortable side effects. There is little information about how much estrogen-laden food a woman must consume (and for how long) to reduce or eliminate the effects of menopause. In other words, adding estrogen-rich foods or supplements to your diet won't necessarily prevent breast cancer, heart attack, osteoporosis, or hot flashes. There are also studies that have shown no improvement or benefit from dietary estrogens (Sources: *Journal of Clinical Endocrinology & Metabolism,* January 2002, pages 118–121; and *Toxicological Science,* February 2002, pages 228–238), although these were hardly sweeping or conclusive reviews.

Clearly, this is a health issue that needs to be examined more closely. But what about plant estrogens used in creams and applied topically? There is no research showing that plant estrogens can provide any benefit when applied topically to skin. But even if there were a benefit, how much would you need to rub on your skin to obtain it? Moreover, when it comes to cosmetics or skin-care products, there is no way to know how much of a plant estrogen extract is being used, or how active it remains in a manufactured product. More to the point, because the cosmetics and natural-supplement industries are not regulated, there is no way to really know what you are getting.

plasticizing agents. Ingredients that place a thin layer of plastic over the skin; typically these are used in facial masks so they can be peeled off the skin. *See* film-forming agent.

plum extract. Extract of *Prunus americana* that may have antioxidant activity when applied topically (Source: *Phytotherapy Research,* February 2002, pages 63–65).

Plumeria alba **flower extract.** Used as a fragrance in cosmetics.

Pogostemon cablin. *See* patchouli.

Polianthes tuberosa **extract.** Limited research has shown that the extract from this tuberous plant can have water-binding and antioxidant properties (Source: *Phytochemistry,* April 1996, pages 1517–1521).

poloxamers. *See* surfactant.

polycaprolactone. Biodegradable thermoplastic polymer derived from the chemical synthesis of crude oil. It may have application in supporting skin-tissue growth for the purposes of skin grafts (Source: *Tissue Engineering,* August 2001, pages 441–455).

polyethylene glycol. Also listed as PEG on ingredient labels, polyethylene glycol is an ingredient that self-proclaimed "natural" Web sites have attempted to make notorious and evil. They gain a great deal of attention by attributing horror stories to PEG, associating it with antifreeze (however, antifreeze is ethylene glycol, not polyethylene glycol), and there is no research indicating that PEG compounds pose any problem for skin. Quite the contrary: PEGs have no known skin toxicity and can be used on skin with great results (Sources: *Advanced Drug Delivery Reviews,* June 2002, pages 587–606; and *Cancer Research,* June 2002, pages 3138–3143). The only negative research for this ingredient indicates that large quantities given orally to rats can cause tumors, but that is unrelated to topical application.

Polyethylene, when it is not combined with glycol, is the most common form of plastic used in the world. It is flexible and has a smooth, waxy feel. When ground up, the small particles are used in scrubs as a gentle abrasive. When mixed with glycol, it becomes a viscous liquid. In the minuscule amounts used in cosmetics, it helps keep products stable and performs functions similar to glycerin. Because polyethylene glycol can penetrate skin, it is also a vehicle that helps deliver other ingredients deeper into the skin. It is even used internally in medical procedures to flush and clean the intestinal tract. *See* glycerin, and propylene glycol.

polyglucuronic acid. *See* film-forming agent.

polyglycerol monostearate. Used as an emollient and thickening agent in cosmetics. *See* glyceryl ester.

polyglycerol polyricinoleate. Used as an emollient and thickening agent in cosmetics. *See* glyceryl ester.

polyglyceryl-2 caprate. Used as an emollient and thickening agent in cosmetics. *See* glyceryl ester.

polyglyceryl methacrylate. *See* film-forming agent.

***Polygonum cuspidatum* root extract.** Extract of the Japanese knotweed plant. When ingested it may have weak estrogenic activity (Source: *Bioorganic and Medicinal Chemistry Letters,* July 2001, pages 1839–1842) and antitumor activity (Source: *Journal of Nutrition,* June 2001, pages 1844–1849). It also has antioxidant properties (Source: *Biological & Pharmaceutical Bulletin,* January 1995, pages 162–166).

polyhydroxy acid (PHA). Because alpha hydroxy acids (AHAs) may be irritating to skin, the search for an effective form of AHA or another ingredient that can enhance performance and reduce irritation is an active issue. Gluconolactone and lactobionic acid are types of PHA that are supposed to be as effective as AHAs but less irritating (Neostrata is the company that holds the patent on glycolic acid as an antiwrinkle agent, as well as a patent for gluconolactone for reducing the appearance of wrinkles). Gluconolactone and lactobionic acid are chemically and functionally similar to AHAs. The significant difference between them is that gluconolactone and lactobionic acid have larger molecular structures, which limits their ability to penetrate into the skin, resulting in a reduction of irritating side effects. This reduced absorption into the skin supposedly doesn't hamper their effectiveness.

Does that mean gluconolactone and lactobionic acid are better for your skin than AHAs in the form of glycolic acid or lactic acid? According to an Internet-published class lecture by Dr. Mark G. Rubin (Source: http://128.11.40.183/lasernews/rubin_lecture/21.html), a board-certified dermatologist and assistant clinical professor of dermatology at the University of California, San Diego, research on gluconolactone demonstrated only a "6% decrease in dermal penetration" in comparison to glycolic acid, which "isn't a dramatic improvement." Gluconolactone may be slightly less irritating for some skin types but this isn't quite the magic bullet for exfoliation that beauty magazines and some cosmetics companies have been extolling. There is no independent research information available about lactobionic acid.

polyquaterniums. Group of ingredients used primarily in hair-care products due to their antistatic and film-forming properties. They can have water-binding properties for skin due to the sheer "plastic" film layer they create on skin. *See* film-forming agent.

polysaccharide. Natural component of skin that can be a good water-binding agent and potentially have antioxidant properties. *See* mucopolysaccharide, and natural moisturizing factors.

polysorbates. Fatty acids that are used as emollients and thickening agents in cosmetics. *See* fatty acid.

polyvinyl alcohol. *See* plasticizing agents.

polyvinylpyrrolidone. Usually listed on ingredient labels as PVP or PVP copolymer, it is one of the primary ingredients used in hairstyling products to hold hair in place. When present in minuscule amounts in skin-care products, it places an imperceptible film over the skin that is considered to be water-binding and that helps give the appearance of firmer skin. It can be a skin sensitizer for some individuals. *See also* film-forming agent.

pomegranate extract. Contains ellagic acid, and is considered effective as an anticarcinogen and antioxidant when taken orally. There is no research showing what effect, if any, this extract can have on skin (Sources: *Journal of Agricultural Food Chemistry,* January 2002, pages 81–86, and 166–171; and *International Journal of Oncology,* May 2002, pages 983–986).

Pongamia glabra **seed oil.** Has antimicrobial properties (Source: *Archives of Andrology,* January-February 2002, pages 9–13).

Pongamia pinnata **extract.** Can have anti-inflammatory properties (Source: *Journal of Ethnopharmacology,* December 2001, pages 151–157).

poppy seeds. Can have analgesic properties when applied topically.

Poria cocos **extract.** Derived from a mushroom, this extract has antioxidant and anti-inflammatory properties (Sources: *Life Sciences,* January 2002, pages 1023–1033; and *Journal of Ethnopharmacology,* November 2000, pages 61–69). Also known as Hoelen and Fu ling.

Porphyra umbilicalis. Form of seaweed. *See* algae.

Porphyridium cruentum. Type of red algae. *See* algae.

Portulaca oleracea **extract.** May have anti-inflammatory or analgesic properties (Sources: *Journal of Ethnopharmacology,* July 2001, pages 171–176, and December 2000, pages 445–451).

potassium. Important dietary element that is present in such fruits as bananas and citrus. It is also common in earth minerals that have absorbent properties and some disinfecting properties, but can also be skin irritants.

potassium cetyl phosphate. Used as a detergent cleansing agent. *See* surfactant.

potassium hydroxide. Also known as lye, it's a highly alkaline ingredient used in small amounts in cosmetics to modulate the pH of a product. It is also used as a cleansing agent in some cleansers. At higher concentrations it is a significant skin irritant.

potassium myristate. Detergent cleansing agent that is a constituent of soap; it can be drying and sensitizing for some skin types. *See* surfactant.

potassium thiocyanate. Chemically, a salt that can be a potent skin irritant, though it can also have antibacterial properties for skin.

Potentilla erecta **root extract.** Can have anti-inflammatory properties, though there is minimal research showing this to be the case (Source: *Natural Medicines Comprehensive Database*, http://www.naturaldatabase.com).

Poterium officinale **root extract.** Derived from the garden burnet plant. *See Sanguisorba officinalis.*

pregnenolone acetate. Precursor to other hormones, it can affect levels of progesterone and estrogen in the body when taken orally. When applied to skin it may work as a water-binding agent. There is no information about whether this can be absorbed through skin.

preservatives. Substances used in cosmetics and other products to prevent bacterial and microbial contamination. While there is definitely a risk of irritation from using these types of ingredients in cosmetics, the risk to skin and eyes from using a contaminated product is considered by many scientists to be even greater. *See also* formaldehyde-releasing preservatives.

prickly pear extract. There is no research showing it to be effective for skin when applied topically, though it may have water-binding properties (Source: *Plant Foods for Human Nutrition*, 1998, volume 52, number 3, pages 263–270).

primrose. *See Primula veris* extract.

Primula veris **extract.** Derived from primrose or cowslip plants. It has no known benefit for skin, though it does contain flavones and may have antioxidant properties (Source: *Journal of Chromatography A*, February 2000, pages 453–462).

pristane. Technically tetramethylpentadecane or pentadecane. It is a component of mineral oil, shark oil, and plant oil. It is used as an emollient in cosmetics.

progesterone USP. A study published in the *American Journal of Obstetrics and Gynecology* (June 1999, pages 1504–1511) states that "In order to obtain the proper (effective) serum levels with use of a progesterone cream, the cream needs to have an adequate amount of progesterone in it [at least 30 milligrams per gram]. Many over-the-counter creams have little [for example, 5 milligrams per ounce] or none at all. The creams that are made from Mexican yams are not metabolized to progesterone by women. The cream used in the above study (Pro-Gest) contains pure United States Pharmacopoeia [USP] progesterone." Dr. John Lee, author and longtime proponent of topically applied progesterone, explains that "The USP progesterone used for hormone replacement comes from plant fats and oils, usually a substance called diosgenin, which is extracted from a very specific type of wild yam that grows in Mexico, or from soybeans. In the laboratory, diosgenin is chemically synthesized into real human progesterone. Some companies are trying to sell … 'wild yam extract' [or other plant extracts] … claiming that the body will then convert it into hormones as needed. While we know this can be done in the laboratory, there is no evidence that this conversion takes place in the human body." Dr. Lee is quick to explain that he doesn't sell any of these products and receives no profit from their sale. He also does *not* recommend the use of natural progesterone creams with any other active hormones or herbs.

prolamine extract. Protein that has water-binding and antioxidant properties.

proline. *See* amino acid.

propagermanium. *See* germanium.

propolis. Brownish, resinous material that is collected by bees and used to construct the hive. It has antibacterial and anti-inflammatory properties for skin (Source: *Antimicrobial Agents and Chemotherapy,* May 2002, pages 1302–1309).

propylene glycol. Along with other glycols and glycerol, propylene glycol is a humectant or humidifying and delivery ingredient used in cosmetics to keep products from melting in high heat and from freezing when it is cold, and to help active ingredients penetrate the skin.

There is a great deal of false and misleading information being presented about propylene glycol on Web sites and via spam e-mails. Some erroneously state that propylene glycol is really industrial antifreeze, that it is the major ingredient in brake and hydraulic fluids, and that it is a strong skin irritant. They further point out that the Material Safety Data Sheet (MSDS) states that users should avoid skin contact because systemically (i.e., in the body) it can cause liver abnormalities and kidney damage. However, as far as the use of propylene glycol in cosmetics is concerned, none of these points holds water, and its use in cosmetics poses no concern to the consumer. First of all, propylene glycol is used only in very small amounts in cosmetics, while the MSDS warnings are based on 100% concentrations (consider that even the MSDSs on water and salt have frightening comments regarding their safety). Thus, in the minute amounts used in cosmetics, propylene glycol is not a concern in the least. Women are not suffering from liver problems because of propylene glycol in cosmetics. Additionally, according to the U.S. Department of Health and Human Servces, Public Health Services Agency for Toxic Substances and Disease Registry, "studies have not shown these chemicals [propylene or the other glycols as used in cosmetics] to be carcinogens" (Source: http://www.atsdr.cdc.gov).

propylparaben. *See* parabens.

proteases. Enzymes that are part of a process that causes the breakdown of amino acids and proteins in skin (Source: http://www.chemistry-info.net/). There is research showing that proteases, when applied topically to skin, can reduce the visible scaling associated with dry, flaky skin (Source: *Archives of Dermatological Research,* November 2001, pages 500–507). Whether proteases can be of benefit for wound healing when applied topically is unclear (Source: *Experimental Dermatology,* October 2001, pages 337–348).

protein. Fundamental components of all living cells that includes a diverse range of biological substances, such as enzymes, hormones, and antibodies, that are necessary for the proper functioning of any organism, plant, or animal. The human body contains perhaps 100,000 different proteins, each composed of an assortment of 20 or so amino acids. The sequence of these amino acids determines the unique properties of each protein, such as, for example, its role as an enzyme acting as a catalyst for a specific biochemical reaction. If even one of the essential amino acids is missing, the protein cannot be formed. This fact is well known to nutritionists because ensuring an adequate supply of essential amino acids is important in determining the nutritional value of proteins in the diet. Components of proteins can have varying benefits for skin, but overall they are used for their water-binding and emollient properties.

Protol. Trade name for mineral oil. *See* mineral oil.

prune seed extract. In large enough amounts can have antioxidant properties (Source: *Journal of Agricultural Food Chemistry,* June 2002, pages 3708–3712).

Prunella vulgaris. See self-heal.

Prunus americana. See plum extract.

Prunus domestica **seed extract.** *See* plum extract.

Prunus dulcis. See almond oil.

Pseudopterogorgia elisabethae. See sea whip extract.

Psidium guajava. See guava extract.

Pueraria lobata. See kudzu root.

pullulan. Produced by black yeast, pullulan is a glucan gum that contains polysaccharides, which makes it a good water-binding agent, thickening agent, and antioxidant. *See* beta-glucan, and mucopolysaccharide.

Punica granatum **extract.** *See* pomegranate.

purified water. *See* deionized water.

PVP. *See* polyvinylpyrrolidone.

PVP copolymer. *See* polyvinylpyrrolidone.

pycnogenol. Plant-derived substance found in everything from pine bark to apples, cocoa beans, unripe strawberries, peanut skin, grape seeds, and red wine. There is a great deal of research on pycnogenol, but most of it dates back to 1990 and earlier (Source: U.S. Patent No. 4,698,360 entitled "Plant Extract with a Proanthocyanidins Content as Therapeutic Agent Having Radical Scavenging Effect and Use Thereof"). There are studies supporting the notion that pycnogenol is a potent antioxidant with strong free radical–scavenging properties (Source: *Free Radical Biology and Medicine,* September 1999, pages 704–724). However, there isn't any research showing that it will have any effect on wrinkles. *See* antioxidant.

pyridoxine hydrochloride. Scientific name for vitamin B6; may have antibacterial and antioxidant benefits for skin when applied topically.

Pyrus cydonia. See quince seed.

Pyrus malus. Is the technical name for apple. The pectin derived from it is used as a thickener in cosmetics.

quaternium-15. Formaldehyde-releasing preservative used in cosmetics. It can be a skin sensitizer, as can all preservatives. *See also* formaldehyde-releasing preservative.

quercus. *See* oak root extract.

Quercus infectoria **extract.** *See* oak root extract.

quillaja extract. Extract of the Chilean soap bark tree. It contains a good amount of saponins, which have cleansing, antimicrobial, and water-binding properties for skin. *See* saponin.

quince seed. Used as a thickening agent in cosmetics, but it also is known to have skin-constricting properties (Source: *Natural Medicines Comprehensive Database,* http://www.naturaldatabase.com) and may cause skin irritation.

quinoa oil. Derived from quinoa grain; it may have antifungal properties (Source: *Journal of Agricultural Food Chemistry,* May 2001, pages 2327–2332). It may also have emollient properties for skin, but there is little research showing this to be the case.

Ranunculus ficaria **extract.** May have antibacterial and antifungal properties and is used in the treatment of hemorrhoids. However, applied topically it can cause skin irritation and may also cause photodermatitis (Source: *Natural Medicines Comprehensive Database,* http://www.naturaldatabase.com).

rapeseed oil. Nonfragrant oil that has emollient and potential antioxidant properties for skin (Source: *British Journal of Nutrition,* May 2002, pages 489–499).

Ravensara **oil.** Plant oil. There is a small amount of research showing it to have antifungal properties, and when tested on insect larvae it showed antimutagenic properties (Sources: *Mutation Research,* January 2002, pages 61–68; and *Phytochemistry,* September 1999, pages 265–269).

red algae. *See* algae.

red clover. Can have antioxidant and anti-inflammatory properties (Source: *Photochemistry and Photobiology,* September 2001, pages 465–470). It is sold as an herbal supplement for relief of menopausal symptoms such as hot flashes and vaginal dryness. Red clover does contain high concentrations of four major isoflavones that have been shown to have estrogenic properties. However, in studies red clover was found to be no better than a placebo for menopausal symptoms (Sources: *Harvard Women's Health Watch,* December 2001, http://www.health.harvard.edu/medline/Women/W1201e.html; and *Natural Medicines Comprehensive Database,* http://www.naturaldatabase.com).

red raspberry extract. Fruit extract that has potent antioxidant properties (Source: *Journal of Agricultural Food Chemistry,* June 5, 2002, pages 3495–3500) and antibacterial properties (Source: *International Journal of Food Microbiology,* May 2000, pages 3–12). It can also cause irritation due to its tannin content.

red sandalwood. Has a phytoestrogen component (Source: *Phytochemistry,* March 2000, pages 605–606), but it can also be a skin irritant (Source: *Contact Dermatitis,* January 1996, page 69). *See* plant estrogen.

reducing agent. Substances that reduce a chemical compound. They have the ability to split or break down the disulfide bonds of hair. Therefore, they are typically used in hair-straightening or hair-waving products and in depilatories. The chemical reaction they generate has antioxidant properties, but they can also be strong skin irritants.

Rehmannia chinensis **root extract.** From the plant also known as Chinese foxglove; there is no research showing it to have benefit for skin.

Rehmannia glutinosa. Chinese herb known as Di huang that has no known benefit for skin.

Renova. *See* Retin-A, and tretinoin.

resorcinol. Considered an effective topical disinfectant in concentrations of 1% to 3% (Source: http://www.fda.gov). However, there is also research showing it to be overly irritating for skin (Source: *Journal of the European Academy of Dermatology and Venereology,* July 1999, pages 14–23). As a result, it is rarely used nowadays for treating blemishes.

respiratory enzyme. Type of enzyme that interacts with several other biological and physiological processes for the activation and use of oxygen in the body. There is no evidence that any respiratory enzyme can do anything topically for skin.

Retin-A. One of several prescription-only drugs (others include Renova, Tazorac, and Avita) that contain tretinoin (technically, all-trans retinoic acid), which is the acid form of vitamin A, as the active ingredient. In skin, tretinoin is the form of vitamin A that can actually affect cell production by binding to the tretinoin receptor sites on the cell. There is a great deal of research establishing that when skin has been damaged (often by exposure to sunlight) tretinoin is effective in improving cell production. Tretinoin is a valid method for addressing wrinkles and, overall, for improving cell production. Applying tretinoin doesn't produce miraculous results, but the positive outcome in terms of skin health is indisputable. However, it is highly possible that using tretinoin on the skin will cause irritation, which is a major drawback of this drug. *See* tretinoin.

retinol. Technical name for vitamin A. There is research demonstrating that retinol can have the same action on skin as tretinoin (a derivative of vitamin A and the active ingredient in Retin-A, Renova, Tazorac, and Avita). In skin, tretinoin is the form of vitamin A that can actually affect cell production by binding to the tretinoin receptor sites on the cell, and, therefore, retinol and retinyl palmitate must *become* tretinoin in the skin if they are to do the same thing. Theoretically, retinol can become tretinoin in the skin, but it is not a direct process. Retinol can be absorbed into the skin and if certain enzymes are present it could be converted to tretinoin. There is research, however, showing that retinol (and retinyl palmitate) can increase epidermal thickness and can indeed function in a manner similar to tretinoin (Sources: *Journal of Investigative Dermatology,* 1998, volume 111, pages 478–484, and September 1997, pages 301–305; *Skin Pharmacology and Applied Skin Physiology,* November-December 2001, pages 363–372; and *Experimental Dermatology,* February 1998, pages 27–34).

Retinol is an unstable ingredient, and therefore its packaging is of vital concern. Any container that allows the product to be exposed to sunlight and air means that the retinol will not be stable for very long, if at all, after it is opened (Source: *Journal of Cosmetic Science,* January-February 2001, pages 77–78). *See also* tretinoin.

retinyl palmitate. Form of vitamin A. It is a combination of retinol (pure vitamin A) and palmitic acid. There is research showing it to be effective as an antioxidant and skin-cell regulator (Source: *European Journal of Medical Research,* September 2001, pages 391–398; and *Journal of Investigative Dermatology,* September 1997, pages 301–305). *See also* retinol.

rhatany. *See Krameria triandra* extract.

Rhus succedanea*. See* Japan wax.

riboflavin. *See* vitamin B2.

ribonucleic acid. *See* RNA.

rice bran oil. Emollient oil similar to other nonfragrant plant oils. There is no research showing this to have superior benefit for skin.

rice oil. Emollient similar to other nonfragrant plant oils. There is no research showing this to have superior benefit for skin.

rice starch. Absorbent substance sometimes used instead of talc. It can cause allergic reactions and, because it is a food derivative (as opposed to a mineral derivative like talc), it can support bacterial growth in pores.

ricinoleate. Glyceryl triester used in cosmetics as a thickening agent and emollient.

Ricinus communis*. See* castor oil.

RNA. **R**ibo**n**ucleic **a**cid is a single strand of molecules, exactly copied from DNA in the cell nucleus, that is required for the body's production of protein. This single strand is a linear, ladder-like sequence of nucleotide bases (chemicals that form its structure) that corresponds precisely to the sequence of bases in the DNA strand (the core of the body's genetic makeup). In a skin-care product, RNA is useless because it cannot affect a cell's genetic elements. The production of DNA and RNA is an extremely complex process that requires a multitude of proteins and enzymes to have its effect on the body's genetic material. It is doubtful that you would ever want to put anything on your skin that could affect your genetic material, and particularly not via a cosmetic that has no safety or efficacy regulations.

***Robinia pseudacacia* extract.** *See* black locust extract.

rockrose oil. *See* labdanum oil.

Rosa canina*. See* rose hip oil.

Rosa centifolia*. See* rose hip oil.

***Rosa damascena* oil.** Very fragrant pink rose, used as fragrance in cosmetics.

Rosa eglanteria*. See* rose hip oil.

***Rosa gallica* flower extract.** Fragrant extract.

Rosa mosqueta*. See* rose hip oil.

Rosa roxburghii **extract.** Extract from the chestnut rose; can be a source of antioxidants for skin, and does not impart fragrance (Source: *International Journal of Clinical Chemistry and Applied Molecular Biology,* November 2001, pages 37–43).

Rosa rubiginosa. *See* rose hip oil.

rose flower. Highly fragrant substance that can be a skin irritant.

rose flower oil. Fragrant, volatile oil that can be a skin irritant and sensitizer. There is no research showing this to have any benefit for skin.

rose hip. Seed-containing part of a rose. *See* rose hip oil, and vitamin C.

rose hip oil. Good emollient oil that has antioxidant properties (Sources: *Journal of Agricultural Food Chemistry,* March 2000, pages 825–828; and *Journal of Nutrition,* March 2002, pages 461–471).

rose of Jericho extract. Extract from an annual desert plant with the scientific name *Anastatica hierochuntica.* It has hygroscopic properties, meaning it can absorb moisture from the air. There is no research showing this extract to have benefit for skin.

rose oil. Fragrant, volatile oil that can be a skin irritant and sensitizer.

rosemary extract. Can have antioxidant benefit for skin (Source: *Journal of Agricultural Food Chemistry,* October 1999, pages 3954–3962), but its aromatic components can cause irritation, sensitizing, or toxic reactions on skin (Source: *Chemical Research in Toxicology,* November 2001, pages 1546–1551).

rosemary oil. *See* rosemary extract.

roseroot. *See Sedum rosea* root extract.

Rosmarinus officinalis **extract.** *See* rosemary extract.

royal jelly. Milky white, thick substance secreted by worker bees that has been shown to have some immune-modulating benefits (Source: *Comparative Immunology, Microbiology and Infectious Diseases,* January 1996, pages 31–38). The myriad other claims about royal jelly being able to prevent wrinkles and heal acne are all anecdotal, and have no research to substantiate them.

Rubus idaeus. *See* red raspberry.

Rubus laciniatus. *See* blackberry.

Rubus occidentalis. *See* black raspberry.

Rubus suavissimus **extract.** Derived from the Chinese blackberry. Most likely, as is true for most berries, this fruit extract has antioxidant properties. However, there is no research proving this to be the case.

Rubus ursinus. *See* marionberry.

Rubus ursinus x idaeus. *See* boysenberry.

Ruscus aculeatus. *See* butcher's broom extract.

rutin. Bioflavonoid extracted from various plants and used as an antioxidant and emollient (Sources: *Cell Biology and Toxicology,* 2000, volume 16, number 2, pages 91–98; and *Life Sciences,* January 14, 2000, pages 709–723). *See* bioflavonoid.

saccharide. *See* mucopolysaccharide.

saccharide isomerate. Good water-binding agent and emollient for skin. *See* mucopolysaccharide.

***Saccharomyces* calcium ferment.** Extract of yeast fermented in the presence of calcium ions. There is no known benefit for skin.

Saccharomyces cerevisiae. *See* yeast.

***Saccharomyces* copper ferment.** *Saccharomyces,* from the Latin, literally means "sugar fungus," and is the scientific name for the yeasts used in fermentation. There are many versions of this fungus fermented with various compounds; this version is fermented in the presence of copper ions. There is no known benefit for skin, though it may have antioxidant properties.

***Saccharomyces* iron ferment.** Extract of yeast fermented in the presence of iron ions. *See Saccharomyces* copper ferment.

***Saccharomyces* lysate.** *See* yeast.

***Saccharomyces* magnesium ferment.** The extract of yeast fermented in the presence of magnesium ions. *See Saccharomyces* copper ferment.

***Saccharomyces* manganese ferment.** Extract of yeast fermented in the presence of manganese ions. *See Saccharomyces* copper ferment.

***Saccharomyces* potassium ferment.** Extract of yeast fermented in the presence of potassium ions. *See Saccharomyces* copper ferment.

***Saccharomyces* silicon ferment.** Extract of yeast fermented in the presence of silicon ions. *See Saccharomyces* copper ferment.

***Saccharomyces* zinc ferment.** Extract of yeast fermented in the presence of zinc ions. *See Saccharomyces* copper ferment.

***Saccharum officinarum* extract.** Derived from the sugarcane plant. Glycolic acid is also derived from sugarcane, but sugarcane extract does not have the same exfoliating properties as glycolic acid. There is no research showing sugarcane extract has any benefit for skin. *See* AHA.

safflower oil. Emollient plant oil similar to all nonfragrant plant oils. Safflower oil can be an antioxidant when consumed in the diet, but whether it retains this benefit when applied topically to skin is unknown. *See* natural moisturizing factors.

sage extract. Can be a potent antioxidant (Source: *Journal of Agricultural Food Chemistry,* March 2002, pages 1845–1851). However, its fragrant camphor and phenol components can also cause skin irritation (Source: *Clinical Toxicology,* December 1981, pages 1485–1498).

salicin. *See* willow bark.

salicylic acid. Referred to as **b**eta **h**ydroxy **a**cid (BHA), it is a multifunctional ingredient that addresses many of the systemic causes of blemishes (Source: *Seminars in Dermatology,* December 1990, pages 305–308). For decades dermatologists have been prescribing salicylic acid as an exceedingly effective keratolytic (exfoliant), but it also is an anti-irritant because salicylic acid is a derivative of aspirin (both are salicylates—

aspirin's technical name is acetyl *salicylic acid*), and so it also functions as an anti-inflammatory (Sources: *Archives of Internal Medicine,* July 2002, pages 1531–1532; *Annals of Dermatology and Venereology,* January 2002, pages 137–142; *Archives of Dermatology,* November 2000, pages 1390–1395; and *Pain,* January 1996, pages 71–82). Another notable aspect of salicylic acid for treating breakouts is that it has antimicrobial properties (Sources: *Preservatives for Cosmetics,* 1996, by David Steinberg, Allured Publishing; and Health Canada Monograph Category IV, *Antiseptic Cleansers,* http://www.hc-sc.gc.ca/english/). It is also well documented that it can improve skin thickness, barrier functions, and collagen production (Sources: *Dermatology,* 1999, volume 199, number 1, pages 50–53; and *Toxicology and Applied Pharmacology,* volume 175, issue 1, pages 76–82).

As an exfoliant, in concentrations of 8% to 12%, salicylic acid is effective in wart-remover medications. In concentrations of 0.5% to 2%, it is far more gentle, and, much like AHAs, can exfoliate the surface of skin. In addition, BHA has the ability to penetrate into the pore (AHAs do not), and thus can exfoliate inside the pore as well as on the surface of the skin, which makes it effective for reducing blemishes, including blackheads and whiteheads. *See also* AHA.

Salix alba extract. *See* willow bark.

Salvia officinalis. *See* sage.

Sambucus canadensis. *See* elderberry.

Sambucus cerulea. Blue elderberry. May have antioxidant properties for skin (Source: *Phytotherapy Research,* February 2002, pages 63–65). *See* elderberry.

Sambucus nigra. *See* black elderberry.

sandalwood oil. Fragrant oil that can cause skin irritation or allergic reactions (Source: *American Journal of Contact Dermatitis,* June 1996, pages 77–83). There is one animal study showing it to have antitumor properties (Source: *European Journal of Cancer Prevention,* October 1999, pages 449–455).

Sang zhi. Derived from twigs of the mulberry tree. It has some effectiveness for reducing skin swelling.

Sanguinaria. *See* bloodroot.

Sanguisorba officinalis. Latin name for salad burnet. There is a small amount of research showing it to have antioxidant properties for skin (Source: *Biological and Pharmaceutical Bulletin,* September 2001, pages 998–1003).

Santalum album. *See* sandalwood oil.

Sapindus mukurossi extract. Derived from a plant indigenous to India, and known for its detergent cleansing properties. *See* saponin.

Saponaria officinalis extract. *See* soapwort.

saponin. Group of natural carbohydrates found in plants that have considerable potential as pharmaceutical and/or nutraceutical agents in natural or synthetic form. Saponins, from a variety of sources, have been shown to have anti-inflammatory and antioxidant properties. (Sources: *Fitoterapia,* July 2002, page 336; *Phytotherapy Research,* March 2001, pages 174–176; and *Drug Metabolism and Drug Interaction,* 2000, volume 17, issue 1-4, pages 211–235).

Sargassum filipendula extract. *See* algae.

saturated fat. Type of fat usually of animal origin. Chemically, when fatty acid chains can't accommodate any more hydrogen atoms, they are considered saturated, as in saturated fatty acids. These are used as emollients in skin-care products.

Saussurea lappa. *See* costus root.

sausurrea oil. Costus oil. Volatile oil and fragrant component used in cosmetics; it can be a skin irritant. It is known to cause contact dermatitis (Source: *Natural Medicines Comprehensive Database,* http://www.naturaldatabase.com)

saw palmetto. Plant extract that, when taken orally, has been shown in short-term trials to be efficacious in reducing the symptoms of benign prostatic hyperplasia (Source: *Annals of Internal Medicine,* January 2002, pages 42–53). It may have an anti-inflammatory effect on skin, but there is little research supporting this. Saw palmetto's reputation is primarily based on the fact that it can reduce the presence of the male hormone dihydrotestosterone, and so it could theoretically reduce hair loss, but this effect has not been proven. There is some anecdotal information that it can also have estrogenic effects; but not only is that unlikely, it is also highly improbable that it could have such effects when applied topically (Source: *Healthnotes Review of Complementary and Integrative Medicine,* http://www.healthwell.com/healthnotes/Herb/Saw_Palmetto.cfm).

Saxifraga sarmentosa extract. *See* strawberry begonia.

sclareolide. Fermented from clary sage and used as a fragrant component in cosmetics.

sclerotium gum. Used as a thickening agent in cosmetics.

scullcap extract. Herbal extract from *Scutellaria baicalensis* that has antioxidant and anti-inflammatory properties for skin (Source: *Life Sciences,* January 2002, pages 1023–1033).

Scutellaria baicalensis extract. *See* scullcap extract.

SD alcohol. *See* alcohol.

sea salt. Can be effective as a topical scrub, but if left on skin it can increase skin sensitivity to UVB radiation (Source: *Der Hautarzt,* June 1998, pages 482–486).

Seamollient. Trade name for an algae extract. *See* algae.

sea whip extract. Extract from a creature that inhabits coral reefs, known for its anti-inflammatory (Source: *Life Sciences,* May 22, 1998, pages 401–407) and antibacterial properties (Source: *Journal of Natural Products,* January 2001, pages 100–102).

seaweed. Group of sea plants (scientific name algae) of all sizes and shapes, and having a gelatin-like consistency. Many seaweeds have antioxidant and anti-inflammatory properties, but many other claims of benefits are not proven. *See* algae.

sebaceous glands. Glands in the skin that open into hair follicles and from which sebum (oil) is secreted.

sebacic acid. Used as a pH adjuster.

Sechium edule **extract.** Extract of the chayote plant. There is a small amount of research showing it to have antioxidant properties (Source: *Free Radical Biology and Medicine,* 1991, volume 11, number 4, pages 379–383).

Sedum rosea **root extract.** Plant extract; there is no research showing this to have any benefit for skin (Source: *Natural Medicines Comprehensive Database,* http://www.naturaldatabase.com).

selenium. Element considered to be a potent antioxidant (Source: *Biomedicine and Pharmacotherapy,* June 2002, pages 173–178). *See* antioxidant.

self-heal. Plant that has antihistamine, anti-inflammatory, antiviral, and antioxidant properties when taken orally (Sources: *Life Sciences,* January 2000, pages 725–735; *Planta Medica,* May 2000, pages 358–360; and *Immunopharmacology and Immunotoxicology,* August 2001, pages 423–435). However, there is no research demonstrating this to be of benefit for skin when applied topically.

Sequoiadendron gigantea **stem extract.** Extract from part of the giant sequoia tree. There is no research showing this extract to have any benefit for skin.

Serenoa serrulata **extract.** *See* saw palmetto extract.

sericin. Scientific name for silk protein. *See* silk protein.

serine. *See* amino acid.

serum protein. *See* protein.

sesame oil. Emollient oil similar to other nonfragrant plant oils. *See* natural moisturizing factors.

Sesamum indicum. *See* sesame seed oil.

sesquioleate. Used in cosmetics as a thickening agent and emollient.

Shao-yao. *See* peony root.

shea butter. Plant lipid that is used as an emollient in cosmetics. *See* natural moisturizing factors.

shikonin. Common name for the Chinese plant Zi Cao, source of a plant extract with supposedly anti-inflammatory properties. There is no research substantiating its effect on skin.

Shorea stenoptera **butter.** Fat obtained from the Borneo tallow nut. It is similar to cocoa and shea butter, and has emollient properties for skin.

Siegesbeckia orientalis. Chinese herb (also known as St. Paul's wort); there is no research showing that it has any benefit for skin.

silanetriol lysinate. *See* silicone.

silica. Mineral found abundantly in sandstone, clay, and granite, as well as in parts of plants and animals. It is the principal ingredient of glass. In cosmetics it is used as an absorbent powder and thickening agent.

silicate. Inorganic salt that has potent absorbing and thickening properties.

silicone. Substance derived from silica (sand is a silica). The unique fluid properties of silicone give it a great deal of slip and in its various forms it can feel like silk on the skin, impart emolliency, and be a water-binding agent that holds up well, even when skin becomes wet. In other forms, it is also used extensively for wound healing and for improving the appearance of scars (Source: *Journal of Wound Care,* July 2000, pages 319–324).

silk. *See* silk protein.

silk protein. Protein substance (also called sericin) formed by converting silk, which is the soft, lustrous thread obtained from the cocoon of the silkworm. Silk protein can have water-binding properties for skin. However, the skin can't tell the difference whether the protein is derived from animals or plants. There is a small amount of research showing silk protein to have topical antioxidant properties (Source: *Bioscience, Biotechnology, and Biochemistry,* January 1998, pages 145–147).

siloxane. *See* silicone.

silver. Metallic element that in cosmetics can have disinfecting properties; however, prolonged contact can turn skin grayish blue. Silver can be irritating to skin, and can cause silver toxicity (Sources: *Annals of Dermatology and Venereology,* February 2002, pages 217–219; and *Critical Reviews in Toxicology,* May 1996, pages 255–260). *See* silver sulfadiazine.

silver chloride. *See* silver sulfadiazine.

silver sulfadiazine. Can be effective for wound healing (Source: *Journal of Vascular Surgery,* August 1992, pages 251–257). However, it is safe for skin only for short-term use, because silver can penetrate abraded skin and cause silver toxicity (Source: *Clinical Chemistry,* February 1997, pages 290–301).

silver tip white tea leaf extract. *See* green tea, and white tea.

***Silybum marianum* extract.** *See* lady's thistle extract.

***Skeletonema costatum* extract.** From a type of marine diatom. There is no research showing it to have benefit for skin.

skin respiratory factor. *See* tissue respiratory factor.

slip agent. Term used to describe a range of ingredients that help other ingredients spread over the skin and help ingredients penetrate into the skin. Slip agents also have humectant properties. Slip agents include propylene glycol, butylene glycol, polysorbates, and glycerin, to name a few. They are as basic to the world of skin care as water.

slippery elm bark. Can be an anti-irritant and anti-inflammatory.

soap. True "soaps" are regulated by the Consumer Product Safety Commission and are not required to list their ingredients on the label. They are made up solely of fats and alkali. Many bar cleansers are not soaps, but contain synthetic detergent cleansing agents and various thickening agents that keep the bar in its bar form. Most soaps are considered very drying and potentially irritating for skin due to their alkaline base (having a pH over 8). Bar cleansers can be more gentle than bar soaps, but are more often than not still drying, depending on their composition (Sources: *Cutis,* December 2001, pages 12–19; *Archives of Dermatologic Research,* June 2001, pages 308–318; and *Dermatologic Clinics,* October 2000, pages 561–575).

soapwort. Plant providing an extract with detergent cleansing properties. There is some research showing it to have antiviral and antibacterial properties (Sources: *Biochemical and Biophysical Research Communications,* May 1997, pages 129–132; and *Phytotherapy Research,* 1990, volume 4, pages 97–100).

sodium ascorbate. *See* ascorbic acid.

sodium bisulfite. Used in acid-type permanent waves to alter the shape of hair. It is less damaging than alkaline permanent waves, but it also has limitations regarding how much change it can effect in hair. It can be a skin irritant.

sodium borate. *See* borates.

sodium C14-16 olefin sulfate. Can be derived from coconut. Used primarily as a detergent cleansing agent, but is considered potentially drying and irritating for skin. *See* surfactant.

sodium carbonate. Absorbent salt used in cosmetics; it can also be a skin irritant.

sodium chloride. Common table salt. Used primarily as a binding agent in skin-care products and occasionally as an abrasive in scrub products.

sodium chondroitin sulfate. *See* glycosaminoglycans.

sodium cocoate. Used as a cleansing agent primarily in soaps. It can be drying and irritating for skin.

sodium cocoyl isethionate. Derived from coconut; it is a mild detergent cleansing agent. *See* surfactant.

sodium hyaluronate. *See* hyaluronic acid.

sodium hydroxide. Also known as lye, it's a highly alkaline ingredient used in small amounts in cosmetics to modulate the pH of a product. It is also used as a cleansing agent in some cleansers. In higher concentrations it is a significant skin irritant.

sodium laureth sulfate. Can be derived from coconut; it is used primarily as a detergent cleansing agent. It is considered gentle and effective. *See* surfactant.

sodium laureth-13 carboxylate. Used primarily as a detergent cleansing agent. *See* surfactant.

sodium lauryl sulfate (SLS). Can be derived from coconut, and is used primarily as a detergent cleansing agent. There has been a great deal of misinformation about sodium lauryl sulfate circulated on the Internet. Although it is a potent skin irritant it is not toxic or dangerous for skin. In concentrations of 2% to 5%, SLS can cause allergic or sensitizing reactions in lots of people. It is used as a standard in scientific studies to establish irritatancy or sensitizing properties of other ingredients (Sources: *European Journal of Dermatology,* September-October 2001, pages 416–419; *American Journal of Contact Dermatitis,* March 2001, pages 28–32; and *Skin Pharmacology and Applied*

Skin Physiology, September-October 2000, pages 246–257). Being a skin irritant, however, is not the same as a link to cancer, which is what erroneous warnings on the Internet are falsely claiming about this ingredient!

According to Health Canada, in a press release of February 12, 1999 (www.hc-sc.gc.ca/), "A letter has been circulating the Internet which claims that there is a link between cancer and sodium laureth (or lauryl) sulfate (SLS), an ingredient used in [cosmetics]. Health Canada has looked into the matter and has found no scientific evidence to suggest that SLS causes cancer. It has a history of safe use in Canada. Upon further investigation, it was discovered that this e-mail warning is a hoax. The letter is signed by a person at the University of Pennsylvania Health System and includes a phone number. Health Canada contacted the University of Pennsylvania Health System and found that it is not the author of the sodium laureth sulfate warning and does not endorse any link between SLS and cancer. Health Canada considers SLS safe for use in cosmetics. Therefore, you can continue to use cosmetics containing SLS without worry." Further, according to the American Cancer Society's Web site (www.cancer.org), "Contrary to popular rumors on the Internet, Sodium Lauryl Sulfate (SLS) and Sodium Laureth Sulfate (SLES) do not cause cancer. E-mails have been flying through cyberspace claiming SLS [and SLES] causes cancer … and is proven to cause cancer…. [Yet] A search of recognized medical journals yielded no published articles relating this substance to cancer in humans." *See* surfactant.

sodium metabisulfite. Reducing agent that is used to alter the structure of hair. It can also be used as a preservative in formulations, and can be a skin irritant. However, it can also be an antioxidant (Source: *Journal of Pharmaceutical Science and Technology,* September-October 1999, pages 252–259). *See* reducing agent.

sodium methyl taurate. Mild surfactant. *See* surfactant.

sodium PCA. PCA stands for **p**yrrolidone**c**arboxylic **a**cid. It is a natural component of skin that is also a very good water-binding agent. *See* natural moisturizing factors.

sodium salicylate. Salt form of salicylic acid (BHA). Because it is not the acid form of salicylate (i.e., salicylic acid), it does not have exfoliating properties.

sodium silicate. Highly alkaline and potentially irritating antiseptic and mineral used in cosmetics (Source: *American Journal of Contact Dermatitis,* September 2002, pages 133–139).

sodium sulfite. Reducing agent that is used to alter the structure of hair. It can also be used as a preservative in cosmetic formulations, and can be a skin irritant. *See* reducing agent.

sodium tallowate. Sodium salt of tallow. *See* tallow.

sodium thioglycolate. *See* thioglycolate.

sodium trideceth sulfate. *See* surfactant.

***Solanum lycocarpum* fruit extract.** Also known as wolf's fruit. There is no research showing this to have benefit for skin, though there is research showing it to have toxic effects when eaten (Source: *Journal of Ethnopharmacology,* July 2002, pages 265–269).

Solanum lycopersicum **extract.** *See* tomato extract.

Solanum tuberosum **extract.** Potato starch; used as a thickening agent in cosmetics.

soluble fish collagen. *See* collagen.

solum fullonum. *See* fuller's earth.

solvent. Large group of ingredients, including water, that are used to dissolve or break down other ingredients in a formulation. Solvents are also used to degrease skin and to remove sebum.

Sonojell. Trade name for petrolatum. *See* petrolatum.

sorbitan stearate. Used to thicken and stabilize cosmetic formulations.

sorbitol. Can be derived synthetically or from natural sources. Similar to glycerin, it is a humectant, thickening agent, and slip agent.

soy extract. Antioxidant and anti-inflammatory agent for skin (Sources: *Cancer Investigation*, 1996, volume 14, number 6, pages 597–608; and *Skin Pharmacology and Applied Skin Physiology*, May-June 2002, pages 175–183). However, there is no research showing that soy extract or soy oil has estrogenic effects when applied to skin (as it can when taken orally).

soy isoflavones. *See* soy extract.

soy oil. Emollient oil similar to all nonfragrant plant oils. *See* natural moisturizing factors, and soy extract.

soy protein. *See* soy extract.

soya sterol. One form of phytosterol. There is no research showing soya sterols to have estrogenic or antioxidant benefit for skin. *See* phytosterol.

spearmint oil. Fragrant, volatile oil that can cause skin irritation and allergic reactions. *See* counter-irritant.

SPF. *See* sun protection factor.

spikenard. Plant that has antibacterial properties for skin.

Spilanthes acmella **extract.** Plant extract that can have antibacterial properties (Source: *Journal of Ethnopharmacology*, February 1998, pages 79–84).

spinach extract. Can have antioxidant properties (Source: *Journal of Agricultural Food Chemistry*, May 2002, pages 3122–3128), but whether benefits can be realized when it is applied topically on skin is not known.

Spiraea ulmaria. *See* meadowsweet.

spirulina. *See* algae.

squalane. *See* natural moisturizing factors, and squalene.

squalene. Oil derived from shark liver or from plants and sebum. It is a natural component of skin and is considered a good emollient that has antioxidant and immune-stimulating properties (Sources: *Lancet Oncology*, October 2000, pages 107–112; and *Free Radical Research*, April 2002, pages 471–477). *See* natural moisturizing factors.

St. John's wort. Contains several components that are toxic on skin in the presence of sunlight (Sources: *Planta Medica*, February 2002, pages 171–173; and *International*

Journal of Biochemistry and Cell Biology, March 2002, pages 221–241). St. John's wort's association with improving depression when taken as an oral supplement is unrelated to its topical impact on skin. However, it does have potent antioxidant properties (Source: *Journal of Agricultural Food Chemistry,* November 2001, pages 5165–5170).

star anise. *See* anise.

steapyrium chloride. Antistatic agent used in hair-care products.

stearalkonium chloride. Antistatic ingredient used in hair-care products to control flyaways and aid in helping a brush or comb get through hair.

stearates. *See* stearic acid.

stearic acid. Fatty acid used as an emollient and as an agent to help keep other ingredients intact in a formulation. *See* fatty acid, and thickening agent.

stearyl alcohol. Fatty alcohol used as an emollient and to help keep other ingredients intact in a formulation. *See* fatty alcohols.

***Stevia rebaudiana* extract.** Plant extract called stevioside, a natural, noncaloric sweetener that has been used as a noncaloric sugar substitute in Japan and South America. It has been shown to have "genuine mutagenic" activity (Source: *Chemical and Pharmaceutical Bulletin,* July 2002, pages 1007–1010). There is no research showing this extract to have any benefit when applied topically to skin.

strawberry begonia. There is no research showing this to have any benefit for skin.

strawberry leaves. Can be a skin irritant and skin sensitizer, with no known benefit for skin.

styrax benzoin. *See* benzoin extract.

subtilisin. Protease enzyme obtained from the fermentation of *Bacillus subtilis. See* proteases.

sucrose. Monosaccharide that has water-binding properties for skin. *See* mucopolysaccharide, and water-binding agent.

sugarcane extract. Ingredients like sugarcane extract, fruit extracts, mixed fruit extracts, and milk solids may claim an association with AHAs, but they are not the same thing nor do they have the same beneficial effect on skin. While glycolic acid can indeed be derived from sugarcane, assuming that sugarcane will net you the same result as glycolic acid would be like assuming you could write on a tree the way you can on paper. Wood is certainly where paper begins, but paper wouldn't exist without the wood undergoing complex mechanical and chemical processes. Similarly, the original forms of these extracts do not have the same effect as the effective ingredients that are derived from them. The same is true for lactic acid, derived from milk. If milk were as acid as lactic acid you would not be able to drink it without serious complications. There is a vast difference between the extracted, pure ingredient and the original form of the source material. *See* AHA.

sulfur. Antibacterial agent (Source: *Applied Microbiology and Biotechnology,* October 2001, pages 282–286). It can be a potent skin irritant and sensitizer. Sulfur also has a high pH, which can encourage the growth of bacteria on skin.

suma. Also known as Brazilian ginseng and *Pfaffia paniculata. See Pfaffia paniculata* extract.

sun protection factor. Most commonly referred to as SPF, it is a number assigned to a product that identifies its ability to protect the skin from sunburn or to protect the skin from turning pink or red when exposed to sun. SPF ratings are regulated by the FDA. It is a measure of the *amount of time* a person can stay in the sun without getting burned if a sunscreen is applied. Since sunburn results from UVB exposure, not UVA radiation, SPF is primarily a measure of UVB protection. At this time, there is no numbering system to indicate the level of protection a sunscreen can provide from UVA radiation, which affects the deeper layers of skin.

A sunscreen with at least an SPF 15 or higher is universally recommended. Sunscreen must be applied liberally and evenly or the sun-protection value of the product will not be achieved and damage to the skin will occur. It is also essential that the sunscreen contain ingredients (chiefly avobenzone, titanium dioxide, and zinc oxide) that protect from UVA damage (Sources: *American Journal of Clinical Dermatology,* 2002, volume 3, number 3, pages 185–191; *Journal of Photochemistry and Photobiology,* November 15, 2001, pages 105–108; *Photodermatology, Photoimmunology, and Photomedicine,* February 2001, pages 2–10; http://www.skincancerprevention.org/prevention_tips.html; The Skin Cancer Foundation, http://www.skincancer.org; and American Academy of Dermatology, http://www.aad.org). *See* sunscreen, and UVA.

sunflower oil. Non-volatile plant oil used as an emollient in cosmetics.

sunscreens. Products strictly regulated by the FDA that provide protection from sunburn and some amount of sun damage. There is a great deal of confusion regarding the efficacy and use of sunscreens. The FDA instituted new regulations that will take effect in 2002 and that will hopefully clarify the issue. According to the FDA's July-August 2002 issue of *Consumer* magazine, "Under the new regulations manufacturers will no longer be allowed to [use] … confusing terms such as 'sunblock,' 'waterproof,' 'all-day protection,' and 'visible and/or infrared light protection' on these [sunscreen] products. In addition to these changes … tanning preparations that do not contain a sunscreen ingredient [are required] to display the following warning: 'Warning: This product does not contain a sunscreen and does not protect against sunburn. Repeated exposure of unprotected skin while tanning may increase the risk of skin aging, skin cancer, and other harmful effects to the skin even if you do not burn.'

"To figure out how much protection a sunscreen provides, most consumers turn to a simple number: the SPF, or sun protection factor, listed on the label. Studies show that most consumers understand that the higher the number, the more the product protects the skin."

The FDA then goes on to say: "Unfortunately, studies also show that people often have the mistaken notion that the higher the SPF number of the sunscreen they use, the longer they can stay—and will stay—in the sun…. Sunscreen should not be used to prolong time spent in the sun. Even with a sunscreen, you are not going to prevent all the possible damage from the sun. Some of the newer research in the last several years shows that [for] the sub-erythemal doses [exposure to the sun that does not cause reddening of the skin], as little as one-tenth the energy needed to get a sunburn, starts the process of skin damage of one sort or another.

"The public under-applies sunscreens by as much as half of the recommended amount, concluded a study published in the *Archives of Dermatology*. Consequently, the study argued, consumers are receiving only half of the SPF protection they believe the product provides." This issue of liberal application has been confirmed in other research as well (Source: *Photochemistry and Photobiology*, July 2001, pages 61–63). *See* sun protection factor, and UVA.

superoxide dismutase. Enzyme considered to be a potent antioxidant in humans (Sources: *Journal of Investigative Dermatology*, April 2002, pages 618–625; *Journal of Photochemistry and Photobiology B*, October 2001, pages 61–69; and *European Journal of Pharmaceutical Sciences*, August 2001, pages 63–67). *See* antioxidant.

surfactant. Acronym for **surf**ace **act**ive **agent**. Surfactants degrease and emulsify oils and fats and suspend soil, allowing them to be washed away, as laundry products do. The term "surfactants"and "detergent cleansing agents" (I refer to them as the latter throughout my writing) are often used interchangeably by chemists and researchers (Sources: Food and Drug Administration, Office of Cosmetics and Colors Fact Sheet, February 3, 1995, http://www.fda.gov; *Dermatology*, 1995, volume 191, number 4, pages 276–280; *Tenside, Surfactants, Detergents,* 1997, volume 34, number 3, pages 156–168; and http://surfactants.net). Surfactants are used in most forms of cleansers and many of them considered gentle and effective for most skin types. There are several types of surfactants that can be sensitizing, drying, and irritating for skin.

sutilain. *See Bacillus subtilis.*

sweet almond oil. Emollient oil. *See* natural moisturizing factors.

***Symphytum officinale* extract.** *See* comfrey.

Szechuan pepper. May have antibacterial properties, but can also be a skin irritant.

Szechuan peppercorn. From a plant native to the Szechuan Province in China. It grows on trees, and so differs from black pepper, which grows on climbing vines. Used extensively in Szechuan cooking, Szechuan pepper is known for the "numbing" sensation it produces on the tongue. It is considered a counter-irritant. *See* black pepper, and counter-irritant.

talc. Finely ground mineral used as an absorbent, and the primary base of most pressed and loose powder. Talc is often criticized and described as a cosmetic ingredient to avoid. The concern about talc is not about it's use in makeup, but rather about the way it was used in pure, large concentrations such as in talcum powder. Part of this story dates back to several studies published in the 1990s that found a significant increase in the risk of ovarian cancer from vaginal (perineal) application of talcum powder (Sources: *American Journal of Epidemiology*, March 1997, pages 459–465; *International Journal of Cancer*, May 1999, pages 351–356; *Seminars in Oncology*, June 1998, pages 255–

264; and *Cancer,* June 1997, pages 2396–2401). However, subsequent and concurrent studies have cast doubt on the way these studies were conducted as well as their conclusions (Sources: *Journal of the National Cancer Institute,* February 2000, pages 249–252; *American Journal of Obstetrics and Gynecology,* March 2000, pages 720–724; and *Obstetrics and Gynecology,* March 1999, pages 372–376). There is no research showing talc to be a problem in cosmetics.

tallow. Substance extracted from the fatty deposits of animals, especially from suet (the fat of cattle and sheep). Tallow is often used to make soap and candles. In soap, because of its fat content, it can be a problem for breakouts.

tamanu oil. From a tree native to Polynesia. It is reputed to have wondrous wound-healing properties, as well as being a cure-all for almost every skin ailment you can think of, from acne to eczema to psoriasis, but all of the miraculous claims hinge on anecdotal, not scientific, evidence. There's no harm in using this oil in skin care because, like most oils, it is composed of phospholipids and glycolipids, and these are natural constituents of healthy skin and are good water-binding agents. Tamanu oil may have anti-inflammatory properties and there is some research showing it has anti-tumor properties, though this has not been proven in any direct research on skin.

***Tambourissa* extract.** Extract of a plant indigenous to Madagascar that has no known benefit for skin. It may contain volatile components that can be skin irritants (Source: *Planta Medica,* April 2001, pages 290–292).

Tanacetum parthenium. *See* feverfew.

tangerine oil. Fragrant, volatile citrus oil that can be a skin irritant.

tannic acid. Potent antioxidant; it may have some anticarcinogenic properties (Sources: *Bioorganic & Medicinal Chemistry Letters,* June 2002, pages 1567–1570; and *Nutrition and Cancer,* 1998, volume 32, number 2, pages 81–85).

tannin. Component of many plants. It can have an antitumor benefit when consumed in tea or foods (Source: *Nutrition and Cancer,* 1998, volume 32, number 2, pages 81–85). There is some research on animals showing that this benefit may translate to skin (Source: *Photochemistry and Photobiology,* June 1998, pages 663–668). Tannins can also have constricting properties on skin, and that may cause irritation with repeated use.

Taraktogenos kurzii. *See* chaulmoogra oil.

Taraxacum japonicum. *See* Japanese dandelion.

Taraxacum officinale. *See* dandelion extract.

Taraxacum platycarpum. *See* Japanese dandelion.

tartaric acid. *See* AHA.

TBHQ. Abbreviation for 2-tert-butylhydroquinone. It is a potent antioxidant (Source: *Journal of Biological Chemistry,* January 2002, pages 2477–2484), though there is no research showing this to be of benefit when applied topically.

tea tree oil. Also known as melaleuca, from the name of its plant source, *Melaleuca alternifolia.* It can have disinfecting properties that have been shown to be effective against the bacteria that cause blemishes. According to *Healthnotes Review of Complementary and Integrative Medicine* (www.healthwell.com/healthnotes/Herb/Tea_Tree.cfm) and the *Medical Journal of Australia* (October 1990, pages 455–458), 5% tea tree oil and 2.5% benzoyl peroxide are effective in reducing the number of blemishes, with a significantly better result for benzoyl peroxide. Skin oiliness was lessened significantly in the benzoyl peroxide group versus the tea tree oil group. However, the tea tree oil had somewhat less irritating side effects. Concentrations of 5% to 10% are recommended. However, the amount found in most skin-care products is usually less than 1% and, therefore, considered not to be effective for disinfecting.

TEA. *See* triethanolamine.

TEA-lauryl sulfate. While there is abundant research showing sodium lauryl sulfate to be a sensitizing cleansing agent, there is no similar supporting research for TEA-lauryl sulfate. However, because the relationship between the two is so close, I decided to recommend against the use of either of them. The basis for this is a judgment call, made from a desire to protect skin from sensitization; however, there are no specific studies I can cite for this recommendation, and there are those who will understandably disagree with my conclusion. *See* sodium lauryl sulfate.

***Tecoma curialis* bark extract.** Potential irritant and sensitizer for skin (Source: *Botanical Dermatology Database,* http://bodd.cf.ac.uk/index.html).

Tepescohuite extract. Spanish name for *Mimosa tenuiflora* extract. *See Mimosa tenuflora* extract.

***Tephrosia purpurea* seed extract.** There is a small amount of research showing this to have antioxidant and anticancer properties when fed to rats and in vitro (Source: *Journal of Pharmacological and Toxicological Methods,* June 2001, pages 294–299), but there is no evidence that this effect can be duplicated when applied topically.

Terminalia catappa. Can be a potent antioxidant (Source: *Anticancer Research,* January-February 2001, pages 237–243).

Terminalia sericea. May have antibacterial properties (Source: *Journal of Ethnopharmacology,* February 2002, pages 169–177), but can also have a high incidence of irritation or contact dermatitis.

tetrahexyldecyl ascorbate. Stable form of vitamin C. *See* vitamin C.

tetrahydrodemethoxycurcumin. *See* curcumin, and turmeric.

tetrasodium EDTA. Chelating agent. It is used to prevent the minerals present in formulations from bonding to other ingredients.

tetrasodium etidronate. Used as a chelating agent in cosmetics to prevent varying mineral components from binding together and negatively affecting the formulation.

***Thea sinensis* extract.** *See* green tea.

thiamine HCL. Vitamin B1. There is no research showing this to be effective when applied topically on skin.

thiazolidine carboxylate. Can have antioxidant properties, but there is no research showing this to be the case when it is applied topically on skin.

thickening agent. Substance that can have a soft to hard waxlike texture or a creamy, emollient feel, and that can be a great lubricant. There are literally thousands of ingredients in this category that give each and every lotion, cream, lipstick, foundation, and mascara, as well as other cosmetic products, their distinctive feel and form.

thioglycolate. Compounds used in permanent waves and depilatories either to alter the structure of hair or to dissolve it. These are potent skin irritants.

thiotaurine. Amino acid. Potentially, it can have antioxidant properties for skin (Source: Shiseido Corporation, http://www.shiseido.co.jp/e/e9608let/html/let00027.htm). *See* amino acid.

threonine. *See* amino acid.

Thuja occidentalis **extract.** Also known as extract of red or yellow cedar. It has antibacterial properties on skin, but it also has constricting properties and can be a skin irritant.

thyme extract. Derived from the thyme plant. It can have potent antioxidant properties (Source: *Journal of Agricultural Food Chemistry,* March 2002, pages 1845–1851). Its fragrant component can also cause skin irritation.

thyme oil. *See* thyme extract.

thymine. Component of DNA that carries genetic information for the cell. *See* DNA.

thymus extract. *See* thymus hydrolysate.

thymus hydrolysate. Form of animal thymus derived by acid, enzyme, or other methods of hydrolysis. It can have water-binding properties for skin but has no other special or unique benefit.

Thymus serpillum **extract.** Extract of wild thyme. *See* thyme extract.

Thymus vulgaris. *See* thyme extract.

Tian men dong. Chinese herbal asparagus extract; it has no known benefit for skin.

Tilia cordata. *See* linden flower extract.

Tinosorb M. *See* Tinosorb S.

Tinosorb S. In Europe there are two sunscreen ingredients, Tinosorb S (bisethylhexyloxyphenol methoxyphenyl triazine) and Tinosorb M (methylene bis-benzotriazolyl tetramethylbutylphenol), that are approved for protection across the entire range of UVA radiation (Sources: *Photochemistry and Photobiology,* September 2001, pages 401–406; and Ciba Specialty Chemicals Corporation, North America, http://www.cibasc.com). Whether they are preferred over the other UVA-protecting ingredients used in sunscreens has not been established. As this book goes to press, neither Tinosorb M nor Tinosorb S has been approved for use in the United States or Canada. *See* UVA.

tissue respiratory factor (TRF). Trade name for a form of yeast suspended in alcohol. There is only one independent study, performed on animals, that showed it to have some wound-healing benefits (Source: *Journal of Burn Care Rehabilitation,* March-April 1999, pages 155–162).

titanium dioxide. Inert earth mineral used as a thickening, whitening, lubricating, and sunscreen ingredient in cosmetics. It protects skin from UVA and UVB radiation and is considered to have no risk of skin irritation (Sources: http://www.photodermatology.com/sunprotection.htm; and *Skin Therapy Letter,* 1997, volume 2, number 5). *See* UVA.

tocopherol acetate. *See* vitamin E.

tocopheryl lineolate. *See* vitamin E.

tocotrienols. Super-potent forms of vitamin E that are considered stable and powerful antioxidants. There is some research showing tocotrienols to be more potent than other forms of vitamin E for antioxidant activity (Source: *Journal of Nutrition,* February 2001, pages 369S–373S), but the studies cited in this review were all performed on animal models or in vitro. According to the University of California at Berkeley's *Wellness Guide to Dietary Supplements* (October 1999), "[Tocotrienol] research in humans is very limited, and the results conflicting." The research that has been done has centered on large doses of oral tocotrienols, animal studies, or test-tube trials. Companies that want you to believe that tocotrienols are now the answer for your skin are only guessing whether or not the laboratory evidence translates to human skin as it exists in the real world (Source: *Healthnotes Review of Complementary and Integrative Medicine,* http://www.healthnotes.com). Full-scale clinical studies on humans to assess the benefits of topical tocotrienols have not yet been performed, so for now (as is true for all antioxidants), choosing it as the "best" one is a leap of faith. *See* vitamin E.

toluene. Solvent used in nail polishes; it is considered toxic with repeated use.

tomato extract. Has weak antioxidant properties (Source: *Free Radical Research,* February 2002, pages 217–233). Tomatoes contain lycopene, which is a significant antioxidant, but it is more bioavailable from tomato paste than from fresh tomatoes (Source: *American Journal of Clinical Nutrition,* 1997, volume 66, number 1, pages 116–122). It can also be a potential skin irritant depending on what part of the tomato is used, but there is no way to know that from an ingredient label. *See* lycopene.

tormentil extract. *See Potentilla erecta* root extract.

tourmaline. Inert, though complex, mineral. One of its unique properties is that it is piezoelectric, meaning that it generates an electrical charge when under pressure. That's why tourmaline is typically used in pressure gauges. Tourmaline is also pyroelectric, which means that it generates an electrical charge during a temperature change (either increase or decrease). One of the results of generating such an electric charge is that dust particles will become attached to one end of the tourmaline crystal. However, none of that can take place in a cosmetic. There is no published research showing tourmaline has any proven effect on skin whatsoever.

tragacanth. Natural gum used as a thickener in cosmetics.

tranexamic acid. Technical name 4-aminomethylcyclohexanecarboxylic acid. When used orally, it is an antihemophilic (stops bleeding) medicine; topically it is an anti-inflammatory agent.

transforming growth factor (TGF). Stimulates wound healing and collagen growth. *See* human growth factor.

transparent soap. Soap that looks milder or less drying than some others because of its unclouded, clear appearance, but many such soaps contain harsh cleansing ingredients, and the ingredients that give the bar its shape can clog pores.

trehalose. Plant sugar that has water-binding properties for skin.

tretinoin. Topical, prescription-only medication that can improve cell production after it has been damaged. It is the active ingredient in Retin-A, Renova, Tazorac, and Avita. One of the more significant problems of sun damage is abnormal and mutated cell growth. An article in *Clinics in Geriatric Medicine* (November 2001, pages 643–659) stated that "Studies that have elucidated photoaging pathophysiology have produced significant evidence that topical tretinoin (all-trans retinoic acid), the only agent approved so far for the treatment of photoaging, also works to prevent it" (Sources: *Cosmetic Dermatology*, December 2001, page 38; and *Journal of Investigative Dermatology*, 2001, volume 111, pages 778–784). Tretinoin affects and improves actual cell production deep in the dermis, far away from the surface of skin (Sources: *Clinical and Experimental Dermatology*, October 2001, pages 613–618; *Clinical Geriatric Medicine*, November 2001, pages 643–659; and *Photochemistry and Photobiology*, February 1999, pages 154–157).

tribenzoin. Used as an emollient and thickening agent in cosmetics. *See* glyceryl ester.

triclosan. Good antibacterial agent used in many products, from those for oral hygiene to cleansers (Sources: *Federation of European Microbiological Societies Microbiology Letter*, August 2001, pages 1–7; and *American Journal of Infection Control*, April 2000, pages 184–196). However, whether triclosan is effective for treatment of acne has not been researched. There is also controversy over whether or not triclosan may contribute to creating strains of bacteria that are resistant to antibiotics owing to its overuse in cosmetic products. Further, there is also concern about whether, in practical use, it can in fact impart the benefits of disinfection indicated on the label (Source: *Journal of Hospital Infection*, August 2001, Supplement A, pages S4–S8).

tridecyl salicylate. Salt form of salicylic acid (BHA). When salicylic acid is converted into a non-acid compound (as here), it no longer has exfoliating properties.

tridecyl stearate. Used in cosmetics as a thickening agent and emollient.

tridecyl trimellitate. Used in cosmetics as a thickening agent and emollient.

triethanolamine. Used in cosmetics as a pH balancer. Like all amines, it has the potential for creating nitrosamines. There is controversy as to whether this poses a real problem for skin, given the low concentrations used in cosmetics and the theory that nitrosamines can't penetrate skin.

Trifolium pratense. *See* red clover.

triglyceride. Used as an emollient and thickening agent in cosmetics. *See* glyceryl ester, and natural moisturizing factors.

Trigonella feonum-graecum. *See* fenugreek.

trilaurin. Group of ingredients that are triesters of glycerin and aliphatic acids, and known generically as glyceryl triesters. They are used in cosmetic products as thickening agents and emollients (Source: *International Journal of Toxicology,* 2001, volume 20, supplement 4, pages 61–94).

trioctanoin. Emollient and thickening agent used in cosmetics. *See* trilaurin.

tristearin. Triglyceride of stearic acid. It is used as an emollient and thickening agent.

Triticum vulgare **oil.** *See* wheat germ oil.

tryptophan. *See* amino acid.

turmeric. Plant source of a spice made from the dried, ground root; its extract is called curcumin. A natural yellow food coloring that has potent antioxidant properties (Sources: *Food Chemistry and Toxicology,* August 2002, pages 1091–1097; and *Planta Medica,* December 2001, pages 876–877). Because it is a potent spice, it may have some irritating properties for skin as well.

Tussilago farfara. *See* coltsfoot.

tyrosinase. Enzyme that stimulates melanin production. *See* tyrosine.

tyrosine. An amino acid in skin that initiates the production of melanin (melanin is the component of skin that gives it "color"). According to information on the FDA's Web site (http://www.fda.gov), tyrosine's "use is based on the assumption that it penetrates the skin, increases the tyrosine content of the melanocytes, and thus enhances melanin formation. This effect has not been documented in the scientific literature. In fact, an animal study reported a few years ago demonstrated that ingestion or topical application of tyrosine has no effect on melanogenesis [the creation of melanin]." Tyrosine is important to the structure of almost all proteins in the body. However, the chemical pathway needed for tyrosine to function is complex and this pathway cannot be duplicated by including tyrosine in a skin-care product or by applying it topically.

ubiquinone. *See* coenzyme Q10.

Ulva lactuca **extract.** Extract of the plant known as sea lettuce. It has some anti-inflammatory and antioxidant properties for skin (Source: *Phytotherapy Research,* December 2000, pages 641–643).

umbilical extract. Obtained from either human or animal umbilical cord. It is used in cosmetics with varying, though unsubstantiated, claims about the effect on skin. Use of animal- and human-derived ingredients is prohibited under the provisions of the European Union Cosmetics Directive. For animal-derived ingredients, this is based on concerns about transmission of bovine spongiform encephalopathy (Mad Cow Disease); for human-derived ingredients the concern is transmission of viral diseases such as human immunodeficiency virus (HIV) (Source: *International Journal of Toxicology,* 2002, volume 21, supplement 1, pages 81–91). There is no way to know from reading a cosmetic ingredient label what the source of the extract is.

Uncaria gambir **extract.** Leaf extract of a shrub from the madder family. Some forms of uncaria have antioxidant properties. There is no research for the gambir variety. However, due to its tannin content, *Uncaria gambir* most likely has antioxidant properties, though the tannin content also makes it a potential skin irritant.

Undaria pinnatifida. Form of seaweed. *See* algae.

urea. Component of urine, though synthetic versions are used in cosmetics. In small amounts urea has good water-binding and exfoliating properties for skin; in larger concentrations it can cause inflammation (Source: *Skin Pharmacology and Applied Skin Physiology*, January-February 2002, pages 44–54).

Urtica dioica. *See* nettle extract.

usnic acid. Antibacterial and possibly anti-inflammatory substance derived from lichens (Sources: *Fitoterapia, September 2000*, pages 564–566; and *European Journal of Pharmaceutical Sciences*, April 1998, pages 141–144). It can also inhibit cell production (Source: *Cellular and Molecular Life Sciences*, August 1997, pages 667–672).

Uva ursi extract. *See* arbutin, and bearberry.

UVA. Ultra-violet A radiation. The sun produces a range of ultra-violet (UV) radiation. Skin damage such as wrinkling, skin discoloration, sagging, and coarse texture is a consequence of unprotected sun exposure due to the cumulative effect of the sun's UV radiation. UVA and UVB radiation are the portions of the sun's rays that cause this damage. UVA rays have wavelengths of 320 to 400 nanometers; UVB rays have wavelengths of 290 to 320 nanometers. UVB radiation causes sunburn, while UVA radiation does not produce any short-term evidence of skin damage. Nonetheless, UVA radiation creates serious cumulative changes in skin that may be far greater than the sunburn caused by UVB radiation. Research has shown that unprotected exposure to UVA rays can, within one week, create distinct injury, such as inflammation, abnormal cell production, stratum corneum (outer layer of skin) thickening, depletion of immune-stimulating cells, and evidence of the possibility of elastin deterioration (Sources: *Journal of the American Academy of Dermatology*, May 2001, pages 837–846; *Bulletin of the Academy of National Medicine*, 2001, volume 185, number 8, pages 1507–1525; *Photodermatology, Photoimmunology, and Photomedicine*, August 2000, page 147; and *Journal of the American Academy of Dermatology*, January 1995, pages 53–62).

To be effective, sunscreens must protect skin from both the sun's UVA and UVB radiation. In the United States, there are only three ingredients that are approved by the FDA that protect across the full UVA range: titanium dioxide, zinc oxide, and avobenzone (also called Parsol 1789 and butyl methoxydibenzoylmethane). Outside of the United States, Mexoryl SX is also used (Sources: *International Journal of Pharmaceutics*, June 2002, pages 85–94; *Photodermatology, Photoimmunology, Photomedicine*, August 2000, pages 147–155 and http://www.photodermatology.com/sunprotection.htm; and *Skin Therapy Letter*, 1997, volume 2, number 5).

The SPF (sun protection factor) number on sunscreens relates only to a product's efficacy against UVB exposure. There is no rating system for UVA protection. The only way to tell if a product can protect skin from UVA radiation is to note that at least one of the ingredients mentioned above is listed among the active ingredients on the label. Because UVA protection is so important, all sunscreen products must contain one or more UVA-protecting ingredient. *See* sunscreen, and sun protection factor.

UVB. Ultra-violet B radiation. *See* UVA.

VA/crotonates. Film-forming agent. *See* film-forming agent.

VA/crotonates copolymer. *See* film-forming agent.

Vaccinium myrtillus. *See* bilberry extract.

valerian. Extract of the common herb valerian *(Valeriana officinalis).* There is definitely research showing that it is effective at improving sleep patterns when taken orally (Source: *Pharmacopsychiatry,* March 2000, pages 47–53). There is no research showing that it has any effect when applied topically on skin.

valine. *See* amino acid.

Vanilla planifolia **fruit extract.** Used primarily as a fragrance and flavoring agent. There is no research showing it to have benefit for skin.

vascular endothelial growth factor (VEGF). Stimulates the growth of blood vessels. *See* human growth factor.

verbena extract. Fragrant extract that can be a skin irritant.

Veronica officinalis **extract.** There is no research showing this extract to have any benefit when applied topically to skin (Source: *Natural Medicines Comprehensive Database,* http://www.naturaldatabase.com).

vetiver oil or extract. Fragrant component in skin-care products that also has some antibacterial properties (Source: *Applied Microbiology,* June 1999, pages 985–990). It can also be a skin sensitizer.

Vinca minor **extract.** *See* periwinkle.

vinegar. Consists of acetic acid and water. The color and flavor of the vinegar is determined by and varies with the alcoholic liquor or juice that is used to ferment the acetic acid (such as apple cider or wine). It does have mild disinfecting and antifungal properties, but according to a study in *Infection Control and Hospital Epidemiology* (January 2000), commercial disinfectants are far more effective in killing germs and bacteria than vinegar. Vinegar can be a skin irritant.

Viola tricolor **extract.** *See* pansy extract.

vitamin A. Considered a good antioxidant in some of its various forms, particularly as retinol and retinyl palmitate. *See* retinol.

vitamin B1. *See* thiamin HCL.

vitamin B2 (riboflavin). There is no research showing this to have any benefit when applied topically to skin. However, there is a small amount of research showing that riboflavin may be photosensitizing and thus cause the breakdown of skin (Sources: *Free Radical Biology and Medicine,* 1997, volume 22, number 7, pages 1139–1144; and *Toxicology Letters,* August 1985, pages 211–217).

vitamin B3. *See* niacinamide.

vitamin B5. Also known as pantothenic acid. *See* pantothenic acid.

vitamin B6. There is no research showing it to have benefit for skin.

vitamin B12. May be effective in the treatment of psoriasis (Source: *Dermatology,* 2001, volume 203, number 2, pages 141–147). Overall there is limited research showing vitamin B12 to have any benefit when applied topically on skin.

vitamin C. Considered a potent antioxidant for skin (Sources: *Journal of Investigative Dermatology,* February 2002, pages 372–379, and June 2001, pages 853–859; and *Toxicology in Vitro,* August-October 2001, pages 357–362). Claims that vitamin C can prevent or eliminate wrinkling are not proven. An article in *Plastic and Reconstructive Surgery* (January 2000, pages 464–465) discussed the issue of vitamin C and concluded that "Vitamin C is a valuable antioxidant and protectant against photodamage that is created by sunlight in both the UVB and UVA bands…. Although oral supplementation may also be useful, topical preparations are able to deliver a higher dosage to the needed area. Topical vitamin C does not absorb or block harmful ultraviolet radiation like a sunscreen. Instead, it augments the skin's ability to neutralize reactive oxygen singlets [free-radical damage] that are created by the ultraviolet radiation, thereby preventing photodamage to the skin. It becomes an integral part of the skin and remains unaffected by bathing, exercise, clothing, or makeup. Used appropriately, topical vitamin C is an important adjunct to the use of sunscreens, an adjunctive treatment to lessen erythema [redness] in skin resurfacing, a helpful adjunct or an alternative to Retin-A in the treatment of fine wrinkles, and a stimulant to wound healing."

vitamin D. Provides no known benefit for skin when applied topically, though it may have antioxidant benefits. Vitamin D, formed in the skin by sunlight or in an oral supplement form, is essential for health.

vitamin E. Considered an antioxidant superstar. Vitamin E is a lipid-soluble vitamin (meaning it likes fat better than water) that has eight different forms, of which some are known for being excellent antioxidants when applied topically to skin, particularly alpha tocopherol and the tocotrienols (Sources: *Current Problems in Dermatology,* 2001, volume 29, pages 26–42; *Free Radical Biology and Medicine,* May 1997, pages 761–769; *Journal of Nutrition,* February 2001, pages 369S–373S; and *International Journal of Radiation Biology,* June 1999, pages 747–755). However, other studies have indicated the acetate form (tocopherol acetate) is also bioavailable and protective for skin (Source: *Journal of Cosmetic Science,* January-February 2001, pages 35–50). And still other research points to tocopherol sorbate as providing significant antioxidant protection against ultraviolet radiation–induced oxidative damage (Source: *Journal of Investigative Dermatology,* April 1995, pages 484–488). Pointing to the significance of vitamin E for skin is an article in the *Journal of Molecular Medicine* (January 1995, pages 7–17), which states: "More than other tissues, the skin is exposed to numerous environmental chemical and physical agents such as ultraviolet light causing oxidative stress [free-radical damage]. In the skin this results in several short- and long-term adverse effects such as erythema [redness], edema [swelling], skin thickening, wrinkling, and an increased incidence of skin cancer.... Vitamin E is the major naturally occurring lipid-soluble ... antioxidant protecting skin from the adverse effects of oxidative stress including photoaging [sun damage]. Many studies document that vitamin E occupies a central position as a highly efficient antioxidant, thereby providing possibilities to decrease the frequency and severity of pathological events in the skin."

In essence, vitamin E functions in the body and on the skin to protect cells against free-radical damage, and an abundant assortment of researchers from diverse medical fields have theorized that this can slow the aging process (Sources: *Skin Pharmacology and Applied Skin Physiology,* November-December 2001, pages 363–372; and *Free Radical Biology and Medicine,* October 1999, pages 729–737). Theory is not fact, yet the research is definitely compelling for this ingredient. Currently, however, we simply don't know how much is needed or how long it lasts, and whether any of the benefit shows up as a reduction of wrinkles.

vitamin E for scars. There is no evidence that vitamin E can help heal scars and, because of skin sensitivity, it can actually impede the healing process for some. A report of research published in *Dermatologic Surgery* (April 1999, pages 311–315), in an article titled "The effects of topical vitamin E on the cosmetic appearance of scars," concluded that the "... study shows that there is no benefit to the cosmetic outcome of scars by applying vitamin E after skin surgery and that the application of topical vitamin E may actually be detrimental to the cosmetic appearance of a scar. In 90% of the cases in this study, topical vitamin E either had no effect on, or actually worsened, the cosmetic appearance of scars. Of the patients studied, 33% developed a contact dermatitis to the vitamin E. Therefore we conclude that use of topical vitamin E on surgical wounds should be discouraged." The study was done double-blind "with patients given two ointments each labeled A or B. A was Aquaphor, a regular emollient, and B was Aquaphor mixed with vitamin E. The scars were randomly divided into parts A and B. Patients were asked to put the A ointment on part A and the B ointment on part B twice daily for 4 weeks." Antioxidants are definitely an option for skin, but for preventing scars vitamin E directly applied on skin does not appear to be one of them.

vitamin F. Name sometimes used to represent essential fatty acids of linoleic acid and linolenic acid. These are considered essential fatty acids (EFA) because they cannot be produced by the body. There are many fatty acids that have benefit for skin, including arachidonic, eicosapentaenoic, docosahexaenoic, and oleic acids to name a few. These all have emollient, water-binding, and often antioxidant properties for skin. *See* gamma linolenic acid, and linoleic acid.

vitamin H. *See* biotin.

vitamin K. Some cosmetics companies sell creams and lotions containing vitamin K, claiming it can reduce or eliminate surfaced spider veins (technically referred to as telangiectasias). These creams can't change spider veins. The only research concerning vitamin K's effectiveness on skin or surfaced spider veins comes from the companies selling these products. There are no published or peer-reviewed studies that add up to results you can even remotely count on (Source: *Archives of Dermatology,* December 1998, pages 1512–1514).

Vitex trifolia **fruit extract.** *See* chaste tree.

Vitis vinifera. Latin name for the vines of wine grapes. *See* grape, and grape seed extract.

Vitreoscilla **ferment.** Made from a bacteria that can help cells utilize oxygen better in vitro (Source: *Journal of Biotechnology,* January 2001, pages 57–66). Whether that effect can be translated to benefit skin cells via a cosmetic formulation is unknown.

volatile oil. Group of volatile fluids derived primarily from plants, and used in cosmetics primarily as fragrant additives. These components most often include a mix of alcohols, ketones, phenols, linalool, borneol, terpenes, camphor, pinene, acids, ethers, aldehydes, and sulfur, which all have extremely irritating and sensitizing effects on skin.

walnut extract. Can have antioxidant properties (Source: *Journal of Nutrition,* November 2001, pages 2837–2842). There is no research showing this to have any benefit for skin.

walnut oil. Emollient, nonfragrant plant oil. *See* natural moisturizing factors.

walnut-shell powder. Abrasive used in scrub products.

water. Most widely used cosmetic ingredient; it is almost always listed first on an ingredient label because it is usually the ingredient with the highest concentration. Yet, despite claims of the skin's need for hydration and the claims regarding the special type of water used, it turns out that water may not be an important ingredient for skin. Only a 10% concentration of water in the outer layer of skin is necessary for softness and pliability in this part of the epidermis (Source: *Skin Pharmacology and Applied Skin Physiology,* November-December 1999, pages 344–351). Studies that have compared the water content of dry skin to that of normal or oily skin don't find a statistically significant difference in moisture levels between them (Source: *Journal of Cosmetic Chemistry,* September/October 1993, page 249). Further, too much water in the skin can be a problem because it can disrupt the skin's intercellular matrix, the substances that keep skin cells bonded to each other (Source: *Contact Dermatitis,* December 1999, pages 311–314). The most significant aspect of the skin's health is the structural organization of the intercellular lipids and the related materials that keep skin intact and prevent water loss (Sources: *Trends in Cell Biology,* August 2002, page 355; and *Journal of the American Academy of Dermatology,* August 2002, pages 198–208). *See* natural moisturizing factors, and oxygenated water.

water-binding agent. Wide range of ingredients that help skin retain water (moisture). Glycerin is one of the more typical and effective water-binding agents used in cosmetics. One group of water-binding agents can mimic the skin's actual structure and can be of benefit in a formulation; these include ceramide, lecithin, glycerin, polysaccharides, hyaluronic acid, sodium hyaluronate, mucopolysaccharides, sodium PCA, collagen, elastin, proteins, amino acids, cholesterol, glucose, sucrose, fructose, glycogen, phospholipids, glycosphingolipids, and glycosaminoglycans. No single one of these is preferred over another because even though they are all effective, none of them can permanently change the actual structure of skin. *See* natural moisturizing factors.

watercress extract. There is some evidence that when consumed in the diet, watercress has some anticancer and antioxidant properties (Sources: *Journal of Nutrition*, March 1999, pages 768S–774S; and *Food Chemistry Toxicology*, February-March 1999, pages 95–103). Whether these properties translate when applied topically is unknown. However, because watercress is a source of mustard oil, it can be a skin irritant.

wheat germ glycerides. Used as emollient and thickening agents in cosmetics. *See* glyceryl ester, and natural moisturizing factors.

wheat germ oil. Emollient plant oil similar to all nonfragrant plant oils. *See* natural moisturizing factors.

wheat protein. *See* natural moisturizing factors, and protein.

whey. Milk contains two primary proteins, casein and whey. When cheese is produced, the more liquid components, casein and whey, are separated from the cheese. When eaten or taken in oral supplements, whey protein can have significant antioxidant properties (Source: *Journal of Dairy Science*, December 2001, pages 2577-2583) as well as anticancer properties (Source: *Anticancer Research*, November-December 2000, pages 4785-4792) because it generates the production of glutathione in the body, which is a significant antioxidant. Whether or not any of those benefits translate to skin is unknown. In skin-care products it is most likely a good water-binding agent.

white camellia extract or oil. Used as a fragrance in cosmetics; it may be a skin sensitizer.

white nettle. Contains components that can have both anti-irritant as well as inflammatory properties (Source: http://www.bastyr.org/academic/botmed/herbs.asp?HerbId=5).

white oak bark extract. *See* oak root extract.

white tea leaf extract. Minimally processed buds and leaves of green tea. There is research showing white and green teas to have the highest concentration of antioxidant properties of all teas, and several in vitro and animal studies have shown green tea and white tea to have anticancer and antimutagenic properties. However, even though tea flavonoids are effective antioxidants, it is unclear to what extent they increase the antioxidant capacity of humans, and there is no research showing what their activity means for skin. If anything, there is a question whether white tea's antioxidant properties (versus those of other teas) might simply be related to white tea's higher caffeine level (Source: Oregon State University Linus Pauling Institute, http://lpi.orst.edu). *See* green tea.

white willow. *See* willow bark.

wild ginger. *See* ginger.

wild yam extract. The roots of wild yams were used in the first commercial production of oral contraceptives, topical hormones, androgens, estrogens, progesterones, and other sex hormones. Diosgenin, a component of wild yam, is promoted as a natural precursor to dehydroepiandrosterone (DHEA). Some wild-yam products are promoted as "natural DHEA." Although diosgenin can be converted to steroidal compounds, including DHEA, in the laboratory, this chemical synthesis does not occur in the human body. So taking wild-yam extracts will not increase DHEA levels in humans (Source: *Natural Medicines Comprehensive Database,* http://www.naturaldatabase.com). There is no research showing wild yam has any effectiveness when applied topically on skin. If anything, the studies that do exist have demonstrated that topical application of wild yam has little to no effect on menopausal symptoms (Source: *Climacteric,* June 2001, pages 144–150). *See* DHEA.

willow bark. Contains salicin, a substance that when taken orally is converted by the digestive process to salicylic acid (beta hydroxy acid). The process of converting the salicin in willow bark into salicylic acid requires the presence of enzymes. The digestive conversion process that turns salicin into saligenin, and then into salicylic acid, is complex. Further, salicin, much like salicylic acid, is stable only under acidic conditions. The likelihood that willow bark in the tiny amount used in cosmetics can mimic the effectiveness of salicylic acid is at best problematic, and in all likelihood impossible. However, willow bark may indeed have some anti-inflammatory benefits for skin because, in this form, it appears to retain more of its aspirin-like composition.

willow herb. *See Epilobium angustifolium* extract.

wintergreen oil. Can be very irritating and sensitizing (Source: *Natural Medicines Comprehensive Database,* http://www.naturaldatabase.com). *See* counter-irritant.

witch hazel. Can have potent antioxidant properties (Sources: *Phytotherapy Research,* June 2002, pages 364–367; and *Journal of Dermatological Science,* July 1995, pages 25–34) and some anti-irritant properties (Source: *Skin Pharmacology and Applied Skin Physiology,* March-April 2002, pages 125–132). However, according to the *Consumer's Dictionary of Cosmetic Ingredients, Fifth Edition,* by Ruth Winter (1995, Random House), "Witch hazel can have an ethanol [alcohol] content of 70 to 80 percent. Witch hazel water … contains 15% ethanol." The alcohol can be an irritant. Witch hazel also has a high tannin content (tannin is a potent antioxidant), which can also be irritating when used repeatedly on skin, though when used for initial swelling from burns it can reduce inflammation.

wormword. Herb that has antioxidant properties (Source: *Journal of Agricultural Food Chemistry,* November 2001, pages 5165–5170).

Wu wei zi. Also known as *Schisandra chinensis,* this herb can have a constricting effect and can be a skin irritant.

xanthan gum. Used as a thickening agent.

Xi xin. *See* ginger extract.

***Ximenia americana* oil.** Plum oil; it can have emollient properties.

xylitol. *See* sorbitol.

xylose. Form of sugar. Similar to other sugars, xylose has water-binding properties for skin.

yarrow extract. There is little research showing yarrow extract to have benefit for skin. What studies do exist were done in vitro and indicate that it may have anti-inflammatory properties (Sources: *Planta Medica,* 1991, volume 57, pages 444–446, and 1994, volume 60, pages 37–40). However, yarrow also has properties that may cause skin irritation and photosensitivity (Source: *Healthnotes Review of Complementary and Integrative Medicine,* http://www.healthwell.com/healthnotes/herb).

yeast. Group of fungi that ferment sugars. Yeast is a source of betaglucan, which is considered a good antioxidant. A simple Internet search for brewer's yeast (Latin name *Saccharomyces cerevisiae*), brings up over 85,000 references. Yeasts are basically fungi that grow as single cells, producing new cells either by budding or fission [splitting]. Because it reproduces well, *Saccharomyces cerevisiae* is the organism that is most widely used in biotechnology. Nevertheless, some forms of yeast are human pathogens, such as *Cryptococcus* and *Candida albicans.*

In relation to skin, there is limited information about how *Saccharomyces cerevisiae* may provide a benefit. Live yeast-cell derivatives have been shown to stimulate wound healing (Source: *Archives of Surgery,* May 1990, pages 641–646), but research like this is scant. Most of what is known about yeast is theoretical, and is about yeast's tissue-repair and protective properties (Source: *Global Cosmetic Industry,* November 2001, pages 12–13) or yeast's antioxidant properties (Source: *Nature Genetics,* December 2001, pages 426–434). As a skin-care ingredient yeast has potential, but what its function may be or how it would affect skin is not understood.

yellow lupine. *See Lupinus luteus* seed extract.

yerba mate extract. Used for the preparation of the most popular tea-like beverage of South America. It has anti-inflammatory and antioxidant properties (Sources: *Fitoterapia,* November 2001, pages 774–778; and *Life Sciences,* June 2002, pages 693–705).

ylang-ylang. Fragrant, volatile oil that can also be a skin irritant. *See* volatile oil.

yogurt. There is no research showing yogurt to be effective when applied topically.

yucca extract. Plant extract that can have anti-inflammatory benefits.

***Zanthoxylum alatum* extract.** Has no known benefit for skin when applied topically (Source: *Natural Medicines Comprehensive Database,* http://www.naturaldatabase.com).

***Zanthoxylum piperitum*.** *See* Szechuan pepper.

zedoary oil. Fragrant oil that can be a skin irritant, though there is also research showing that components of zedoary can have anti-inflammatory and antioxidant properties (Source: *Inflammation Research,* December 1998, pages 476–481).

zeolite. One of a group of minerals used as an absorbent in cosmetics. It has been shown to have anticancer properties (Source: *Journal of Cancer Research and Clinical Oncology,* January 2002, pages 37–44).

zinc. Studies in the 1970s linked zinc with a positive effect on acne, but those studies were never duplicated and zinc is not considered to have any real significance for skin. Taken orally, zinc may have positive effects for wound healing and other health benefits, but these are not experienced when it is applied topically. It can be a skin irritant.

zinc carbonate. *See* calamine.

zinc gluconate. Combination of zinc with a form of glucose (a sugar) that is commonly used in cold lozenges for its antiviral effects. A study reported in *Dermatology* (2001, volume 203, issue 2, page 40) evaluated "the place of zinc gluconate in relation to antibiotics in the treatment of acne vulgaris. Zinc was compared to minocycline [an antibiotic] in a multicenter randomized double-blind trial. 332 patients received either 30 milligrams elemental zinc or 100 milligrams minocycline over 3 months. The primary endpoint was defined as the percentage of the clinical success rate on day 90...." The study concluded that "Minocycline and zinc gluconate are both effective in the treatment of inflammatory acne, but minocycline has a superior effect evaluated to be 17% in our study." Whether or not this relates to topical applications is unknown. **Note:** High doses of zinc can be toxic. Avoid taking more than 100 mg of zinc per day from a supplement (Source: http://www.drweil.com). It is also recommended that you take a daily multivitamin with minerals, because increased levels of zinc mean that the body requires more copper and manganese.

zinc oxide. Inert earth mineral used as a thickening, whitening, lubricating, and sunscreen ingredient in cosmetics. One manufacturer of zinc oxide has heavily promoted this ingredient as being the only option for broad-spectrum sun protection, but this has not been proven from other independent research. Along with titanium dioxide, zinc oxide is considered to have no risk of skin irritation, though both of these minerals may clog pores. *See* UVA.

zinc phenolsulfonate. Antimicrobial agent that can also be a skin irritant.

zinc sulfate. Chemical resulting from the interaction of zinc with sulfuric acid. There is little research showing this to be beneficial for skin. The little information there is shows it doesn't help skin healing (Source: *Acta Dermato-Venereologica,* Supplemental, 1990, volume 154, pages 1–36) and it can be a skin irritant. There is no research showing it to be effective for treating acne (Source: *International Journal of Dermatology,* April 1985, pages 188–190). It can be a skin irritant. *See* zinc.

***Zingiber officinale* Roscoe.** *See* ginger.

Zingiber zerumbet. *See* ginger.

Zingiberaceae. *See* ginger.

Ziziphus jujube. Chinese jujube, *Ziziphus jujuba,* is one of the five major fruits of China, where some 300 varieties are grown. There is no research showing it to have benefit on skin.

CHAPTER EIGHT

Animal Testing

The National Anti-Vivisection Society (NAVS) is a not-for-profit educational group that opposes the use of animals for any purpose, whether in product testing, research, education, or food. While I find some of their policies and agendas rather extreme and radical, I still support many of their efforts to stop unnecessary animal testing and prevent animal cruelty in all forms. NAVS and I differ in that I do not oppose the use of animal testing for health-care research of afflictions such as breast cancer, Alzheimer's, and heart disease, and I am not vegan (NAVS and PETA, People for the Ethical Treatment of Animals, are both opposed to the use of animals for any medical or food use). However, I do oppose the inhumane treatment of animals (no animal should suffer in the effort to help humankind), as well as the testing of standard cosmetic formulations and ingredients on animals. In this regard, NAVS and I agree.

The definitive book on the issue is NAVS's *Personal Care for People Who Care,* now in its tenth edition. This 200-page book lists which cosmetics companies do and do not test on animals, and is a must-read source for any consumer interested in purchasing products that have not been tested on animals. You can obtain the book by calling NAVS at (800) 888-NAVS, by communicating via e-mail at navs@navs.org, or by writing them at P.O. Box 94020, Palatine, IL 60094-9834. The cost is $10 per book plus shipping and handling. Visit their Web site at www.navs.org.

Please note: When a product's label states that the company that made it doesn't test on animals, and the company reports this information to NAVS for the listing they ultimately use in their book *Personal Care for People Who Care,* there is every reason to believe that information is correct. However, it is naïve to assume that this general information means animal testing information was not an integral part of creating the product. For example, all sunscreen ingredients and almost all of the new antioxidant ingredients currently used in cosmetics, including vitamin C, vitamin A, and most plant extracts, have all been tested on animals. In reality, what we know about the efficacy of these ingredients was first obtained from animal testing. I have broached this apparent double standard with NAVS several times but they refuse to acknowledge the challenge to their criteria. So, while the label on a skin-care product may indeed be accurate in regard to the particular product and the company's policy of animal testing, what it does not represent is the vast group of ingredient manufacturers and university research facilities that use animal testing to determine the basic efficacy of cosmetic ingredients that we all use.

The August 1999 issue of *Cosmetics & Toiletries* magazine reported on a new in vitro testing alternative that can further reduce the need for animal testing. It was approved by the Inter-Agency Coordinating Committee for the Validation of Alternative Methods (ICCVAM). The new "Corrositex assay [test] determines skin corrosivity of a chemical by placing it on a layer of collagen, the same material that holds skin together. As the chemical penetrates the collagen barrier, a material underneath changes color. Corrosivity is rated according to the time it takes the chemical to penetrate and by the color change of the material beneath the barrier."

I am proud to say that my skin-care company, Paula's Choice, does not test any aspect of its products on animals, and I donate a portion of my company's earnings to The Humane Society of the United States (HSUS) every year, particularly during the month of April, which is officially Prevention of Cruelty to Animals month. Please check out HSUS's Web site at www.hsus.org. Their mailing address is: The Humane Society of the United States, 2100 L Street NW, Washington, DC 20037 (they can use your financial help as well). HSUS's approach to the issue of animal rights and animal testing is one I agree with most strongly. The spring 1998 issue of *HSUS News* stated that "The HSUS shares with these scientists [the many who are opposed to or are uncomfortable with animal testing] the desire to eliminate the harmful use of animals in laboratories. In the meantime The HSUS is planning a campaign to urge the scientific community to adopt, as a priority goal, the elimination of all animal pain and distress in the laboratory. The HSUS believes that an emphasis on humane issues will lead to good science and will benefit, rather than harm, the advance of human knowledge."

COMPANIES THAT DO NOT USE ANIMAL TESTING ON THEIR FINISHED PRODUCTS

Aesop	California Baby	Jason Natural
Almay	Chanel	Kiehl's
Aramis Lab Series	Christian Dior	Kiss My Face
Arbonne	Clarins	L'Occitane
Astara	Clinique	L'Oreal
Aubrey Organics	Decleor Paris	La Mer
Aveda	Dermalogica	La Prairie
Avon	DHC	Lancome
Bath & Body Works	Dr. Hauschka	Little Forest Baby Care
BeautiControl	Elizabeth Arden	Lush
Beauty Without Cruelty	Estee Lauder	M.A.C.
BeneFit	Exuviance by Neostrata	Marcelle
Bioelements	Giorgio Armani	Mary Kay
Biore	H_2O+ Skin Care	Maybelline
BioTherm	Helena Rubinstein	Mustela
Bobbi Brown	Hydron	N.V. Perricone, M.D.
Burt's Bees	Jane	Neostrata

Ole Henriksen Skin Care
Ombrelle
Origins
Orlane
Paula Dorf Cosmetics
Paula's Choice &
  Paula's Select
PEDIAM
Phytomer

Prescriptives
Prestige Cosmetics
ProActiv
Ralph Lauren Polo Sport
Revlon
Sense Usana Skin Care
Serious Skin Care
Seventh Generation
Stila

Sue Devitt Studio Makeup
Thalgo
The Body Shop
Tony & Tina
Urban Decay
Vichy
Zirh Men's Skin Care

COMPANIES THAT CONTINUE TO USE ANIMAL TESTING

Baby Magic
Banana Boat
Calvin Klein
Chubs (Playtex)
Clearasil
Colgate Shaving Care
Cover Girl
Diaparene (Playtex)
Dove
Edge Pro Gel
Eucerin

Gillette
Huggies (Kimberly-Clark)
Lac-Hydrin
Max Factor
MetroGel, MetroLotion,
  and MetroCream
Moisturel
Nivea Visage
Noxzema
Olay

Old Spice
Pampers (Procter &
  Gamble)
Pond's
Sea Breeze
Shiseido
Skin Bracer by Mennen
Suave
Wet Ones (Playtex)

COMPANIES WITH UNKNOWN ANIMAL TESTING STATUS

Acne-Statin
Adrien Arpel's Signature
  Club A
Ahava
Alexandra de Markoff
Aloette
Alpha Hydrox
Anna Sui Cosmetics
Annemarie Borlind
Anthony Logistics
Aqua Velva
Artistry by Amway
Aveeno Facial Care
Awake
B. Kamins Skin Care
Bain de Soleil
bare escentuals

Basis
BioMedic
Black Opal
BlissLabs
Blistex
Body & Soul
Bonne Bell
Borghese
California North Men's
  Skin Care
CamoCare
CARGO
Caudalie
Cellex-C
Cetaphil
Chantal Ethocyn
Chantecaille

Cle de Peau Beaute
Clean & Clear (Johnson &
  Johnson)
Clientele
Clinac
Club Monaco
Complex 15
Coppertone
Corn Silk
Crabtree & Evelyn
Darphin
Dermablend
Desitin (Pfizer)
Diane Young
Doctor's Dermatologic
  Formula (DDF)
Dr. Dennis Gross, M.D.

Dr. Jeannette Graf, M.D.
Dr. LeWinn's Private
   Formula
Dr. Mary Lupo Skin Care
   System
Elizabeth Grant
Ella Bache
Ellen Lange Skin Care
English Ideas and Lip Last
Epicuren
ERA Face Foundation
Erno Laszlo
Esoterica
FACE Stockholm
Fashion Fair
Flori Roberts
Gatineau
Gerber
Givenchy
Glymed Plus
G.M. Collin
Gold Bond (Chattem)
Guerlain
Guinot
Hard Candy
IGIA
Illuminare
Iman
I-Iman
Jafra
Jan Marini Skin Research
Jane Iredale
Joey New York
Johnson & Johnson
Jurlique International
Karin Herzog Skin Care
Kinerase
Kiss Me Mascara
La Roche-Posay
Lancaster
Laura Mercier
Linda Sy
Lip Ink

Liz Earle Naturally Active
   Skin Care
Lorac
Lubriderm
M.D. Formulations
M.D. Forte
Make Up For Ever
Marilyn Miglin
Mario Badescu
Mederma
Merle Norman
Morgen Schick
Murad
Nad's Gel Hair Removal
NARS
Natura Bisse
Neutrogena
Neways Skin Care
Noevir
Nu Skin
Nutrifirm Isomers
N.Y.C.
Obagi Nu-Derm
Ocean Potion
Osmotics
Oxy Balance
PanOxyl
Parthena
Peter Thomas Roth
Pevonia
Pharmagel
philosophy
pHisoDerm
Physician's Choice
Physicians Formula
Pola
Porcelana
Posner
Prada
Principal Secret
PropapH
Purpose
Quo Cosmetics

Rachel Perry
Re Vive
Rejuveness
Rejuvenique
Remede
Reversa
Rimmel
RoC
Sage Skin Care
Sephora
Shaklee
Shu Uemura
Sisley
SkinCeuticals
smashbox
Sonia Kashuk
Sothys Paris
St. Ives
Stri-Dex
T. Le Clerc
Tend Skin
Three Custom Color
Tri-Luma
Trish McEvoy
Trucco
Ultima II
University Medical
   Skin Care
Uvavita
Vaniqa
Versace
Victoria Jackson
   Cosmetics
Victoria's Secret Cosmetics
Vincent Longo
Wet 'n' Wild
Yon-Ka Paris
Youngblood
Yves St. Laurent
Z. Bigatti Skin Care
ZAPZYT
Zia Natural Skin Care